Musculoskeletal Disorders

Contributors

Daniel R. Benson, M.D.
Assistant Professor, Department of Orthopaedic Surgery, University of California, Davis School of Medicine, Davis, California

Henry H. Bohlman, M.D.
Assistant Professor Orthopedic Surgery, Case Western Reserve University School of Medicine; Chief, Spinal Cord Injury Service, Veterans Administration Hospital, Cleveland, Ohio

Paul W. Brown, M.D.
Chairman, Department of Surgery, St. Vincent's Medical Center, Bridgeport, Connecticut; Assistant Clinical Professor of Orthopaedic Surgery, Yale University School of Medicine, New Haven, Connecticut; Consultant in Hand Surgery, Veteran's Administration Hospital, West Haven, Connecticut

Robert G. Chuinard, M.D.
Associate Professor, Chief, Hand and Upper Extremity Service, Department of Orthopedic Surgery, Louisiana State University School of Medicine in New Orleans, New Orleans, Louisiana

Robert D. D'Ambrosia, M.D.
Professor and Chairman, Department of Orthopedic Surgery, Louisiana State University School of Medicine in New Orleans, New Orleans, Louisiana

Albert B. Ferguson, M.D.
Formerly Orthopedic Roentgenologist, Boston University Hospital, Boston, Massachusetts; Formerly Orthopaedic Roentgenologist, New York Orthopaedic Hospital, New York, New York

William M. Fowler, Jr., M.D.
Professor and Chairman, Department of Physical Medicine and Rehabilitation, University of California, Davis School of Medicine, Davis, California

Stanley L. James, M.D.
Senior Clinical Instructor, Department of Orthopedics, University of Oregon School of Medicine, Portland, Oregon; Orthopedic Staff Physician, Sacred Heart General Hospital; Adjunct Associate Professor, Department of Physical Education and Orthopedic Consultant, Department of Athletics, University of Oregon, Eugene, Oregon

Richard S. Riggins, M.D.
Associate Professor, Department of Orthopaedic Surgery, University of California, Davis School of Medicine, Davis, California

Hiromu Shoji, M.D.
Associate Professor, Department of Orthopedic Surgery, Louisiana State University School of Medicine in New Orleans, New Orleans, Louisiana

Robert G. Taylor, M.D.
Associate Professor, Department of Physical Medicine and Rehabilitation, University of California, Davis School of Medicine, Davis, California

Musculoskeletal Disorders

Regional Examination and Differential Diagnosis

Robert D. D'Ambrosia, M.D.

Professor and Chairman
Department of Orthopedic Surgery
Louisiana State University
School of Medicine in New Orleans
New Orleans, Louisiana

with

Ten Contributors

J. B. Lippincott Company
Philadelphia • Toronto

ISBN 0-397-50373-3

Library of Congress Catalog Card Number 77-8562

Printed in the United States of America

3 5 4 2

Library of Congress Cataloging in Publication Data

Main entry under title:

Musculoskeletal disorders.

Bibliography: p.
Includes index.
1. Musculoskeletal system—Diseases—Diagnosis. I. D'Ambrosia, Robert D. [DNLM: 1. Bone diseases—diagnosis. 2. Muscular diseases—Diagnosis. 3. Musculoskeletal system—Physiopathology. WE141 M985]
RC925.7.M87 616.7'07'5 77-8562
ISBN 0-397-50373-3

To my wife, Barbara,
and Lisa, Chris, Matt, and Peter

Foreword

I was highly honored to be asked by Dr. D'Ambrosia to write the foreword of this book. When he, the editor as well as the author of two of the chapters, began his academic career, we discussed the need for a comprehensive text devoted to diagnosis rather than to treatment of diseases which primarily involve the musculoskeletal system.

The outstanding chapter written by Albert B. Ferguson, Sr., M.D., the father of Dr. D'Ambrosia's chief while in residency, was probably the last of his many significant writings before his death. The contributions to Orthopaedics by this world-renowned radiologist serve to perpetuate his memory.

Most of the chapters were written by young musculoskelotologists. It is they, because of their recent experiences in medical school and residency, who should know best what is necessary and desired by today's students, residents, fellows, and practitioners.

Any medical text written by multiple authors is bound to reflect differences in approach, emphasis, opinion, and content. This book is no exception. The lack of stereotypy, in my opinion, makes for more interesting reading and study. Almost without exception, the authors of the various chapters have supplied excellent references.

Hopefully, all who use this text will be better able to arrive at a logical diagnosis after considering all the possibilities concerned with the patient's musculoskeletal complaint. It has been estimated that 25 per cent of visits to practitioners of medicine are because of complaints related to the musculoskeletal system. If we, the practitioners, accurately diagnose the etiology of these complaints, we can then—and only then—offer rational and scientific alternatives for treatment. Otherwise, we become dogmatists or cultists.

It is my belief that this text fills a real need. I hope that you, the readers, will agree. If you do, the many hours expended by Dr. D'Ambrosia, his co-authors, and supporting staff will be justified.

PAUL R. LIPSCOMB, M.D.

Foreword

Anyone interested in the medical care of functioning people has to be awfully glad that this book has been written. All treatment that is to be successful must start with accurate diagnosis. The teaching of the art and science of diagnosis of the musculoskeletal system suffers in medical education. This book will provide a solid base for the student, family physician, and specialist and try to make up for this deficiency. Important information that makes accurate diagnosis possible is within these covers and must live again through daily use if patient care is to be improved.

The entire volume is dominated by the tone set by Robert D'Ambrosia in the first chapter—namely that there is logic that must be adhered to in order to make an accurate diagnosis. The copy is so clearly written that it is a delight to follow it. The information is so well correlated and so relevant that it is hard to stop reading; and as time wears on, one is anxious to return to it again (unusual for a medical book).

Robert D'Ambrosia had an outstanding career in medical school and developed a background in his training in Pittsburgh beyond the ordinary level and into the exceptional. He can write clearly and definitely about many phases of medicine, as is evident in this book. His teaching experience at the University of California at Davis led him into contact with many of his fellow authors, who have a concept of clarity and logic in diagnosing a problem and an extensive background that makes them experts. There is a unified approach in the book, not so clearly evident in most multi-author books.

Essentially the book answers the question, "What tools do we have?" It then begins with physical diagnosis but then goes into depth on laboratory procedures, the radiographic examination, and electrical diagnosis. When regions are examined, then further depth is entered into for all these modalities. The approach is unique; the information gathered in one place will save untold hours for the practitioner. It is surprising that it has not been done this well before—or with such a clear view of the objective.

When regions are presented, the salient features of anatomy and various syndromes make it a ready reference for the puzzled practitioner. The expertise of each of the authors is clearly evident.

The thinking that led to the creation of this book recognized a need, and the authors have performed well to serve the underlying philosophy.

The book will live on merit and usefulness. It will make a major contribution to the improvement of medical care of the musculoskeletal system, and patients will benefit greatly because it exists.

ALBERT B. FERGUSON, JR., M.D.

Preface

When confronted with the task of performing a musculoskeletal examination, medical students and even first-year residents frequently find themselves in a totally perplexing situation. They usually don't know where to begin, where to end, or how to put it all together. The aim of this book is to present a systematic and logical approach to musculoskeletal disorders.

Before any disease can be treated effectively, an accurate diagnosis must first be established. The question is, of course, how does one go about making a specific diagnosis? Physicians must have thorough knowledge of the applied anatomy, and of equal importance, they must be able to put the patient's symptoms, physical findings, and the result of laboratory and roentgenographic examinations in the proper framework and in a logical sequence. With this in mind, it is hoped that this book will aid the student of the musculoskeletal system in making an accurate diagnosis earlier in the disease process so that treatment might be initiated sooner and subsequent deformity prevented.

ROBERT D. D'AMBROSIA

Acknowledgments

The collation and editing of a manuscript such as this is always a time-consuming task, not only for the editor, but for all of the people on whom he depends for contributions and preparation. This was begun during my tenure on the faculty of the School of Medicine at the University of California at Davis. I wish to thank the School of Medicine for providing me the time and opportunity to begin my labors. I am especially grateful to my associates in the Department of Orthopaedics at Davis, Drs. Paul Lipscomb, Richard Riggins, Robert Chuinard, Hiromu Shoji, and Daniel Benson, each of whom not only wrote for the text but unselfishly provided me with the time to compile and edit the book. I am also indebted to Drs. Henry Bohlman, William Fowler, Robert Taylor Paul Brown, Stanley James, and the late Albert Ferguson, Sr., for authoring chapters in the text. The advanced perspective on regional examination and differential diagnosis detailed in this book is a direct benefit of the expertise of the contributing authors.

My deepest gratitude is extended to the dedicated women in the Department of Orthopaedics of the University of California, School of Medicine at Davis, who helped prepare and type the manuscript: Nancy Willis, Loral Gord, Pat Carr, Janice Coleman, Jane Schroeder, and Paula Dunning; and especially to Lois Faulkin who guided and directed the project.

My deepest gratitude is also extended to Vicki Saeto for her constructive criticism and copy editing; her aid was invaluable. The efforts of the members of the Medical Illustration Department, especially Hal Pullum, who drew most of the illustrations contained in the text, are also appreciated.

I have been very fortunate, since my arrival at Louisiana State University Medical Center in New Orleans, to have another excellent group of people assisting me in the completion of the project. Myrna Gemelli, Gloria Worrell, Charles Chapman, copy editor, and the Medical Illustration Department have helped in the re-editing process, and the administration of the Louisiana State University Medical School has provided their ongoing support without hesitancy.

I wish to thank Dr. Albert Ferguson, Jr. and Dr. Paul Rodgers Lipscomb for their encouragement and guidance while preparing this text and for allowing me the opportunity to be associated with them.

Last, but not least, I wish to thank Lewis Reines, Editor-in-Chief, Medical Books Division, J. B. Lippincott Company, who saw the need for such a book, and by whose aid and guidance this manuscript came to fruition.

Contents

1 Evaluation of the Patient

Robert D. D'Ambrosia, M.D.

A patient seeking a physician knowledgeable in musculoskeletal disorders most often is looking for treatment of a specific problem. The obvious is not always the correct diagnosis, and good physicians should not concentrate immediately on their initial assumption without first giving sufficient thought to the other possible diagnoses. Too often, a hasty diagnosis is not accurate, and it is impossible to institute the appropriate form of treatment without first having an accurate diagnosis. An accurate diagnosis is obtained only by thinking through a systematic and logical sequence of ideas and thoughts in an orderly manner. Evaluations which are hasty and careless often lead to incorrect diagnosis and improper treatment. For example, a child presenting with intoeing may be hastily misdiagnosed as having metatarsus adductus and casted or given corrective outflare shoes. However, in actual fact, most intoeing is caused by an anteversion deformity of the neck of the femur and not the foot. Therefore, it is imperative to approach musculoskeletal disorders in an orderly manner with a logical sequence of thoughts to arrive at an accurate diagnosis. The main areas which require evaluation are: knowledge of the regional anatomy, an accurate history taken from the patient, a thorough clinical examination, appropriate laboratory tests and other special tests for verification of clinical findings, specific roentgenograms of the involved area, and awareness of the disease possibilities in the differential diagnosis. Only when the data from these areas are available can physicians synthesize their thoughts and arrive at an accurate diagnosis and institute proper treatment. If data from any area are sketchy or not available, the musculoskeletal evaluation will result in unfavorable circumstances for both patient and physician.

ANATOMY

There is no substitute for a thorough knowledge of anatomy when evaluating a musculoskeletal problem. In 1543, Vesalius wrote that anatomy is "the firm foundation of the whole art of medicine." Some specialties of medicine may disagree with this statement but not a physician who deals on a daily basis with musculoskeletal problems. Chapters 6 through 12 deal with the regional areas, and the beginning of each region is devoted to the surface and functional anatomy of that particular area. The physician dealing with musculoskeletal problems must have a knowledge of the surface, function, and radiologic anatomy as they relate to that specific area. It would be impossible to begin patient evaluations without it.

There are certain anatomical terms which refer to position and direction that the reader must be familiar with as they will be constantly referred to throughout this text. *Anterior* or *ventral* is that part nearest the front of the body. *Posterior* and *dorsal* is that part nearest to the back. In the upper extremity *palmar* or *volar* is synonymous with anterior, and in the lower extremity *plantar* refers to the *inferior* surface. Also in reference to the extremities *proximal* means that part closest the root of the attached limb, and *distal* is that part farthest from the root. *Medial* and *lateral* are used in reference to the median plane; the former is closest to the median plane, and the latter is farthest from it. *Medial* in the upper limb is often substituted by *ulnar* and in the lower limb by *tibial. Lateral* in the upper limb is often substituted by *radial* and in the lower extremity by *fibular* or *peroneal.*

HISTORY

The history can be extremely valuable if it is taken carefully and accurately without suggesting words and thoughts to the patient being interviewed. The patient must be able to tell his own story with his emphasis on specific points. Your job is only to lead and be sure that the patient does not leave out important aspects of the history which may have been forgotten or put aside because he feels they do not relate or are unimportant.

An orthopaedic history is subdivided into five parts: chief complaint, present illness, review of systems, past history, and family history. When you first ask the question "What appears to be the problem?" the focus is immediately on a single area of the musculoskeletal system, for example, the neck, back, shoulder, hand, hip, knee, or foot. Each area is unique and requires a specific history and examination particular to the region. However, the focus may be on multiple joints in many regions and be indicative of a generalized systemic disease, such as rheumatoid arthritis.

Chief Complaint

The chief complaint is the symptom or symptoms for which the patient has sought out your services. It usually is pain, but it may be deformity, neurologic loss, weakness, swelling, loss of function, or some other disability. It focuses on a definite part of the musculoskeletal system where the symptoms are occurring.

Pain, the most common orthopaedic complaint, is difficult to define and measure quantitatively. Pain thresholds vary from person to person, and what may only be an annoyance to one person may be intolerable to another. A physician should not place himself in a position of judging when pain is severe enough to require his services for he may be wrong, and it may prove disastrous. The patient who was recently casted for a supracondylar fracture of the elbow and who returns because of pain with finger extension may have an impending Volkmann's ischemic contracture which, if neglected, could cause loss of function of that extremity.

Pain has a particular onset, certain vague characteristics, and usually is in a specific location, and all aspects are important to the physician. Record accurately the date of onset and whether the pain presented insidiously or suddenly. Did a particular injury or illness precede the symptoms, such as streptococcal infection of the throat present four weeks prior to a painful migratory polyarthralgia which would be indicative of rheumatic fever? Pain has certain characteristics, such as being sharp, dull, boring, shooting, burning, aching, throbbing, or crampy, and these characteristics help differentiate the site of origin. Bone pain is usually described as dull, deep, and having a boring quality; fracture pain is usually described as sharp; muscle pain usually as crampy; and joint pain is usually described with multiple adjectives because of the complex and varied tissues involved. The relation of the pain characteristics to rest and motion are also important. Most musculoskeletal pain is relieved by rest, and when it is not, it denotes something more serious. An active osteomyelitis which is under pressure becomes progressively more painful even with rest. The location of pain is important particularly if there is radiation with the pain. Pain may be localized, diffuse, radicular, or referred. Whether it is localized to a specific area or diffuse can supply useful information. Radicular pain refers to pain radiating in the distribution of a particular nerve, like the sciatic, and is often associated with sensory and motor changes. Referred pain is that felt in an area remote from the actual pathological condition. Areas to which pain is commonly referred should have a *special imprint in the mind of the examiner.* Hip joint pain is commonly referred to the knee, especially in children because similar nerves supply a portion of both joints. What effect coughing, sneezing, weather, or change of position has on the pain should be asked. Is the pain worse at night, and does such medication as aspirin relieve the pain? An osteoid osteoma has characteristic night pain which is relieved by aspirin.

Deformity. The patient or parents may be aware of some defect in the general appearance of the extremities or back. For instance, idiopathic scoliosis, when discovered at puberty, is first noticed as one breast being larger, one shoulder or hip being higher

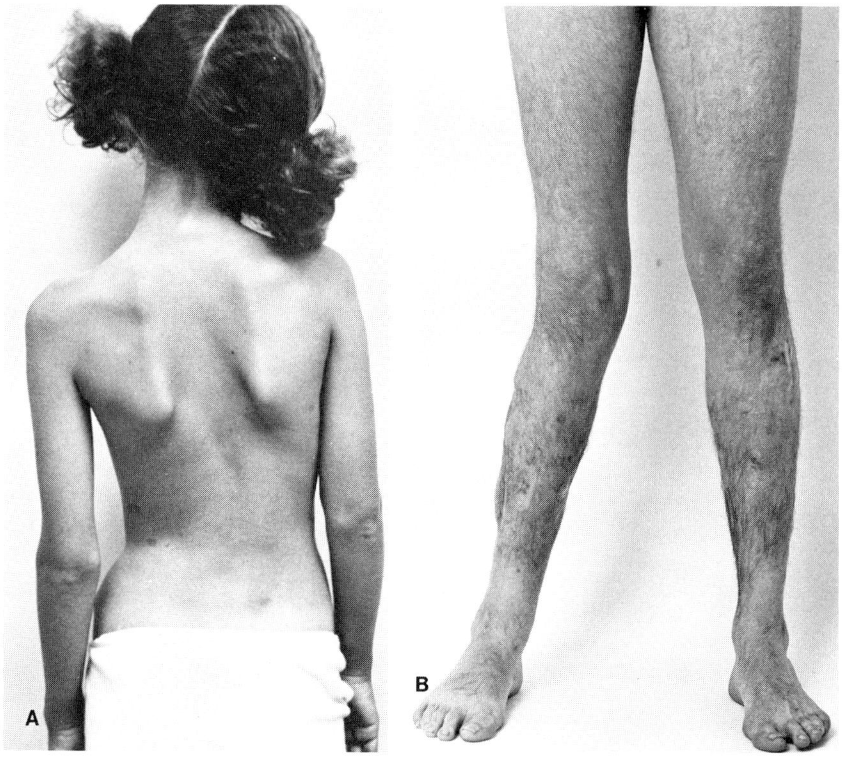

Fig. 1-1. Deformities. (*A*) Idiopathic scoliosis presenting with one shoulder being higher. (*B*) Valgus deformity at knee secondary to malunion of fracture.

(Fig. 1-1A), or the dress length being irregular. The deformity may be in the limbs and may be angular (Fig. 1-1B) or rotational and be marked by leg length discrepancy, atrophy, or a limp or gait abnormality resulting from one of the above physical defects.

Whatever the deformity, certain facts about it must be asked. What characteristics does it have, such as inflammation, swelling, tenderness, and is the muscle contracture or stiffness associated with it? When and by whom was the deformity first noticed, and did it come on gradually or suddenly? Did the deformity develop after an injury? An epiphyseal fracture may have caused premature closure of one side of the epiphysis, but the deformity usually is not noticed for six months or longer. Is the deformity increasing, improving, and what disability is it causing?

Neurological loss is usually described as a sensory or motor deficit. The sensory loss may produce hypoesthesia, paresthesia, or hyperesthesia and be related as pain or numbness over a specific area. The motor deficit may be described as a weakness, stiffness, or more commonly difficulty in walking far, running, or jumping. If there is outright paralysis, was it sudden or insidious in onset, and did it result in a flaccid or spastic extremity? Flaccidity is associated with lower motor neuron disorders and spasticity with upper motor neuron damage. Have the symptoms increased or decreased, and what disability is it causing the patient? Is there loss of sphincter control in the bladder or rectum?

Miscellaneous. Other presenting symptoms may be loss of function, swelling, or disability. Loss of function or motion in a joint may be expressed in various ways, such as stiffness, but more commonly it is expressed as inability to tie one's shoes or cross one's legs. An osteoarthritic patient with a stiffening hip quickly becomes aware of inability or great difficulty in the tying of shoes. Swelling at a joint may be secondary to rheumatoid arthritis or occur in the adjacent soft tissues as a result of an expanding tumor. Disability is expressed as decreased ability in walking, running, working, or playing. Disability must always be evaluated accurately in terms of performance for individuals of the same sex and age doing the same activity.

Review of Systems

Although not always important, a thorough review of systems should never be overlooked. As a physician becomes busy and more harried with a thriving practice, he inevitably takes shortcuts. It is the routine elicitation of a systems review which may save him from making an improper diagnosis by providing an important link. For example, arthritis of the heel associated with urethral discharge may elicit a diagnosis of Reiter's syndrome. A systematic review includes all systems beginning with the head and neck proceeding down through the nervous system. In orthopaedics, special emphasis must always be placed on areas which may be a focus of infection, such as the ears, tonsils, teeth, sinuses, and genitourinary tract.

Medical History

A complete and accurate history, including previous illnesses, injuries, or operations, may add real significance to the present illness. The history begins at birth and progresses chronologically through adulthood. Birth injury may result in a brachial paralysis or a less obvious case of cerebral palsy manifesting later in childhood. Diet history as well as changes in weight and sleeping patterns all may be extremely significant in the final evaluation.

Family History

Many congenital deformities such as clubfoot, congenital dislocated hip, and scoliosis are inherited and are often found to have expression in other members of the family. A parent or sibling may have tuberculosis which has been transmitted to the patient. Many musculoskeletal diseases, although having no direct hereditary pattern, have patterns of incomplete penetrance, or constitutional abnormalities may be present in the family which may give significant clues to the patient's present problem.

PHYSICAL EXAMINATION

The Whole Patient

There are two parts to a musculoskeletal physical examination: examination of the patient as a whole and the musculoskeletal examination proper. A complete physical examination of the patient as a whole should be done with the patient undressed and under good lighting conditions. Describe any positive physical findings and any negative findings which may have diagnostic significance. Always begin the examination with the patient's age, sex, apparent age, race, body development, a general statement of his health, and if he appears acutely or chronically ill. Pulse, respiration, and blood pressure are recorded. During the examination, constantly be aware of the emotional and mental status of the patient and make note of it at the completion of your examination. Is the patient introspective or extrovertive? How attentive, alert, and cooperative is he? What is his motivation? These questions are important in the final evaluation of the patient because often patients seeking musculoskeletal consultation require reconstructive surgery, and if they are not motivated toward pursuing a cooperative postoperative course, any surgical procedure may prove to be a disaster. It is not uncommon for a rheumatoid patient to withdraw and become catatonic following a technically flawless reconstructive procedure on one of the major joints. A patient like this becomes a disaster in the postoperative period because of total withdrawal and lack of cooperation.

Proceed as in a general physical examination, evaluating the skin, glands, eyes, ears, nose, throat, neck, chest, abdomen, genital organs, rectum, and nervous system. When going through these organ systems, always remember inspection, palpation, percussion, and auscultation when appropriate.

Musculoskeletal Examination

This examination is highly dependent on the observing powers of the physician. Inspection and palpation are the cornerstones of the orthopaedic examination. Auscultation and percussion play minor roles except in rare instances. Percussion is important when evaluating a muscle for pain, and auscultation is important in listening for crepitation in a joint or a bruit in an extremity. The examination varies slightly according to the area in question, and this is the reason for dividing our text into regional areas of examination. Each regional area will be covered in detail later. There are some general features common to all regions, but all are not necessarily applicable to every area in the body. A check list should be available for evaluating an orthopaedic problem in a sequential fashion. The areas covered include: inspection, palpation, deformity, measurement, range of motion, muscle testing, neurological status, posture and gait, stability, vascular status, and special functional tests peculiar to each region.

Inspection. The musculoskeletal examination begins with careful inspection. It is both an evaluation of the body as a whole and its individual mechanical units. Observe the patient as he walks, undresses, and moves from chair to examining table. Examine the skin for marks and color. The skin of a rheumatoid patient is often tissue paper thin with hemorrhagic areas. Patients with neurofibromatosis have skin with areas of light brown pigmentation (cafe au lait spots) throughout the body (Fig. 1-2). Note any scars, draining sinuses, or previous surgical incisions. Accuracy in inspection will usually differentiate between apparent or real limb length discrepancies or atrophy of particular muscle parts. Note any masses, swellings, or deformities that may require your closer attention later in the examination.

Palpation. Any area that seemed to be suspicious should be palpated directly and carefully. Palpate with a kind, gentle, warm hand, and avoid unnecessary roughness because more will be felt in a relaxed than in a tense patient, both in children and adults. Palpation enables you to evaluate skin temperature, soft tissues, bones, and specific areas of local tenderness. Feel for increased warmth and when in doubt compare the identical area on the opposite extremity. Increase in warmth usually denotes an increase in vascularity. This is usually from inflammation, but a rapidly growing neoplasm also has accentuated hyperemia. When evaluating soft tissues, direct special attention to the muscles and joint tissues. Evaluate the tone and bulk of the muscles to determine if spasm or atrophy is present. If the joint is swollen, is it secondary to fluid within the joint or due to a thickened synovial membrane? When palpating the bones, evaluate general contour, abnormal prominences, and the presence of local landmarks. If tenderness is elicited, map out the exact location and attempt to correlate it with a particular structure.

Deformity. Deformity is noted at the time of inspection. It is placed in a special category because of its importance, and careful documentation is necessary for any deformity. Deformity may be shortening, atrophy, or hypertrophy of an extremity. It may be marked by asymmetry or the presence of an abnormal swelling or mass. It may be abnormal curves in the back, such as scoliosis or kyphosis (Fig. 1-3). It may be increased anteversion or retroversion in the hips (see Chapter 10) or external torsion of the tibia (see Chapter 11). The deformity of the foot may be pes cavus or pes planus (see Chapter 12). The usual deformity in an extremity is an abnormal angulation at a particular joint. Angulatory deformities of joints are expressed as either varus or valgus. Angulation toward the midline is known as varus while angulation away from the body is called valgus. A decrease in the normal carrying angle of the elbow is known as cubitus varus, and an increase in the normal carrying angle is called cubitus valgus (Fig. 1-4). A decrease in the neck-shaft angle of the hip below 130 degrees is coxa vara, and an increase in the neck-shaft angle of the hip above 130 degrees is coxa valga (see Fig. 1-4). Medial angulation at the knee joint is genu varum (bowleg) and lateral angulation at the knee is genu valgum (knock-knee) (see Fig. 1-4). Medial angulation at the heel is heel varus (inversion), and lateral angulation at the heel is heel valgus (eversion) (see Fig. 1-4). An adduction deformity of the great toe at the metatarsophalangeal joint is hallux varus, and an abduction deformity is hallux valgus (see Fig. 1-4). An adduction deformity of the forefoot's relation with the hindfoot is metatarsus varus (see Fig. 1-4).

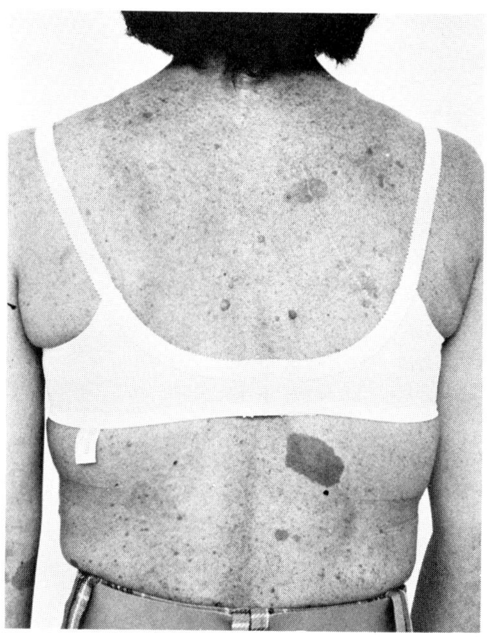

Fig. 1-2. Areas of light brown pigmentation known as cafe au lait spots should alert the examiner to the possibility of neurofibromatosis.

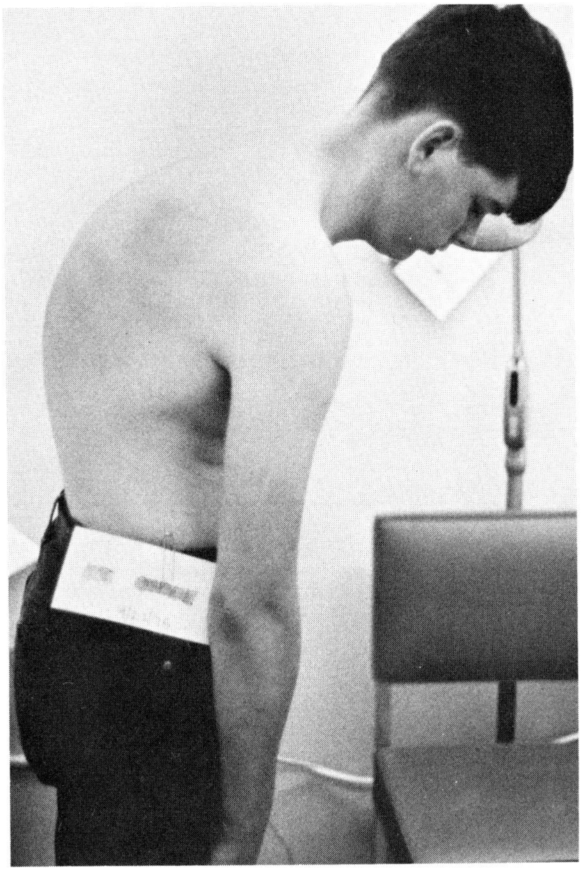

Fig. 1-3. Kyphosis or postural roundback is an abnormal curvature of the spine with the convexity backward.

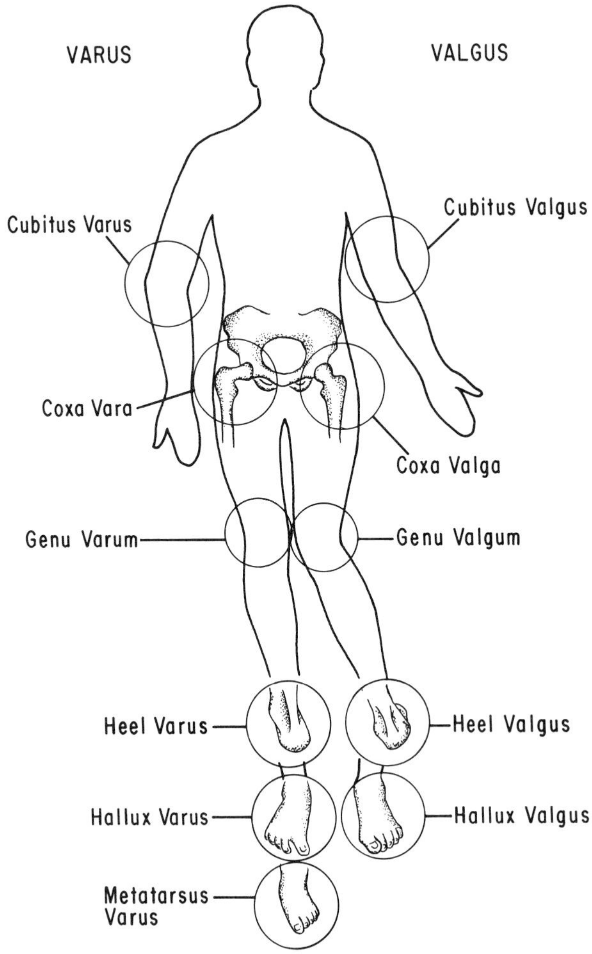

Fig. 1-4. Varus and valgus deformities. Angulation toward the midline is known as varus while angulation away from the body is called valgus.

Measurement. Accurate measurement of extremities is vital, especially in the lower extremity. Apparent shortening as opposed to true shortening is evaluated (see Fig. 10-12). If shortening is present in the lower extremity from the anterior iliac spine to the medial malleolus, then what part is shortened? Is it between the anterior iliac spine and greater trochanter, denoting a pathological condition at the hip, or is it in the femur or tibia? A measurement taken at the medial joint line of the knee is, thus, important. If abnormalities are found with tape measurement, then a special limb length roentgenographic study should be performed. This is done with a ruler alongside the roentgenogram. Measurement of the circumference of a particular limb segment, as the calf, is an index of muscle wasting, soft tissue swelling, or bony thickening. Common measurements of the upper extremity are at midarm, above elbow, elbow, midforearm, and wrist. Measurements of the lower extremity include thigh, above knee, knee, calf, above ankle, and ankle.

Range of Motion. When examining movements of a joint, evaluate both active and passive motion. Active motion is motion which the patient performs and is the result of the functioning of his musculature, while passive motion is the motion elicited by the examiner and is the result of an external force outside the patient. Passive motion is usually equal to active motion but exceeds it in two instances: if the muscles responsible for the movement of the joint are paralyzed or if the muscles or tendons about the joint are damaged or torn. When placing a joint through a range of motion, it is important to note if pain or crepitation is present, and if so at what point in the range. The individual motions of each joint will be commented upon separately in the forthcoming sections, but there are basically six types of motion described: (1) flexion and extension (2) dorsiflexion and plantar (palmar) flexion, (3) abduction and adduction, (4) inversion and eversion, (5) internal and external rotation, and (6) pronation and supination.

Flexion and extension are observed at most joints. Flexion is motion away from the zero position, and extension is the return motion to the zero starting position (see Fig. 11-12). If the motion goes beyond the zero starting position, it is known as hyperextension which often occurs at the elbow and knee.

Dorsiflexion and plantar (or palmar) flexion occur at the ankle (see Fig. 12-8), toes, wrist, and fingers. Dorsiflexion is movement of the ankle and toes or wrist and fingers in the direction of the dorsal surface. Plantar flexion is movement of the foot or toes in the direction of the plantar surface, and palmar flexion is movement of the wrist and fingers in the direction of the palmar surface.

Adduction and abduction occur at the shoulder (see Fig. 8-7), hip, metacarpophalangeal, and metatarsophalangeal joints. Abduction is movement away from the midline of the body, and adduction is movement toward the midline. In the foot and hand, the midline is a line drawn through the middle finger or middle toe.

Inversion (adduction) and eversion (abduction) occur as a result of combined motion in the subtalar and midtarsal joints of the foot (see Fig. 12-8). Inversion is the turning of the plantar surface of the foot inward with relation to the leg. Eversion is turning of the plantar surface of the foot outward in relation to the leg.

Internal and external rotation occur at the shoulder and hip (see Figs. 10-19, 10-20) and to some degree at the knee; they are accentuated in the pathological state. Internal rotation is the turning of the anterior surface of the limb inward, and external rotation is the turning of the anterior surface of the limb outward.

Pronation and supination occur at the forearm (see Fig. 9-10) and in the foot. Pronation of the forearm is rotation of the forearm between the wrist and elbow so that the palmar surface of the hand is directed downward. Supination of the forearm is rotation of the forearm between the wrist and elbow so that the palmar surface of the hand is directed upward. Pronation of the foot is its rotation into eversion, and supination is its rotation into inversion. Pronation and supination should really be eliminated as descriptive terms in the foot because inversion and eversion are more specific and descriptive.

Muscle Testing. Muscle testing is part of the neurological examination but is listed separately to emphasize its importance. There are six grades of muscle power: (1) Grade 0 in which there is no power and no evidence of muscle contraction. (2) Grade 1 in which there is a flicker or *trace* of power under 10 percent and some evidence of muscle contraction but no measureable joint motion. (3) Grade 2 which is *poor* with 25 percent power; the joint can go through a complete range of motion if gravity is eliminated. (4) Grade 3 which is *fair* with 50 percent power; the joint can go through a complete range of motion against gravity. (5) Grade 4 which is *good* with 75 percent power; the joint can go through a complete range of motion against gravity with some but not full resistance. (6) Grade 5 which is *normal* or 100 percent power; the joint can go through a complete range of motion against gravity with full resistance.

Neurological Status. In addition to muscle testing, the neurological examination provides an evaluation of the reflexes. The superficial reflexes tested are the biceps (Fig. 1-5A), triceps (Fig. 1-5B), brachioradialis (Fig. 1-5C), knee jerk (Fig. 1-5D), and ankle jerk (Fig. 1-5E). Abdominal and cremasteric reflexes are also evaluated and graded on a scale of 1 plus (+) to 4 plus (++++). Evaluate for tremors (choreiform movements), ataxia (Romberg test), and pathological reflexes. Pathological reflexes will be determined by the Hoffman and Babinski tests and the presence of clonus. Clonus may be patellar or ankle and be either sustained or unsustained. Coordination movements such as finger to nose, heel down shin, bicycling movements, and foot circles should be accomplished. Evaluation of proprioception, vibratory sense, and response to hot and cold should be performed. Neurological examinations of the back and other specific regions will be described in the individual chapters.

Gait. The patient's gait refers specifically to disorders of the lower extremity. Gaits are peculiar to

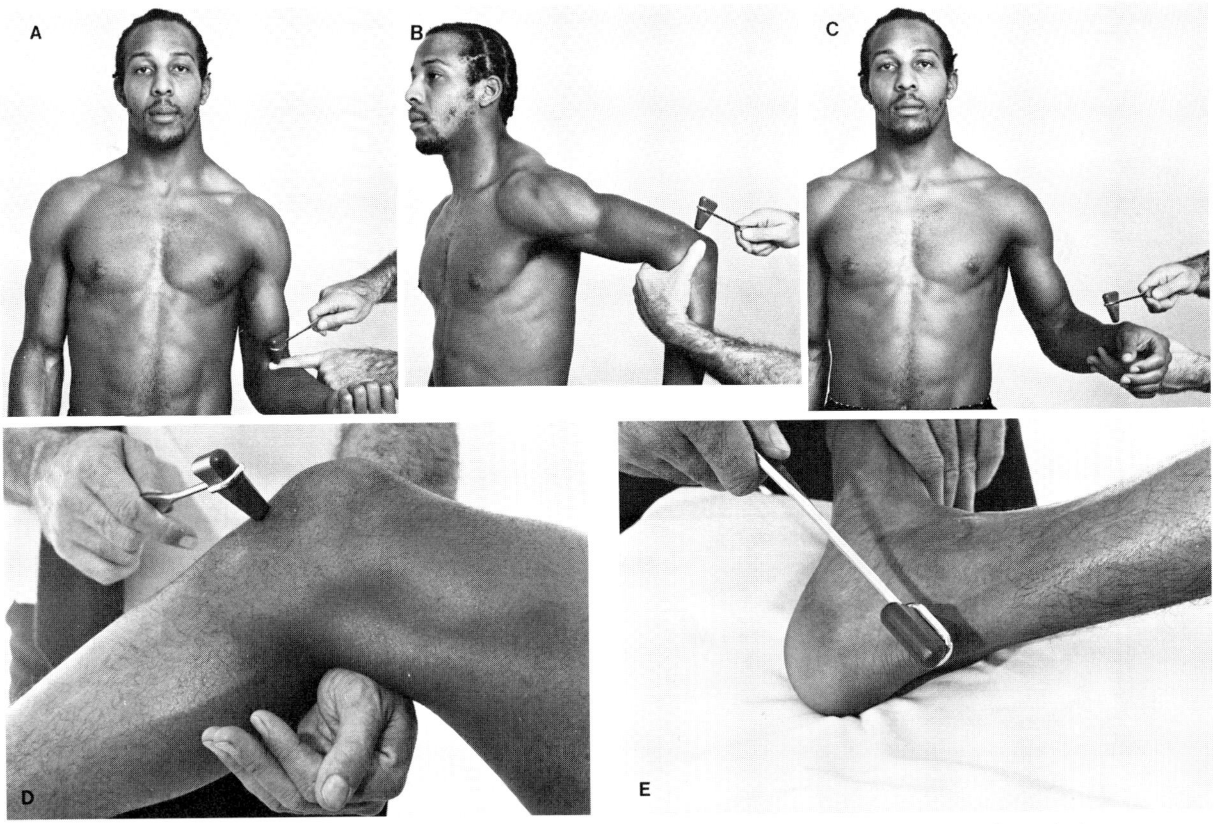

Fig. 1-5. Elicitation of superficial reflexes. (*A*) Biceps reflex. (*B*) Triceps reflex. (*C*) Brachioradialis reflex. (*D*) Knee jerk. (*E*) Ankle jerk.

even normal individuals, and differences are seen in speed, rhythm, smoothness, balance, and coordination. Some gaits are specific for the hip, some are specific to the foot and ankle, and others are more general. An antalgic gait may indicate a disorder in any part of the lower limb. It produces a short stance phase and is protective. The weight of the body is applied gently to the foot of the involved extremity and quickly removed.

A short gait causes the pelvis to dip as the weight of the body is transferred to the short leg. The dip is produced so the foot can reach the floor. The patient may avoid this dip by either placing the foot of the involved extremity in equinus or by flexing the opposite knee or hip. The gait is eliminated with a built-up shoe.

Ankylosed joints produce distinctive gaits which implicate hip and knee. A stiff hip has more swing of the pelvis and abduction of the extremity because the lumbar spine moves more to compensate for the stiffness of the hip. An extremity with a stiff knee and no shortening is abducted to the side or the pelvis is elevated to enable the foot to clear ground in the swing phase of gait. The gait resulting from a stiff ankle is not as characteristic and is often difficult to distinguish from normal. This gait lacks spring and becomes discernible when the patient jumps up and down.

Muscle weakness causes characteristic gaits. The most characteristic muscle weakness gait is gluteal weakness which produces a Trendelenburg gait. The weak abductors cannot keep the pelvis level, and to avoid taxing them, the pelvis drops and the body sways to the side of the weak muscle to maintain the center of gravity over the hip. Weakness of the gluteus maximus has a characteristic thrusting forward of the pelvis and thrusting backward of the upper torso as the foot is placed on the ground to decelerate the extremity an activity that the gluteus maximus formerly performed. Quadriceps weakness results in giving way of the knee and causes unwanted flexion when weight is placed on the knee. This tendency is counteracted by contracting the gastrosoleus muscle and maintaining the foot in equinus, both of which thrust the knee backward so that the weight thrust is in front of the knee. It is also counteracted by contraction of the gluteus maximus, which extends the thigh and keeps the knee extended. Anterior tibial and toe extensor muscle weakness from peroneal nerve injury results in a drop foot gait, and the patient will either drag the foot or the knee will be lifted higher so it clears the ground. Weakness of the gastrosoleus complex results in a calcaneal gait.

The most characteristic neurological gait is the spastic gait. Spastic muscles result in muscle imbalance around the hip and knee, causing them to respond more slowly and with less precision, and the resulting spastic gait lacks rhythm and coordination. Strong tibial muscles may pull the foot into varus, strong hamstrings hold the knee in flexion, strong internal rotators at the hip rotate the extremity internally, and strong adductors at the hip adduct the thigh. This gait is known as a *scissors gait* (Fig. 1-6) and is stiff and awkward with very poor balance while walking. An athetoid gait is very uncoordinated with movements which are lacking in precision and effectiveness. An ataxic gait is unsteady and the result of severe muscle balance disturbance. There are many abnormal gaits associated with neurological diseases but they are beyond the scope of this text. There are also peculiar gaits associated with deformities or limited motion at certain joints.

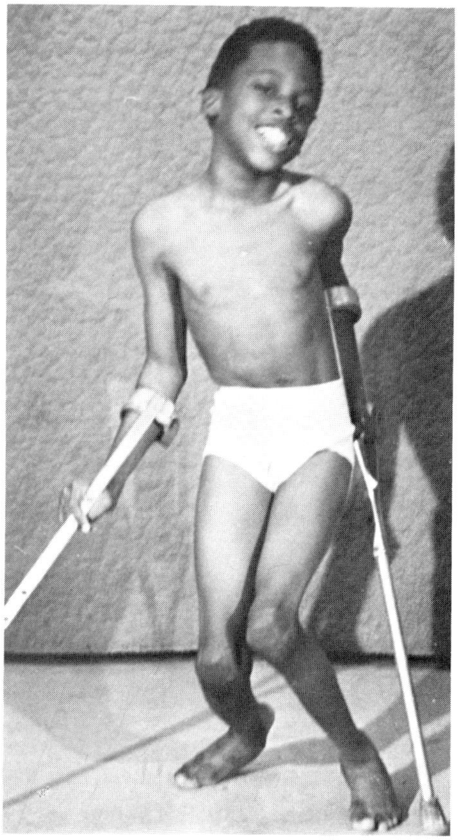

Fig. 1-6. Spastic scissors gait of cerebral palsy.

Stability. The stability of a joint is dependent on the congruity of its articulating surfaces and of the surrounding ligaments of the joint. Rheumatoid arthritis and syphilis can also destroy cartilage, rendering a joint totally unstable and useless. Ligaments may be lax because of previous injury, usually athletic, or from an inherited disorder such as Ehlers-Danlos syndrome. If a joint is unstable, it has abnormal mobility.

It is important to relax the muscles about a joint when testing for stability because a strongly contracted muscle will conceal ligamentous instability. Instability occurs most often at the knees, ankles, and fingers, but no joint is immune. Instability of joints will be discussed in the specific chapters.

Vascular Status. Symptoms in the upper and lower extremity are often associated with some impairment of the arterial circulation. Examine the color and temperature of the skin and nails of both extremities. Palpate the radial, brachial, and axillary pulses in the upper extremity. It is not unusual to see a pulse obliterated from pressure by a cervical rib or other cause. Palpate the femoral, popliteal, dorsal pedal, and posterior tibial pulses in the lower extremity. The dorsal pedal pulse is felt on the dorsum of the foot between the first and second metatarsals. The posterior tibial pulse is felt approximately 2 cm. posterior and slightly below the medial malleolus.

Special Signs and Functional Tests. There are many special tests which should be performed when indicated. If fluid is present, does it fluctuate, is it ballotable, and is there a fluid wave? If an aneurysm or vascular tumor is present, it should be evaluated for a bruit, thrill, or pulsation. Masses in the soft tissues should be transilluminated. A lipoma (fat mass) or ganglion (liquid mass) transmits light whereas fibrous tissue and vascular masses do not.

Many special tests have been developed and are applicable to specific regions of the body, for example, the McMurray test for evaluation of a meniscus injury (Fig. 11-28) or the Trendelenburg test (Fig. 10-22) for evaluation of the hip abductors. Special tests appropriate to a region will be discussed in that specific section of the text.

LABORATORY TESTS

Musculoskeletal specialists do not use the laboratory as fully or as often as practitioners of internal medicine, but in many instances the diagnosis is confirmed in this area. The laboratory examinations most useful in evaluating musculoskeletal disorders are those involving blood, synovial fluid, cerebrospinal fluid, urine, biopsy specimens, skin, abnormal fluids in soft tissues, bursas, and muscle function.

Blood

A complete blood count (CBC) should be done routinely on every patient. It includes a hemoglobin, hematocrit, red blood cell count, white blood cell count, and microscopic examination. The reasons for obtaining a CBC should be obvious, as it aids in diagnosing infections, arthritides, and certain tumors.

The sedimentation rate of erythrocytes is a nonspecific study but is a commonly used index of musculoskeletal dysfunction. It begins with rouleaux formation followed by settling and packing of the red blood cells. Altered electrical charge on the surfaces of erythrocytes is the principal cause of increased sedimentation. The test is simple to perform and read, but it has inherent complexities with many sources of technical error. It is only roughly quantitative; therefore, minor variations from normal are of little significance. It is variable with age and sex, being higher in children and women, regardless of the technique used—Westergren, Cutler, or Wintrobe-Landsberg. Clinically, it is a nonspecific test and is used mainly as an index of tissue injury and in differentiating functional diseases and neuroses from organic diseases. It is used as a general screening test for musculoskeletal disorders, and elevation in a patient with musculoskeletal complaints warrants closer investigation. The sedimentation rate is elevated in any condition which is actively destroying bone, cartilage, or soft tissues (Table 1-1). It is often used as a guide in treating infections of bone. Some physicians continue to use antibiotics in treating osteomyelitis until the sedimentation rate returns to normal. It is also used as an index of activity of rheumatic fever or rheumatoid arthritis.

The blood glucose level is the most commonly used indicator of carbohydrate metabolism. The two common methods in use are the Folin-Wu and True methods (see Table 1-1). The former gives higher values because it measures some nonglucose elements like glutathione, ergothioneine, and uric acid which can account for 15 to 40 mg./100 ml. of whole blood. The newer methods, of which there are many, determine the true glucose level in the blood with a high degree of accuracy. The values given in Table 1-1 are normal fasting values. More sophisticated evaluation of glucose metabolism is done with a glucose tolerance test.

Calcium is not only an electrolyte but is important in calcium-phosphorus metabolism. Ninety-nine percent of calcium occurs in bones, with adults requiring 10 to 15 mg. per kilogram of body weight and children, 45 mg. per kilogram. It is absorbed in the intestine with the aid of vitamin D, fat, soluble salts, and normal pH. The total plasma calcium is composed of ionized or diffusible calcium and nondiffusible calcium bound to plasma proteins. Both forms are in a state of equilibrium influenced by parathyroid hormone. The normal serum calcium level is 9 to 11.5 mg./100 ml. in the adult and is slightly higher in children. Elevation of serum calcium is known as hypercalcemia, and depression is called hypocalcemia. Elevation or depression of serum calcium is diagnostically and clinically significant in a number of metabolic diseases.

Phosphorus is an important buffer in the blood in addition to playing an active role in calcium-phosphorus metabolism. It occurs as an inorganic phosphate. Eighty percent of body phosphorus is in bone matrix complexed as an insoluble calcium salt. It is regulated by the effect of parathyroid hormone on phosphorus excretions at the kidney level and calcium mobilization from bones. It is also influenced by vitamin D, growth hormone, kidney diseases, and the serum concentration of calcium. An increase in phosphorus is known as hyperphosphatemia, and a decrease constitutes hypophosphatemia. It is intricately related to calcium metabolism, and abnormalities suggest a disorder of the normal homeostasis.

Alkaline phosphatase is an enzyme occurring in the osteoblasts of bone, but it is also present in intestinal mucosal cells, renal tubular cells, adrenal glands, spleen, lungs, mammary gland, leukocytes, and seminiferous tubules. Its level does not vary with sex but is higher in children because of actively growing bones. The serum alkaline phosphatase value (see Table 1-1) is elevated in any disease of bone involving increased osteoblastic activity. The highest levels are seen in Paget's disease. It is not specific for bone disease because obstructive diseases of the liver and bile ducts will also cause an inordinate elevation.

Acid phosphatase is produced primarily by the acinar cells of the prostate with smaller amounts produced by erythrocytes. It is also produced by carcinomatous cells of the bladder, bronchi, bones, and stomach, primarily when metastatic. Serum acid phosphatase (see Table 1-1) is the same in adults and children of both sexes. Increased levels of acid phosphatase in a patient over age 50 strongly suggest the diagnosis of metastatic carcinoma of the prostate gland.

Uric acid is the end product of purine metabolism formed by the degradation of nucleoproteins found in all body cells. The chemical methods for its estimation are nonspecific, and 10 percent of the expressed total amount is not uric acid. Its level is highest in men and found in decreasing concentrations in women and children (see Table 1-1). Increased blood uric acid is known as hyperuricemia, and it can be caused by a primary enzyme defect causing increased production which is hereditary or it can be secondary from decreased excretion. It is rare for verified instances of untreated gout to occur with a serum urate of less than 7 mg./100 ml. However, an elevation in itself is not diagnostic of gout.

The globulins in the serum are now determined by an electrophoretic method separating it into the different fractions: alpha, beta, and gamma globulin. The alpha globulin averages from 0.7 to 1.3 and the beta fraction, from 1.0 to 1.2 g./100 ml. The different fractions are elevated in specific disease states: alpha globulin is usually increased in chronic infections and rheumatoid arthritis, whereas the beta and gamma fractions are elevated in multiple myeloma.

Creatine phosphokinase (CPK) is a measure of a particular enzyme which leaks into the serum when muscle fibers are damaged. It is a very sensitive indicator of early muscle damage and is even increased in 70 percent of the female carriers of the sex-linked recessive gene.

Rheumatoid Factor. The serums of most patients with rheumatoid arthritis contain anti-gamma globulin antibodies. These anti-gamma globulin antibodies are called rheumatoid factors. They are not unique to rheumatoid arthritis patients, but most adults with rheumatoid disease do exhibit them. These tests may be elevated in juvenile rheumatoid arthritis, but this is not likely unless the disease has been present for many years. Therefore, they are not very useful as a diagnostic aid in children. The most common tests performed for evaluation of rheumatoid factor are the sheep-cell agglutination and the latex fixation and bentonite tests.

Lupus Erythematosus Prep. Positive LE cell tests are found in about 80 percent of patients with systemic lupus erythematosus (SLE). A negative test does not rule out the diagnosis, and a positive test is not in itself diagnostic. It confirms the clinical diagnosis.

Total antinucleoprotein (ANA), if positive, is not specific as it is seen in a variety of chronic diseases. If negative, it rules strongly against the diagnosis of SLE.

Anti-DNA. This is the antibody to native DNA, and a positive test is essentially diagnostic of SLE. It indicates the probability of nephritis. A negative study is not particularly helpful.

HL-A Typing. Brewerton first noted a 95 percent incidence of HL-A antigen of the W-27 type in ankylosing spondylitis. Subsequently, it has been found in 76 percent of those with Reiter's syndrome. It has also been found in a high percentage of patients with sacroiliitis associated with inflammatory bowel diseases. In psoriasis, there appears to be an increased incidence of A-13 and W-17 antigens, but not the W-27 type. However, in those with psoriatic arthritis, it is seen in a high percentage. Therefore, if a patient has psoriasis and a W-27 antigen, there is a strong likelihood he will develop arthritis.

Venereal Disease Research Laboratories Test. Since Wassermann first discovered the complement fixation test for syphilis, there have been

Table 1-1. Common Blood Chemistries Used in Differentiating Musculoskeletal Disorders

	Normal Value	Increased		Decreased
Sed. rate	1-7 men 4-11 women (Westergren)	Osteomyelitis Septic arthritis Gout Infections, acute and chronic Multiple myeloma	Lead poisoning Rheumatoid arthritis Rheumatic fever Collagen diseases All bone malignancies (leukemia, metastatic, primary)	Sickle cell anemia
Glucose	80-120 mg./100 ml. (Folin-Wu) 60-100 mg./100 ml. (True)	Diabetes mellitus Hyperthyroidism Acromegaly (early) Hemochromatosis	Adrenal tumors Strenuous exercise Severe infections Steroid administration	Addison's disease Acromegaly (late) Hypothyroidism Muscular dystrophies
Calcium	9-11.5 mg./100 ml.	Hyperparathyroidism Hypervitaminosis D Hypophosphatasia (or normal) Multiple myeloma	Addison's disease Osteogenic sarcoma Sarcoidosis	Hypoparathyroidism (tetany) Childhood rickets (or normal) Renal rickets (or normal) Osteomalacia Hypovitaminosis D Osteogenesis imperfecta (or normal) Pseudohypoparathyroidism
Phosphorus	2.5-4.5 mg./100 ml. (adults) 4-6 mg./100 ml. (children)	Renal rickets (or normal) Hypoparathyroidism (tetany) Pseudohypoparathyroidism		Hyperparathyroidism Rickets
Alkaline phosphatase	4-10 K.A.U. 1-6 Bod. units (adult) 10-20 K.A.U. 1-15 Bod. units (child)	Paget's disease Gaucher's disease Leukemia Myeloma Osteogenic sarcoma Sarcoidosis Rickets Hyperparathyroidism Osteoblastic bone metastases	Healing fractures Hyperphosphatasia Polyostotic fibrous dysplasia (or normal) Osteogenesis imperfecta (or normal) Osteomyelitis Osteomalacia	Hypophosphatasia Osteoporosis (or normal) Hypothyroidism in children

Acid phosphatase	0-4 K.A.U. 0-1 Bod. U.	Metastatic carcinoma of prostate Gaucher's disease (or normal) Myeloma Paget's (or normal)		Male castration
Uric acid	3-6 mg./100 ml. (men) 2-5 mg./100 ml. (women) 1-4 mg./100 ml. (children)	Gout Leukemia Myeloma		Administration of uricosuric drugs (aspirin, Benemid, colchicine)
Globulin (electrophoresis)	2.5-3.5 gm./100 ml.	Multiple myeloma Sarcoidosis Osteomyelitis Chronic infectious disease (tuberculosis, syphilis, malaria) Rheumatoid arthritis Systemic lupus erythematosus		Administration of nitrogen mustard
CPK		Strenuous exercise Muscular dystrophy Diseases actively destroying muscle (dermatomyositis)		

(Modified from Fox, T. [ed.]: Manual of Orthopaedic Surgery. American Orthopaedic Association, 1963; and Yater, W. M.: Fundamentals of Internal Medicine, ed. 4. New York, Appleton-Century-Crofts, 1954.)

innumerable specific diagnostic tests for syphilis including serologic tests like the VDRL and many treponemal antibody tests.

Synovial Fluid

The technique of aspirating specific joints to obtain synovial fluid for study may be found in standard orthopaedic and arthritis texts. Always keep in mind the insertion of a needle into a joint has the potential for carrying bacteria into the area. Therefore, all aspirations for synovial fluid must be carried out under sterile conditions. A betadine prep which is allowed to dry for several minutes is adequate. A 20-gauge needle or larger is required to aspirate the fluid.

Synovial fluid is a transudate which is a dialysate of blood plasma. There are five factors to study grossly: volume, color, clarity, viscosity, and the formation of a mucin clot. The color of normal fluid is straw and almost colorless but changes in disease states (Table 1-2). Normally, it is transparent and clear enough to read a printed page through a test

Table 1-2. Synovial Fluid Analysis

	Gross Appearance				*Microscopically*				*Special Tests*		
	Color	*Clarity*	*Viscosity*	*Mucin Clot*	*WBC* (mm^3)	*Predominant Cell*	*Crystals*	*Bacteria*	*Sugar mg. %*	*Total Protein mg. %*	*Complement*
Normal	Straw	Transparent	High	Good	10-150	Mono	0	0	90	1.7	
					Noninflammatory						
Osteoarthritis	Amber-yellow	Transparent	High	Good	800	Mono	0	0	90	3.0	
Neuropathic Charcot joint	Yellow	Transparent	High	Good	800	Mono	0	0	80	3.4	
Osteochondritis dissecans	Yellow	Transparent	High	Good	500	Mono	0	0	90	2.0	
					Hemorrhagic						
Hemophilic arthritis	Red	Turbid	High	Good	5,000	RBC	0	0	60	6.0	
Traumatic arthritis	Red	Turbid	High	Good	1,500	RBC	0	0	90	4.0	
Pigmented villonodular synovitis	Brown to red	Turbid	Moderate	Poor to good	3,000	RBC	0	0	70	4.2	
					Inflammatory						
Rheumatoid arthritis	Yellow-green	Turbid	Low	Poor	15,000	Poly	0	0	80	4.7	Reduced
Gout	Milky-yellow	Turbid	Low	Poor	15,000	Poly	+ Urate	0	85	4.0	
Pseudogout	Yellow	May be cloudy	Moderate	Poor to good	3,000	Poly	+ Calcium pyrophosphate	0	85	3.0	
Reiter's syndrome	Yellow	Mildly turbid	Moderate	Poor to good	20,000	Poly	0	0	80	4.4	High but serum also high
Systemic lupus erythematosus	Straw	May be cloudy	High	Good	5,000	Poly	0	0			Reduced
Rheumatic fever	Yellow	Turbid	Low	Good	50,000	Poly	0	0	90	3.5	
					Septic						
Bacterial	Grey-brown	Very turbid	Low	Poor	100,000 plus	Poly	0	+	20	5.0	
Tuberculous	Yellow	Turbid	Low	Poor	25,000	Poly	0	+	25	5.5	
Gonococcal	Yellow & brown	Turbid	Low	Poor	50,000 plus	Poly	0	+	30-80	5.5	

(Modified from Ropes, M. W., and Bauer, W.: Synovial Fluid Changes in Joint Disease. Cambridge, Mass., Harvard University Press, 1953; and Jessar, R. A.: The study of synovial fluid, pp. 67–81. *In* Hollander, J. L., and McCarty, D. J., Jr., [eds.]: Arthritis and Allied Conditions, ed. 8. Philadelphia, Lea & Febiger, 1972.)

tube. One can measure viscosity precisely with a viscosimeter, but this is not normally done. Instead, if it is dripped slowly from the aspirating syringe drop by drop, a rough quantitation may be made. In very viscous fluids, the drops may form a string several inches long, and in low viscous fluids, it will drop like water. The other method used is to place a drop of fluid between the thumb and forefinger and then to separate them. In very viscous fluids it may string for more than 1 inch. The mucin clot test is an indicator of the protein-polysaccharide complex. It can be performed by adding glacial acetic acid drop by drop to synovial fluid or conversely by adding synovial fluid drop by drip to a beaker of 5 percent acetic acid. Normal fluids form a firm, white, ropy clot (Fig. 1-7), and the fluids of patients with rheumatoid arthritis or septic conditions are loose and friable.

The microscopic examination of the joint fluid consists of a cell count with identification of specific cells, plus Gram stain or other special stains for bacteria, and examination for formed elements, such as crystals. The white blood cell count is performed in the standard counting chamber except that the ordinary white cell counting solution is changed. Normal sodium chloride solution is substituted to prevent mucin clot formation. If the fluid is bloody, a hypotonic saline solution (0.3 percent) is used. If the fluid sediment is stained with Wright's, the predominant cell can be identified. In the majority of patients with lupus, a LE cell can be seen. Cell counts above 25,000 with a shift to the left (immature polymorphonuclear cells) indicate infectious arthritis, and appropriate bacterial stains and cultures are indicated. Partially treated infections and low virulent organisms will give counts below 25,000 and can be a source of great confusion.

The formed elements to be looked for are usually crystals, such as urate, calcium, pyrophosphate, or cholesterol, but cartilage debris and the so-called *rheumatoid arthritis cell* may be seen. A polarizing light microscope aids in the identification of specific crystals. If unavailable, it can be improvised by inserting Polaroid disks into the eyepiece and condenser of a standard microscope. The crystals are rod shaped with a strongly negative birefringence and are pathognomonic for gout (Fig. 1-8). Chondrocalcinosis or pseudogout exhibits calcium pyrophosphate crystals which are rod-like or rhomboid shaped with sharp corners and under polarization are weakly positive birefringent. Cholesterol crystals which are flat with notched corners have been seen in rheumatoid arthritis. Steroid crystals may be seen in joints previously injected with corticosteroids. Other formed elements identified include metallic fragments from total joints and cartilage debris found in osteoarthritis, Charcot joints, and osteochondritis

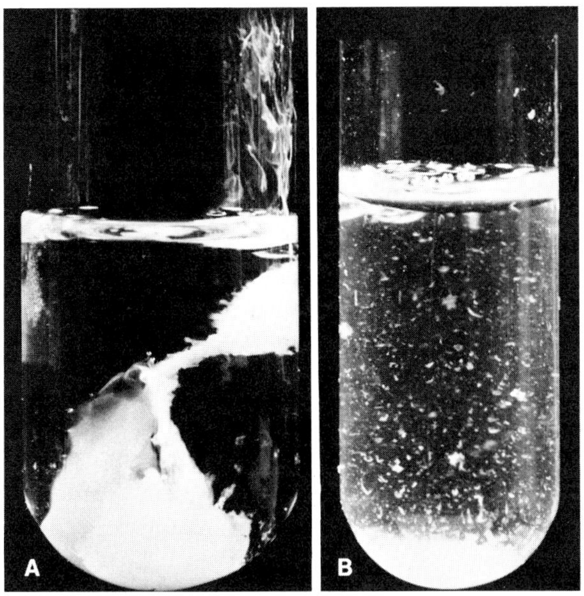

Fig. 1-7. Mucin clot test. (*A*) Normal fluids form a firm white ropy clot. (*B*) Loose and friable clots are seen in rheumatoid arthritis or septic joints.

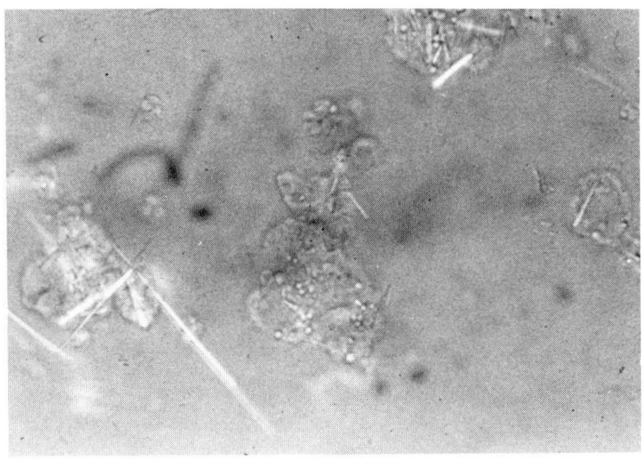

Fig. 1-8. Sodium urate crystals in a patient with gout. The crystals are rod-shaped with a strongly negative birefringence and are pathognomonic for gout.

dissecans. A special cell known as the *rheumatoid arthritis cell* is a leukocyte with dark granules which are cytoplasmic inclusions and can be identified by special staining techniques.

Several special tests can be performed on synovial fluid including determination of sugar, protein, and complement levels. Sugar is normally 90 mg./100 ml. and less than 10 mg./100 ml. below the normal blood level. In most disease conditions, it is decreased less than 10 mg./100 ml. but is 20 mg./100 ml. lower in hemorrhagic conditions and 60 mg./100 ml. lower in septic conditions. The total protein is normally one third that found in the blood but approaches and surpasses this level in septic conditions.

Evaluation of complement in synovial fluid has been helpful in differentiating rheumatoid arthritis and systemic lupus erythematosus. In these two diseases, immune complexes are formed in the joint which activate and fix complement causing a decrease in joint fluid complement compared with serum levels. The complement system plays an important role in blood vessel permeability, attracting neutrophils for phagocytosis and ultimate rupture of the neutrophils with subsequent liberation of lysosomal enzymes which destroy cartilage. When inflammation occurs in a joint, there is increased permeability with resultant increase in complement, but this parallels serum levels. Usually, the synovial fluid complement is 10 percent lower than serum levels except in rheumatoid arthritis and systemic lupus erythematosus in which it is markedly reduced. Reiter's syndrome has marked elevation of synovial fluid complement, but this is also paralleled with an elevation in serum complement activity.

Cerebrospinal Fluid

Cerebrospinal fluid is formed as a blood plasma dialysate filtered by the choroid plexuses, primarily in the lateral ventricles. Smaller quantities are secreted by the ependymal cells of the plexuses and minimal quantities by the perivascular spaces of the spinal cord. This fluid serves as a mechanical buffer which protects the brain and spinal cord from sudden trauma. It also equalizes pressure within the various compartments, removes wastes, and forms an alkali reserve between the blood and central nervous system.

The technique of spinal fluid collection is described in detail in most texts. It can be done with the patient in the sitting or recumbent position, but the latter is preferred. It should be done in a hospital under sterile conditions with a 20-gauge needle. The puncture is best performed between the third and fourth or fourth and fifth lumbar vertebrae. The fluid is collected in three tubes of approximately 3 to 4 ml. each. It is important for the patient to stay at bedrest on his back for 24 hours to reduce the risk of post-spinal-tap headache.

The examination of the fluid falls into three categories: physical appearance, microscopic examination, and changes in blood chemistry. Under physical appearance, the color, clarity, specific gravity, pressure, and presence of coagulum or xanthochromia are evaluated. The fluid is normally colorless and transparent, with a specific gravity of 1.006 to 1.008. In encephalitis and meningitis, it is cloudy grey and purulent and possibly bloody. In subarachnoid hemorrhage, it will be bloody and when spun down xanthochromic. A coagulum will be present in tumors, meningitis, and like conditions which cause increase in spinal fluid protein. It is important to realize that in many diseases, especially early in the course, the spinal fluid is clear. Normal spinal fluid pressure in adults is 80 to 140 mm. of water or 6 to 10 mm. of mercury in the recumbent position. It is moderately elevated in the sitting position and approximately 3 mm. of water lower in children. It becomes increased in the presence of a ruptured cerebral aneurysm, encephalitis and meningitis, or cerebral trauma. It is decreased in hydrocephalus, dehydration, or with blockage from a tumor. The pressure should be checked before and after the fluid is collected. A drop of water pressure less than 20 mm. suggests a large reservoir, as in hydrocephalus, and an excessive drop suggests a small reservoir caused by some obstructive lesion. Queckenstedt developed a test for evaluating the presence of a partial or complete block of the subarachnoid space. When the jugular veins are compressed in the neck, there is immediate increase in spinal fluid pressure from venous congestion and a subsequent increase in spinal fluid pressure in the lumbar region. Normally, the pressure will rise 40 mm. in 20 sec. and return to the original level in another 20 sec. If the block is complete, as in fracture-dislocations of vertebrae or in spinal cord tumor, a rise in pressure does not occur, and, if partial, it is delayed and does not reach as high a level. This test is dangerous, especially in diseases which produce high pressure because the brain may herniate downward through the foramen magnum with fatal results.

The microscopic examination includes a total cell count, identification of predominant cells, and presence of red blood cells. In normal individuals, the total cell count is under 8 per $mm.^3$ in adults and up to 10 per $mm.^3$ in children. The cells are usually lymphocytes and occasionally mononuclear. Normally, erythrocytes are not present unless from a traumatic tap or some disease process which has caused them to enter the fluid. The total cell count is increased in all infectious processes plus tumors and multiple sclerosis. The polymorphonuclears are predominant in cerebral tumors and in early encephalitis, meningitis, and poliomyelitis, but in the later stages of these diseases the lymphocytes predominate. The lymphocyte is the prominent cell in multiple sclerosis. Erythrocytes are seen in spinal cord injuries and birth injuries.

The blood chemistries that can be performed on serum can also be performed on spinal fluid. The most commonly evaluated are glucose, protein, chloride, colloidal gold, and VDRL. Glucose normally is 40 to 70 mg./100 ml. in adults and 70 to 90 mg./100 ml. in children. It is roughly 70 percent of the serum value. Marked depression is characteristic of the acute stages of purulent meningitis, with increases in acidosis or diseases producing hyperglycemia. Total protein varies between 15 to 45 mg./100 ml., and electrophoresis will determine if a specific component like gamma globulin is elevated which is helpful in the diagnosis of multiple sclerosis. Total protein is increased in the acute stage of meningitis and encephalitis with lesser increases later in the disease, and increases are seen in both spinal and cerebral tumors. Cerebrospinal fluid chloride is decreased in purulent meningitis, especially tuberculosis. In various diseases, but particularly tabes dorsalis, the spinal fluid will precipitate gold, characteristically in three different zones. Syphilis characteristically precipitates in zone I, and multiple sclerosis also precipitates in this zone in half of the cases. The diseases which precipitate in zone II include congenital syphilis, tabes dorsalis, viral encephalitis, cerebral hemorrhage, spinal cord and cerebral tumors, poliomyelitis, lead encephalopathy, transverse myelitis, and rarely multiple sclerosis. The epidemic encephalitides, aseptic and purulent meningitis, and poliomyelitis precipitate in zone III. The VDRL test for syphilis can be performed on spinal fluid similar to serum from the blood. Many sophisticated examinations for gamma globulin fractions, like immune electrophoresis, can be performed to identify diseases affecting specific globulin fragments, such as multiple sclerosis.

Abnormal Fluids

Any fluid collection in any area of bone, soft tissue, or bursa in the musculoskeletal system should be examined grossly, microscopically, and with blood chemistries much as synovial and cerebrospinal fluids are examined.

Urine

A urinalysis should be done on each patient including specific gravity, sugar, protein, acetone, and microscopy. When indicated, culture and sensitivity of the urine should be performed. If a bone marrow disturbance is suspected, the diagnosis of multiple myeloma can be made by evaluation for Bence Jones protein. Urine protein electrophoresis may also be used in the diagnosis of multiple myeloma. Urine cultures may reveal the presence of tuberculous bacilli. The reasons for doing a urinalysis are obvious, especially if an orthopaedic operation is planned and the patient has a urinary tract infection.

Biopsy Specimens

The musculoskeletal specialist works closely with a pathologist when examining soft tissues and bone, particularly in diagnosing and differentiating musculoskeletal neoplasms and infections. These biopsies may be aspirated from the sternum or iliac crest or a punch biopsy may be performed. Usually in the case of a tumor an open biopsy is performed in the surgical theater. It is beyond the scope of this text to go into the pathology of orthopaedic diseases, and the reader is referred to Aegeiter and Kirkpatrick's text.[1]

Skin

Skin tests are important in diagnosing certain infectious diseases which affect bone, such as tuberculosis, coccidioidomycosis, and histoplasmosis. When suspicions are aroused from these tests, further investigations should be done with microscopy, sputum smears, and gastric washings.

ELECTROMYOGRAPHY

Electromyography is important in diagnosing musculoskeletal disease, and Chapter 3 is devoted to this technique and its application to the musculoskeletal examination.

ROENTGENOGRAPHY

The roentgenographic examination is extremely valuable in differentiating musculoskeletal disorders, and Chapter 2 is devoted to the interpretation of musculoskeletal roentgenograms. As important as it is, it does not take the place of a careful history, physical examination, and laboratory studies, but instead is used in close conjunction with them. The proper roentgen views for specific areas and special roentgenographic techniques like arthrography and myelography are described when applicable for specific body regions.

DIFFERENTIAL DIAGNOSIS

To diagnose is to recognize a disease from its symptoms. To differentiate is to distinguish by a specific difference, characteristic, or symptoms. Therefore, when one is asked to elaborate on a differential diagnosis of a particular symptom complex like painful hip with temperature elevation in a child, immediately a number of specific diagnoses should come to mind: pyogenic arthritis, nonpyogenic arthritis, osteomyelitis of the proximal femur, transient synovitis, pauciarticular arthritis, and rheumatic fever. Only by thinking of all possible diagnoses while assimilating the data can the physician be sure that he does not overlook the diagnosis. Chapters 6 through 12 deal with the specific regional areas of the musculoskeletal system. The last part of each of these chapters has a differential diagnosis section. Diseases which present in a particular manner are grouped together and discussed with their particular characteristics.

SUGGESTED READINGS

1. Aegeiter, Ernest, and Kirkpatrick, John A., Jr.: Orthopedic Diseases. ed. 2. Philadelphia, W. B. Saunders Company, 1975.
2. American Rheumatism Association, Arthritis Foundation: Primer on the Rheumatic Diseases. JAMA, *224*:5, 1973.
3. Crenshaw, A. H.: Campbell's Operative Orthopaedics. ed. 5. St. Louis, C. V. Mosby Company, 1971.
4. Ducroquet; Robert: Walking and Limping: A Study of Normal and Pathological Walking. Philadelphia, J. B. Lippincott, 1968.
5. Gardner, Ernest; Gray, Donald J.; and O'Rahilly, Ronon: Anatomy. Philadelphia, W. B. Saunders Company, 1975.
6. Hollander, Joseph L., and McCarty, Daniel J.: Arthritis and Allied Conditions. ed. 8. Philadelphia, Lea & Febiger, 1972.
7. Kolmer, John A.: Clinical Diagnosis by Laboratory Examinations. ed. 3. New York, Appleton-Century-Crofts, Inc., 1961.
8. Manual of Orthopaedic Surgery. American Orthopaedic Association, 1966.
9. Ropes, Marian W., and Bauer, Walter: Synovial Fluid Changes in Joint Disease. Cambridge, Harvard University Press, 1953.

2 Roentgenogram Interpretation

Albert B. Ferguson, M.D.

It is not the purpose of this chapter to discuss all the special radiological techniques but to offer to the student of orthopaedics an organized method of study of films to achieve rapid and efficient extraction of the information which can be useful in differentiating various diagnoses.

HOW TO APPROACH READING ROENTGENOGRAMS

The state of mind in which one approaches inspection of orthopaedic roentgenograms has much to do with successful observation, interpretation, and deduction.

The able examiner proceeds in an orderly manner to consider all facts which may be helpful. Students should become familiar with those facts so that they can do likewise and acquire a habit which will lead them successively through the signs whose presence, absence, and significance should become discernible. Little time should be spent on shadows which are not yet known to have significance. The purpose of this chapter is to outline a method for such analysis.

It is not necessarily the task of the roentgenographic examiner to arrive at a precise diagnosis; that task belongs to the physician who is responsible for the patient. The orthopaedic surgeon inspecting the roentgenograms may be that physician, but he is momentarily in the position of the examiner of the roentgenograms. The more he can temporarily divorce himself from the diagnostic responsibility, the more readily he can concentrate on gleaning from the roentgenograms all of the information which is available and relevant. Thereafter comes the time to consider the data from all other examinations and facets of the case and get down to the serious matter of decision on diagnosis, prognosis, and treatment.

Consistent with that statement of the situation, the examiner of the roentgenograms may more freely and fully glean available information if the nature and clinical history of the patient are not yet known. However, the orthopaedist is not often without such knowledge. The orthopaedist must try to avoid the trap which is waiting for him if he has an opinion about what is wrong with the patient, sees something which confirms that opinion, and leaps to the conclusion that the roentgenogram has supplied the corroboratory evidence. If this happens, other facts which may put a different interpretation upon the observation or indicate another and possibly important additional condition may be missed.

The examiner should not feel uneasy because of lack of familiarity with the roentgenographic signs which must be interpreted. If a shadow has size, shape, position, and relations which are consistent with an organ or part normally present or with a feature with which he is familiar, the shadow should be assumed to represent that organ, part, or feature. This deduction should be correct most of the time.

Often, an eye-catching, outstanding feature will be recognizable at first glance, visible at a distance, and indicative of the nature of the lesion or disease. Lacking an outstanding feature of such utility, look for other features which will identify a condition. Such a search is needed even though there is one characteristic outstanding feature; otherwise, a second important condition may be overlooked.

The abundance of features whose presence should be confirmed or eliminated might make this task seem difficult or even impossible. Some means of simplifying the procedure is needed if the examination is to be speedy and accurate. Such a means is available. It should be learned and followed.

The first step is to become familiar with the appearance of normal bones and tissues. They are characterized by clarity, contrast, and transparency of the structures as opposed to the haziness, indistinctness, and translucency associated with diseased tissues. Healthy bones and tissue are further characterized by evenness and regularity of outline, structure, and density.

One should be able to recognize healthy tissue at a glance. The way to do this is to spend time examining groups of films of both normal and abnormal conditions.

Clinical Facts Required Before Interpretation of a Roentgenogram

There are some clinical facts which are essential and should be known about the patient before one starts to examine a roentgenogram.

Sex

Some lesions, such as metastatic carcinoma of the prostate, occur only in one sex, but there may be lesions in females which present some similarity. Accurate, rapid reading of a roentgenogram is promoted if the sex is known. The relative development of bones and muscles which may be typical in one sex may be atypical in the other.

Age of the Patient

One may develop skill at judging the age of the patient by examination of roentgenograms. Nevertheless, the age should be known by inquiry. Development may be inconsistent with the actual age. Bones appearing as those of a child may be recognized as those of a cretin if the age is known. Some lesions tend to appear within a restricted age period. When appearances suggest a lesion at an unusual age, one should be alerted to that fact and be careful that nothing has been missed or misinterpreted. A lesion which, for example, suggests Ewing's sarcoma in patients past the age of 40 is likely to be a hemangioendothelioma. Conversely, a typical lesion at an apparently impossible age may actually be present because of an unusual cause for its presence; such a possibility should be investigated. An example is postmenopausal osteoporosis with collapsing vertebrae; there have been rare occurrences in childhood following circumstances which produced an untimely menopause.

Displacement in spondylolisthesis tends to increase before the age of 30, but there is little such trend thereafter unless there is an unusual cause, such as lifelong fatigue effects in the Eskimo due to an habitual form of labor in an unusual posture.

Increase of the sagittal diameter of the first sacral surface in spondylolisthesis occurs during teenage growth. Its presence in an adult dates the lesion from childhood instead of from some recent injury.

Sex-Age Interrelationships

Skeletal structures develop about two years earlier in females. Rapid growth in height in the spine may be over at 13 in girls but, normally, not before 16 in boys. This has a profound effect upon the expectation of progressive changes in scoliosis.

Age may have a controlling effect upon the sex incidence of some lesions, and this phenomenon should be well understood by the orthopaedist. The affliction of the tibial tubercle at the point where the patellar tendon inserts (Osgood-Schlatter's disease) often begins in males in their fourteenth year, but it is not common in females because the causative factors have not developed sufficient intensity at age 12 when rapid growth in the length of the female femur is nearly over.

Comparing two young groups with differences in age, sex, or both, it can be seen that the same causes may produce different effects or different causes produce similar lesions. Synovitis potentially preliminary to Legg-Calvé-Perthes disease may produce that condition when the age and sex are suitable and slipped capital femoral epiphysis at a later period.

Legg-Calvé-Perthes disease, for example, is not as common in the female except as a complication of other conditions because the circulation for the head of the femur becomes more stable at an earlier age before other etiological factors for the condition have become sufficiently potent. Also, slipped capital femoral epiphysis at the head of the femur will probably occur a year or two earlier in females because the most rapid growth in that area comes earlier.

The rate and duration of growth have great influence upon the results produced by other factors. The orthopaedist must acquire understanding of such influences. Such understanding develops for those who associate what they see in a roentgenogram with the actual age and sex of the patient.

Duration of the Complaint

Different causes may produce similar changes in varying lengths of time. One may list, for example, the individual features which appear in a roentgenogram of a tuberculous joint, and the same list might be duplicated with gonococcal arthritis. A big difference is that the gonococcal lesion produces those features in a month or two while the tuberculous condition takes several years. True, a skilled examiner might be able to judge this difference in timing from the relative degree of the various features, but it is far better, especially for those who are still unskilled, to know the actual apparent duration.

Calcareous reactions take time to develop. In spite of the absence of such reactions in the first 10 to 20 days after an injury or onset of an infection, the possibility of such an occurence should not be disregarded. The timing of the complaint should be known.

Previous Treatment of the Lesion

One should not spend time seeking a cause for absence of substance when it could be known that it was removed surgically. Aspiration may make effusion less prominent than would be expected for a typical lesion of the known duration. The use of antibiotics may have inhibited the development of soft tissue reactions which might otherwise be the only evidence of infection in the first few days of the disease or, later, be the evidence of activity of the lesion.

Apparent Virulence of the Lesion

With tuberculosis, there tends to be progressive effusion and decalcification about a joint. These may be much less than is expected when the lesion has been so avirulent that clinical symptoms have been very minor for a period of years.

Examination of the Films

Roentgenograms may be used for a record, fluoroscopy for function, study of a contemplated field for operation, or for mensuration and are best considered in connection with the part of the body which is concerned. They will be left to the discussion of particular areas by the authors of regional essays in this volume.

The examiner of films for diagnosis, prognosis, and selection of treatment may accumulate a mass of noted detail, much of which will consume time and be irrelevant to the purpose. An approach which combines usefulness, speed, and accuracy is needed. It is found in a search for the few relevant features which serve to classify the abnormalities and then a search for those specific details which will enable distinction of the presenting lesion from others in the same class. The examiner must look at both the soft and osseous tissues, preferably the soft tissues first, because subtle changes that may give the precise diagnosis to the osseous disease are often overlooked.

DIFFERENTIATING SOFT TISSUE DISORDERS

It commonly happens that lesions confined to the structural, nonosseous tissues present few or no roentgenographic features suitable for our classification except in the case of some degenerative lesions. Roentgenography does not always aid in diagnosis, for example, lesions of the breast and carcinoma of the skin. For those reasons, we consider it advisable to discuss the identifiable features of extraosseous lesions first and also because it will facilitate introducing you to some features which may also be seen at lesions arising in bone. This will enable us to familiarize you more gradually with the radiologically descriptive terms which we use for those features.

Specific technical terminology is needed for description of roentgenographic features. We can only obtain it by defining the exact meaning of each term for use in this chapter.

Descriptive Technical Terms of the Soft Tissues

Muscle Density

The density exhibited in those areas of a film which are mostly occupied by muscle without shadows of bone or gas (Fig. 2-1).

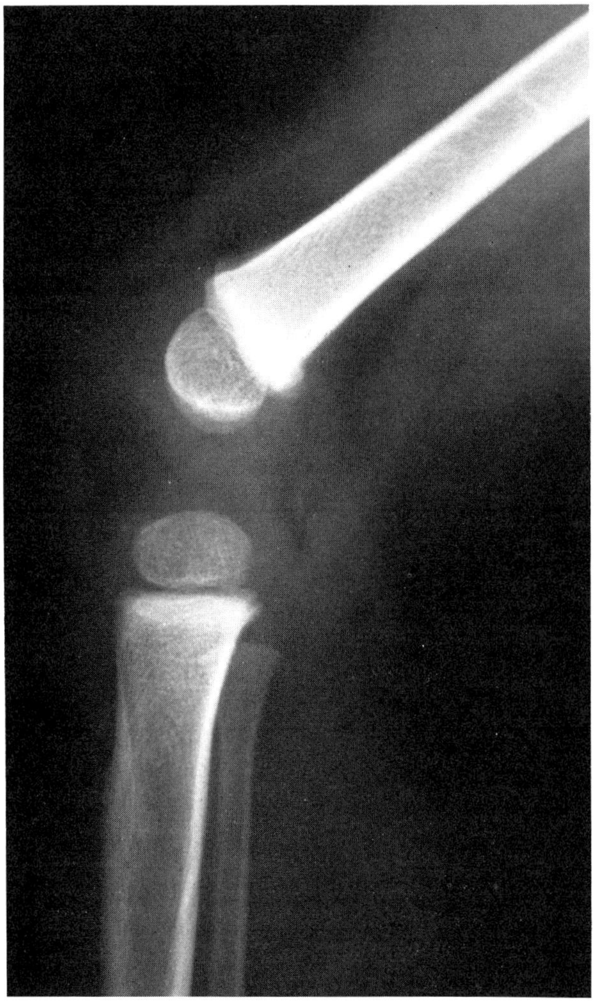

Fig. 2-1. Normal calcareous density, muscle density, and fat density. The fat pads at the knee help to outline tendons and articular cartilage. The bones and tissues have the transparent clarity of healthy tissues.

Calcareous Density

A density so much greater than muscle density that it necessarily must represent a material of substantially greater density, such as bone (see Fig. 2-1).

Metallic Density

A density so much greater than calcareous density that it necessarily represents a material of much greater specific gravity than bone. It is exhibited by the metallic markers which are used for identification of a roentgenogram. It identifies metallic foreign bodies and opaque materials injected in sinus tracts (Fig. 2-2).

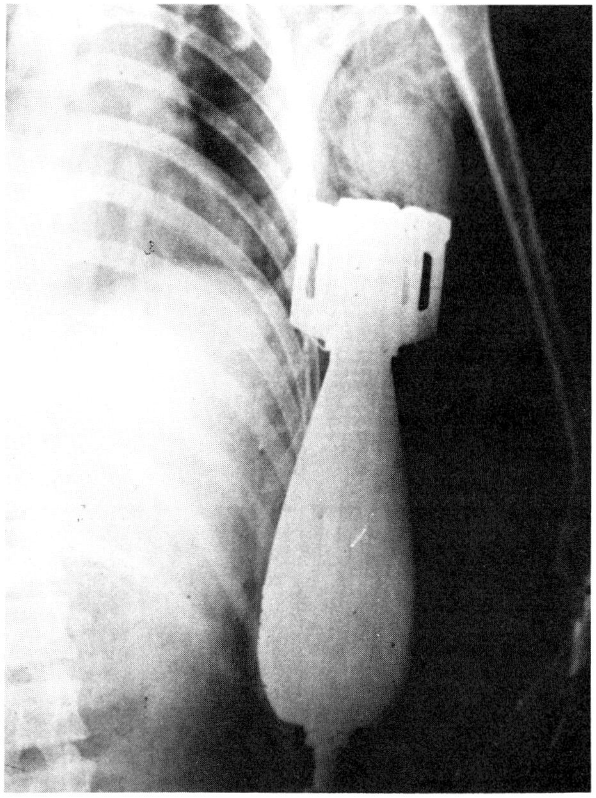

Fig. 2-2. Anteroposterior chest radiograph revealing a metallic density. A South Vietnamese soldier presented to the casualty unit, Naval Support Activity, DaNang with a left chest mass. The mass, a live mortar round, had entered superiorly, fracturing the left clavicle, and lodged subcutaneously in the left chest wall. After the round was removed surgically, the patient recovered without sequelae. The operating surgeon received the Navy Cross for his effort. (Courtesy Dr. Daniel Benson.)

Fat Density

A density so much less than muscle density that it necessarily represents a material of substantially less specific gravity, such as fat. It is seen in the subcutaneous areas and in fat pads about joints, but it is observable in fatty tumors and in fatty degeneration of muscle (see Fig. 2-1).

Gas Density

Darkness representing a density so much less than fat density that it must represent something of much less specific gravity than fat. It is observable in the areas of the film beyond the outlines of the skin and is seen in the areas of the lungs, the air passages of the neck, the intestinal shadows, and in sinuses. It is

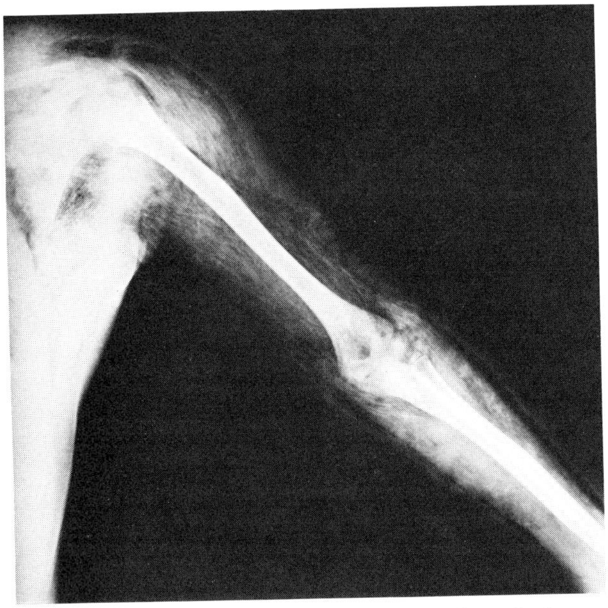

Fig. 2-3. Gas density. There is darkness in the soft tissues caused by a density much less than fat tissue. This patient was noted to have a gas bacillus secondary to an open wound. (Courtesy R. D. D'Ambrosia.)

detectable in gas bacillus infection (Fig. 2-3), open wounds, conditions which tend to produce a vacuum in a joint, air infections, and at excessively degenerated articular cartilage or intervertebral disks.

It should be evident that one should learn to recognize at a glance the nature of substances which are visible in a roentgenogram. Judgment of density is a relatively new experience for the eyes of a neophyte and time should be devoted to acquiring this ability.

Abnormalities confined to the soft tissues may reveal significant alterations of density, structure (in subcutaneous stroma, fat masses, and striation of muscles), continuity, positional relations, bilateral symmetry, length, breadth, or cartilaginous joint space. When these are not accompanied by changes in the bones, the condition is an affection of a soft tissue structure or a portion of one or more of them.

Differentiating Specific Features

Ossification

One must first differentiate ossification as contrasted to calcification. Ossification is accumulation of material of calcareous density which shows osseous structure at the time it is laid down. Osseous structure is evidenced by internal reticulation, smoothly rounded corners, and at least a thin line of continuous calcareous density at the periphery representing cortex.

Calcification

Calcification is accumulation of material of calcareous density which initially is amorphous and only slowly and indirectly develops osseous structure. One should always be able to locate some area at the periphery which is still amorphous. The distinction between these two processes, as we have defined them, is a helpful aid in identifying and understanding the roentgenographic features of many lesions (Fig. 2-4).

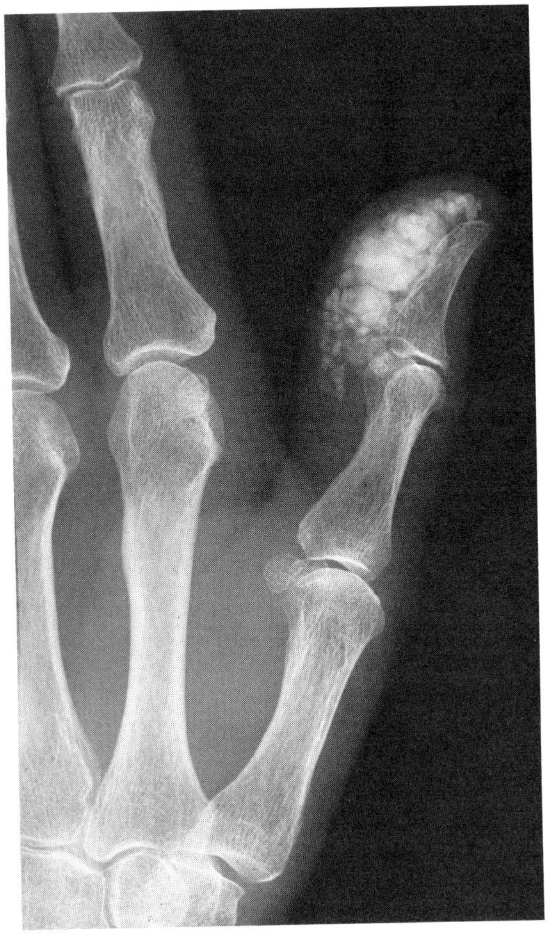

Fig. 2-4. Calcification. There are rounded masses of calcareous density in the soft tissue area. They show no internal structure, no suggestion of cortex at the periphery. They are of various sizes. A very few tiny thin short rods are visible and are indicative of calcified fat. Because most of the masses are rounded and some are large, recurring occupational trauma is the suggested cause. The bones are not affected and appear healthy.

Mass

A soft tissue mass is enlargement of a portion of a soft tissue. It tends to have a spherical outline and an identifiable limit which distinguishes it from the remainder of that tissue (Fig. 2-5).

Swelling

Swelling differs from mass in that it tends to be elongated and finally merges into unswollen tissue without demarcation at the ends (Fig. 2-6).

Inert Swelling

Inert swelling tends to show a recognizable peripheral limit unless its density is exactly equal to that of the adjacent tissue.

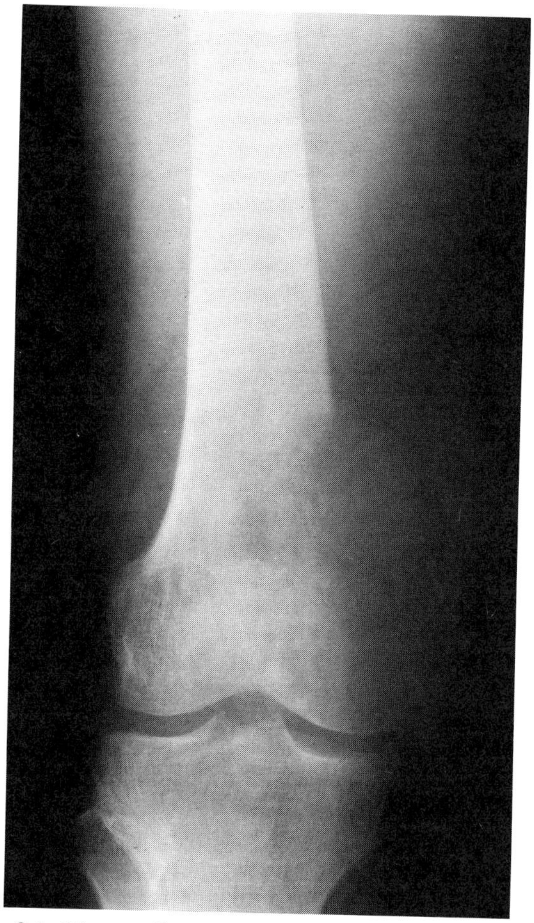

Fig. 2-5. Giant cell tumor of distal femur. There is an associated soft tissue mass which has a spherical outline and definite limits separating it from the remainder of the soft tissues. (Courtesy R. D. D'Ambrosia.)

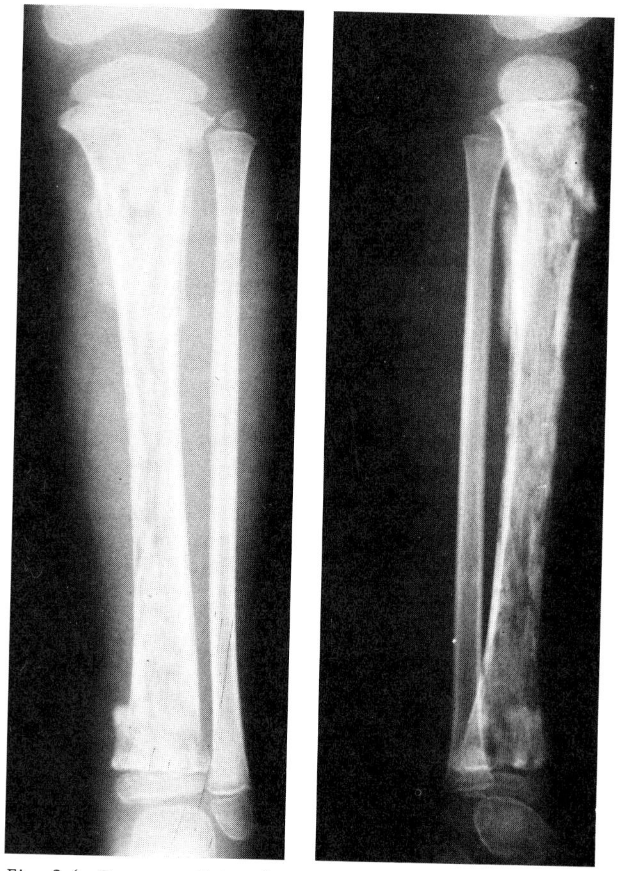

Fig. 2-6. Osteomyelitis of tibia. In distinction to a mass which has definite soft tissue limits, swelling secondary to infection is elongated and merges into the unswollen tissue with poor demarcation of its sides. (Courtesy R. D. D'Ambrosia.)

Reactive Swelling

Reactive swelling is characterized by poor demarcation of its sides due to increase of vascularity fading peripherally in adjacent tissue and reaction to the irritation by the adjacent infection (see Fig. 2-6). It is most evident when subcutaneous fat is adjacent to the periphery of the swelling. The abundant minute vessels in the deep half of that tissue, normally invisible, develop visibility which imparts an impression of faint and nearly perpendicular striation in the deep half of that tissue.

Effusion

Effusion is visible distention of the capsule of a joint by material with muscle density accumulated within its confines (Fig. 2-7). The material may be

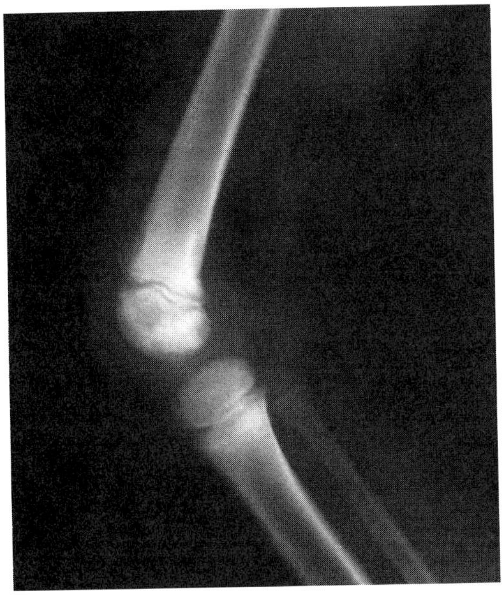

Fig. 2-7. Effusion of knee with distended capsule secondary to osteomyelitis of the distal femoral epiphysis. The joint is distended with fluid of a muscle density. (Courtesy R. D. D'Ambrosia.)

fluid of various types, synovial thickening, villi, or the tumor tissue of synovioma. The last may impart a nodular contour to the capsular outline. The distended capsule is most clearly outlined at joints well supplied with fat pads, such as the knee or ankle. The fat pads also enable easier determination as to whether the effusion is inert or reactive.

Fat Pads

Fat pads enable clear visualization of some tendons, especially the patella and calcaneal tendons. This aids detection of rupture or stenosing tenosynovitis (see Fig. 2-1). Fat pads also tend to outline the contour of adjacent articular cartilage clearly and, thus, enable observation of its thickness and smoothness. This is especially important when a portion of the cartilage is affected by abnormal development produced by a process analogous to the production of a sesamoidoma or by generalized disturbance of development in chondrodystrophy or other conditions.

Calcified Fat

Calcified fat is rare but its usual site is fat pads about a joint. The fat contains multiple minute amorphous calcifications which appear as thin rods. They become more nodular with increased duration, but some tiny rods should still be visible. The condition is posttraumatic. If a question of tumor formation has been raised it may be advisable to make additional films with and without a small area of pressure at some accessible aspect of the lesion. Lack of rigidity should be demonstrable.

Fusiform Effusion

Fusiform effusion at the proximal interphalangeal joints of the fingers is centered on the joint and symmetrical on the two sides. It indicates rheumatoid diathesis even though clinical symptoms and changes in osseous tissues are not yet present. The effusion can be detected clinically by palpation (Fig. 2-8).

Alteration of Cartilaginous Joint Space

This is the area between the bone attachments of adjacent articular cartilages. It may be thin, wide, or

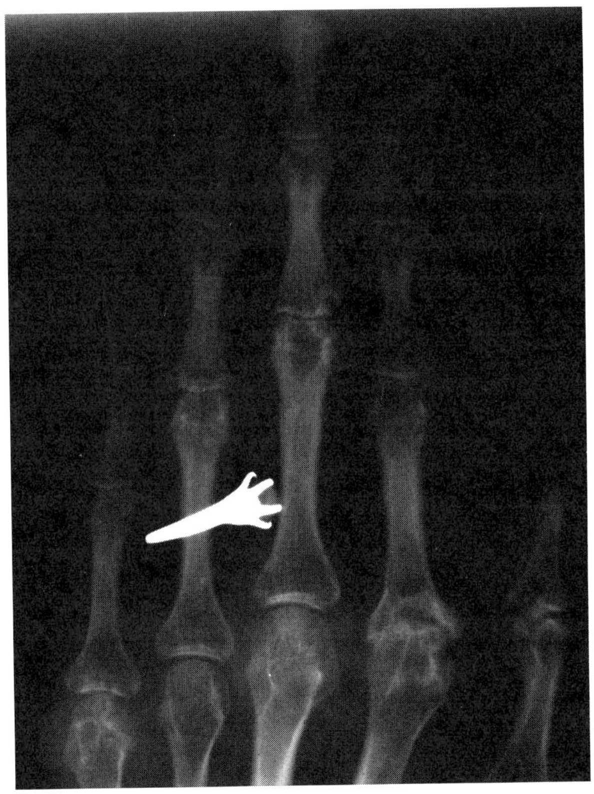

Fig. 2-8. Fusiform effusion of the proximal interphalangeal joints of the fingers in rheumatoid arthritis. It is most pronounced in the long and ring proximal interphalangeal joints. (Courtesy R. D. D'Ambrosia.)

unbalanced. Variation in depth of articular cartilage may be noted by means of visibility of its outline or by abnormality of the space between the osseous shadows. The cartilage may be diminished by underdevelopment, atrophy, or destruction. It may be increased by overdevelopment of cartilage, tumor-like development of a portion of it, or delayed conversion of cartilaginous to osseous structure. Its space may be increased by sufficient distention of the capsule by tumor mass or effusion. Function is an important factor in alteration of thickness of cartilage. Diminution of motion results in thinness by underdevelopment or atrophy, and overdevelopment may result from increase of motion or frequency of movement.

Unbalanced Joint Space

Unbalanced joint space may be seen at the knee. The space may be abnormally thin medially and abnormally deep laterally or vice versa (Fig. 2-9). It indicates derangement of the meniscus on the thin side if no other feature has been produced. Some conditions producing osseous changes, such as neurotrophic arthritis, may disorganize the joint and imitate the unbalanced space.

Calcifications in Soft Tissues

There are many types of calcification present in the soft tissues. Most calcareous densities in affections of the soft tissues are abnormal. They may be ossifications in the cases of sesamoid bones, accessory bones, and sesamoidomas. Others are almost always calcifications. Some of them have significance which it is useful to note here.

Calcareous loose bodies may be present in a joint with or without effusion. They are calcifications although they may have existed long enough to show considerable conversion to ossification (Fig. 2-10). It cannot be said that they are free within one joint unless convincing change of position is demonstrated by successive examinations. The tissue in which calcification occurs is usually attached to the capsular structures. Many of them are accompanied by osseous changes produced by the underlying disease. Fragments arising from fracture of cartilage are rarely visible unless they have suffered some calcification.

Chondromatosis produces effusion and multiple rounded loose bodies in various stages of development. It may occur without the osseous changes of osteoarthritis of which it may be a variant. The number of loose bodies, usually 10 or more, is generally diagnostic. Rarely do more than two or three loose bodies form from other causes which do not visibly affect the bones (Fig. 2-11).

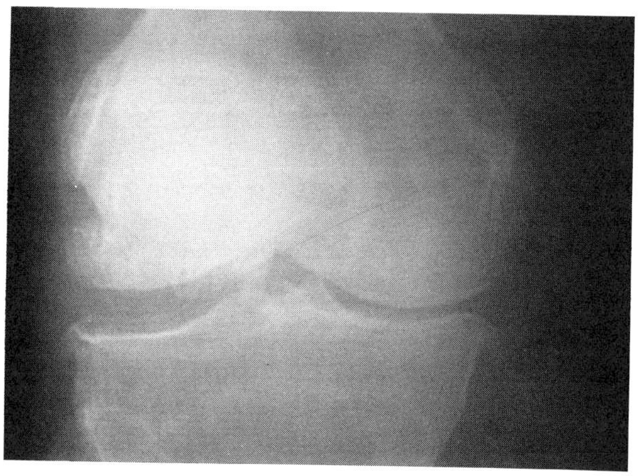

Fig. 2-9. Unbalanced joint space with abnormal thinness medially, abnormal depth laterally. The joint appears otherwise normal except for slight osteoarthritic degenerative lipping which commonly develops in the presence of abnormal stress after age 16. Medially deranged meniscus is indicated.

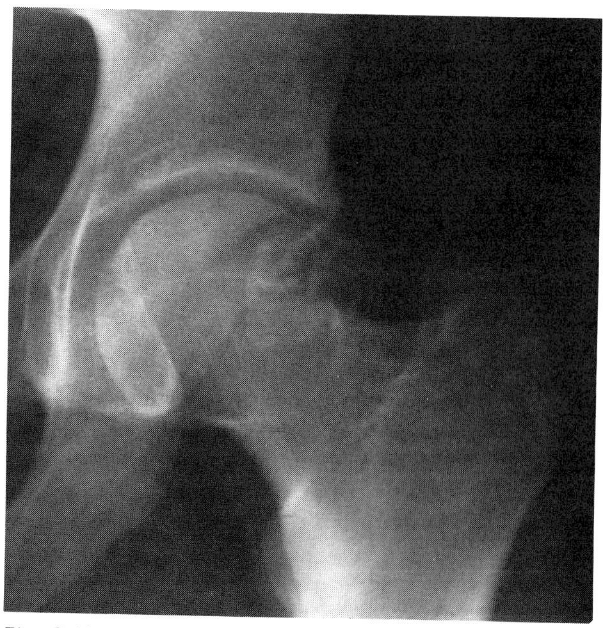

Fig. 2-10. Calcareous loose body within the hip joint. Occasionally they are free within the joint, but more often they are attached to the capsular structures. (Courtesy R. D. D'Ambrosia.)

Arteriosclerosis is diagnosed by calcifications present in the walls of arteries which outline the sides of specific arteries in more or less interrupted lines. There may be some degree of calcareous density between the lines.

Phleboliths are rounded or oval calcifications in the walls of veins although there may be some degree of calcareous density centrally. They are constantly present near the floor of the pelvis; they are not uncommon in subcutaneous tissue, especially in the legs; and they may be numerous, as in hemangiomas.

Varicose veins become recognizable by increase of width of their muscle density amid surrounding fat. Tortuosity should be clearly evident.

The vascular features which have just been mentioned should always be looked for. The state of circulation which they may suggest may affect development of certain features of lesions involving bone. Particularly subject to such influence are calcareous reactions, either productive or decalcifying, and growth.

Calcification in soft tissue occurs in masses, such as angioma, hematoma, and distended bursae; in abnormal tracts, such as subsiding abscesses, wounds, or sinuses; and in posttraumatic conditions, including calcified fat and calcifying myositis or fibrositis.

Calcification in a bursa distended by fluid or granulations tends to occur as a diffuse amorphous mass or in small discrete nodules of varying density, or both.

Posttraumatic calcifications in soft tissues tend to result from stagnation of fluid in muscle or fibrous tissue. The deposit is diffuse and amorphous at first. It tends to become more dense, more sharply defined, and contracted. When resorption follows, the deposit loses density and disappears. It may persist and gradually develop osseous texture if it is subject to the stresses of functioning.

In calcifying myositis the posttraumatic calcification in areas of stagnation of blood or lymph is confined to the involved muscle or muscles, tends to be distributed axially therein, and frays out in the direction of the muscle fibers when recently formed but is more sharply defined and contracted when mature.

Calcified hematoma, in contrast to calcifying myositis, is a more or less rounded or oval mass in muscle or other tissue. The size, shape, and position of the mass are not consistent with an organ or part normally present, although a distended bursa may be simulated. Calcification is confined to the mass and is diffuse or flocculent, irregular, and amorphous. There is little tendency to form discrete nodules, such as may be seen in calcification in a bursa or in an *ichor* pocket dependent from a tuberculous lesion. In the latter, the nodules are affected by gravity and may tend to settle toward the bottom of the ichor pocket.

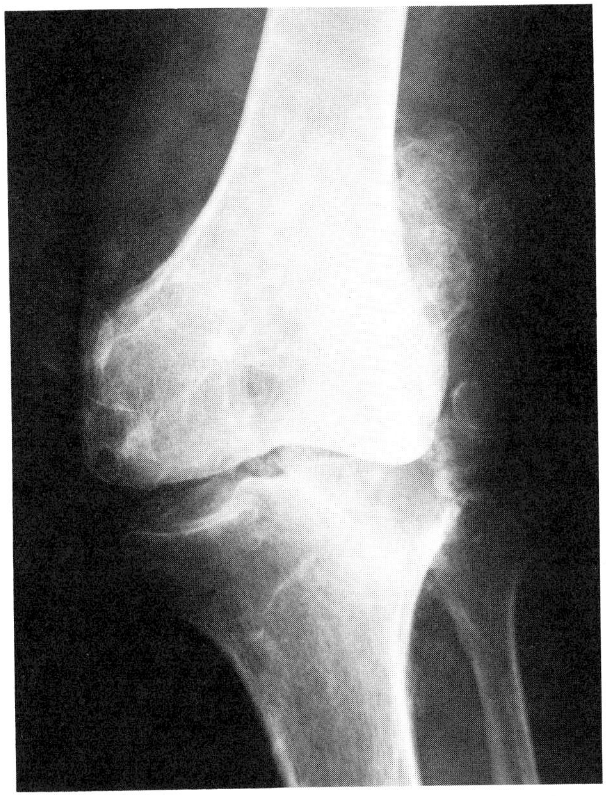

Fig. 2-11. Chondromatosis of the knee. Multiple loose bodies in various stages of development are present. (Courtesy R. D. D'Ambrosia.)

Reparative calcification may occur in the healing of soft tissues after inflammation. Calcification at a subsided pyogenic abscess is more irregular and more dense than at a hematoma or calcifying myositis. Sclerotic tissue may delay osseous change in the calcification but healthy tissues may promote it. In calcification following tendinitis of the patellar tendon, for example, osseous conversion of the calcification may occur promptly and eventually become complete.

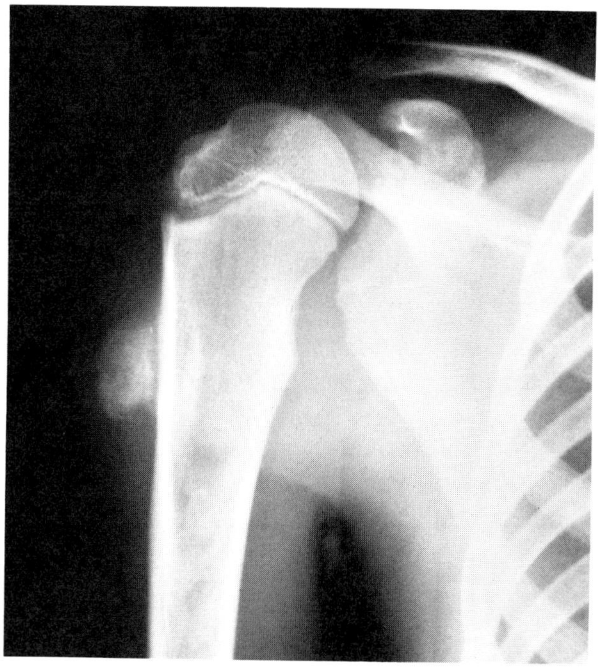

Fig. 2-12. Benign osteochondroma of proximal third of humerus. (Courtesy R. D. D'Ambrosia.)

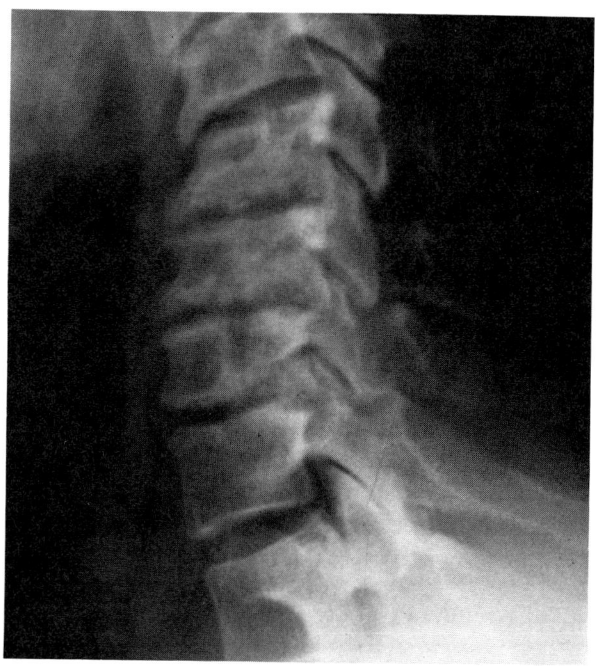

Fig. 2-13. Degenerative arthritis of the cervical spine secondary to old trauma. Note the lipping and spur formation at fibrous tissue attachments. (Courtesy R. D. D'Ambrosia.)

DIFFERENTIATING BONE AND JOINT DISORDERS

The abnormal conditions of the bones and joints can be grouped into a few classes, and each can be identified by the presence of a few certain specific features. One can easily acquire sufficient familiarity with them so that they become efficient tools for the second step of the examination, classification of the lesion. Further examination of that lesion can then be confined to our third step—the search for features which have been found to be useful for specific identification within the specified class. Thus, the diagnostic study becomes confined to a small significant portion of the vast number of features which may be present. If further information is wanted for prognosis or treatment, one knows what to look for.

Classes of Lesions

The lesions are listed in such an order that the features which identify a class do not tend to appear in a class subsequently listed except as a complication or secondary condition. Each of these conditions is known to be present when its characteristic feature is seen.

Benign Bone-Forming Tumor

Benign bone-forming tumor is indicated by adventitious ossification which is ossification outside of the reasonably expectable limits of the bone outlines. There is no change indicating any other class of lesion unless two conditions are present. The common examples are sesamoidoma, osteoma, and osteochondroma (Fig. 2-12). The latter may be capped by a thin mass having muscle density caused by the presence of cartilage not yet ossified.

Degenerative Disease

Degenerative disease at the bones and joints is practically limited to osteoarthritis involving many joints or posttraumatic degenerative arthritis confined to a joint which has been injured or is under chronic stress. Those are characterized by lipping and spur formation at the attachment of fibrous tissues, usually at the joint margins (Fig. 2-13). Such changes are calcifications within the fibrous tissue. They may be broader than the normal width of the tissue because the calcification is the end result of degenerative inflammation which may have produced swelling of the tissue before calcification. Secondary features may be present, such as effusion, fibrocystic degeneration of articular bone, or deformity due to previous injury.

We have already noted the possible presence of some degenerative conditions in the soft tissues, such as arteriosclerosis. Some noncalcareous degenerations may also be seen: fatty degeneration, fibrous degeneration, and, in the bones, fibrocystic degeneration. These appear as features secondary to other conditions rather than as specific diseases.

Active Infection

The designation of this class emphasizes that it deals with infections which are active or have an active area (Fig. 2-14). Infections which are no longer active and present a healthy appearance are classified as deformity residual from previous infection.

There are a number of features any one of which may be indicative of the presence of active infection. There are certain characteristics of infection which fall into four general areas and serve to differentiate and diagnose this condition. These are: *calcification,* which is subperiosteal; *soft tissue reaction,* i.e., reactive swelling and effusion; *bone destruction,* i.e., reactive area within bone; and *infiltrative active destruction.*

Calcification—Subperiosteal. Subperiosteal calcification is seen in many conditions including scurvy, posttraumatic subperiosteal hemorrhage, stasis, malignant tumor, and subperiosteal shell of a benign giant cell tumor. These are inert subperiosteal calcifications. Obviously, it is essential to establish a definite distinction between inert subperiosteal calcification and that which is of the infectious type (see Fig. 2-14).

Calcification beneath the periosteum is identified by the fact that its distribution is limited by the periosteum on the one hand and by the bone on the other. The character of the calcification is affected by the state of the periosteum.

Inert calcification develops beneath healthy periosteum and conforms to its outline. It is fusiform in shape, smooth in outline, and even in density except in the first few days of its formation. It is demarcated from the cortex by a thin dark line which may be merely an optical effect. This line is an important identifying feature.

Calcifications of the infectious type develop beneath diseased periosteum and are affected by its condition. They are uneven in outline, depth, and density. They tend to fuse with the cortex, especially near the ends, instead of being completely demarcated by a thin dark line. They indicate that infection is or has been present but do not necessarily indicate that the disease is active. They may persist after infection has subsided and, thus, determine the cause of the residual deformity.

Note that the thin dark line which has been described is a definite means of distinction between inert subperiosteal calcification and that of the infectious type. Fortunately, it is an easily identifiable feature.

Other forms of calcareous productive reaction occur in infections, but they also occur in other

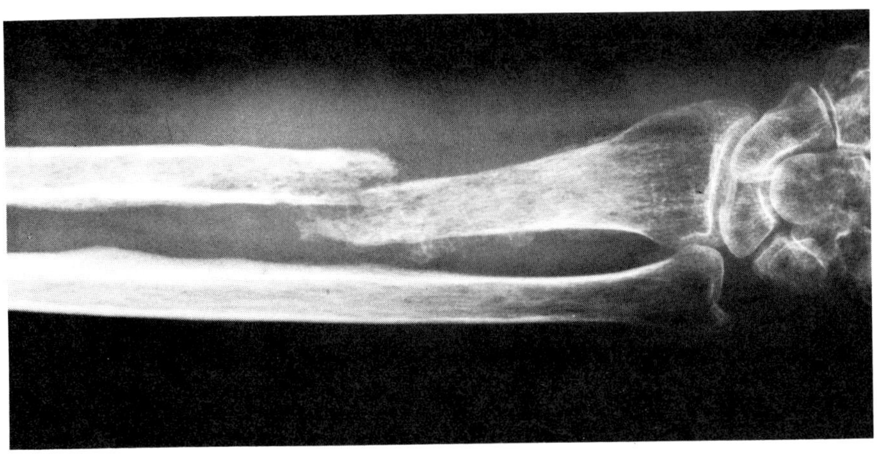

Fig. 2-14. Infection. Infiltrative active destruction affects the shaft of the radius. There is dense reactive swelling laterally which gradually fades at the ends with no outline of a spherical mass. Traces of irregular subperiosteal calcification of infectious type are present. Light density of those calcifications suggest tuberculosis, which is further suggested by general decalcification and soft tissue atrophy indicating a chronic long-standing lesion.

conditions and do not serve to identify any one class. The same may be said of decalcification which is decrease of calcareous density as visualized on a roentgenogram.

Soft Tissue Reactions. Active infection at a bone or joint may produce swelling and effusion but not a mass (see Fig. 2-7). If a mass is simulated, it will lack spherical shape because of the effect of gravity and the confining pressure of fascial planes; it will change its shape if pressure is applied.

Evidence of an active infection may be visible if the state of the circulation in tissues adjacent to the lesion produces an identifying reaction. The features referred to are described as reactive swelling, reactive effusion, and reaction area (see Fig. 2-14).

Swelling and effusion are reactive and indicate an active infection when the sides of the shadow have become indistinct because of engorgement of tiny capillaries at its surface which fade out into adjacent normal tissue. It is most clearly shown when the surface of the swelling or effusion is adjacent to subcutaneous fat or a fat pad at a joint. At the subcutaneous fat, for example, minute vessels normally not visible have become visible at least to the extent of imparting slight increase of density with faint, more or less perpendicular striation in the deep half of that tissue.

A reaction area is a highly important indicator of active infection. About such a lesion in bone there is a more or less extensive area in which there is considerable congestion and stagnation of fluid. This region is usually visible as an area of increased soft tissue density within bone. It is the reaction area. The shadow differs from that produced by overlying soft tissue masses or swelling and from the more dense harsh shadow resulting from calcareous reactions.

The reaction area has a peculiar soft hazy quality which is not duplicated by other shadows. This quality cannot be appreciated from the study of illustrations, but it can readily be recognized by comparison of several roentgenograms known to represent active infection in bone with several others known to represent other conditions, providing that the roentgenograms have been made to exhibit soft tissues as well as bone. This method is recommended as a means for gaining familiarity with several features because it is very efficient for the purpose. The bone in the reaction area is hazy, translucent, and obscured by a soft density which renders detail indistinct. Other conditions in which the bone structure appears hazy or dense tend to harshness, contrast, and transparency instead of softness, flatness, and translucency.

The underlying cause of the presence of a reaction area is resorption of medullary fat under pressure and its replacement by fluid which has muscle density. This reduces the contrast between calcareous trabeculae and the density of the medullary tissue which is seen in the interstices. The reduction of contrast by increased density of the soft tissue elements produces the translucency.

The reactive features of soft tissues, whether reactive swelling, effusion, or reaction area, have importance in addition to identifying the class of the lesion. They are a means of judging the course of the disease as to whether it is subsiding or continuing. They may be the only roentgenographic means of locating a spot or area which is the site of reactivity of an infection which had been quiescent or subsided. They may be the only roentgenographic evidence that the condition present is an active infection in the first few days of the disease before other changes have developed sufficiently to be visible. One must make sure that they have not been prevented or inhibited by use of any effective antibiotic.

Bone Destruction. An area of deficiency of a portion of bone should not be judged to represent an area of destruction until one has reason to think that bone was present there at a previous time. The words to use initially are "lack of substance." It may represent congenital absence, developmental deficiency in conversion of cartilage to bone, surgical removal, or some other state.

An area of lack of substance may show details which indicate that destruction of bone previously present is occurring or has occurred and not yet reached the stage of repair. The picture is that of active destruction. It concerns us at the moment because it indicates that the lesion is either an active infection or a malignant tumor. No lesion of any other class exhibits this feature (see Fig. 2-14).

As bone is being resorbed at the surface of an area of active destruction, the resorption is not uniform. Some spicules of bone reticulum remain projecting at the surface, and one must look further from the surface to encounter the full calcareous density of the bone. The fading of the density and the spiculated surface characterize active destruction.

The depth to which the surface shows decreased density varies with the activity and the type of the lesion. It may be very shallow in a slowly growing tumor, such as myeloma, or very deep in a persistently active tumor, such as hypernephroma.

Infiltrative Active Destruction. This condition in the bone may be characterized by the irregular spreading of the disease along bone channels, thus forming a number of more or less closely connected areas of active destruction. It is seen only in active infections (see Fig. 2-14).

Localized lesions lacking this evidence of infiltration may present invasive active destruction which is present in malignant tumors but may be simulated by some localized osteal or subperiosteal abscesses. The area of destruction tends to be spherical except on an aspect which may be flattened because it has approached an area where blood is less available for growth as at cartilage or dense fascia. When the lesion is actually an infection, the area involved is apt to be less truly spherical and is accompanied by adjacent swelling which is not a feature of malignancy unless there is secondary infection.

Malignant Tumor

A malignant tumor involving bone is indicated by the presence of invasive active destruction without the soft tissue or calcifying reactions of infections; destruction with a soft tissue mass but no swelling; or with certain forms of calcareous reaction (Fig. 2-15). The only calcareous reaction which is sufficiently unique to indicate a malignant lesion is a periosteal cuff. The lesion may occur in the presence of disease of some other class, such as osteitis deformans which is classed as a trophic disease, or osteochondroma which is a benign bone-forming tumor.

In order for a cuff to be indicative of malignancy, there must be inert subperiosteal calcification and a soft tissue mass which is destroying the calcification from the middle portion outward.

The calcification tends to be fusiform in shape with evenness of both density and the periosteal surface. It exhibits active destruction on a blunt surface which abuts upon the soft tissue mass which has invaded the calcification. Such a cuff is common in osteogenic sarcoma and in Ewing's sarcoma. It may be suggested with some infectious lesions, but there must be swelling, no mass, a calcification of the infectious type with irregularity of outline and density, and no demarcation from the cortex by a thin dark line.

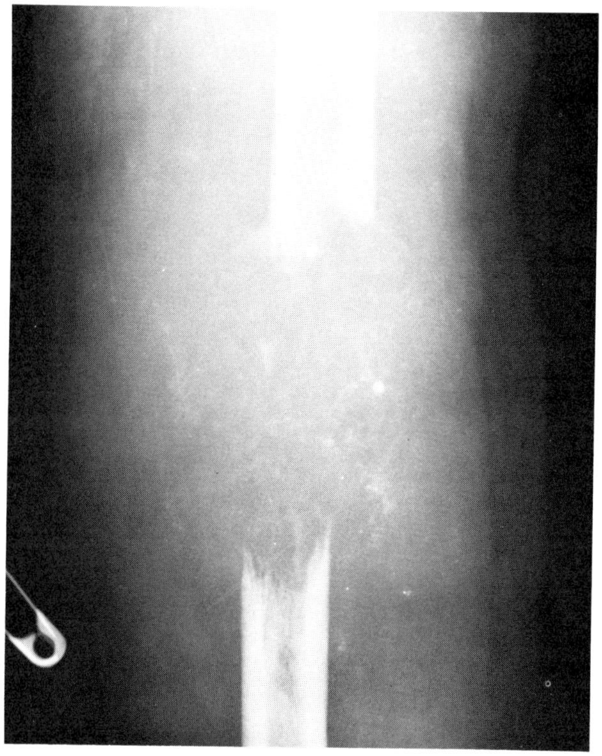

Fig. 2-15. Metastatic hypernephroma. Malignancy is indicated by invasive active total destruction, spherical soft tissue mass rather than elongated swelling, and absence of reaction area within the bone. Scattered traces of calcareous material persist in the soft tissue mass, but there is no tendency to calcifying reaction in this malignancy. The lesion is central in the midportion of the shaft rather than near a metaphysis.

Benign Tumor at Bone

Most of the lesions which are commonly designated as benign tumors within bone or at the parosteal areas develop as defects of formation of bone from cartilage in chondrodysplasia with roentgenographic features of trophic disease rather than as tumors exhibiting autonomous growth. Osteoid dysplasia, often called osteoid osteoma, is also classified as a trophic disturbance of the reparative process (Fig. 2-16). Some benign tumors identifiable by unique characteristics do exhibit autonomous growth. They are giant cell tumor, xanthoma, angioma, neurofibroma, and parosteal osteoma. Sometimes there is autonomous growth at the cartilaginous cap of an exostosis, osteoma, or osteochondroma. There is no feature which can be said to identify the class rather than the individual lesion. We will return to them when we discuss features which separate lesions within a class or you may encounter them in other portions of this book.

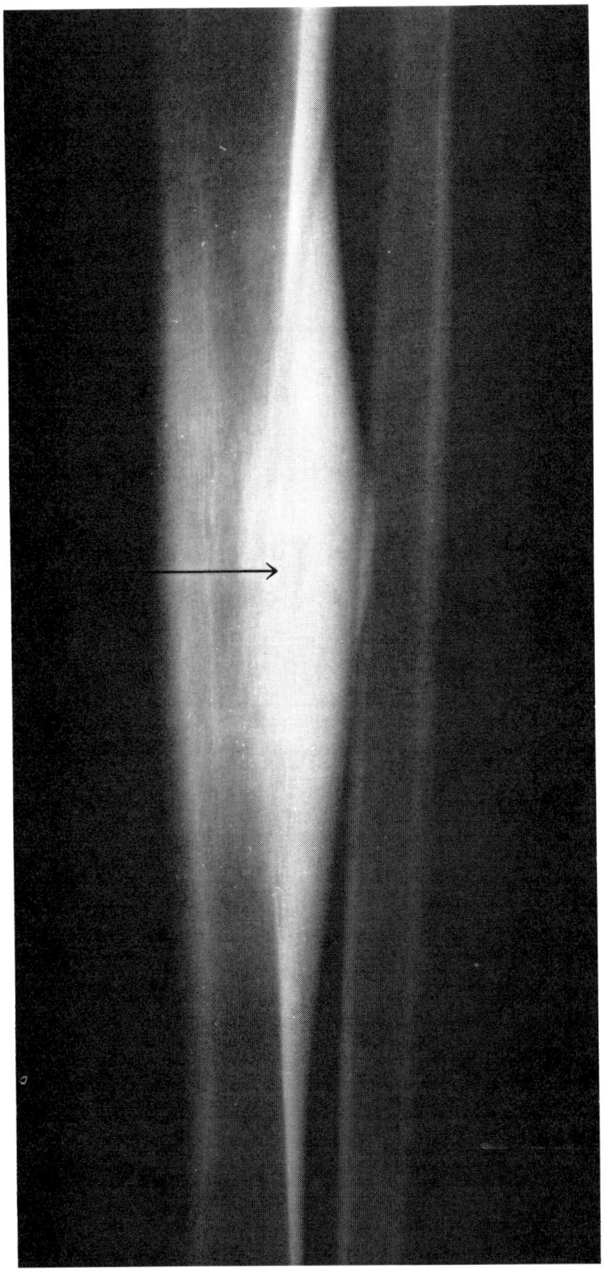

Fig. 2-16. Osteoid osteoma of midshaft of tibia. Within the area of reactive new bone formation there is a small radiolucent nidus lesion (*arrow*). (Courtesy R. D. D'Ambrosia.)

Deformities

Deformities as a class are characterized by the presence of healthy bone and the absence of evidence of some other class of lesion or of a particular lesion within one of those classes. An abnormality consists wholly or essentially of a physical change, such as division, failure of division, loss of continuity, angulation, displacement, dislocation, and subluxation (Fig. 2-17).

Posttraumatic inert swelling and inert calcification beneath the periosteum or as callus may be present. Deformity residual from previous disease should present the appearance of health with repair. Deformity may be present with other conditions, such as fracture in osteitis deformans or in osteogenesis imperfecta.

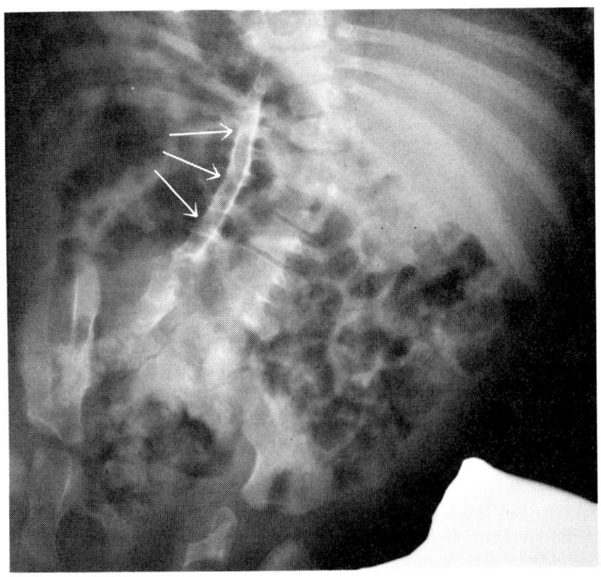

Fig. 2-17. Scoliosis of the thoracic lumbar spine. The angulation of the spine is produced by a unilateral bar (*arrows*) secondary to failure of segmentation. (Courtesy R. D. D'Ambrosia.)

Trophic Disease

Lesions not yet classified form a miscellaneous group in which the diagnostic indications are peculiar to each disease or small subgroup of diseases. They do not exhibit the characteristic features of lesions in other classes and differ from deformity in that there is alteration of character of tissues instead of mere physical change. Most of the lesions are metabolic or trophic disturbances, and the group is, therefore, referred to as the trophic class. Differentiation of and within this class will require, in general, acquaintance with and identification of the features of each disease.

DIFFERENTIATION OF COMMON INFECTIOUS LESIONS

A number of common lesions appear in several of the classes. This is especially true in active infections, malignant lesions, and trophic diseases. Identification of particular lesions within the classes usually requires the ability to recognize and make use of variations of features which have been described and familiarity with some features which have not yet been mentioned.

A particular infectious disease may be identified by certain peculiarities. Useful considerations for this purpose may exist in the degree of density of calcareous reactions, peculiarities of effusion, or the relation of features to each other which expresses the timing of the lesion.

Calcareous Reactions

The degree of density of subperiosteal calcification of the infectious type may be judged by its relation to the density of cortex. In the *pyogenic infections* the calcifications approach the density of normal cortex but do not quite equal it. The cortical outline can be detected through the shadow of the calcifications. That is properly designated pyogenic density. It may become more dense in longstanding lesions which gradually accumulate a greater concentration of calcareous molecules (see Fig. 2-6).

Syphilitic density which tends to identify a syphilitic lesion is present when the calcifications equal or exceed the density of cortex. The cortex cannot be distinguished or can be identified only with difficulty through the calcifications (Fig. 2-18).

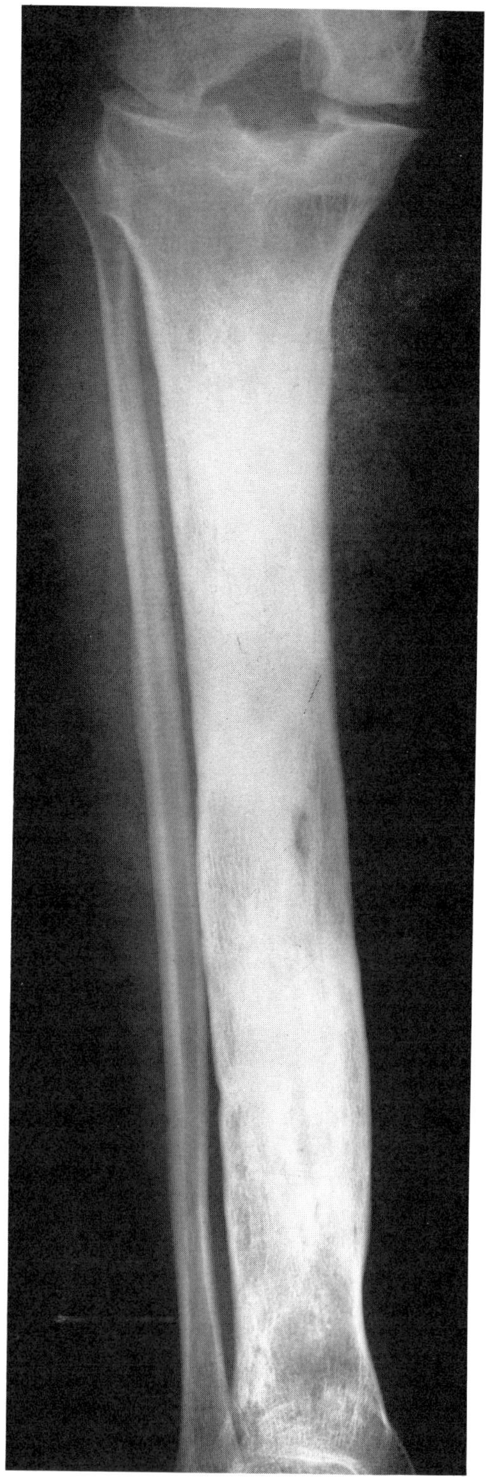

Fig. 2-18. Leutic periostitis of the tibia. The cortex of the tibia cannot be identified through the calcification. (Courtesy R. D. D'Ambrosia.)

Tuberculous calcareous reactions tend to be of light, even faint, density. The density of existing bone about the lesion may be decreased. There is a theory that body fluids about tuberculous lesions contain a product of activity of the disease which tends to dissolve precipitated calcareous molecules or inhibit their deposit (Fig. 2-19).

Decalcification

Decrease of density of calcareous structures caused by less than normal concentration of calcium salts within them is decalcification. It differs from lack or loss of substance and from decrease of size of those structures by underdevelopment, atrophy, or other forms of narrowing. There are three principal types.

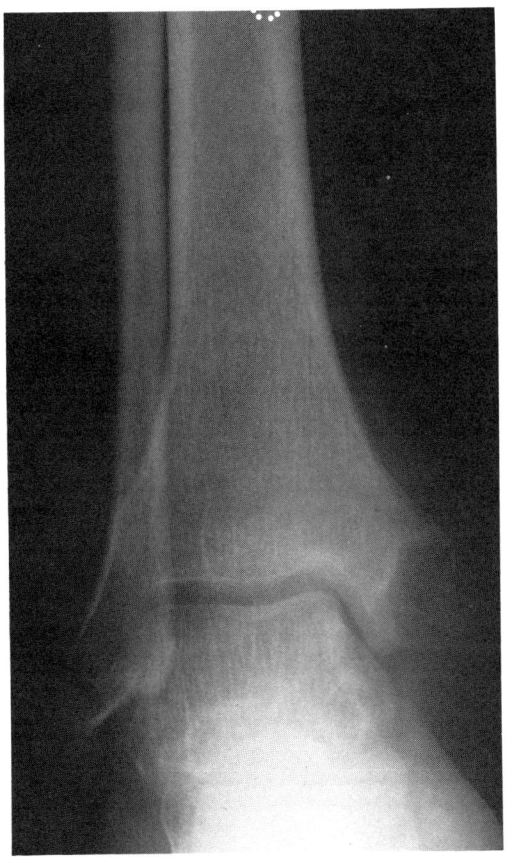

Fig. 2-19. Tuberculous osteitis of the ankle. The calcareous reaction at the medial malleolus is light and faint. (Courtesy R. D. D'Ambrosia.)

General Decalcification

General decalcification is deficient density which is widespread about a joint or lesion, especially distally. General decalcification may be present at and distal to some infections as a result of chronic limitation of activity. It is to be expected at and distal to *tuberculous lesions* and suggests that condition when there is evidence of infection (see Fig. 2-14).

Systemic Decalcification

Systemic decalcification appears in some trophic conditions. It differs from general decalcification in its extensive systemic distribution. It is not established by roentgenogram unless a sufficient number of areas are depicted.

Local Decalcification

Local decalcification has many varieties. They appear in various classes of lesions. They are characterized by decalcification in a limited well-circumscribed area. They are usually the result of sufficient circulatory or nutritional disturbance in the affected area or areas (Fig. 2-20).

Local decalcification of small masses, such as at epiphysis or carpal bones, occurs in many condi-

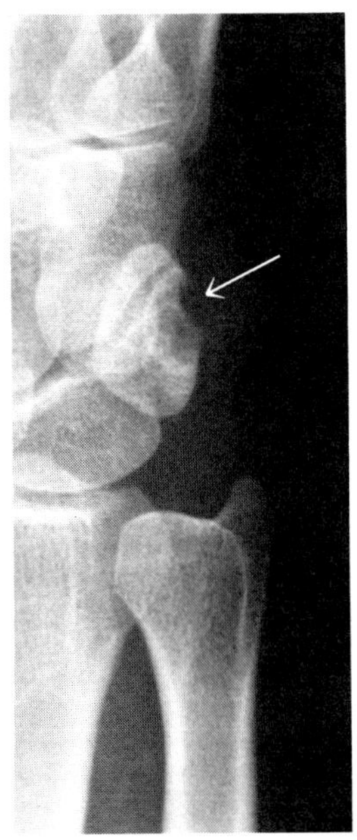

Fig. 2-20. Decalcification of triquetrum. At surgery the ganglion mass was peeled from the eroded surface of the triquetrum (*arrow*). (Courtesy R. D. D'Ambrosia.)

tions. It is usually present at *tuberculous lesions.* It develops rapidly in *gonococcal arthritis* but decreases in a few months as the disease subsides; it is often intense enough to be called acute decalcification. There are three types of local decalcification: superficial, cortical, and metaphyseal.

Superficial decalcification is decalcification at a narrow saucer-shaped area at the surface of cortex. It is the result of vascular disturbance which may be caused by hypervascularity about a sufficiently active infection, such as swelling at a pyogenic subperiosteal abscess. Such hypervascularity also produces the changes at the surface of swelling or effusion which class those features as reactive. Such changes are more obvious with active pyogenic infections, less so with tuberculous lesions, and they may be faint or undetectable with syphilitic disease.

Cortical decalcification is decreased density of the thin line of articular cortex. It is common in tuberculous arthritis and may appear as an early feature of pyogenic arthritis. The decrease of density may extend further as a thin line of subcortical decalcification of the medullary structure immediately adjacent to the articular cortex.

Loss of density by cortical decalcification of the thin opaque line of cortex beneath articular cartilage is not the same as subcartilaginous decalcification of the adjacent bone in which the line of cortex maintains its density. It has a specific significance. It indicates the presence of active infection in the joint. This may be particularly helpful in the spine in determining whether thinning of a disk is due to infection, trauma, or degeneration.

Metaphyseal Decalcification. Disturbance of circulation in the area of infection in a diaphysis, epiphysis, or joint may produce metaphyseal decalcification which appears as a transverse band of decreased density adjacent to metaphyseal cartilage or its site, but it may also appear in several other conditions. Return of density after any decalcification should be considered an indication of improvement.

EFFUSION

A variety of features of effusion are notable. It may be *reactive.* Its outline may be clearly defined or obscured by adjacent swelling. Its contour may be *nodular* due to tumor, blood clots, or gout. It may be distributed throughout the joint or limited to a portion of it. Effusion which does not appear in all compartments of the joint in which it might have been detectable is rarely due to infection. Such disease spreads throughout the joint and effusion develops in all parts of it. *Distribution of the effusion* may be uneven when it is fluid and tends to collect in areas least under pressure, such as the suprapatellar pouch at the knee. More viscous material is less apt to be affected by this factor. The density of effusion is commonly that of adjacent muscle or tendon shadows. It may be more dense if purulent, hemorrhagic, or massive, and it will be less dense if serous or in the first few days of acute infection. Calcareous loose bodies may be present, or osseous detritus may be distributed to its periphery. The joint space may be shallow, deep, or unbalanced.

Of these features, the ones most apt to be useful in infection are the reactive character which may be the available means of classifying the disease, distribution pervading the whole joint, smoothness of outline, density which may be greater than usual when the effusion is not massive in purulent pyogenic lesions or less than usual in tuberculous lesions over a considerable period of time or in the first few days of pyogenic infection, and disturbance of the joint space.

THE CARTILAGINOUS JOINT SPACE

The joint space as defined for our purposes is the area between the bone attachments of adjacent articular cartilages plus the articular cortex. It may be increased in depth because of distention of the capsule by massive effusion or by overdevelopment of cartilage or delay in its conversion to osseous structure. Overdevelopment of the cartilage may be localized in a limited area. The space may be shallow because of underdevelopment of cartilage, excessively rapid conversion to osseous structure, or destruction caused by infection, fibrous degeneration, or atrophy. When fibrous degeneration occurs with chlorosis, a thin line or area of gas density may appear between the cartilages. Accumulation of gas from the body fluids is caused by the effect of leverage produced by traction directly applied or resulting from leverage effects accompanying repeated motion.

An unbalanced joint space is one which is deeper than it should be on one side and thinner than it should be on the other. It occurs at the knee. When there is no other feature except effusion, it indicates derangement of the cartilage on the thin side. It is sometimes suggested in other conditions when other features are present.

Timing of the Lesion

We have not presented a picture for any one lesion of which we can say "this is the picture on which diagnosis of this infection is made." The reason is that the appearance of the various infections is influenced by factors in the particular case, such as the extent and degree of soft tissue atrophy, reactive swelling, local and general decalcification, activity of destruction, repair accompanying destruction, and other features which yield impressions as to the duration and virulence of the disease and picture the timing of the lesion which leads to the possible diagnosis. One should not feel that the diagnosis must be made from the roentgenogram alone. All of the facts, features, and possibilities derived from all of the means of examination should be considered together for that purpose.

Tuberculosis, for example, may be described as a disease which gradually but progressively produces effusion or swelling, or both, with local and general decalcification, soft tissue atrophy, underdevelopment, and, eventually, destruction. Thinning of articular cartilage appears slowly but it may be a prominent feature because it is not obscured by dense calcifying reactions. It may be present when tuberculous arthritis is first seen because symptoms have existed for months before the patient sees a doctor. Features which indicate such a course are consistent with tuberculosis (see Fig. 2-14).

Gonococcal arthritis, on the other hand, may be described as a disease which deals a devastating blow very rapidly. When effusion, thinning of cartilage, and marked local decalcification in the absence of general decalcification and soft tissue atrophy indicate severe, rapid damage, the picture is consistent with the active stage of gonococcal arthritis.

Remote subperiosteal calcification of the inert type removed from the actual infection but in an area of disturbed circulation may accompany these infections, especially tuberculosis.

Pyogenic infection which is not gonococcal tends to have some rather obvious features, but the particular bacterium involved may remain uncertain. Aspiration and culture of swelling, effusion, or a bone lesion are desirable for more assured identification of the organism.

The early features of these infections are reaction area and prompt development of soft tissue reaction as reactive swelling or reactive effusion. The reactive character may become quite obvious. Alterations of bone density or structure take longer. Local decalcifications of various types may appear and become marked, but general decalcification is not a usual feature. Evidence of active destruction of bone may require 10 to 20 days to become visible but then may increase rapidly. The typical destruction is infiltrative, and this may isolate areas of intact bone which eventually become sequestra. The destruction is invasive at a bone abscess.

Calcifying reactions tend to pyogenic density which is only slightly less than cortical density. It may increase with duration of the lesion, exceed cortical density, and eventually approach syphilitic density with sufficient duration.

Subperiosteal calcification is often the most prominent feature. It is of the infectious type. It may persist after the disease has subsided, especially so when some of it is subject to stresses of function. Pneumococcic infection has some tendency to produce voluminous subperiosteal calcification, but it may be slight or even absent when the organism is streptococcus or meningococcus. Tuberculosis may be complicated by features of secondary pyogenic infection.

This may be summarized briefly by stating that pyogenic infections as a group are characterized early by soft tissue reactions and later by subperiosteal calcifications of the infectious type, other calcifications, and active destruction of bone (see Fig. 2-6).

In lesions of the spine, a period of observation may be required for distinguishing the roentgenogram features of pyogenic infection from tuberculosis, especially if the pyogenic infection happens to be brucellosis. If there are indications of a short course and a tendency to ankylosis or other calcifying reactions have appeared, the diagnosis of pyogenic infection may be favored.

Syphilitic lesions tend to be either gummatous and destructive or mostly productive of subperiosteal calcifications of syphilitic density (see Fig. 2-18).

Parasitic infections are usually suggestive of tumor because of one or more areas of invasive destruction, but sufficient soft tissue reaction in the form of swelling or reaction area should be evident to indicate the type of lesion.

DIFFERENTIATION OF COMMON MALIGNANT TUMORS

There are a great many varieties of malignant tumor. The picture of any one of them may vary considerably depending on the age of the patient, the site, and duration of the lesion. A picture common for one tumor at one age may be similar to that of a different tumor at a different age. One does not encounter enough examples of a rare tumor to make generalizations.

Two needs are evident. There is the constant need to be aware of the possibility that a malignant lesion may be present. There is also the need to simplify the problem. That can be accomplished, but even so, one should maintain the attitude that the diagnosis, even though highly probable, does not become established until the tissue is actually examined.

Although it may be said that any metastatic tumor may appear in bone, this is true for many tumors only when they have existed long enough and are in the terminal stage. They should have been recognized much earlier and no longer present a diagnostic problem. Several of the tumors are so rare that the whole group represents less than 2 percent of the cases involving structural tissues.

An effort to identify them by roentgenogram is not likely to be rewarding because the examiner has not seen a sufficient number of each particular tumor and because a picture rarely seen is more likely to represent an unusual variation of a common tumor than a tumor which is actually rare.

These considerations serve to reduce the list of malignant lesions for practical consideration to more than 13 varieties, and two of these, metastatic carcinoma of the breast and prostate, are differentiated by the sex of the patient.

THE THIRTEEN COMMON LESIONS

1. Neuroblastoma
2. Ewing's sarcoma
3. Lymphoma
4. Primary osteogenic sarcoma or chondrosarcoma
5. Secondary osteogenic sarcoma or chondrosarcoma

   Metastatic carcinoma of:

6. Thyroid
7. Breast in females
8. Prostate in males
9. Bronchus
10. Kidney
11. Hypernephroma
12. Myeloma
13. Neurogenic sarcoma

These few lesions can be separated into conveniently small groups when the usual age of onset of the particular disease is considered. We will discuss them in such groups. A lesion is very important when it is a common one within its age group. Such lesions should comprise individually more than 20 percent of the group and in total more than 60 percent. Occasional lesions should comprise individually 2 to 20 percent of the group and in total less than 40 percent. Uncommon lesions should comprise individually less than 2 percent of the group and in total less than 5 percent. Since rare lesions have a tiny incidence in a group, and all of them together total less than 2 percent of all malignant tumors, they will not be considered further in this discussion.

Further progress toward determining the most probable malignant tumor in a given instance is made by applying the facts of distribution of particular malignant conditions. For example, carcinoma of the breast or prostate is quite uncommon below the knee or elbow; carcinoma of the prostate is not apt to be seen in other bones before there are numerous lesions in or near the pelvis; osteogenic sarcoma is uncommon at any age in the hands, feet, and spine; neuroblastoma distributes itself in bilateral symmetrical lesions which characterize the disease; hypernephroma tends to produce marked active invasive destruction in single lesions in the diaphysis of a long bone; and myeloma may be large and solitary, but it usually exhibits multiple small lesions of various sizes in the bones of the trunk, including ribs and clavicles, and in adjacent long bones of the limbs and in the skull.

DIFFERENTIATION BY AGE GROUP

The limits of age chosen for the age groups are not determined by decades or equal years but by periods which do represent areas of change of frequency for their more common lesions.

Age 0 to 8 Years

1. Neuroblastoma
2. Ewing's sarcoma

3. Lymphoma
4. Osteogenic sarcoma

Neuroblastoma and Ewing's sarcoma are common. Lymphoma is occasional. Osteogenic sarcoma is uncommon.

Neuroblastoma is rare after age 8. Bilaterally symmetrical lesions near the metaphyses of long bones are typical. Absorption of bone within the area of invasive active destruction tends to be uneven. This may impart a spotty appearance which is seen in many malignant conditions. Inert subperiosteal calcification is apt to be prominent. Soft tissue mass eventually extends beyond the cortex.

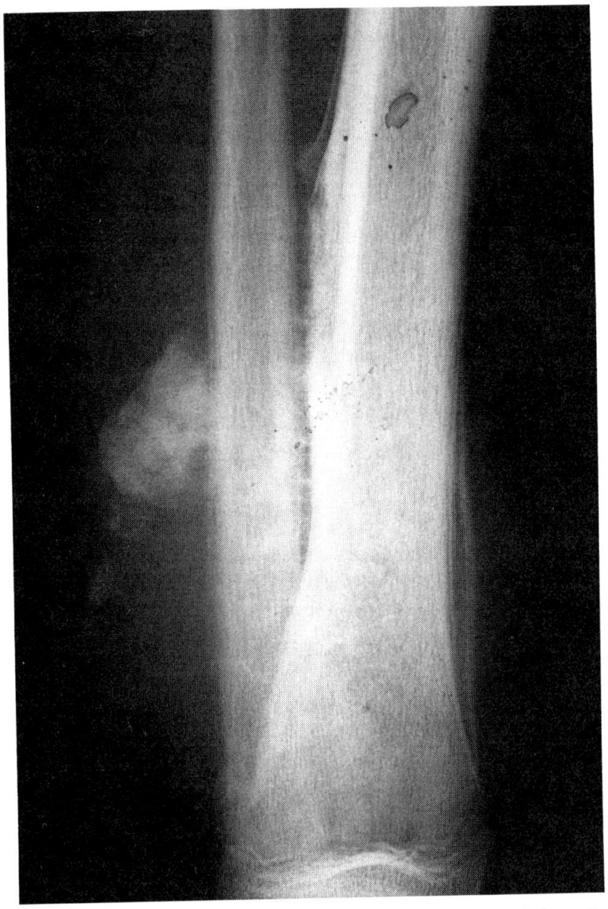

Fig. 2-21. Malignancy arising centrally in the distal fourth of the shaft but not very close to the metaphysis. A large soft tissue mass contains calcareous material which is probably subperiosteal rays displaced by growth of the mass. Active destruction is lagging, with no areas of total resorption although involvement is extensive. Destruction does not reach the metaphysis although a transverse band of metaphyseal decalcification is present because of impairment of circulation. There are inert subperiosteal calcifications with subperiosteal cuff proximally abutting on the mass. The calcifications anteriorly exhibit six or seven very thin layers, which are sufficient to indicate Ewing's sarcoma (endothelioma).

Ewing's sarcoma may be seen up to age 40, but the diagnosis is subject to suspicion thereafter (Fig. 2-21). It is common before the age of 9 but not because of its more frequent occurrence but because of scarcity of other malignant lesions. Pulmonary metastasis occurs early. It often may be present when the patient is first seen. It may appear in small bones but usually arises in the diaphysis of a long bone near but not close to the metaphysis. Its origin is central within the bone. A single lesion is usual but more bones may soon become involved. The lesion has usually become elongated because of delay in penetrating the cortex. It lacks power to penetrate cartilage because nourishment is deficient in that direction. At least a thin area of intact bone tends to persist between the lesion and metaphyseal cartilage. Inert subperiosteal calcification tends to develop in thin layers. More than three such layers are practically indicative of this tumor. Absorption of bone at the lesion is sometimes total, especially when the site is a small bone, but it is often spotty. Most often it is so slow that it is lagging. The area visibly affected by the tumor may be elongated before the bone is completely absorbed in any portion of the area.

Lymphomas is a term applied to many diseases. Most of them produce clinical enlargement of lymph nodes which may sometimes be noted in the roentgenogram as masses in consistent locations. Bone lesions may be a feature in leukemia, lymphosarcoma, reticulum cell sarcoma, and a few cases of Hodgkin's disease. These appear occasionally in every age period.

Leukemia of sufficient duration may produce general or systemic decalcification with unusual width of long bones resulting from lack of remodeling during growth. Such bones have a thin cortex.

The bone lesion of lymphosarcoma is usually single. It may have lagging destruction as in Ewing's tumor, but the lesion may be eccentric or even peripheral rather than central. The affected area is not necessarily near a metaphysis. Calcareous reactions are usually not prominent. There is no tendency for subperiosteal calcifications to develop in layers.

Reticulum cell sarcoma is usually a single lesion

which is central or somewhat eccentric. Generally, it is not far from a metaphysis. Absorption of bone in the area of active destruction may exhibit a network pattern such as may also be seen in bone not yet absorbed in neuroblastoma and in metastases of renal cell carcinoma. Subperiosteal calcification may be prominent.

Hodgkin's disease in bone is usually single but does not have a distinctive pattern. Destruction may appear spotty because of uneven absorption of affected bone. Prominence of subperiosteal calcification is variable from case to case as in many other malignant conditions, for example, metastatic carcinoma of the breast.

Age 8 to 40 years

1. Osteogenic sarcoma
2. Chondrosarcoma
3. Ewing's sarcoma
4. Lymphoma
5. Secondary osteogenic or chondrosarcoma
6. Metastatic carcinoma of the thyroid
7. Metastatic carcinoma of the breast

This period is characterized by the great predominence of osteogenic sarcoma and chondrosarcoma.

Occasional lesions are Ewing's sarcoma, lymphoma, secondary osteogenic or chondrosarcoma, and carcinoma of the thyroid. Metastatic carcinoma of the breast is occasional in 30 to 40 year olds but uncommon in 8 to 30 year olds.

A feature which may be seen is subperiosteal calcareous ray formation in osteogenic sarcoma, chondrosarcoma, or Ewing's sarcoma. The mass of a malignant tumor may tighten and straighten blood vessels between elevated periosteum and cortex. Calcification may appear in the most avascular area of the stroma between the vessels. The result is a thin, calcareous line nearly perpendicular to the shaft extending from near the cortex toward the periosteum. Such rays may be slightly curved. They may be displaced from the cortex by central growth of the tumor and become less perpendicular to the shaft. When sufficiently numerous they may form a dense mass. They have been seen in invasion of a pubic bone by extension of carcinoma of the bladder. Other calcareous deposits which are irregularly linear and curved may develop in the stroma of malignant tumors which have a period of sufficiently slow growth to permit their appearances; they may be described as tumor bone.

Since the features of osteogenic sarcoma and those of chondrosarcoma are the same, they will be considered together.

Osteogenic sarcoma begins as a single lesion. Metastasis does not occur quickly in bones, lymph nodes, or lungs in most of the untreated persons. The preferred site of the disease is the diaphysis of a long bone close to a metaphysis which has had a period of rapid growth. The lesion may be central but is most often eccentric, even cortical. Few lesions are entirely free of calcareous reactions. Inert subperiosteal calcification, cuff, and rays appear after the tissue mass has reached the periosteal surface. They are often prominent. Rays may be sufficiently numerous to form a dense mass. A cortical lesion may be made obvious by subperiosteal calcification with a cuff when the mass and erosion of the cortex have not yet become prominent. The axial length of visibly involved bone is not much greater than the diameter of the tumor. Spherical growth proceeds without much hindrance by adjacent poorly nourished tissue, such as cartilage, because the tumor forms its own blood sinuses as it grows.

Bone may be produced by cellular activity of the tissue of osteogenic sarcoma. It must be distinguished from calcification and from remnants of preexisting bone. For definite identification, it is necessary that the material have some visible osseous texture and a size between 2 and 10 millimeters in diameter. The fragments, ossa, are not continuous with other calcareous material, are irregular, somewhat angular in outline with some evidence of spiculation at the periphery, and they are situated within the tumorous tissue.

Ewing's sarcoma often has rays and a cuff which make it resemble a typical picture of osteogenic sarcoma. It rarely begins at a site so close to the metaphysis, the axial length of visibly involved bone is greater than the diameter of the tumor, it does not extend to metaphyseal cartilage, and ossa are not present. A study of cases in the Registry of Bone Sarcoma revealed a few instances in which we were unable to distinguish osteogenic sarcoma from Ewing's sarcoma on roentgenogram evidence before we looked for the presence of ossa. Their presence or absence resolved the problem with much certainty (Fig. 2-22).

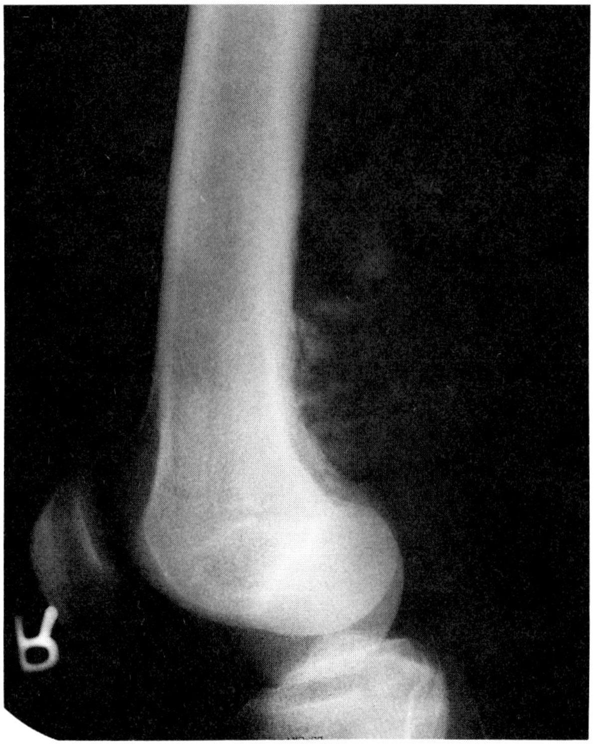

Fig. 2-22. A peripheral lesion in the metaphyseal area with slight destruction of cortex and a large soft tissue mass. Calcareous material in the mass consists of numerous nodules which tend to angular outlines. They are not amorphous. Their size varies in the range of 2 to 8 mm. They are consistent with ossa. They indicate osteogenic sarcoma although they are not always present in that condition.

Secondary osteogenic sarcoma and chondrosarcoma are distinguished from the primary types by evidence of the presence of a preexisting lesion. Examples of such conditions are osteoma, osteochondroma, and osteitis deformans.

Carcinoma of the thyroid tends to have metastasized by the time the patient appears for examination. The site is central. There is little or no tendency to calcifying reactions. The nature of the tumor is often suggested by a degree of density of the tissue mass exceeding nearby muscle density.

Age 40 to 55 Years

1. Secondary osteogenic sarcoma
2. Secondary chondrosarcoma
3. Multiple myeloma
4. Metastatic carcinoma of the breast
5. Primary osteogenic sarcoma
6. Neurogenic sarcoma

This is a transitional period in which frequency of lesions encountered earlier is changing while other lesions not yet seen appear. The common lesions are secondary osteogenic sarcoma, chondrosarcoma, multiple myeloma, and metastatic carcinoma of the breast in the female.

Primary osteogenic sarcoma has become uncommon. Neurogenic sarcoma is also uncommon and remains so until age 65 when it becomes rare. Neuroblastoma and Ewing's sarcoma should not be expected. All other lesions listed are occasional, including lymphoma.

The occurrence of multiple lesions is notable. They are represented by multiple myeloma and by carcinoma of the breast in the female or of the prostate in the male.

Later Ages 55 to 75 Years

1. Metastatic carcinoma of the breast
2. Metastatic carcinoma of the prostate
3. Secondary osteogenic sarcoma
4. Secondary chondrosarcoma
5. Multiple myeloma
6. Other metastatic tumors

Changes in incidence of these various lesions occur in later years.

At age 55 to 65, carcinoma of the breast in the female is joined by carcinoma of the prostate in the male as a common malignant condition in bone. Secondary osteogenic sarcoma or chondrosarcoma and multiple myeloma have become occasional. Carcinoma of the thyroid is unexpected in this age group.

At age 65 to 75 carcinoma of the prostate continues to be the common lesion among males, but there is no outstanding common lesion among females. Secondary osteogenic sarcoma, chondrosarcoma, and multiple myeloma have become uncommon. Neurogenic sarcoma and carcinoma of a bronchus are no longer expectable.

It is unlikely that a new malignant disease of bone will arise after age 75.

Metastasis of carcinoma of the breast is the only lesion of the late age periods which often produces enough calcareous reaction to resemble some lesions of osteogenic sarcoma, but the lesions are commonly multiple and not all alike. They are most apt to be seen in the bones of and adjacent to the trunk. They have no predilection for the area close to a metaphysis in the diaphysis of a long bone.

Other multiple lesions are multiple myeloma and metastases of carcinoma of the prostate. Multiplicity may be exhibited as to the number of bones involved or the number of lesions in an individual bone.

Metastases of prostatic carcinoma occur centrally in the bones of the trunk and adjacent long bones. Lesions elsewhere are not apt to occur before the pelvis and adjacent bones are involved. The lesions tend to distinguish themselves by dense calcareous condensation at the periphery of the mass or masses within the bones. This may make the perception of loss of substance at the lesion difficult.

The multiple lesions of myeloma have practically no tendency to calcifying reactions. They are central or eccentric. Their distribution is general. It commonly includes the pelvis, ribs, and skull. The number of individual lesions is usually small. A diameter of 3 to 10 mm. is common enough to be called typical. Each lesion may appear round unless it is flattened by contact with the cortex. A solitary lesion is rare and may be large. Spread of individual lesions is slow. Spiculation at an area of active destruction may be minute and difficult to identify.

The remaining varieties of malignant tumors do not tend to produce prominent calcifying reactions and show no great tendency to appear in a specific area although the most distal parts of the extremities are not apt to be affected.

Metastasis of bronchial carcinoma suggests itself by unusual clarity at an invasively destructive lesion. The cellular mass of the tumor is so nearly identical with neighboring muscle density that the calcareous structure of the bone simply appears to have been removed without any other change (Fig. 2-23).

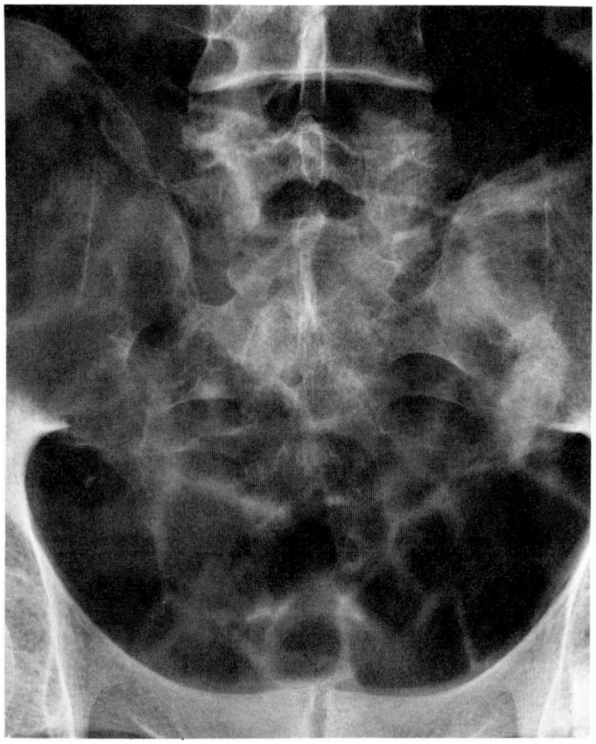

Fig. 2-23. There is complete lack of bone structure at one wing of the first sacral vertebra. The margins of the area are obscured by other bones, but some active destruction can be identified. There is no increase of soft tissue density to outline a mass. This remarkable clarity of muscle density in the area of invasive active destruction indicates a need for investigation for possible bronchial carcinoma.

Metastasis of renal cell carcinoma has a tendency to maintain a network pattern of bone not yet absorbed or of calcification in stroma in the area of invasive active destruction.

Hypernephroma commonly locates centrally in the diaphysis of a long bone not close to a metaphysis. It is characterized by the length of spiculation at the area of invasive active destruction. This may be due to streaking of actively invasive tissue. There is no tendency to calcifying reaction. There often is more than one bone lesion (see Fig. 2-15).

Neurogenic sarcoma tends to be characterized by the large size of the soft tissue mass. Its limits may be obscured by streaking into adjacent tissue. The bone may be only slightly affected or the involvement may be small in relation to the soft tissue mass. This tumor is not expectable after age 65.

There are some rare lesions which also are characterized by large size of their soft tissue mass without calcifying reactions. They are rhabdomyosarcoma, neurofibrosarcoma, and periosteal fibrosarcoma. The latter tends to be round and well defined; bone may be saucer-shaped by the circulatory effects of pressure at the periphery of the mass adjacent to bone. Bone may be slightly eroded or invaded (Fig. 2-24).

DIFFERENTIATION OF BENIGN TUMORS AND TROPHIC DISEASE (CHONDRODYSPLASIA)

A variety of lesions are commonly classed as benign tumors when they do not present evidence of autonomous growth. Radiographically, these are bet-

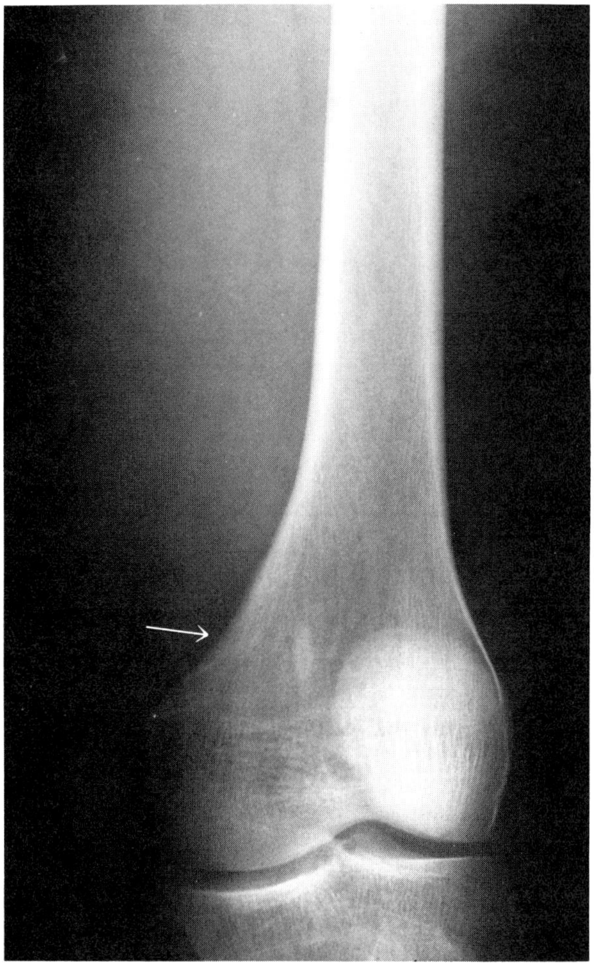

Fig. 2-24. Neurofibrosarcoma in a patient with von Recklinghausen's disease. The distal cortex of the femur is eroded (*arrow*) from pressure on the bone. (Courtesy R. D. D'Ambrosia.)

ter classed as a form of trophic disease under the designation of chondrodysplasia.

Chondrodysplasia is defined for our purposes as an abnormality affecting cartilage which normally produces bone. It suffers a disturbance of conversion of cartilage to bone causing a permanent defect or defects in the bone which is formed (Fig. 2-25). This contrasts with chondrodystrophy in which the disturbance of formation of cartilage or of the time it takes to convert to bone does not produce lasting defects in the bone which is formed.

Chondrodysplasia may result from one or more of a variety of causes affecting the cartilage. They include inherited factors, trauma, blebs, capillary breakdown at the metaphysis, other hemorrhage, endocrine disturbances, and unknown possibilities. The contents of a resulting defect have no constant relation to the causative agent. They may be any derivative of fibroblastic cells including cartilage, calcified material lacking osseous structure, fibrous tissue, and fluid cysts. Metaphyseal cartilages which have the faster rate of growth are most commonly affected. Each defect left in the growing bone continues to lengthen in the axis of growth as long as defective conversion of cartilage to bone continues (Fig. 2-26).

The defects may be single, multiple, or widely distributed. Not all defects in a given case have the same appearance. They may be intermittent if the duration of their formation ended with return to

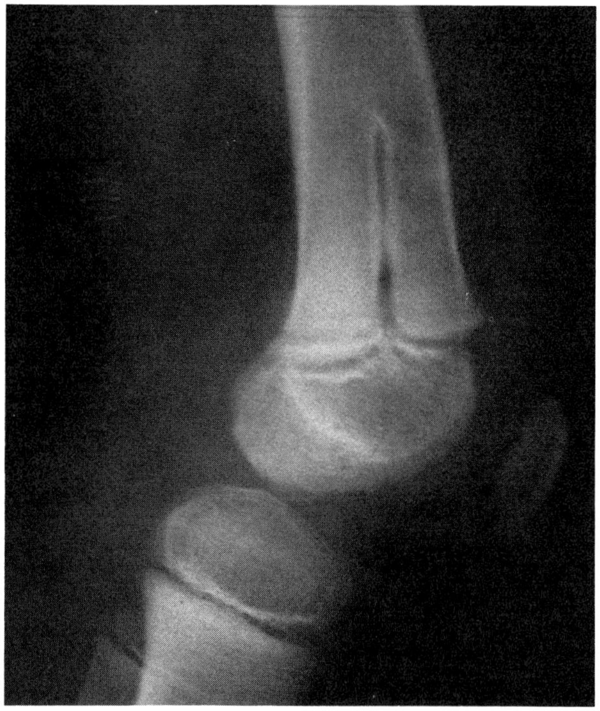

Fig. 2-25. An interesting example of development of a defect in chondrodysplasia from a known cause. Some years previously, a drill hole for a pin for traction had been made in the plane of the metaphyseal cartilage. No further production of growth cartilage or bone occurred at that spot. As the femur became elongated by growth at the metaphysis, an axial defect containing some noncalcareous derivative of fibroblasts was left in the growth line of that spot, and the present length of the defect is clearly visible.

normal bone formation thereafter. They may be continuous if that has not occurred. They may be broad or narrow. The material present may vary in different portions of the same defect.

The situation of the defect in the transverse diameter of the cartilage has a profound effect upon the eventual features of the lesion. If the lesion is central, it may not be visible for years because of its situation in the cross section of the bone where medullary structure normally becomes too scant to present an identifiable deficiency. The tissues of such a defect may eventually undergo nodular calcification of its cartilage or fibrous tissue and, thus, become visible.

If the lesion is in the submarginal area of a long bone it becomes more distant from the cartilage in the axis of growth. Remodeling of the diaphysis by subperiosteal resorption brings the cortex to the axis in which the defect is situated, and it then appears as a defect in or even projecting beyond the cortex.

If the lesion is peripheral at the time it is formed, it remains in the axis of growth while remodeling of the diaphysis is inhibited by the nonosseous material of the defect so that it projects as an exostosis or osteoma even though it has never grown autonomously since it was formed.

Since all of these features may appear in any combination, the apparent variety of possible conditions is innumerable.

A cartilaginous cap is frequently present at the crest of an exostosis, osteoma, or osteochondroma (see Fig. 2-12). When this is in a position where it is subject to irritation by stress or repeated friction with adjacent parts, there may be some physiologic continuation of growth of that cartilage with some formation of additional bone. Sometimes such growth does become autonomous, causing extension well beyond the axis of growth, and indicates the presence of an actual osteochondroma. In rare cases it becomes massive. Such lesions eventually may be the site of secondary chondrosarcoma with development of active destruction and soft tissue mass.

A broad central defect containing fibrous tissue or fluid deprives the bone structure of some of its ability to meet stress and bear the weight which increases with growth. This results in inhibition of the resorption necessary for normal remodeling and the result is a thin cortex at an abnormally broad portion of the bone (see Fig. 2-26). This is not actual expansion but false expansion by nonresorption. As weight increases there may be slight axial compression of the weak, affected area with a trace of actual expansion and of decreased addition to length by growth.

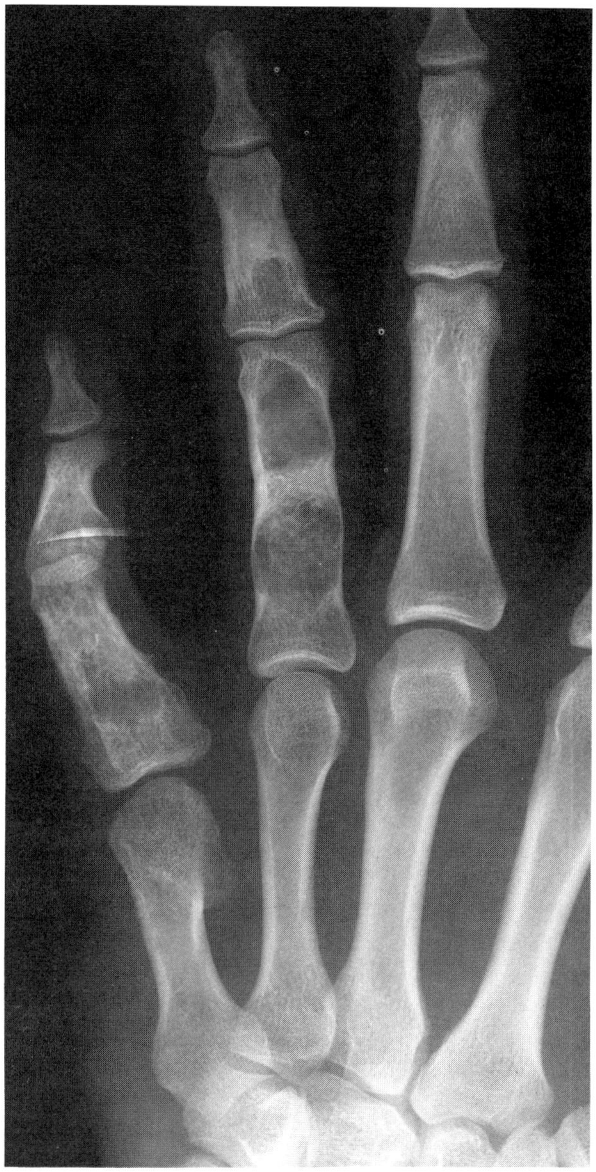

Fig. 2-26. Failure of conversion of cartilage to bone has left areas of lack of bone substance in the phalanges. The bones appear healthy. No form of active destruction or calcareous or soft tissue reaction is seen. This form of multiple chondrodysplasia in the hands is commonly called multiple enchondromatosis although the defects may be occupied by derivatives of fibroblasts other than cartilage.

These lesions may have similarity to areas of osteitis fibrosa in parathyroidism, but that condition is a transformation in formed bone and is accompanied by systemic decalcification.

Chondrodysplasia not complicated by fracture, infection, or malignancy has no tendency to decalcification, soft tissue masses, swelling, other soft tissue reaction, or calcifying reactions other than the nonreticulated calcareous material which may be produced within the defect.

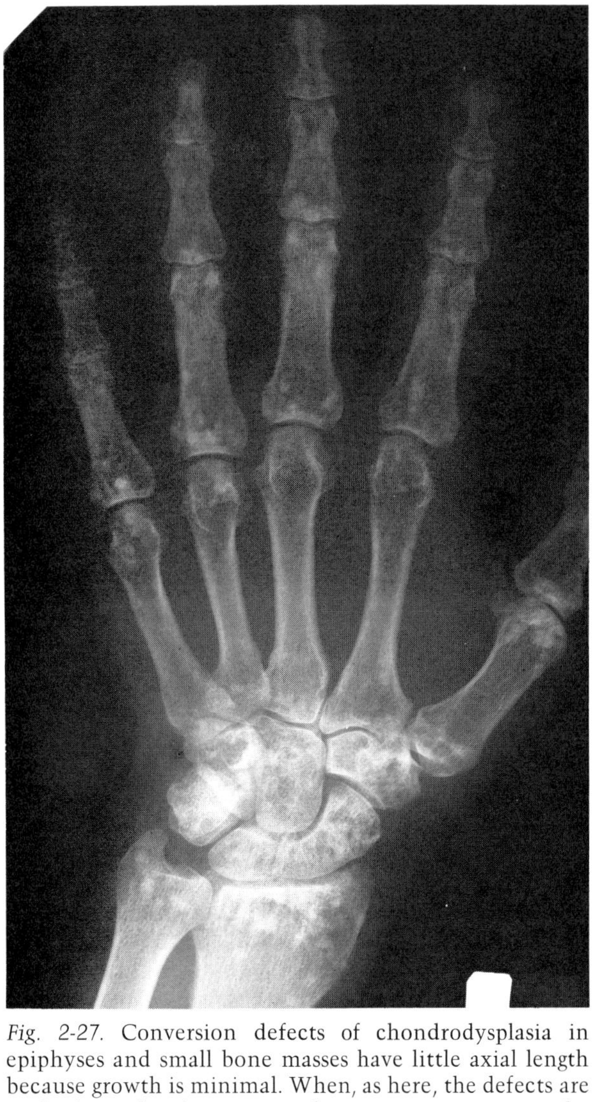

Fig. 2-27. Conversion defects of chondrodysplasia in epiphyses and small bone masses have little axial length because growth is minimal. When, as here, the defects are multiple and calcareous without osseous texture, the condition is commonly called *osteopoikilosis.* The bones appear healthy without the soft tissue or calcifying reactions of infections or tumors.

Single or multiple central defects containing some irregularly amorphous calcareous material sometimes need to be distinguished from lesions of caisson disease which is a transformation of formed bone in patients old enough to have been exposed to it. That disease does not show true or false expansion. The lesions may involve the portion of the diaphysis formed from fetal cartilage, an unexpectable feature for chondrodysplasia. The history should be subject to inquiry.

Some calcareous nonreticulated defects which continue to develop in the submarginal area for a sufficient time may cause the cortex of the diaphysis to appear thick, dense, and irregular. That is melorheostosis. The defect may include the area developed from fetal cartilage.

Articular cartilage and epiphyses grow slowly. The defects formed from them have a short axial diameter. They are apt to be so small that they will not become visible unless they contain calcareous material. Calcareous nonreticulation defects are dense and sharply defined against a background of healthy bone which shows no reaction of any sort. The defects of osteopoikilosis (Fig. 2-27) are of this character and so is the broad band type defect of marble bones.

Fibrous tissue of the capsular structure at a joint attaches at the periphery of the epiphyseal cartilage. This cartilage is destined to produce bone. As the fibrous tissue grows in accord with growth in depth of the epiphysis, some area of it may fail to produce the needed fibrous tissue. A portion of the cartilage then remains in situ in the fibrous tissue while it increases its distance from the metaphysis by greater development of cartilage or becomes entirely separated from it. The latter forms a sesamoidoma; the former deforms a portion of the epiphysis by overdevelopment. Since the displaced cartilage is subject to stresses and friction at the joint, it may become larger by continued growth which should eventually convert to bone. These defects may affect more than one joint or be multiple at a single joint.

Obviously, the concept of chondrodysplasia which we have described enables understanding as well as recognition of a large variety of lesions. Otherwise, an individual conception of its nature and cause would need to be sought for each of them.

Some of the many names suggestive of benign tumors and other conditions which are commonly applied to defects of chondrodysplasia are: exostosis, osteoma, osteochondroma, diaphyseal aclasia, bone cyst, osteitis fibrosa, nonosseous fibroma, melorheostosis, osteopoikilosis, and sesamoidoma.

LESIONS WITH SPECIAL FEATURES

One trophic disease and three benign tumors which do have autonomous growth have special features which should be discussed. We hope to emphasize a point that already should be evident. It is that attention to detail, even minute detail, of a roentgenogram which can lead to the correct interpretation and identification of the disease process.

Osteitis Deformans

Osteitis deformans (Paget's disease) often affects the skull where it thickens the bone and causes disorganization of its structure such that the affected area shows only mottled remnants of calcareous material which no longer have identifiable texture.

The characteristic changes of the disease, however, appear in the diaphyses of long bones, starting in the metaphyseal area and spreading the length of the bone in sudden spurts at irregular intervals. Affected bone appears dense because of increased size although the calcareous elements which remain are usually less dense. The thickened cortex develops longitudinal striation, and the texture of the medullary reticulum shows large spaces between remaining trabeculae which are thick and cross each other at broad angles.

An element in the increase in size of the bone is interstitial growth which increases length as well as breadth and contributes to bowing which is common. Spontaneous fracture tends to occur in long bones which have become bowed (Fig. 2-28).

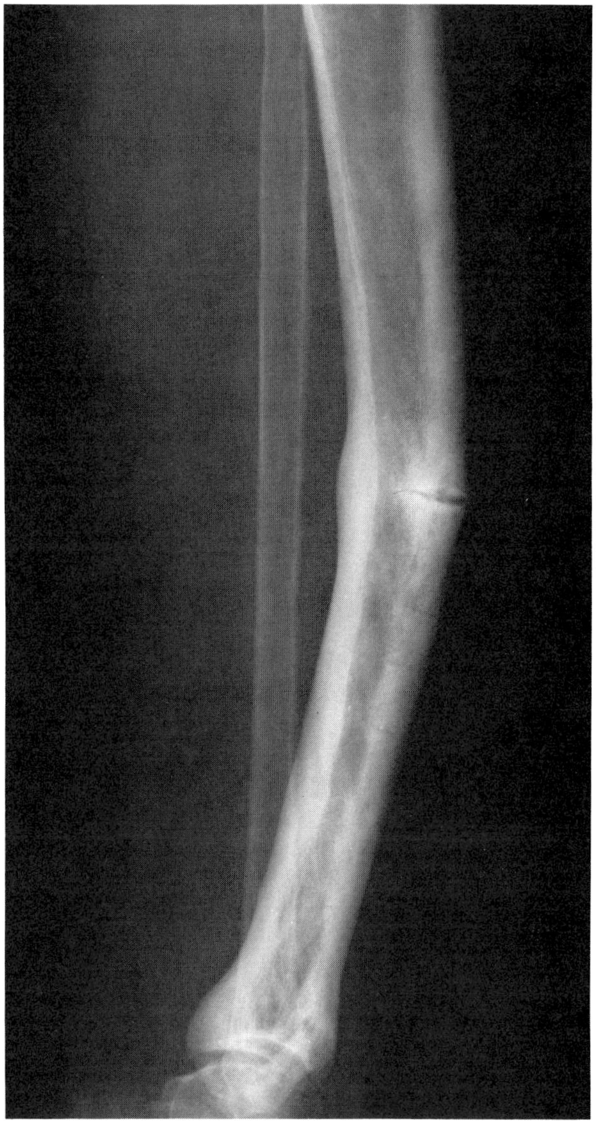

Fig. 2-28. Alteration of structure, thickness of cortex, and narrowed medullary canal with bowing due to osteitis deformans. Tension on the convexity of the curved bone may develop fatigue fracture which gradually extends transversely until "spontaneous" fracture may occur.

The special feature which we want to mention is to be seen in a good view of the junction of affected with unaffected cortex. The affected cortex with its decreased density extends into the unaffected area in a wedge which is rounded, not pointed, at its termination. The unaffected cortex on the peripheral aspect extends further than that on the endosteal side with the termination of the wedge nearer the endosteal surface. Such a picture is practically indicative of the disease.

Much of the calcareous density of the bone often disappears when the periosteum is torn by fracture or otherwise. This is sometimes interpreted as a surge of activity of the disease, but the affected area has not extended and does not do so at that time. The change seems to be due to release of body fluids which have been under pressure within the bone with washing out of some of the calcareous salts in the process.

The quick washing out of calcium salts which are

in solution or not firmly incorporated in living bone is not confined to osteitis deformans. It is a feature of osteochondrosis and aseptic necrosis as in Legg-Calvé-Perthes (Fig. 2-29), Kienboeck's or Freiberg's disease. Some calcareous material is held diffused in fluids where there is a marked degree of stasis due to impaired circulation. The calcareous density is sufficient throughout the affected area to hide the loss of substance which has occurred. When circulation improves, the salts are washed out rapidly, and the impaired bone structure becomes visible. This often is accepted as a sign of activity of the disease, but actually it indicates the onset of the reparative stage which begins with improvement of circulation.

Benign Giant Cell Tumor

A typical junction of affected cortex with that of unaffected bone is also seen in benign giant cell tumor. The tumor begins at or adjacent to metaphyseal cartilage or, occasionally, at other cartilage. It is not seen in bones of the skull which are formed in fibrous tissue. It usually is eccentric rather than truly central. Extension of the area of destruction is slow, and it does not produce spiculation. A network of delicate calcareous strands forms in the stroma of the tumor within the bone, but it is temporary and, later, is absorbed.

The cartilage of growth disks is readily destroyed, and the tumor continues to progress in a more or less spherical mass in the diaphysis and epiphysis. It may extend entirely up to articular cartilage although that is rarely penetrated.

The cortex becomes absorbed from the endosteal surface over the tumor. The thinning cortex does not show expansion but becomes evident as the cortex is replaced at the periphery of the tumor tissue by a subperiosteal calcareous shell. This shell is a special feature. It is a thin layer of calcareous material deposited beneath the periosteum in the area where cortex is absent. It is irregular in outline and has perceptibly less density than cortex. The junction with normal cortex is characteristic. That cortex narrows to a point on the peripheral aspect. The shell does not continue from that point but covers the peripheral aspect of the cortex from which it is distinguishable by lesser density. This junction is characteristic for the tumor and is still so when the tumor has become massive and much of the shell has been destroyed over it (Fig. 2-30).

A shell may also be seen at the pelvic aspect of the acetabulum in protrusio acetabuli. It forms over and eventually replaces the cortex which is resorbed during the inward displacement of the acetabulum (see Fig. 2-35).

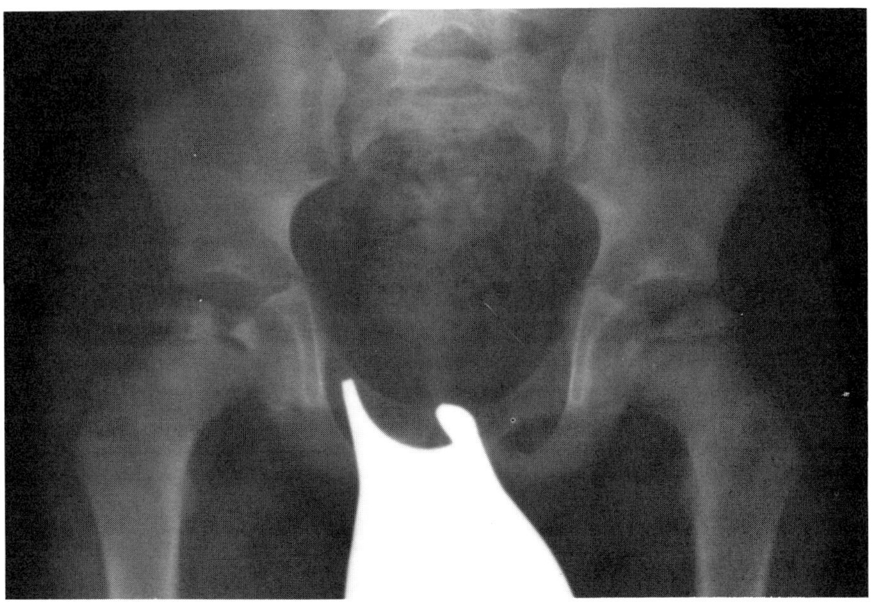

Fig. 2-29. Bilateral Legg-Calvé-Perthes in a patient in the reparative stages of the disease. The washed-out areas of the femoral head are the result of revascularization.

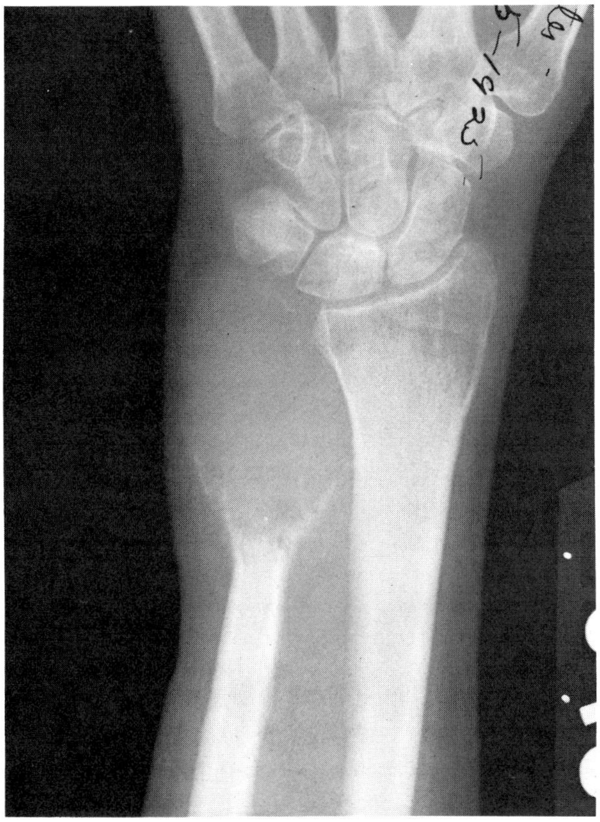

Fig. 2-30. Benign giant cell tumor occupies the distal 2 inches of the ulna. Resorption of bone has crossed the site of the metaphysis and extends completely to the articular cartilage. Growth of the tumor mass has expanded the periosteum with development of some subperiosteal calcareous material forming an incomplete shell. The shell is less dense and less smooth than cortex. The defective cortex is beveled with the point peripherally. The shell does not continue from that point but from the peripheral surface. A junction of shell and cortex of this character, when visible, identifies the benign giant cell tumor.

Aneurysmal Bone Cyst

The aneurysmal bone cyst (Fig. 2-31) is an uncommon lesion which may be easily mistaken for osteogenic sarcoma or chondrosarcoma. It occurs in the peripheral area of metaphyseal bone in young teenagers. The cortex is absorbed, and the soft tissue mass projects from the bone. There is inert subperiosteal calcification over it which may be incomplete or resorbed toward the metaphysis. It is smooth in outline and approaches cortical density. It may strongly suggest a cuff and, hence, malignancy, but there is no active destruction at the surface which abuts on the mass, and it tends to narrow peripherally to a thin line which extends at least a short distance over the mass. It neither suggests nor imitates expansion of the cortex.

Parosteal Osteoma

Parosteal osteoma presents a unique appearance. There is a spherical soft tissue mass adjacent to bone. Within the mass, calcification may have developed in the stroma in the interrupted concentric circles between the center and the periphery of the mass, but it does not involve either of them.

The reaction at the periosteal surface of the bone is also characteristic. There is some saucerization by pressure resorption with calcareous condensation extending into the bone where it fades into normal structure. There is subperiosteal calcification which is dense enough to be not clearly distinguishable from cortex. This calcification participates in the saucerization and appears to extend it.

These calcifications at and in the bone have much importance. There is argument whether this is a sarcoma from the start, but it appears to us to be

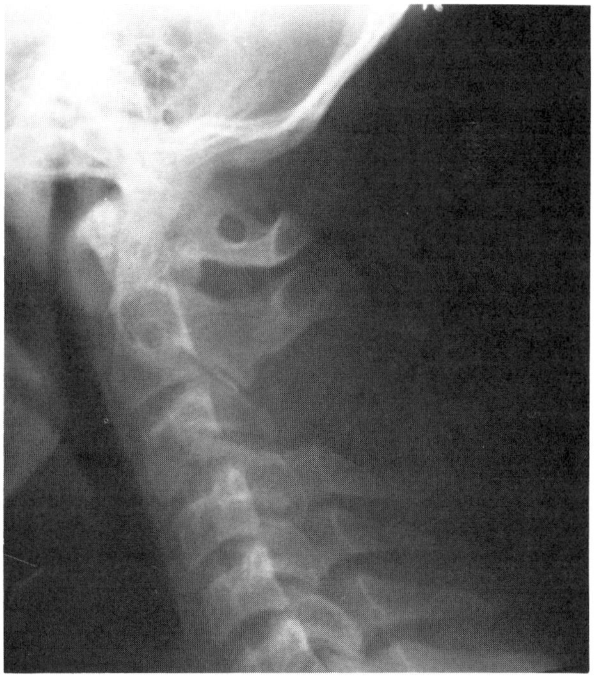

Fig. 2-31. Aneurysmal bone cyst of the spinous process of C3. The cortex has been absorbed and a large soft tissue mass is present. (Courtesy R. D. D'Ambrosia.)

benign because there is no active destruction, no invasion, and no metastases in persons not yet treated or injured. The important thing is that surgical removal of the tumor in less than a complete block which includes all of the area of calcareous deposit subperiosteally and in adjacent bone is destined to be followed by recurrence. Each successive removal has an increasingly greater chance of recurrence of a definitely malignant sarcoma with metastases.

DIFFERENTIATION OF TROPHIC DISEASES CAUSING LOSS OF SUBSTANCE

It is nearly impossible to generalize about the trophic diseases as a class, but there are some small subgroups in which the lesions have in common a feature not yet mentioned. When loss of bone substance previously present occurs, it may be due to some form of atrophic loss of substance.

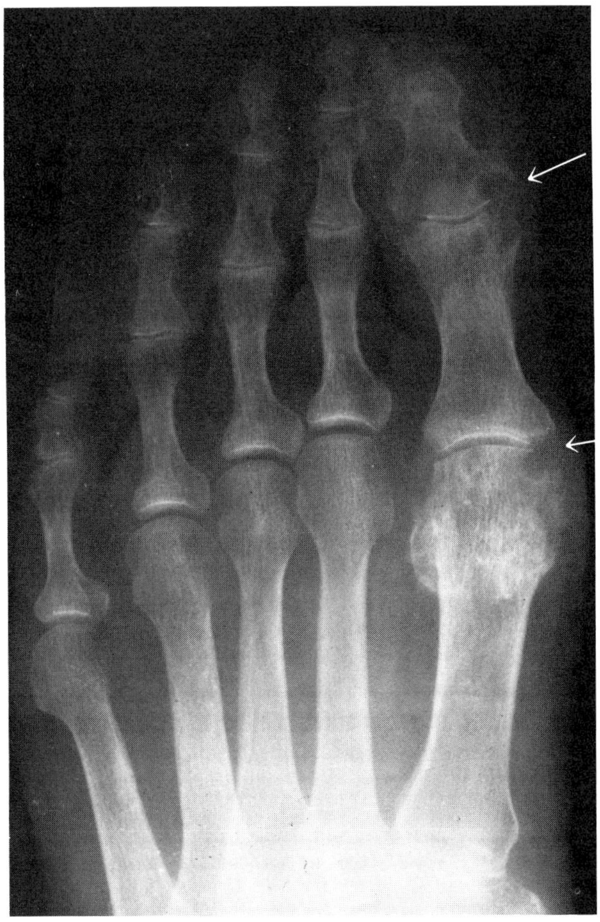

Fig. 2-32. Atrophic bone loss (*arrows*) in the foot secondary to gout. (Courtesy R. D. D'Ambrosia.)

Rheumatoid Arthritis and Gout

The punched out area of atrophic loss of bone substance appears in *rheumatoid arthritis* at the margin of articular cartilage (see Fig. 2-8) and in *gout* at a less limited portion of the periphery of the bone (Fig. 2-32). It is definitely round and usually small, sometimes minute. It seems to be a form of pressure atrophy caused by expansion of a tophus in gout or of synovial villi or granulations in rheumatoid arthritis. Adjacent bone appears healthy and shows no reaction except a thin repair line of calcareous density at its surface.

In rheumatoid arthritis, it is preceded or accompanied by some degree of systemic decalcification greater toward the distal end of the extremities and by variable intermittent distention of the capsule of the joint by synovial productive reaction. Inert swelling may also be present.

In gout, there is a rounded soft tissue mass corresponding to the site of loss of substance (Fig. 2-32). Hopefully, the outline of the mass will be visible. There is no tendency to decalcifications.

Charcot Joint

Neurotrophic loss of substance is an atrophic phenomenon seen in neurotrophic arthritis, such as Charcot's joint. The area of loss of substance is at the articular surface of the bone and is flat. It maintains a plane at right angles to the line of weight thrust. Calcareous condensation becomes marked at bone adjacent to the loss of substance and gradually fades into slightly more remote bone. There is no tendency to decalcification. Effusion and disorganization of the joint are present (Fig. 2-33). If calcareous detritus is distributed to the periphery of the effusion within the capsule it is practically indicative of the disease.

That fact that neurotrophic arthritis is a form of pressure atrophy of bone which is nutritionally disturbed is indicated by the flat surface, its plane, and the condensation in adjacent bone. Pressure atrophy occurs in other conditions besides those with abnormally close relation of parts of adjacent bones.

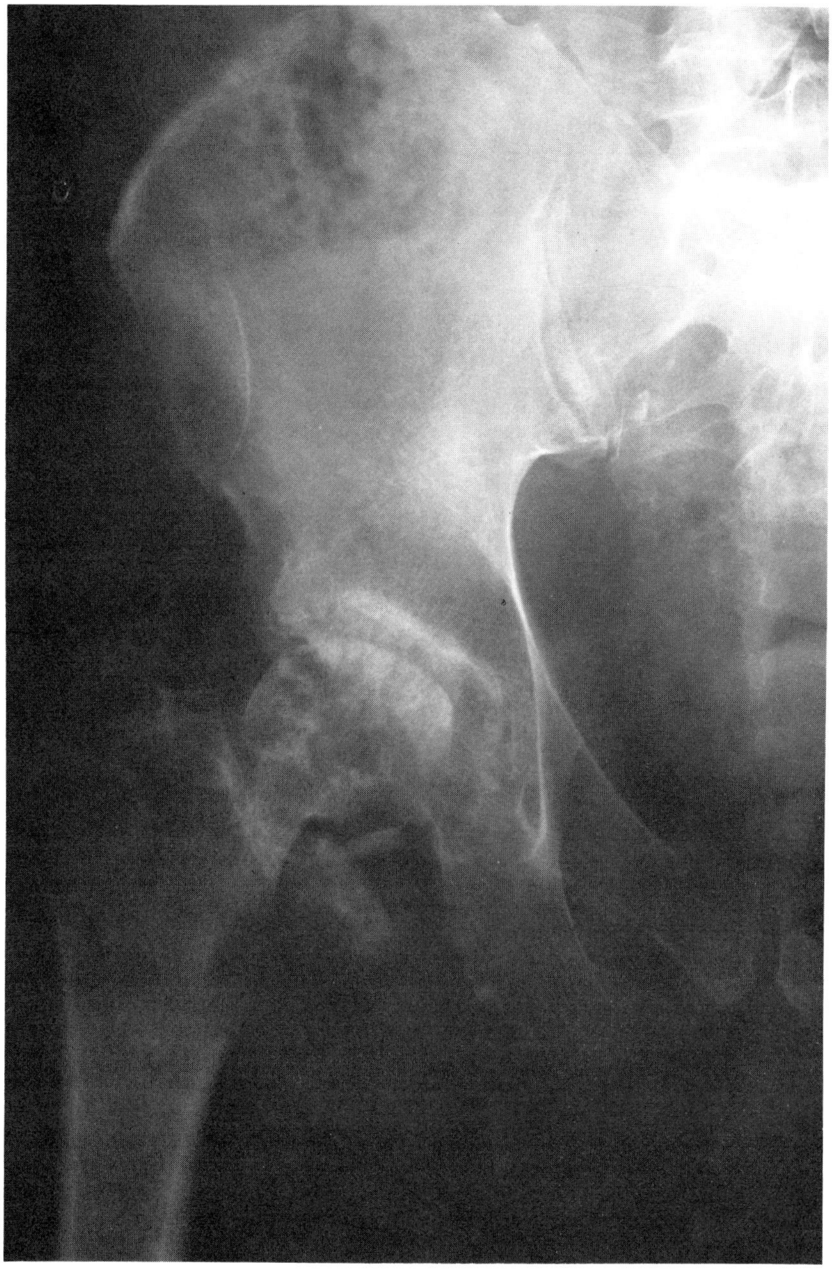

Fig. 2-33. Charcot's joint in the hip. Gross disorganization with calcareous detritus is present. The patient had a positive VDRL. (Courtesy R. D. D'Ambrosia.)

Neurofibroma

Neurofibroma adjacent to bone produces pressure atrophy. The bone is saucer-shaped peripherally, and the cortex is thickened endosteally by calcification in the same area. The soft tissue about the tumor is fibrosed axially. This dense tissue is resistant to elongation by growth of the bones and, therefore, tends to produce bowing with the concavity at the affected side. An important fact about this tissue is that it is not well vascularized, and nonunion is apt to result from this after fracture or osteotomy unless measures are taken to promote improvement of nutrition in the area. When a neurofibroma is adjacent to the side of a vertebra it is likely to produce a short, sharp, rapidly progressing lateral curve which resists correction (Fig. 2-34).

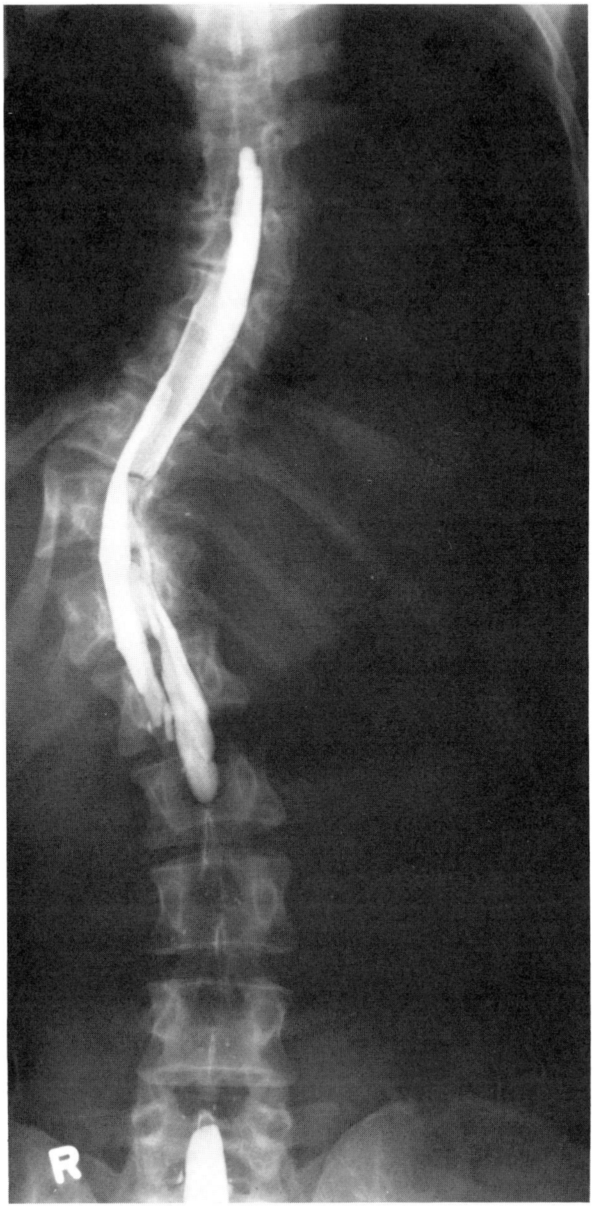

Fig. 2-34. Neurofibromatosis producing a short, sharp lateral curve. There is scalloping of the vertebrae, particularly T11, with indentation of the dye column from the neurofibroma mass. Also note the feathering of the ribs.

DIFFERENTIATION OF EPIPHYSEAL CARTILAGE ABNORMALITIES

Each epiphyseal and apophyseal cartilage and bone adjacent to it merits inspection. Diseases involving the area include *chondrodystrophy* and *chondrodysplasia* which have been described, and *osteochondrosis, epiphysiolysis* (slipped capital femoral epiphysis), *aseptic necrosis, rickets, scurvy, congenital syphilis, trophic osteitis,* and *developmental coxa vara.* Features include local decalcification and excesses, deficiencies, and irregularities of conversion of cartilage to bone and of formation of cartilage.

Osteochondroses and aseptic necrosis result from trauma or inflammation of soft tissues at the joint (or covering a small bone mass) which produce effusion, sclerosis, and impairment of circulation in the involved bone. When the effusion is at the hip and is accompanied by decalcification at the metaphysis of the femur as well as an increase of epiphyseal and articular cartilage by delayed conversion to bone, the condition is recognizable as synovitis potentially preliminary to epiphysiolysis or coxa plana. Aseptic necrosis becomes evident at such bone when a diffuse, amorphous area of increased density appears at a portion or all of the small bone mass. After circulation has improved, the diffuse density is washed out, and irregular loss of substance of the underlying bone becomes visible. Still later, reparative bone production may proceed.

Multiplication of muscle or tendon cells would merely form a mass rather than an elongated organized part were it not for growth of the bones which increases the distance between attachments of a long soft tissue part and forces its elongation. Whatever amount of force is exerted in this process it is equaled by force resisting elongation of the bones by growth. The direction of growth and the amount of elongation are affected by these forces.

In poliomyelitis affecting the thigh sufficiently the muscles resist elongation less and the neck of the femur grows more erect in a valgus deformity. Lack of normal balance of the forces on opposed sides of the bone may cause angulation of epiphyseal growth toward the side where resistance is increased or away from the side where it is decreased. Genu varum or genu valgum can result from soft tissue imbalance affecting the proximal metaphysis of the tibia in bones apparently healthy with apparently healthy cartilage. Weight thrust acting obliquely on epiphyseal cartilage can cause enough tension to result in elongation of the cartilage and consequently of bone in the direction of the thrust. This effect is seen, for example, at the elongated anterior lip of the first sacral vertebra in spondylolisthesis during the growth period.

Both of these effects of forces accompanying growth are acting in developmental coxa vara to produce a striking deformity. The normal plane of the proximal metaphysis of the femur is somewhat inclined medially. It does not meet the weight thrust squarely. When the epiphyseal cartilage is weak or the medial soft tissues resistant, varus deformity increases during growth. When it is sufficiently great, the epiphyseal cartilage and the bone it produces are elongated medially downward. The deformity may become very great but an identifying detail of the process is that the superior lateral surface of the neck of the femur, normally concave, becomes convex as an effect of continuous change in the direction of metaphyseal growth.

Growth effects act in still another way to contribute to the features of a trophic disease in medial protrusion of the acetabulum into the pelvis without obvious cause. The remodeling of the pelvic bones by accretion laterally and resorption medially during growth to produce a male or a female pelvis is under genetic control. When the genes are mixed, there may be little accretion laterally as in the male type but marked resorption medially as in the female type. The result is a form of arthrokatadysis (Otto pelvis) with medial protrusion of the acetabulum and thinning of its floor during growth (Fig. 2-35). When the floor is sufficiently deficient, a thin shell of cal-

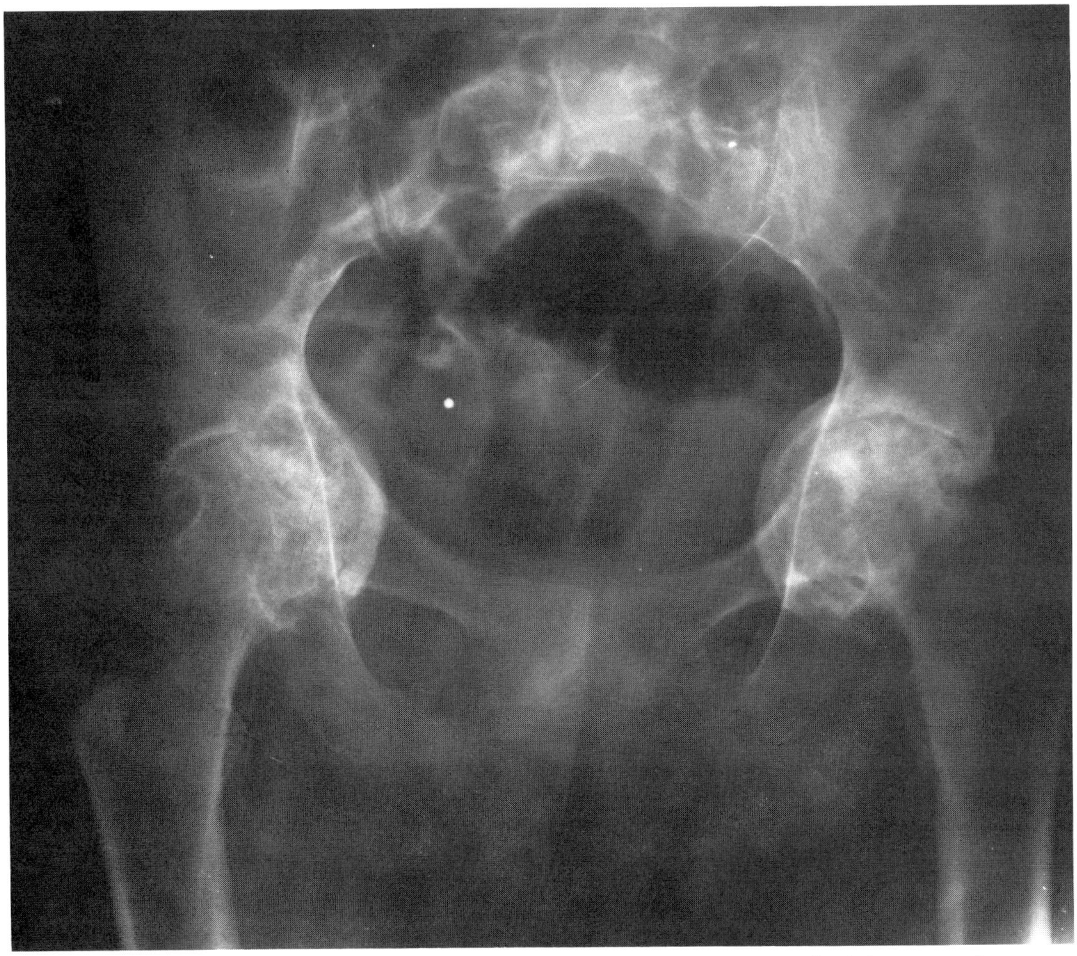

Fig. 2-35. Otto pelvis in a 70-year-old man with a 20-year history of pain in both hips secondary to osteoarthritis. There is medial protrusion of the acetabulum, and a thin, weak shell of calcareous material has taken the place of the resorbed bone. (Courtesy R. D. D'Ambrosia.)

careous material tends to take the place of resorbed bone, but it is less dense than cortex, less smooth in outline, and much less strong.

Softening of the bones in the presence of general or systemic decalcification is malacia. It may be found in rickets, postmenopausal osteoporosis of vertebrae, osteogenesis imperfecta, and hyperparathyroidism. In advanced cases of the latter two, medial protrusion of the acetabulum is produced as part of general collapse of the pelvis, but the shell which we have just described does not appear.

In postmenopausal osteoporosis with collapsing vertebrae, there is general decalcification. Malacia becomes evident when the disks become spherical because their elasticity exceeds the ability of the vertebral bone to meet this expansible force. The disks become more spherical at the expense of the adjacent bodies which become concave on the surface toward the disk. The bodies may also become wedged anteriorly. The picture is unique and diagnostic.

DIFFERENTIATING THE FRACTURE LINE

Lack of continuity of bone and spiculated surfaces of the fragments usually make a fracture obvious. A problem may arise, however, when the division in the bone might be a normal, accessory, or unusual cartilage line. A standard is needed for their identification.

The cartilage line tends to have an even width throughout its length. Bone surfaces abutting upon the line tend to be smooth and fairly straight. Bone at the ends of the line tend to be rounded rather than angular (Fig. 2-36A).

The fracture line tends to be wider at one end than at the other. Bone at the surfaces of the line tends to be sharply irregular or jagged. Bone at the peripheral margins of the fracture tends to be definitely angular instead of rounded (Fig. 2-36B).

Such standards are most helpful in the presence of a cartilage line in an unexpected place, such as divi-

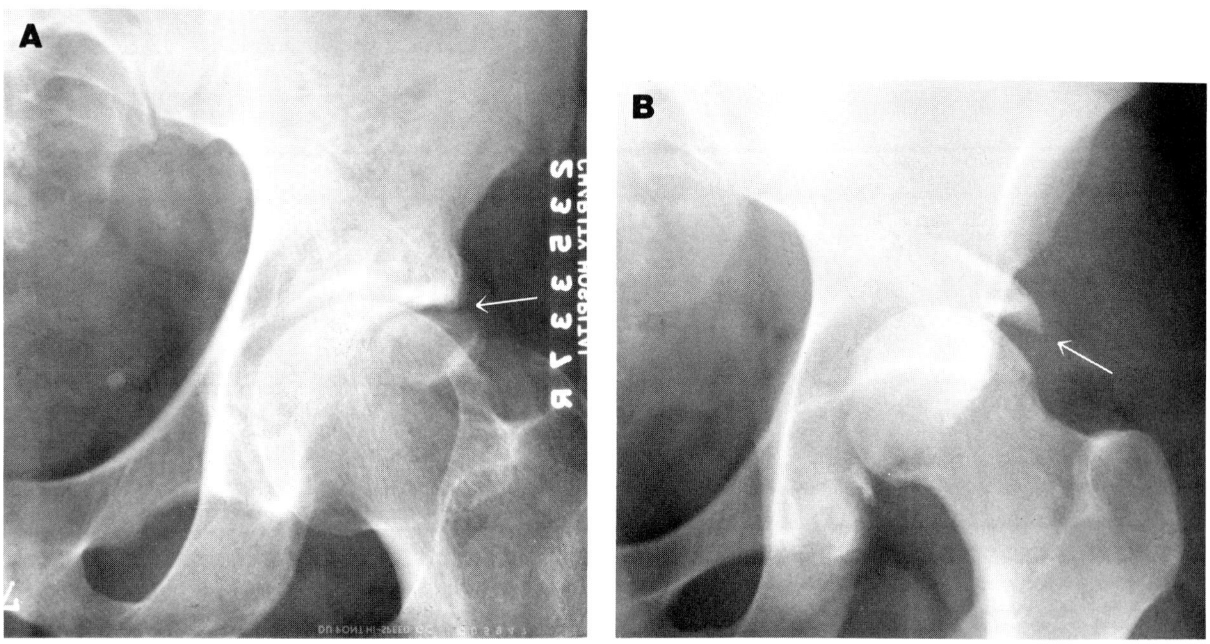

Fig. 2-36. (*A*) Os acetabuli in a 57-year-old man. This secondary center of ossification is separated from the main portion of the acetabulum by a cartilage line (*arrow*). It has an even width, and the bone at the ends of the line tend to be rounded rather than angular. (*B*) Fracture of acetabulum. Bone at the surface of the line (*arrow*) is jagged and very irregular. The bone at the ends of the fracture is definitely angular rather than rounded. (Courtesy R. D. D'Ambrosia.)

sion of a small bone, an adventitious epiphysis, an accessory ossification center, and some developmental lines in diaphyseal bone. Division may be multiple in the patella but is rare elsewhere.

Old fracture lines may be smooth and their margins rounded, but this occurs only with some reparative change and sclerosis which do not normally accompany healthy cartilage lines.

The two bone elements at an accessory ossification center have the additional feature that they cannot be visualized as fitting together to form a bone of normal size and outline.

Incomplete segmentation of bone units causes a persisting cartilage line which is narrow because of absence of motion and presence of underdevelopment of the cartilage. A feature is that the termination of the line at the unsegmented area is smoothly rounded instead of tapered to a point as would be expected at an incomplete fracture.

Certain transverse lines of cartilage or fibrous tissue appear in diaphyses of long bones as a result of certain forces or processes. Examples are not rare in Paget's disease or chondrodysplasia.

A long bone, such as the femur or tibia, which is bowed as a result of Paget's disease is the site of tension stresses on the convexity of the curve. Fatigue fracture may develop (see Fig. 2-28). It starts from the convex surface and extends increasingly toward the concavity in a thin transverse line of resorption of calcareous structure with fibrous tissue persisting. This has the appearance of a cartilage line. It is visible before it has extended sufficiently to be completed by spontaneous fracture and is the reason why fractures in bowed bones in this disease typically are transverse although a small area at the concavity does not truly continue in that plane.

In some cases of chondrodysplasia a broad plane of failure of cartilage to convert to bone may be present. When such a plane is central without reaching the periphery and is continuous only for a relatively short distance, a thin plane of fibrous tissue or cartilage is left behind by the growing metaphysis. It does not deprive the bone of enough calcareous structure to be visible at once, but the submarginal area will eventually become peripheral because of remodeling of the shaft during growth. The cortex, thus, becomes deficient at the affected plane, and a transverse line similar to a cartilage line is visible parallel to the plane of the metaphysis from which the defect was derived. The only clinical significance of such a line is possible liability to fracture under normal stresses if the defective plane is sufficiently extensive. Such lines may be multiple, especially if a genetic disturbance contributed to their production.

DIAGNOSING BONY UNION OF A FRACTURE

There is hemorrhage at fragments of bone resulting from fracture or surgery, and some swelling soon becomes detectable. Callus becomes apparent as it calcifies. It may be visible at about 10 days in young children or at 3 or more weeks in elderly adults (Fig. 2-37). It is a calcification of posttraumatic type. If it is subperiosteal, it has the characteristics of inert subperiosteal calcification. If it is exuberant, it will appear flocculent and amorphous at first but will become dense. After weeks or months, the exuberant callus begins to resorb. It continues to do so until the portion which is not involved in functioning has disappeared.

The speed with which callus develops varies greatly. It is accelerated by youth, apposition of fragments, minimal hematoma, adequate circulation, normal local calcium content, immobilization, early use after there is some union, and by absence of disease. It is delayed by conditions adverse to those factors.

If one adopts the view that useful union is not present until new calcareous trabeculae are visibly incorporating fragment with fragment, most fracture patients will be without function for a considerable time. A state more difficult to judge but present in a shorter time is clinical union. Clinical union is when there is sufficient firmness of callus to hold the fragments together and permit functional weight-bearing.

Skill in judging the presence and strength of clinical union is developed from recognition of the presence of a situation in which union is expectable and of changes in the picture at the fracture line which indicate that a course toward union rather than nonunion and pseudoarthrosis is being pursued within a normal range of timing. It is worthy of note that a unilateral handstand as performed by an acrobat demonstrates that the strength supplied by the

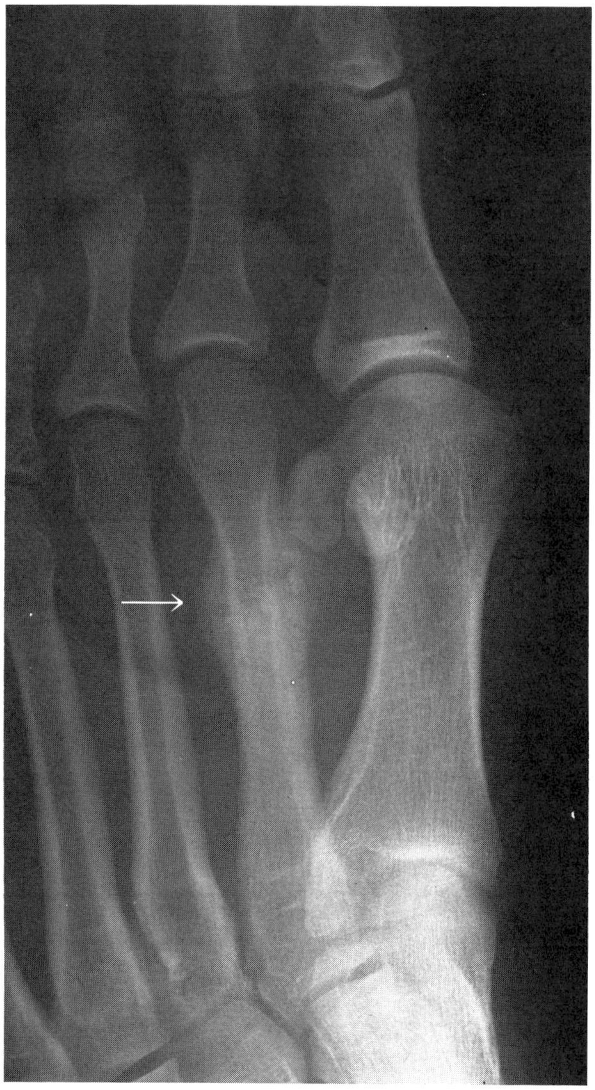

Fig. 2-37. March fracture of the second metatarsal in an Army recruit (*arrow*). The fracture was initially unrecognized but at three weeks there is extensive subperiosteal calcification of the callus. (Courtesy R. D. D'Ambrosia.)

small amount of bone at the neck of the radius is ample for bearing the direct weight thrust of the entire body although not necessarily the greater impact in walking or jumping.

The features to be noted are these: calcareous density quickly decreases in a thin area at the surface of a fracture line; it demonstrates adequate circulation for washing out that calcium; density begins to be recovered within a few days if conditions are normal; and bony union derives from extension of osseous trabeculae from fragment to fragment. If the course is not normal this does not occur and a thin line of calcareous material develops connecting adjacent trabeculae on each individual surface until nonunion or pseudoarthrosis is present (Fig. 2-38).

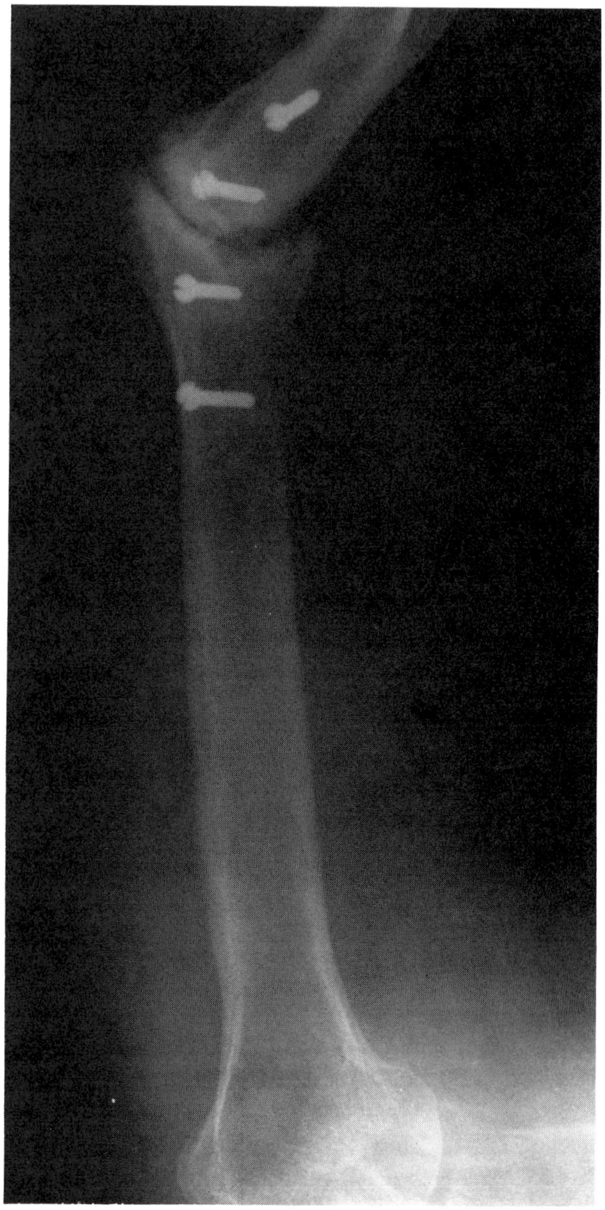

Fig. 2-38. Pseudarthrosis of the humerus. The bony trabeculae have failed to cross the fracture fragments, and instead a dense calcareous line has connected the trabeculae on the opposing services; nonunion is the result. (Courtesy R. D. D'Ambrosia.)

A most important factor is the amount of space between the fragments. When they are fully apposed or impacted, especially if there is some interlocking of trabeculae clinical union may become fairly firm within 2 or 3 weeks. If the space is as much as 1 mm., the needed time may be as much as 2 or 3 months. With a 2 mm. space, the needed time runs some months longer. With greater space, there is increasing probability for failure of union.

When clinical union is present, minimal function, as by use of gradually increased direct axial pressure, can be started. This stimulates strengthening of union but when applied before clinical union, it may be a deterrent.

Judgment that clinical union is present may be made in the normal expectable time since fracture in view of the apposition of the fragments or the space between them has about elapsed without evidence of a tendency to failure of union which would be shown by extension of decalcification or even resorption of bone at a fracture surface or by development of a thin reparative line of calcareous density at one or both of those surfaces, with or without condensation in adjacent bone.

3 Electrodiagnosis of Musculoskeletal Disorders

Robert G. Taylor, M.D., and William M. Fowler, Jr., M.D.

The measurement of nerve conduction velocity was first reported in 1852, and electromyography was first recognized and used experimentally about 1907.[25] Clinical interest in electrodiagnostic techniques did not occur, however, until World War II. This interest was the result of the large number of nerve injuries inflicted during that conflict, and research in the electronic field during and following that period produced significant improvements in instrumentation. As a result, the procedures have now become reliable and the results reproducible.

Electroneuromyographic tests either measure the response of nerves and muscles to electrical stimulation or record bioelectrical potentials from muscles and nerves. The purpose of these procedures is to determine if there is any abnormal physiological involvement of the motor unit. When such involvement produces an abnormal response to electrical stimulation or abnormal bioelectrical potentials, anatomical localization of the lesion is then often possible.

The major symptoms and signs of neuromusculoskeletal disease are: pain and tenderness; fatigue, weakness, hypotonia, paresis, and atrophy; limitation of movement and/or deformity; stiffness; muscle spasm, contracture, or cramps; and sensory loss. Since weakness is the predominant finding in diseases of the motor unit, the greatest value of electroneuromyographic procedures is in the differential diagnosis of fatigue, weakness, hypotonia, paresis, and atrophy. Because electrodiagnostic tests only evaluate the functional status of the motor unit, they are not capable of defining the specific etiological diagnosis. As with all laboratory tests, they merely assist the clinician in arriving at a diagnosis, and the findings must be integrated with the results of other tests, the clinical examination, and the history.

INDICATIONS FOR ELECTRODIAGNOSTIC TESTS

Detection of Functional Damage to the Motor Unit

Electrodiagnostic procedures are concerned primarily with diagnosis of disease or dysfunction of the motor unit. They rarely contribute, except in a negative way, to diagnosis of disease within the central nervous system. The motor unit consists of the motor neuron cell body (anterior horn cell), its axon, the myoneural junctions, and all the muscle fibers supplied by the terminal branches of the axon. The cell body, its axon, and terminal branches comprise the lower motor neuron (Fig. 3-1). At times, the clinician is not certain as to whether or not weakness or some other motor dysfunction is the result of disease of the motor unit or is solely due to pain, hysterical conversion reactions, malingering, or disease. At other times, a disease may be in an early stage or be so mild that there is no objective finding of dysfunction of the motor unit. Under these circumstances electroneuromyographic evidence of normality or abnormality of the motor unit is of considerable value.

Three clinical electrodiagnostic tests are available in most medical centers. Although there is considerable overlapping, each procedure has a specific purpose in identifying abnormalities occurring in the major subdivisions of the motor unit. The *electromyogram* is usually considered as a screening procedure since it can detect abnormalities in all of the divisions of the motor unit. In many circumstances it is not, however, very selective. As an example, lesions of the anterior horn cells, the ventral roots, the nerve plexus, and the peripheral nerves often result in identical electromyographic findings. *Nerve conduction tests,* motor and sensory, represent the best method for evaluating the functional status of the peripheral nerves and can assist in distinguishing conditions affecting axons from those affecting the anterior horn cells. *Repetitive nerve stimulation* studies are of primary value in evaluating suspected abnormalities of the myoneural junction.

The first indication, therefore, for obtaining an electrodiagnostic test is to determine the presence or absence of motor unit disease and to localize the level of the physiologic abnormality within the motor unit. The second indication is to determine the stage and extent of the lesion since the clinician is often expected to prognosticate the recovery from muscular weakness. We now have a third indication for obtaining an electrodiagnostic test to determine the anatomical site of a lesion once functional damage has been established.

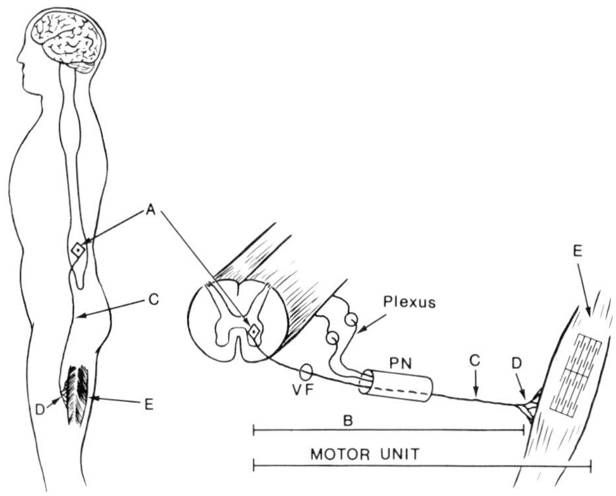

Fig. 3-1. Concept of the motor unit. The figure (*left*) illustrates the role of the motor unit in the organism as a whole; (*right*) the elements of the motor unit are defined. The signal for *voluntary* muscle contraction originates in the brain and is transmitted down the spinal cord to the central element of the motor unit (A), the motor nerve cell body (anterior horn cell). The lower motor neuron (B) consists of the anterior horn cell (A) plus its axon (C) which proceeds distally in the peripheral nerve (PN). The neuromuscular junction (D) is where the terminal elements of the axon synapse with the muscle fiber (E) indicated as a whole muscle. The sarcomere (*inset*) represents the contractile elements of the muscle fiber. From its origin, the axon proceeds in a peripheral direction, passing through the vertebral foramen (VF), and merges with axons from other segmental levels in the plexus before forming the peripheral nerve which ultimately reaches the muscle.

Determination of Anatomical Site of Lesion Within the Motor Unit

If there is functional involvement of any of the divisions of the motor unit resulting in an abnormality of one or more of the electrodiagnostic tests, anatomical localization of the lesion is then often possible. There are six anatomical sites along the motor unit pathway where specific pathological processes may produce electroneuromyographic abnormalities (Fig. 3-2): (1) *anterior horn cell,* (2) *ventral root,* (3) *plexus,* (4) *peripheral nerve* (sensory and motor components), (5) *myoneural junction,* and (6) *muscle fibers.* In addition, a systematic investigation of the various segments of the nerve often allows precise localization of the site of the lesion or entrapment of the peripheral nerve.

Identification of the anatomical site of the lesion usually requires two or more electrodiagnostic tests and a thorough knowledge of the patient's history and physical examination. In most cases, standard electromyography can distinguish neuropathic disorders affecting the lower motor neuron from myopathic diseases. The greatest difficulty is in separating out lesions affecting the anterior horn cell, root,

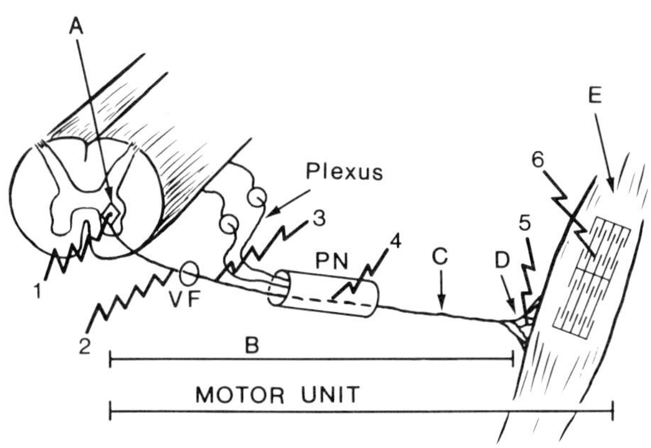

Fig. 3-2. Sites within the motor unit that are vulnerable to disease or injury and which can be localized by appropriate electrodiagnostic tests. (1) Anterior horn cell. (2) Ventral root. (3) The nerve plexus. (4) The peripheral nerve. (5) Myoneural junction. (6) The muscle fiber.

plexus, and peripheral nerve. A relatively simple example of this is the differential diagnosis of weakness of the tibialis anterior muscle since this condition can result from compression of the peroneal nerve or a lesion of the L4 root. With root involvement, the peroneal nerve conduction velocity will be normal. Since the *major* root innervation to the tibialis anterior is L4, with compression of this root the electromyogram will usually show marked evidence of denervation in the tibialis anterior, occasional mild findings of denervation in the tensor fascia latae (L4 L5 S1), and little or no abnormal findings in the quadriceps (L2, 3, 4). In addition, denervation is also usually present in the posterior primary division (rami) paraspinal muscles. Examination of the muscles of the back is especially valuable in differentiation of a plexus from a root lesion since the plexus forms from the most distal portion of the anterior primary division. If the posterior division axial muscles are involved, the lesion must be proximal.

Classification of the Disease Most Likely to Produce the Lesion

Electrodiagnostic tests are not capable of determining specific etiological diagnoses nor will they always neatly compartmentalize myopathies and neuropathies. Many disorders, however, can be clustered into various clinical symptom-sign combinations, and there are often specific electrodiagnostic patterns for each of these combinations as well as within groups.

An example of this is the several syndromes characterized by myotonia. Common to all are the electromyographic findings of high frequency repetitive discharges which increase rapidly in frequency and amplitude and then rapidly diminish. Patients with congenital myotonia, paramyotonia, and hyperkalemic periodic paralysis usually do not have significant muscle fiber involvement, and only demonstrate electrical myotonia. Myotonic muscular dystrophy, on the other hand, is characterized by marked muscle fiber changes. The electromyogram often demonstrates fibrillation potentials at rest, in addition to myotonia, and the motor unit action potentials during contraction are usually reduced in amplitude with brief duration.

In summary, the clinical indications for electrodiagnostic procedures are:

Detection of functional damage to the motor unit. Is the patient's symptom of fatigue or sign of weakness the result of disease of the motor unit or is it due to pain, conversion reaction, malingering, disuse, or a lesion of the upper motor neuron?

Determination of the degree of functional damage. Is peripheral nerve palsy due to neurapraxia, axon stenosis, axonal cachexia, or axonotmesis?

Determination of the anatomical site of the lesion. Is the patient's weakness due to involvement of the anterior horn cell, ventral root, plexus, peripheral nerve, myoneural junction, or the muscle fibers?

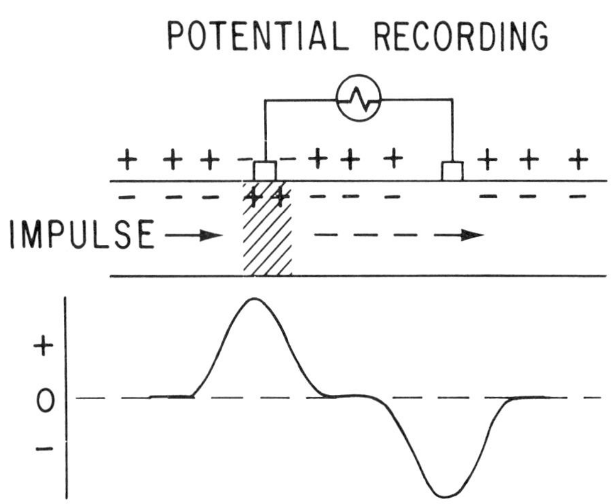

Fig. 3-3. Origin of the biphasic action potential. The recording electrodes are adjacent to the cell membrane, and the wave of depolarization (impulse) is moving from the left to right. As the depolarized region passes under the primary electrode, the oscilloscope records the electrical potential moving in one direction, which is reversed as the depolarization passes under the reference electrode.

NEUROPHYSIOLOGY

The electromyograph (EMG) is merely a sophisticated and complicated voltmeter which has been adapted to measure the electrical activity of muscle. Muscle, like nerve, is a polarized tissue which has a large resting membrane potential. This resting membrane potential is a result of the ionic imbalance across the muscle fiber membrane which is maintained by the active, coupled, sodium potassium pump. When an appropriate signal is received membrane conductance for these ions is altered (Fig. 3-3). A brief but rapid migration of these ions occurs, and the resting electrical potential is lost with a slight overshoot. This depolarization produces a brief change in the electrical environment surrounding the muscle fiber which can be recorded as an electrical action potential. It is not a localized phenomenon and once started is transmitted as a wave of depolarization over the full length of each muscle fiber. The trigger for this coordinated electrical activity originates at the skeletal neuromuscular junction in response to a stimulus traveling down the nerve.

The origin of the willed impulse for contraction of a muscle is in the motor area of the brain. This originates as depolarization of the appropriate nerve cells in the motor cortex and is transmitted down the axons of the pyramidal (corticospinal) and extrapyramidal tracts to the anterior horn cells. These tracts of the brain stem and spinal cord behave as cable conducting systems carrying the signal to the next relay station which in this case is the anterior horn cell at the appropriate segmental level. The anterior horn cell receives a barrage of impulses coming from segmental as well as suprasegmental levels. These impulses can be inhibitory as well as facilitory. As a result, there is a definite element of information processing occurring at the anterior horn cell. When the total sum of the facilitory and inhibitory segmental and suprasegmental influences reaches threshold level for the anterior horn cell, it will depolarize. Information received by way of the spinal cord tracts from suprasegmental levels directly to the anterior horn cells is primarily facilitory. The anterior horn cell also receives information from suprasegmental levels indirectly via the gamma (fusimotor) system to the muscle spindles which are the stretch receptor organs for the muscles. These impulses influence the fusimotor muscle fibers to increase or decrease resting tension on the muscle spindles thereby adjusting their sensitivity to a stretch stimulus. Input to anterior horn cells from the annulospiral receptors of muscle spindles from the homonomous muscle is always facilitory, and input from or to its synergists is usually facilitory. Annulospiral input from or to antagonist muscles is usually inhibitory. Input to the anterior horn cell from spindles of muscle of the contralateral extremity is usually reciprocal to that originating from the ipsilateral extremity. When stimulated, the muscle stretch receptors can signal the muscle to contract via the segmental monosynaptic or polysynaptic reflex arcs. The monosynaptic reflex arcs are the ones activated when testing for the deep tendon reflexes. The motor unit is the final effector in the neural regulation of muscular activity. It is this basic functional structure that we are most concerned with in clinical electromyography. The motor unit is defined as the anterior horn cell, its axon, and the many muscle fibers it controls (see Fig. 3-1). The soma or cell body of the anterior horn cell is located in the grey matter of the anterior columns of the spinal cord. Its axons are the large alpha motor neurons, with diameters ranging from 3 to 20 microns. The alpha motor neurons are myelinated, and since they have both large diameter and saltatory conduction, the conduction velocity for these axons is very fast. There is a direct relationship between the conduction velocity of a nerve and its diameter. The Hursh factor estimates that the conduction velocity of a nerve fiber, expressed in meters per second, is equal to the diameter of the nerve including its myelin sheath, expressed in microns, times the constant factor six.[15] As a nerve continues distally, the diameter of its axon will gradually decrease. As the nerve approaches the muscle, the individual axons will decrease rapidly in size so that by the time the individual axons near their myoneural junctions, they usually have been reduced to diameters approaching 1 micron. As would be expected from the aforementioned relationship, the conduction velocity for these very small terminal branches is extremely slow. When an anterior horn cell is activated, the impulse will travel down its axon and activate most, if not all, of the muscle fibers innervated. The size of the motor units are variable and range from 100 to 200 muscle fibers per axon for the intrinsic muscles of the hand to as many as 1,500 to 2,000 muscle fibers per axon in the very large muscles such as the gastrocnemius.

Another structure which is an integral part of the motor unit is the myoneural junction. The skeletal neuromuscular junction (Fig. 3-4) converts the electrical signal received from the nerve to a chemical message for transmission to the muscle fiber where it is again converted to an electrical signal. The neuromuscular junction is primarily composed of three elements: the presynaptic membrane, which is a contribution from the terminal axon of the nerve fiber; the postsynaptic membrane, a part of the muscle fiber membrane specialized to receive the chemical message and reconvert it to an electrical signal by altering its ionic conductance so that an electrical

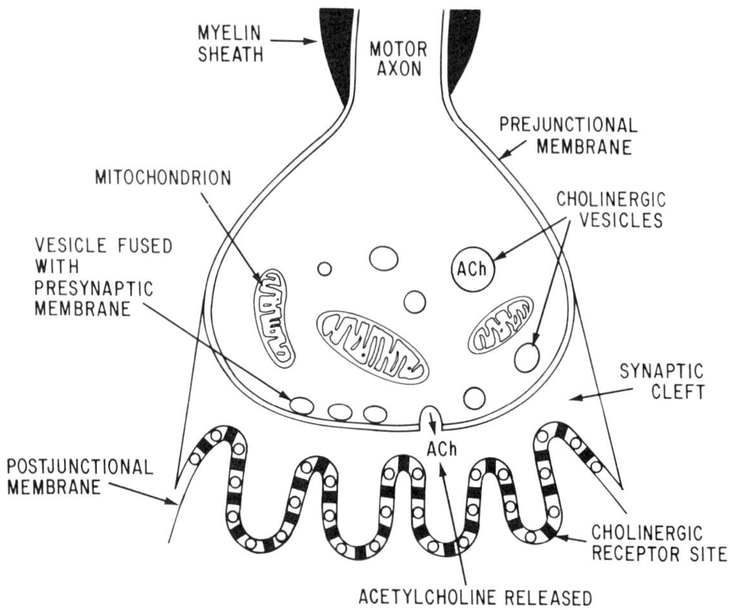

Fig. 3-4. Schematic representation of the elements and function of the skeletal neuromuscular junction. The electrical impulse is received in the nerve terminus where it stimulates release of acetylcholine (ACh) from the prejunctional membrane into the synaptic cleft, converting the electrical to a chemical transmission. The ACh receptor complex alters ionic conduction of the postjunctional membrane, producing electrical potential which starts a propagated impulse in the muscle fiber membrane. (Rosenberg, R. N. and Campbell, J.: Myasthenia gravis. Calif. Med., *118:*18, Jan. 1973.)

potential is generated; and the synaptic cleft which is the space that separates the two membranes. This specialization of the neuromuscular junction by which it converts the electrical to chemical and then back to electrical signal permits it to function as a one-way gate so that the message travels from the nerve to the muscle in a one-way direction only.[14] It is possible that if it were not for this one-way gate, an electrical to electrical connection could establish a reverberating circuit so that it would continue to fire until all energy supply had been exhausted. The terminal portion of the axon produces acetylcholine (ACh) which is stored in membrane-bound packets called quanta. A *quanta* is defined as the amount of ACh contained in one vesicle or packet. Calcium ions, present in this region, assist these quanta or packets of ACh to fuse with the presynaptic membrane in preparation for release into the synaptic cleft. Fluctuations in the amount of calcium ions available in this area will alter the ability of the ACh vesicles to fuse with the presynaptic membrane. Fusion of the ACh vesicles with the presynaptic membrane is necessary before they can be released.[14] When the electrical signal is received, the presynaptic membrane releases several quanta of ACh into the synaptic cleft. The ACh molecules cross the synaptic cleft by diffusion. When they reach the postsynaptic membrane, they complex with a receptor substance in the postsynaptic membrane. This ACh-receptor complex brings about a brief alteration in the ionic permeability of the postsynaptic membrane so that potassium ions flow out and sodium ions flow in through the sarcolemmal membrane at very rapid rates.[14] This movement of ions produces an electrical potential change from resting levels, and when this change reaches threshold values, a propagated spike or action potential occurs. The electromyograph is capable of measuring this propagated action potential. Under normal circumstances, it is the motor unit that fires, and the EMG records the electrical activity of all of the muscle fibers in an individual motor unit occurring simultaneously.

From a physiological standpoint, an individual muscle fiber can be divided into four major functional compartments: the excitation-impulse conduction system; the excitation-contraction coupling mechanism; the contractile mechanism; and the energy supply mechanisms.

Excitation-Impulse Conduction System

This function is primarily the responsibility of the sarcolemmal membrane. When the signal for depolarization is received by the postsynaptic membrane, the electrical activity is carried as a wave of electrical activity, depolarization, along the full length of the muscle fiber in both directions from the myoneural junction. To facilitate this signal so that it can reach the deeper, more central parts of the muscle fiber there is a specialized structure, the transverse tubules, which conducts the signal to each myofibril and sarcomere. When the signal is received at the sarcomere level, it then becomes the trigger for the excitation-contraction coupling mechanism. It is the electrical activity of this excitation-impulse conduction that is recorded by the EMG system.

Excitation-Contraction Coupling Mechanism

The structure specialized for excitation-contraction coupling is the sarcoplasmic reticulum. This is a group of membranous sacs which are arranged around each sarcomere. These sacs are specialized to release calcium ions on signal from the excitation-impulse conduction system. The sarcoplasmic reticulum has a tremendous affinity for calcium ions, and once calcium is released, it immediately starts to resequester these ions. The flow of the calcium ions in this direction is against a concentration gradient, requiring an energy system to move the calcium back into the sarcoplasmic reticulum. The primary energy source for this activity is adenosine triphosphate (ATP).

Contractile Mechanisms

A muscle fiber is further subdivided into parallel bundles of myofibrils, and the myofibrils are subdivided along their longitudinal axis into sarcomeres. The sarcomere is the basic functional unit of a muscle (Fig. 3-5). It consists of the thin actin myofilaments which are attached to the Z bands. Suspended between the Z band myofilament complexes are the "thick" myofilaments which are composed primarily of myosin with a high level of myosin ATPase activity. The thin filaments are composed primarily of actin molecules; however, another important protein in the thin filaments is troponin. Actin and myosin have an inherent affinity for each other, and when this actin-myosin interaction occurs, the result is contraction. The troponin molecules in the thin filaments have an inhibitory effect on the actin-myosin interaction, and in normal situations this prevents the actin and myosin from interacting so that muscle relaxation can occur.

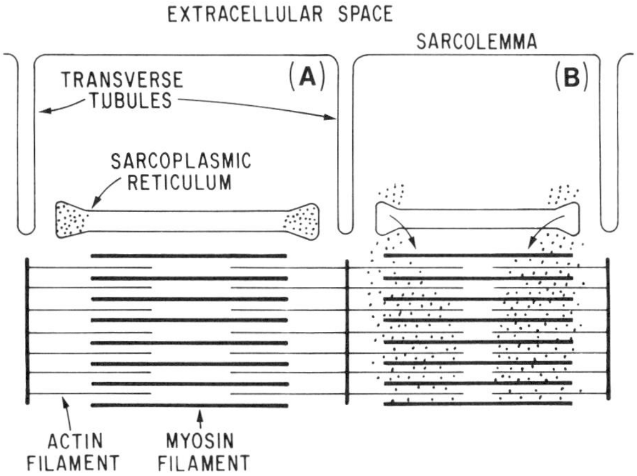

Fig. 3-5. Diagrams of a sarcomere in the relaxed state (*A*) and in the shortened or contracted state (*B*). The calcium ion (small dots) concentration is high in the sarcoplasmic reticulum and low in the sarcoplasm. On signal via the transverse tubules, the sarcoplasmic reticulum releases calcium ions into the sarcoplasm, permitting interaction between the actin and myosin myofilaments and shortening of the sarcomere (*B*). The process is reversed and relaxation occurs.

When calcium ions are released from the sarcoplasmic reticulum, they combine with the troponin molecules and cancel the inhibitory effect that troponin has on the actin-myosin interaction. When this occurs, the actin and myosin interact causing the sarcomeres to shorten and produce tension. The sarcoplasmic reticulum resequesters the calcium at a rapid rate, and once the level of the calcium ions in the sarcoplasm is reduced to a certain critical level, its bonds with the troponin molecules are released, the troponin molecules re-exert their inhibitory effect on the actin-myosin interactions, and muscle relaxation occurs. The actual processes of muscle contraction and relaxation are nonelectrically mediated and are electrically silent on the electromyogram. It is only the electrical activity of the excitation-impulse conduction system that can be observed by the EMG.

Energy Supply Mechanisms

In general, there are two energy supply mechanisms for muscle: aerobic and anaerobic. The aerobic system is the basic Krebs cycle mechanism and is dependent on a supply of oxygen adequate to meet the energy requirements of the muscle. The anaerobic system utilizes the reserve mechanisms of the

Embden-Meyerhof pathway to permit energy to be released from the stored glycogen. It is inefficient, however, and creates an oxygen deficit which must later be compensated for by the basic and more efficient mechanism. The anaerobic system is the primary mechanism for supply of energy to the membrane of the muscle and nerve fibers.

The electromyogram provides a Cartesian (x,y) plot of the electrical activity of the excitation-impulse conduction system (the sarcolemmal membrane) as a function of time. With this as a basic concept, it can be seen that there are only a few variables that can be examined by electromyography:

1. Electrical silence at rest
2. Voluntary motor unit action potentials
   a. Amplitude of the potentials
   b. Duration of the potentials
   c. Shape of the potentials
   d. Numbers of action potentials
   e. Recruitment pattern
3. Insertional activity
4. Repetitive discharges

ELECTRODIAGNOSTIC PROCEDURES

Traditional Electrodiagnostic Tests

Although the clinical use of the electroneuromyographic tests of electromyography and nerve conduction is a relatively recent development, other simpler but less sensitive electrodiagnostic procedures have been available for many years. These include measurements of reaction of degeneration, rheobase, chronaxy, strength-duration curves, and the tetanus twitch ratio.[25]

Rheobase and Chronaxy. The minimal amount or intensity of current which will stimulate a muscle when the current is permitted to flow for an infinite period of time is called the rheobase and is synonomous with threshold. Infinite time is considered to be 300 m.s. of current flow. The chronaxy is the duration of flow of a current twice the intensity of the rheobase that is required to stimulate a muscle.

Strength-Duration Curve. Since intensity of current and the duration required to stimulate muscle are inversely related, plotting the duration of current flow against the intensity of current results in the strength-duration curve (Fig. 3-6). Either the voltage or current may be plotted as the intensity of stimulus, depending on the instrument available. The chronaxy is one point on the strength-duration curve.

Reaction of Degeneration. Nerve tissue is inherently more excitable than muscle tissue. Hence, when an electrical stimulus is applied to a muscle with an intact nerve supply, it is the small terminal nerve fibers that are activated by the current. In addition, innervated muscle also responds best when stimulated at its motor point. When a muscle has lost its nerve supply, it is necessary to stimulate it directly. Since denervated muscle fibers then become less excitable than nerve tissue, the duration of current flow must be prolonged but at similar intensities in order to produce a muscle contraction. Direct (galvanic) current permits stimulus flow of prolonged duration.

Reaction of degeneration is muscle contraction in response to stimulation with galvanic but not faradic current. Unlike muscle with an intact nerve supply, denervated muscle responds equally to the stimulus applied anywhere over the muscle, and the resulting twitch is slow and "worm-like" since muscle tissue, rather than nerve, is the conducting medium. In addition, while the cathode closing current is the most effective in stimulating nerve tissue, it has no such ability for denervated muscle. When the muscle is only partially denervated, the muscle twitch would be diminished in response to a current flow of short duration in proportion to the number of de-

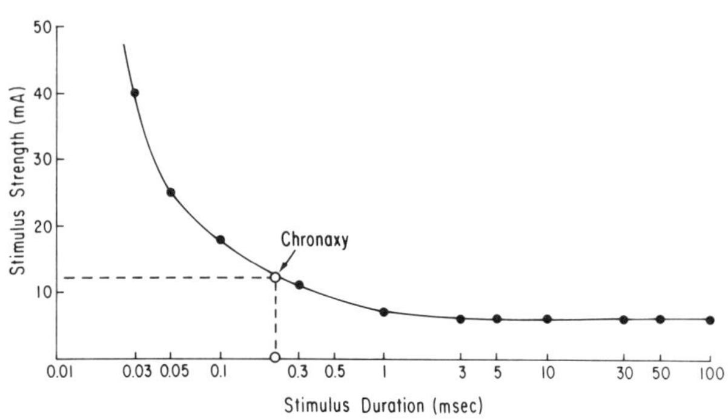

Fig. 3-6. The strength-duration curve is a graph of the intensity (strength = volts or milliamps) and duration (msec.) that a stimulating current must flow to produce contraction of a muscle. Following denervation, the muscle fibers must be stimulated directly, and this requires currents of longer duration, causing a marked shift of the curve to the right and a marked increase in chronaxy.

nervated muscle fibers since they would be unable to respond. This is termed partial reaction of degeneration.

Many factors, such as the location of the underlying muscle, skin resistance, and the visible recognition of a minimal twitch, compound the variability to these traditional electrodiagnostic tests and, hence, cloud their significance. They have, for the most part, been supplanted by the more sensitive and objective electromyographic and nerve conduction techniques.[12,20,25,29,31,33,37] It should be noted, however, that such procedures as the strength-duration curve may give evidence of denervation following nerve injury or denervation in the early stage when spontaneous fibrillation is difficult to detect.

ELECTROMYOGRAPHY AND NERVE STIMULATION PROCEDURES

Instrumentation

The essential components for electromyography and nerve conduction studies include electrodes, a preamplifier, an audioamplifier and loudspeaker, an oscilloscope, and a physiological stimulator (Fig. 3-7). Permanent records of the displayed electrical activity can be made by utilization of a magnetic tape recorder or by photographic recorders.

Many types of electrodes are available for clinical electromyography. Surface electrodes on the skin are used primarily for indifferent (reference) and ground purposes. The two electrodes used most frequently for exploration are the monopolar and concentric needle electrodes. The monopolar electrode consists of a piece of stainless steel wire coated, except at the tip, with insulating material. The concentric type consists of a wire located within but insulated from a hypodermic needle; only a surface ground electrode is required. Other less frequently used electrodes in electromyography are the bipolar, multielectrode "Janus," and flexible wire implanted electrodes.

The electrical potentials observed in electromyography are usually small in amplitude and, hence, must be amplified to a level that can be conveniently handled by the other apparatus. The amplifier, therefore, should have the following characteristics: uniform and high voltage gain for all frequencies and a frequency range of 2 to 10,000 Hz.; differential input; high input impedance and low input capacities; low inherent noise; and high common-mode rejection. Variations in electric potentials between the uninsulated tip of the exploring electrode in the muscle and the reference electrode are amplified up to 1 million times (from microvolts to volts) and displayed on the oscilloscope. For both nerve conduction and electromyography, sweep speeds will range from 2 to 30 m.s. per centimeter.

For nerve conduction studies, it is desirable to have the time base on the oscilloscope independent of the sweep speed; for complete accuracy in the perception of small signals, an electronic averager is necessary. The physiological stimulator, usually a rectangular pulse wave generator isolated from ground by an isolation transformer, should be capable of delivering voltages up to 150 volts in amplitude at durations of 0.05 to 2 m.s. and at variable frequencies up to 50 Hz. The stimulator triggers the sweep for nerve conduction studies, and the time base is matched to the sweep start. Either surface or needle electrodes may be used for recording the response to stimulation.[5,12,29,33]

Electromyography

Electromyography (EMG) should be performed by a physician since a neurological history and examination are necessary for planning purposes. The plan must usually be modified as the findings unfold, and the displayed electrical activity depends on the actions of the electromyographer at any particular moment as well as on the location of the electrode.[20] Medical training is an essential background if the patient and the illness are to be viewed in an integrated perspective.[12]

The examination begins with the introduction of the electrode into the muscle. Adequate exploration of each muscle examined usually requires at least 5 to 10 needle advancements at several locations in each muscle. Sweep speeds vary from 5 to 20 m.s. per division, and the gain is usually held at 50 to 100 μv. per division except during maximal muscle contraction when it is moved to 500 to 1000 μv. per division. With the needle inserted in the muscle, observations are made of the electrical activity evoked in the resting muscle by insertion and movement of the electrode; the activity of the resting muscle with the needle undisturbed (spontaneous activity); and the activity of the motor unit action potentials during minimal and maximal muscle contraction.

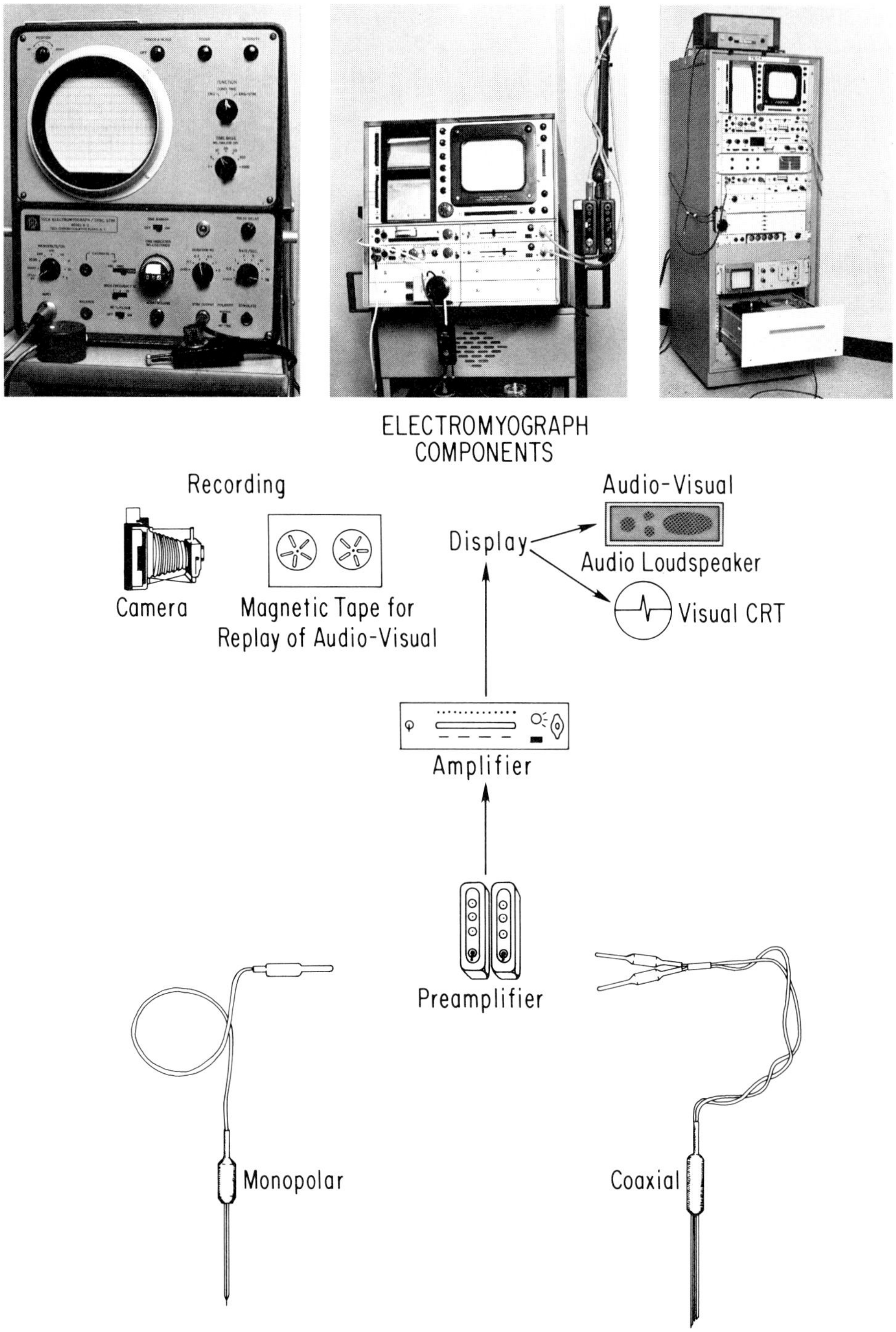

Fig. 3-7. Electromyographical equipment. (*Upper left*) a simple single channel unit; (*upper center*) a more complex dual channel unit with capacity for photographic and/or magnetic tape recording; and (*upper right*) complex unit designed for research and teaching purposes. In the schematic drawings, electrical activity from the electrodes is led via the preamplifier to the amplifier and from there to the audiovisual display system (loudspeaker and cathode ray tube, oscilloscope). To the left of the display system are illustrated the photographic and magnetic tape recording units.

As the electrode penetrates the resting muscle or is moved within the muscle, fibers are mechanically stimulated and injured producing a brief burst of electrical discharges lasting 10 to 300 m.s. (Fig. 3-8). This is called *insertional activity* and should not be confused with spontaneous activity. The absence of insertional activity indicates that there are no functioning muscle fibers or that the electrode is not in muscle tissue. When muscle atrophies after denervation or is replaced by fat and fibrous tissue, as in muscular dystrophy, it becomes increasingly difficult to locate muscle tissue. On occasion, it is difficult to tell when insertional activity ceases and spontaneous activity starts. In patients with inflammatory myopathy, for example, the muscle fibers are hyperirritable, giving rise to exaggerated bursts of electrical activity following movement of the electrode. These bursts of activity usually exceed 300 m.s. in duration.

Normal muscle at rest is electrically silent following a brief burst of insertional activity (see Fig. 3-8). The EMG registers only voltage changes, and when muscle is at rest there is no electrical change even though there is a resting membrane potential. In practice, of course, it is often difficult to obtain a completely relaxed muscle. Exceptions to the finding of no activity at rest in normal muscle are the two types of so-called end-plate "noise" (see Fig. 3-8). On occasion, normal spontaneous discharges may be found in the muscles' zone of innervation. They occur at a fairly regular frequency; have short dura-

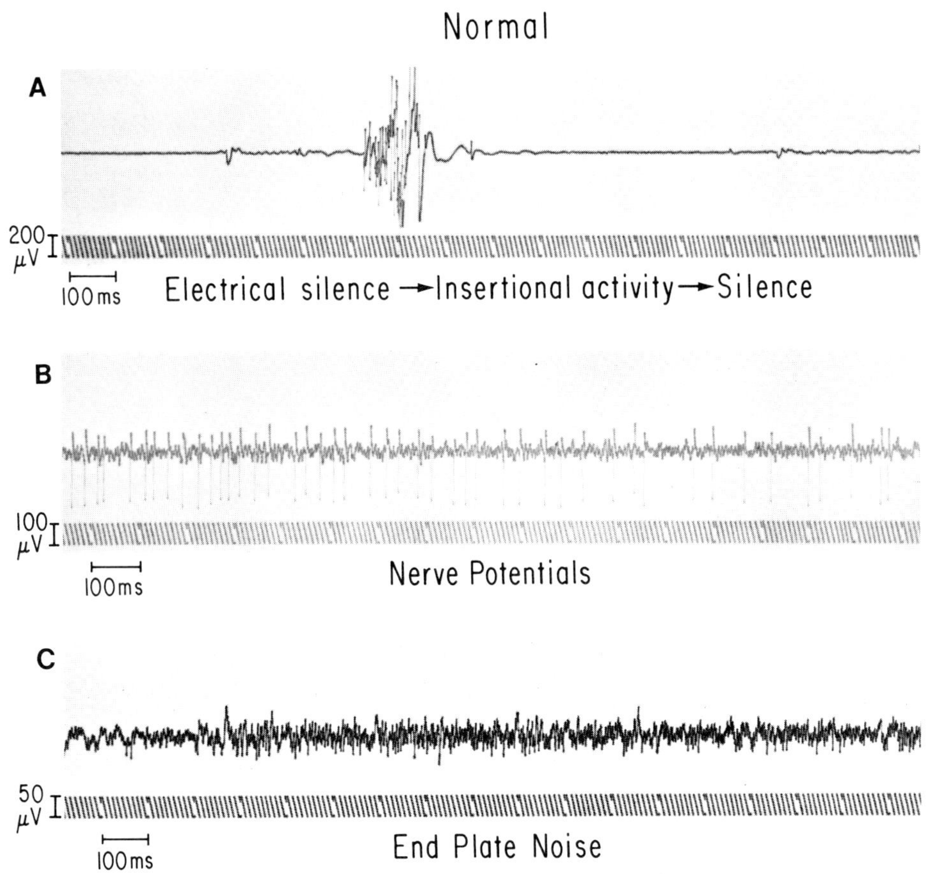

Fig. 3-8. (*A*) Electrical silence at rest with a brief burst of insertional activity following movement of the needle electrode; note the prompt return to electrical silence with the electrode at rest. (*B*) Nerve action potentials are high frequency discharges observed in the vicinity of a small nerve or motor point. Factors which distinguish these potentials from fibrillation potentials are the rapid rate of firing and the initial negative deflection of the nerve potentials. (*C*) End plate noise is of low amplitude and high frequency, considerably greater than baseline electronic noise.

tions (3 to 5 m.s.) and low amplitudes (up to 200 μv.); and the initial phase is negative followed by a positive deflection (diphasic) (see Fig. 3-8). Since the patient usually complains of pain at the time these potentials are seen, they have been assumed to originate from irritation of small intramuscular nerves and, hence, are referred to as nerve potentials. Their only clinical significance is that they are occasionally confused with fibrillation potentials, although the latter have an initial positive phase. High frequency spontaneous potentials, ranging from 10 to 100 μv. in amplitude and 1 to 2 m.s. in duration, may also be found in the region of the end-plate (see Fig. 3-8). Negative in deflection, they sound like a seashell held to ear and disappear with slight movement of the needle. They probably represent the summated activity of nonpropagated potentials and correspond to the miniature end-plate potentials recorded experimentally with microelectrodes.[12]

With the muscle at rest, spontaneous activity detected away from the end-plate zone is usually indication of abnormality. There are four types of spontaneous potentials: fibrillation, positive sharp waves, fasciculation, and several types of "high frequency discharges" (Fig. 3-9).

Under normal circumstances, a functioning nerve brings a muscle fiber under its control so that it is not capable of activity except under direction of the nerve. When the neural control of the muscle fiber is lost, the muscle fiber is then released from this control and returns to its basic pattern of "uninhibited" contraction. Each muscle fiber then contracts at its own rate or rhythm and is recorded by the EMG since it is a change in electrical activity representing the depolarization of a single muscle fiber. These spontaneous diphasic or triphasic waves with an initial positive deflection are referred to as *fibrillation potentials.* Their duration ranges from 1 to 5 m.s., the amplitude from 20 to 300 μv., and the frequency of firing is usually <2/sec. The rhythm may be regular or irregular, and the sound resembles "rain on a tin roof" or "frying eggs." To be significant, these potentials should be recorded at several sites of the muscle outside the end-plate zone. They are definitely spontaneous since they can be recorded subcutaneously and most likely originate from a single muscle fiber. Many mechanisms have been proposed to explain the occurrence of fibrillation potentials. There is good evidence to suggest that, at least following denervation, the motor end-plate region of the muscle fiber develops pacemaker characteristics which serve as their point of origin.[1,3] Since the suppression of the fibrillation potentials with curare is associated with tension production, it would appear that denervated end-plates have been so altered that the combination with curare produces depolarization.[2,35]

For many years, fibrillation potential was considered synonomous with "denervation potential." More recent studies have shown that these potentials are found in conditions in which the lower motor neuron still has anatomical continuity with the muscle fiber, such as myopathies,[3,8] cerebral vascular accidents,[22] and spinal cord lesions.[34] These spontaneous discharges are also observed in botulism, and in this condition, the nerve maintains its normal contact with the muscle fiber but has lost its ability to release acetylcholine at the neuromuscular junction.[9,21] In view of the aforementioned, it is no longer possible to consider the term fibrillation potentials as synonomous with lesions of the anterior horn cell or peripheral nerve. Only when found in a pattern compatible with a peripheral neuropathy or a specific myotome and associated with abnormal motor unit action potentials is it possible to state that they represent denervation.

Positive sharp waves are diphasic potentials appearing at irregular intervals and are characterized by

Fig. 3-9. The classic abnormal potentials observed on EMG fall into three categories: spontaneous at rest, spontaneous high frequency discharges at rest, and induced high frequency discharges. (*A*) Fibrillation potential. The initial deflection of the fibrillation potential is positive, and the rate of firing of spontaneous fibrillation potentials is less than 3 per second. (*B*) Positive sharp wave potentials. The initial positive deflection is followed by a relatively prolonged low amplitude negative deflection. (*C*) Fasciculation potentials are spontaneous firing of individual motor units. (*D* and *E*) Spontaneous high frequency discharges, at rest. (*D*) In the Schwartz-Jampel syndrome, muscle fiber activity is continuous, even with the patient asleep. Amplitude and duration of these potentials are less than for normal MUAP. (*E*) The neuromyotonias represent acquired abnormalities of the peripheral nerves. (*F* and *G*) Induced high frequency discharges. (*F*) Electrical myotonia is believed to originate from abnormality of the muscle fiber membrane. (*G*) Bizarre high frequency discharges originate from muscle in which there is abnormal irritability.

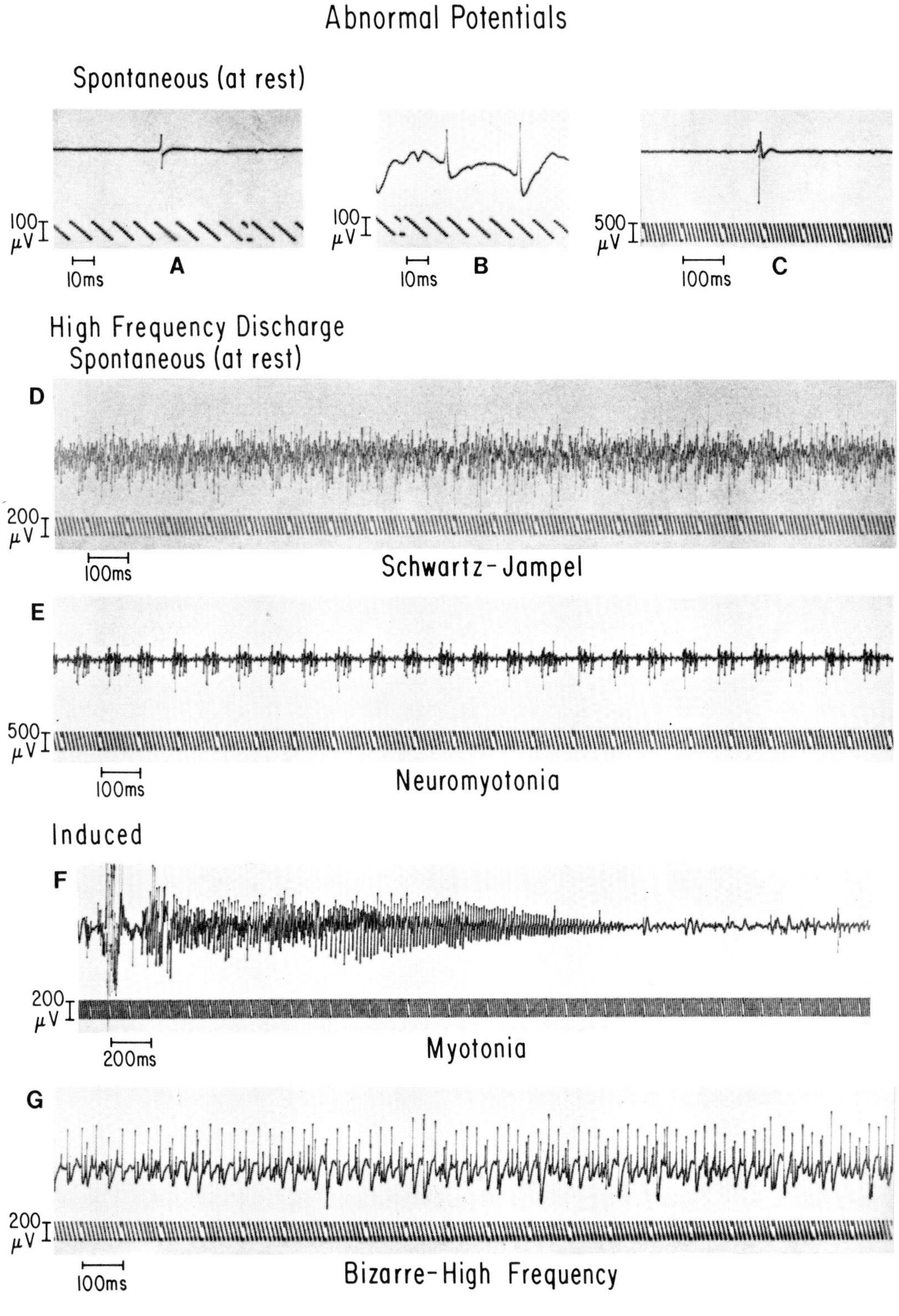
Abnormal Potentials
Spontaneous (at rest)
100 μV
10ms
A
100 μV
10ms
B
500 μV
100ms
C
High Frequency Discharge
Spontaneous (at rest)
D
200 μV
100ms
Schwartz-Jampel
E
500 μV
100ms
Neuromyotonia
Induced
F
200 μV
200ms
Myotonia
G
200 μV
100ms
Bizarre-High Frequency

a sharp initial positive deflection and a long duration, lower amplitude negative phase. The amplitude may range from 50 μv. to 1 mv., the total duration usually exceeds 10 m.s., and the frequency of discharge varies from less than 2/sec. to 100/sec. They are considered to be abnormal only if they persist after the electrode movement stops and are usually found in conjunction with fibrillation potentials. Positive sharp waves are, like fibrillation potentials, considered to originate from single muscle fibers, although the high amplitude in some suggests the synchronized firing of several muscle fibers.

Clinically, *fasciculation* is the spontaneous nonvolitional twitching of a group of muscle fibers and may be visible through the skin. On the EMG, the wave form may be diphasic, triphasic, or polyphasic. The duration and amplitude of this potential resemble single motor unit potentials. Irregularity of rhythm is characteristic and varies considerably. Fasciculation does not always indicate disease since it has also been observed in normal individuals. In active degenerative lesions of the anterior horn cell, however, fasciculation potentials apparently originate from the muscle fibers since they persist for several days after transection of the peripheral nerve in patients with amyotrophic lateral sclerosis. Some investigators believe that they represent synchronized fibrillation potentials occurring within a single motor unit; the fibrillations are synchronized into fasciculations by antidromic impulses from the myoneural junction firing in an axon reflex fashion.

There are several types of so-called *high frequency discharges* occurring in the absence of voluntary muscle contraction (see Fig. 3-9). Some are not really spontaneous, and in others the muscle is not actually at rest but is in a state of continuous contraction. Electrical activity in the first type is characterized by high frequency discharges consisting of trains of potentials of various durations, amplitudes, and wave forms. The discharges are actually not present at rest and, hence, are not spontaneous but evoked by muscle contraction, muscle percussion, and needle movement. The biphasic spikes or positive waves increase rapidly in frequency and amplitude and then rapidly diminish (wax and wane). This type of high frequency discharge is observed in patients with myotonic muscular dystrophy, congenital myotonia, and paramyotonia; it has also been reported in patients and animals receiving anticholesterol drugs as well as in dystrophic chickens and dystrophic mice. Microelectrode studies have shown spontaneous rhythmic depolarizations. The discharges apparently originate from an unstable muscle fiber membrane acting as pacemaker tissue and producing a generator potential capable of depolarizing the muscle fiber membrane in a repetitive manner. Curare reduces but does not abolish the electrical activity indicating that there may also be a neural component.

The second type of high frequency potentials is characterized by intense, highly repetitive discharges that continue for long periods of time (see Fig. 3-9). The electrical activity is present at rest, the potentials do not "wax and wane," and it is observed in patients with the neuromyotonia and Schwartz-Jampel syndromes (see Chap. 4). The electrical activity is abolished by curare but not by general anesthesia or peripheral nerve block. The discharges probably originate from the muscle fiber membrane in the Schwartz-Jampel syndrome and in the peripheral nerve in the syndromes of neuromyotonia.

The third type of high frequency potentials is brief discharge occurring at a fairly constant frequency and is occasionally observed in patients with acute, rapidly progressive disease of the anterior horn cells, peripheral nerves, and muscle fibers or in patients with metabolic disease such as hypothyroid myopathy.

Electrical activity in the fourth type of high frequency potentials has all the characteristics of motor unit action potentials. Indeed, it is found in those diseases of the central nervous system (tetanus and stiff-man syndrome) and peripheral nerve (tetany) in which one of the predominant findings is involuntary cramps, stiffness, or muscle contraction. The classic example of this type of activity is the synchronous high frequency discharges found in idiopathic muscle cramps.

The final step in the EMG examination is the evaluation of the voluntary motor unit action potentials (MUAP) during minimal and maximum muscle contraction (Fig. 3-10). These are evaluated in terms of the parameters of *amplitude, duration, wave form,* and *number of potentials recruited* during contraction.[12,31] Some of the physical and biological determinants affecting the parameters of the MUAP are the type and size of the recording electrodes; distance between the electrode and the active motor unit; number of activated fibers (fiber den-

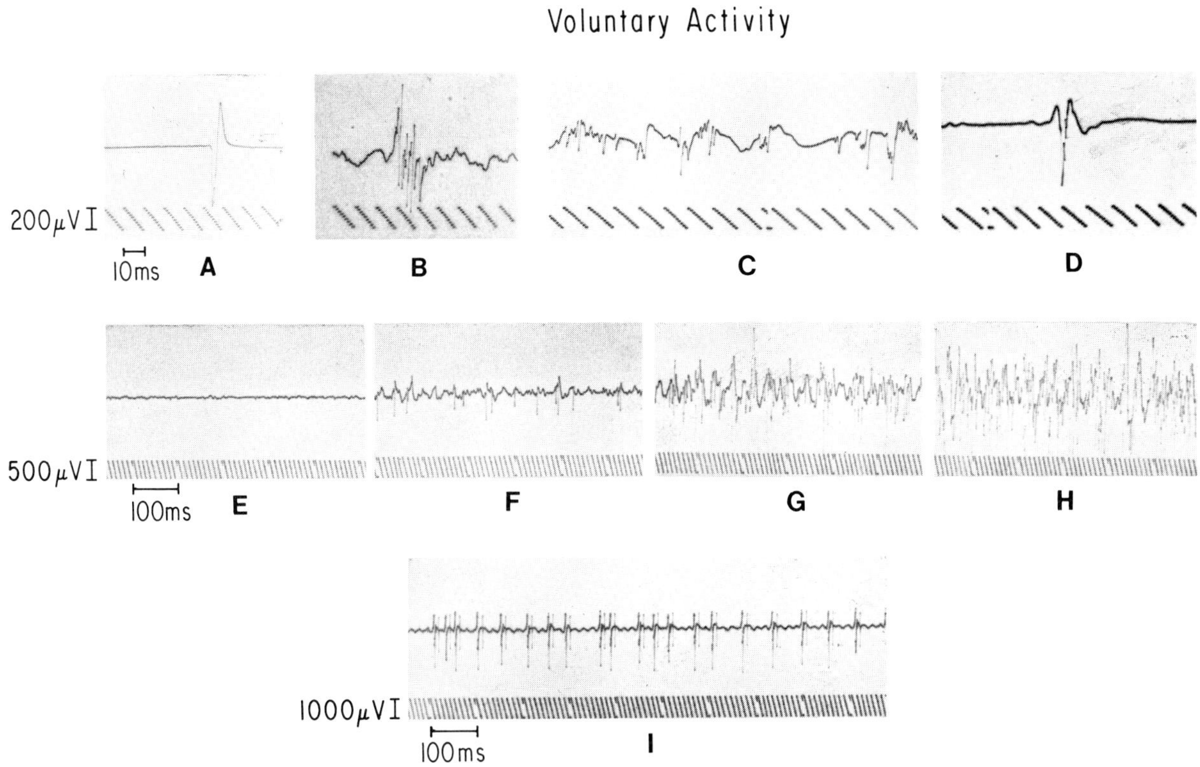

Fig. 3-10. Voluntary activity. (*A*) Normal motor unit action potential (MUAP) during minimal to mild voluntary contraction. (*B*) Polyphasic MUAP with prolonged duration (> 20 msec.). (*C*) Small amplitude, brief duration MUAPs, indicating reduction in size of the motor unit. (*D*) Large amplitude MUAP with prolonged duration, indicating enlargement of the motor unit. Height of time base for (*D*) is 2000 μV., therefore, amplitude of this MUAP is 8000 μV. with duration ~ 20 msec. (*E, F, G,* and *H*) Progression from the normal electrical silence at rest (*E*) to a few potentials of relatively low amplitude at slow firing rates with minimal voluntary contraction. As strength of contraction is increased to moderate (*G*) and maximum (*H*), both amplitude and rate of firing of MUAP increase. (*I*) Reduced numbers of MUAP on attempt at maximum voluntary contraction. In this example only one MUAP is firing.

sity) lying close to the tip of the electrode; differences in conduction velocity of the action potentials over individual muscle fibers and the spatial distribution of motor end-plate for different fibers of the motor unit; size of the muscle (proximal vs. distal); and fiber type (predominantly type I or II). Physiological variables affecting the MUAP include age, temperature of the muscle, strength of the muscle contraction, and fatigue.

With so many complex variables, it is obvious that there is a wide range of normal values for MUAP durations, amplitudes, wave forms, and rates of firing. The normal muscle potentials are usually diphasic or triphasic with a duration of 5 to 15 m.s. and an amplitude of 300 to 5,000 μv. (see Fig. 3-10). The rate of firing varies from 6 to 12/sec. during a weak muscle contraction to 20 to 50/sec. during maximal muscle contraction. Electrical activity as detected in the EMG during contraction is produced by depolarization of the muscle fibers. The nerve impulse at the myoneural junction triggers the action potentials of the muscle fiber at the motor end-plate. The potential sweeps down the muscle fiber in both directions from the end-plate at about 4 meters/sec., exciting the contractile mechanism of the fiber. Polarization exists at rest and is momentarily abolished during muscle contraction. This depolarization produces the action potentials.

The origin of the single MUAP is still not resolved. It was originally thought that single potentials were derived from 10 to 30 muscle fibers, indicating that a motor unit consisted of several subunits of approximately 10 fibers each. More recent investigations, however, cast doubt on the existence of subunits and indicate that the origin of the single MUAP is the motor unit.

One or two single motor units can be observed when a weak voluntary contraction is initially recruited. The rate of discharge of these motor units increases with increased effort, and additional motor units are recruited (partial interference pattern), resulting in a recording of many MUAP firing asynchronously (see Fig. 3-10). The additionally recruited motor units fire at a rate only slightly lower than that of the initially recruited units. As greater tension is produced, more and more motor units are recruited, each firing at a high frequency, thus, interfering with one another so that single potentials can no longer be seen. This is called a complete interference pattern, and the smoothness of the muscle contraction is primarily due to the asynchronous discharge of the motor units (see Fig. 3-10). If each motor unit within a specific muscle is regarded as being capable of producing a unit amount of force, the number of motor units firing in any contraction will be proportional to the strength of that contraction. This is, of course, an oversimplification because motor units vary in size as well as in physiological characteristics. If the muscle fiber population of the individual motor units has been reduced, as in the case of a primary myopathy, the number of motor units that must fire to produce a specific amount of force will be increased. When a partial neuropathy has been present long enough to cause enlargement of the motor unit, an individual motor unit will have increased its total number of muscle fibers and, thus, be capable of producing more force than the original motor unit. In this situation, the number of motor units required to produce a specific amount of force is reduced compared with normal. In the case of upper neuron lesions, the size of the motor unit remains normal; thus, even though the number of motor units that can be fired may be reduced, the numbers firing remain proportionate to the strength of the contraction.

In producing force, normal muscle follows a specific pattern of recruitment (see Fig. 3-10). When the needle electrode is located in an area where only one motor unit is firing, that motor unit will start firing at a frequency of about 6 to 9 per second. As more force is required, the motor unit will increase its rate of firing. When the initially recruited motor unit reaches a firing rate of about 10 to 12/sec., a second motor unit will be recruited to assist in production of the force required. When it is called into action this second motor unit will start to fire at a rate only slightly lower than that of the initially recruited unit rather than at the original slow rate.[30] Warmolts and Engel also suggest there is a difference in the firing rate and in the ability to sustain contraction of the two basic muscle types.[40] Aerobic (type I or beta red) muscle fibers have slow contraction characteristics and are the motor units recruited for low level force requirements and for sustained contraction. Anaerobic (type II or alpha white) motor units are capable of producing brief but unsustained large amounts of force. The range of firing rates for the aerobic motor units is 6 to 20/sec., while the anaerobic motor units may reach firing rates as high as 50/sec., but only in relatively brief unsustained bursts of activity. Based on these observations, there is validity to the concept that maximum voluntary contraction is not being attempted by the patient unless rates of firing are 20/sec. or greater. This observation is of considerable value in attempting to identify uncooperative or malingering patients; however, it must be remembered that appropriate rates of firing will not be achieved if maximum effort by the patient is limited by pain. The patient with hysterical weakness will often give a submaximal contraction with low firing rates and will commonly produce cog-wheel type bursts of activity. In patients with incomplete upper motor neuron lesions, maximum rates of firing of those motor units still under voluntary control should be normal.

The amplitude of the MUAP cannot be satisfactorily evaluated with clinical equipment at submaximal levels of contraction because of the extreme variability of these amplitudes. At present, the only satisfactory clinical estimate of amplitude is to measure the height of the MUAP on attempts at maximum voluntary effort (contraction). By this maneuver, with the monopolar electrode technique, maximum amplitudes should be within the range of 2,000 to 4,000 μv. for the more proximal muscles and should still be considered within normal limits at amplitudes as high as 5,000 μv. for small muscles, such as the intrinsic muscles of the hand. Amplitude recorded will vary with the different types of electrodes that may be used. The EMG tracing on voluntary contraction represents a summation of the electrical activity of the many motor units that are firing within the range (volume of tissue) of the electrode used. This EMG activity is modified because of the interdigitation of muscle fibers from many motor units within the area being sampled by the examining electrode.[40] If one thinks in terms of motor units, it is easier to understand how variations in amplitude can occur in abnormal conditions. In the case of total denervation (loss of all motor neurons), there is complete loss of voluntary control and, thus, no MUAP on attempts at contraction of the muscle. When some of the motor neurons regenerate, the pattern is similar to partial denervation. In partial denervation, the healthy motor neurons that survived will undergo terminal branching to bring some of the muscle fibers that have lost their nerve supply into that motor unit; this results in enlargement and concentration of the motor unit territory.[40] In this situation the examining electrode "sees" a concentration of electrical activity, and when it is close to these enlarged units the amplitudes are increased, usually in the range of 5,000 to 8,000 μv. with monopolar electrodes but occasionally might be higher. Atrophy of the denervated muscle fibers probably facilitates the concentration of the surviving motor units. In the case of upper motor neuron lesions, the muscle fibers retain their peripheral nerves, and, thus, there is no terminal branching. In this situation any motor units which remain under voluntary control or can be fired by reflex activity will have normal characteristics. In the case of a primary muscle disorder (myopathy), individual muscle fibers are dying or dropping out of the motor unit. This will result in reduction of the total number of muscle fibers in these motor units, and the amplitude of the MUAPs seen on voluntary contraction will be reduced. In this situation, maximum amplitudes are below 2,000 μv. and commonly below 1,000 μv.

Duration of the MUAP follows a pattern closely resembling that of the amplitude. With nerve regeneration following total denervation or with terminal branching of surviving axons following partial nerve injury, the motor unit is enlarged by inclusion of the muscle fibers which have lost their nerve supply. The area of the remaining or regenerating motor units is also concentrated as a result of atrophy of the intervening muscle fibers which have lost their nerve supply and are no longer functional. The end result is that with partial denervation or reinnervation the durations of the MUAP of the individual motor units may become increased. This outgrowth or branching from the surviving or regenerating axons requires time. As a result, an increase in duration of the MUAP will not be observed in the early months following nerve damage. In upper motor neuron lesions, the muscle fibers retain their axons, and there is no stimulus for terminal branching. In this condition those motor units that remain under voluntary control or can be activated by reflex activity are normal. With a primary muscle disorder, the number of muscle fibers in the motor unit has been reduced, thus the duration of the MUAP from these units is reduced. The limits of normal for duration of the MUAP is 5 to 15 msec.

A normal MUAP is usually biphasic or triphasic. When a MUAP crosses the baseline more than four times, it is referred to as a polyphasic or multiphasic action potential. A normal MUAP can appear polyphasic when the electrode is not in optimum position for recording from that motor unit. When a MUAP is thought to be polyphasic the recording electrode should be readjusted to assure optimum positioning for recording that motor unit before calling the potentials polyphasic. Polyphasic MUAP can occur as a result of neuropathy or a primary disease of muscle. These are most commonly seen as the large polyphasic action potentials observed in patients with lower motor neuron dysfunction, such as anterior horn cell disease or partial nerve injury. In these conditions the MUAP will usually become increased in amplitude and/or duration in addition to the change in shape. The enlargement of the motor unit is a slow process requiring outgrowth of new sprouts from the axon, and this requires time. The large polyphasic MUAP will rarely be seen in the first six months following partial denervation. In upper motor neuron lesions the muscle fibers retain their axons and polyphasic potentials are rare. Polyphasic MUAP are also observed in patients with primary diseases of muscle. These "myopathic" polyphasic MUAP differ from those of neuropathy in that they are usually of low amplitude and brief duration since the total size (number of muscle fibers) of the motor unit has been decreased. As previously described, polyphasic MUAP are usually associated with changes in amplitude and/or duration, and if these are present, it is easy to attach significance to them. Polyphasic potentials are frequently observed in normal patients. These potentials are usually of normal amplitude and duration, and they can only be considered significant when they are found only in the distribution of a specific peripheral nerve or myotome pattern or when they represent a significant proportion (greater than 15%) of the total MUAP observed.[25]

Nerve Conduction

The presence of three types of nerve fibers permits testing of motor nerve conduction, the monosynaptic reflex, and sensory nerve conduction. Physiological functions which, therefore, may be evaluated include: the excitability of the peripheral neuromuscular system; motor and sensory conduction velocity or time; abnormalities and changes of the evoked action potential; the duration and amplitude of the evoked action potential; and the abnormal fatigability of the peripheral neuromuscular system on repetitive stimulation.[12,33]

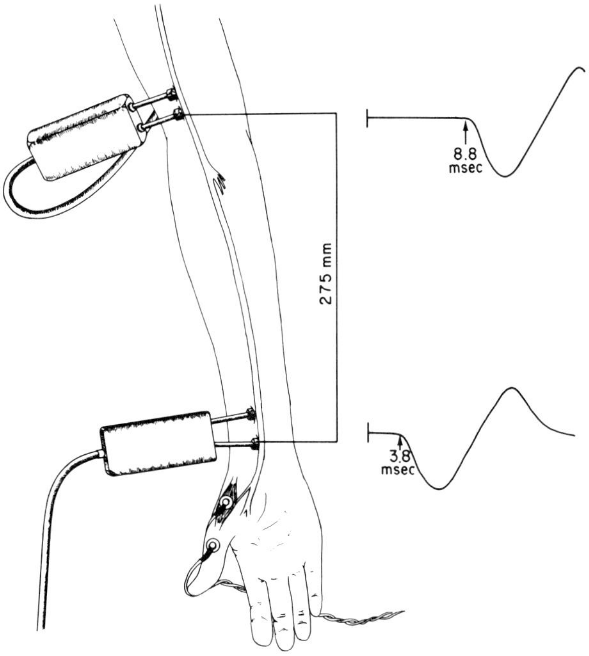

Fig. 3-11. Motor nerve conduction study. In this example the median nerve is stimulated at the wrist and elbow. Pickup is by surface electrode from the thenar muscles, and the time from delivery of stimulus to *onset* of the M wave is illustrated.

$$\text{Velocity (M./sec.)} = \frac{\text{distance (mm.)}}{\Delta \text{ time (ms.)}}$$

$$= \frac{275}{5} = 55 \text{ M./sec.}$$

Motor Nerve Conduction. From a practical standpoint, this procedure is limited to those nerves which are accessible to stimulation. These include the median, ulnar, radial, tibial, peroneal, and facial nerves. While less frequently evaluated, studies have also been done on the sciatic, femoral, recurrent laryngeal, as well as the accessory and phrenic nerves. The time between the delivery of the stimulus and the initial deflection of the evoked muscle action potential is the *conduction or latency time.* The motor nerve is stimulated at two points in order to eliminate the delay caused by end-plate conduction and conduction through the muscle fibers. The distance between these two points is measured, and the time taken by the impulse traveling between these points is the difference between the two times. *Conduction velocity* (meters/sec.) is the distance (mm.) of the segment between the two stimulation points divided by the time difference (m.s.) (Fig. 3-11). The distance between the site of stimulation and the recording electrode divided by the time taken by the impulse to cover the distance is the *latency rate;* it is occasionally used when only one point of stimulation is available. To measure conduction velocity, the oscilloscope must have a calibrated sweep triggered by the stimulation pulse and a variable delay circuit to observe the artifact on the scope. The active pickup electrode is placed on the belly of the muscle near the end-plate cluster, with the indifferent electrode located 2 to 4 cm. distal to the muscle; the ground electrode is placed at a convenient point, relatively remote to the stimulating electrode. The stimulating electrodes are placed as close to the nerve trunk as possible, and the intensity of the stimulus is increased until a maximal response is obtained. A maximal response is obtained when there is no further increase of amplitude or decrease in latency with moderate increases in stimulation intensity. The muscle response is a muscle action potential with an onset corresponding to the take-off of the negative deflection. The onset of the potential reflects the onset of excitation in the innervation zone and the initial deflection on the oscilloscope is

Table 3-1. Normal Motor Nerve Conduction Values: Adults

	Response Evoked From	Velocity (M./sec.)		Distal Latency (msec.)	
		Mean ± 1 S.D.	Lower Limit of Normal	Mean ± 1 S.D.	Upper Limit of Normal
Ulnar	Abductor dig. minimi	56 ± 5	45	2.9 ± 0.4	4
Median	Opponens	57 ± 4	47	3.8 ± 0.5	5
Radial	Extensor indicis	58 ± 7	45	2.4 ± 0.5	4
Peroneal	Extensor dig. brevis	50 ± 7	40	5 ± 1	7
Posterior Tibial	Abductor hallucis	50 ± 5	37	5 ± 1	7
Facial	Orbicularis oris	—	—	3.4 ± 0.8	5

negative. When the electrode is at a distance from the activation site of the end-plate zone, the initial component will be positive.

Normal values for motor nerve conduction latencies and velocities are summarized in Tables 3-1 and 3-2.[10,11,16,18,27,37] Even in adults under carefully controlled laboratory conditions, there is a wide range of normal. Moreover, the various parameters of nerve conduction are, like the EMG, affected by various technical and biological variables. For a detailed review of the former, the reader is referred to other sources.[33] Major biological and physiological variables include: age, temperature, number of motor units activated, the muscle selected for the pickup, and double innervation to a muscle. Despite the marked possibility of errors, the average velocities are usually consistent. In the upper extremities, a range of 45 to 75 M./sec. is considered normal. In general, the conduction velocity is faster in proximal segments of nerves than in distal segments.[37] In the lower extremities, the normal range is 38 to 55 M./sec.

Sensory Nerve Conduction. The methods of measuring sensory conduction are either by direct determination by recording nerve potentials through the skin or by needle electrodes or by indirect determination. Direct determinations may be done by either the orthodromic or antidromic techniques (Fig. 3-12). In the orthodromic method, also called the direct neurographic technique, the measurements are obtained by stimulating the digital nerves in fingers (index finger for the median and little finger for the ulnar) and recording the nerve action potentials at the wrist, elbow, and axilla. Surface electrodes are adequate for recording at the wrist, but recording of potentials at the elbow usually requires the use of needle electrodes and/or an electronic averaging technique. In the antidromic technique, the median and ulnar nerves, for example, are stimulated at the wrist and the responses recorded with finger electrodes. In both techniques, latency is determined by measuring the time to the peak of the major negative deflection.

Orthodromic conduction means impulse propagation along an axon in the normal direction. Hence, this relates to impulses traveling from distal to proximal for sensory fibers. Antidromic conduction denotes nerve impulses propagating in a direction op-

Table 3-2. Normal Motor Nerve Conduction Values: Children

	Velocity (M./sec.)			Mean ± 1 S.D.		
	Birth to 1 week	1 week to 4 months	4 months to 1 year	1 year to 3 years	3 years to 8 years	8 years to 16 years
Ulnar	32 ± 4	42 ± 8	50 ± 7	60 ± 8	65 ± 8	67 ± 6
Median	29 ± 4	34 ± 9	40 ± 5	49 ± 6	58 ± 5	64 ± 6
Peroneal	29 ± 4	37 ± 7	48 ± 8	54 ± 8	57 ± 7	57 ± 7

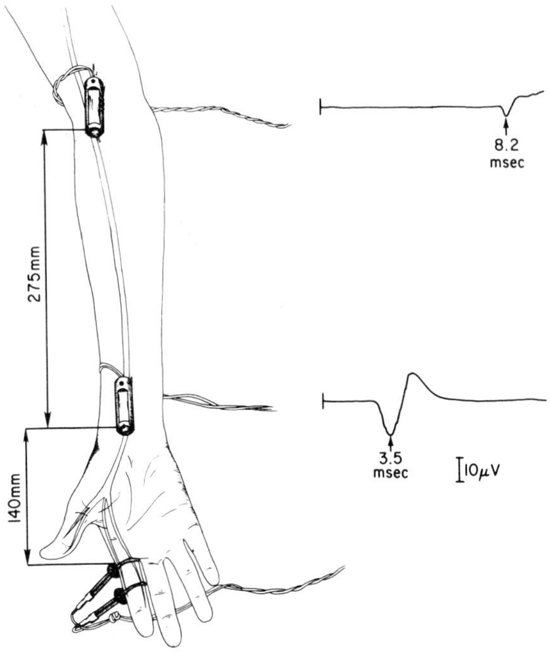

Fig. 3-12. Sensory nerve conduction study of the median nerve. For orthodromic technique, the stimulus is delivered to the digital nerves distal to any motor branches and only sensory fibers are activated. Velocity is calculated in the same manner as for the motor response.

posite to normal or in the case of sensory conduction, proximal to distal. In the antidromic technique, both motor and sensory fibers are stimulated, but only the sensory action potentials are recorded. Usually a higher amplitude response is obtained with the antidromic method. Sensory potentials can also be evoked for the radial, tibial, and sural nerves. Sensory nerve examination is, however, more difficult and less reliable in the lower extremities because of anatomic differences, low amplitude signals, and volume conduction motor responses. Normal values for some sensory nerve examinations are summarized in Table 3-3.[26,28,32,38] Velocities between 45 and 75 M./sec. in the upper extremities and 2 to 4 msec. for distal latency are considered normal.

The indirect determinations are essentially experimental and, hence, will not be discussed in detail. One method which is used to elicit H and F waves (reflex technique) primarily evaluates the sensory fibers which arise from the muscle; it does not evaluate the rapidly conducting skin sensory fibers. Another method is to stimulate proximal and distal nerve points and record the evoked potentials on the contralateral parietal areas of the skull (cerebral or cortical evoked somatosensory techniques).

General Clinical Considerations. Partial injury to a nerve may involve the motor, sensory, or more commonly both nerve fiber types. Depending on the degree of denervation, motor conduction velocity and latency may be normal since those motor fibers which were not damaged would conduct normally. The amplitude of the response is, however, usually decreased and the duration prolonged. If the large diameter fibers have been injured, a slower conduction rate is often found over the damaged segment. Sensory response is usually abolished.

Nerve compression is secondary to a stenosing or inflammatory processes and is most often confined to the nerve segments where they are restricted in an inelastic fibro-osseous space. Therefore, certain anatomical locations predispose nerves to potential entrapment and compression. Examples of this are: compression of the median nerve in the carpal tunnel (Fig. 3-13) or between the two heads of the pronator teres; compression of the ulnar nerve in the cubital tunnel or beneath the pisohamate ligament;

Table 3-3. Normal Sensory Nerve Conduction Values: Adults

		Velocity (M./sec.)		*Distal Latency (msec.)*	
	Type	*Mean ± 1 S.D.*	*Lower Limit of Normal*	*Mean ± 1 S.D.*	*Upper Limit of Normal*
Ulnar	Orthodromic	57 ± 4	45	3 ± 0.2	4
Digits IV & V	Antidromic	55 ± 4	45	3 ± 0.3	4
Median	Orthodromic	58 ± 5	47	3 ± 0.2	4
Digits II & III	Antidromic	57 ± 4	47	3 ± 0.2	4

compression of the radial nerve in the axilla, the spiral groove, or the proximal portion of the forearm; compression of the posterior tibial nerve in the popliteal space or the tarsal tunnel, and compression of the peroneal nerve as it winds superficially over the neck of the fibula. Whenever segmental involvement is suspected, studies should be performed at several points along the involved nerve and the conduction velocity for each segment established (Fig. 3-14). In compression of the peripheral nerves there are various degrees of involvement of the nerve fibers. Neurapraxia is a local interruption of the nerve fiber conductivity; stimulation below the block produces a normal motor reaction, and latencies are also normal. Axonal stenosis is a local attenuation in axon caliber; the conduction velocity is reduced over the involved portion but is normal or near normal below it. Axonal cachexia is a reduction of axon caliber over the entire distal segment of the nerve; a decrease in conduction velocity exists over the entire involved portion. Neurotmesis is a complete discontinuity of the nerve, and there would be no response to nerve stimulation. When a nerve is completely cut, the distal portion undergoes wallerian degeneration. By stimulating the distal portion of the nerve, potentials may be evoked from the muscles but for no more than seven days after nerve section. Conduction latencies along the distal segment are essentially normal during this period of time so that the amplitude of the evoked response is a better indication of abnormality as it gradually decreases. During the early stage of regeneration, stimulation at or distal to the nerve lesion will not produce a response. Conduction velocity during the period of nerve regeneration is extremely slow and may not return to normal values until long after recovery of voluntary movement.

It must also be kept in mind, of course, that various generalized systemic diseases often affect the peripheral nerves. Abnormal nerve conduction is often the main finding in an early polyneuropathy due to diphtheria, alcohol, lead, thallium, sulfur, carbon monoxide, triorthocresylphosphate, and idanthoine. Abnormal conductions are also usually found in such neurological diseases as the Guillain-Barré syndrome, Charcot-Marie-Tooth disease, and interstitial neuritis, and in such metabolic diseases as diabetes mellitus, porphyria, uremic states, hypoglycemia, amyloidosis, and myxedema. It should also be remembered when nerve conduction studies indicate a segmental localized lesion that entrapment of peripheral nerves often occurs in generalized disease, such as myxedema, diabetes, and tumors.

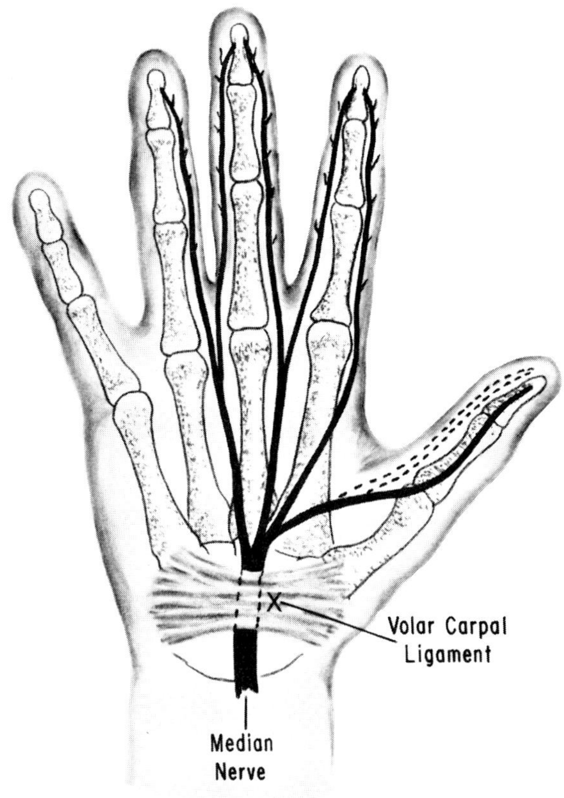

Fig. 3-13. The anatomical location of the median nerve at the wrist makes it vulnerable to entrapment. The most sensitive tests to detect this problem are the nerve conduction studies, with sensory nerve conduction studies detecting the abnormality earlier than the motor nerve conduction studies.

Repetitive nerve stimulation studies are primarily used to determine abnormal fatigability of the neuromuscular unit. Such fatigability is reflected by a progressive decline in the amplitude of the response to repetitive supramaximal stimulation applied to the distal portion of a peripheral nerve (Fig. 3-15). The amplitude of the negative spike of the action potential is evaluated in terms of frequency, continuous or intermittent mode of shock application, duration of the individual shocks, and the time during which the stimuli are applied; the stimulus intensity is consistent and is at supramaximal inten-

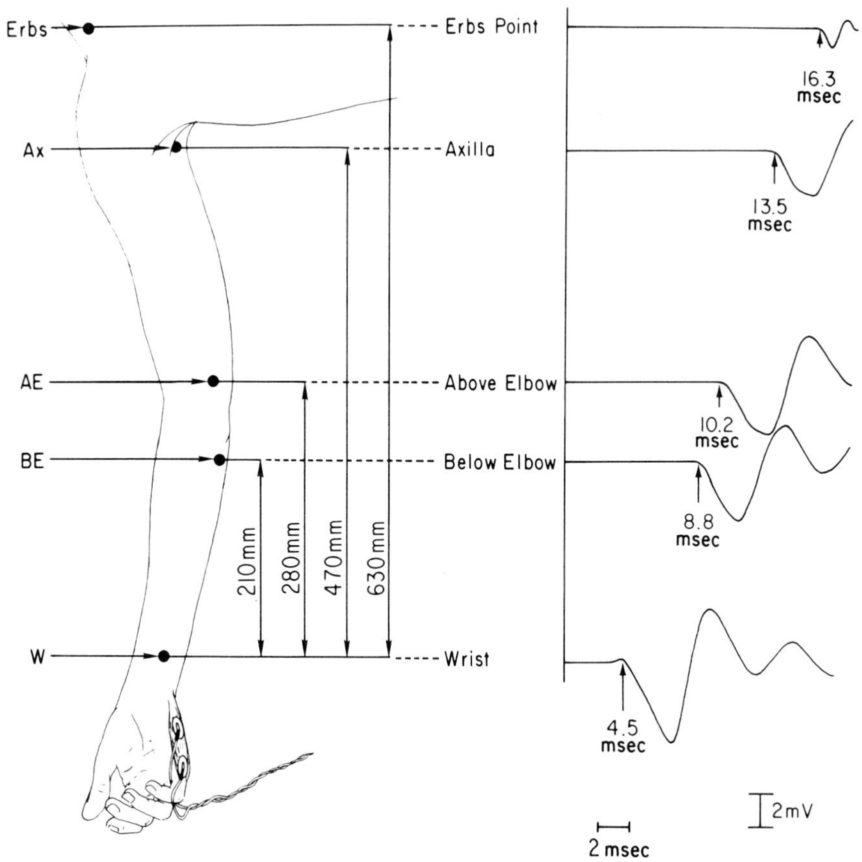

Fig. 3-14. Segmental motor nerve conduction study of the ulnar nerve. The ulnar nerve, because of anatomical reasons, is particularly vulnerable to entrapment at several levels (p. 74). Its anatomy also permits study of this nerve over several segments. This method allows calculation of velocities for seven segments: below elbow to wrist, above elbow to wrist, axilla to wrist, Erb's point to the wrist, across elbow segment (AE—BE), brachial segment (Ax—AE), and segment through thoracic outlet (Erb's—AE). In this case the value of 4.5 msec. for the distal latency is above the upper limits of normal for this nerve (4 msec.).

sity. The amplitude of the normal action potential does not significantly change when the stimulation rate is 1 to 10/sec. and can be maintained at that rate for several minutes. At 10 to 30/sec. the amplitude can be maintained for 0.5 to 1 minute, although there may be a small decrement in amplitude after 1 minute. At a frequency of 50/sec., the decrement may be as much as 50 percent after a 30 second interval in normal individuals.

Two methods have been used in repetitive nerve stimulation studies. The first is the response to pairs of stimuli. The first (conditioning) tetanizing stimulus is separated from the second (test) stimulus by varying rest intervals. In a normal subject the responses to the test stimuli show neither significant posttetanic facilitation nor post-activation exhaustion. In a disease like myasthenia gravis, however, there is transient, brief initial facilitation of neuromuscular transmission producing an increase in amplitude of about 20 percent. This is rapidly followed by a decrement which continues for several minutes and is then followed by a recovery period in which pretest levels are obtained in 10 to 15 minutes. The second method is evaluating the response to 3/sec. supramaximal stimulation before and at 3 sec., 2 min., and 10 min. after a condition tetanus. Muscle action potentials may be superimposed on the record so that a fall in amplitude can be easily seen.

When a decrement in amplitude of the muscular response to repetitive nerve stimulation is observed, there is often a problem of differentiating between myasthenia gravis, which responds to anticholinesterase drugs, and myasthenic syndrome which does not. Therefore, the use of Tensilon has become a routine part of most evaluations of the neuromuscular unit. Some of the diseases that often show abnormalities with repetitive nerve stimulation are myasthenia gravis, the myasthenic syndrome, hyperthyroidism, diabetes, and some types of muscle diseases.

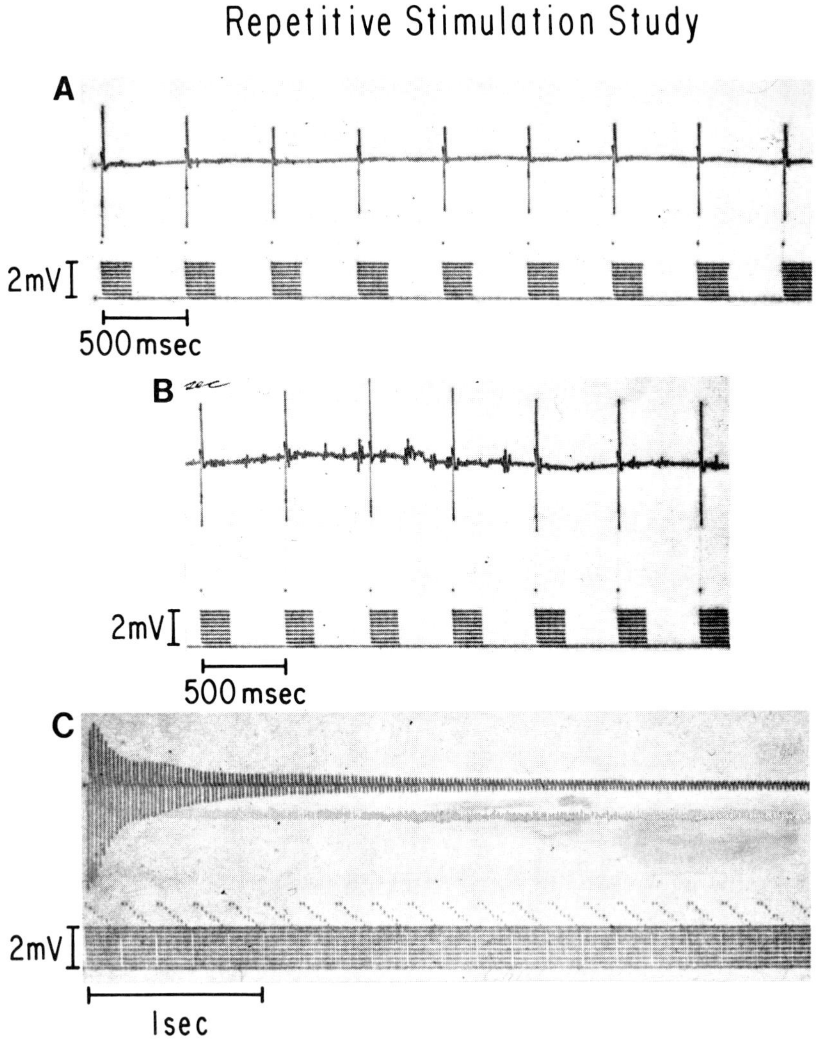

Fig. 3-15. The most common use of the repetitive stimulation study is to assist in identification of patients with myasthenia gravis. (*A*) Response in a patient with myasthenia gravis demonstrating a severe decrement in amplitude, 64 percent of the initial response by the fourth stimulus, at the slow stimulus frequency of two pulses per second. A normal individual would show no evidence of decrement (decrease in amplitude of the response) at this slow stimulus frequency. (*B*) Repeat study on same patient five minutes after the intravenous administration of 10 mg. of edrophonium chloride. The decrementing response has been corrected. (*C*) Another patient with severe myasthenia gravis demonstrating a marked decrementing response at a stimulus frequency of 20 pulses per second.

Other Less Frequently Used and Experimental Procedures

"H" Reflex. This electrically induced equivalent of the monosynaptic stretch reflex is induced by stimulation of a peripheral nerve with a low intensity current. This results in excitation of the afferent nerve fibers arising from the muscle spindle with exclusion of the large efferent motor fibers. Using the "H" reflex, sensory nerve conductions of the fibers arising from the muscle spindle can be measured.

Refractory Period and Conduction Velocity of Muscle Fibers. The electrical activity of single muscle fibers can be evaluated by stimulation through a bipolar electrode inserted into the muscle outside the end-plate zone. The conduction velocity is recorded from between two electrodes separated by a distance of about 5 mm. The refractory period, a measure of the gradual recovery of the surface membrane after the passage of an action potential, is studied by applying paired stimuli to the fiber; an initial conditioning is followed by a test stimulus. The refractory period is the shortest time interval at which the test stimulus evokes an action potential following the conditioning stimulus. The refractory period has been reported to be shorter than normal in patients with muscular dystrophy, increased in denervated muscle, and normal in muscle of patients with severe atrophy secondary to motor neuron disease. The conduction velocity of the muscle fiber action potential is reduced in denervated muscle and unchanged in muscular dystrophy.[4]

Motor Unit Territory and Muscle Fiber Density. Although primarily an experimental procedure, several spike potentials can be recorded simultaneously at different transverse distances by utilizing a multielectrode and, thus, estimating the territory in a given cross-section of a muscle occupied by that motor unit. In muscular dystrophy and polymyositis, the motor unit territory and fiber density are diminished while they are increased in atrophied muscles secondary to involvement of the peripheral nerves and anterior horn cells.[4]

Measurement of Contractile Properties of Muscle. Still an experimental procedure, such *in situ* measurements show great promise for more clearly identifying the pathophysiological characteristics of neuropathies and myopathies. By recording isometric force (myogram) and the accompanying action potentials (electrogram) produced by nerve stimulation, such parameters as twitch time, tension, and relaxation time can be measured.[6] Automatic computer analysis of the parameters of the EMG is also being explored in various laboratories.[24] It is anticipated that these advanced quantitation techniques will make examination of the motor unit more valid and reliable in the future.

Regional Neuromuscular Block with Curare. The technique of regional neuromuscular block permits useful clinical neurophysiological studies to be made without subjecting the patients to the risks of the systemic administration of drugs like curare.[36] While still not available in most clinical electrodiagnostic laboratories, neuromuscular block with curare provides valuable assistance in locating the area of motor unit involvement in disorders characterized by persistent muscular contraction.[23,35] It has been proved to be a safe test for the diagnosis of myasthenia gravis.[7]

LOCALIZATION OF LESIONS BY ELECTRODIAGNOSTIC FINDINGS

At this point, it must be reemphasized that the activity recorded on EMG and the motor nerve conduction studies is the electrical activity of the muscle. Muscle is dependent upon the central nervous system and its peripheral nerve supply for control; however, it is dependent upon its energy (vascular) supply for survival. Any conclusions regarding the cause or location of a lesion are based on the anatomical distribution of the abnormal findings.

Abnormalities of function of muscle result from injury to or disease of:

1. The upper motor neuron—brain or spinal cord injury or disease.
2. Lower motor neuron
   a. The cell body in the anterior columns of the spinal cord—poliomyelitis and the spinal muscular atrophies.
   b. The axon—nerve injury, entrapment neuropathies, and systemic peripheral neuropathies.
3. The neuromuscular junction—myasthenia gravis, myasthenic syndrome, electrolyte abnormalities, botulism, and poisoning with curare or other blocking agents.
4. Muscle is divided into its significant functional compartments:
   a. Excitation impulse conduction system; the sarcolemmal membrane and T tubules—myotonia.
   b. Excitation-contraction coupling mechanism; the sarcoplasmic reticulum—malignant hyperpyrexia and hypothyroid myopathy.
   c. Contractile elements; the sarcomere—the primary muscle diseases.
   d. The aerobic and anaerobic energy supply mechanisms contained within the muscle fiber—the mitochondrial and metabolic myopathies.
5. Vascular supply to the nerve and muscle.
   a. Small vessel disease—vasculitis, such as the collagen vascular disorders.
   b. Large vessel occlusion—obliteration of blood supply to a region with resulting necrosis of the tissues.

Upper Motor Neuron Lesions

1. Cerebrovascular accidents (strokes)
2. Spinal cord injury (paraplegia, quadriplegia)
3. The CNS degenerative disorders

In the past, it was thought that the only EMG abnormality that resulted from upper motor neuron lesions was loss of MUAP in the involved muscles. The typical upper motor neuron lesions (Fig. 3-16)

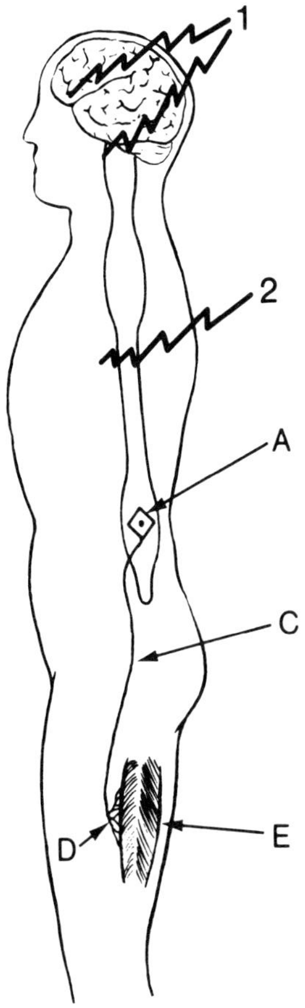

Fig. 3-16. Upper motor neuron lesions result from (1) damage to the brain (trauma or stroke), or (2) from spinal cord injury or disease (paraplegia, quadriplegia). In this situation, integrity of the motor unit is preserved; however, voluntary control of activity is lost.

are cerebrovascular accidents (strokes) and spinal cord injury (paraplegia and quadriplegia). Recent studies have shown that in addition to loss of voluntary control, fibrillation and positive sharp wave potentials are commonly observed in patients with upper neuron lesions.[22,34] On occasions, this will pose some difficulty in deciding whether the abnormal findings on EMG are a result of the primary upper motor neuron lesion or secondary to a superimposed lower motor neuron injury or disease. If the pattern of abnormal findings is diffuse, it should be interpreted as secondary to the upper motor neuron lesion. If the pattern of abnormal findings is localized to the distribution of a single peripheral nerve or myotome, then the findings should be interpreted as representing a segmental or localized lesion.

Lower Motor Neuron Lesions

1. Poliomyeletis
2. Trauma to spinal cord
3. The spinal muscular atrophies
4. Syringomyelia
5. Herniated intervertebral disk

The cell body of the lower motor neuron is located in the anterior columns of the spinal cord, and its axon conducts the impulse originating in the anterior horn cell to the periphery. This complex of the anterior horn cell and its axon is commonly referred to as the final common pathway as it is the last, or final, pathway in transmission of the signal for voluntary contraction to the muscle, which is the final effector of the motor system (Fig. 3-17).

One concept that is basic to the interpretation of EMG findings in lesions of the lower motor neuron is that the spinal nerve, as it exits from the neural foramen, divides into an anterior and a posterior primary division. The posterior primary division

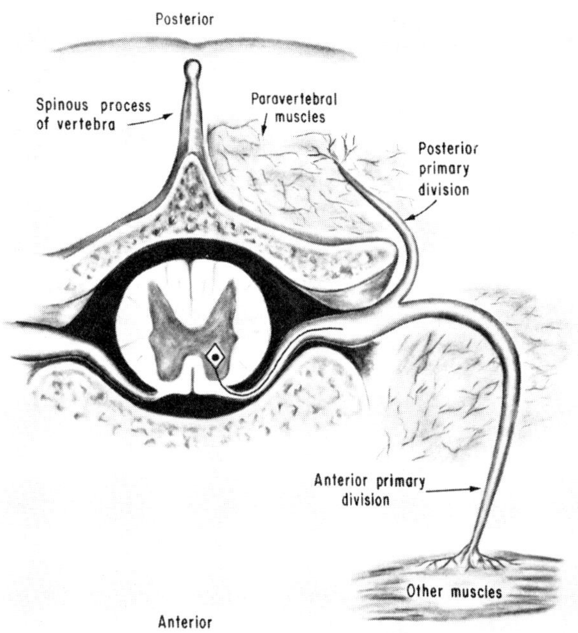

Fig. 3-17. Lower motor neuron lesions. As the ventral root exits from the vertebral (neural) foramen it divides into an anterior and a posterior primary division. If abnormality is observed in muscles innervated by the anterior *and* posterior primary divisions, then the lesion must be at or proximal to the vertebral foramen.

supplies sensation and motor control to the erector muscles of the spine (paravertebral) and to most of the skin overlying this posterior group of muscles. The anterior primary division of the spinal nerve supplies sensation and motor control to the remainder of the body. If abnormal EMG findings are present in muscles from the anterior and posterior primary divisions, the lesion must be at or proximal to the neural foramen. The conditions which would permit these findings are the infectious diseases of the anterior horn cell, such as poliomyelitis, local trauma, myelopathic diseases, syringomyelia, trauma to a nerve from a herniated intervertebral disk, or upper motor neuron lesions. In poliomyelitis, the disease affects the anterior horn cell, producing denervation of the involved motor units. The EMG findings are fibrillation and positive sharp wave potentials plus reduced numbers of voluntary action potentials in the involved muscles. The involved muscles are usually too diffuse and asymmetrical to fit the pattern of a peripheral nerve or a pattern that would be confused with one of the hereditary nerve or muscle disorders. By contrast, the myelopathic diseases, such as syringomyelia or transverse myelitis, would show fibrillation potentials localized to the involved myotomes. If these lesions produced a complete lesion of the spinal cord, there would be loss of voluntary control below the level of the lesion.

The spinal muscular atrophies (Werdnig-Hoffmann disease and Kugelberg-Welander disease) are genetically transmitted disorders in which there is degeneration of the anterior horn cells. The involvement is widespread with clinical and EMG evidence of involvement of all segments of the spinal cord. The EMG findings are fibrillation and positive sharp wave potentials present in almost all muscles examined. The voluntary motor unit action potentials are reduced in number, and the individual action potentials are the large amplitude, long duration, neuropathic potentials. Fasciculation potentials are common in these conditions. Amyotrophic lateral sclerosis is a spinal muscular atrophy of unknown cause. The EMG findings in this condition are similar to the other spinal muscular atrophies. In addition, fasciculation potentials may occasionally occur in trains, particularly trains of doublets which is almost never seen in the other spinal muscular atrophies.

Lesions of the Axons

1. Laceration
2. Blunt trauma
3. Gunshot wounds
4. Hereditary peripheral neuropathies
5. Entrapment neuropathies (including herniated intervertebral disk)

It is this group of lesions for which the EMG can be of greatest assistance in localizing the area of abnormal function. These problems usually result from trauma which can be acute or chronic and mild or severe. If a peripheral nerve has been completely severed (Fig. 3-18) all of the muscles supplied by that nerve will be denervated, and after a brief period of time (10 to 21 days) will show fibrillation potentials. Complete nerve lesions can be diagnosed by a history of specific open trauma and clinical findings of paralysis of all muscles innervated by that nerve distal to the lesion plus anesthesia in the appropriate sensory distribution. In such an obvious case, electrodiagnostic testing is probably not necessary for diagnosis; however, many physicians will request EMG and nerve conduction studies for laboratory confirmation of their clinical findings. These studies can, however, be of considerable value in monitoring return of function. In less severe closed cases, electrodiagnostic testing can be of significant assistance in determining the site of the lesion (root, plexus, or peripheral nerve) and its degree of completeness or severity. In the case of a complete lesion, neurotmesis, there is flaccid paralysis with fibrillation and positive sharp wave potentials on EMG associated with absence of muscle response to stimulation of the nerve. If the lesion is neurapraxia, there is flaccid paralysis, usually without fibrillation or positive sharp wave potentials on the EMG, and the muscle will respond in a nearly normal manner when its nerve is stimulated distal to the area of the block.

It is this process of elimination that allows the electromyographer to suggest the location of a lesion. For this reason, it is necessary that the routine EMG examination must include muscles from each myotome plus other muscles from the same myotome but innervated by different peripheral nerves. A routine EMG examination of an upper extremity would include the following muscles as a minimum study: deltoid, biceps, triceps, extensor carpi radialis, flexor carpi radialis, flexor carpi ulnaris, abductor digiti quinti, and the thenar muscle group. This routine provides at least two muscles with different peripheral nerve supply for each myotome distribution. Tables 3-4 and 3-5 summarize the usual peripheral nerve supply and myotome distribution for the accessible muscles in the upper and lower extremities that can be used to provide localization of a lesion.

Trauma is probably the most common cause of interruption of function of a peripheral nerve; however, the entrapment neuropathies are now being recognized with increasing frequency. There are three typical EMG findings in entrapment neuropathies: reduced numbers of voluntary motor unit action potentials in the muscles distal to the entrapment; the action potentials may be increased in amplitude and/or duration if the condition has been present long enough for these changes to occur; and fibrillation and positive sharp wave potentials will be present in the muscles distal to the lesion if the pressure has been adequate to cause degeneration of some of the axons. The muscles proximal to the level of the entrapment are, of course, normal. The muscles with the most proximal innervation from the spinal nerves are the erector spinae muscles innervated by the posterior primary division of the spinal

Table 3-4. Myotome and Peripheral Nerve Distribution of Muscles Frequently Sampled During EMG Examination of the Upper Extremity

	Myotome	*Peripheral Nerve*
Rhomboid	C4,5	Dorsal scapular
Infraspinatus	C5	Suprascapular
Supraspinatus	C5,6	Suprascapular
Deltoid	C5,6	Axillary
Teres minor	C5,6	Axillary
Biceps	C5,6	Musculocutaneous
Brachioradialis	C5,6	Radial
Supinator	C5,6	Radial
Triceps	C6,7,8	Radial
Extensor carpi radialis	C6,7,8	Radial
Flexor carpi radialis	C7,8	Median
Extensor digitorum communis	C7,8	Radial
Flexor digitorum superficialis	C7,8,-T1	Median
Flexor digitorum profundus	C7,8,-T1	Median and ulnar
Flexor carpi ulnaris	C8,-T1	Ulnar
Thenar muscles	C8,-T1	Median
Dorsal interossei	C8,-T1	Ulnar
Hypothenar muscles	C8,-T1	Ulnar

Table 3-5. Myotome and Peripheral Nerve Distribution of Muscles Frequently Sampled During EMG Examination of the Lower Extremity

	Myotome	*Peripheral Nerve*
Quadriceps	L2,3,4	Femoral
Adductor group	L2,3,4	Obturator
Gluteus medius	L4,5,-S1	Superior gluteal
Hamstrings	L4,5,-S1	Sciatic
Tibialis anterior	L4,5	Peroneal
Peroneus longus	L5,-S1	Peroneal
Extensor digitorum brevis	L5,-S1	Peroneal
Gastrocnemius	L5,-S1,2	Sciatic
Gluteus maximus	L5,-S1,2	Inferior gluteal

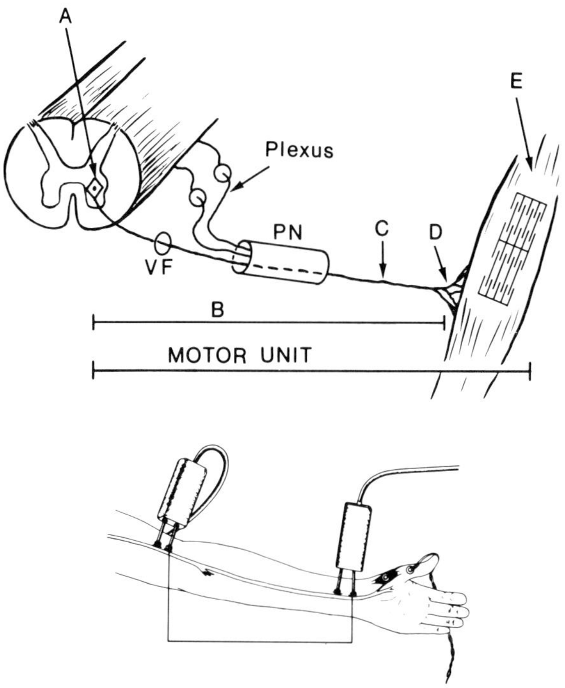

Fig. 3-18. Lesions of axons. For problems occurring at a myotome or proximal plexus level, the EMG provides the most reliable information. The EMG permits identification of abnormal function in the distribution of a specific myotome or peripheral nerve. If the peripheral nerve is involved, nerve conduction studies can usually localize the involved region.

nerve. Abnormal findings would be present in these muscles if the pressure on the nerve is from a herniated intervertebral disk.

The clinical condition for which EMG is requested most commonly is the "disk syndrome." This condition is an entrapment neuropathy as the nerve root is trapped or compressed by the herniated intervertebral disk prior to its exit through the neural foramen. This represents a truly segmental lesion with the abnormal findings localized to a specific myotome. As an example, if the lesion involved the C7 nerve root, the routine EMG study for the upper extremity would reveal fibrillation and positive sharp wave potentials in the triceps, extensor carpi radialis, and the flexor carpi radialis. Two of these muscles are innervated by the radial nerve; however, one is innervated by the median nerve. Since the other muscles innervated by the median nerve are normal, the lesion must be of the C7 nerve root or the middle trunk of the brachial plexus. In order to localize this lesion more specifically, it would be necessary to examine the erector spinae muscles. If there is evidence of abnormality in these muscles (see Fig. 3-17) on the involved side but not the asymptomatic side, then the lesion must be at or proximal to the neural foramen. The most common clinical condition for these findings would, of course, be entrapment of the C7 nerve root by the herniated disk. If the involvement was of the L5 nerve root, abnormal findings would be present in the gluteus medius, tibialis anterior, peroneus longus, and the erector spinae muscles for that segment. With all other muscles on the involved side and all muscles on the contralateral side normal, the conclusion would be entrapment of the L5 nerve root and this is most common just prior to the exit of the nerve root from the neural foramen.

Study of the other muscles listed in Table 4 is of value when it is necessary to separate an involvement in the brachial plexus from involvement of peripheral nerves or spinal nerve roots. For example, if the lesion was of the upper trunk of the brachial plexus, all muscles innervated by the fifth and sixth cervical myotomes, except for the rhomboids and erector spinae muscles, would show abnormal findings. The erector spinae muscles would be spared because the lesion is distal to the division of the spinal nerve into its anterior and posterior primary divisions. The rhomboids would be spared because the dorsal scapular nerve to this muscle is formed at root levels, before the C5 and 6 roots combine to form the upper trunk of the brachial plexus. The anatomy of the brachial plexus is relatively constant, and many muscles are available in the upper extremity so that this process of elimination can be used to fairly well localize the level of a lesion in this plexus. We are not so fortunate in the lower extremity. The distribution is not as specific and distinct so that we are usually only able to indicate that a lesion is proximal or distal in location. For example, if abnormal findings were present in the gluteus medius, medial hamstrings, tibialis anterior, and peroneus longus muscles and normal in the remainder of the muscles examined in the lower extremity, the lesion would have to be at or proximal to the point of origin of the superior gluteal nerve from the sacral plexus. If the erector spinae muscles for these segments were abnormal, it would suggest the lesion was due to nerve root injury or abnormality of the spinal cord for those segments (fifth lumbar myotome). If the posterior muscles were normal, then the lesion would have to be in the plexus.

All peripheral nerves are subject to entrapment, and it is appropriate to mention a few of the more common entrapment neuropathies. This condition is more common in the upper than in the lower extremities. Perhaps the most common entrapment neuropathy is the carpal tunnel syndrome. In this syndrome, the median nerve is damaged by pressure from the deeper structures pushing it against the inelastic volar carpal ligament (see Fig. 3-13). This condition is seen most frequently in patients with systemic disease, such as rheumatoid arthritis or diabetes mellitus. The EMG abnormalities in this condition are limited to the thenar muscles and consist of reduced numbers of motor unit action potentials on voluntary contraction; some of these potentials may have increased amplitude and duration. Fibrillation and positive sharp wave potentials are also usually seen. The more important test for this condition is the nerve conduction study. The ability of the nerve to transmit its signal across the trapped segment is impaired, and as a result, there is slowing for this segment, resulting in prolonged motor and sensory distal latencies. In the carpal tunnel syndrome, the sensory nerve conduction studies are slightly more sensitive than the motor studies and show earlier evidence of abnormality.

The upper limit of normal for a sensory nerve distal latency for the median nerve at the wrist is 4 msec. and for the motor distal latency it is 5 msec. In addition to the prolonged distal latency, the amplitude of the evoked muscle or nerve action potential is usually reduced. During the period of recovery following appropriate conservative or surgical treatment, the amplitude of the evoked response frequently shows evidence of improvement before there is return toward normal of the distal latencies. Thus, the nerve conduction studies can be used as a monitor of recovery after treatment as well as for diagnosis.

The median nerve can also be trapped as it passes between the humeral and ulnar heads of the pronator teres. Repetitive supination and pronation at the forearm can produce hypertrophy of the pronator teres and potential damage to the median nerve. The ulnar nerve, by contrast, has four potential sites of entrapment: at the wrist as it crosses lateral to the pisiform bone (in Guyon's canal); just distal to the elbow, as it passes through the yoke formed by the two heads of the flexor carpi ulnaris; at the elbow, in the ulnar groove; and as the ulnar nerve passes through the intermuscular fascia in the distal portion of the brachial segment. The anatomy of the ulnar nerve allows a segmental evaluation of four major segments (see Fig. 3-14): below elbow to wrist; above elbow to wrist; axilla to wrist; and Erb's point (at the base of the neck, over the lower trunk of the brachial plexus) to the wrist.[17] This method also allows for calculation of the conduction velocities for the intermediate segments across the elbow, axillae to above elbow, and Erb's point to axilla. In the case of entrapment of the ulnar nerve at the wrist, the EMG findings show abnormalities limited to the ulnar intrinsic muscles of the hand. The nerve conduction studies show prolonged motor and sensory distal latencies at the wrist. The conduction velocities for the forearm segment are usually normal but may be slightly slowed if the condition has been present for a significant period of time. In the case of entrapment at the elbow, the findings are usually more specific. The motor nerve for the flexor carpi ulnaris branches off of the main trunk of the ulnar nerve after it exits from the ulnar groove under the medial epicondyle. If the ulnar nerve has been damaged in the ulnar groove, abnormal findings will be present in all muscles innervated by it. If the damage is at the yoke formed by the two heads of the flexor carpi ulnaris, there will be no abnormal EMG findings in the flexor carpi ulnaris since the branch for this muscle originates before the nerve penetrates the muscle. If the entrapment is at the point where the ulnar nerve penetrates the intramuscular fascia in the brachium, all muscles innervated by the ulnar nerve will show abnormal findings. The nerve conduction studies, performed in the segmental manner previously described, would show slowing for the segment through the brachium or across the elbow.

In recent years, segmental examination of the ulnar nerve has been stated to be of value in diagnosing the thoracic outlet syndrome. In this condition, there would be slowing of the conduction velocity for the segment from Erb's point to the axilla. Measurement of motor nerve conduction velocity for this segment is not difficult; however, repeat studies on the same patient, by the same or different examiners, may give conflicting and confusing results. A normal study definitely does not rule out the possibility of a thoracic outlet syndrome, and slowed conduction velocities for this segment serve only to show that there is something wrong in this region and will not determine the underlying cause. If the studies are abnormal, it is also not possible to determine if these findings are a result of a recent or old lesion. In addition, there is considerable disagreement as to what the range of normal values is across this segment. As a result, it is necessary to compare both sides before saying that there is an abnormality.

In the absence of direct trauma, the only usual, but not very common, site for entrapment of the radial nerve is where its deep branch penetrates the two layers of the supinator muscle. Since it is the superficial branch of this nerve that carries sensation to the hand, the findings in this case are motor rather than sensory so clinical findings are usually confusing: pain and weakness in the absence of sensory loss. In this case, the EMG findings are usually more valuable than the nerve conduction studies. The EMG would show abnormal findings in all muscles innervated by the radial nerve distal to its branch to the supinator muscle, e.g., the extensor carpi radialis and supinator muscles would be normal, but there would be abnormal findings in the extensor digitorum communis and all muscles innervated by the radial nerve distal to that muscle. Motor nerve conduction studies of the radial nerve are possible for confirmation of entrapment; however, technical difficulties are common with motor nerve conduction studies of this nerve.

The common entrapment neuropathies in the lower extremity are rare. They include entrapment of the posterior tibial nerve as it passes through the roofed canal behind the medial malleolus, the tarsal tunnel syndrome; the common peroneal nerve in the popliteal space or as it passes around the neck of the fibula; and the sciatic nerve as it exits from the pelvis through, or over the sciatic notch. In the tarsal tunnel syndrome, abnormal findings on EMG would be limited to the intrinsic muscles of the foot supplied by the tibial nerve, with the exception of the extensor digitorum brevis. The nerve conduction studies would demonstrate a prolonged distal latency for the tibial nerve at the ankle and possibly a reduced amplitude of the M wave if the lesion had been present long enough for any change to occur.[19] The nerve conduction velocity for the tibial nerve for the segment through the leg will usually be normal or possibly slowed in chronic cases.

Entrapment of the common peroneal nerve in the popliteal space or at the head of the fibula is commonly referred to as crossed leg palsy. This condition can result from any chronic or repeated mild trauma to the common peroneal nerve. In this condition, the EMG would show abnormal findings in all of the muscles of the anterior and lateral compartments of the leg plus the extensor digitorum brevis. Conduction studies of the peroneal nerve will usually show slowed motor nerve conduction velocity. This nerve can also be studied for the segment through the popliteal space, and this may occasionally delineate abnormality.

Even though the sciatic nerve has its own intrinsic blood supply, it is not exempt from possible entrapment. The sciatic nerve is vulnerable to entrapment at the point where it crosses the sciatic notch as it exits from the pelvis. In this condition, abnormal findings on EMG would be present in the hamstring muscles and all muscles distal to the knee. Motor nerve conduction studies would not be abnormal unless the condition was severe or had been present for a significant period of time, since the available sites for testing are distal to the point of entrapment.

To prove that a nerve has been trapped at a specific point, it is necessary to demonstrate that the velocities for that nerve are normal proximal to the point of entrapment, slowed through the area of entrapment, and normal or only slightly slowed for the segment distal to the point of entrapment. Entrapment neuropathies, exclusive of those due to local trauma, appear to be more common in patients with an underlying systemic disease, such as the collagen vascular diseases or diabetes. Systemic peripheral neuropathies are common to these conditions, and the possible increased susceptibility of the nerves to minor trauma has been discussed by Upton and McComas.[39] For this reason, it is always advisable to perform studies on the contralateral extremity when evidence of entrapment neuropathy is found in a nerve in the absence of a clearcut history of specific trauma.

The systemic peripheral neuropathies can be congenital or acquired. The EMG abnormalities in these conditions are almost always symmetrical and about equal in intensity bilaterally. The findings are usually more severe in the distal muscles, with the proximal muscles becoming involved only late in the disease. The nerve conduction velocities are slowed in these conditions.

Neuromuscular Junction

1. Myasthenia gravis
2. Myasthenic syndrome (facilitating—occasionally seen with pulmonary malignancy)
3. Electrolyte abnormalities
4. Botulism
5. Drugs—curare, succinylcholine, anticholinesterase compounds

The next structure along the motor unit is the skeletal neuromuscular junction (see Fig. 3-4). The diseases which occur at the neuromuscular junction are myasthenia gravis and the myasthenic syndrome. The EMG findings are usually normal in myasthenia gravis; however, there may be evidence of an abnormal fatigue pattern as the patient attempts to sustain a voluntary contraction (Fig. 3-19). Patients with the myasthenic syndrome may occasionally show an incomplete interference pattern at the start of a voluntary contraction, and as the contraction is sustained, the interference pattern will become normal. The nerve conduction velocities are normal in both conditions. The M wave amplitude is normal in myasthenia gravis but is definitely reduced in myasthenic syndrome. The repetitive nerve stimulation studies are helpful in differentiating these condi-

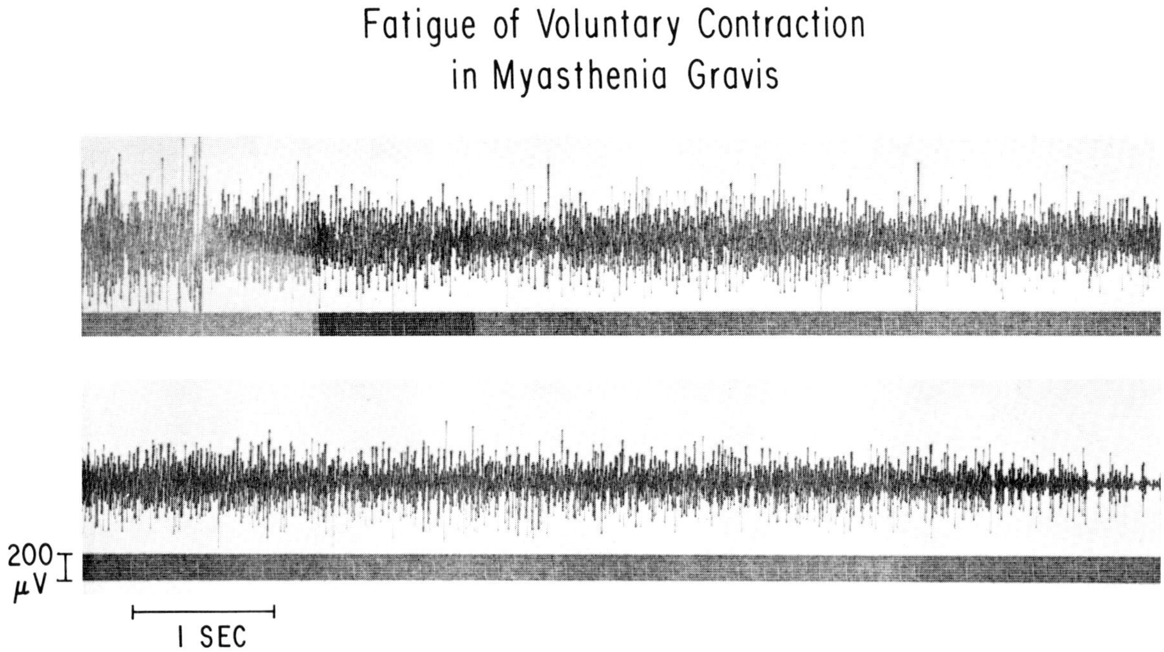

Fig. 3-19. Evidence of abnormal fatigability in a patient with myasthenia gravis. The lower tracing is a continuation of the upper tracing, demonstrating the abnormal, progressive decline in amplitude of the voluntary potentials with sustained contraction, total duration 16 seconds.

tions. In myasthenia gravis, the amplitude of the response will decrease (decrement) slightly, then recover at the slow frequency of 2 stimuli per second. At higher frequencies, 20 to 50 stimuli per second, the amplitude of the response will start to decline (decrement) during the first second of stimulation and in some severe cases may decrease to as low as 25 percent of the initial response (see Fig. 3-15). In the myasthenic syndrome, there is usually no change in the amplitude of the response at the slow frequencies, and at the high frequencies the amplitude of the response increases (increments) markedly. In severe cases, it may then start to decrement after a few (1 to 5) seconds and may even cease to respond. Therefore, in myasthenia gravis, the M wave amplitude is normal; at slow stimulus frequencies it will decrement slightly and then recover; and at higher frequencies it will decrement and not recover like an exaggeration of the fatigue pattern of normal muscle. In the myasthenic syndrome, the M wave is small; there is no change at the slow stimulus frequencies; and there is a definite incrementing response at the higher frequencies.

Abnormalities of function of the neuromuscular junction can also occur as a result of electrolyte abnormalities. Calcium ion (Ca^{++}) is necessary in the region of the neuromuscular junction in order for the acetylcholine molecules to be bound into the packets or quanta which facilitates its release. Reduced levels of Ca^{++} inhibit release of acetylcholine, and elevated levels of Ca^{++} accelerate its fusion with the presynaptic membrane and release into the synaptic cleft. Magnesium, on the other hand, has an action that is almost reciprocal to the effect of Ca^{++}.

Proper attention to the care of meat and the handling of canned food stuffs has all but eliminated botulism as a clinical problem. Yet in spite of this, individual cases or local epidemics of botulinum intoxication still occur. The action of the botulinum toxin is to prevent the release of acetylcholine from the nerve terminal. If this block is complete, stimulation of the nerve will produce no response from the muscle. If the block is sustained for an adequate period of time, fibrillation and positive sharp wave potentials will become profuse.[9] Repetitive stimulation studies will demonstrate abnormal fatigability of the neuromuscular junction.

Several drugs have a significant effect on the

neuromuscular junction. One of these, curare, has been used as a provocative test for myasthenia gravis[7] and has also been used for pharmacological dissection of the motor unit in certain neuromuscular problems.[35] The anticholinesterase drugs inhibit the destruction of the acetylcholine after it is released from the nerve terminal. At present, the only diseases attributed to this type of compound are acute problems secondary to exposure to pesticides. EMG is rarely of value in these acute cases. Some patients do, however, develop neuromyotonia or myokymia. Electrodiagnostic testing can be of value in helping to determine if the abnormal electrical discharges originate from the peripheral nerve or the muscle fiber. The clinical anticholinesterase drugs can also be of value in the differential diagnosis between myasthenia gravis and myasthenic syndrome. Electrodiagnostic studies on repetitive stimulation show marked improvement in patients with myasthenia gravis following the administration of Tensilon while patients with the myasthenic syndrome show no effect.

Muscle

1. The muscular dystrophies
2. The inflammatory myopathies
3. The myotonias
4. The congenital myopathies

The EMG findings in the muscle diseases are almost always symmetrical and of about equal intensity bilaterally. The EMG abnormalities are usually low amplitude, brief duration motor unit action potentials. These findings are more marked in the proximal muscles, with the distal muscles becoming involved only late in the disease. Fibrillation and positive sharp wave potentials may be found in patients with the more rapidly progressive Duchenne type muscular dystrophy or polymyositis but are rarely present in the other dystrophies. The nerve conduction studies in these patients reveal normal motor nerve conduction velocities, and the M wave is usually normal until late in the disease when the distal muscles become involved. In myotonic muscular dystrophy, the pattern of involvement is different with the more distal muscles being involved earlier than the proximal muscles. The EMG findings are the low amplitude, brief duration potentials, characteristic of myopathy, with the pattern of involvement greater distally than proximally. In addition to the potentials described, the EMG will have the high frequency myotonic electrical discharges which are characteristic of this disease. The nerve conduction velocities are normal, but since the distal muscles are involved early the M wave will be reduced. In myotonia congenita the only abnormality is the electrical evidence of myotonia on EMG; the results of all other tests will be normal. Since electrical myotonia originates from the muscle fiber membrane, these discharges are not abolished by the administration of curare.

Vascular

1. Acute arterial occlusion
2. Small vessel disease; arteriosclerosis; collagen vascular diseases

As stated earlier, muscle is dependent on its peripheral and central nervous supply for control, but it is dependent upon its vascular (energy) supply for survival. Total interruption of the vascular supply to a region will result in necrosis of the nerves and muscles in this region. A clinical example of this would be the anterior tibial compartment syndrome. In the early period there would be loss of voluntary control, and movement of the needle electrode reveals normal or slightly reduced insertional activity. When the condition has been present for a longer period of time even this insertional activity will disappear. After this point, it is probable that decompressive procedures will not prevent necrosis of the nerves and muscles.

The most common causes of small vessel disease are arteriosclerosis and the collagen vascular diseases. Hathaway and Engel[13] demonstrated that microembolization will produce histological changes in muscle that are comparable to those seen in myopathic diseases. This is acute obstruction of small vessels; and the clinical conditions are chronic and usually slowly progressive. The collagen vascular diseases may have periods of acute flare-up, and during these periods, they are relatively rapidly progressive. In this case the EMG findings would be myopathic in nature, resembling polymyositis. The nerve conduction studies would show normal or slightly slowed velocities, and the M wave would probably be reduced slightly. In the slowly progressive arteriosclerosis, EMG studies are rarely performed. The changes would be very slow and would represent loss of individual muscle fibers from the motor units as well as loss of small nerve fibers. The EMG findings would be mixed myopathic and neuropathic, with some large amplitude and some small amplitude, brief duration motor units; fibrillation potentials would be a rare finding.

Another form of vascular insult that is being seen with increasing frequency occurs as a result of accidental intraarterial injection of drugs. This causes an acute chemical vasculitis with rapid loss of random muscle fibers and small nerve fibers. The EMG findings are reduced numbers of motor unit action potentials and those potentials which are present are usually low amplitude and of brief duration. The reduced numbers suggest neuropathic changes, while the low amplitude, brief duration potentials suggest myopathic changes. Fibrillation potentials are present early in this condition, and disappearance of these potentials on serial studies probably indicates destruction and replacement of the muscle fibers with fibrous tissue rather than reinnervation. The nerve conduction velocities are usually normal or slightly slowed. The M wave amplitude can be used to monitor the progress of the disease process. If the M wave remains normal on serial studies, it indicates that the muscle and nerves have been only slightly damaged and should recover. If the M wave is small or diminishes in size with serial studies, it indicates that the ischemic process is still active and destroying nerve and muscle.

In review, localization of lesions of nerve or muscle by EMG findings depends on the accurate determination of the pattern or distribution of the abnormal findings. The abnormal findings may then be categorized as neuropathic (large amplitude, long duration potentials in reduced numbers) or myopathic (small amplitude, brief duration potentials increased in numbers proportionate to strength of contraction). The physiological explanation for the small amplitude, brief duration potential is loss of muscle fibers resulting in reduction in size of the individual motor units. The large amplitude neuropathic potential results from an increase in the size of the surviving motor units. This occurs as a result of terminal branching of the surviving axons to bring some of the denervated muscle fibers under their control. Fibrillation potentials are always abnormal but do not by themselves provide etiological insight as to whether or not the cause is neuropathic or myopathic. Further conclusions are based on the anatomical distribution of the abnormal findings to decide whether the lesion is of the peripheral nerve, the plexus, or represents a myotome distribution.

DISORDERS WITH SYSTEMIC SYMMETRICAL CLINICAL FINDINGS

Unlike segmental localized lesions of the roots, plexus, and nerves, many neuromuscular disorders affect one or more of the divisions of the motor unit in a systemic symmetrical manner. Whether neuronal diseases, polyneuropathies, or primary muscle diseases, these disorders, many of which are poorly understood, can be best classified according to their predominant clinical findings as follows: weakness and/or hypotonia; cramping, myotonia, and stiffness; flaccid paralysis; and fatigue.

A pedagogic description of the electrophysiological characteristics of neuromuscular diseases and the unequivocal differentiation of primary neuropathic from myopathic disease is often not possible. Myopathic histological findings have been well documented in diseases of the anterior horn cells and peripheral nerves, while neuropathic biopsy findings have been reported in diseases long considered to be myopathies. The congenital and early onset disorders of skeletal muscle clearly document the growing realization that the classic concept of a clearcut separation of myopathies and neuropathies is no longer valid and that both nerve and muscle are apparently involved in many of these diseases.[8] Whatever the basic mechanism may be, neurotrophic regulation of muscle or simultaneous direct involvement of both nerve and muscle, the evidence now indicates that these disorders can no longer be placed into the simple categories of myopathies and neuropathies. The interpretation of the electrodiagnostic tests, therefore, must be carried out with the realization that the electrophysiological observations play a counterpoint role to the lack of absolute specificity of histology and pathophysiology.[12] Regardless, certain electrodiagnostic patterns have been observed for many of these disorders, and keeping these patterns in mind, the clinician can still effectively utilize the electrodiagnostic data.

Weakness and/or Hypotonia as the Predominant Clinical Finding

Depending on several factors, such as the length of time of the disease, the location of the muscle examined, degree of progression, and degree of inflammation, most disorders identified clinically as primarily involving the muscle fibers will usually have EMG motor unit action potentials which are reduced in amplitude and duration but which have a normal pattern of recruitment with an increased incidence of polyphasic potentials. Both motor and sensory nerve conduction velocities are usually normal.

While often variable, the findings in diseases which are predominantly neuropathic can usually be related to the presence of axonal failure, primary damage to myelin, a combination of both lesions, or anterior horn cell disease.[12] In general, demyelination results in a defect in conduction, while axonal and anterior horn cell damage produce changes in the action potentials and denervation findings. In peripheral neuropathy and anterior horn cell disease, the duration of the motor unit action potential is usually increased while the amplitude is normal or increased. In both peripheral neuropathy and anterior horn cell disease, there is a reduced interference pattern. Nerve conduction velocity is usually reduced in peripheral neuropathy and normal in anterior horn cell disease. In lesions of the muscle fiber, peripheral nerve, and anterior horn cell, an increased incidence of polyphasic potentials will usually be found. Sharp waves, fasciculation potentials, and fibrillation may also be seen in lesions of all three of the divisions of motor unit. In general, however, fasciculation potentials are more commonly found in anterior horn cell lesions, and the incidence of fibrillation potentials is much less in most diseases of the muscle fiber.

EMG Action Potentials Usually Reduced in Amplitude and Duration. (1) The primary disorders of muscle. As mentioned, most myopathies have action potentials which are reduced in amplitude and duration depending upon the type and degree of muscle fiber involvement. The duration and amplitude of the action potentials are reduced to a greater degree in Duchenne dystrophy, acute polymyositis, centronuclear myopathy, and Pompe's disease than in the slowly progressive or static facioscapulohumeral and limb-girdle dystrophies, central core disease, and nemaline and mitochrondrial myopathy. In Pompe's disease (Alpha, 1, 4-glucosidase deficiency), centronuclear myopathy, and acute polymyositis, there are usually also spontaneous high frequency discharges, frequent and marked positive sharp waves, and fibrillation potentials. Duchenne dystrophy is occasionally associated with scattered areas of sharp waves and fibrillation potentials, especially midway in the course of the disease and in the proximal muscles, while this spontaneous activity is rare in the slowly progressive dystrophies, thyroid myopathy, central core disease, and mitochondrial myopathy. Nerve conduction studies are usually within normal limits in these disorders.

EMG Action Potentials Usually Increased in Duration and Amplitude. As mentioned previously, potentials with an increased amplitude as well as an increased duration are usually found in patients with anterior horn cell disease, such as progressive spinal atrophy, amyotrophic lateral sclerosis, infantile spinal muscular atrophy (Werdnig-Hoffmann and Kugelberg-Welander diseases), syringomyelia, and poliomyelitis. Spontaneous sharp waves, fibrillation potentials, and, especially, fasciculation are usually seen. Again, the findings depend upon the type and degree of muscle fiber damage. In infantile spinal muscular atrophy, for example, only about 50 percent of the patients will have spontaneous EMG activity.[8]

EMG Action Potentials Usually Increased in Duration but Normal or Reduced in Amplitude. (1) Peripheral neuropathies; (2) incomplete peripheral nerve injury or nerve regeneration. In general, motor unit action potentials are increased in duration and normal, increased, or even reduced in amplitude in patients with widespread systemic peripheral nerve disease depending on whether there is primary axonal failure or primary myelin degeneration. In demyelination alone, the only abnormality may be a defect in nerve conduction velocity and the amplitude of the evoked response, especially in the sensory fibers. Early or mild axonal failure may show motor unit potential changes at the lower limits of normal and marked EMG spontaneous activity with normal nerve conduction velocities. Late or total axonal degeneration may demonstrate no EMG spontaneous activity, motor unit action potentials reduced in amplitude and number, and normal in duration. Examples of diseases in which demyelination is usually predominant are lead intoxication, mild or moderate diabetic neuropathy, early alcoholic neuropathy, metachromatic leukodystrophy, and Refsum's disease. Those conditions with a predominant effect on the axon include Furadantin, triorthocresyl phosphate, isoniazid, and thalidomide toxicity; acute onset diabetes; porphyria; and chronic alcoholic neuropathy. Neuropathy secondary to neoplasms, uremic polyneuropathy, Guillain-Barré syndrome, peroneal muscular atrophy, Dejerine-Sottas neuropathy, idiopathic polyneuropathy, leprosy, and rheumatoid neuropathy appear to result in both axonal failure and myelin degeneration. Therefore,those diseases in which demyelination neuropathy predominates will usually demonstrate slowed nerve conduction velocities long before the EMG becomes abnormal. Those patients in whom axonal failure predominates will usually have abnormal EMGs and essentially normal nerve conduction velocities, at least in the early stages of the disease. Those with both axonal failure and myelin degeneration will often have both abnormal EMGs and nerve conduction studies. It would also be noted that some diseases, such as diabetes, rheumatoid arthritis, and alcohol abuse, often directly affect the muscle fiber so that the EMG may show reduced duration as well as reduced amplitude action potentials. Entrapment neuropathies also often occur in rheumatoid arthritis, diabetes, and leprosy.

Myotonia, Myokymia, and Cramping as the Predominant Clinical Finding

(1) Myotonic muscular dystrophy; (2) congenital myotonia; (3) paramyotonia; (4) hyperkalemic periodic paralysis; (5) toxic involvement of myoneural junction; (6) metabolic myopathies.

Persistent involuntary muscle contraction, with or without continuous muscle fiber electrical activity (high frequency discharges), could result from abnormalities in any one of the many steps leading to muscle contraction and relaxation.[23] At the one end of the spectrum, persistent contractile responses could occur in the contraction process itself secondary to failure of the sarcoplasmic reticulum to accumulate calcium and/or the abnormal interaction of actin and myosin. This mechanical shortening of the muscle fiber is not, however, accompanied by electrical activity and is contracture rather than a contraction. Examples of this are the phosphorylase, phosphofructokinase, and phosphohexoisomerase deficiencies in which there is electrical silence in the shortened, cramped muscles. Since the structure of the muscle fiber is not significantly disturbed and there is no nerve or anterior horn cell involvement, both the nerve conductions and the EMG are normal during rest or minimal muscle contraction. During strenuous, maintained, maximal contraction, especially ischemic work producing muscular spasm and cramps, the amplitude of the action potentials rapidly drops, resulting in electrical silence in one to two minutes even though the muscle remains tightly contracted. Combined tension-myography and electromyography during ischemic exercise show a progressive decline in the amplitude of the action potentials and the force of the voluntary contraction while the baseline tension of the muscle progressively increases. Supramaximal repetitive nerve stimulation at over 18 per second will often produce a rapid decrement in the evoked potential despite any muscle cramp or contraction; stimulation at rates two to five per second do not produce any change from normal.

High Frequency EMG Discharges Which "Wax and Wane." (1) The myotonias. Clinical and electrical myotonia may be observed in myotonic dystrophy, congenital myotonia, paramyotonia, and hyperkalemic periodic paralysis as well as after the long-term use of drugs which interfere with the synthesis of cholesterol, such as diazacholesterol. Electrical myotonia is induced by needle insertion, percussion, or volitional activity and is characterized by high frequency repetitive discharges which increase rapidly in frequency and amplitude and then rapidly diminish. Nerve conduction studies are usually normal, and repetitive nerve stimulation does not produce a significant prolongation of relaxation, at least in myotonic dystrophy. The myotonia is not abolished by nerve block or blockade with curare. Since there is usually marked structural degeneration of the muscle in myotonic dystrophy, the EMG motor unit action potentials are often reduced in duration and amplitude, and there are occasionally sharp waves and fibrillation potentials. In congenital myotonia, however, action potentials are usually normal, and there are no sharp waves or fibrillation potentials since the only significant structural change in the muscle fibers is usually hypertrophy. In hyperkalemic periodic paralysis with myotonia, abnormal action potentials may be observed late in the course of the disease since a vacuolar myopathy often develops. Although clincial myotonia does not occur in Pompe's disease, high frequency repetitive EMG discharges which may "wax and wane" have been reported.

Continuous High Frequency Repetitive EMG Discharges. (1) Neuromyotonia (toxic); (2) Schwartz-Jampel syndrome (see Chap. 4). These discharges may be seen in irritative lesions of the anterior horn cells, peripheral nerves, or muscle fibers. In most of these lesions, such as in polymyositis and peripheral nerve damage, the discharges are brief and are usually evoked by needle insertion. In the Schwartz-Jampel and neuromyotonia (myokymia, Armadillo syndrome, pseudomyotonia, and quantal squander) syndromes, however, the discharges are intense and continuous for long periods of time. Patients with both syndromes have persistent contraction of the muscle at rest, delayed relaxation of voluntary contraction, and the electrical activity is abolished by the administration of curare but not by anesthesia or peripheral nerve block. In the Schwartz-Jampel syndrome, the discharges probably originate from the muscle component of the neuromuscular junction, the peripheral nerves do not appear to be involved, and there is only minimal disturbance of the muscle fiber structure. Nerve conduction velocities are normal, and the only other EMG abnormality may be a tendency for the voluntary motor unit action potentials to be of small amplitude and brief duration. The pathogenesis of neuromyotonia appears to be overactivity of the motor nerve fibers secondary to demyelination and axonal swelling of the peripheral nerves. Muscle fiber structure is often disturbed to a greater degree than in the Schwartz-Jampel syndrome. Motor nerve conduction velocities are often slowed, and the EMG may reveal voluntary motor unit action potentials of varying size associated with irregular bursts of fibrillation potentials. In addition, unlike the Schwartz-Jampel syndrome in which the muscle is hyperirritable, muscle membrane irritability to direct stimulation is lacking, and transient electrical silence follows the after-discharges precipitated by voluntary contraction.

High Frequency Repetitive EMG Discharges with the Appearance of Voluntary Motor Unit Action Potentials. (1) Tetany; (2) tetanus; (3) stiff-man syndrome; (4) idiopathic muscle cramps. In the stiff-man syndrome, tetanus, and tetany, the continuous EMG electrical activity is usually indistinguishable from voluntary activity. In the stiff-man syndrome and tetanus, the stiffness, electrical activity, and spasm, thought to be due to loss of inhibitory postsynaptic potentials in the spinal cord or hyperactivity of the fusimotor system, are reduced by sleep or general anesthesia and abolished by both nerve block and blockade with curare. In tetany, the probable cause is a low threshold of the motor nerve fibers, and it is not usually associated with cramps or stiffness at rest. The EMG electrical activity often persists during sleep, narcosis, or nerve block but is abolished by blockade with curare. In tetany, the EMG activity consists of regularly repetitive motor-unit discharges in doublets or triplets at about 15 per second. In tetanus and the stiff-man syndrome, there are persistent motor unit discharges at rest which are heightened during spasm. Since there is no significant disturbance of the motor unit, sharp waves and fibrillation potentials are not seen.

In ordinary idiopathic muscle cramps, the EMG activity is one of irregular, high-frequency, high-amplitude profuse burst of motor unit action potentials. Progressive muscle cramping is also a predominant finding in idiopathic paroxysmal myoglobinuria. This disorder is not homogeneous so electromyographic findings will vary considerably since histological findings, regardless of the duration of the disorder, range from no abnormalities to extensive necrosis of the muscle fiber.

Flaccid Paralysis as the Predominant Clinical Finding

(1) Poliomyelitis; (2) systemic peripheral neuropathy (Guillain-Barré syndrome); (3) periodic paralyses.

Poliomyelitis and the Guillain-Barré syndrome often present with weakness varying from paresis to paralysis during the acute stages. In the former, a typical neuronal disorder, nerve motor conduction velocity may be normal in a partial lesion in which some residual motor units are intact; with severe destruction there may be no response at all. Normal sensory nerve action potentials are usually found.

The EMG of partially denervated muscle shows action potentials increased in duration and amplitude with fibrillation potentials occurring 3 to 4 weeks after the onset of the disease. The muscles which are affected reflect the irregular segmental pattern in which poliomyelitis attacks various levels of the spinal cord and the unpredictable degree of destruction of the motor neurons.[12] During the usual course of recovery, long duration polyphasic potentials appear associated with a progressive decrease in fibrillation potentials.

The Guillain-Barré syndrome can be considered as a *polyradiculoneuropathy* since the electrodiagnostic findings depend on the site of involvement of the lower motor neuron.[12] With proximal neuronal lesions, the EMG findings are indistinguishable from poliomyelitis. When the lesion is isolated to the level of the roots and consists of local demyelination without axonal degeneration, conduction velocities may be normal and EMG abnormalities sparse or absent. In most patients, however, there is diffuse demyelination of the peripheral nerve resulting in slowed motor nerve conduction velocities.

Periodic attacks of flaccid paralysis occur in both hyperkalemic and hypokalemic periodic paralysis. In both types, nerve conduction studies are normal between attacks. In hypokalemic paralysis, the action potentials may be reduced in duration between attacks, but there are rarely any fibrillation potentials, sharp waves, or high frequency discharges. During paralysis, there is complete electrical silence, no response to electrical stimulation of the nerve or muscle, and the muscle refractory period, reduced between attacks, shows a slight additional reduction. In hyperkalemic periodic paralysis, positive sharp waves, fibrillation potentials, and myotonic discharges are often seen between attacks. During attacks, the motor unit action potentials are usually reduced in duration, and the muscle refractory period, reduced between attacks, increases.

Diseases with Fatigue as the Predominant Clinical Finding

(1) Functional (hysterical); (2) exercise; (3) myasthenia gravis; (4) myasthenic syndrome.

Fatigue is primarily a subjective complaint and, hence, may be a symptom of either organic disease or functional emotional impairment. During muscle fatigue secondary to exercise, EMG grouping of motor unit potentials has been observed, and frequency analysis has shown a total increase in the EMG level, an increase in the amplitude of the low frequency components, and a decrease in the high frequency components.

In weakness secondary to a hysterical conversion reaction, nerve conduction velocities, repetitive nerve stimulation studies, and electromyograms are obviously normal. Occasionally, during attempts at maximal muscle contraction, a periodic "cog-wheel" response will be observed in the EMG action potentials. The two organic conditions in which fatigue is a predominant clinical finding, myasthenia gravis and the myasthenic syndrome, have been described previously.

SUGGESTED READINGS

1. Belmar, J., and Eyzaguirre, C.: Pacemaker site of fibrillation potentials in denervated mammalian muscle. J. Neurophysiol. *29*:425, 1966.
2. Bowman, W. C., and Raper, C.: Spontaneous fibrillary activity of denervated muscle. Nature (Lond.) *201*:160, 1964.
3. Buchthal, F., and Rosenfalck, P.: Spontaneous electrical activity of human muscle. Electroencephalogr. Clin. Neurophysiol. *20*:321, 1966.
4. Buchthal, F.: Electrophysiological differences between myopathy and neuropathy. *In* Milhorat, A. T. (ed.): Exploratory Concepts in Muscular Dystrophy and Related Disorders. pp. 207–216. New York, Excerpta Medica Foundation, International Congress Series No. 147, 1967.
5. Cohen, H. L., and Brumlik, J.: A Manual of Electroneuromyography. New York, Harper and Row, 1968.
6. Desmedt, J. E.: The isometric twitch of human muscle in the normal and dystrophic states. *In* Milhorat, A. T. (ed.): Exploratory Concepts in Muscular Dystrophy and Related Disorders. pp. 224–231. New York, Excerpta Medica Foundation, International Congress Series No. 147, 1967.
7. Foldes, F. F., Klonymus, D. H., Maisel, W., and Osserman, K. E.: A new curare test for the diagnosis of myasthenia gravis. JAMA *203*:649, 1968.
8. Fowler, W. M., Jr., Taylor, R. G., and Munsat, T. L.: Electromyographic characteristics of congenital and early onset motor unit diseases. Arch. Phys. Med. *52*:343, 1971.
9. Fusfeld, R. D.: EMG abnormalities in a case of botulism. Bull. Los Angeles Neurol. Soc. *35*:164, 1970.
10. Gamstorp, I.: Normal conduction velocity of ulnar, median, and peroneal nerves in infancy, childhood and adolescence. Acta Paediatrica (Suppl.) *146*:68, 1963.
11. Gilliatt, R. W.: Nerve conduction in human and experimental neuropathies. Proc. Roy. Soc. Med. *59*:989, 1966.
12. Goodgold, J., and Eberstein, A.: Electrodiagnosis of Neuromuscular Diseases. Baltimore, Williams and Wilkins, 1972.
13. Hathaway, P. W., Engel, W. K. and Zellweger, H.: Experimental myopathy after microarterial embolization. Arch. Neurol. *22*:365, 1970.
14. Hubbard, J. I.: Mechanism of transmitter release. Prog. Biophys. *21*:33, 1970.
15. Hursh, J. B.: Conduction velocity and diameter of nerve fibers. Am. J. Physiol. *127*:131, 1939.

16. Jebsen, R. H.: Motor conduction velocity in proximal and distal segments of the radial nerve. Arch. Phys. Med. *47*:597, 1966.
17. Jebsen, R. H.: Motor conduction velocity in the median and ulnar nerves. Arch. Phys. Med. *48*:185, 1967.
18. Johnson, E. W., and Olsen, K. J.: Clinical value of motor nerve conduction velocity determination. JAMA *172*:2030, 1960.
19. Johnson, E. W., and Ortiz, P. R.: Electrodiagnosis of tarsal tunnel syndrome. Arch. Phys. Med. *47*:776, 1966.
20. Johnson, E. W.: Electrodiagnosis. *In* Krusen, F. H., Kottke, F. J., and Ellwood, P.M., Jr. (eds.): Handbook of Physical Medicine and Rehabilitation. ed. 2. pp. 222–256. Philadelphia, W. B. Saunders, 1971.
21. Josefsson, J. D., and Thesleff, S.: Electromyographic findings in experimental botulinum intoxication. Acta Physiol. Scand. *51*:163, 1961.
22. Kruger, K. C., and Waylonis, G. W.: Hemiplegia: lower motor neuron electromyographic findings. Arch. Phys. Med. *54*:360, 1973.
23. Layzer, R. B., and Rowland, L. P.: Cramps. N. Engl. J. Med. *285*:31, 1971.
24. Lenman, F. A. R.: Integration and analysis of the electromyogram and related techniques. *In* Walton, J. N. (ed.): Disorders of Voluntary Muscle. ed. 2. pp. 843–876. London, J&A Churchill Ltd., 1969.
25. Licht, S. (ed.): Electrodiagnosis and Electromyography. ed. 3. Baltimore, Waverly Press, 1971.
26. Mavor, H., and Libman, I.: Motor nerve conduction velocity measurement as a diagnostic tool. Neurology (Minn.) *12*:733, 1962.
27. McQuillen, M. P., and Gorin, F. J.: Serial ulnar nerve conduction velocity measurements in normal subjects. J. Neurol. Neurosurg. Psychiat. *32*:144, 1969.
28. Melvin, J. L., Harris, D. H., and Johnson, E. W.: Sensory and motor conduction velocities in the ulnar and median nerves. Arch. Phys. Med. *47*:511, 1966.
29. Norris, F. H.: The EMG: A Guide and Atlas for Practical Electromyography. New York, Grune and Stratton, 1963.
30. Petajan, J. H., and Philip, B. A.: Frequency control of motor unit action potentials. Electroencephalogr. Clin. Neurophysiol. *27*:66, 1969.
31. Report of Sub-Committee of the Pavia Committee on Terminology on Electromyography. Bull. Am. Assn. Electromyogr. Electrodiag. *14*:34, 1967.
32. Shahani, B., Goodgold, J., and Spielholz, N. I: Sensory nerve action potentials in the radial nerve. Arch. Phys. Med. *48*:602, 1967.
33. Smorto, M. P., and Basmajian, J. V.: Clinical Electroneurography. An Introduction to Nerve Conduction Tests. Baltimore, Williams and Wilkins, 1972.
34. Taylor, R. G., Kewalramani, L. S., and Fowler, W. M. Jr.: Electromyographic findings in lower extremities of patients with high spinal cord injury. Arch. Phys. Med. *55*:16, 1974.
35. Taylor, R. G., Layzer, R. B., Marta, J. A., and Fowler, W. M. Jr.: Motor unit study by regional intravenous perfusion with curare. Arch. Phys. Med. *55*:152, 1974.
36. Torda, T. A. G., and Klonymus, D. H.: Regional neuromuscular block. Acta Anesth. Scand. *2A*:177, 1966.
37. Trojaborg, W.: Motor nerve conduction velocities in normal subjects with particular reference to the conduction in proximal and distal segments of median and ulnar nerve. Electroencephalogr. Clin. Neurophysiol. *17*:314, 1964.
38. Trojaborg, W., and Sindrup, E. H.: Motor and sensory conduction in different segments of the radial nerve in normal subjects. J. Neurol. Neurosurg. Psychiat. *32*:354, 1969.
39. Upton, A. R. M., and McComas, A. J.: The double crush in nerve-entrapment syndromes, Lancet *7825*:359, 1973.
40. Warmoltz, J. R, and Engel, W. K.: Open-biopsy electromyography. I. Correlation of motor unit behavior with histochemical muscle fiber type in human limb muscle. Arch. Neurol. *27*:512, 1972.

4 Differential Diagnosis of Muscle Diseases

William M. Fowler, Jr., M.D., and Robert G. Taylor, M.D.

The differential diagnosis of muscle disorders is primarily concerned with weakness, atrophy, and cramps. Because muscle is anatomically and physiologically dependent upon the remainder of the motor unit, a differential diagnosis of weakness must also consider the anterior horn cells, the peripheral nerves, and the myoneural junctions.

This chapter is designed to acquaint the reader with a differential diagnosis of disease. Various factors, both normal and pathological, modify muscle function, and clinical and laboratory findings reflect the interaction of disease and the motor unit. Like all other organ systems, muscle can be affected by a multitude of disorders, primary and secondary, many of which are extremely rare. In an attempt to identify the disease immediately, the inexperienced physician can easily get lost among the many diseases. If, on the other hand, clinical and laboratory findings are grouped according to the predominant clinical finding and placed in their appropriate motor unit compartment, the physician will soon learn that only a few disorders exist for each part of the motor unit. Moreover, each disorder usually has a specific pattern as to time of onset, progression, distribution of weakness, and age prevalence. When this information is available, it is then relatively easy to arrive at a diagnosis.

NORMAL STRUCTURE AND FUNCTION OF SKELETAL MUSCLE

The mobility provided by muscles by their action across joints is one of the major distinguishing features between animal and the lower forms of life. In the human, there are approximately 434 skeletal muscles; combined, these account for 40 to 45 percent of the total body weight.[4,5] Muscle is also unique as it can almost instantaneously convert from a basal level to a very high level of energy consumption. The work performed by muscle makes it the major consumer of our daily caloric intake.

The primary function of muscle is to contract and, thus, produce tension and shortening of the muscle length. In order for this to be functionally useful, the muscle must also be able to relax rapidly on command. The amount of shortening and tension a muscle can produce is determined, in part, by its size and anatomical organization at a macroscopic level. Muscles which have myofibers parallel to the long axis of the muscle belly (sartorius and biceps) produce significant lengthening or shortening. Other muscles, however, have an oblique structural arrangement which permits the production of greater amounts of force but at the sacrifice of the distance traveled. These oblique muscles are called penniform and are referred to as unipennate (flexor pollicis longus), bipennate (rectus femoris), multipennate (deltoid), and circumpennate (tibialis anterior).[4,5]

Skeletal muscle cannot function without control from the central and peripheral nervous systems. Groups of muscle fibers are organized into their basic functional unit, the motor unit, by the axon and anterior horn cell that control them. These motor units are regulated at segmental levels as well as from suprasegmental levels. The neurophysiology of the motor unit is reviewed in detail in Chapter 3, as are the functional physiological compartments of the muscle fiber (Table 4-1), the excitation-impulse conduction system of the sarcolemmal membrane, the excitation-contraction coupling mechanism of the sarcoplasmic reticulum, the contractile mechanisms of the sarcomere, and the energy supply systems.[6,7,9]

Individual muscle fibers are grouped together into fascicles, with several fascicles forming an entire muscle. Each muscle has a tendon of origin and insertion and is surrounded by or covered with a fibrous sheath, the epimysium or, as it is sometimes called, the external perimysium. The muscle is subdivided by *septa* of connective tissue which form the perimysium surrounding the fascicles. The individual muscle fibers are encased in a delicate reticulum of connective tissue, the endomysium, or internal perimysium.[4,5]

Morphological changes in the perimysium and individual muscle fibers, as well as vascular and other connective tissue structures, can be observed with conventional light microscopic techniques. Newer histological staining methods now permit a histochemical classification of muscle based on characteristics of the contractile elements and energy supply mechanisms (Table 4-2). Fibers which stain dark with alkaline myosin ATPase represent fast-twitch Type II or alpha fibers. The lighter staining fibers are slow-twitch Type I or beta fibers.[11]

According to the sliding filament theory, the basic contractile unit is the sarcomere, and the contractile elements are the actin and myosin myofilaments. These myofilaments are organized in a parallel fashion with the larger myosin filaments interdigitated between the small actin filaments in a specific geometric arrangement. The actin filaments slide along the surface of the myosin filaments because of cross-bridges originating from myosin. The cross-bridges represent the heavy meromyosin subunits of the myosin molecules and are thought to make and break contact with the thin filaments as a result of conformational changes induced during hydrolysis of adenosine triphosphate (ATP). Regulation of this contractile mechanism is by the excitation-contraction coupling mechanism of the sarcoplasmic reticulum through its ability to control the amount of free calcium ions in the sarcoplasm of the sarcomere.

Table 4-2. Muscle Fiber Types

ATPase Reaction	*Energy Type Based on SDH Reaction*	*Fiber Type*	*Contractile Characteristics*
Low	Oxidative	I Beta red	Slow twitch, fatigue resistant
High	Oxidative	I Alpha red	Fast twitch, fatigue resistant
High	Anaerobic	II Alpha white	Fast twitch, fast fatigue

Table 4-1. Major Subcellular Compartments in Skeletal Muscle

Compartment	*Major Biochemical Contents*	*Function*
Membrane (sarcolemma and basal lamina)	Lipoprotein structure with variable selective permeability for ions	Excitation and impulse conduction
Sarcotubular system (T system and sarcoplasmic reticulum)	Active concentration and release of calcium ions	On-and-off control of the active state
Mitochondria	Enzymes of oxidation and phosphorylation	Steady-state aerobic activity or recovery from oxygen debt
Nuclei, ribosomes, lysosomes, and lipid granules	Acid and neutral proteases, triglycerides, DNA, and RNA	Protein synthesis, growth, and maintenance of muscle
Myofibrils	Contractile and regulatory proteins	Contraction
Sarcoplasm	Enzymes and substrates of carbohydrate metabolism	Glycolysis

When the signal for contraction reaches the sarcomere level, via the transverse tubules, calcium is released into the sarcoplasm of the sarcomere. The calcium ions diffuse through the sarcoplasm and attach to an active site on the troponin molecules on the thin actin myofilaments. The calcium-troponin complex then blocks the inhibitory effect of troponin on the interaction of actin and myosin allowing this reaction to occur, thereby producing shortening of the sarcomere. If no further signal for contraction is received, calcium is actively pumped out of the sarcoplasm by the sarcoplasmic reticulum. This allows the inhibitory effect of troponin to again be exerted and bring about relaxation.[6,9]

At the sarcomere molecular level, the energy requirements for the contractile elements and sarcoplasmic reticulum are supplied by the high energy compound ATP. ATP can be produced by aerobic or anaerobic pathways. The simplest but least efficient pathway is via the anaerobic or glycolytic system which serves as a preparatory phase for the aerobic system. The glycolytic pathway utilizes glucose which has been released from glycogen stores and produces a net of two ATP molecules for each molecule of glucose plus the metabolic by-products lactate and/or pyruvate. The more efficient aerobic or oxidative pathway is via the Krebs citric acid cycle contained in the mitochondria. This system produces a net of 36 molecules of ATP from the two molecules of lactate or pyruvate that were formed from the original glucose molecule. In addition, the mitochondria are able to use lipids and amino acids as fuel for the production of ATP.[6,9]

The metabolic character of muscle fibers is apparently neuron-regulated and subject to alterations with change in innervation. The exact mechanism regulating the enzyme profile of muscle fibers is unknown although it has been proposed that the pattern of efferent activity is responsible for the metabolic differences among fibers of normal muscle. It seems likely that this coding of efferent activity is also responsible for the metabolic conversion and functional redifferentiation in muscle fibers that have been reinnervated by alien neurons. Studies of nerve cross innervation, limb bud transplants, and axoplasmic flow in nerves indicate that the energy metabolism of the muscle fibers is dependent upon and determined by the nerve supply within a single muscle, the metabolism of individual muscle fibers can be differentiated in opposite directions by different types of nerves, the pattern of innervation of muscle fibers during development differs from that which occurs with nerve regeneration, and motor units are probably histochemically homogeneous. The actual neurotrophic mechanism, however, remains unknown.

ADAPTATION OF SKELETAL MUSCLE TO PHYSIOLOGICAL FACTORS

As with all other organ systems, skeletal muscle is affected by normal physiological as well as pathological factors. The former includes the adaptations and responses of muscle to maturation, nutritional requirements, hormonal influences, and exercise. A general knowledge of the effects of these factors on muscle is desirable since many of the pathological responses appear to be either due to deficiencies in these otherwise normal factors or are modified by them.

Maturation

The number of muscle fibers increases throughout fetal life with relatively little change in the diameter. After birth, the growth of the muscle results from an increase in the length and thickness of its fibers, without any further increase in number. The diameter of limb muscle fibers increases steadily throughout childhood while in other muscles, such as the extrinsic eye muscles, there is relatively little change. During early development, growth in the length of the muscle fibers results from an increase in the number of sarcomeres; later it is due to an increase in the length of each sarcomere. The number of fiber nuclei also increases during growth. Postnatal maturation of muscle fibers is concerned with the development of a preprogrammed potential for growth, contraction, and energy generation. Each of these is a multifaceted trait, and optimal expansion depends upon correct environmental interactions with genetically determined potential.[4,5]

The development of aerobic or oxidative metabolic capacity precedes the development of anaerobic capacity so that initially all fibers can be described as being red. The beta fiber population never develops any substantial capacity for anaerobic metabolism and so remains red throughout their life-span. They also remain relatively small in diameter and are supplied with a liberal number of capillaries. The alpha fiber population begins to exhibit an increasing capacity for anaerobic metabolism near birth. This increase is more rapid in some of the alpha fibers than in others and is accompanied by a rapid increase in fiber growth and a dilution of mitochondrial density. The specific activity and the pattern of the mitochondrial enzymes also change and the morphology of the organelles is altered during this transformation of alpha red to alpha white fibers. While the regulatory signals and mechanisms which induce this transformation are still unknown, it appears likely that it occurs in alpha fibers in which functional activity occurs at a level below that required to maintain a high aerobic capacity.

Although the development of specific fiber types occurs at different ages in different species, fetal muscle fibers are initially indistinguishable from each other. This is especially apparent with regard to energy metabolism since all fibers are initially red, with the subsequent development of alpha white from alpha red fibers occurring in most species just before or after birth. However, distinct alpha and beta fiber populations can be observed during the early stages of myogenesis, well before any substantial amount of muscular activity. Therefore, the differentiation of alpha and beta fibers does not appear to be related to the quantity of muscle contraction.

The beta fibers apparently act as primary myotubes and serve as a structural framework upon which myoblast proliferation and fusion continue with the subsequent generations of secondary myotubes. These secondary generations of myotubes are designed to be the alpha fiber population and are progressively formed, released, and displaced outward. Thus, the first alpha fibers formed in fetal muscle are those which commonly reside on the periphery of fiber bundles in mature muscle. The beta fiber population is completed in a relatively short period of time, precedes the formation of the alpha fiber population, and serves some yet undefined role in the organization of muscle fiber bundles. Beta fibers serving as "nuclei" for the development of alpha fibers explains the internal location of beta red fibers in adult fiber bundles.

There is a growing awareness that many of the congenital myopathies probably occur as a result of some biochemical abnormality in fetal fiber type maturation. The fiber abnormalities (rods, central cores, and central nuclei) in some appear to affect red (Type I) fibers selectively while in others the muscle appears to be undifferentiated. Arrest of fiber type maturation at various stages in fetal life could well lead to the development of these disorders.

Hormonal and Nutritional Effects

Although every endocrine gland has, at one time or another, been implicated as possibly causing a myopathy, our knowledge of the direct effect of the various hormones on normal skeletal muscle is scattered and fragmentary. This is due not only to the complex relationship between the various hormones but also because the primary areas of investigation in the past have been directed toward endocrine control of muscle growth and development or the effects of the hormones on general metabolism.

Androgens

The relation of the testes to muscular development and strength in the male has been known for some time. Castrated or hypogonadal males usually have smaller muscles while, conversely, the musculature is often unusually well developed in females receiving androgens. The effects of testosterone and the synthetic anabolic steroids on muscle have been studied primarily in relation to nitrogen and protein metabolism. In both female and male animals, androgens induce nitrogen retention and protein synthesis even in the absence of the pituitary gland, adrenal glands, thyroid, or testes. In the absence of the pancreas, however, androgens will not induce nitrogen retention unless insulin is also given. The nitrogen retention induced by androgen differs from that induced by growth hormone since in the former there is a prompt rebound of nitrogen excretion when the administration of androgen is terminated. In the castrated or eunuchoid animal, therefore, the gain in nitrogen is not consolidated. The amounts of nitrogen retained by castrated animals receiving androgens are far greater than can be accounted for by the growth of the secondary sexual apparatus. The effect is more general but the direct role of the androgens or anabolic steroids on muscle strength or size has still not been clarified fully, especially in the human.

In male animals, skeletal muscle mass decreases following the removal of the testes or hypophysis, is restored by replacement androgen therapy, and can be increased by excesses of testosterone. In untrained male animals, adult or growing, anabolic steroids result in skeletal muscle and fiber hypertrophy with biochemical adaptations similar to those found with some types of exercise training. These changes, however, are not necessarily reflected in increases in strength, in vitro tetanic tension, or performance, and the effect of the steroid is not significantly intensified by the addition of exercise training.

In female animals, anabolic steroids result in the same biochemical and morphological changes, but, in addition, these changes are associated with increases in in vitro tetanic tension, strength, and performance. Changes are intensified by the addition of exercise training. In the young adult human, these steroids apparently only produce increases in strength when used in combination with a very vigorous, high resistive (weight lifting) exercise training program and only in previously trained subjects (weight lifters). Apparently, in young male humans, these drugs only produce increases in strength in situations in which the subjects are persistently in negative nitrogen balance. In prepubertal males and in men over 60, at a time when testosterone levels are relatively low, anabolic steroids alone may result in increases in strength.

There are no known disorders of the motor unit attributable to deficiencies or excesses of testosterone or the anabolic steroids. A general knowledge of the androgens, especially the anabolic steroids, is of importance because of their widespread use among athletes seeking to increase muscle strength. This is a practice that every physician should be aware of and condemn. Not only is there little evidence that the anabolic steroids have a significant effect on increasing muscle strength in young human males, but there is no doubt that these drugs also have serious toxic side-effects. This is especially true at the dosage and duration used by most athletes.

Adrenomedullary Adrenocortical Hormones

Although the adrenomedullary hormones do not have as great an effect on skeletal muscle as on cardiac and smooth muscle, epinephrine can modify the contractile responses of skeletal muscle to direct stimulation under certain conditions. The contractile response to stimulation is prolonged, and epinephrine also increases the ability of fatigued muscle to respond to continued stimulation by increasing the tension. Epinephrine apparently prolongs and maintains the active state of contraction although neuromuscular transmission is also altered. However, the primary site of action of epinephrine in the responses of fatigued or working muscle appears to reside in the muscle fiber itself, probably through facilitation of glycogenolysis, since it inhibits the inactivation of phosphorylase and hastens its reactivation during recovery.[7] Although epinephrine has not been implicated in any of the myopathies and neuropathies, recent evidence suggests that norepinephrine and some of the other catecholamines may be involved in the pathogenesis of Duchenne muscular dystrophy. Histochemical studies, for example, have shown an increased amount of catecholamines at the end-plate level in dystrophic skeletal muscle, and the administration of serotonin to normal animals produces muscular contractile changes and pathological lesions similar to those found in Duchenne dystrophy.

One of the symptoms of both adrenocortical deficiency and hyperfunction is weakness or easy fatigability of the muscles which can readily be prevented by suitable treatment. The mechanisms concerned are not clear and are very complex in view of the relationships of the adrenocortical hormones with insulin, growth hormone, and epinephrine. The defect responsible for the weakness in both deficiency and hyperfunction appears to be due to the inability of the muscle to continue responding to repeated stimulation. During direct and indirect stimulation, the maximal tension is essentially normal but tends to decline rapidly, especially during and after brief periods of repetitive, nontetanic stimulation. This defect which reduces the contractility of muscle fibers, especially white fibers, is probably due to a change at the level of the contractile proteins.[7]

Muscle involvement associated with disorders of the adrenal gland includes an occasional mild myopathy in Cushing's disease, a moderate to severe myopathy in some patients treated with corticosteroids, and an occasional mild myopathy and skin pigmentation after adrenalectomy. Contractures of the lower extremities have also been observed in Addison's disease, and periodic paralysis sometimes occurs with hyperaldosteronism.[1,20]

Thyroid Hormone

Although weakness of skeletal muscles and a mild myopathy are common in thyroid disease, only during the past few years has the nature of the physiological defect been clarified. Skeletal muscle weakness, tremor, and a shortened duration of the deep tendon reflexes are frequently seen in hyperthyroid patients while a prolongation of the reflexes and a slowness of muscle contraction are found in myxedematous patients.

Recent studies in animals and humans have shown that maximum isometric tension at high stimulation rates is normal in hyperthyroid muscle and reduced in hypothyroid muscle. The rate of tension development is increased in hyperthyroid muscle and normal in hypothyroid while the duration of the active state is shortened in hyperthyroid muscle and prolonged in hypothyroid states. The mean rate of isometric relaxation is increased in hyperthyroid and slowed in hypothyroid muscle. In hyperthyroid muscle, fusion frequency is increased at high stimulation rates while tension is reduced at low stimulation rates. Hyperthyroid and myxedematous states result in profound alterations in the intrinsic contractile properties of skeletal muscle. The reduction in duration of the active state in the hyperthyroid muscle may lower tension by preventing complete fusion of the contractile events while in myxedematous muscle, tension is reduced as a consequence of lowered intensity of the active state.

Although actual histopathological findings are nonspecific and mild, many patients with chronic thyrotoxicosis have profound muscular weakness. Weakness, fatigue, and a slowness of muscle contraction also occur in patients with myxedema, but histologically, there are usually no or few pathological findings.[1,20]

Nutrition

Muscle comprises approximately one half of the total body weight. In addition, the complexity of metabolic interactions and structural organization for maintenance and functional activity is greater than for any other organ system. In spite of this, muscle fibers are remarkably resistant to undernutrition and to specific nutritional deficiencies which exert profound effects upon other body tissues and organs.

Chronic undernutrition due to a deficient caloric intake results in a general decrease in the size of muscle fibers, and deficiencies of essential nutrients leading to general debility may likewise result in simple muscular atrophy. However, nutritional deficiencies specifically affecting human skeletal muscle are very unusual. Muscle wasting due to a deficient caloric intake can hardly be regarded as myopathic, but that due to protein deficiency, as in kwashiorkor, is more specific. Vitamin E deficiency affecting human skeletal muscle occurs but apparently only in association with other diseases, such as cystic fibrosis or biliary atresia. Vitamin D deficiency secondary to malabsorption has also been reported in association with the myopathy of osteomalacia. Degeneration of skeletal muscle has long been recognized as a feature of human scurvy but is considered to be secondary to intramuscular hemorrhage, trauma, or cachetic atrophy rather than to any direct action of vitamin C on muscle. The apparent resistance of human skeletal muscle to nutritional deficiencies is especially surprising since many myopathies have been produced in experimental animals. These include vitamin E, selenium, vitamin C, vitamin B_6, choline, potassium, and magnesium deficiencies.[7,20]

Exercise

The responses of human movement which determine physical performance may be divided into two major areas: neuromuscular and cardiovascular-pulmonary. Each area can be further subdivided into several subfactors. In skeletal muscle, the major concern is with two types of exercise: high intensity and high repetitive.[28]

High intensity, low repetitive exercise training refers to the contraction power and endurance of the skeletal muscles and is characterized by maximal or near maximal contractions of a few muscles for relatively brief periods of time, such as in weight lifting. The primary objective is the development of muscular strength. Physiological adaptations occur primarily in skeletal muscle, and the biochemical adaptations are mostly in anaerobic metabolism. High intensity exercise may be either static (isometric) or dynamic (isotonic). During static high intensity exercise, the muscles work against an immovable resistance with little or no angular motion of the lever arm. Dynamic work is characterized by movement of a lever arm around its joint axis, and a weight is moved through a given distance. The major and most often used type of dynamic work is progressive resistive exercise training. There are also several other types of dynamic work which are mostly of academic interest: concentric or positive work, eccentric or negative work, and isokinetic work. During a concentric contraction, there is increased shortening of the muscle and an increase in the number of active muscle fibers. Eccentric work is controlled lengthening of a muscle in which a decrease in the number of active muscle fibers takes place. Isokinetic or accommodating resistance exercise resembles the dynamic contraction since the joint moves through a range of motion. However, the speed of movement is held constant so that there is increased resistance throughout the full range of movement.

High repetitive, low intensity exercise training is characterized by moderate contractions of many muscle groups for relatively long periods of time, such as in running or swimming. The primary objective is the development of endurance. Physiological adaptations occur in the cardiovascular and respiratory systems, and the biochemical adaptations in skeletal muscle are primarily in aerobic metabolism. This type of exercise training is often confused with exercise testing on the bicycle ergometer or treadmill. Exercise testing is a single-bout situation in which neuromuscular training may occur but with little or no metabolic adaptations.

During exercise it is well established that protein is not used as a fuel to any appreciable extent when the caloric supply is adequate. The choice of fuel for the working muscle is limited to carbohydrate or fat. The percentage participation of these two fuels in energy metabolism depends upon the diet and the duration and intensity of the work in relation to the individual's total work capacity. The more inadequate the oxygen supply, the higher the carbohydrate utilization, and the ability to perform heavy prolonged exercise is directly related to the initial glycogen stores of the working muscle. In general, during light or moderate muscular work, the energy is supplied by fat and carbohydrate, mainly glycogen, in about equal amounts. As the work increases, fat contributes in an increasing amount to the energy fuel. During heavy muscular work, the major source of energy fuel switches back to glycogen.

High Intensity Exercise Training

Dynamic exercise training clearly increases muscular strength. All of the various training regimens have been shown to be equally effective although an optimum progressive resistive exercise program would appear to be six repetitions for three sets, three times a week. The basic principles of using heavy weights with few repetitions for muscle strength and light weights with many repetitions for muscle endurance have been reasonably well documented. The slope gradient of the training curve varies with the magnitude of the imposed stress, the frequency of the training sessions, and the duration of the overload effort. The amount of work done per unit time appears to be the critical variable, and mere repetitions of contractions which place little stress on the neuromuscular system have little effect on the functional capacity of skeletal muscle. Dynamic exercise training also increases muscle bulk and appears to have some effect on modifying other areas of motor performance but does not significantly affect cardiovascular or respiratory performance. It effectively develops muscular endurance with a relatively rapid recovery from muscular fatigue, and muscle blood flow is uniformly modified.

At a biochemical level, dynamic exercise training develops increases in both the glycolytic and oxidative enzymes in skeletal muscle as well as in the energy-rich phosphates. Depending on the intensity and duration of the exercise period, one or the other adaptation will predominate although most of the changes are usually in anaerobic metabolism.

Static exercise training also increases muscular strength, but the amount of increase is usually not predictable. In general, the increase in muscle force is related to the number of contractions used, and overloading appears to increase the strength gains. The amount of tension applied to be effective may vary from 50 to 100 percent of the individual's maximum strength for a five second contraction once a day. Static exercise training produces little or no increase in muscle bulk and does not significantly modify muscular endurance, other areas of motor performance, or cardiovascular-respiratory endurance. There is a slow recovery from muscular fatigue following static training, the muscle oxygen debt is quite large with a relatively small oxygen consumption, and in strong contractions the muscular circulation is occluded, thereby interfering with the oxygen supply to the contracting muscles.

At the biochemical level, static exercise training promotes a high turnover of ATP per unit of time. For brief periods, this turnover can be covered by the muscle's creatine phosphate reserve. The major adaptation at the muscle fiber level appears to be an increased content of energy-rich phosphates and of the enzyme necessary for their transformation. The changes, therefore, are primarily in anaerobic metabolism.

A comparison of these two types of high intensity exercise training indicates that: (1) both improve muscular strength although there are usually greater gains with dynamic exercise; (2) muscular endurance is more effectively developed through dynamic exercise, and recovery from muscular fatigue is more rapid; (3) dynamic exercise appears to have a more generalized effect in developing strength as well as modifying other areas of motor performance; (4) with static exercise, muscle oxygen debt is greater, and the muscular circulation to the contracting muscles is occluded; (5) neither type of training significantly modifies cardiovascular or respiratory performance; (6) in both types, muscular strength, once gained, will persist for several months before gradually returning to pretraining levels; (7) the major adaptations at the biochemical level are primarily in muscle fiber anaerobic metabolism and (8) dynamic exercise training increases muscular bulk to a greater degree than static exercise. However, it should be noted that correlations between increases in muscle girth and strength are very low. It has been clearly shown that muscle strength can increase without any significant hypertrophy of muscle fiber. Moreover, actual decreases in muscle tension per muscle or fiber cross-sectional area can occur in exercise-produced hypertrophy.

High Repetitive Exercise Training

Individuals who have adapted to this type of training have an increase in maximal oxygen uptake capacity. When compared with untrained subjects, they also have lower blood lactate levels and a lower respiratory quotient during actual bouts of exercise since they derive a greater percentage of their energy from oxidation of fatty acids. Trained individuals show during exercise testing improved pulmonary ventilation and blood flow with a lower alveolar-arterial oxygen gradient. Training also appears to result in an increase in red blood cell mass and total blood volume. There does not, however, appear to be an increased delivery of blood and oxygen to the working muscles or an increased oxygen utilization. Muscular blood flow increases which occur during exercise testing are essentially the same in trained and untrained subjects although there is a more rapid return to resting levels in trained individuals. Muscular blood flow at rest is the same in trained and untrained subjects, and there is no clear-cut evidence that training produces any increase in the actual number of muscle capillaries. Training may, however, activate capillaries which are usually not used in the nontrained individual. It would appear that the working muscles in trained subjects compensate for the lower blood flow and are more efficient at extracting more oxygen, since muscle trained with high repetitive exercise has a higher myoglobin content, more efficient mitochondrial system, and more functional capillaries per muscle fiber.

High repetitive exercise training does result in an increase in the average size of the muscle fibers although the increase is much less than with high resistive training. Histochemical studies performed after training have clearly indicated an increase in the oxidative potential of both fiber types, with an increase in the glycolytic activity of Type II fibers only. Some studies have even shown a conversion of Type II to Type I fibers. At the biochemical level, there is an increase of the constituents of the mitochondrial respiratory chain as well as increases in the size and number of mitochondria. An increased rate of conversion of long chain fatty acids to CO_2 takes place during bouts of exercise with a greater release of fatty acids from adipose tissue. There is a slower glycogen depletion in trained muscle during exercise testing with an increased capacity to oxidize pyruvate. This type of training develops an increased aerobic capacity since the organ systems associated with oxidative supply are required to adapt.

It must, of course be recognized that the various types of exercise training represent a spectrum in which both aerobic and anaerobic adaptations occur. Depending upon the type of exercise, the intensity, and the duration, one adaptation may predominate but rarely to the complete exclusion of the other. In general, however, the predominant adaptation in high resistive exercise training is an anaerobic metabolism.

REACTION OF SKELETAL MUSCLE TO PATHOLOGICAL FACTORS

Various classifications have been applied to the diseases and syndromes that affect the motor unit.[1,14,22] The simplest, however, and of greatest significance to the clinician are those based upon clinical symptoms and physical findings. Whether anterior horn cell diseases, polyneuropathies, or primary muscle diseases, these disorders, many of which are poorly understood, can be best classified according to the predominant clinical finding:

1. Weakness or hypotonia (Table 4-3).
2. Periodic paralysis (Table 4-4).
3. Fatigue (Table 4-5).
4. Cramping, stiffness, muscle contractions, and myotonia (Table 4-6).

The unequivocal differentiation of diseases considered to be primarily neuropathic (anterior horn cell or peripheral nerve) from those traditionally considered to be myopathic (primary muscle disease) is impossible. So-called myopathic histological

Table 4-4. Disorders with Periodic Paralysis as the Predominant Finding

Primary	*Secondary*
Hypokalemic	Hyperthyroidism
Hypokalemic with myotonia	Renal disease
Hyperkalemic	Hyperaldosteronism
Hyperkalemic with paramyotonia congenita	Pleoconial myopathy
Normokalemic	

Table 4-5. Disorders with Fatigue as the Predominant Finding

Myasthenia gravis	*Myasthenic syndrome*
Transient neonatal	Malignant disease (Eaton-Lambert)
Congenital and juvenile	Symptomatic myasthenia
Associated with thymic tumor	Lupus erythematosus
	Polymyositis
Associated with thyrotoxicosis	Anterior horn cell disease
	Chronic polyneuropathy
	Neurasthenia
	After bilateral adrenalectomy
	Hysteria

Table 4-3. Disorders with Widespread Weakness or Hypotonia as the Predominant Finding

Anterior Horn Cells	*Motor Nerve Roots and Peripheral Nerves*	*Myoneural Junction, Muscles, and Uncertain Origin*
Genetically determined: Infantile spinal muscular atrophy, arthrogryposis due to anterior horn cell disease, familial spinal muscular atrophy, scapuloperoneal spinal muscular atrophy and familial motor neuron disease	Genetically determined: Peroneal muscular atrophy, hypertrophic interstitial neuropathy, neurofibromatosis, Refsum's syndrome, leukodystrophy, amyloidosis, and porphyria	Myasthenia gravis with myopathy
Congenital: Hydromyelia, spinal dysraphism, syringomyelia, and aplasia of spinal cord	Traumatic	Tick paralysis
Traumatic: Physical and toxic	Toxic: Chloroquine, cytotoxic agents, iproniazid, isoniazid, nitrofurantoin, streptomycin, sulphanilamide, heavy metals, phosphorus	Cholinergic paralysis
Infective amyotrophy: Poliomyelitis, encephalitis	Infective and inflammatory: Botulism, diphtheria, leprosy, syphilis, Guillain-Barré syndrome, chronic progressive polyneuropathy, sarcoidosis, and neuropathy with collagen vascular disorders	Genetically determined: Muscular dystrophies, arthrogryposis due to congenital myopathy, "benign congenital hypotonia," central core disease, nemaline myopathy, centronuclear myopathy, mitochondrial myopathies, disordered lipid metabolism, glycogen storage diseases, and generalized myositis ossificans
Amyotrophy of unknown etiology: Progressive muscular atrophy and amyotrophic lateral sclerosis	Metabolic: Nutritional, diabetic, uremic, and alcoholic	Physical
Amyotrophy in malignant disease	Carcinomatous neuropathy	Toxic: Steroid, chloroquine; and colchicine
	Idiopathic polyneuropathy	Infective and inflammatory: Viral, bacterial, fungal, and parasitic, polymyositis, dermatomyositis, myosclerosis, and myositis with other collagen vascular diseases
		Metabolic and endocrine: Thyrotoxicosis and myxedema, alcoholic, nutritional, osteomalacia
		Amyloidosis
		Disuse atrophy

Table 4-6. Disorders with Cramping, Stiffness, Muscle Spasm, and Myotonia as the Predominant Finding

Central Nervous System	*Anterior Horn Cells and Peripheral Nerves*	*Myoneural Junction, Muscle, and Uncertain Origin*
Tetanus Stiff-man syndrome	Tetany Myokymia and neuromyotonia	Muscle contracture: Myophosphorylase, phosphofructokinase, and phosphohexoisomerase deficiencies Myotonia: Myotonic dystrophy, congenital myotonia, paramyotonia and hyperkalemic periodic paralysis, and drug induced myotonia Schwartz-Jampel syndrome Malignant hyperpyrexia Myoglobinuric myopathies Defect in relaxing factor myopathy Some of the mitochondrial disorders

and electromyographic findings have now been well documented in diseases of the anterior horn cells and peripheral nerves, while classic neuropathic biopsy and electromyographic findings have been described in disorders long considered to be primary muscle diseases. There is a growing realization that the classic concept of a clearcut separation of myopathies and neuropathies is no longer valid, that both nerve and muscle are apparently involved in many of these diseases, and that it may not be possible to separate the components of the motor unit. Whatever the basic mechanism may be, neurotrophic regulation of muscle or simultaneous direct involvement of both nerve and muscle, recent studies clearly indicate that many of these disorders can no longer be placed into the simple categories of myopathies and neuropathies. Regardless, most of these diseases or syndromes can be clustered into various clinical symptom-sign combinations, and there are usually specific clinical and laboratory patterns for each of these combinations as well as within groups. Hence, until more is known about the etiology of these diseases, a clinical classification is not only the simplest but probably the most relevant.

Clinical and Laboratory Examination of Skeletal Muscles

Although there are many disorders of the motor unit, there are only a few symptoms and signs: pain or tenderness and weakness being the most frequent with fatigue, wasting, spontaneous movements, palpable lumps, and contractures being of lesser importance.[14] While information from laboratory tests is often valuable, the differential diagnosis of neuromuscular diseases depends primarily on a careful clinical history and physical examination.[13] The history should include a thorough family survey in search of any similar conditions, detailed information about the age of onset, as well as the rate and mode of progression of the weakness. Clinical assessment should stress the distribution of weakness and any associated findings, such as hypertrophy, fasciculations, muscular tenderness, upper motor neuron signs, contractures, myotonia, and nonmuscular symptoms and signs.

Whenever possible, each clinical and laboratory finding should be categorized in terms of its possible neuroanatomical site (Table 4-7). Weakness due to lesions in the upper motor neuron, at least in adults, is rarely confused with weakness resulting from lesions of the lower motor neuron or muscle since the presence of other signs of brain or spinal cord damage are readily recognized. Disorders of the anterior horn cells are usually characterized by fasciculation, hypoactive or absent deep tendon reflexes, and a distal or generalized distribution of weakness and atrophy. Associated sensory findings are commonly present when the peripheral nerves are involved, fasciculations are unusual, and the weakness and atrophy are usually distal. Deep tendon reflexes are, of course, hypoactive or absent. Diseases primarily affecting the muscles, such as muscular dystrophy, endocrine myopathies, and myositis, are also characterized by hypoactive or absent reflexes. Fasciculations are rare, and the weakness and atrophy are usually most severe in the proximal musculature. Other disorders primarily affecting muscles, such as the congenital myopathies, frequently have associated congenital defects, and the weakness and atrophy are often generalized and include the facial muscles. Myasthenia gravis, the only significant disorder associated with dysfunction of the myoneural junction, is usually characterized by early involvement of the extraocular and bulbar musculature.

Table 4-7. Evaluation of Weakness by Anatomical Area

Clinical Findings	*Laboratory Findings*
Corticospinal Pathway Involvement	
Hyperactive stretch reflexes. Increased resistance to passive motion. Abnormal reflexes. Sensory abnormalities. Weakness usually greater than atrophy.	*CPK* levels usually normal with exception of moderate increases in spinal cord injury and severe cerebral hemorrhage. *Nerve conduction normal. EMG* usually normal with exception of occasional sharp waves and fibrillation potentials in acute spinal injury and cerebral vascular accidents. *Biopsy* essentially normal.
Anterior Horn Cell Involvement	
Hypoactive or absent stretch reflexes. Muscle fasciculations often present. Weakness distribution usually generalized and occasionally distal. Degree of atrophy usually in proportion to degree of weakness.	*CPK* levels usually normal but may be slightly elevated in rapidly progressive weakness. *Nerve conduction* usually normal. *EMG* usually abnormal. *Biopsy* usually abnormal.
Peripheral Nerve Involvement	
Hypoactive or absent stretch reflexes. Muscle fasciculations occasionally present. Weakness distribution usually distal and occasionally generalized. Degree of atrophy usually in proportion to degree of weakness. Sensory changes or paresthesia usually present.	*CPK* levels usually normal but may be slightly elevated in rapidly progressive weakness. *Nerve conduction* usually abnormal. *EMG* usually abnormal. *Biopsy* usually abnormal.
Myoneural Junction Involvement	
Normal stretch reflexes. Muscle fasciculation rarely present. Fatigue, rather than weakness following muscle contraction with strength increase after rest. Extraocular musculature often involved first. Usually variable and fluctuating course.	*CPK* levels usually normal. *Nerve conduction* usually normal but *repetitive nerve stimulation* study usually abnormal. *EMG* usually normal. *Biopsy* usually normal.
Muscle Fiber Involvement	
Hypoactive or absent proximal stretch reflexes; distal reflexes often normal. Fasciculations rarely present. Weakness distribution usually proximal. Degree of atrophy usually in proportion to degree of weakness.	*CPK* levels usually elevated. *Nerve conduction* usually normal. *EMG* usually abnormal. *Biopsy* usually abnormal.
Functional Involvement	
Normal stretch reflexes. No fasciculations. No atrophy. Cogwheel responses. Inconsistencies. Slowness of motion. Overflow of activity. Hoover sign.	*CPK* levels normal. *Nerve conduction* normal. *EMG* normal. *Biopsy* normal.

There is rarely any atrophy, and rapid fatigue occurs following prolonged muscle contractions with a return of strength following rest. Because of its variable course, it may be mistaken for a psychogenic disturbance.

Indeed, the words weakness, tiredness, and fatigue are quite vague and nonspecific. They do not necessarily denote a disorder of the neuromuscular system but may relate to a conversion reaction, depression, or malingering. Psychogenic weakness, however, is usually accompanied by specific physical responses and inconsistencies.[29] A ratchet or cogwheel response is often found during muscle testing. In true neuromuscular weakness, the patient exerts maximal effort throughout the test, and the weak muscles give way smoothly. Inconsistencies also become apparent during the examination. For example, during muscle testing in the recumbent position, the patient will be unable to resist a few pounds of force applied to the knee and hip flexors and extensors but is able to carry out deep-knee bends without difficulty. Muscles which are apparently flaccid may suddenly contract when the patient performs functional or unusual movements, such as crawling or walking backwards. The patient with a conversion reaction may also perform physical activities in a slow and laborious manner and frequently carries out simple acts with an overflow of activity into unrelated areas.

Clinical Examination

Evaluation of weakness includes a thorough history and careful observation of the patient in a variety of positions and activities as well as an evaluation of individual muscle strength and joint range of motion. A knowledge of functional anatomy is necessary since the patient with a slowly progressive neuromuscular disorder has often learned to substitute normal for weak muscle groups. The resulting activity pattern will often appear to be completely normal to the inexperienced observer. In the following review, symptoms and signs will usually be discussed together.

The *familial* occurrence of a disease can obviously be of diagnostic assistance[7,17] (Table 4-8). However, it should be noted that in some disorders the course of the disease may differ greatly in different members of a family. This is especially true in infantile and familial (juvenile) spinal muscular atrophy and the various glycogen storage diseases of muscle in which slowly progressive proximal weakness in one sibling may often bear little resemblance to the severe and rapidly fatal disease in another. In other

Table 4-8. Types of Inheritance in Some of the More Common Neuromuscular Disorders

Anterior Horn Cells	*Peripheral Nerves*	*Myoneural Junction Muscles and Uncertain Origins*
	Autosomal Dominant	
Familial spinal muscular atrophy Scapuloperoneal spinal muscular atrophy	Peroneal muscular atrophy Hypertrophic interstitial neuropathy	Facioscapulohumeral dystrophy Limb girdle dystrophy Distal myopathy Ocular myopathy Oculopharyngeal dystrophy Nemaline myopathy Central core disease Centronuclear myopathy Myotonic dystrophy Generalized myositis ossificans Potassium periodic paralysis Congenital myotonia
	Autosomal Recessive	
Infantile spinal muscular atrophy Familial spinal muscular atrophy Amyotrophy with arthrogryposis	Peroneal muscular atrophy Metachromatic leukodystrophy	Limb girdle dystrophy Congenital muscular dystrophy with arthrogryposis Most mitochondrial myopathies Most glycogen storage diseases Paroxysmal myoglobinuria
	Recessive X-Chromosomal	
		Duchenne dystrophy Becker dystrophy
	Dominant X-Chromosomal	
	Peroneal muscular atrophy	

disorders, such as peroneal muscular atrophy, autosomal dominant, autosomal recessive, and even X-linked recessive patterns of transmission have been reported. In general, it is among the X-linked and dominant conditions that the family history is most helpful. A clearcut family history of an X-linked recessive pattern of transmission in a child with proximal weakness is an obvious help in the early diagnosis of the Duchenne or Becker types of muscular dystrophy.

Muscle pain or painful muscular contraction at rest is probably the most common musculoskeletal symptom.[14] Painful muscle spasm often accompanies joint disease, and pain may be referred to muscle from other sites. *Cramps* which are transient and involuntary, and often associated with painful muscular contractions may result from uremia, tetany, sodium depletion, amyotrophic lateral sclerosis, and unaccustomed exertion but are much more often unexplained. In upper motor neuron lesions, *flexor spasms* due to spasticity may also be very painful. Neuralgic amyotrophy often begins with severe aching pain, and painful polyneuropathies are usually those associated with alcoholism, porphyria, arsenic poisoning, polyarteritis nodosa, and diabetic amyotrophy. In both poliomyelitis and the Guillain-Barré syndrome, the muscle weakness may be preceded by pain; visible fasciculations are often seen at this stage in the former. *Myalgia*, an aching type of pain, is common in viral infections and varies in severity from that found in influenza to the rather severe diaphragmatic pain of coxsackie B myalgia (Bornholm disease). *Muscle pain on exertion* is usually attributable to muscle ischemia, as experienced in the intermittent claudication resulting from atherosclerotic occlusion. In myophosphorylase (McArdle's disease), phosphofructokinase, and phosphohexoisomerase deficiencies, the earliest symptom is usually an aching sensation in the calves during walking which becomes more painful and cramp-like with anaerobic activity. The ill-differentiated group of conditions collectively known as paroxysmal myoglobinuria is also characterized by acute attacks of cramp-like muscle pain and tenderness.

Palpation of the muscles is important in the assessment of muscle tone, atrophy, hypertrophy, or weakness.[14] It is also important in locating local or general areas of *tenderness*. Pain and generalized tenderness are common in poliomyelitis and the Guillain-Barré syndrome. Tenderness may also be elicited in acute polymyositis and the polyneuropathies due to vitamin B_1 or B_{12} deficiency. Palpable local masses in muscle are usually areas of local spasm, posttraumatic hematoma, or a muscle hernia although myositis ossificans or a rhabdomyosarcoma can occasionally be felt.

Careful observation for *spontaneous involuntary movement* is also important since *fasciculation* and *myokymia* often signify neuromuscular disease.[14,18] Both are painless contractions of small groups of muscle fibers which may be felt by the patient and which cause visible movement of the overlying skin but not of the neighboring joints. Fasciculations are brief twitches of the fibers of single motor units and are best seen where the muscle is close to the skin, as in the hands or especially in the tongue. They can often be induced by percussing or pinching the muscle and may either involve the same motor unit repetitively over short periods or be totally irregular. Fasciculation occurs in acute degenerative disorders of the anterior horn cells, such as in amyotrophic lateral sclerosis, familial, and infantile spinal muscular atrophy, although spontaneous benign fasciculations are not uncommon in normal individuals. In the latter, however, it is usually seen in the calf or small muscles of the hand after movement or a strong contraction and, of course, is not associated with weakness. Fasciculation may also occur in nerve root lesions where it repetitively involves larger fasciculi during minimal contraction but not during complete relaxation. Myokymia is a slower contraction of independent small bands or strips of muscle fibers; there is an undulating or rippling appearance to the overlying skin, and movement is usually in the direction of the muscle fibers. It is rare and is seen in occasional cases of thyrotoxicosis or may be associated with neuromyotonia. Facial clonic spasm, sometimes confused with myokymia, is a recurrent twitch of part of the musculature supplied by the facial nerve. Movements are stereotyped but irregular in timing. Cramps, also a form of spontaneous involuntary movement, have been discussed above. *Involuntary muscle movement* can also be produced by muscle contraction or stimulation. *Myotonia* is characterized by a failure of the muscles to relax immediately after voluntary contraction has ceased and a tendency for a dimple to persist for a few seconds after percussion of the muscle (Fig. 4-1). Patients complain of stiffness of the limbs, difficulty in walking, inability to relax the grip, and difficulty in opening the eyelids after forceful closure (Fig. 4-2). In general, myotonia improves after repeated contraction and is worse in the cold. Myotonia is found in myotonic dystrophy, congenital myotonia, paramyotonia, and hyperkalemic periodic paralysis, and may be confused with *myoedema* which is an electrically silent ridge induced by percussion of atrophic muscles in wasting conditions, such as tuberculosis and malabsorption. Other types of movement induced by muscle contraction or stimulation are *tetany, tetanus,* and the *cramp contracture* seen in myophosphorylase deficiency. The pathophysiology and electrodiagnostic characteristics of fasciculation, myokymia, myotonia, tetany, tetanus, cramp contracture, and cramps are discussed in greater detail in Chapter 3.

Contracture is a state of shortening of a muscle not caused by active contraction.[14] It may be acute and spontaneously reversible with electrical silence, as in myophosphorylase, phosphofructokinase, and phosphohexoisomerase deficiencies. More often, however, it is the result of the rearrangement of collagen fibrils within the muscle over a longer period of time, tightness of soft tissues, or joint ankylosis. In the early stage of rearrangement of collagen fibrils, a contracture can be reversible by repeated stretching. Later, fibrosis usually takes place. The failure of a muscle to grow in length when its action is not opposed by a sufficiently powerful antagonist can also result in a contracture. Palpation of the muscles during passive movement at the affected joint will usually distinguish contracture caused by ankylosis from active contraction. Fixed, severe, chronic contractures are common in the syndrome of arthrogryposis multiplex congenita (Fig. 4-3), progressive myosclerosis, and Duchenne muscular dystrophy (Fig. 4-4), but are unusual or mild in most other diseases of the motor unit.

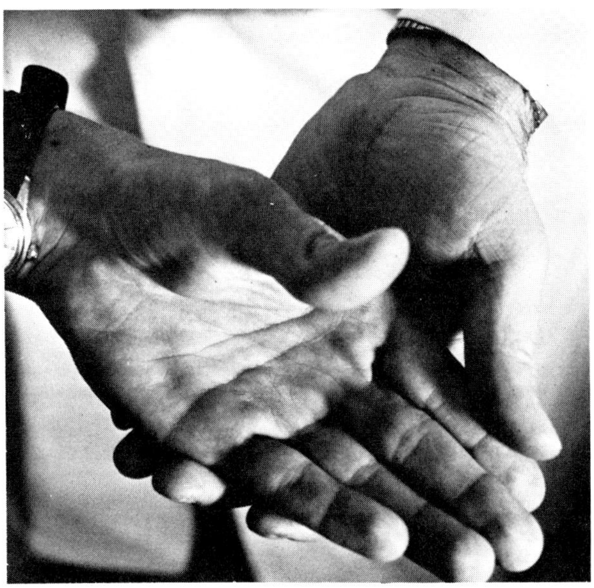

Fig. 4-1. Myotonic response of the thenar muscles produced by percussion in a 17-year-old patient with congenital myotonia of 15-years' duration.

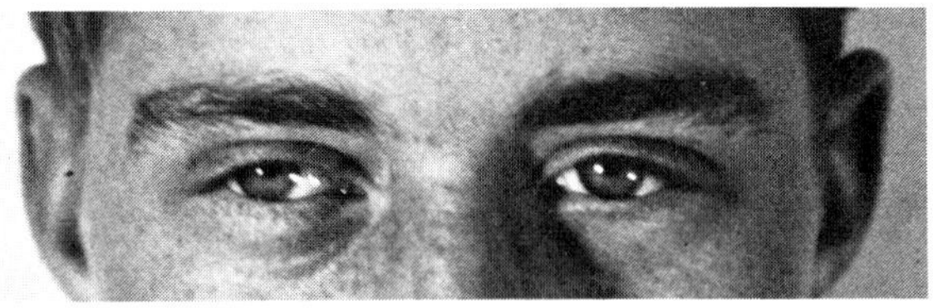

Fig. 4-2. Myotonic response of the eyelids in a 17-year-old boy with congenital myotonia produced by forceful closure of the lids.

Weakness, used in the global sense of the word, is actually a spectrum ranging from the vague complaint of fatigue through frank outright paralysis. *Fatigability,* which has already been discussed briefly, is characteristic of myasthenia gravis when it is variable and made worse by repeated muscle contraction.[14] It must be distinguished from simple fatigue due to constant slight muscular weakness, stiffness, or pain induced by exercise, conversion reaction, and the myasthenic syndrome associated with carcinoma (Eaton-Lambert syndrome). Fatigue, usually in the lower extremities, which improves during the first few contractions following a period of inactivity is characteristic of the myasthenic syndrome.

Muscle tone, primarily a clinical term, is dependent upon the viscoelastic properties of muscle, joint, and tendon resistance as well as on the tonic stretch reflex, and can be evaluated in various ways. *Consistency* of a muscle may be tested by palpating it laterally or by shaking the limbs; *extensibilité* by slow movement of joints through their full range; and *passivité* by measuring the amplitude of a flapping movement when the proximal part of a limb is shaken.[2] The *recoil* of a muscle suddenly released

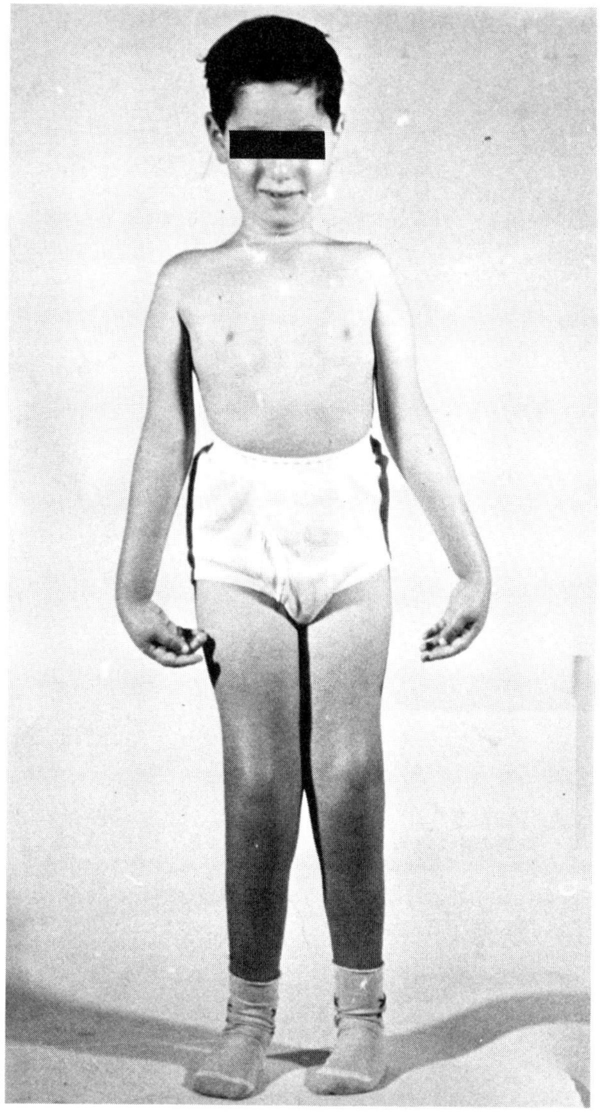

Fig. 4-3. Fixed chronic flexion contractures at the wrists, hips, and knees in a 10-year-old boy with arthrogryposis multiplex congenita since birth secondary to congenital muscular dystrophy. Patient also has a superior rectus paresis and a mild pectus excavatum.

from a fully stretched position is another measurement of tone. Tone is obviously increased in lesions of the upper motor neuron resulting in spasticity, rigidity, and dystonia. Hypotonia, the major finding in the "floppy infant," is usually defined as that state in which the resistance to passive motion of the limbs at absolute rest is less than normally anticipated for the age of the child. Muscular weakness and hypotonia are not always distinguishable since weakness due to a lesion of the motor neuron or of the muscle fiber is usually accompanied by hypotonia. This is, however, only true at rest, and there is usually a considerable difference in muscle strength between, for example, the child with infantile spinal muscular atrophy and the patient with muscular dystrophy. In muscle disease *consistency* and *passivité* are often more abnormal than *extensibilité*.[2,14] Other useful signs of hypotonia are the hanging posture of the head and limbs when an infant is lifted supine (Fig. 4-5) and the tendency to slip through the hands when held under the axilla. It is also important to remember that muscle tone normally decreases from birth until the second to sixth month of life and then gradually increases again in later childhood.

Different patterns of *deep tendon reflex* changes are often observed in otherwise similar disorders.[14] They are usually abolished early in peripheral neu-

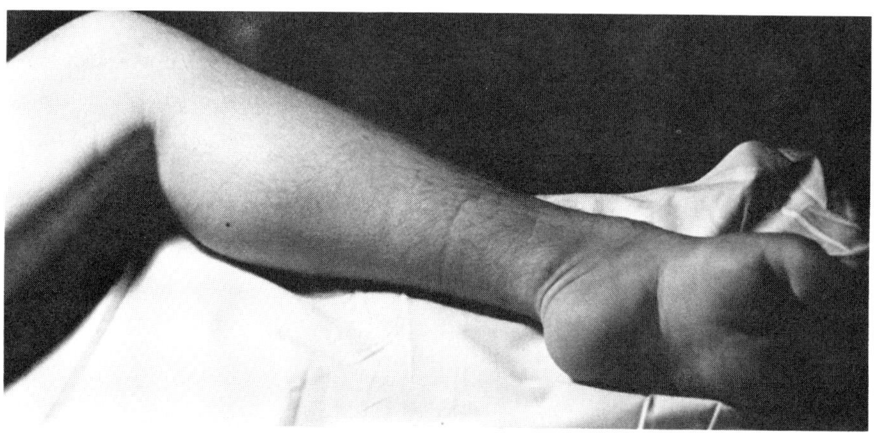

Fig. 4-4. Contractures at the hips and knees with tightness of the heel cords and early talipes equinovarus in a 12-year-old boy with Duchenne muscular dystrophy of 10-years' duration.

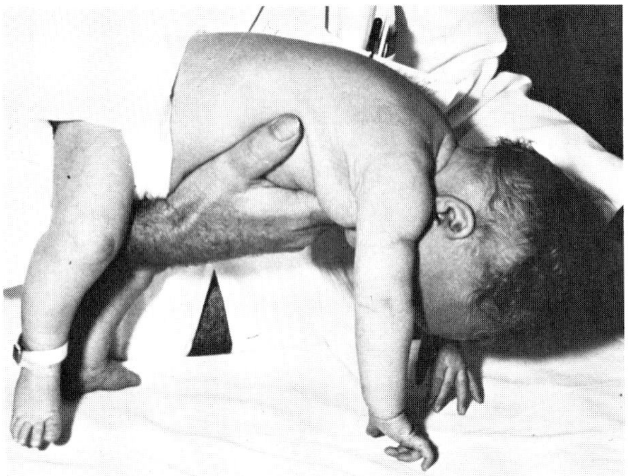

Fig. 4-5. Hanging flaccid posture of head and extremities in a hypotonic one-month-old child with infantile spinal muscular atrophy since birth.

ropathies and are often absent in muscles which are otherwise unaffected. In the dystrophies, the loss of the deep tendon reflex tends to follow closely the degree and location of the weakness. Hence, at least early in the disease, the distal reflexes are usually relatively well preserved. In anterior horn cell disease, however, brisk deep tendon reflexes may be found in muscles with marked wasting and weakness. They usually tend to be preserved in the weak muscles of patients with polymyositis and osteomalacia. In myasthenia gravis, the tendon reflexes are usually retained while they are lost in carcinomatous myasthenia. It is, of course, well known that in hypothyroidism the rates of contraction and relaxation of the reflex response are slow with an often excessively brisk response in thyrotoxicosis. Plantar responses are usually flexor or absent in muscle diseases and the polyneuropathies. The observation of extensor plantar responses, especially in patients with proximal muscle weakness, should arouse suspicions of anterior horn cell disease in which evidence of pyramidal tract involvement is also present.

Weakness can be considered as a symptom as well as a physical finding.[14] Few individuals use their muscles to full capacity, and marked weakness may go unnoticed especially if the patient has learned to substitute normal for weak muscles. Difficulty in running, in climbing stairs, or in arising from low chairs are often the early symptoms of proximal lower extremity weakness while shoulder girdle weakness, equally severe, may be asymptomatic. On the other hand, individuals whose occupations involve lifting heavy objects may notice upper extremity weakness first. Quadriceps weakness usually leads to sudden falls due to the resulting instability of the knees while distal lower extremity weakness, especially of the dorsiflexors, often results in tripping over stairs and curbs. Hand weakness is often first described as clumsiness or difficulty in unscrewing the lid from a jar while patients who complain of difficulty in walking down stairs often have spasticity or cerebellar ataxia of the legs. The mode of onset and progression of weakness should also be noted. For example, a rapid onset after a febrile illness may indicate poliomyelitis or the Guillain-Barré syndrome. Rates of progression are reviewed in Table 4-9.

Weakness as a physical finding can be evaluated in three ways: watching the patient in action, evaluation of functional activities, and by lengthy detailed manual muscle testing. A discussion of formal tests of functional activities and muscle testing is beyond the scope of this chapter, and the reader is referred to other sources.[10,26] A great deal can be learned about the degree of severity of muscle weakness and its location by observing the patient during various physical activities: walking, hopping, jumping, getting up from a chair or the floor, climbing stairs, combing the hair, and writing.[13,14] Indeed, in examining children this may be the only approach possible.

Observing the *facial expression* can often provide a valuable clue to the diagnosis as in myotonic dystrophy in which baldness, apathy, atrophy of temporal and sternomastoid muscles, masseter weakness, ptosis, cataract, and drooping of the cheeks and lower lip are immediately evident (Fig. 4-6). In facioscapulohumeral dystrophy, the lips are in an everted position, there is a lack of facial lines, the patient is unable to whistle, and the shoulders have a sloping posture with elevation of the scapula when the arm is abducted (Fig. 4-7).

Winging of the scapula at rest is seen in palsies of the serratus anterior and in limb-girdle dystrophy, but winging in the other dystrophies can usually only be obtained by putting the serratus into action (Fig. 4-8). *Kyphoscoliosis,* seen early in Friedreich's ataxia, the Levy-Roussy syndrome, and neurofibromatosis, does not occur until late in the course of the disease in the muscular dystrophies (Fig. 4-9).

Evaluation of *gait* can be helpful in confirming the

Table 4-9. Examples of Neuromuscular Disorders by Usual Rate of Progression of the Weakness or Paralysis

Progressive	*Static or Very Slowly Progressive*	*Variable Progression*
Dystrophies	Congenital myopathies	Myoglobinuric myopathies
Duchenne	Nemaline	Amyloid myopathy
Becker	Central core	Sarcoidosis
Facioscapulohumeral	Centronuclear	Myositis ossificans
Limb-girdle	Mitochondrial	Myasthenia gravis
Myotonic	Endocrine myopathies	Infantile spinal muscular atrophy
Distal	Thyroid	
Ocular and oculopharyngeal	Parathyroid	
Inflammatory myopathies	Adrenal	
Known etiology	Pituitary	
Bacterial, parasitic	Glycogen storage diseases	
Fungal, viral	Acid alpha-1, 4-glucosidase	
Unknown etiology	Branching enzyme	
Polymyositis	Debranching enzyme	
Dermatomyositis		
Myositis with neoplasm		
Myositis with other connective tissue diseases		
Toxic myopathies		
Deficiency states:		
Postgastrectomy and tocopherol		
Exogenous:		
Steroid, chloroquine, and alcohol		
Periodic paralysis		
Myasthenic syndromes		
Tumors of muscle		
Spinal muscular atrophy, adult		
Familial spinal muscular atrophy		
Amyotrophic lateral sclerosis		
Syringomyelia		
Poliomyelitis		
Idiopathic polyneuropathy		
Peroneal muscular atrophy		
Hypertrophic interstitial neuropathy		
Rheumatoid neuropathy		
Amyloid neuropathy		
Diabetic neuropathy		
Exogeneous toxic neuropathies		

presence of weakness and its approximate distribution. Gait patterns, are, however, usually nonspecific, and it is incorrect to assume that any abnormal gait is pathognomonic of a specific neuromuscular disease. In disorders primarily affecting the distal muscles, the patient often has foot drop and a steppage gait, and even mild weakness of the dorsiflexors can be easily detected by having the patient walk on his heels. In disorders primarily affecting the proximal muscles, a waddling lordotic gait is usually seen (Fig. 4-10). In early and doubtful cases of proximal weakness, it is important to watch the patient running and going up stairs. Attempts to run often resemble a racing walk, and the patient will often push up on the knees or pull on the hand railing to assist him in rapidly climbing stairs.

Gowers' sign is also valuable in identifying lower extremity proximal weakness, but it is not pathognomonic of Duchenne muscular dystrophy. In this maneuver, the patient arises from a chair or the floor by pushing up on his knees with his hands (Fig. 4-11). Having the patient sit up from a lying position will also often identify weakness of the anterior neck muscles since the head will lag instead of being the first part to be lifted. In the case of weakness of either hip flexion or the abdominal muscles, the patient

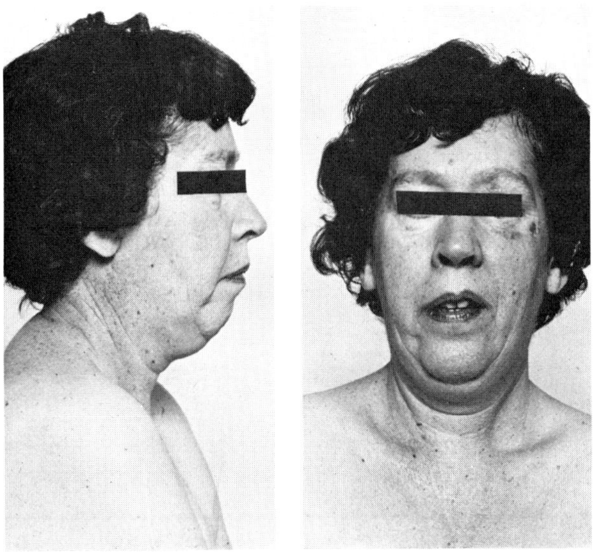

Fig. 4-6. Weakness of the temporal, sternomastoid, and masseter muscles, mild ptosis, and drooping of the cheeks and lower lip in a 45-year-old female with myotonic dystrophy of 35-years' duration. Early mild frontal baldness is also evident.

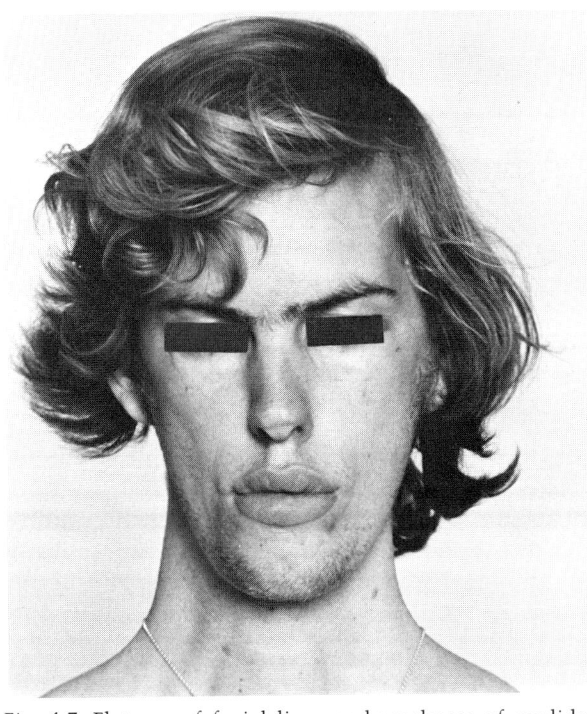

Fig. 4-7. Flatness of facial lines and weakness of eyelids and lips in an everted position in a 19-year-old male with facioscapulohumeral dystrophy of 14-years' duration.

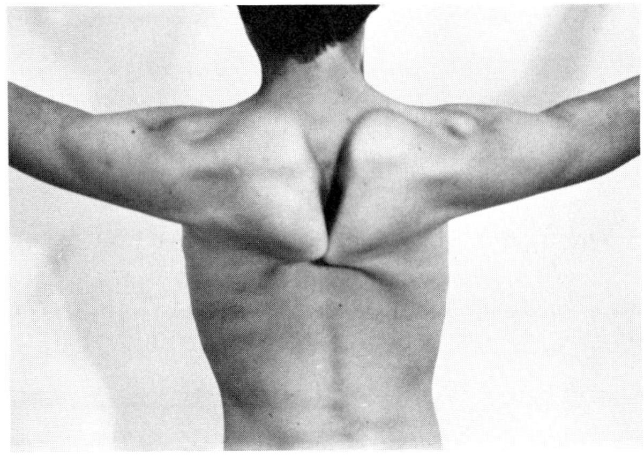

Fig. 4-8. Severe bilateral winging of the scapulae in a 14-year-old boy with myotonic dystrophy of 12-years' duration.

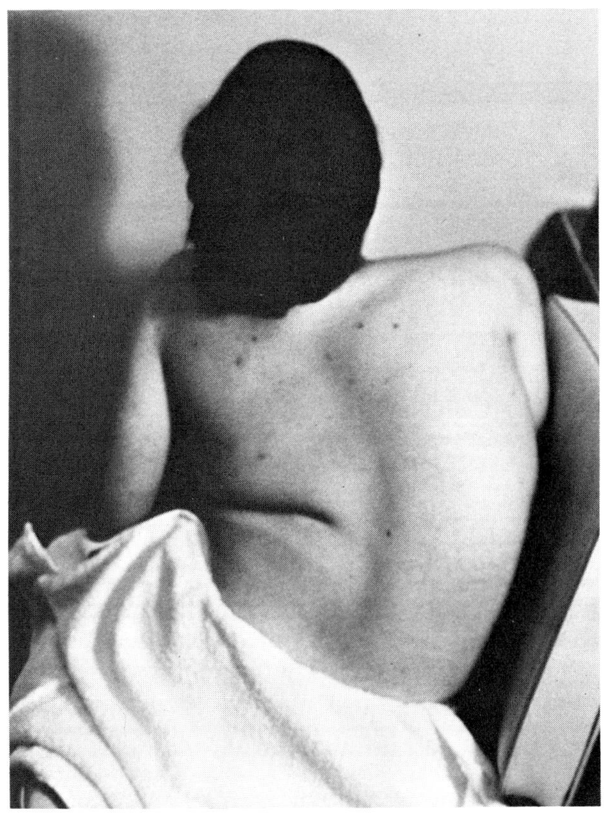

Fig. 4-9. Marked kyphoscoliosis in a 15-year-old boy with Duchenne muscular dystrophy of 13-years' duration.

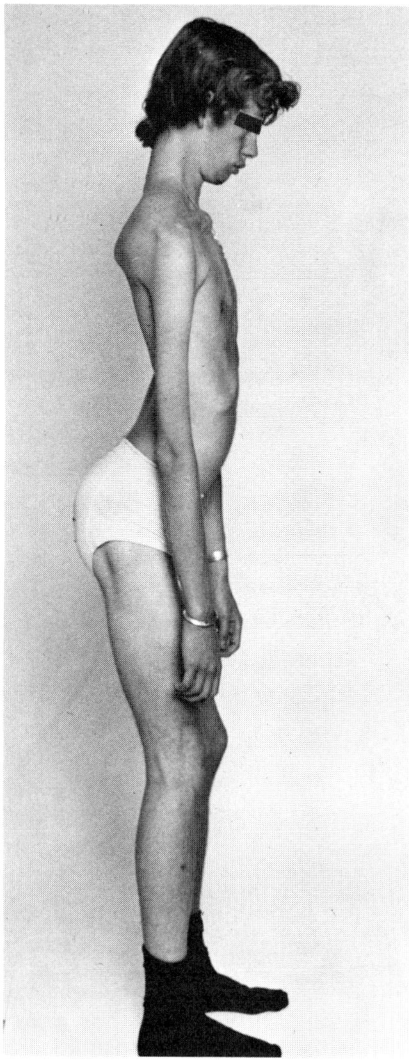

Fig. 4-10. Marked lordosis, forward tilt of the pelvis, tightness of the hip flexors, and winging of the scapulae in a 19-year-old male with facioscapulohumeral dystrophy of 14-years' duration.

may actually not be able to sit up at all, and localized weakness of the upper or lower abdominal muscles will cause a shift of the umbilicus. Early paraspinal muscle weakness can often be detected by asking the patient to lift the head and shoulders from the prone position.

In evaluating weakness, the observer should be aware of several pitfalls. Spasticity, rigidity, or akinesia often gives an initial impression of weakness. Pain due to joint disease can be confused with weakness especially in the lower extremities. The diagnosis of hysterical weakness or malingering, already discussed, depends primarily on the identification of inconsistencies in the examination. Localized weakness in a single limb is usually neurogenic although muscle trauma or tendon rupture should be considered. When localized weakness appears not to

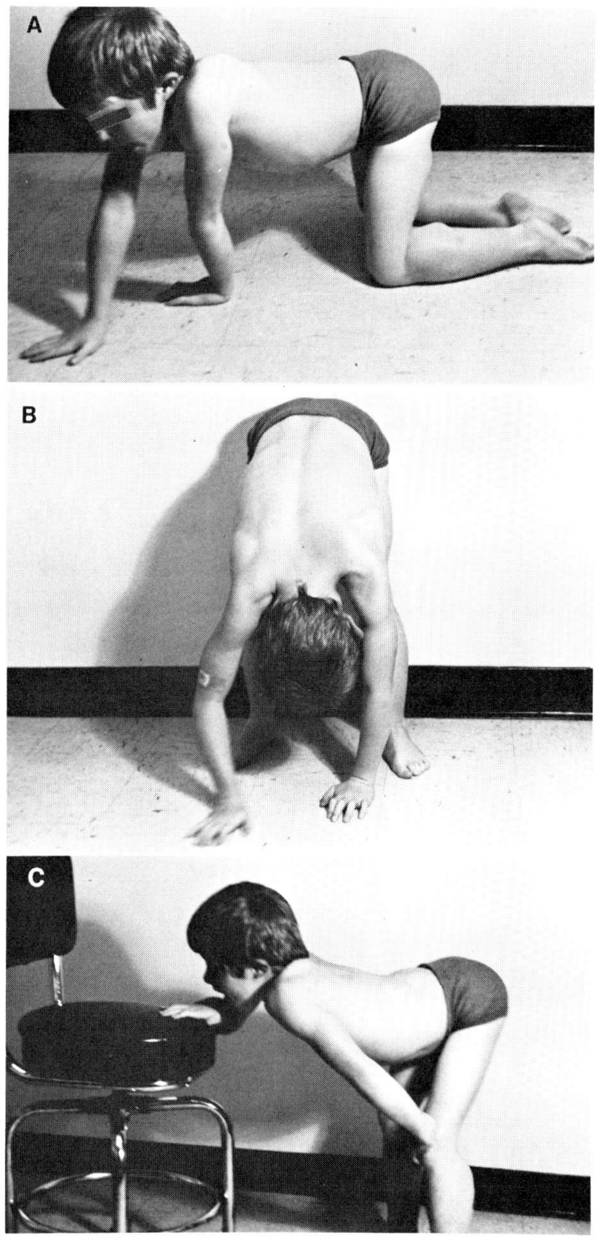

Fig. 4-11. Gowers' sign in a 5-year-old boy with Duchenne muscular dystrophy.

fit into an anatomical pattern, poliomyelitis and early motor neuron disease are the most likely possibilities. A selective, symmetrical, proximal pattern of weakness is typical of muscular dystrophy although spinal muscular atrophy may imitate this. The information presented in Table 4-10 can be helpful as an approximate guide as long as it is understood that patterns of weakness are not diagnostic without cor-

Table 4-10. Examples of Neuromuscular Disorders by Usual Patterns of Weakness or Fatigue and Atrophy

	Usual Site of Weakness			*Location*	
	Generalized	*Mainly Distal*	*Mainly Proximal*	*Symmetrical*	*Asymmetrical*
Anterior horn cells	Infantile spinal muscular atrophy Poliomyelitis Scapuloperoneal atrophy Amyotrophy with arthrogryposis	Amyotrophic lateral sclerosis	Familial spinal muscular atrophy	Infantile spinal muscular atrophy Scapuloperoneal atrophy Familial spinal muscular atrophy Amyotrophic lateral sclerosis	Poliomyelitis
Peripheral Nerves		Peroneal muscular atrophy Hypertrophic interstitial neuropathy Diabetic neuropathy			Peripheral neuropathy
Myoneural junction, muscles and uncertain origin	Myasthenia gravis* Myasthenic syndrome* Periodic paralysis* Hypothyroidism* Steroid myopathy* Generalized myositis ossificans Congenital dystrophy with arthrogryposis Congenital myopathies: Nemaline, central core disease, centronuclear myopathy	Distal myopathy Myotonic dystrophy Ocular myopathy	Polymyositis Muscular dystrophy: Duchenne, facioscapulohumeral, limb girdle, Becker Thyrotoxic myopathy Glycogen storage disease	Muscular dystrophy: Duchenne, facioscapulohumeral, limb-girdle, Becker, and distal Thyrotoxic myopathy Ocular myopathy Glycogen storage disease Polymyositis Congenital myopathies	Periodic paralysis*

*With little or no wasting.

Table 4-11. Examples of Neuromuscular Disorders in Which Weakness Is the Predominant Finding by Usual Age at Onset

Anterior Horn Cells	*Peripheral Nerves*	*Myoneural Junction: Muscles and Uncertain Origins*
	Birth	
Infantile spinal muscular atrophy Amyotrophy with arthrogryposis Aplasia of spinal cord	Hypertrophic interstitial neuropathy	"Benign congenital hypotonia" Congenital muscular dystrophy with arthrogryposis Nemaline myopathy Central core disease Centronuclear myopathy Glycogen storage diseases
	Early Childhood	
	Peroneal muscular atrophy Guillain-Barré syndrome Metachromatic leukodystrophy	Duchenne dystrophy Generalized myositis ossificans Mitochondrial myopathies
	Late Childhood and Adolescence	
Scapuloperoneal spinal muscular atrophy Familial spinal muscular atrophy Syringomyelia	Peroneal muscular atrophy Guillain-Barré syndrome	Limb girdle dystrophy Facioscapulohumeral dystrophy Myotonic dystrophy Potassium periodic paralysis Becker dystrophy Mitochondrial myopathies
	Adults	
Amyotrophic lateral sclerosis Progressive muscular atrophy	Guillain-Barré syndrome Carcinomatous neuropathy Alcoholic neuropathy	Limb-girdle dystrophy Facioscapulohumeral dystrophy Myotonic dystrophy Sarcoid myopathy
	Any Age	
Poliomyelitis Traumatic: physical and toxic	Toxic neuropathies Botulism neuropathies Nutritional, diabetic and uremic neuropathy Neuropathy with collagen vascular disorders	Thyrotoxic myopathy Dermatomyositis and polymyositis Myasthenia gravis Drug-induced toxic myopathies Bacterial, fungal, parasitic, and viral myositis Disuse atrophy

relation with other points such as the age of onset (Table 4-11), duration, rate (see Table 4-9) and mode of progression, and the presence of other muscular and nonmuscular findings (Table 4-12).

A thorough evaluation of the *muscles supplied by the cranial nerves* is also important.[14] Pareses of the *external ocular muscles* which do not conform to the pattern of single or multiple nerve palsies suggest

Table 4-12. Findings Often Associated with Disorders in Which Weakness Is the Predominant Finding

Fasciculations	Anterior horn cell disease
Congenital absence of muscles	Muscular dystrophy
Congenital defects	Nemaline and centronuclear myopathy
Congenital contractures	Arthrogryposis
Myotonia	Myotonic dystrophy, congenital myotonia, hyperkalemic periodic paralysis
Frontal baldness, cataracts, and testicular atrophy	Myotonic dystrophy
Mental retardation	Duchenne dystrophy, myotonic dystrophy
Hypertrophy	Duchenne dystrophy
Muscle cramping	Phosphorylase syndrome, myoglobinuria
Muscle tenderness	Dermatomyositis and polymyositis, poliomyelitis, Guillain-Barré syndrome
Dermal lesions	Dermatomyositis
Myoedema	Myxedema
Hypertrophied nerves	Hypertrophic interstitial neuropathy

a local muscular disorder, an expanding orbital lesion, or a generalized myopathy. Ptosis usually occurs before ocular pareses or diplopia in the ocular, oculopharyngeal, and myotonic muscular dystrophies, and ocular myopathy may progress to complete external ophthalmoplegia. Myasthenia gravis is the great imitator of ocular palsies, and maintaining upward gaze for a minute or so will usually induce ptosis. Mobius' syndrome is characterized by bilateral facial weakness with bilateral sixth nerve palsy and is often confused with early facioscapulohumeral or myotonic dystrophy. The *muscles of mastication* are often involved early in myasthenia gravis and myotonic dystrophy in which wasting of the temporal and masseter muscles and drooping of the jaw also occur. The *facial muscles* are also commonly involved in myopathies but are rare in progressive muscular atrophy; a brisk jaw jerk will usually distinguish the latter. *Dysarthria and dysphagia* are common in myasthenia gravis and polymyositis while dysphagia alone is more frequent in the myotonic and oculopharyngeal muscular dystrophies. Bulbar involvement is, of course, characteristic of poliomyelitis, motor neuron disease, and acute polyneuritis. *Weakness of neck flexion or extension* is usually prominent in myotonic dystrophy, polymyositis, and myasthenia gravis. The *tongue* is important because of the ease with which it shows the fasciculation commonly present in anterior horn cell diseases. Few of the myopathies affect the tongue.

Evaluation of weakness in infants and young children is especially difficult and involves a thorough knowledge of normal growth and development.[2,16,25] Weakness or hypotonia due to lesions in the corticospinal pathways, cerebellum, and brain stem is not always accompanied in early life by exaggerated tendon reflexes, spasticity, or pathological reflexes. Examples of such lesions are early atonic diplegia and congenital athetosis or cerebellar ataxia. Before the examination, it is necessary to put the child in such a position that the muscle group being tested can lift the appropriate part of the body against gravity. In addition, the muscle group must be made to contract or move spontaneously. During the first six months of life, the various attitudinal reflexes may be utilized to elicit the desired muscle function. The asymmetrical tonic neck reflex demonstrates knee and elbow flexion and extension weakness; Landau's reflex will elicit weakness of the hip, neck, and trunk extensors, the grasp reflex can be used to determine weakness of finger flexion, and the Moro reflex will indicate the involvement of one extremity. If motor activity is not spontaneously present, noxious stimuli may be used to produce withdrawal. When motor activity is present, relative weakness may be determined by several methods. The weak extremity will often resist movement with less force when rapid alternating passive movement is superimposed on spontaneous activity. Information may be obtained by restraining the spontaneous activity of an extremity and noting the force which tends to continue the motion. The shoulder adductors and scapular stabilizers can be tested by lifting the infant under the axilla, since the normal spontaneous response is to push down against the examiner's fingers with surprising force. Arm and neck weakness may be determined by pulling the infant from a supine to a sitting position. The weak extremity will straighten out while the normal arm will flex at the elbow. Ambulation and locomotion patterns should also be observed.[13] When ambulation is delayed, abnormal patterns of locomotion, such as rolling, asymmetric crawling, scooting, and hitching, are often used to substitute for normal walking. Close observation of these patterns may help in more precise identification of areas of weakness. Hitching, for example, can be performed only with stability of the trunk and upper extremities.

Atrophy, a physical sign of motor unit disease, is second in importance only to weakness, and it is helpful to compare the degrees of atrophy and weakness in the affected muscle.[14] Although atrophy can usually be recognized, it is sometimes difficult to assess especially in infants, women, and in the obese. Measurement of limb girth, palpation of muscles during contraction, and soft tissue radiography are often helpful when asymmetry is suspected. Atrophy is sometimes confused with congenital absence of muscles, most commonly the pectoralis major, since it may only involve part of a muscle. The latter often occurs in limb-girdle dystrophy in which the upper part of the deltoid is wasted while the lower portion may be soft and bulky or even hypertrophic. The other major cause of focal atrophy of a muscle is infarction. In most disorders of the lower motor neuron and in many myopathies, the muscle wasting is in proportion to the weakness. In general, there tends to be proportionately more wasting in anterior horn cell disease, tuberculosis, malnutrition, carcinomatosis, and simple atrophy due to aging, while in muscular dystrophy there is proportionately more weakness. There are also several myopathies in which severe weakness may occur with very little atrophy early in the course of the disease: myasthenia gravis, polymyositis, periodic paralysis, and the myopathy of osteomalacia. It is also important to remember that when the weakness is recent, atrophy may not have had time to develop.

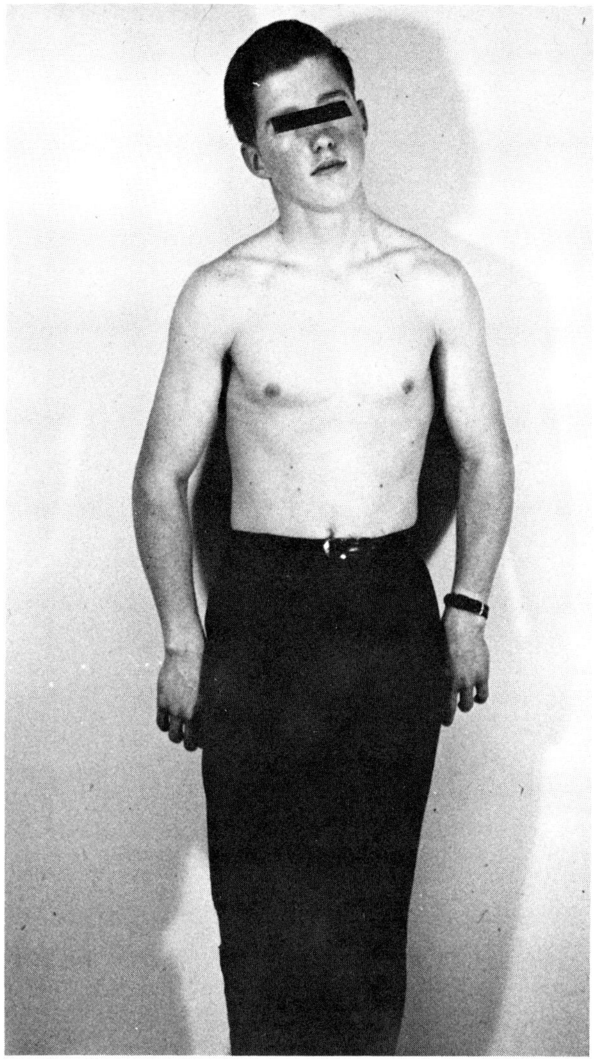

Fig. 4-12. Mild generalized muscular hypertrophy in a 17-year-old boy with congenital myotonia of 15-years' duration. The myotonia is also reflected in his stiff posture.

Muscular hypertrophy and pseudohypertrophy are common in several diseases. The latter is the replacement of muscle fibers within a muscle with fat and connective tissue at a level whereby the bulk of the muscle is maintained. Hypertrophy has been considered by some in terms of physiological or pathological changes, although others believe that it is doubtful whether increasing muscle bulk is ever a primary pathological phenomenon. Of all the disorders affecting the motor unit, it is most striking in congenital myotonia (Fig. 4-12) and the Schwartz-Jampel syndrome (Fig. 4-13) in which the hypertrophy occurs in essentially all muscles. In these two conditions, the strength of the muscles is consistent with their bulk, and it is most likely that the continual muscle fiber activity produces a true work hypertrophy. The enlarged and relatively strong calf muscles seen in the early stages of the Duchenne (Fig. 4-14) and Becker types of dystrophy are, of course, well known. Early in the stage of the disease, this is probably due to true work hypertrophy. Later, with replacement with fat and connective tissue, there is pseudohypertrophy. About one third of the young patients with limb-girdle dystrophy also have calf muscle hypertrophy. Localized muscular hypertro-

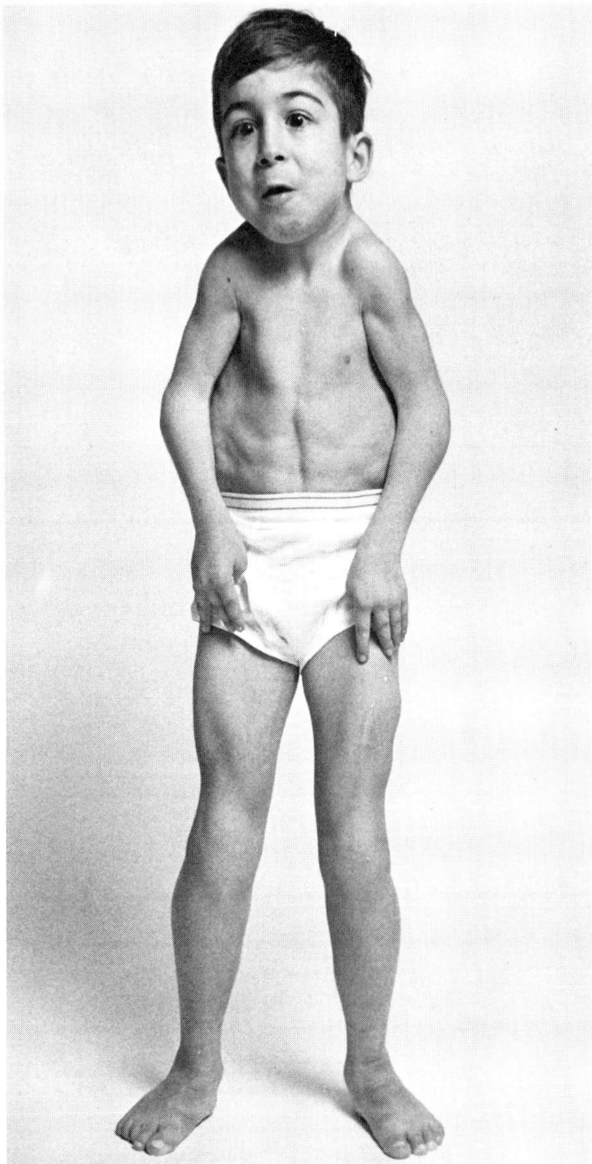

Fig. 4-13. Marked generalized muscular hypertrophy in an eight-year-old boy with Schwartz-Jampel syndrome. Also note the flat expressionless face, puckered mouth, short neck, pectus carinatum, forward shoulders, and flaring of the lower rib cage. Abnormal stance primarily due to continuous muscle contractions rather than to contractures. (Fowler, W. M., Jr.: J. Neurol. Sci., *22:*127, 1974)

phy in areas other than the calf muscles may also occur in other diseases of the motor unit, while generalized hypertrophy has been reported in hypertrophy musculorum vera, de Lange's syndrome, and hypothyroidism.

As noted in Table 4-12, there are several *nonmuscular findings* which can be of considerable importance.[14] The presence of a skin rash, Raynaud's phenomenon, and dysphagia, for example, can be very helpful in diagnosing polymyositis or dermatomyositis. Vascular changes in the capillaries of the nail beds are often found early in many of the collagen vascular disorders (Fig. 4-15) as are anemia, proteinuria, arthropathy, pleurisy, or splenomegaly. Sarcoid myopathy is often associated with uveitis, erythema nodosum, or pulmonary infiltration; systemic sclerosis with a tight shining skin over the face or fingers, and osteomalacia or hyperparathyroidism with steatorrhea, uremia, and bony tenderness. In all these disorders, the myopathy may be the presenting feature before the more classic symptoms become obvious. Myoglobinuria is, of course, associated with

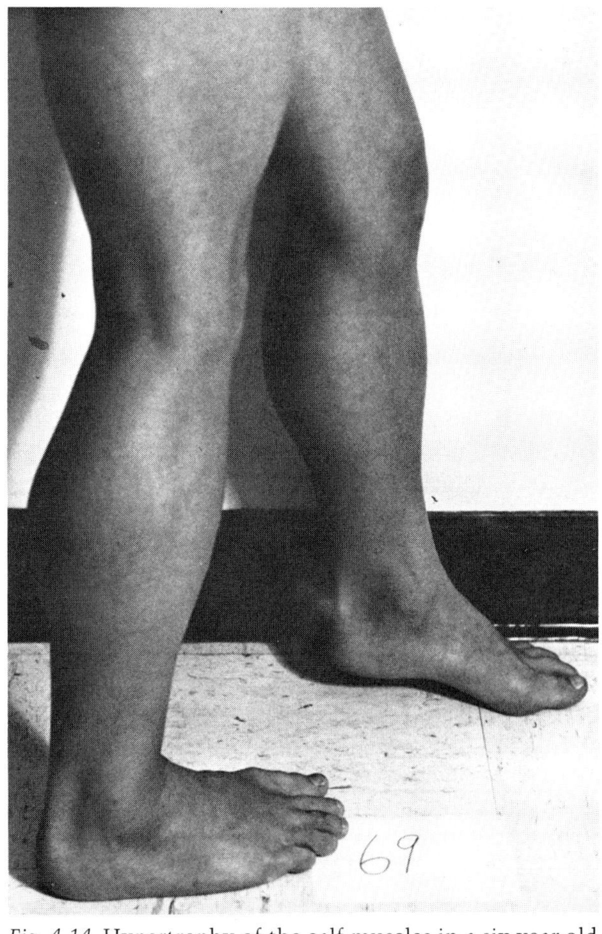

Fig. 4-14. Hypertrophy of the calf muscles in a six-year-old boy with Duchenne muscular dystrophy.

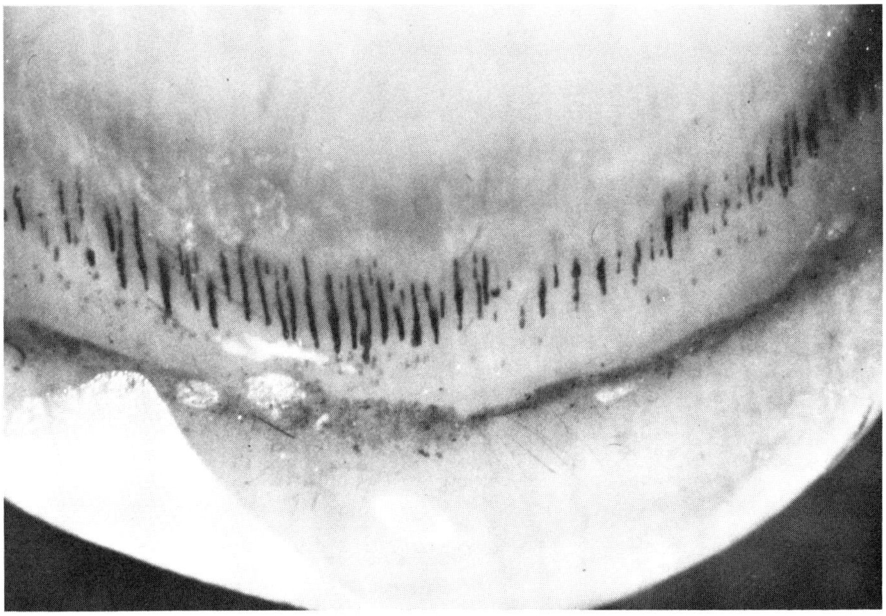

Fig. 4-15. Splinter hemorrhages in the nail beds of a patient following the intraarterial injection of secobarbital.

severe necrotizing myopathy in polymyositis, acute alcoholism, after exercise in the anterior tibial syndrome, and in myophosphorylase deficiency. The genetically determined myopathies are often associated with other congenital abnormalities; a high arched palate (Fig. 4-16), long face, protruding jaw and dental malocclusion in nemaline myopathy, hepatic involvement in Types II and III glycogen storage disease, and cardiac, cerebral, and spinal cord involvement in Type II glycogen storage disease.

Laboratory Evaluation

Following the clinical evaluation, a general laboratory survey is indicated especially with reference to endocrine dysfunction, serum potassium abnormalities, and the response of any weakness to Tensilon. The major diagnostically useful laboratory tests are electromyography, nerve conduction, serum enzyme levels, and muscle biopsy. Measurement of serum enzymes and the electrodiagnostic tests should be done before the biopsy.

Enzymes, such as the transaminases (GOT and GPT), lactic dehydrogenase (LDH), aldolase and creatine phosphokinase (CPK), are normally present in muscle and other tissues.[21] Increased levels in the serum merely reflect an accelerated release from

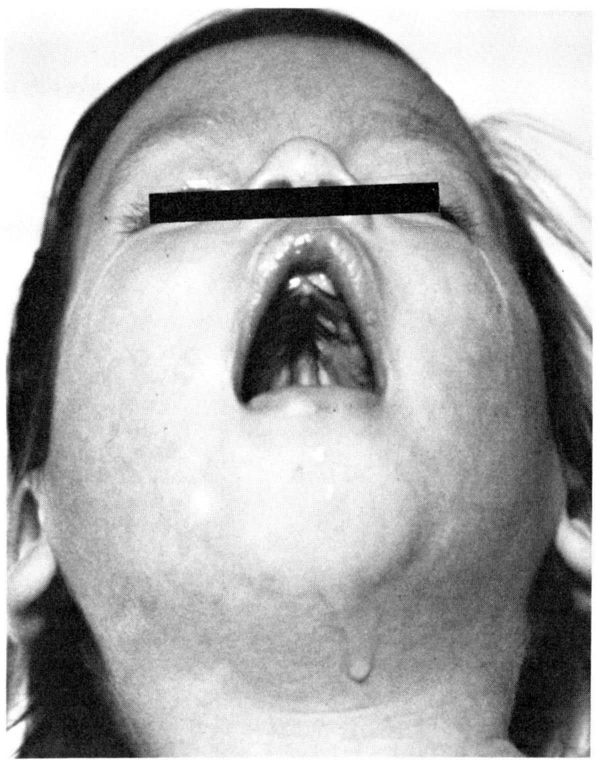

Fig. 4-16. High arched palate in a one-year-old child with nemaline myopathy since birth.

Table 4-13. Disorders and Situations in Which CPK Levels May Be Elevated

Anterior Horn Cells	*Peripheral Nerves*	*Myoneural Junction: Muscles and Uncertain Origins*
	Mild	
Amyotrophic lateral sclerosis Syringomyelia Poliomyelitis	Some toxic neuropathies	Facioscapulohumeral dystrophy Oculopharyngeal dystrophy Distal dystrophy Bacterial, fungal, parasitic, and viral myositis Sarcoidosis myopathy Nemaline myopathy Central core disease Centronuclear myopathy Mitochondrial myopathy Thyroid myopathy Amyloid myopathy Pompe's disease Congenital myotonia Psychoses, acute Postpartum Hypoxia Dilantin Succinylcholine
	Moderate	
Progressive spinal muscular atrophy Juvenile spinal muscular atrophy Infantile spinal muscular atrophy	Guillain-Barré syndrome	Adult limb-girdle dystrophy Some toxic myopathies Steroid myopathy Myotonic dystrophy Myokymia Spinal cord injury, acute Tetanus Tetany Convulsions Delirium tremens Exercise Prolonged exposure to cold Lidocaine
	Marked	
		Duchenne dystrophy Becker dystrophy Juvenile limb-girdle dystrophy Polymyositis and dermatomyositis, acute Myoglobinuria, acute Malignant hyperpyrexia Traumatized muscle Myocardial infarctions Cerebral infarctions

damaged or diseased tissues. The value of serum enzymes for the diagnosis of muscular diseases depends upon the integrity of other organs since most enzymes are not specific to muscle and can be elevated in many other diseases and conditions. CPK, therefore, has emerged as the most reliable and sensitive indicator of muscle fiber breakdown. Its main advantage is its limited distribution in the human body since it is found in far greater quantity in striated and cardiac muscle and central nervous system tissue than in other organ systems. Although it may be slightly or moderately elevated in a variety of situations and diseases (Table 4-13), the only other common sources of marked elevation in the serum are acute myocardial disease, acute cerebral hemorrhage, and early in the course of spinal cord injury.

The electromyogram and nerve conduction, when abnormal, also provide valuable information about the etiology of the weakness (Table 4-14). Electrodiagnostic tests are covered in detail in Chapter 3.

Although not always necessary to arrive at a diagnosis, the muscle biopsy is the most valuable test in the differential diagnosis of weakness. The significance of the biopsy, however, depends completely on the care exercised in selecting the muscle to be biopsied, the surgical technique employed, the size of the specimen, and the methods by which the tissue is processed for histologic examination.[11] While a relatively simple procedure, it is frequently poorly done.

Prior to the biopsy, a full clinical assessment of the

Table 4-14. Comparison of Electrodiagnostic Findings in Some of the More Common Neuromuscular Disorders

		EMG				
		Activity at Rest		*Motor Unit Action Potentials*		
Disorder	*Nerve Conduction Velocity*	*Fibrillation Potential and/or Sharp Waves*	*Other*	*Amplitude*	*Duration*	*Other*
Motor neuron diseases (ALS, ISMA), acute	Normal	Frequent	Occasional high frequency repetitive discharges	Usually increased	Usually increased	Fasciculation potentials common; reduced interference pattern; short duration, low amplitude polyphasic units
Peripheral neuropathies, acute	Slowing	Frequent	Occasional high frequency repetitive discharges	May be increased, decreased, or normal	Usually increased	Reduced interference pattern; increased duration polyphasic units
Myasthenia gravis	Normal Repetitive nerve stimulation abnormal	Absent	None	Normal	Normal	Normal interference pattern but amplitude drops off with contraction of muscle
Muscular dystrophy	Normal	Occasional	Rare high frequency repetitive discharges	Usually reduced	Usually shortened	Normal interference pattern; short duration, low amplitude polyphasic units
Myotonic dystrophy	Normal	Occasional	Frequent high frequency repetitive discharges which wax and wane	Usually reduced	Usually shortened	Normal interference pattern; short duration, low amplitude polyphasic units.
Congenital myotonia	Normal	Absent	Frequent high frequency repetitive discharges which wax and wane	Normal	Normal	Normal interference pattern
Inflammatory myopathies (polymyositis and dermatomyositis), acute	Normal	Common	Common high frequency repetitive discharges	Usually reduced	Usually shortened	Normal interference pattern; short duration, low amplitude polyphasic units
Congenital "nonprogressive" myopathies	Normal	Rare except in centronuclear myopathy	Rare high frequency discharges except in centronuclear myopathy	Occasionally reduced	Occasionally reduced	Normal interference pattern; occasionally polyphasic units

patient is essential. The selection of the muscle to be biopsied is based on the distribution of weakness since it is important not to select either a muscle which is so severely involved that it will be largely replaced by fat or connective tissue or, on the other hand, a muscle which is completely unaffected. In general, when the weakness is primarily proximal, the rectus femoris or vastus lateralis in the leg or the biceps in the arm are selected. When the distribution of weakness is mainly distal, a more distal limb muscle is selected. It should also be remembered that a muscle which is relatively little involved usually shows the most diagnostic changes in a chronic disease, such as dystrophy of longstanding. A more severely involved muscle is usually selected in an acute disease, such as polymyositis, since the process has not had time to progress to extensive destruction. Biopsies should also be limited to muscles with which the pathologist is familiar since fiber sizes and types show marked variations between different muscles. One should also avoid sampling any muscle which has been the site of an injection or electromyography since needling can produce changes in the muscle which are indistinguishable from inflammatory disease.

It is usually preferable to do muscle biopsies under local anesthesia, thus eliminating the risks attached to general anesthesia which are particularly hazardous in patients with neuromuscular disease because of poor respiratory function. The skin is infiltrated with 1 percent Xylocaine without adrenaline. The muscle itself should not be infiltrated since the purpose of the biopsy is to isolate a portion of the muscle with as little trauma as possible. The incision of about 1½ inches is made over the belly of the muscle in the direction of the fibers. The fascia is then incised to expose the muscle fascicles following retraction of the skin. A strip of muscle, about an inch long by a quarter of an inch wide, is then removed together with the sutures. The muscle may then be stretched on a wooden tongue depressor by securing the sutures over the ends. Maintaining the muscle at a slightly stretched length is critical for electron microscopy. For routine histologic evaluation and for histochemistry, there is no real need to maintain the muscle under stretch although it does help to preserve the orientation of the muscle fascicles. If intravital staining of nerve terminals is desired, the biopsy should be done near the motor point of the muscle as determined by the site of maximum response to an electrical stimulus. After the muscle is removed, the fascia is sutured with absorbable material to prevent muscle herniation and the skin closed. The procedure is usually painless, and patients can use the extremity immediately after the biopsy. The use of percutaneous needle biopsy has recently been advocated. While simple and easily repeatable, only a small sample can be obtained, and there is often difficulty in obtaining a proper orientation of the sample. It may be reasonably reliable when the pathological changes are diffusely distributed, but it usually misses focal changes, such as in denervation processes, and is not a satisfactory alternative to open biopsy.

A review of the preparation of the specimen and the desirable histologic and histochemical stains is beyond the scope of this discussion. For histologic and histochemical studies, however, specimens should be frozen as soon as possible after removal to prevent the loss of soluble enzymes. For electron microscopy, the specimen is placed in 4 percent glutaraldehyde. While probably not necessary for the diagnosis of the more common neuromuscular disease, histochemical studies and electron microscopy are essential for the diagnosis of many of the congenital myopathies. For routine histologic examination, the five stains routinely used are hematoxylin and eosin (H&E), Verhoeff-van Gieson (VVG), modified Gomori trichrome, Sudan black B, and phosphotungstic acid-hematoxylin (PTAH). These will reveal basophilic fibers, proliferation of collagen and lipids, and cytoplasmic structures, such as the rods seen in nemaline myopathy. The major histologic findings found in some of the more common neuromuscular diseases are reviewed in Table 4-15.

Muscle usually responds to pathological circumstances by either hypertrophy, atrophy, or degeneration. While hypertrophy can represent an increase in total muscle volume, the word should be used to indicate an increase in cross-sectional area or the diameter of the muscle or the individual muscle fiber. Atrophy should also be used in a specific sense since it actually refers to a reduction in the size of the individual muscle fibers. However, it is more commonly used clinically to describe reduced total muscle volume. Another word that requires clarifi-

Table 4-15. Comparison of the Major Histological Findings in Some of the More Common Neuromuscular Disorders

Disease	*Changes in Fiber Size*	*Abnormalities of Fiber Distribution*	*Changes in Sarcolemmal Nuclei*	*Degeneration and Regeneration*	*Cellular Reactions*	*Changes in Cytochemical Architecture*
Motor neuron disease (ALS, ISMA)	Small angular fibers Type I and II fiber atrophy Type II fiber hypertrophy	Small group fiber atrophy				
Chronic peripheral neuropathies (peroneal muscular atrophy)	Small angular fibers Type II fiber atrophy Type I fiber hypertrophy	Small group fiber atrophy Fiber type grouping Type I fiber type predominance	Internalization Pyknotic Clumps			
Acute or subacute neuropathies	Small angular fibers Type I and II fiber atrophy	Small group fiber atrophy				Targetoid fibers
Duchenne muscular dystrophy	Type II fiber hypertrophy	Type I fiber type predominance Type II fiber type deficiency	Internalization	Necrosis Basophilia Phagocytosis	Inflammatory Fibrosis	
Limb-girdle dystrophy	Type I and II fiber atrophy Type I and II fiber hypertrophy	Type II fiber type deficiency	Internalization	Necrosis Fiber splitting	Fibrosis	Motheaten and ring fibers
Facioscapulo-humeral dystrophy	Small angular fibers Type II fiber hypertrophy			Necrosis	Inflammatory	Motheaten fibers
Myotonic dystrophy	Type I fiber atrophy Type II fiber hypertrophy	Type II fiber type deficiency	Internalization Pyknotic clumps			Motheaten and ring fibers
Inflammatory myopathies: polymyositis/dermatomyositis	Type I and II fiber atrophy		Internalization	Necrosis	Inflammatory	Motheaten fibers
Congenital "Non-progressive" myopathies	*General:* Occasional small fibers or variation in fiber size and internalization of nuclei. *Specific:* 1. *Central core disease:* Central areas within fibers which stain blue with Gomori trichrome in contrast to red-staining outer myofibrils. Central cores devoid of oxidative enzymes and phosphorylase, mitochondria, and sarcoplasmic reticulum. Usually selectively affects Type I fibers. 2. *Nemaline myopathy:* Red rods within fibers with Gomori trichrome. May selectively affect either Type I or Type II fibers. Rods have a lattice pattern of consistent periodicity and in continuity with Z lines. 3. *Centronuclear myopathy:* Centrally placed nuclei. Myofibrillar ATPase lacking in central zones. May be with or without Type I fiber atrophy. 4. *Congenital fiber type disproportion:* Small Type I and large Type II fibers.					

cation is degeneration, the changes that occur in muscle fibers as they are being destroyed to such an extent that the tissue may, at times, no longer be recognized as muscle.

In summary, the evaluation of the patient with weakness includes a thorough family survey, detailed information concerning the rate, mode of progression and distribution of weakness, and the age at the time of onset. Associated findings such as tenderness, myotonia, and dermal lesions should also be noted. The major diagnostically useful laboratory tests are electromyography, nerve conduction, serum enzyme levels, and muscle biopsy.

Neuromuscular Disorders

In the following discussion, the general format outlined in Tables 4-3 to 4-6 will be followed as closely as possible. Disorders of muscle will be stressed, and only the more common diseases will be described.

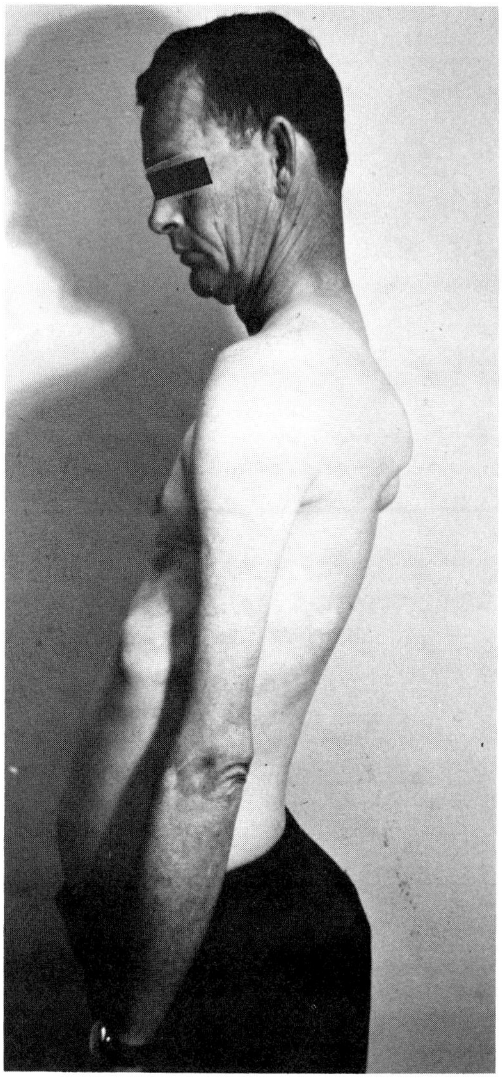

Fig. 4-17. Forty-five-year-old male with limb girdle muscular dystrophy of 35-years' duration.

Weakness or Hypotonia as Predominant Clinical Finding

As outlined in Table 4-3, there are many diseases and syndromes which have weakness as the predominant clinical finding. As summarized in Table 4-9, some are characterized by a rapidly progressive course while others are either static or slowly progressive. Among the more common are the dystrophies, especially Duchenne dystrophy; the inflammatory myopathies, especially the polymyositis syndrome; the toxic and nutritional neuropathies and myopathies; and some of the other peripheral nerve and anterior horn cell diseases, such as amyotrophic lateral sclerosis, infantile spinal muscular atrophy, and the Guillain-Barré syndrome.

Genetically Determined and Congenital Myopathies. The genetically determined and congenital myopathies include the muscular dystrophies, the congenital nonprogressive myopathy syndromes, generalized myositis ossificans, congenital absences of muscle, arthrogryposis, and the glycogen storage diseases. The more common neuropathies include infantile spinal muscular atrophy, familial spinal muscular atrophy, and peroneal muscular atrophy.

Muscular Dystrophies. There are at least nine types of muscular dystrophy each with different clinical and genetic patterns.[1,27] In general, however, the dystrophies may be divided into two major categories (Table 4-16). The first are those characterized by a relatively mild, slowly progressive, restricted course and include the limb-girdle (Fig. 4-17), facioscapulohumeral (Fig. 4-18), myotonic (Fig. 4-6 and 4-19), distal, ocular and oculopharyngeal, and Becker dystrophies. The second category contains those characterized by a relatively severe, rapidly progressive, generalized course. These include the Duchenne (Fig. 4-4, 4-9, 4-11) and congenital dystrophies. The major clinical and laboratory characteristics of each type are reviewed in detail in Tables 4-17 to 4-24.

The diagnosis of muscular dystrophy is never justified unless the patient's clinical features and genetic history clearly place him in one of the above categories. The clinical diagnosis of established cases is rarely difficult especially in the Duchenne, facioscapulohumeral, and myotonic types. The greatest difficulty is in distinguishing the limb-girdle type from chronic polymyositis. Dystrophy in childhood is more common in males while polymyositis is seen

Table 4-16. Dystrophic Myopathies

Slowly progressive	*Rapidly progressive*
Limb-girdle	Duchenne
Facioscapulohumeral	Congenital
Myotonic	
Distal	
Ocular	
Oculopharyngeal	
Becker	

more frequently in females. Dystrophy is an inherited disease usually affecting more than one member of a family. In polymyositis, the progress of the disease is more rapid, and weakness generally affects all proximal muscles equally. Weakness of the neck muscles is more common in polymyositis, dysphagia is frequent, atrophy is less severe than would be expected from the degree of weakness, hypertrophy is rare, and the deep tendon reflexes tend to be spared longer.

In Duchenne dystrophy, carrier detection is important for genetic counseling. The female carrier of the Duchenne dystrophic gene can affect 50 percent

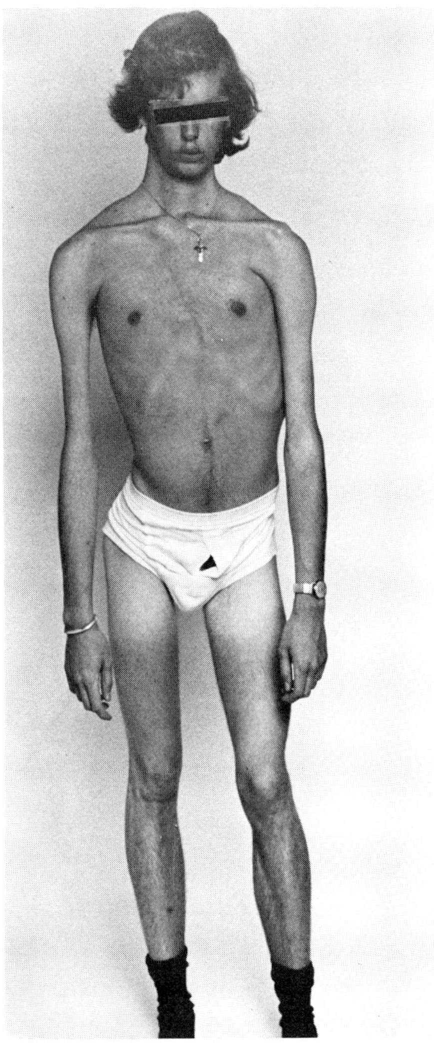

Fig. 4-18. Nineteen-year-old male with facioscapulohumeral muscular dystrophy of 14-years' duration.

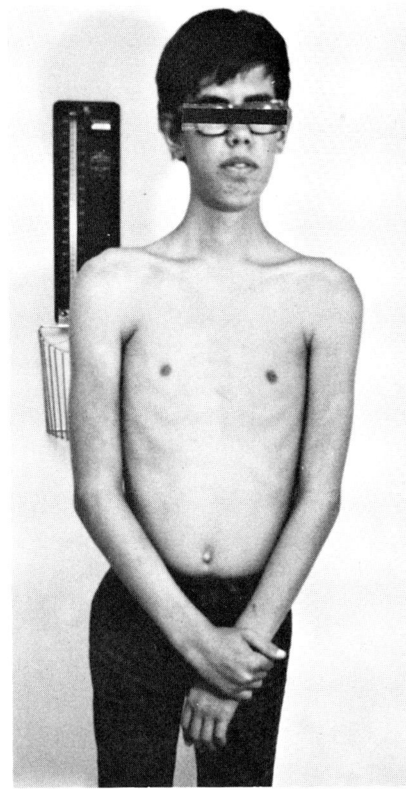

Fig. 4-19. Fourteen-year-old boy with myotonic dystrophy of at least 12-years' duration.

of her sons with the disease and each of her daughters has a 50 percent risk of becoming a carrier. All true carriers of the Duchenne gene probably have a slight degree of myopathy which is usually subclinical, and 60 to 75 percent of definite carriers can be detected by serum creatine phosphokinase levels. Carrier detection by enzyme analysis should be done as early as possible because the reliability of the test decreases markedly with increasing age.[21] For a more detailed discussion of the genetic aspects of the dystrophies the reader is referred to other more comprehensive sources.[11,17,27]

Table 4-17. Limb-Girdle Dystrophy

Onset:	Variable; late in first decade to adult life but usually in second or third decade.
Genetics and Incidence:	Usually autosomal recessive (59%); rarely as autosomal dominant. Abortive cases are uncommon. Expression is in either sex. Incidence

Table 4-17. (*Continued*)

Genetics and Incidence:	rate for autosomal recessive trait of 468×10^{-7} to 385×10^{-7} with a prevalence rate of 142×10^{-7} to 118×10^{-7}. Incidence rate for sporatic cases ranges from 326×10^{-7} to 268×10^{-7} with a prevalence rate of 99×10^{-7} to 82×10^{-7}.
Rate of Progression:	Extremely variable. Severe disability usually occurs 10 to 20 years after the onset, especially when the onset is in the first decade of life (childhood muscular dystrophy with autosomal recessive inheritance). In some cases with late onset, however, there may be periods of apparent arrest. Life expectancy is often shortened by 10 to 20 years.
Distribution of Weakness:	Primary involvement of either shoulder or pelvic girdle muscles with spread to other muscles after a variable period of time. Dorsiflexors are rarely involved early.
Clinical Characteristics:	Muscles in upper extremities most often affected early are the serratus, trapezius, rhomboids, latissimus, and pectoralis major with occasional involvement of the neck muscles; deltoids are often spared until quite late. In the lower extremities, the hip flexors, extensors, and adductors and the knee extensors are usually affected early. Weakness and atrophy are sometimes asymmetrical. Contractures and deformity are rare until late in the disease. Hypertrophy of the calves and lateral vastus occur in about one third of the cases. Clinical cardiac involvement is rare. Prognosis is better in those cases in which the shoulder girdle muscles are first involved.
Laboratory Characteristics:	Serum enzymes may be markedly elevated in patients with an early onset and normal or only slightly elevated in cases with a late onset. EMG is usually abnormal with a normal nerve conduction.
Differential Diagnosis:	Polymyositis, scapuloperoneal atrophy, muscle glycogenosis, sarcoid myopathy, and the myopathies of thyrotoxicosis and osteomalacia, central core disease, nemaline myopathy, carnitine deficiency, and mitochondrial myopathy.

Table 4-18. Facioscapulohumeral Dystrophy (Landouzy-Dejerine)

Onset:	Insidious; early childhood to adult life but usually in the second decade.
Genetics and Incidence:	Usually autosomal dominant occasionally with apparent sex limitations in some families. Abortive or mildly affected cases are quite common. Rarely inherited as an autosomal recessive trait. Expression is in either sex. Incidence rate ranges from 92×10^{-7} to 38×10^{-7} with a prevalence rate of 56×10^{-7} to 23×10^{-7}.
Rate of Progression:	Usually very benign. Considerable variation, however, from one family to another and even within the same family. No apparent progression for several years in some cases. Essentially normal life expectancy.
Distribution of Weakness:	Initial involvement of face and shoulder girdle muscles and early involvement of foot dorsiflexors with subsequent spread to pelvic girdle muscles.
Clinical Characteristics:	Unlined face, pouting appearance of lips and transverse smile. Difficulty in closing eyes and inability to whistle. With advanced weakness unable to pronounce labials and often have indistinct speech. Pattern of muscular involvement is similar to limb-girdle dystrophy but with a characteristic difficulty in elevation of the scapula when the arms are abducted. Asymmetry of weakness and atrophy and occasional absence of muscles in some cases. Muscular hypertrophy is uncommon, and it is rare that any contractures and deformity are present. Clinical cardiac involvement is uncommon.
Laboratory Characteristics:	Serum enzymes are usually normal or slightly elevated. EMG is usually abnormal with a normal nerve conduction.
Differential Diagnosis:	Early: ocular and oculopharyngeal myopathy, myotonic dystrophy, myasthenia gravis, congenital ptosis, and congenital facial diplegia. Late: limb-girdle dystrophy and polymyositis. Some cases have been reported to show inflammatory changes in muscle resembling polymyositis.

Table 4-19. Myotonic Dystrophy (Steinert)

Onset:	Variable; birth to fourth decade.
Genetics and Incidence:	Autosomal dominant with complete or almost complete penetrance. Diversity of findings suggests the pleiotropic effects of a single autosomal dominant gene. Expression is in either sex. Incidence ranges from 120×10^{-5} to 5×10^{-5}.
Rate of Progression:	Variable; adult type usually quite gradual.
Distribution of Weakness:	Weakness and atrophy usually generalized but primarily proximal in the early stages. Clinical myotonia is primarily found in the hand, ocular muscles, and tongue and often occurs before the onset of weakness.
Clinical Characteristics:	Marked heterogeneity of expression of various traits and symptoms with multiple organ involvement including skeletal, smooth, and cardiac muscle, cataracts, testicular atrophy with diminished fertility, baldness, and mental retardation. Types can be grouped as follows: Adult onset either with or without 1. Cardiovascular features 2. Pulmonary and respiratory muscle involvement 3. Visceral or smooth muscle involvement 4. Various endocrinopathies Early onset with positive family history in adults 1. Myotonia as only early feature 2. Onset in infancy with hypotonia and facial diplegia 3. Occult myotonia with speech abnormalities and mental retardation
Laboratory Characteristics:	Usually normal or slightly elevated serum enzymes. EMG always abnormal with a normal nerve conduction. EKG is usually abnormal.
Differential Diagnosis:	Congenital myotonia, hyperkalemic periodic paralysis, Schwartz-Jampel syndrome, and facioscapulohumeral dystrophy.

Table 4-20. Distal Dystrophy (Gower)

Onset:	Usually between ages of 30 and 40.
Genetics and Incidence:	Dominant. Expression is in either sex but is more common in men. Very rare.
Rate of Progression:	Very slow and comparatively benign. Essentially a normal life expectancy.
Clinical Characteristics:	Usually begins in the hand muscles and spreads to the plantar and dorsiflexors of the feet.
Laboratory Characteristics:	Serum enzymes usually within normal limits. EMG of distal muscles often abnormal with a normal nerve conduction.
Differential Diagnosis:	Peroneal muscular atrophy and distal chronic spinal muscular atrophy.

Table 4-21. Ocular Myopathy

Onset:	Early childhood to adult life but usually in childhood.
Genetics and Incidence:	Most are sporadic but may also be dominant. Expression is in either sex. Very rare.
Rate of Progression:	Variable; essentially normal life expectancy.
Clinical Characteristics:	Weakness of external ocular muscles. Some facial weakness is often present and 25 percent have a slight degree of skeletal muscle weakness elsewhere. Frequent association with clinical features of central nervous system involvement, retinal pigmentation, heart block, growth failure, and deafness.
Laboratory Characteristics:	Serum enzymes usually within normal limits. EMG of external ocular muscles may be abnormal. EKG may show a heart block.
Differential Diagnosis:	Oculopharyngeal myopathy, myotonic dystrophy, Refsum's syndrome, myasthenia gravis, congenital ptosis, and congenital facial diplegia.
Oculopharyngeal Myopathy:	Ocular myopathy plus dysphagia with a later onset and a dominant inheritance.

The etiology of the muscular dystrophies remains unknown, and there is probably a different biochemical lesion for each type. Current evidence indicates, however, that they may not be primary degenerative myopathies. The primary lesion in some, such as myotonic dystrophy, now appears to reside in the membrane of several body tissues. In all types there is evidence of involvement of multiple organ tissues, including the nervous system. In all probability, the etiology will most likely be a genetically determined biochemical defect with a pleiotropic effect and multiple organ involvement. It is beyond

Table 4-22. Becker Dystrophy (Benign X-Linked)

Onset:	Between 5 and 25 years of age.
Genetics and Incidence:	Expression in males. Sex linked recessive with transmission of the disorder by affected males through carrier daughters to their grandsons. Lower mutation rate than with Duchenne dystrophy. Incidence rate estimated at 279×10^{-7} to 92×10^{-7} with a prevalence rate of 56×10^{-7} to 23×10^{-7}.
Rate of Progression:	Relatively gradual with inability to walk 25 years after the onset. Often a normal life span.
Clinical Characteristics:	Wasting of pelvic and later of the shoulder girdle muscles. Hypertrophy of calf muscles less common than in Duchenne dystrophy. Normal mentation. Contractures are rare in most cases. Rarely cardiac involvement.
Laboratory Characteristics:	Serum enzymes moderately elevated. EMG usually abnormal with a normal nerve conduction. EKG occasionally abnormal.
Differential Diagnosis:	Duchenne dystrophy, limb girdle dystrophy of early onset, and some of the congenital myopathies.

Table 4-23. Duchenne Dystrophy (Severe X-linked)

Onset:	Almost always between 18 months and 4 years.
Genetics and Incidence:	Sex-linked recessive with a high mutation rate. Expression is in males although female carriers may be rarely involved. Abortive cases rarely occur, if ever. Estimates of incidence range from 251×10^{-6} to 160×10^{-6} with a prevalence rate of 59×10^{-6} to 38×10^{-6}. One third of the new mutants have a previous family history and one third are born to unwitting and often mutant carriers.
Rate of Progression:	Relentlessly progressive weakness leading to inability to walk within 7 to 11 years of life with death in the second or third decade from cardiac or respiratory failure.
Distribution of Weakness:	Selective involvement of the pelvic girdle muscles rapidly followed by weakness of the shoulder girdle muscles.
Clinical Characteristics:	Unless there is mental retardation, developmental landmarks are normal followed by clumsiness in walking and especially in running or climbing stairs. Child then usually walks with a waddle, protrudes the abdomen with lordosis, and rises on the toes. At ages 4 or 5 years, growth may outstrip the progress of the disease leading to a false impression of improvement. Rapid increase in weakness may follow bed rest. Weakness in the lower extremities usually begins in the hip flexors and extensors and the knee extensors and rapidly spreads to foot dorsiflexors. In the upper extremities the serratus, pectoralis, and latissimus and later the elbow flexors are first involved. Calf and neck muscles remain relatively strong for many years. Usually a symmetrical involvement. Hypertrophy of the calf muscles and often of other muscles. Rapidly progressive muscular contractures and early skeletal deformity, especially scoliosis. Some become very thin while others are very obese. Mental retardation occurs in about one third of the cases. Cardiac involvement always occurs.
Laboratory Characteristics:	Serum enzymes are markedly elevated until late in the disease. EMG always abnormal with a normal nerve conduction. EKG usually abnormal.
Differential Diagnosis:	Congenital dystrophy, limb-girdle dystrophy of early onset with calf hypertrophy, and some of the congenital myopathies.

the scope of this book to discuss the management of diseases so the interested reader is referred to other sources for a discussion of the detailed management of the dystrophies.[26] Suffice it to say at this time that the physician can only offer these individuals the physical and surgical treatment of complications and psychological support.

Congenital Nonprogressive Myopathies and Related Diseases. These disorders, several of which now appear to have a neuropathic component, are quite rare (Table 4-25). Their major importance is that they are usually nonprogressive or at times very slowly progressive and, hence, must be considered in

Table 4-24. Congenital Dystrophy

Onset:	Birth.
Genetics and Incidence:	Usually recessive. Expression is in either sex. Very rare.
Rate of Progression:	Variable; ranging from severe but relatively nonprogressive weakness to rapidly progressive weakness and death at 6 to 12 months.
Clinical Characteristics:	Essential features are severe hypotonia from birth with variable progression of weakness. High association with arthrogryposis. Syndrome overlaps with benign congenital myopathy.
Laboratory Characteristics:	Serum enzymes are usually normal to slightly elevated. EMG is usually abnormal with normal nerve conduction.
Differential Diagnosis:	Arthrogryposis of neurogenic origin, infantile spinal muscular atrophy, benign congenital hypotonia, and autosomal recessive childhood dystrophy.

Table 4-25. Congenital and Related Myopathies

Congenital nonprogressive myopathy syndrome
Central core disease
Nemaline myopathy
Centronuclear myopathy
Mitochondrial diseases
Type I fiber hypotrophy
Reducing body myopathy
Cytoplasmic inclusion myopathy
Fingerprint body myopathy
Multicore disease
Lipid metabolism disorders affecting muscle: carnitine myopathy
Myositis ossificans
Arthrogryposis multiplex congenita
Congenital defects in muscle
Idiopathic—"benign congenital hypotonia"

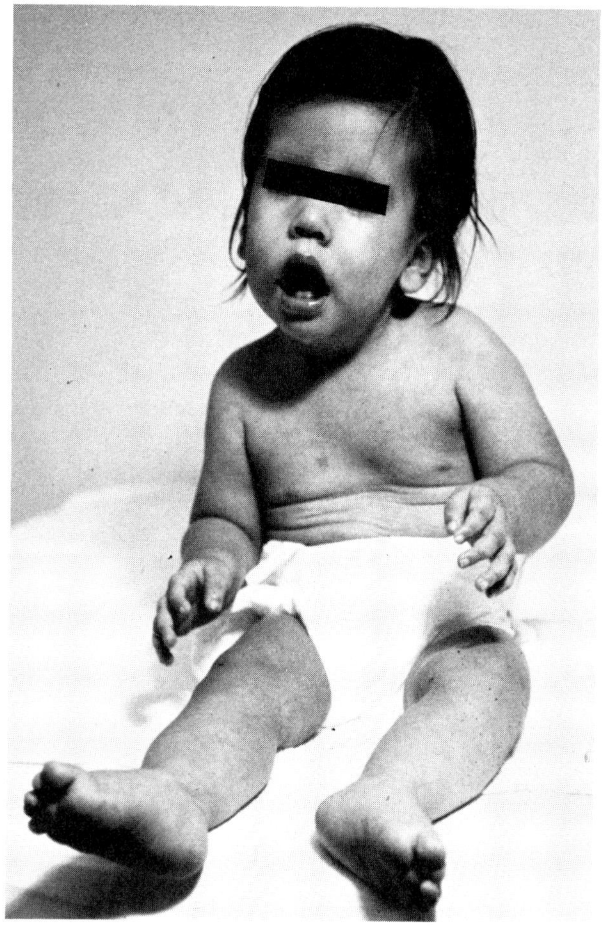

Fig. 4-20. One-year-old child with nemaline myopathy. Child was hypotonic since birth.

the differential diagnosis of the progressive nontreatable diseases like muscular dystrophy.[12,22,25]

The first group, sometimes called the congenital nonprogressive myopathy syndrome, includes central core disease, nemaline or rod body myopathy (Fig. 4-20), centronuclear myopathy, and mitochondrial disease. Their clinical characteristics are reviewed in Table 4-26 and their histologic findings in Table 4-15. The mitochondrial disorders are not a homogeneous group and include various types, such as megaconial myopathy, pleoconial myopathy, hypermetabolism due to deficient mitochondrial respiratory control, and myopathies with inclusions in the mitochondria. Some are related to the various disorders of lipid metabolism affecting muscle, and mitochondrial abnormalities have also been reported in myotonic dystrophy and the periodic paralyses.[22] The others in this syndrome have specific pathological characteristics.

Most of the other disorders listed in Table 4-25 are extremely rare. There are two types of myositis ossificans—progressive myositis ossificans (fibrodysplasia ossificans progressiva) and traumatic ossifying myositis (myositis ossificans circumscripta). In progressive myositis ossificans there is widespread generalized sclerosis of muscle connective tissue followed by the deposition of bone. It is usually associated with a congenital anomaly of the great toes or other digits and appears to be transmitted by a

Table 4-26. Congenital Nonprogressive Myopathy Syndrome

Onset:	Birth or shortly thereafter.
Genetics and Incidence:	Autosomal dominant-central core, nemaline, and centro-nuclear myopathies. Autosomal recessive—most mitochondrial myopathies. All quite rare.
Rate of Progression:	Nonprogressive or very slowly progressive.
Distribution of Weakness:	Diffuse, mainly proximal, symmetrical, and with frequent involvement of the cranial musculature.
Clinical Characteristics:	Delayed achievement of developmental landmarks. Often associated with other congenital deformities, such as a cleft palate.
Laboratory Characteristics:	Serum enzymes are usually normal or slightly elevated. EMG is often abnormal with a normal nerve conduction.
Differential Diagnosis:	Other congenital myopathies, infantile spinal muscular atrophy.

dominant gene. Ultimately, large groups of muscles become ossified leading to an early death from terminal asphyxia.[1] Another congenital defect is congenital absence of muscles which includes several syndromes such as congenital ptosis, congenital facial diplegia, and congenital contractures of muscles.[1] The latter includes the syndromes of congenital clubfoot, congenital torticollis, Sprengel's deformity, and arthrogryposis.

Arthrogryposis multiplex congenita is a syndrome characterized by joint contractures present at birth in at least two different areas of the body, no evidence of progressive neurological disease, and evidence of muscle wasting with fusiform joint configuration.[1,12,25] There are often grotesque deformities of joints but no bony ankylosis. In a typical case there is talipes equinovarus deformity of the feet, the hips are either abducted and flexed or extended, the knees and elbows are extended, the forearms pronated, and the hands flexed with a claw-like apposition of thenar and hypothenar eminences (see Fig. 4-3). Based upon a number of reports it would appear that arthrogryposis is not a single entity but rather a clinical syndrome that originates from a number of different pathological processes causing immobilization of the limbs during or shortly after the embryonic formation of joints. It has been reported in patients with neuropathic diseases, such as loss of anterior horn cells, atrophy of the corticospinal tracts, and a nodular fibrosis of the anterior spinal roots, as well as in patients with myopathic diseases, such as congenital muscular dystrophy and glycogen storage disorders. It has also been observed in patients with disseminated lipogranulomatosis (Farber's disease) and in embryonic failure of muscle development.

Glycogen Storage Diseases. While interesting in that the enzyme abnormality has been identified in most types, these diseases representing specific biochemical defects in carbohydrate metabolism are quite rare (Table 4-27).[27] All glycogen storage diseases do not affect the skeletal muscles. Children with Pompe's disease, branching enzyme deficiency, and debranching enzyme deficiency usually have marked hypotonia with remorseless deterioration, although a relatively benign course has been reported in adults. Other organs are also involved. Myophosphorylase, phosphohexoisomerase, and phosphofructokinase deficiencies are characterized by muscular pain, cramps, and stiffness during anaerobic exercise.

Neuropathies. These disorders often have a variable clinical course and are often confused with the muscular dystrophies. Although only the infantile, familial (juvenile), and scapuloperoneal spinal muscular atrophies and peroneal muscular atrophy will be discussed, this category includes other disorders, such as familial motor neuron disease, amyotrophy in some of the upper motor neuron disorders and in syringomyelia as well as some of the rare childhood peripheral nerve diseases like leukodystrophy, hypertrophic interstitial neuropathy, and neurofibromatosis.[8,19]

The spinal muscular atrophies outlined in Table 4-28 are a group of inherited disorders in which the primary defect is degeneration of the anterior horn cells and, in some, of the bulbar motor nuclei. The

Table 4-27. Glycogen Storage Diseases

Pompe's disease
Branching enzyme deficiency
Debranching enzyme deficiency
Phosphoglucomutase deficiency
Myophosphorylase deficiency
Phosphohexoisomerase deficiency
Phosphofructokinase deficiency

Table 4-28. Inherited Spinal Muscular Atrophies

Proximal
Infantile
Intermediate
Juvenile
Adult
Distal
Juvenile Progressive Bulbar Palsy
Scapuloperoneal Muscular Atrophy
Facioscapulohumeral

occasional instances of genetic heterogeneity and the variable course in many support a unitary hypothesis and suggest that phenotypic variation may result from the effect of modifier genes. There is a tendency for the clinical course to follow certain patterns which are often repeated when more than one member of a family is affected. The distribution of weakness is symmetrical and predominantly affects either the proximal or distal limb muscles. Sensory loss is rare. Spinal muscular atrophy can produce its effects at any time from embryonic life to middle age. If occurring in the embryonic period, the baby is often born with arthrogryposis; if in the fetal period, a reduction of normal fetal movements may often be noted; if at birth, profound hypotonia is usually found; if in infancy, delay in postural control and weakness are often the presenting signs; and in later childhood and adult life, fatigue, weakness, and atrophy develop. In general, the spinal muscular atrophies are progressive and usually the earlier the onset the swifter is the downhill course. All appear to be genetically determined, and those that are fatal in early childhood usually show an autosomal recessive inheritance. In the more benign forms, autosomal dominant as well as autosomal recessive inheritance occur. In those with an autosomal recessive inheritance, males are usually more severely affected than females.[19,25]

The clinical and laboratory characteristics of infantile spinal muscular atrophy (Werdnig-Hoffmann disease) (see Fig. 4-5 and 4-21) are summarized in Table 4-29. Werdnig-Hoffmann disease is considered by some authors to exist as two types: acute and chronic. The latter in this review is considered as the intermediate type of spinal muscular atrophy and is characterized by a later onset in infancy, up to two years, and a known mean survival beyond 10 years.

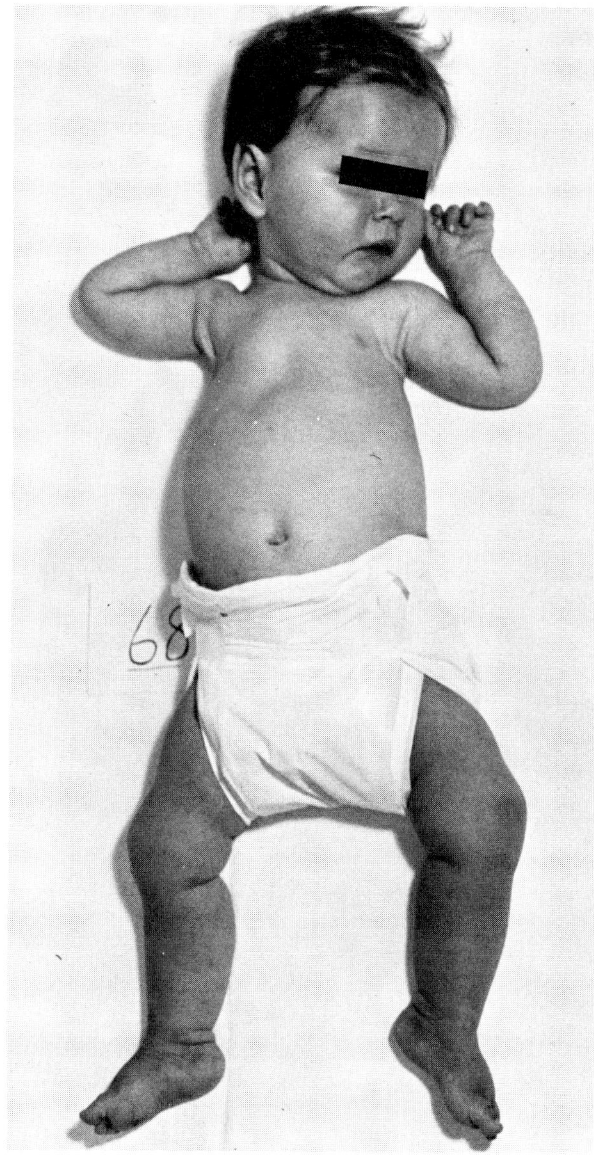

Fig. 4-21. One-month-old child with infantile spinal muscular atrophy and hypotonia since birth.

Inheritance is also usually autosomal recessive. Weakness is usually generalized but initially may be primarily evident in the proximal muscles of the lower extremities. Motor milestones are delayed, the cranial nerves are less severely affected than in the acute form, fasciculations of the tongue usually develop, and progression is relatively slow. Disability in later life ranges from moderate to severe.[19-25] Juvenile proximal muscular atrophy (Kugelberg and

Table 4-29. Infantile Spinal Muscular Atrophy

Onset:	Birth to six months. In about one third decreased fetal movements occur.
Genetics and Incidence:	Autosomal recessive. Expression is in either sex with the risks of involvement in a sibling being one in four. Incidence is one in 20,000 births.
Rate of Progression:	Rapidly progressive with early intercostal weakness accompanied or followed by progressive bulbar weakness and increasing respiratory difficulties. About 50 percent die before the age of 18 months.
Distribution of Weakness:	Severe generalized muscle involvement which is often greater in the proximal muscles.
Clinical Characteristics:	Delayed motor developmental milestones. Early involvement of cervical and trunk musculature. Profuse hypotonia with abducted limbs in "frog" position, expressionless face, and open mouth. Paradoxical respiratory movements, bell-shaped chest, and severe intercostal muscle weakness. Total tendon areflexia. No corticospinal or sensory changes. Tongue fasciculation in at least 50 percent. Some have dysphagia. In spite of massive hypotonia, the baby is usually alert in contrast to cases of hypotonia of cerebral origin.
Laboratory Characteristics:	Serum enzymes are usually normal or slightly elevated. Normal nerve conductions and abnormal EMG.
Differential Diagnosis:	Congenital muscular dystrophy, myotonic dystrophy, congenital myopathies, glycogen storage diseases, neonatal myasthenia gravis, birth trauma, flaccid forms of cerebral palsy, leukodystrophy, acute neuropathies, and benign congenital hypotonia.

Welander) and scapuloperoneal atrophy are much less common, and the others listed in Table 4-28 are quite rare. In juvenile proximal muscular atrophy, the onset occurs between 2 and 17 years of age, and most cases have an autosomal recessive pattern of inheritance. Its principal characteristics are a slowly progressive, symmetrical, proximal limb weakness commencing in the lower extremities and the frequent occurrence of fasciculations in the limb muscles but rarely in the tongue. Hypertrophy of the calves occurs frequently, thus, it is often mistaken for Duchenne muscular dystrophy. The disease may have an abrupt onset related to a febrile illness or may show a stuttering course. Most patients have a normal life span.[19,25] Scapuloperoneal atrophy, often confused with muscular dystrophy, is characterized by an onset in adult life although sporadic cases with an onset in infancy have been reported. It is usually autosomal dominant and the presenting symptoms are symmetrical weakness and atrophy of the long extensor muscles of the feet. After several years, the shoulder girdle muscles become involved (Fig. 4-22), and the leg weakness spreads to involve the calf and proximal thigh muscles.[19,25]

The only relatively common inherited peripheral nerve disease is peroneal muscular atrophy (Charcot-Marie-Tooth disease) (Fig. 4-23). Inheritance is variable, including autosomal dominant and sex-linked recessive patterns. There are various expressions so only the more common type with dominant inheritance will be described. The earliest signs are pes cavus and gait disturbances which usually appear

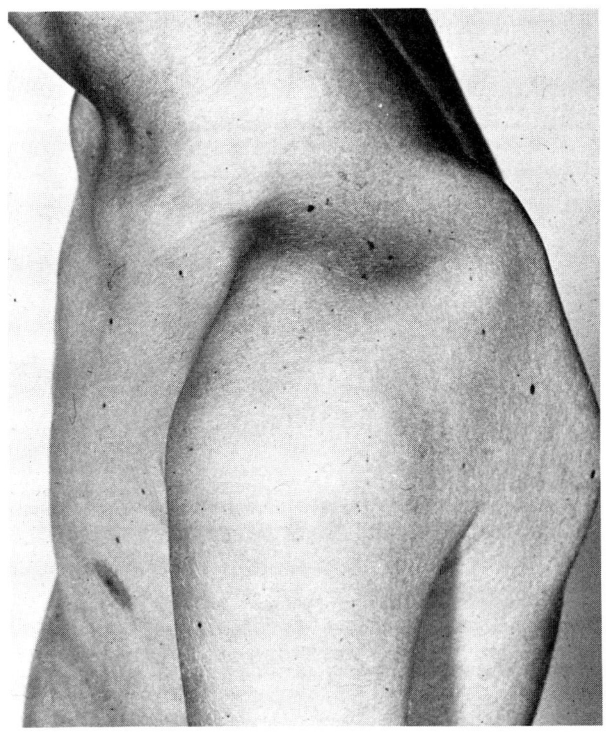

Fig. 4-22. Marked atrophy of the shoulder girdle muscles in a 35-year-old male with scapuloperoneal atrophy of about 10-years' duration.

by the second decade due to progressive weakness of the dorsiflexors of the feet. A progressive foot drop develops with later involvement of the hands. Sensory impairment may appear late. A number of relatives may be without symptoms but will often have marked slowing of nerve conduction velocities. It is usually slowly progressive, and most patients can still ambulate with braces long after the onset. Other types of this variable disorder have been observed, and peroneal muscular atrophy may also occur in other diseases such as in the Roussy-Levy syndrome and Friedreich's ataxia.[8]

Infectious and Inflammatory Myopathies and Neuropathies. *Myopathies.* As can be seen in Table 4-30, these myopathies can be divided into two major areas: infectious diseases of known etiology affecting muscle and the inflammatory myopathies of unknown etiology.

The two most important types of *bacteria myositis* are acute suppurative and clostridial.[1] Acute myositis with pus formation may occur with blood stream infections, follow crush or infected bullet wounds, or be associated with infectious arthritis, pleuritis, or decubitus ulcers from which it arises by direct extension. The most common causative organisms are staphylococcus and streptococcus. The rarity of abscess formation in muscle, even in the face of overwhelming septicemia, indicates that muscle does not provide a suitable medium for the growth of most bacteria. *Streptococcus pyogenes* may produce local gas formation and general toxemia resulting in a condition closely resembling clostridial myositis. Trauma to muscle leading to necrosis renders it susceptible to infection, especially *clostridium welchii.* Saprophytic bacteria cause rapid decomposition of the tissue with the formation of gas bubbles and edema. This produces the characteristic finding in

Table 4-30. Infectious and Inflammatory Myopathies

Known etiology
Bacterial
Fungal
Parasitic
Viral
Unknown etiology
Polymyositis syndrome
Myositis with connective tissue disorders
Disseminated lupus erythematosus
Rheumatic fever
Rheumatoid arthritis
Scleroderma and/or systemic sclerosis
Scleroderma with myopathy
Ocular myositis
Polyarteritis nodosa
Sjögren's disease
Werner's disease
Myositis in malignant disease
Sarcoidosis with myopathy
Granulomatous myopathy
Polymyalgia rheumatica
Localized myositis ossificans
Fibrositis and nodular fasciitis
Myopathy in relapsing panniculitis
Myopathy in psoriasis

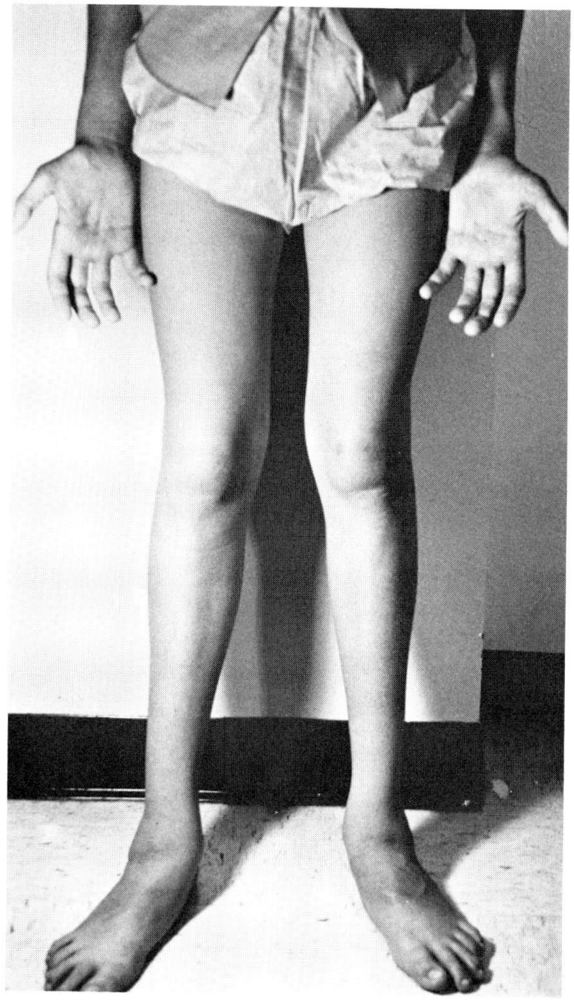

Fig. 4-23. Pes cavus and atrophy of the muscles below the knee in a 15-year-old child with Charcot-Marie-Tooth disease.

gas gangrene of a watery discharge and crepitus to palpation. Other bacterial infections involving muscle are tetanus, tuberculous myositis, syphilitic myositis, and leprous myositis. Presumed *viral infections* of muscle include Bornholm disease and epidemic torticollis and some occur following influenza. The viruses of the Coxsackie Group B have been implicated in patients with these diseases.

Parasitic type organisms affecting skeletal muscle include *Toxoplasma gondii, Trypanosoma cruzi, Cysticercus,* and *Trichinella spiralis.* The causal agent of trichinosis, *Trichinella spiralis,* is a nematode which frequently infects the hog, rat, and human as result of the ingestation of raw or poorly cooked pork. The symptomatology of trichinosis in humans is variable and depends on the number of viable ingested parasites. Three clinical stages are recognized. The first, intestinal stage, appears from the second to seventh day after ingestion as a mild gastroenteritis. The second stage, muscular invasion, begins at about the end of the second week and lasts about five weeks. Symptoms during this period are due to the effects on the tissues of the embryo trichinae: chilliness, low grade fever, pain and tenderness in the trunk and extremities, edema of the conjunctival and orbital tissues, fatigue, and weakness. Unusually heavy infestations may provoke disorders of the central nervous system, involvement of the myocardium, and a skin eruption. Eosinophilic leukocytosis, sensitivity to the trichinae antigen, and the appearance of antibodies aid in the diagnosis. The third stage of convalescence is indicated by the subsidence of symptoms and usually occurs during the second month of the infection. Trichinosis is seldom fatal, but there is a high incidence in the United States estimated at 18 to 22 percent of the adult population. Muscle weakness can be accounted for by the effect of an interstitial inflammatory reaction.[1]

There are a number of conditions in which nonsuppurative inflammation occurs. Prominent in this group is the polymyositis syndrome in which weakness occurs to some degree in every case (Table 4-31).[23] The general characteristics of the typical adult type are reviewed in Table 4-32. Pathologically, inflammatory and degenerative changes are found in the muscles. About one half of all the cases included in the polymyositis syndrome are linked with one of the collagen tissue disorders or with a malignant

Table 4-31. Polymyositis Syndrome

Polymyositis in adults	Childhood dermatomyositis
Dermatomyositis in adults	Acute myolysis
Myositis with malignancy	

Table 4-32. Polymyositis and Dermatomyositis in Adults

Onset:	Polymyositis—third to fifth decade usually with an insidious onset. Dermatomyositis—second to seventh decade usually with an acute onset.
Incidence:	Five new cases/million population/year. More common in females.
Rate of Progression:	Variable but usually rapidly progressive in acute polymyositis. Exacerbations and remissions may occur.
Distribution of Weakness:	Primarily proximal but, in addition, weakness of the anterior neck and pharyngeal muscles is very common. Usually symmetrical.
Clinical Characteristics:	No initiating cause evident in most cases. The first symptom is muscular weakness in about 42 percent of all cases, a skin rash in 25 percent, and joint or muscular pain in 15 percent. Early clinical picture, rate of onset, and progression of symptoms is quite variable. At some time, however, weakness is present in all cases, pain or tenderness in over 50 percent, dysphagia in 54 percent, Raynaud's phenomenon in 33 percent, and arthritic features in 33 percent. Contractures and atrophy except in cases of long-standing are rare. In subacute or chronic cases, the weakness may come on slowly and closely resemble muscular dystrophy. The typical rash of dermatomyositis, a dusky erythematous eruption on the face, periorbital regions, neck, shoulders, and upper chest, occurs in about 40 percent of the patients. Other common skin manifestations include the thickening also seen in systemic sclerosis, dermal atrophy (poikilohyperemia) about the base and along the side of the fingernails and on the ends of the fingers. On the upper eyelids a dusky lilac suffusion can often be seen called a heliotrope which is pathognomonic for dermatomyositis. Occasionally, there is cardiac interstitial fibrosis and pneumonitis.

Table 4-32. (*Continued*)

Laboratory Characteristics:	Serum enzymes and sedimentation rate are usually elevated at least in acute cases. Abnormality of serum proteins and positive tests for circulating rheumatoid factor occur in 50 percent of all cases. EMG is usually abnormal with a normal nerve conduction. Pharyngeal weakness and hypomotility of the esophagus can often be demonstrated roentgenographically.
Differential Diagnosis:	Chronic cases often confused with limb-girdle dystrophy and acute cases with other collagen diseases.

tumor. Dermatomyositis and occasionally polymyositis with malignancy, usually a carcinoma, occur most commonly after 40 and are slightly more frequent in men. Proximal weakness is the rule, and dysphagia is common. Response to corticosteroid therapy is generally poor in contrast to that noted in polymyositis or dermatomyositis in adults. Childhood dermatomyositis shows either an acute or a chronic course and often results in severe contractures, skin ulceration, and calcification in the affected muscles. Subcutaneous calcinosis and ulcerations over bony prominences which extrude calcium are prominent features. Pathologically, marked vascular changes occur. It may run a self-limiting course, and some patients do not respond to corticosteroid therapy. Acute myolysis is also more common in children and can recur. Whether this is a true variant of polymyositis or a separate necrotizing myolysis of unknown origin is not clear.

Although still not confirmed, clinical and pathological findings as well as experimental evidence indicate an immunological pathogenesis for the polymyositis syndrome. The onset is often preceded by viral infection, and viral particles in the muscle have been reported in some cases, suggesting a mechanism of hypersensitivity. Neoplasia may be another precipitant. The association of the polymyositis syndrome with other connective tissue disorders is also significant since there is considerable evidence for an immunological basis in these conditions. Corticosteroid therapy has proved the first and virtually the only form of effective therapy and is capable of suppressing activity and altering the natural course of the disorder. Although not yet well documented, immunosuppressive drugs may be required in those patients who do not respond to steroid therapy. Physical and surgical treatment are rarely needed except in patients with a chronic course.

Other types of inflammatory myositis, outlined in Table 4-30, include focal nodular myositis in systemic lupus erythematosus, rheumatoid arthritis, Sjögren's disease, scleroderma, acute rheumatic fever, vacuolar myopathy in systemic lupus erythematosus, muscular involvement in polyarteritis nodosa, Werner's disease, psoriasis, relapsing panniculitis, sarcoidosis of muscle, polymyalgia rheumatica, and neuromyositis. These are either extremely rare or else occur primarily as an incidental finding in skeletal muscle.[1,23] One which is very common, however, is interstitial myofibrositis (myogelosis, fibromyositis) which is a diffuse, poorly defined syndrome, presumed to be an inflammation of the interstitial connective tissue elements of muscle. Cold, dampness, and especially trauma are predisposing factors, and the syndrome consists of pain and stiffness often of acute onset in and around a group of muscles. The neck and shoulder are the most common sites of involvement, and firm, tender nodules are found in most cases. Low grade fever may occur at the onset of the illness which is self-limiting. Muscular strength is usually good although a mild atrophy may be present. Careful deep palpation of the muscles usually reveals evidence of a localized edema. Histologic changes include the presence of a metachromatic mucoid substance in the nodular areas with mast cells and platelet clots. The cause is assumed to be trauma which leads to extravasation of blood, release of serotonin, vasoconstriction, edema, degranulation of the mast cells, and release of histamine and heparin to counteract the vasoconstriction and clotting.[3]

Neuropathies. The infectious and inflammatory neuropathies include the anterior horn cell amyotrophies of poliomyelitis and encephalitis and the peripheral nerve diseases associated with diphtheria, leprosy, syphilis, sarcoidosis, the collagen vascular disorders, and the Guillain-Barré syndrome.[8,19] The characteristics of the latter are outlined in Table 4-33.

Endocrine and Related Myopathies and Neuropathies. Only the muscle disorders associated with disturbances of thyroid function and steroid myopathy have clinical significance (Table 4-34). Muscular weakness and wasting are frequent

Table 4-33. Guillain-Barré Syndrome

Onset:	Peak of involvement up to two weeks following the onset of weakness. Fifty percent have a history of some preceding viral infection two to four weeks prior to the onset of the weakness.
Incidence:	Quite common and occurs in all age groups.
Rate of Progression:	Variable; ranges from the acute with a relatively poor prognosis to the subacute and chronic cases with a worsening of the prognosis.
Distribution of Weakness:	Diffuse in 50 percent. In the remainder, there is a spread from the lower limbs to involve the arms, the respiratory system, and then the bulbar muscles.
Clinical Characteristics:	About one-fourth begin with paresthesias in the feet spreading proximally and then involving the hands. Over a third have moderately severe pain and tenderness in the back and limbs. Sensory loss is usually slight or absent. Paresis is usually maximum for one to four weeks with a gradual recovery over a three to six week period. About 25 percent require artificial respiration.
Laboratory Characteristics:	Albuminocytologic dissociation in the cerebrospinal fluid. Serum enzymes may be slightly elevated in severe cases. EMG and nerve conduction usually abnormal.
Differential Diagnosis:	Poliomyelitis, encephalitis, diphtheria neuropathy, and polymyositis.

Table 4-34. Endocrine and Related Myopathies

- Associated with diseases of the thyroid gland
  - Thyrotoxic myopathy
  - Thyrotoxicosis and periodic paralysis
  - Hyperthyroidism and myasthenia gravis
  - Exophthalmic ophthalmoplegia
  - Hypothyroidism
- Associated with diseases of the parathyroid gland
  - Hyperparathyroidism and osteomalacia
  - Hypoparathyroidism
- Associated with diseases of the pituitary and suprarenal glands
  - Acromegaly and hypopituitarism
  - Cushing's syndrome
  - Steroid myopathy
  - Addison's disease
  - Primary hyperaldosteronism

features of chronic thyrotoxicosis. Although pain is not common, muscle aching may occur. Atrophy and weakness are mainly proximal with the extensor muscles more commonly affected. In contrast to most other myopathies, the reflexes remain essentially unchanged, and in some cases extensive fasciculation has been reported. Pathological changes in the muscles are mild and nonspecific although electromyographic abnormalities are frequent. Adequate treatment of thyrotoxicosis usually results in full recovery. The myopathy is thought to be due to either uncoupling of oxidative phosphorylation in the mitochondria or an increased number of mitochondria. Hyperthyroidism has also been reported to be associated with periodic paralysis and myasthenia gravis and is the cause of exophthalmic ophthalmoplegia. In hypothyroidism, the major symptoms and findings are weakness, cramps, aching, painful muscles, sluggish movements and reflexes, myoedema, and an occasional increase in muscle bulk. Recent evidence suggests that the contractile mechanism of the muscle is involved. Muscular hypertrophy associated with weakness and slowness of movement is called the Debré-Semelaigne syndrome and occurs primarily in cretinous children. When accompanied by painful spasms, slow relaxation, and myoedema, it is called Hoffmann's syndrome and is primarily found in myxedematous adults. Pathological and electromyographic findings are mild and nonspecific. Recovery usually follows appropriate treatment.[20]

Muscular weakness with atrophy in patients under treatment with corticosteroids is relatively common especially since the advent of steroids with a fluorine atom in the 9-alpha position. The pelvic girdle and thigh muscles are most involved, and the reflexes remain relatively normal. Histochemically, there is selective atrophy of the Type II fibers, and the myopathy is reversible on withdrawal of the steroid.[20]

Neuropathies. Peripheral nerve involvement may occur in hypoglycemia, myxedema, and acromegaly; the carpal tunnel syndrome is relatively common in myxedema and acromegaly. Of the endocrine and related disorders, however, polyneuropathy in diabetes mellitus is the most common. In most cases this is primarily a distal, symmetrical, sensory polyneuropathy, but some patients may also have a proximal acute mononeuropathy with weak and wasted knee extensors secondary to motor involvement of the femoral nerve. Nerve entrapment is also quite common in diabetes.[8,20]

Toxic and Nutritional Myopathies and Neuropathies. A tremendous number of drugs, inorganic and organic substances, toxins from bacteria, and nutritional deficiencies have been reported to affect the motor unit. Some occur quite frequently, and most affect only the peripheral nerves. For a discussion of the general findings and the pathophysiology of peripheral nerve damage, the reader is referred to other sources.[1,8]

Of the drugs commonly used in medicine, the following have been reported to cause peripheral nerve damage: barbiturates, chloroquine, vincristine, emetine, iproniazid, isoniazid, nitrofurantoin, phenytoin, streptomycin, and sulfanilamide. Of these, chloroquine, emetine, and vincristine may also produce muscle fiber damage. In addition, the corticosteroids, diazocholesterol, clofibrate, carbenoxolone, amphotericin B, Anodiaquine, and colchicine may also affect the skeletal muscle fiber. None of these drugs has been reported to cause any significant damage to the anterior horn cells. Care is required before accepting a report of neuropathies or myopathies due to drugs or any toxic substances. The disorder may actually be due to the underlying disease for which the drug was first given, and allergic immunological reactions to almost any agent can occur. Other idiosyncratic reactions may indicate an underlying metabolic abnormality. Isoniazid intoxication, for example, occurs in slow inactivators of the drug, a tendency inherited as a genetic trait. In most cases of toxic neuropathies, the agent acts primarily on the axon producing axonal degeneration, especially the distal parts of the largest fibers. The presence of a toxic neuropathy may also predispose to the development of an entrapment neuropathy.[8,12,14,19]

The various inorganic and organic substances causing peripheral nerve damage include arsenic, bismuth, copper, lead, mercury, phosphorus, acrylamide, alcohol, carbon tetrachloride, carbon monoxide, dinitrophenol, dinitrobenzol, dichlorodiphenyltrichloroethane, triorthocresylphosphate, and organic chlorine derivatives. Only alcohol significantly affects the muscle. Lead intoxication and magnesium deficiency may cause damage to the anterior horn cells, and the latter has also been reported to affect the myoneural junction. Alcoholics frequently have a peripheral neuropathy similar to patients with thiamine deficiency and have been shown to have deficiencies of thiamine, folic acid, pyridoxin, pantothenic acid, and riboflavin. Their high caloric intake in the form of alcohol with deficiency of thiamine may be responsible for the nerve damage in many. Two types of clinically distinct myopathy, acute and subacute, occur in chronic alcoholics. The acute type, occurring after a bout of heavy drinking, is characterized by severe pain, tenderness, and edema of the muscles. Myoglobinuria occurs in those severely affected. In the subacute type, symmetrical proximal weakness without significant atrophy or reflex alterations develops. Findings in both types are usually reversible within two or three months after withdrawal of alcohol.[8,12,14,19]

Toxins from bacteria will also cause damage to the motor unit. Botulinus toxin can affect the anterior horn cells and the myoneural junctions as well as the peripheral nerves. Tetanus toxin may involve the anterior horn cells while diphtheria and dysentery are restricted mostly to the peripheral nerves.[8,12,14,19]

Specific nutritional deficiencies affecting peripheral nerves are cyanocobalamin and folic acid deficiencies. Nutritional involvement of the peripheral nerves, probably B_1, B_2, and B_6 vitamin deficiency, has also been implicated in chronic alcoholism, beriberi, pellagra, and gluten-sensitive enteropathy. In the latter condition, as in osteomalacia, malabsorption often leads to a vitamin D deficiency which, in turn, can result in muscle involvement. The only other deficiencies known to affect muscle are the protein deficiency of kwashiorkor and the vitamin E deficiencies of cystic fibrosis and biliary atresia. Various general medical diseases may also affect the nerves and muscles as with the neuropathies associated with renal, thyroid, and liver disease and some of the blood dyscrasias.[8,12,14,19]

Tumors and Malignant Diseases Affecting the Motor Unit. Muscular tumors can be divided into two general categories, those that are primary and develop from a constituent element of muscle proper and those that are secondary arising either as distant metastases or direct extension from an adjacent tumor.[1] Tumors of mesenchymal or mesodermal origin which differentiate into striated muscle cells are exceedingly uncommon. The three types of tumors derived from myoblastic tissue are rhabdomyomas, rhabdomyosarcomas, and granular cell myoblastomas. Teratomas also frequently contain striated muscle fibers, such as in rhabdomyoma and rhabdomyosarcoma of the genital organs and adenomyosarcoma of Wilms. Tumors of blood vessels and supporting tissues which are occasionally present in skeletal muscle include lipomas, fibromas, neuromas, synoviomas, and, especially, angiomas and desmoid tumors. The more common malignant tumors of the human body seldom spread to skeletal muscle, and carcinomas are more apt to involve muscle by direct extension from an adjacent tumor than by metastases, thus causing simple compression atrophy of surrounding muscle fibers. Tumors arising from elements of striated muscles are very uncommon but usually highly malignant. Tumors arising from the supporting tissues of muscle are less rare but are usually benign.[1,15]

The muscular wasting commonly found in patients with malignant disease is due to a variety or combination of factors including cachexia, malnutrition, disease, infection, and arthropathy. Muscular atrophy and weakness deriving from involvement of the anterior horn cells and peripheral nerves are relatively rare as are the myopathies, such as the myasthenic syndrome. The relationship of polymyositis and carcinoma has already been discussed. In the myopathy of malignant cachexia, there is a great loss of subcutaneous fat, atrophy is associated with widespread symmetrical weakness, and myoedema may be present. The most common type of peripheral nerve lesion encountered in malignant disease is compression or infiltration of nerves or plexuses by neoplastic tissue from neighboring growths. Occasionally, diffuse infiltration of the spinal nerve roots or peripheral nerves or intraspinal metastases may occur in myeloma, leukemia, or the reticuloendothelioses. The terms carcinomatous neuropathy and neuromyopathy have been used to describe involvement of the central or peripheral nervous system and muscle by nonmetastatic processes in patients with cancer presumably by some immune mechanism. These include a peripheral, subacute, and sensorimotor neuropathy and encephalomyelitis with oat cell bronchial carcinoma.[15]

Other Myopathies and Neuropathies. Other uncommon diseases affecting muscle are sarcoidosis and amyloidosis. Traumatic and circulatory disorders affecting muscle, senile muscular atrophy, and the effects of chronic infectious diseases and cachexia have already been discussed.

Other relatively common anterior horn cell diseases are progressive muscular atrophy (Aran-Duchenne) and amyotrophic lateral sclerosis. These, along with progressive bulbar palsy, are often called the classic motor neuron diseases, and represent degeneration of the motor neurons at all levels.[19] Adult motor neuron disease is a worldwide sporadic disorder with an incidence of about 1 in 100,000 population per year. Between 5 and 10 percent of the cases are familial with an autosomal dominant pattern of inheritance. There is now little doubt that they are all part of a disease spectrum dependent on the site of neuronal involvement and the degree of upper or lower motor neuron disease. The characteristics of classic amyotrophic lateral sclerosis are outlined in Table 4-35. The major differences between it

Table 4-35. Amyotrophic Lateral Sclerosis

Onset:	Adult life.
Rate of Progression:	Steadily progressive with a mean survival of about three years.
Distribution of Weakness:	In most cases the disease is asymmetrical with patchy atrophy early, which then becomes generalized and severe.
Clinical Characteristics:	Weakness, atrophy, and fasciculations of the muscles of the hand and arm associated with stiffness, usually of the legs, and in some cases with affection of speech and swallowing. Occasionally, generalized spasticity may be prominent with only mild wasting or the presenting feature may be spasticity of speech and swallowing. Cramps, usually in the legs and at night, are common. Hands tend to show guttering early. The tongue often shows wasting and fasciculation, and there is dysarthria. Jaw jerk and facial reflexes are very brisk, the tendon reflexes are exaggerated, and the plantar reflexes are extensor.
Laboratory Characteristics:	Serum enzymes are usually normal or slightly elevated. Nerve conduction is normal, and EMG is usually abnormal.
Differential Diagnosis:	Other motor neuron diseases, distal muscular dystrophy, and other polyneuropathies.

and progressive muscular atrophy are the absence of upper motor neuron signs, a greater degree of sensory symptoms, and a more rapid, fatal course in the latter.[19]

Other peripheral nerve diseases not already mentioned include that associated with porphyria, radiation neuropathy, idiopathic and chronic polyneuropathy, and mononeuropathies associated with trauma.[8]

Other rare syndromes are neuromyositis and idiopathic noninflammatory neuromyopathy. The former has been reported in the collagen vascular diseases, especially in polymyositis, in which histological inflammatory changes are found in the large peripheral nerve trunks. The latter is characterized by concomitant lower motor neuron and myopathic dysfunction. These two syndromes plus an increasing number of reports showing neuropathic findings in a number of disorders always felt to be primary muscle diseases indicate that it now seems justified to at least recognize the clinical existence of simultaneous dysfunction of nerve and muscle.

Floppy Baby Syndrome. Until recently, the differential diagnosis of hypotonia was confusing since several disorders had been grouped under the general heading of amyotonia congenita. Infantile spinal muscular atrophy, a disease of the anterior horn cells, was first described in the late 1800s by Werdnig and Hoffmann. In 1900, Oppenheim described a series of patients with a similar clinical picture but whose findings gradually improved with age. This syndrome was then given the name amyotonia congenita or Oppenheim's disease. In the 1950s, reexamination of the cases reported by Oppenheim as well as several new clinical reviews clearly indicated that this condition did not represent any clearly definable disease. Therefore, it is now recommended that the term amyotonia congenita no longer be used. In most infants with hypotonia, a specific disease can be identified, usually infantile spinal muscular atrophy. Those for which a diagnosis cannot be made are now usually called benign congenital hypotonia.

Periodic Paralysis as the Predominant Clinical Finding

The various disorders with periodic paralysis are outlined in Table 4-4. The primary ones are quite rare and will only be described briefly.[20] Familial or hypokalemic periodic paralysis is characterized by attacks of flaccid quadriplegia and a low serum potassium level. It is usually inherited as an autosomal dominant trait. Attacks in most families begin in the second decade, are most frequent between the ages of 20 and 35 years, and then tend to decrease in number and severity. Most attacks occur in the early morning and can either be prevented or reduced by potassium chloride.

Hyperkalemic periodic paralysis is characterized by attacks of paralysis usually occurring about midday and a high serum potassium level. It is usually inherited as a single autosomal dominant trait, is usually first detected in infancy, and attacks become most frequent in childhood after exercise and then tend to decrease in number and severity with the avoidance of exercise. In most cases, the attacks can be reduced by diuretics. Myotonia is found in many of the reported cases, thus linking it with paramyotonia congenita.

The third type of hereditary periodic paralysis, normokalemic, is similar to hyperkalemic periodic paralysis, but the attacks may last for days or even weeks, are usually more severe, and occur mainly at night. The serum potassium levels are not affected. As summarized in Table 4-4, periodic attacks of paralysis may also occur in other systemic diseases.

Fatigue as Predominant Clinical Finding

Fatigue is a difficult symptom to evaluate especially when it is not associated with any objective findings. The fatigability associated with myasthenia gravis or the myasthenic syndrome must first be distinguished from the subjective feeling of tiredness expressed in patients with hysteria or depression and from simple fatigue due to constant slight muscular weakness or from stiffness and pain induced by exercise. Disorders with fatigue as the predominant symptom are outlined in Table 4-5.

Myasthenia gravis is characterized by the development of an abnormal amount of muscular weakness following repetitive muscle contractions or prolonged tension with a marked tendency to recover strength after rest. It is relatively common with estimates of prevalence in the population ranging from 1 in 10,000 to 1 in 50,000. Females are affected twice as often as males, and the ocular muscles are less often involved.[24] The electrodiagnostic features of both

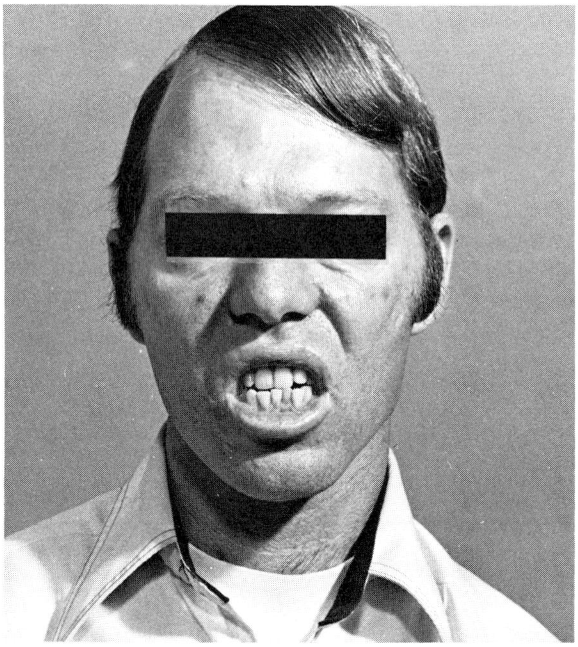

Fig. 4-24. So-called myasthenic snarl in a 30-year-old male with myasthenia gravis.

myasthenia gravis and myasthenic syndrome are reviewed in Chapter 3.

Cramping, Stiffness, Continuous Muscle Contractions, and Myotonia as Predominant Clinical Finding

Most of these disorders (Table 4-6) have already been discussed in this chapter or in Chapter 3. The stiff-man syndrome is characterized by a progressive, fluctuating, painful muscle rigidity and spasm and tends to affect middle-aged males. The muscles may actually become boardlike and rigid, and attempts at motion will precipitate excruciatingly painful muscle spasms with extension rigidity. Relaxation occurs during sleep, and the spasms are abolished by peripheral nerve blocks and myoneural blocking agents and relieved by diazepam.[12]

The myotonic disorders are characterized by the continued active contraction of a muscle which persists after the cessation of voluntary effort or stimulation. Clinically, it can be demonstrated as a slowness in relaxation of the grip or by a persistent dimpling ("hillock") after a sharp blow on the muscle belly (see Fig. 4-1). It appears to be due to an abnormality of the muscle fiber, probably the sarcolemma, since it persists after curarization. Myotonia occurs in three hereditary disorders, myotonic dystrophy (see Table 4-19), congenital myotonia, and paramyotonia congenita and can also be induced by some drugs, such as diazocholesterol. Myotonic dystrophy and the relationship of paramyotonia congenita to hyperkalemic periodic paralysis have been discussed. Congenital myotonia, or Thomsen's disease, usually begins at birth although symptoms may be delayed to the end of the first decade. The myotonia is more widespread than in myotonic dystrophy and characteristically causes a generalized painless stiffness which is accentuated by rest and cold and gradually relieved by exercise. Diffuse hypertrophy of the muscles usually persists during life although the myotonia tends to gradually diminish.[27]

Malignant hyperpyrexia is of great interest to all clinicians, especially surgeons and anesthesiologists. In susceptible individuals, a fulminating rise in temperature develops during anesthesia accompanied by massive muscular rigidity, tachycardia, tachypnea, cyanosis, and acidosis. Only one third of the patients survive. While most general anesthetics and muscle relaxants can precipitate the reaction, halothane and succinylcholine are most commonly implicated. Clinical or subclinical evidence of a myopathy is present in the susceptible, and predisposition can often be shown by elevated serum CPK levels. Susceptibility may be associated with a number of different myopathies so there are probably several metabolic defects.[12]

Injury, Denervation, and Disuse[1,2,8]

Injury to muscle can be either direct or indirect. Direct injury is easier to comprehend and will be described first. Examples of direct injury are laceration and crush or thermal (burning or freezing) wounds. All of these result in destruction of all or part of an individual muscle with the degree of loss directly proportional to the severity of the insult. In the past, it was thought that muscle was not capable of regeneration and that healing of direct injury to muscle was only a fibroblastic repair with noncontractile, connective tissue scar formation. More recent studies have shown that muscle does have the capacity for regeneration and repair in response to direct injury. The key element of the regenerative process is the reserve myoblasts called satellite cells. Following trauma, the injured muscle fibers degenerate back for a short distance from the point of injury, and the necrotic tissue is removed by macrophages and other phagocytic cells. In this stage, the histological pattern shows the area of injury plus associated phagocytic and inflammatory activity. In the surviving portion of the muscle fibers, on both sides of the injury, myoblastic activity is seen as the reserve myoblasts become activated. This stage is followed by a period of rapid cell proliferation with the myoblasts fusing to form small myotubes which ultimately fuse to reform the muscle fiber. Once the sarcolemma is restored, the regenerated or repaired muscle fiber is again capable of contraction. Such a complicated repair mechanism is, of course, capable of bridging only relatively small local injuries. If several centimeters of muscle are avulsed or destroyed, the repair process will be incomplete, and healing will be primarily by scar tissue. This repair system is also incomplete when regeneration is inhibited by systemic disease, vascular insufficiency, or nerve injury.

Most other types of injury to muscle can be classified as indirect. The classic indirect injuries to muscle are a result of paralysis which may be secondary to either an upper or lower motor neuron lesion or to ischemic changes resulting from vascular insufficiency. In contrast to direct injury, there is a reduced capacity for regeneration and repair. In addition to the classic indirect injuries, there are injuries which result from disuse or misuse of muscle. Many of these are far more common than the classic indirect injuries.

The classic indirect injury to muscle is denervation secondary to lesions of the peripheral nerves or anterior horn cells. These changes are summarized and compared with disuse in Table 4-36. Following complete section of the nerve, the muscle is no longer capable of voluntary contraction. The paralysis is flaccid, and the muscle is areflexic. The individual muscle fibers atrophy at a rapid rate, and gross or clinical atrophy occurs very early. The electrodiagnostic changes can be reviewed in detail in Chapter 3. There is no response to stimulation of the nerve after wallerian degeneration has occurred. Therefore, nerve conduction studies are not possible. The muscle will contract with the reaction of degeneration in response to direct stimulations using currents of long duration but will show no response to currents of brief duration. The histological pattern in denervation is rapid atrophy of all muscle fibers. Histochemical studies, however, show a preferential rate of atrophy with the Type II fibers having the most rapid rate of atrophy and the Type I fibers demonstrating a slightly greater resistance. There is no evidence of regeneration in these muscles, and the muscle fibers are ultimately replaced by fat and/or fibrous connective tissue. Electron microscopic studies demonstrate reduction in size of the individual myofibrils as a result of loss of myofilaments. In normal muscle, the muscle fiber is sensitive to acetylcholine only in the region of the neuromuscular junction. However, following denervation this sensitivity to directly applied acetylcholine spreads so that the entire sarcolemma becomes sensitive within a few weeks. In vitro studies with denervated muscle have also demonstrated marked alterations in the contractile characteristics so that tetanic tension and the rate of tension development are reduced.

Indirect damage to muscle as a result of upper

Table 4-36. Comparison of Atrophy of Denervation with Disuse Atrophy

	Denervation	*Disuse*
Gross	Rapid reduction in gross muscle volume	Less rapid reduction in volume
Muscle strength	No voluntary contraction	Mild to moderate reduction in muscle strength. Paralysis in upper motor neuron lesions.
Tendon reflexes	Absent	Normal—hyperactive after period of initial shock with upper motor neuron lesions
EMG	Abnormal	Normal, but will show some spontaneous potentials in upper motor neuron lesions
Nerve conduction	No response	Normal
Response to direct stimulation of muscle	No response to stimuli of brief duration (less than 1 m./sec.)	Normal
Histology		
Routine studies	Rapidly progressing atrophy	Atrophy mild and slowly progressive
Fiber typing	Atrophy Type II Type I	In early stage atrophy primarily of Type II fibers
Electron microscopy	Rapid reduction in number of myofibrils	Less rapid change
Physiological	Spread of sensitivity to ACh	ACh sensitivity normal
	In vitro contractility altered	In vitro contractility normal

The model for denervation in this table is total (complete) denervation, e.g., section of peripheral nerve.

motor neuron lesions is seen most commonly in patients with paralysis secondary to cerebrovascular accidents or spinal cord injury. In these conditions, when paralysis is complete, atrophy of muscle occurs at a slower rate than in patients with denervation. Since the paralysis is complete, the muscle is not capable of voluntary contraction. Muscle contraction will occur in response to tendon tap (reflex stimulation), after the initial areflexia which occurs during the period of spinal shock, and the reflexes become hyperactive. Histological studies show generalized atrophy occurring at a much slower rate than with denervated muscle, and histochemical studies demonstrate preferential atrophy of the Type II fibers. There are no histological or electron microscopic changes characteristic for upper motor neuron paralysis. Since the axon and neuromuscular junction remain intact, there is no spread of sensitivity to acetylcholine, and contractile studies do not show abnormal changes other than those that would be expected as a result of reduced muscle bulk and reduced activity.

Indirect damage to muscle can occur as a result of vascular problems and these may be due to complete or incomplete loss of vascular supply. The most common lesions would be from decreased arterial perfusion of muscle as a result of myocardial decompensation or generalized atherosclerosis. Since atherosclerosis only involves the larger intramuscular arteries, this condition or myocardial decompensation result in a reduced energy supply to the muscle secondary to the decreased perfusion. The symptoms are reduced strength and easy fatigability as a result of the diminished energy supply. In time, occasional muscle fibers may die and degenerate; however, there are no specific histological or electrodiagnostic changes for this condition.

Ischemic damage to muscle can also be sudden and severe, as in the case of occlusion of a major artery to an extremity. If the occlusion is complete and beyond recovery through collateral circulation, dry gangrene will occur, and the tissues of the limb will die back to the level at which circulation is still intact. The tissues deprived of blood become dry and mummified. In the area deprived of blood supply, the dead cells rapidly lose all identifying characteristics. The tissues at the margin of the lesion, where circulation remains, show phagocytosis of necrotic material and activation of the repair and regeneration mechanisms. Gangrene is also common in patients with widespread atherosclerosis, such as in diabetics. The same processes occur only at a much slower rate.

Small vessel disease of muscle is seen with the small vessel infarcts associated with polyarteritis nodosa as well as with the chemical vasculitis and microarterial infarcts that occur with accidental intraarterial injection of medications or street drugs (see Fig. 4-15). In these conditions, small nerves as well as muscle fibers are lost. Hence, the histological picture is mixed with both small and large group atrophy of muscle fibers as well as random muscle fiber atrophy plus evidence of damage to small vessels and arterioles.

Other types of indirect injury to muscle are disuse and misuse. Disuse is best typified by prolonged bed rest or immobilization of a body part by a cast. This situation could also occur during periods of prolonged weightlessness as during space flight. The "misuse" category includes the variety of injuries that occur to muscle as a result of abnormal activity, such as excessive or unaccustomed exercise or closed trauma.

The word disuse is used to indicate periods of prolonged muscle inactivity in the absence of other direct or indirect injuries to muscle or nerve. In this condition, there is moderately rapid atrophy, with reduction in muscle weight as great as 25 percent by six weeks. There is reduction in muscle strength proportionate to the degree of atrophy. The tendon reflexes remain normal. Histological studies only show evidence of slight reduction in muscle fiber diameter. Again, the more energy expensive Type II fibers are the ones most susceptible to atrophy. There are no significant changes seen on electron microscopic examination. If the period of immobilization is relatively brief, there are no detectable changes in muscle contractility. However, in time, total tension and rate of tension development become reduced.

In the "misuse" category of injuries to muscle we have all experienced the pain and tenderness which follows a period of intense and unaccustomed effort. By contrast, severe exertion of muscle or externally applied force can occasionally result in rupture of a muscle, its tendon, or the fascial supporting structures. These injuries were not listed in the category of direct injuries as that term usually carries with it the concept of externally applied violence or visible insult to the muscle. Since this type of injury most commonly results from excessive, unaccustomed, or violent activity, the term *misuse of muscle* is more appropriate.

Rupture of a muscle will occasionally occur as a result of sudden overloading. It is usually associated with an audible snap, pain, swelling, and a local bulge in the involved muscle at the opposite end from where the rupture occurred. The rupture may initially be incomplete but becomes complete after about 24 hours. Reflex response to tendon tap is usually lost. However, the muscle belly will respond to percussion with the usual myotactic response. Histological studies show attempts at regeneration and repair along the margins of the rupture.

Fascial tears can occasionally result from direct trauma, violent physical effort, bullet or stab wounds, or surgical procedures. The underlying muscle belly will usually bulge or herniate through the fascial defect. The bulge will increase when the muscle contracts and reduce when the muscle relaxes. Reduction of the muscle hernia is facilitated if the relaxed muscle is passively stretched by the examiner. Muscle hernias are usually more a curiosity than a problem. If the fascial defect is small, the herniated muscle might possibly strangulate with resultant muscle necrosis. The diagnosis is clinical, and electrodiagnostic or histological testing is rarely indicated.

Hemorrhage into a muscle can result from trauma, rupture of a blood vessel, or coagulation defects. The muscle fibers are damaged by pressure from the hematoma and from the inflammatory reaction that results from the accumulation of blood in the tissues. These conditions are always painful, and the tender swelling can be palpated if the muscle is superficial. Muscle strength is reduced due to pain but will usually recover. The histological pattern usually shows marked inflammatory reaction, destruction of muscle fibers in the area of the hemorrhage, and evidence of regeneration and repair on the viable margins. Because it is usually associated with relatively remote complications, hemorrhage into the iliopsoas muscle requires special mention. This condition occurs most commonly in patients receiving anticoagulant medication or with hemorrhagic disorders. The complications result from the fact that the femoral nerve passes through the fibers of the psoas muscle. Therefore, femoral motor and sensory neuropathy can result from a bleed into this muscle.

Shin splints is a syndrome frequently seen by physicians. The presenting complaint is pain and tenderness of the pretibial or posttibial muscle groups sometimes associated with swelling and occurs after unaccustomed or strenuous exercise. The pretibial or posttibial muscle groups may be firm to palpation, and active or passive movement of the ankle may be restricted because of the pain. Some think it is the result of overactivity of unconditioned muscles. Despite the severity of the symptoms, the discomfort will usually resolve completely in a few hours, or, at most, a few days with rest and limited activity. This syndrome is seen most often in the "weekend athlete" or at the beginning of the training season in athletes. Shin splints can be significant, however, because of the need to differentiate this benign condition from the destructive compartment syndromes.

Some think the anterior tibial compartment syndrome is an extreme version of shin splints in which the muscles undergo necrosis. The anterior tibial compartment is a rigid compartment, formed by the tibia, fibula, and interosseous membrane behind and the tough anterior tibial fascia in front. The dorsiflexor muscles of the ankle and toes are contained within. When these muscles are traumatized by excess effort or by direct trauma, hemorrhage and/or swelling will occur. The swelling in this dense fascial compartment increases pressure which occludes venous return. This causes further swelling until tissue pressures approximate arterial systolic pressure. The tissues are deprived of adequate vascular perfusion and are probably also damaged by the direct effects of pressure and the accumulation of toxic metabolic by-products. This results in necrosis of all of the muscles and nerve tissue contained in the anterior compartment, thus producing foot drop and sensory loss in the distribution of the deep branch of the peroneal nerve. If the syndrome is diagnosed early, anterior tibial fasciotomy can relieve the pressure, restore circulation, and decrease or prevent loss of muscle and/or nerve. Histological studies show destruction and necrosis of all muscle except that immediately adjacent to the anterior tibial fascia which survives presumably by nutrition through the fascia.

Clinical damage to muscle can occur as a result of exposure to cold. The typical example is frostbite.

However, since frostbite usually involves only the digits, muscle is involved only to a minor degree. When the damage extends more proximally, the muscle in the damaged area undergoes changes similar to those seen with gangrene. Muscle can also be damaged as a result of prolonged exposure to cold and does not necessarily result in frostbite. This occurs as a result of prolonged exposure to cold water as in trench foot. After exposure, the extremity becomes warm and may become cyanotic with the development of cutaneous bullae. Pain may be intense, and sensory impairment is common. If the limb survives, the histological changes in muscle can vary from normal to areas of necrosis or fibrosis depending on the time of injury.

Damage to muscle has also been described as a late and rare effect of severe carbon monoxide poisoning. However, this seems to be more a result of vascular occlusion or direct pressure on the tissues resulting from prolonged periods of unconsciousness.

Volkmann's ischemic contracture usually occurs as a result of arterial occlusion secondary to tight bandages or casts. This condition is more common in injuries of the upper extremity. Onset of symptoms is usually a few hours or days following injury and is characterized by burning pain in the distal portion of the extremity, usually associated with swelling, cyanosis, or pallor and reduced temperature of the involved parts. The muscles become incapable of contraction in response to voluntary effort, reflex, or electrical stimulation. At this stage, the muscle is rapidly replaced by fibrous connective tissue in a position of contracture. Clinically, the upper extremity assumes a position of flexion as a result of firm contractures of the muscles, with the wrist and elbow in flexion.

Muscle can react to damage in a variety of ways. However, none are more confusing than the conditions of myositis ossificans or ectopic ossification. The generalized form, myositis ossificans progressiva, has already been discussed. Ectopic ossification can also occur as a late result of trauma to muscle, and this condition has been termed traumatic myositis ossificans or ossifying hematoma. The muscle which most commonly undergoes ossification is the brachialis. On rare occasions, ossification may occur in a muscle following a single injury, and again, the brachialis is the most common muscle involved.

Perhaps the most frustrating example of myositis ossificans is the rapid ectopic ossification that can occur in patients with upper motor neuron lesions producing tetraplegia and paraplegia. In these patients, the most common areas of ectopic ossification are the muscles about the hip. In most cases, the involvement is mild and produces no impairment to passive motion; in other cases, the ectopic ossification may be extreme, totally prohibiting passive motion to the joint to the point that even sitting is no longer possible. Even though there is no evidence of trauma to the muscle, histological changes still occur. The tissues organize into osteoblastic activity and osteoid is formed. This is rapidly followed by mineralization (calcification) of the osteoid to form typical bone. The newly formed bone is usually of the cancellous type and resembles the bone of callus formation in the healing of fractures. Signs accompanying ectopic bone formation in these patients are swelling and/or increased temperature in the local area, elevated erythrocyte sedimentation rate, and elevated serum alkaline phosphatase activity. In the early stages, the osteoblastic activity is not visible roentgenographically but can be identified by radioactive scan techniques specific for osteoblastic activity. Ossification of the osteoid becomes obvious about two to three weeks following identification of the active areas by scanning methods. The etiology of myositis ossificans is unknown as these lesions are usually symmetrical and cannot be explained on the basis of local trauma. Treatment is equally frustrating as excised bone is often reformed at a more rapid rate than the original formation.

SUGGESTED READINGS

1. Adams, R. D., Denny-Brown, D., and Pearson, C. M.: Diseases of Muscle: A Study in Pathology. New York, Harper & Row, 1962.
2. André-Thomas, Chesni Y., and Dargassies, S. S.-A.: The neurological examination of the infant. *In* MacKeith, R. C., Polani, P. E., and Clayton-Jones, E.: Little Club Clinics in Developmental Medicine, No. 1. London, National Spastics Society, 1960.
3. Award, E. A.: Interstitial myofibrositis: Hypothesis of the mechanism. Arch. Phys. Med. Rehabil. *54*:449, 1973.
4. Bourne, G. H. (ed.): The Structure and Function of Muscle, Structure Part I. ed. 2. vol. I. New York, Academic Press, 1972.
5. Bourne, G. H. (ed.): The Structure and Function of Muscle, Structure Part 2. ed. 2. vol. II. New York, Academic Press, 1973.
6. Bourne, G. H. (ed.): The Structure and Function of Muscle, Physiology and Biochemistry. ed. 2. vol. III. New York, Academic Press, 1973.

7. Bourne, G. H. (ed.): The Structure and Function of Muscle, Pharmacology and Disease. ed. 2. vol. IV. New York, Academic Press, 1973.
8. Bradley, W. G.: The neuropathies. *In* Walton, J. N. (ed.): Disorders of Voluntary Muscle. pp. 804-851. London, Churchill Livingstone, 1974.
9. Carlson, F. D., and Wilkie, D. R.: Muscle Physiology. Englewood Cliffs, Prentice-Hall, Inc., 1974.
10. Daniels, L., and Worthingham, C.: Muscle Testing. Techniques of Manual Examination. ed. 3. Philadelphia, W. B. Saunders, 1972.
11. Dubowitz, V., and Brooke, M. H.: Muscle Biopsy: A Modern Approach. Philadelphia, W. B. Saunders, 1973.
12. Foster, J. B.: The clinical features of some miscellaneous neuromuscular disorders. *In* Walton, J. N. (ed.): Disorders of Voluntary Muscle. pp. 886-906. London, Churchill Livingstone, 1974.
13. Fowler, W. M., Jr.: Muscle Weakness and Atrophy. Clinical and Laboratory Evaluation. Calif. Med. *108:*24, 1968.
14. Gardner-Medwin, D., and Walton, J. N.: The clinical examination of the voluntary muscles. *In* Walton, J. N. (ed.): Disorders of Voluntary Muscle. pp. 517-560. London, Churchill and Livingstone, 1974.
15. Henson, R. A.: Neuromuscular disorders associated with malignant disease. *In* Walton, J. N. (ed.): Disorders of Voluntary Muscle. pp. 760-774. London, Churchill and Livingstone, 1974.
16. Johnson, E. W.: Examination for muscle weakness in infants and small children. JAMA, *168:*1306, 1958.
17. Kloepfer, H. W.: Genetic aspects of neuromuscular disease. *In* Walton, J. N. (ed.): ,Disorders of Voluntary Muscle. pp. 852–885. London, Churchill Livingstone, 1974.
18. Layzer, R. B., and Rowland, L. P.: Cramps. N. Engl. J. Med. *285:*31, 1971.
19. Liversedge, L. A., and Campbell, M. J.: The central neuronal muscular atrophies and other dysfunctions of the anterior horn cells. *In* Walton, J. N. (ed.): Disorders of Voluntary Muscle. pp. 775-803. London, Churchill and Livingstone, 1974.
20. McArdle, B.: Metabolic and endocrine myopathies. *In* Walton, J. N. (ed.): Disorders of Voluntary Muscle. pp. 726-759. London, Churchill and Livingstone, 1974.
21. Munsat, T. L., Baloh, R., Pearson, C. M., and Fowler, W. M., Jr.: Serum enzyme alterations in neuromuscular disorders. JAMA *226:*1536, 1973.
22. Pearson, C. M., Coleman, R. F., Fowler, W. M., Jr., Mommaerts, W. F., Munsat, T. L., and Peter, M. B.: The UCLA Interdepartmental Conference. Skeletal muscle: Basic and clinical aspects and illustrative new diseases Ann. Intern. Med. *67:*614, 1967.
23. Pearson, C. M., and Currie, S.: Polymyositis and related diseases. Walton, J. N. (ed.): Disorders of Voluntary Muscle. pp. 653-692. London, Churchill and Livingstone, 1974.
24. Simpson, J. A.: Myasthenia gravis and myasthenic syndromes. *In* Walton, J. N. (ed.): Disorders of Voluntary Muscle. pp. 653-692. London, Churchill and Livingstone, 1974.
25. Tizard, J. P. M.: Neuromuscular disorders in infancy and early childhood. *In* Walton, J. N. (ed.): Disorders of Voluntary Muscle. pp. 693-725. London, Churchill and Livingstone, 1974.
26. Vignos, Jr., P. J.: Rehabilitation in muscular dystrophy. *In* Licht, S. (ed.): Rehabilitation and Medicine. pp. 584-642. Baltimore, Waverly Press, 1968.
27. Walton, J. N., and Gardner, Medwin, D.: Progressive muscular dystrophy and the myotonic disorders. *In* Walton, J. N. (ed.): Disorders of Voluntary Muscle. pp. 561-613. London, Churchill and Livingstone, 1974.
28. Wilmore, J. H. (ed.): Exercise and Sport Sciences Reviews. vol. 1. New York, Academic Press, 1963.
29. Worden, R. E., Johnson, E. W., and Burk, R. D.: Diagnosis of hysterical paralysis. Arch. Phys. Med. *42:*122, 1961.

5 Peripheral Nerve Lesions

Paul W. Brown, M.D.

STRUCTURE AND FUNCTION OF PERIPHERAL NERVE

General Structure

Nerves are composed of two types of tissue: the functional element or neural tissue called axoplasm and the supporting element of connecting tissue. Axoplasm has little tensile strength and depends on surrounding connective tissue for structural integrity. Each nerve fiber is an axoplasmic extension or axon of a nerve cell located in the anterior horn cell of the spinal cord, in the sympathetic ganglia, or in the ganglia of the posterior root. The axon is surrounded by connective tissue called endoneurium which forms the endoneurial tube and which is attached by loose connective tissue to its neighboring endoneurial tubes. Groups of nerve fibers form bundles called funiculi or fascicles which, in turn, are surrounded by connective tissue sheaths of perineurium. The clusters of funiculi are contained within a connective tissue sheath of epineurium and form a nerve trunk which contains dozens of funiculi and thousands of individual nerve fibers.

The Nerve Fiber

The nerve fiber has a core of viscous axoplasm, the axon, which is an extension of the cell body and is surrounded by a multilayered connective tissue sheath called endoneurium. Continuity between the entire length of the axoplasm and the nerve cell body is a prerequisite for nerve fiber function. Surrounding the axon is a network of Schwann cells with or without a layer of myelin, a lipoprotein. Myelinated axons are segmented longitudinally into nodes, each of which has a single Schwann cell nucleus. The Schwann cell layer is also called the neurilemma, and external to it is the endoneurium, a sheath or tube of delicate connective tissue.

Nerve fibers range from 2 to 30 microns in diameter and vary in length from a few millimeters to over 1 meter. They have one of three different physiological functions: motor, sensory, or sympathetic. Motor fibers originate from the anterior horn cells of the spinal cord; carry neural impulses peripherally and, hence, are known as efferent fibers; and terminate in the neuromuscular endings of skeletal muscle. Sensory fibers carry the axons (technically the dendrites) of the posterior root nerve cells, are mainly nonmyelinated, and carry impulses proximally from various types of sensory end-organs and are, therefore, called afferent. Sympathetic fibers are generally nonmyelinated and are the extensions of neurons in the ganglia of the sympathetic trunk. The sympathetic fibers accompany cutaneous nerves to skin structures, and they accompany deep branches of the main nerve trunks to deeper structures. The concept of correlating fiber function with fiber size and degree of myelinization is no longer valid.

The Nerve Trunk

A funiculus—also called fasciculus—is a bundle of nerve fibers surrounded by a thin sheath of connective tissue, the perineurium. Each funiculus usually includes all three types of fibers—motor, sensory, and sympathetic—to varying degrees, and the number of funiculi in a single trunk varies from one to many. There is a longitudinal plexus formation of the funiculi within the trunk with groups of fibers crossing over from one funiculus to another so that the cross-section of the same nerve trunk varies considerably at different levels in respect to the number, size, and arrangement of the funiculi.

Surrounding the funiculus is a discrete sheath of perineurium formed of elastic and collagenous fibrils which makes a major contribution to the elasticity and tensile strength of the nerve trunk. Usually, the larger the funiculus, the thicker the perineurium, although the funiculi of the nerve roots are devoid of perineurial sheaths.

Surrounding the groups of funiculi which form the trunk is an investing sheath of longitudinally-oriented collagen and elastic fibrils. This sheath is condensed around the periphery of the trunk and also extends out from the trunk to connect it loosely to its surrounding structures; it also extends inward as interfunicular areolar tissue filling the areas between the individual funiculi. This nerve trunk sheath with both its peripheral and inward extensions is the epineurium. Contained within it in the interfunicular regions are varying amounts of adipose tissue. The relative amount of epineurium varies with the individual nerve and its level but generally makes up more than half of the mass of the trunk.

Nutrition is supplied to the nerve trunk from numerous branches of neighboring arteries that contribute arterioles which form a complex interfunicular and intrafunicular network of arterioles, capillaries, and vessels running throughout the length of the trunk. Only the median and sciatic nerves contain vessels larger than arterioles.

The Anatomy of Innervation

Innervation Patterns. The arrangements and branching of the brachial plexus and of the lumbosacral plexus as well as the involved progression of axons from nerve roots through trunks to cords and finally to individually named peripheral nerves must be learned. Keep in mind that nerve fibers from a single cord segment pass to several different muscles and that each muscle is usually innervated from more than one level of the cord.

It is important to have access to diagrams of the sensory and muscular innervation as dermatomes (Fig. 5-1A) and myotomes. Dermatomes are diagrammed showing the segmental regional innervation of both the spinal segments and the peripheral nerves whereas myotomes are presented as a table of individual muscles along with their segmental innervation (see Chap. 3). Knowledge of the common single nerve root syndromes in the lower cervical and lumbosacral areas is also important (Fig. 5-1B).

The Level of Disease. It is essential for both diagnosis and treatment to establish not only the distribution but also the level of the lesion involving the peripheral nerve or nerves, and this is true for either disease or injury of the nerve. On the motor side, the levels to be considered are the anterior horn cell, the nerve root, the nerve itself, the motor nerve terminal, and neuromuscular junctions. On the sensory side, one must attempt to localize the pathological condition within the spinal cord, the posterior root, the posterior root ganglion, the sensory nerve itself, or the sensory terminals.

Anterior horn cell and motor nerve terminals and neuromuscular involvement will be affected by neurological diseases, such as acute anterior poliomyelitis for the former and toxic neuropathies and myasthenia gravis in the latter. The nerve trunk itself and the nerve roots may be affected by either neuropathy or trauma. The same schema is applicable to the sensory side of the loop. Within the cord, the posterior root may be affected by multiple sclerosis, the posterior root itself by either trauma or arachnoiditis, the posterior root ganglion by a familial sensory neuropathy, the sensory peripheral nerve trunk by trauma or disease, and the sensory terminal by toxic neuropathy.

METHODS OF TESTING AND EXAMINATION

History

When the patient with a peripheral nerve disability and the physician first come together, the patient tends to assume the physician already knows what has gone on before, and he will, if permitted, concentrate on the most troublesome and obvious aspects of his problem. The physician can easily be led along an erroneous course as he is eager to get to the specific physical findings of the lesion. The patient with a median nerve entrapment may start by describing his present symptoms and will present the troublesome hand to the physician who may then be led to start an examination of the hand before a proper history is taken. It is proper, of course, to have the patient start by giving his chief complaint; then, the physician must learn the occupation of the pa-

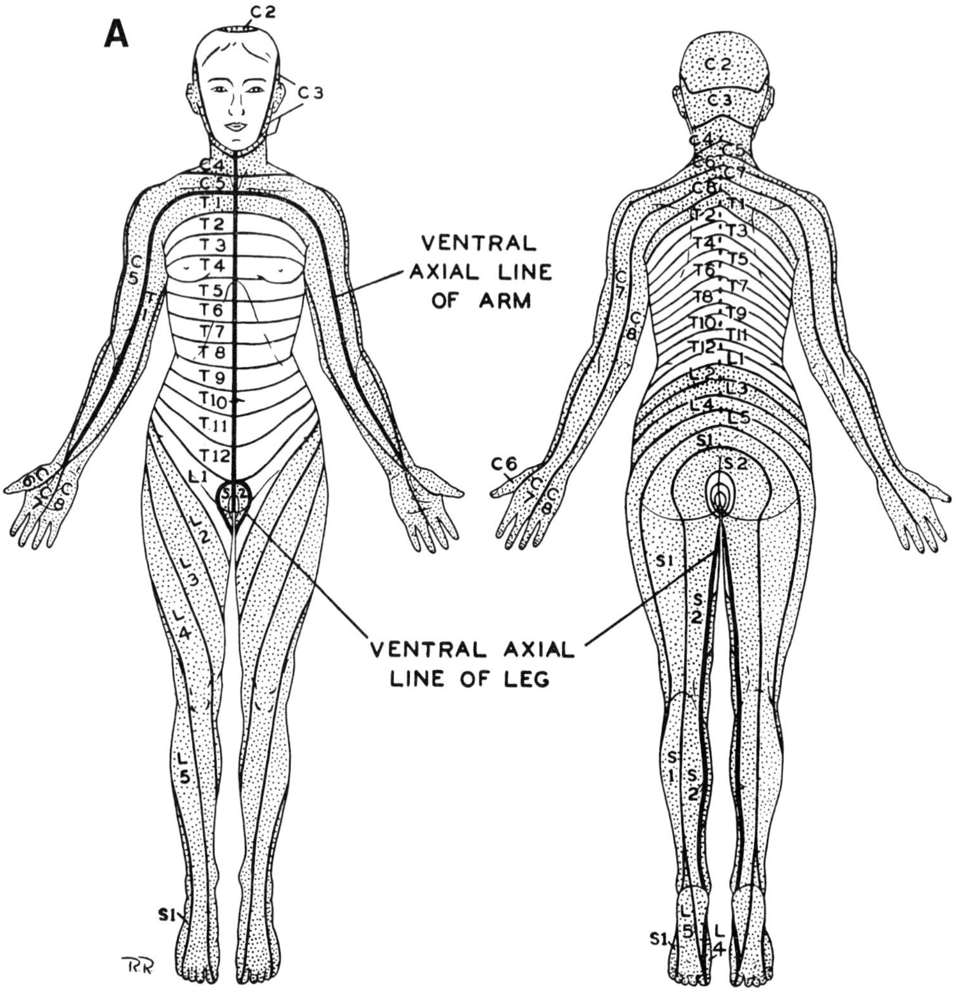

Fig. 5-1. (*A*) Sensory dermatome distribution with new patterns in the extremities based on single nerve root syndromes. (*B, Opposite*) Common single nerve root syndromes. (Keegan, J. J., and Garrett, F. D.: Anat. Rec. *102*:411, 1948)

tient, what specialized functional requirements he has of his hand or foot, and which is the dominant extremity. The physician must then obtain a detailed, chronological description of the development and nature of the symptoms. A simple but effective aid to this is to seat the patient out of reach or even across the room; one will be less tempted to skip the history which may be considerably more illuminating than the physical findings. Methods for good history taking must be developed early in one's clinical career and must be adhered to until they become not an effort but a habit. The effective clinician will invariably be a good historian and will be less likely to jump to conclusions and less likely to get started down the wrong path.

One would like to know what the patient first experienced, when it started, what it was like, what functional loss was noted, and how the trouble has progressed. One must know the qualitative and quantitative aspects of the symptoms as well as the rate of progression, regression, or intermittency. The significance of a carpal tunnel syndrome due to myxedema is far different from that due to localized trauma; the treatment is quite different as is the prognosis, but without proper history, an incorrect or only partially correct diagnosis will be made, inade-

B

LOWER CERVICAL

FIFTH CERVICAL

PAIN UPPER BORDER SCAPULA.

TENDERNESS OVER TRANSVERSE PROCESS C4–5 VERTEBRAE.

RADIATION OF PAIN TO ANTERO-LATERAL ARM.

NUMB SENSATION ANTEROLATERAL FOREARM.

HYPOALGESIA AS OUTLINED, MORE EVIDENT DISTALLY.

REFLEX OF BICEPS TENDON REDUCED.

MOTOR WEAKNESS & ATROPHY OF SERRATUS MAGNUS (WINGED SCAPULA) AND ANTERIOR DELTOID MUSCLES.

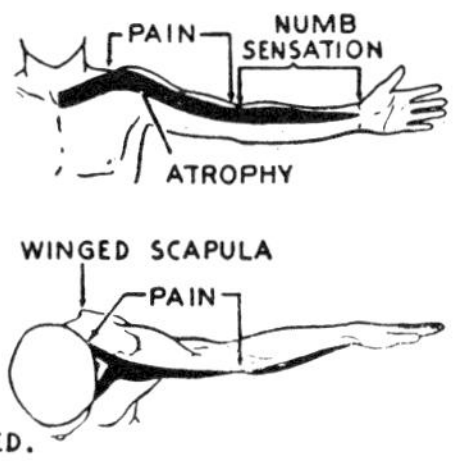

SIXTH CERVICAL

PAIN UPPER MEDIAL SCAPULA.

TENDERNESS OVER TRANSVERSE PROCESS OF VERTEBRA.

RADIATION OF PAIN TO LATERAL ARM.

NUMB SENSATION OF THUMB.

HYPOALGESIA AS OUTLINED.

REFLEX OF BICEPS TENDON REDUCED OR ABSENT.

MOTOR WEAKNESS & ATROPHY OF THUMB, BICEPS AND SCAPULAR MUSCLES.

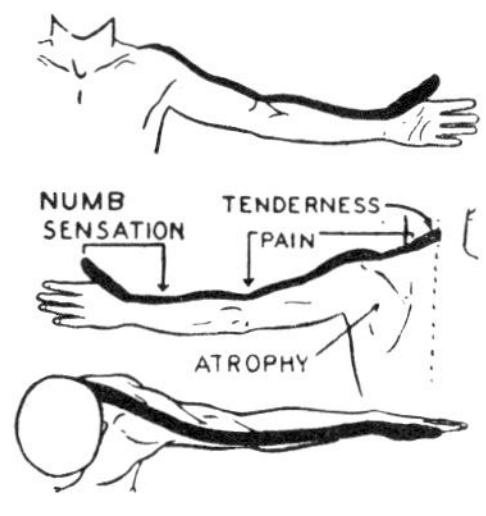

SEVENTH CERVICAL

PAIN UPPER MEDIAL SCAPULA.

TENDERNESS OVER TRANSVERSE PROCESS OF VERTEBRA.

RADIATION OF PAIN TO POSTERO-LATERAL ARM.

NUMB SENSATION 2ND & 3RD DIGITS.

HYPOALGESIA AS OUTLINED.

REFLEX OF TRICEPS TENDON REDUCED OR ABSENT.

MOTOR WEAKNESS & ATROPHY OF TRICEPS MUSCLE.

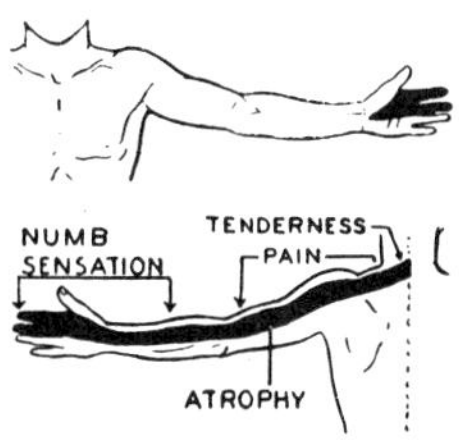

EIGHTH CERVICAL

PAIN OVER MEDIAL SCAPULAR SPINE.

TENDERNESS OVER TRANSVERSE PROCESS OF VERTEBRA.

RADIATION OF PAIN TO POSTERO-MEDIAL ARM.

NUMB SENSATION 4TH & 5TH DIGITS.

HYPOALGESIA AS OUTLINED.

REFLEX NO CHANGES RECOGNIZED.

MOTOR WEAKNESS & ATROPHY OF INTRINSIC MUSCLES OF HAND.

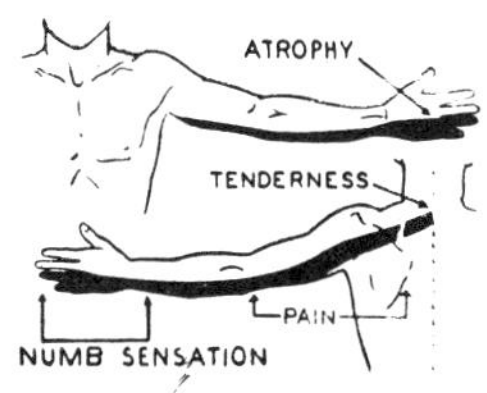

LUMBOSACRAL

FOURTH LUMBAR

PAIN IN GLUTEAL (HIP) REGION OVER TROCHANTER

TENDERNESS OVER TRANSVERSE PROCESS OF VERTEBRA

RADIATION OF PAIN TO ANTERIOR THIGH & LEG

NUMB SENSATION ANTERIOR LEG, GREAT TOE

HYPOALGESIA AS OUTLINED

REFLEX OF PATELLAR TENDON REDUCED OR ABSENT

MOTOR WEAKNESS & ATROPHY OF QUADRICEPS MUSCLE

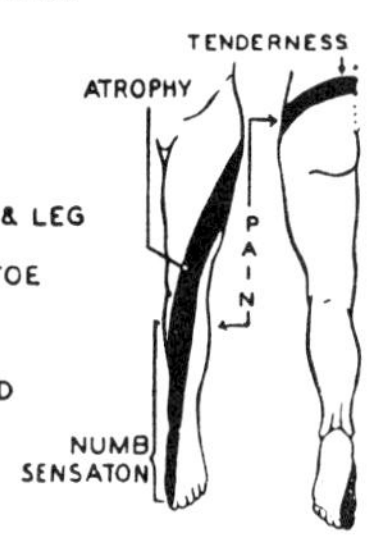

FIFTH LUMBAR

PAIN IN GLUTEAL (HIP) REGION BETWEEN ISCHIAL TUBEROSITY & GREATER TROCHANTER

TENDERNESS OVER TRANSVERSE PROCESS OF VERTEBRA

RADIATION OF PAIN TO LATERAL THIGH AND LEG

NUMB SENSATION LATERAL LEG, THREE MIDDLE (OR GREAT) TOES

HYPOALGESIA AS OUTLINED

REFLEX USUALLY NO ALTERATION

MOTOR WEAKNESS & ATROPHY OF DORSAL FLEXORS OF ANKLE AND TOES

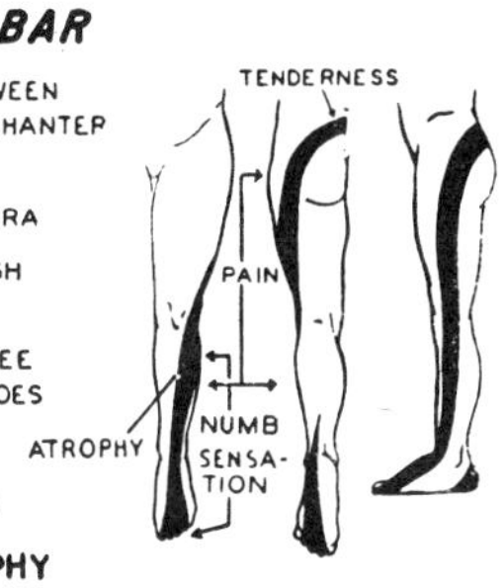

FIRST SACRAL

PAIN IN MEDIAL GLUTEAL (HIP) REGION (OVER ISCHIAL TUBEROSITY)

TENDERNESS OVER TRANSVERSE PROCESS OF VERTEBRA

RADIATION OF PAIN TO POSTERIOR THIGH & LEG

NUMB SENSATION POSTERIOR LEG, LITTLE TOE

HYPOALGESIA AS OUTLINED

REFLEX OF ACHILLES TENDON REDUCED OR ABSENT

MOTOR WEAKNESS & ATROPHY OF PLANTAR FLEXORS

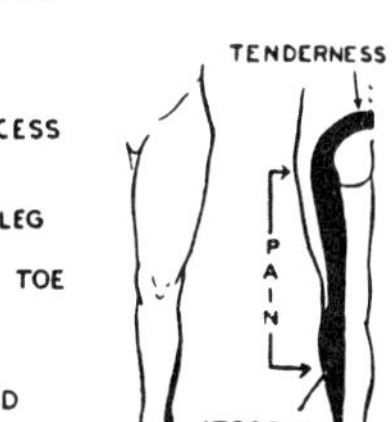

SECOND SACRAL

PAIN IN MEDIAL GLUTEAL FOLD

TENDERNESS OVER UPPER LATERAL SACRUM

RADIATION OF PAIN TO POSTERO-MEDIAL THIGH, LEG AND HEEL

NUMB SENSATION MEDIAL GLUTEAL FOLD, LABIUM MAJUS OR SCROTUM

HYPOALGESIA AS OUTLINED

REFLEX PLANTAR FLEXION RESPONSE REDUCED

MOTOR WEAKNESS NONE RECOGNIZED

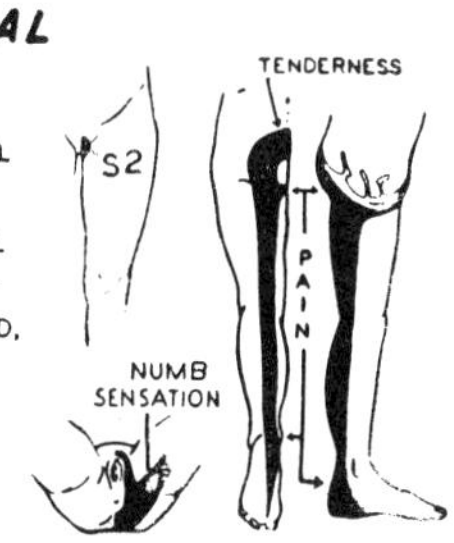

quate treatment instituted, and a poor result obtained.

Even in apparently obvious episodes of trauma, specifics are necessary. What were the details of the accident, under what circumstances, in what environment, and what first aid and subsequent treatment are given? Did the trouble start with an injection or a specific traumatic episode? The young man with a wrist drop secondary to a motorcycle accident may have an irreversible stretch palsy or a simple neurapraxia of the radial nerve due to a contusion. If one knows what forces were involved, how long ago, what the initial symptoms were, or something of the development of the palsy, the proper therapeutic course may reveal itself even as the history unfolds.

A clear description of pain or sensory aberration is difficult to put into words, and what is one patient's agony may be another's annoyance. The historian must adhere to simple language. Terms, such as "paresthesias" or "lancinating," may establish one's erudition but will not contribute much to understanding, whereas "pins and needles" or "shooting pains" are easily understood. Pain is difficult to describe as is alteration of normal sensation or diminution in feeling, and each patient will describe these symptoms differently. Pain exists in many degrees and variations; an uncomfortable feeling may not necessarily be painful, and one would like to know if the feeling is one of discomfort or pain, increased sensation, decreased sensation, or combinations of any of these.

Allowing for differing individual reactions to alterations in normal sensation, differing personalities, and the difficulties in verbalization and description, the examiner must put together the symptom picture. As the picture takes form, a skeleton differential diagnosis should begin to appear, and with it should appear leads to explore by means of more specific questions to the patient. Guiding the patient in giving his history can be overdone and may tempt the examiner to ask leading questions. The malleable or insecure patient or the one overanxious to please may be talked into relating an erroneous history if led by the examiner. For example, it is better to ask, "Do you have any unusual sensations in your hands?" rather than, "Do your fingertips tingle?" The latter may lead the patient to conclude that the examiner's "tingle" is really referring to the decreased sensation he experiences, and he may well answer honestly but erroneously in the affirmative.

A relationship of anatomical position of the extremity to the onset or aggravation of symptoms may be established by careful history-taking. Similarly, a particular activity or function may be found to either cause or modify a neurological symptom. Exposure to temperature extremes may be discovered, e.g., exacerbation of the dysesthesias of a neuroma when groping in the refrigerator. Symptoms may wax or wane nocturnally, seasonally, climatically, or with mood change. An examination will never reveal these points but a good history will. A review of symptoms is a part of every good history and will often lead to a diagnosis of systemic disease of which the neurological manifestations are only a part.

Clinical history taking is both an art and a discipline; it is clinical detective work in which clues may be abundant or sparse or misleading or false. The physician must be able to persuade the patient into revealing all and at the same time hold him to the theme. Some patients indulge in a barrage of non sequiturs, and some are reluctant to part with information, and some even look with suspicion at the whole process. With experience, one learns to deal with the different patient personalities and have the problem revealed—and within a reasonable time. In the process, the physician has the opportunity to establish communication and rapport with the patient, and by the time the physical examination commences, the patient should already have decided that his doctor is not only competent but, even more important, interested.

Examination

Appearance. The experienced clinican is a trained observer and has disciplined himself to use his eyes. Many peripheral nerve lesions may be diagnosed simply by the appearance of the patient's hand, not forgetting that the history may have indicated where to look for further clues or to confirm an historical impression. The visual examination really has four phases. It starts when the patient enters the room, and this first phase consists of a cursory assessment of gait, stance, and demeanor. Does the patient limp? Is he willing to shake hands or does he protect his right hand? Is he tense or nervous? Does he show outward evidence of pain? The second part of the visual examination is conducted during the history taking wherein the examiner observes how the patient sits, how he moves his extremities, and whether or not he uses his hands in communication. Phase three starts at the end of history taking and is a preliminary to the more formal and systematic physical examination; in this phase, the examiner systematically observes and records gross abnormalities, color, motion, abnormalities of hair growth, skin texture, evidence of wounds, nail changes, and visible sweating. All this can be done before the patient is touched, and this is reassuring to the patient with a painful lesion. He becomes more willing to cooperate in the examination as he realizes the physician is not going to seize the painful part roughly or abruptly.

Phase four consists of observation of function. The patient is asked to perform motor activities, finger flexion, wrist extension, thumb opposition, coordinated movements, and the like. The performance of specific tasks, such as removing a jacket, tying a shoelace, holding a pen, or turning pages of a book, may give an excellent picture of the type and degree of functional impairment. By this time, the patient should be working as a partner with the physician in an attempt to make the picture clear.

Tactile Examination. Following the visual examination, the physician then touches the involved extremity for the first time. He wishes to learn through his own tactile sensation about skin temperature, moisture, and texture (Fig. 5-2). This really represents an objective sensory examination inasmuch as no response from the patient is required, and often an accurate appraisal can be made of the area and degree of sensory disability through the examiner's own sensory information. The tactile pads of normal fingers have a well-defined texture due to the rugal folds of the fingerprints. Among the trophic changes resulting from loss of sensibility is a flattening of these rugas which may be mild in degree in the hypoesthetic finger or have progressed to the point where the skin is smooth and shiny in the case of complete anesthesia. This objective sensory examination may be the only sensory examination possible on infants, unconscious patients, or uncooperative patients, and it is of obvious value in the patient in whom malingering or exaggeration is suspected.

Motor Examination. Active motion implies motion initiated by the patient whereas passive motion is that caused by an outside force, such as the examiner's hands or a dynamic splint. Except for assessing joint stiffness or spasticity, passive motion is of little significance in a neurological examination. One is interested instead in the voluntary response of muscles: to what degree and with what strength. The distinction between flaccid and spastic paralysis is also a part of the motor examination. Although it seems to the beginner a monumental task to assess *all* of the muscles of the involved extremity, it is often essential for accurate diagnosis. Nevertheless, the majority of peripheral nerve motor lesions can be quickly and accurately recognized and catalogued with a few simple tests which will be explained later in the section on specific nerve lesions. In examining the motor response, the concept of the closed loop must be understood. In response to efferent cerebral command, the muscle belly is stimulated to contract; shortening of the muscle belly is relayed through the tendon across a joint or joints to cause one bone to move on another. When the desired motion is accomplished, the information is relayed through proprioceptive sensation via the afferent sensory fibers back to the brain, and the loop is, thus, completed. Not only are the primary muscles of action stimulated but also a reciprocal adjustment is necessary and is accomplished automatically in antagonistic muscles; the net result is a controlled and coordinated response.

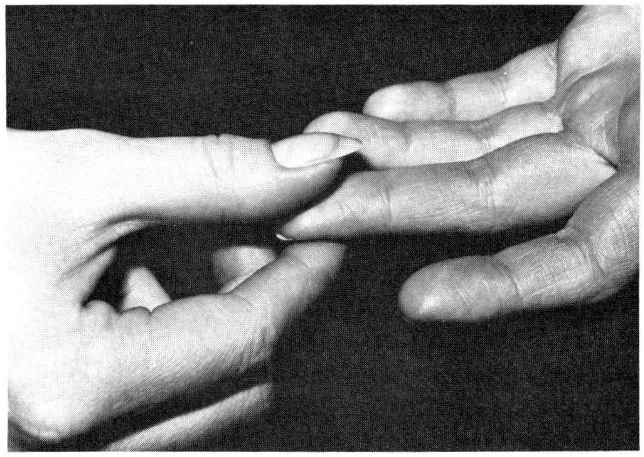

Fig. 5-2. Objective tactile testing. It is the examiner's tactile sensation which allows him to assess smoothness and dryness of the patient's fingers. It is useful in the established nerve lesion but not informative in the recent injury.

Atrophy of muscles may be detected visually and may be due to disuse or paralysis (Fig. 5-3). Muscle

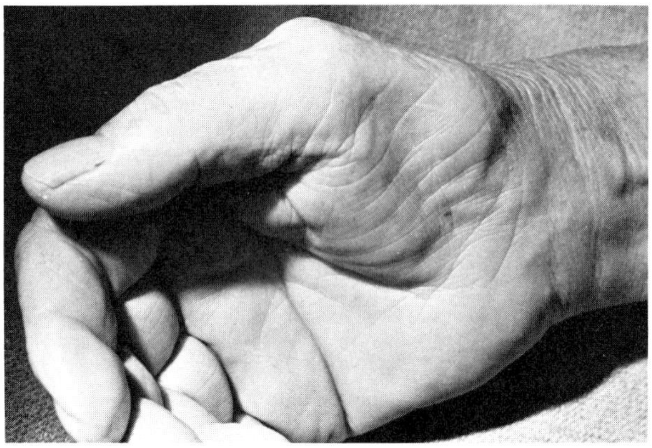

Fig. 5-3. Paralytic atrophy of the median innervated thenar muscles. The concavity is due to atrophy of the abductor pollicis brevis and the opponens pollicis. The ulnar-innervated portion of the flexor pollicis brevis appears normal and is able to give fair opposition to this thumb.

examination is accomplished not only through this observation but also by palpation of the muscle belly as well as testing the muscle's strength against resistence. Muscle strength is graded from total paralysis to normal strength either as zero through five or, descriptively, as zero, trace, poor, fair, good, or normal. "Zero" implies no muscle response at all. "Trace" is only a flicker of contraction. "Poor" means active motion is possible when gravity is eliminated. "Fair" means active motion is possible against gravity but not against added resistence. "Good" means motion is possible against both gravity and added resistence but not to a normal degree. "Normal" is determined by comparison with the opposite extremity if uninvolved or compared, if possible, with the patient's prepathological state. Elaborate rating charts are available for all of the skeletal muscles in the body, and although these are occasionally useful in the more complex lesions, more often a simple notation of a few key muscles is adequate.

Muscle fasciculation, fine irregular twitching of portions of a muscle, may be either observed in a muscle at rest or may be provoked by percussing the muscle. Tendon reflexes test both the efferent and afferent components and are depressed or absent in peripheral nerve disease when muscle power may still be intact. Tendon reflexes are subject to much individual variation; some normal persons lack them almost completely whereas with anxiety or stress the reflexes may be abnormally hyperactive.

Some patients develop, either deliberately or unconsciously, substitute or trick motions to overcome motor loss. Gravity is often used for elbow extension when there is paralysis of the triceps. If paralyzed muscles are put on a stretch, they may act as check reins which may create a spring or rebound effect. A tenodesis effect can be demonstrated in a radial palsy in which strong wrist flexion may cause the paralyzed finger extensors to become stretched thereby causing some finger extension.

Deviation from the textbook description of muscle innervation, particularly in the hand, is common and must be suspected when the results of motor examination are not consistent with the preliminary diagnosis. Common examples of this are seen in the variations in innervation of the thenar muscles in which the flexor pollicis brevis may act as a fair substitute for opposition and may be innervated entirely by the median nerve, by the ulnar nerve, or by contributions from both.

Supplementary activities of other muscles may also give motion which seems inconsistent with some nerve lesions. Extension of the distal joint of the thumb may result from an anomalous insertion of the abductor pollicis brevis in radial palsy even though there is complete loss of the extrinsic thumb extensors.

Sensory Examination. Thorough sensory examination of an extremity is a time-consuming and exacting procedure, and because it is at least in part subjective, the results may vary with the patient's mood, fatigue, or degree of pain. Generally, the simplest testing methods are best, and in many instances, the examiner's objective tactile examination will suffice. Nevertheless, one will want to know at least roughly what the levels of sensibility to the more basic stimuli are. Pain can be tested for by pinprick and should be done in a relatively painless manner. Tactile sensibility, i.e., touch, both fine and gross, can be tested for by the patient's verbal response to the examiner's stroking finger or with wisps of cotton or a special examining instrument, such as a von Frey hair. Testing for vibration sensation is done with a tuning fork and is of more value for the neuropathies of interest to the neurologist than for the peripheral nerve lesions which generally involve the surgeon.

Most revealing in the fingertips is the test for two point discrimination, the ability to distinguish more than one pressure sensation at one time. Normal fingertips should be able to detect points of pressure 2 to 3 mm. apart, and the ability is most highly developed in the tactile pads of the thumb and index fingers. Two point discrimination of greater than 10 mm. in a fingertip represents marked impairment of useful sensation. The examination must be carried out without visual assistance, i.e., the patient is not allowed to watch the examination. A caliper with two blunt points may be used, but simpler, and always available, is a paper clip which can be bent to fit the purpose, the distance between the two points being easily adjusted and varied (Fig. 5-4). Some patients try hard to please and some wish to score high on any test, and it is, therefore, wise to vary the task by touching with only one point sporadically throughout the test. The test should not be painful, and only light pressure is required.

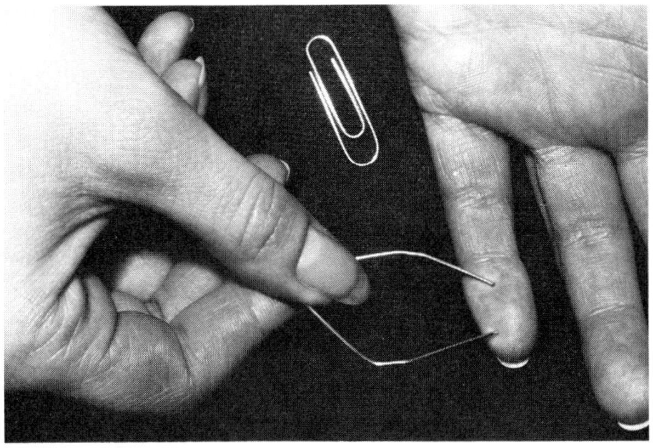

Fig. 5-4. Two-point discrimination testing. The distance between the blunt points of the paper clip is easily varied. Only light pressure is necessary.

Autonomic and Nutritional Changes. Sweating, i.e., pseudomotor function, can be qualitatively and simply tested for by observation and by palpation with one's own fingers. More specific and quantitative tests can be done with various chemicals, but they rarely yield enough practical clinical information to warrant the required time and resultant mess. Skin temperature, as detected by the examiner's fingers, is of some value in autonomic assessment, the affected part usually being colder to the touch than normally innervated skin. Color changes, such as redness and cyanosis or blotchiness, may also indicate autonomic denervation. Denervated skin is usually smoother than normal, but on occasion there may be hyperkeratinization. There may also be nail changes with transverse ridging, overgrowth or undergrowth of nails, and the disappearance of cuticle. Ulcers and blisters may be seen and are usually due to injury to an anesthetic part. Atrophy of denervated digits is common but not consistent or predictable.

Other Tests. Roentgenograms are mainly of value in demonstrating bone or joint injury or deformity which may be the underlying cause of nerve damage. Laboratory studies of value are those which may indicate systemic disease of which the neuropathy is a secondary manifestation. Electrodiagnostic studies are covered in Chapter 3, and although they may be informative in gauging the rate and degree of regeneration, they are in no way a substitute for the simpler, quicker, and cheaper methods outlined here. There is an unfortunate tendency to slight the physical examination in favor of electromyograms and nerve conduction studies, and it should be emphasized that electronic gadgetry is no substitute for a trained eye and a knowledgeable motor and sensory examination.

Tinel's Test. This is a test of regeneration, the importance of which has been exaggerated but which is, nevertheless, of some practical value in *qualitatively* detecting return of function in a sensory nerve. Light percussion over the tip of a regenerating sensory axon will be felt as a tingling or shock-like sensation in the *peripheral* distribution of that axon. It is best elicited by light fingertip percussion over the digit which should progress proximally until the patient notices paresthesias in the finger or toe. Percussion over a neuroma will give similar sensations either at the site of the neuroma or in the distal distribution of a nerve, and this response tells one nothing of regeneration. It is, therefore, important to damp out vibratory transmission from the percussing finger to the neuroma by applying digital pressure over the nerve between the neuroma and the level of percussion, as in the accompanying figure (Fig. 5-5). Tingling sensations felt at the site of the neuroma on percussion are not Tinel's sign and give little information about the process of regeneration.

Central Nervous System and Psychic Factors. Hysteria, although the term is decried by psychiatrists, is nevertheless a real and common clinical

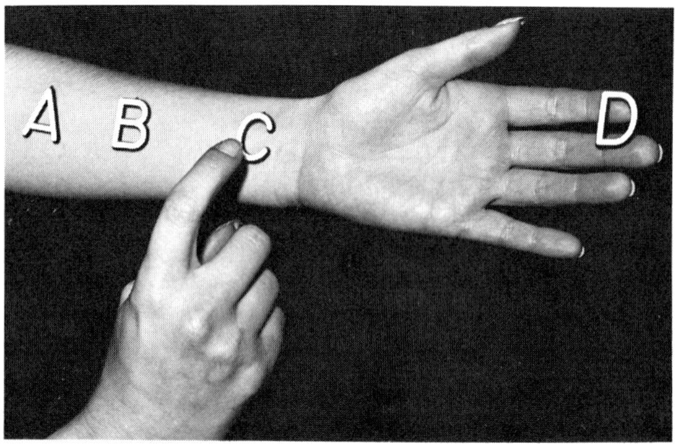

Fig. 5-5. Tinel's test. Light percussion over the nerve (C) distal to the nerve lesion (A) while blocking out vibrations of the neuroma with digital pressure at (B) will cause shock-like or tingling sensations in the distal distribution of the nerve (D). Percussion should start at (D) and progress proximally up the nerve. The point at which paresthesias are elicited marks the most distal level of axon regrowth.

condition, and its more advanced forms may present marked aberration from normal neurological function manifested by total paralysis or anesthesia and shading over into very mild variations which are more the product of mood swings, personality differences, or ethnic traits than of actual neurological disease. The examiner must be alert to suggestions that symptoms may be psychogenic and must attempt to prove or eliminate this conjecture during the examination. The classic glove anesthesia of overt hysteria is seldom seen and presents little diagnostic problem when it is present. More common and more difficult to recognize is the marginal type of hysteria based on motivation or secondary gain. Common in this category is the patient with minimal injury who consciously or unconsciously exaggerates or modifies symptoms in order to increase a compensation award. Malingering in its pure, i.e., dishonest, form is very rare; more often the patient has convinced himself that his minor symptoms are really major. Once this pattern is established, objectivity is lost and the patient's desires become the opposite of his physician's with the latter wishing to diagnose and improve whereas the compensation-oriented patient really wants obfuscation and exaggeration of the problem. Do not expect to prove this to this type of patient as he will neither wish to understand it nor admit it.

The symptoms of central nervous system disease and those of psychic origin may mimic each other, and the diagnosis can only be unraveled by careful objective neurological examination. Central nervous system disease may also give rise to motor or sensory symptoms masquerading as peripheral nerve lesions. Multiple sclerosis is such a disease, and diagnosis will depend on the accuracy of detail of the neurological examination and the integration of the physical findings with the innervation patterns of dermatomes, myotomes, and the muscle innervation tables. Diseases that affect both central and peripheral nervous systems, such as Vitamin B_{12} deficiency and focal cord lesions involving nerve roots, confuse the picture further.

Putting It All Together. The complete neurologic examination may take hours and is a trial for both patient and physician. One must learn to separate quickly the inconsequential from the significant and to exploit leads which appear as the history and examination progress. The history will generally give the examiner clues to follow in defining the lesion, and the examination should then establish the location and level of the lesion. As history and examination proceed, the examiner builds his diagnosis on the scaffolding of his knowledge of neuroanatomy and, as the picture develops, is able to take many shortcuts and eliminate much of what would be tedious and uninformative. The history of the injury of the motorcyclist may suggest a traction injury of the brachial plexus, but if all abnormalities are limited to the distribution of one of the peripheral nerves, the localization of the lesion becomes clearer. Loss of extrinsic finger and thumb extensors with an intact radial wrist extensor immediately localizes the lesion in the dorsal interosseous nerve and eliminates higher radial nerve damage. In the following section on specific nerve lesions, a few key physical findings will be illustrated. These should not lead one to jump to conclusions but can be of immense help as signposts to point the way to quick diagnosis. Lesions involving a plexus, or more than one nerve, will, of course, be more difficult to sort out, and anatomical anomalies may also confuse the picture; but with increasing knowledge of neuroanatomy and growing clinical experience, the diagnostic process will become evermore efficient, accurate, and rewarding.

DEGENERATION AND REGENERATION

Types of Injury

Conduction Loss Without Interruption of the Axoplasm or Histological Change in the Fiber. Such loss is generally due to transient ischemia or pressure on the nerve, causing loss of transmission of impulse. This lasts anywhere from a few minutes to a few weeks and is followed by complete recovery of function. Neurapraxia is a clinical term implying a loss of nerve function followed by spontaneous recovery which usually occurs within a few hours, days, or weeks of injury.

Axonotmesis Damage to the Axoplasm Without Loss of Continuity of the Endoneurium. With this condition, there is histological change in the axon and a reaction of degeneration followed by regeneration of the axon and restoration of function.

Neurotmesis Damage to Both Axon and Endoneurium. In this injury, both the neural and connective tissue elements of the fiber are disrupted. If the damage is localized and there is still continuity of the epineurium, there may be spontaneous regeneration leading to recovery of function, but when there is severance of the entire nerve trunk, regeneration may be impossible without some type of surgical repair, and even this is not always successful.

Degeneration

Damage to the nerve fiber causes changes in the fiber both distal and proximal to the point of injury. Distally, there is a fragmentation of the axoplasm and its myelin sheath, and within a few weeks there is complete disappearance of both elements through microphage activity. The distal endoneurial tubes shrink to a fraction of their original size, and the investing perineurium decreases in volume over a three to six month period with resultant loss in diameter of the nerve trunk. A similar dissolution of axon and myelin sheath, called wallerian degeneration, as well as a concomitant shrinkage of the connective tissue elements occurs proximal to the interruption; the degeneration extends proximally to the next node of Ranvier. There may also be central changes within the nerve cell body itself depending on the degree of violence sustained by the nerve and in inverse proportion to the distance between the site of injury and the cell body.

Regeneration

When the neuron has recovered from the effects of retrograde degeneration, regrowth of the axon begins. This regrowth occurs within a few days when the injury has been slight but will take several weeks or even months in cases of severe trunk injury. The rate of regeneration varies with numerous factors, such as the level and nature of the injury and the age of the patient, and the classic rule of 1 mm. of axonal regrowth per day, although a rough approximation, is still useful.

If the endoneurial tube is intact, the axon crosses the site of injury without delay, proceeds distally to the end-organ, and function is reestablished. When the endoneurium has been disrupted, the regenerating axon may successfully find its way across the gap, may find another endoneurial tube in which to regenerate, or may become snarled in the fibroblastic build-up of connective tissue at the injury site thereby forming a neuroma.

Regeneration on the distal side of the interruption is limited to the connective tissue elements which form a nodule smaller than the neuroma; this is called a glioma and is devoid of neural tissue. Except when there has been a segmental loss of nerve trunk, as in severe gunshot wounds, the neuroma and glioma are usually in continuity forming a dumbbell-shaped mass. Some axons may successfully penetrate this mass depending on its density; if they find their way into foreign endoneurial tubes—cross shunting—a distorted pattern of innervation may result and seriously impair function.

Tinel's sign, more properly called the Hoffman-Tinel sign, is elicited by percussion over the regenerating tip of a sensory axon which produces a tingling sensation in the distal cutaneous distribution of that axon, and this is of some use in following the rate and pattern of regeneration of less severe nerve injuries. It should not be confused with the paresthetic or dysesthetic sensations elicited by tapping over the neuroma. The importance of Tinel's sign has been exaggerated, and it is of little value in cases of severe injury to the nerve trunk.

DISEASES OF THE PERIPHERAL NERVES

There are several hundred types and causes of diseases and disorders of the peripheral nerves. Of major interest to readers of this text are the traumatic and compression lesions which will be covered in detail later on. These are manifested by axonal division or degeneration, one of the two major types of nerve disease; the other is segmental demyelinization. One or the other, or combinations of the two, are represented by the diseases outlined in the following. The classification of neurological conditions is complex and, at best, arbitrary as often cause and effect are not understood. The groupings which follow are on the basis of etiology, and only the highlights of diagnosis will be mentioned.

Infection

Leprosy. Leprosy is the most common cause of serious peripheral nerve disease in the world. Infection with *Mycobacterium leprae* most commonly involves cutaneous nerves causing anesthesia resulting in ulcers, infection, Charcot's joints, and loss of digits. Involvement of nerve trunks gives mixed motor and sensory loss of either individual nerves or combinations of nerves. The ulnar nerve is most commonly involved. In the lepromatous type, many leprosy bacteria are found in the nerves, hypertrophic skin lesions are common, and the nerve involvement is generally sensory and symmetrical. In the tuberculoid form of leprosy, the bacilli are absent from the nerve, and diagnosis is confirmed with a skin test in contrast to the nerve biopsy which is positive in the lepromatous type. In the tuberculoid form, many types of sensory and motor deficits are possible, and depigmentation and atrophy of the skin are common.

Diphtheritic Neuropathy. The neurotoxin of *Corynebacterium diphtheriae* does not cause clinical signs until a month or two after the onset of the pharyngitis. It may cause a progressive paralysis of all peripheral nerves, both motor and sensory, and may lead to death by respiratory paralysis. The segmental demyelinization reverses itself, and unless death ensues from paralysis or cardiac involvement, remyelinization and recovery occur within another month.

Guillain-Barré Syndrome. Although the exact nature and cause of this disease is not understood, and since it often follows within a few weeks of a viral infection, it is classified herein with the infectious neuropathies. It may start with paresthesias and dysesthesias of feet or hands spreading proximally and followed by muscle weakness in the extremities and severe back pain. In severe cases, respiratory muscle weakness may be life-threatening. The nerves involved have decreased conduction velocity, and the cerebrospinal fluid has an elevated level of protein. After one to several weeks, the progress of symptoms ceases, and the majority of patients recover normal function within several months.

Metabolic

Diabetes causes the most common of the metabolic neuropathies, and most prominent in this type is sensory loss, usually distal and symmetrical. The diabetic with nerve loss often first notices burning feet and tender calves, although sometimes the hands are similarly affected. When autonomic dysfunction, poor blood supply, and sensory loss are combined, persistent ulcers, gangrene of the toes, Charcot's joints, and loss of proprioception may result. Loss of tactile sensation, pain, and vibratory sensation is common and more so in diabetes of long-standing or the diabetic in poor control. Weak and atrophied quadriceps femoris muscles are fairly frequent in severe diabetes but other motor loss is uncommon.

Acute porphyria may cause psychiatric disturbances and both central and peripheral nervous system disorders. The peripheral neuropathy is usually severe and predominantly motor and most often causes muscle weakness in the upper extremities. Sensory loss occurs in some, and recovery may be complete, partial, or not occur at all.

Renal, hepatic, and thyroid diseases may all cause peripheral neuropathies. Uremic peripheral nerve involvement is common in patients sustained by dialysis and is manifested by burning and numbness of the feet and hands, often with some slight motor loss. Liver failure more commonly involves the central nervous system, but distal sensory and motor loss may also occur. Hyperthyroidism and hypothyroidism can also cause peripheral nerve loss in both sensory and motor components. Nerve entrapment—particularly the carpal tunnel syndrome—is common in myxedema.

Several vitamin deficiencies cause peripheral nerve changes; these may be due to deficiency in thiamine (B_1), pyridoxine (B_6), or nicotinic acid or, more commonly, malnutrition due to inadequate diet, alcoholism, or to the diseases of malabsorption. The symptoms are predominantly sensory and are similar to those of diabetic neuropathy, but motor loss in all extremities may occur also. Vitamin B_{12} deficiency gives a mixed picture of central nervous system and both sensory and motor loss in the periphery; the peripheral changes respond quickly to replacement therapy, whereas the cord changes do not.

Toxic Neuropathies

There are hundreds, probably thousands, of organic and inorganic compounds, drugs, industrial chemicals, solvents, and insecticides which can poison nerves. Some substances, harmless to most, may cause an immunologic or allergic reaction in some patients and may lead to nerve damage. Other toxins, by damaging kidneys or liver, may be indirect contributors to neuropathy. Such nerve involvement is manifest by mixed motor and sensory loss, with the sensory dysesthesias and paresthesias having the most common complaints. Lead poisoning is well known for its paralytic signs of wrist and foot drop.

Ischemic Conditions May Cause Local or Diffuse Peripheral Nerve Disease

The local changes occur on a traumatic or thromboembolic basis, and the diffuse changes are most often due to occlusive vascular disease. Arteriosclerosis often first manifests itself through sensory complaints of burning sensations or numbness in the feet and hands and also by pain and weakness in muscles. Some of the symptoms will be attributable to muscle ischemia, but definite degenerative changes in both sensory and motor nerves are also found. Related to ischemic changes are the neuropathies associated with the aging process, and it is impossible to dissociate the two types. Although there is much individual variation, there is a general progressive degeneration of both motor and sensory nerves with slowed conduction times and often histological evidence of demyelinization and axonal degeneration as the aging process proceeds.

The collagen diseases, such as scleroderma, dermatomyositis, and polyarteritis nodosa, may also result in ischemic peripheral neuropathy. More common are the nerve changes of rheumatoid arthritis, many of which are due to compression but some of which are ischemic in nature and secondary to arteritis from rheumatoid involvement.

Neoplastic Neuropathies

These may be due to the secondary effects of carcinoma or to primary involvement by nerve tumors per se. Carcinomatous neuropathy is most common with carcinoma of the lung, breast, and stomach and seems to be associated with the wasting seen with cancer and is manifested by a distal and symmetrical degeneration of both sensory and motor elements. Primary nerve tumors consist of benign overgrowths of Schwann cells or fibroblasts and are variously called schwannomas, neurilemomas, or neurofibromas. These tumors are usually solitary and may involve any of the peripheral nerves, causing pressure which may lead to axonal degeneration.

Multiple neurofibromatosis or von Recklinghausen's disease is a hereditary disease in which there are widespread skin, bone, and nerve abnormalities. The latter consist of many neurofibromas of several or many nerve trunks, particularly involving cutaneous nerves, and may cause pain and loss of both sensory and motor function depending on the distribution and degree of involvement. The skin changes are often startling and range from the well known café-au-lait spots to the pedunculated skin lesions called molluscum fibrosum. The neurofibromas may form plexuses which are palpable and visible subcutaneously. The tumors grow slowly causing focal enlargment of the nerve trunk but seldom cause paralysis except in the young patient.

Hereditary Diseases of Peripheral Nerves

There are many inherited or congenital neuropathies, many that are familial, and some which are ethnic or racial in background. Patients with congenital insensitivity to pain have otherwise normal sensation, but the loss of pain as a protective mechanism leads to recurrent injury, infection, ulceration, and mutilation. In other types of congenital sensory neuropathy, all types of sensation may be lost but with no or slight motor involvement. In some, all abnormalities are peripheral, and in others, autonomic and central nervous system dysfunctions of different combinations may exist. The sensory impairment may be apparent at birth or appear later in life and be progressive.

Charcot-Marie-Tooth disease or peroneal muscular atrophy is characterized by progressive distal muscle atrophy appearing in adolescence; it first presents as pes cavus followed by progressive atrophy of the leg muscles giving the appearance of "bird legs" and later spreading to the hands. There may or may not be sensory changes, but these are less severe than the muscle atrophy. There are several different familial types which occur in various degrees; most are slowly progressive, but some lead to severe crippling early in life.

Amyloidosis neuropathy is also familial and may vary from mild to life-terminating by age 30. Symptoms usually appear at age 25 to 30, and the initial picture is often that of a carpal tunnel syndrome or other compression neuropathy. Decompression of the involved nerve may give temporary improvement, and the endoneurium will be found to contain masses of amyloid. Shooting pains and paresthesias of both lower and upper extremities may occur as well as progressive loss of pain and temperature sensation, changes in autonomic function leading to distal autonomic changes and ulceration, and systemic autonomic symptoms, such as gastrointestinal disturbances, impotence, and cardiac problems. The Andrade type of amyloidosis found in some Portugese families is the most severe and is usually fatal by age 50. Other types are seen in Swiss, German, and British families and may have similar but less severe or progressive changes.

Recurrent, Chronic, and Idiopathic Neuropathies

Some of these may be seen in association with the hereditary neuropathies or with metabolic disorders; others appear to have no relationship to any other disease picture and as the cause is unknown, are truly idiopathic. Attacks may be acute and self-limited followed by complete recovery, or they may be repeated and with or without residuals. Sensory and/or motor symptoms and signs may be present and to all degrees of severity. One type is the brachial plexus neuropathy. This starts with severe shoulder pain which lasts for several days and is followed by motor and sometimes sensory loss in the distribution of one or more regions of the brachial plexus, particularly involving the shoulder girdle. Paralysis of the serratus anterior muscle may result from isolated involvement of the long thoracic nerve. Recovery is spontaneous but may take many months.

Radiation Neuropathy

Therapeutic radiation in the range of 5,000 rads or more may cause peripheral nerve damage in the regions of the brachial or lumbosacral plexus, and these changes are usually irreversible.

DISEASES OF THE PERIPHERAL NERVE CELL BODY

These are often inseparable from diseases of the peripheral nerve trunks and fibers, and one may—and usually does—lead to the other. Anterior horn cell disease is predominantly motor in nature whereas disorders of the posterior root ganglia are primarily sensory.

The anterior horn cells may be damaged by infections, as in acute anterior poliomyelitis or rabies, or by progressive idiopathic degeneration, as in amyotrophic lateral sclerosis and the hereditary spinal muscular atrophies. The anterior horn cells may also be damaged by various central nervous system lesions and such diseases as syphilis, thromboses, and spinal cord tumors.

The most common posterior root ganglion disease is herpes zoster or shingles, a virus infection in which pain appears more or less in the distribution of one or more of the sensory nerve roots on one side of the chest followed in a few days by vesicle formation. There may be complete and spontaneous resolution within a few days, or a postherpetic neuralgia may develop which may be chronic and very severe. Sensory changes of hypoesthesia, dysesthesia, or hyperesthesia may accompany the symptoms.

NERVE ROOT INVOLVEMENT: RADICULOPATHY

Spinal nerve root disease or lesions produce sensory changes in a dermatome distribution and motor changes, according to a myotome pattern; when specific roots are involved, the neurological examination will be specific for localization of the disease. The radicular pattern will be much less definite when both cord and root are involved. Roentgenograms of the spine and examination of cerebrospinal fluid may aid in the neurological examination.

Most common are the mechanical lesions of compression from bulging or ruptured cervical or lumbosacral intervertebral disks; the neurological signs and symptoms may appear acutely when prolapse of the disk is sudden and traumatic, or they may appear insidiously in the case of degenerative disk disease. The acute onset presents a radicular distribution of pain which may be severe and increased with motion. Various degrees of paresthesias, sensory and motor loss, and areflexia may then follow depending on the degree of compression. Most common is disk prolapse in the fifth lumbar interspace causing unilateral sciatica, loss of ankle jerk, sensory diminution about the foot, and weakness of muscles innervated by roots at the fifth lumbar and first sacral levels. For the latter, the extensor hallucis longus and the extensor digitorum brevis are easy to examine for weakness. The herniated disk of the fourth lumbar interspace (i.e., L-4, 5) will also cause sciatica, and the only physical sign may be weakness of the extensor hallucis longus. A disk of the second or third lumbar interspace will more likely cause pain radiating into the thigh or knee, and there will be loss of the knee jerk. Various combinations of signs and symptoms are common, and myelographic confirmation of the level may be necessary.

Chronic disk degeneration, osteophyte formation about the nerve root foramen, and spinal stenosis may cause symptoms similar to acute disk prolapse but usually have a more protracted onset and respond better to conservative treatment. Roentgenograms and myelograms of the lumbar spine may help in demonstrating the nature and level of the lesion.

Intraspinal tumors, such as neurofibromas, meningiomas, and lipomas, as well as secondary tumors, such as carcinoma, may cause many combinations of symptoms and signs. When these involve the cauda equina, sphincter impairment and loss of the anal reflex become important diagnostic signs.

Chronic meningitis or granulomas caused by tuberculosis, syphilis, and sarcoidosis may cause nerve root disease, and one theory has it that the findings of syphilitic tabes dorsalis—loss of position and deep pain sensation—are more due to degeneration of the posterior nerve roots than to the posterior columns of the cord.

MUSCLE DISEASE

Myasthenia gravis is a disease of impaired neuromuscular transmission in which repetitive actions become progressively weakened. It is purely motor and most commonly involves the muscles about the face, head, and neck and leads to difficulties in chewing or holding the eyelids open or the head erect. Also involved are the proximal muscles of the extremities; the patient may have trouble lifting the arms, walking, or climbing stairs, particularly at the end of the day. It is twice as common in women and usually appears at about age 20. It is diagnosed by repetitive electrical nerve stimulation and anticholinesterase testing.

There are many diseases of skeletal muscle, and although confusing and complex, it is not difficult to separate them from the true peripheral neuropathies as the muscle disorders manifest no sensory or reflex abnormalities and often have a typical progression of symptoms, helpful electrodiagnostic findings, and a familial history of the disease. They include the primary muscular dystrophies, the myotonias, periodic paralysis and polymyositis, as well as many myopathies resulting from toxins and metabolic and endocrine disorders. In myotonia congenita and pseudohypertrophic muscular dystrophy, groups of muscles, particularly in the calf, may be bulky in mass but weak or relatively unresponsive. Polymyositis, of which there are several types, is an inflammatory condition activated by an autoimmune reaction, and its differentiation from peripheral neuropathy may be more difficult because of pain and sensory changes that may accompany the muscular weakness.

Confusion between muscle disease and peripheral neuropathy arises when the neuropathy is only manifested by motor changes, such as in lead intoxication and some types of Guillain-Barré syndrome.

TRAUMATIC NERVE LESIONS

Peripheral nerves may be traumatized by acute or chronic compression, traction, or severance. Also included in this classification is the peripheral neuropathy caused by direct injection of nerve trunks with drugs. Interruption of axonal flow may be due to transsection of the nerve fibers, a stretching of the fibers with relative loss of continuity or ischemia.

Nerve Compression

Compression of the nerve can occur from an outside force, such as a blow or repetitive pressure; from the local pressure of tumors, exostoses, or hematomas; or by entrapment of the nerve within surrounding anatomical structures.

A sharp blow to the nerve may cause sensory paresthesias in the distal distribution of the nerve, such as the tingling and sometimes pain one experiences when the ulnar nerve at the elbow is smartly struck; these may be called "funny-bone" paresthesias. Somewhat more extensive symptoms can result from "toilet-seat paralysis" in which both sensory and motor changes occur from pressure on the sciatic nerve. These changes are reversible within a few minutes and whether due to primary alteration of the axon or the secondary influence of ischemia on the nerve is not clear.

More prolonged pressure from crutches may cause a brachial plexus palsy with both motor and sensory changes, and this may or may not be transient. The pressure of another's body on the outstretched arm for several hours causes the "Saturday night palsy," which represents a neurapraxia of the radial nerve that can take weeks or months to reverse itself.

Occupational palsies occur from repetitive pressure or blows to a nerve over a prolonged period of time. An example of this is the digital neuropathy seen in cloth cutters, tailors, and seamstresses who use scissors for many hours a day. An extreme example is the median or ulnar neuropathy seen in the operators of pneumatic jackhammers.

Entrapment neuropathies occur where peripheral nerve trunks pass through a potentially restricted tunnel or space; swelling of the nerve or other structures within the space creates a compression of the nerve which, if protracted, may lead to intraneural changes. These entrapment neuropathies are outlined below.

Carpal Tunnel Syndrome. This is by far the most common nerve entrapment, is seen most often in middle-aged women, and is sometimes associated with rheumatoid tenosynovitis, amyloidosis, myxedema, tumors, or anatomical abnormalities within the carpal tunnel, but it is frequently idiopathic, i.e., due to no apparent pathological disorder (see Fig. 3-13). The symptoms consist of paresthesias and dysesthesias in the median distribution of the hand manifested by numbness and tingling in the fingertips, often at night or after manual work. When the condition has existed for several years, motor weakness will be reflected in complaints of loss of strength and easy fatigability. A common complaint of "clumsiness" in such everyday but, nevertheless, complex acts such as buttoning a shirt or tying shoelaces is a manifestation of the diminution of tactile sense and is often accompanied by median intrinsic motor loss. Thenar atrophy and weakness of thumb abduction and opposition is seen in severe cases. Usually the symptoms are readily brought on by the patient holding the wrist acutely flexed for 20 to 30 seconds. They may also be reproduced with a tourniquet test in which a sphygmomanometer cuff inflated to 250 mg. of mercury will cause median paresthesias within one minute. Sensory examination will show diminution of two point discrimination often to greater than 1 cm. In severe cases, there will be a smoothness and dryness of the tactile pads of the fingers which represent trophic changes of sensory impairment.

The carpal tunnel syndrome is most common in the dominant hand, is often bilateral, and may also be associated with symptoms and signs of ulnar nerve involvement as well as median involvement. Electrodiagnostic studies show slowed sensory and motor conduction velocities and signs of denervation of the median innervated thenar muscles. Usually the history is pathognomonic, and the physical examination is sufficiently confirmatory to make electrical studies unnecessary.

There is an acute form of carpal tunnel syndrome which may follow reduction of a Colles' fracture with immobilization in the wrist flexion position. This should be suspected when there are unusual complaints of pain in the wrist and hand and particularly if there is sensory diminution in the thumb, index finger, or middle finger. Prompt release of wrist flexion is necessary to avoid irreversible median nerve damage.

Pronator Entrapment. The median nerve may also be compressed where it perforates the pronator teres muscle in the proximal forearm. In this case, weakness of wrist pronation and occasionally of thumb flexion will be added to the distal sensory and motor changes seen in the carpal tunnel syndrome.

Ulnar Entrapment. This is most commonly seen in the form of a tardy ulnar palsy in which there are symptoms of paresthesia and dysesthesia in the ulnar sensory distribution in the hand, often nerve tenderness in the ulnar groove at the elbow, and eventually motor signs of a high ulnar palsy. The condition may be occupational as in the writer who puts pressure on the elbow for many hours a day or may result from elbow deformity resulting from a childhood fracture. The nerve changes may progress slowly for many years before the patient seeks medical attention, and by then they can be irreversible.

The ulnar nerve may also be compressed in the canal of Guyon at the wrist. In this condition, the ulnar symptoms and signs in the hand are the counterpart of median nerve entrapment within the adjacent carpal tunnel. This is often an occupational development of motorcyclists, leather workers, and gardeners and may also be caused by the pressure of a ganglion.

The posterior interosseous nerve may be entrapped by the supinator muscle where the nerve winds about the neck of the radius, although more frequently problems with this nerve are the result of wounds or direct blows.

Nerve compression of the brachial plexus by cervical ribs, the first rib, or the anterior scalene muscle, although overdiagnosed in the past, does occur and is manifested by pain in the arm, weakness of grasp, ulnar paresthesias, increased sweating, and sometimes vascular impairment in the hand.

Tarsal Tunnel Syndrome. Entrapment of the posterior tibial nerve in the tarsal tunnel causes sensory changes over the toes and sole of the foot. There are seldom any motor changes, but often there is tenderness over the nerve posterior to the medial malleolus.

Common Peroneal Entrapment. Compression of the common peroneal nerve over the head of the fibula may cause not only paresthesias over the dorsum of the foot but also weakness of the peroneal musculature. Pressure on this nerve may be caused by careless positioning of the anesthetized patient on the operating table or by sitting for long periods with the legs crossed.

Morton's Toe. Morton's metatarsalgia is caused by a neuroma of the plantar digital nerve between metatarsals three and four. The burning pain from this neuroma is usually felt in the fourth toe although the third toe may also be painful. The neuroma may be palpable.

Meralgia Paresthetica. This is a poorly understood entrapment of the lateral femoral cutaneous nerve where it leaves the pelvis beneath the inguinal ligament and perforates the sartorius muscle to a canal running through the fascia lata. The burning pain in the distribution of this nerve can be severe and increased by standing or walking. There may be decreased loss of sensation and hair growth in its distribution.

Traction Injuries

Nerve trunks are quite resistent to traction as the fibrous connective tissue elements of the epineurium impart considerable tensile strength and elasticity which give resistance to longitudinal stress. The intertwining and cross-over of the individual fascicles within the trunk probably also impart a resiliency or helical spring action. It has been estimated by some that a nerve trunk can be stretched or elongated more than 10 percent beyond its normal length before axonal transmission is seriously disrupted. This helps to explain the relative resistance to damage by nerve trunks to missile injury in contrast to the shattering of bone and the disruption of muscle. Bunnell has likened increasing traction on a nerve to that on a manila rope; the structure will accept considerable stretch, even to the point where many individual fibers are damaged, before irreversible changes or complete disruption occurs. In the case of the pulled nerve, when structure changes do occur they are usually severe, often extend over a long segment, and are generally irreversible. Thus, traction may cause a lengthy spectrum of changes from very slight to severe and irreversible, depending on the degree of force expended and perhaps to its duration.

The most common traction injuries to nerves are those which occur in conjunction with dislocations and fractures. The brachial plexus is the most vulnerable and may be injured in difficult or inept deliveries giving rise to birth palsies. The proximal or Erb's type of palsy shows damage to the upper trunk of the plexus and presents a picture of adduction contracture of the shoulder secondary to loss of abduction and external rotation. In the distal or Klumpke type, the lower trunk of the plexus is injured causing paralysis of the forearm flexor muscles and loss of intrinsic muscles and sensation in the hand. Traction injuries of the brachial plexus may also be caused by passive wide abduction of the upper extremity in positioning the anesthetized patient.

The brachial plexus may also be injured by forced depression of the shoulder when an opposite force is applied to the neck, as happens when a motorcyclist is thrown through the air and lands on his shoulder. Isolated traction paralysis of the axillary nerve may occur with dislocation of the shoulder, although the nerve loss is usually a neurapraxia from which full recovery may be expected.

Injection Neuropathies

These unfortunate injuries are caused by the careless or inadvertent injection of a drug directly into or around a nerve trunk. There is immediate and severe burning pain followed by nerve loss which may or may not be complete depending on the nature of the medication, its amount, and location. Most commonly affected is the sciatic nerve, particularly in children or slightly muscled or wasted individuals who receive injections in the buttock. The radial nerve may be injured by injections into the midbrachium.

Causalgia

This painful condition is usually caused by incomplete injury to a nerve trunk, although it occasionally originates from the neuroma of a completely severed nerve. Weir Mitchell based his description of this condition on his observations of wounds incurred in the American Civil War; his work is classic and is recommended reading for all physicians. The condition consists of intractable burning pain which may radiate both distally and proximally from the site of injury. The pain may also be described as twisting, cramping, or aching, or may be severe enough to cause complete disability of the extremity and eventually totally disable the patient. Severe cases may lead to personality changes and even suicide. The pain is aggravated by such stimuli as loud noises, cold, or dryness, and the patient will go to extremes to protect the involved extremity even to the point of keeping it continuously covered by moist towels or not allowing it to be touched by an examiner or clothing. The condition is difficult to understand and frustrating to treat, and is frequently overlain with personality changes which may be secondary to the nerve lesion or which may be primary and contribute to the extreme symptomatic response.

Nerve Trunk Severance

The Challenge of Nerve Repair. It is only in time of war that large numbers of nerve injuries are seen, and it is from our military experience that we have obtained much of our information about peripheral nerve injuries, their diagnostic and prognostic problems, and how to repair them. Successful nerve repair requires accurate approximation of the severed ends of the nerve to allow regenerating axons to grow across the anastomosis and into the empty endoneurial tubes from which the degenerated distal axonal material has been phagocytized. The sucess of nerve suture—neurorrhaphy—is dependent on many factors too complex to be elaborated on here. Suffice it to say that success is greatest when there is minimal damage to the tissues surrounding the nerve, when there is minimal loss of nerve substance, when there is absence of infection, and when there has been a meticulous surgical approximation of the nerve ends with an accurate matching or orientation of the fascicles. The younger the patient and the more distal the lesion, the better the result. Only small defects in the nerve trunk can be overcome by end-to-end suture; a segmental loss of more than 3 or 4 cm. must be replaced with an autogenous nerve graft, usually taken from the sural nerve of the calf or the antebrachial cutaneous nerve of the forearm.

The timing of repair is a difficult problem. The sooner it is done the better the result, but it may have to wait until other injuries are taken care of first, and long delays may be encountered while infection is cleared, fractures are stabilized, and skin coverage is obtained. This presents the surgeon with a frustrating dilemma as it may well be that it is the nerve injury which will give the greatest disability but which may have to wait for repair until a proper surgical stage is set. Primary neurorrhaphy, nerve repair done on the day of injury, gives better results than delayed or secondary repair but only when ideal conditions are met, i.e., when the wound is not extensive, when contamination is minimal, and when the surgical technique for the repair has been of the highest order. The war-time injury due to shell fragments or high velocity missile injuries in which there is widespread contamination and tissue damage does not lend itself to primary nerve repair whereas the relatively clean wound of a simple laceration does.

The regenerative potential of the nerve cell body progressively declines after a few months, and nerve repair is seldom successful after a year or more from the time of injury. On the other hand, if nerve repair is done in the face of infection, skeletal instability, or in a bed of poorly vascularized tissue, or by an inexpert surgical team, the result will not be good.

The Diagnosis of Nerve Injury. Rarely will the patient with a fresh injury of a peripheral nerve complain of that injury or even be aware of it. He will be more concerned with the appearance and bleeding of the wound and with pain or anxiety. A fracture will cause obvious deformity, but the signs of associated nerve injury are at first obscure. As a result, many nerve injuries are missed by the examining physician because they were not obvious, because their likelihood did not occur to him, and because he neglected to examine the injured extremity adequately. The nerve injury will always become apparent later on, but by then the opportunity for ideal treatment may have been lost. On the day after the fracture has been reduced, the wound sutured, and the extremity dressed, it is embarrassing, to say the least, to have the patient point out to the physician that he has no sensation in the thumb, index finger, or middle finger, or that he cannot extend his fingers. Even worse, is to see an ulnar claw-hand deformity appear and become progressively worse over the ensuing weeks.

The physician must check nerve status in every injured extremity he examines. A few simple motor and sensory tests suffice and can be done in a few minutes. In old injuries, pinprick and tactile sensation is a sufficient preliminary sensory examination, but in fresh injuries, these modalities are undependable, and a quick two-point discrimination test is best. Motor loss in the hand can be quickly detected by wrist, finger, and thumb flexion and extension, as well as observation and palpation of a few key intrinsic muscles. In the lower extremity it is even simpler: sensation in the toes, sole, and dorsum of the foot; knee, ankle, and toe flexion and extension; and eversion of the ankle. If the patient is unconscious, an infant, or uncooperative, the problem is more complex, but at least the appearance and location of the wound, coupled with some idea of the mechanism of injury, can give a hint of the probability of nerve injury.

UPPER EXTREMITY NERVE LESIONS

The primary purpose of the bones, joints, muscles, and nerves of the upper extremity is to place the hand in a position in which its sensory and motor capabilities can be used. From the standpoint of function, then, any injury to a nerve of the upper limb or to the plexus from which it originates represents a hand injury, and the ultimate use of the hand will be the yardstick by which the success or failure of the diagnosis and treatment of peripheral nerve injuries will be judged.

Brachial Plexus Injuries

Attempts to classify plexus lesions help clarify one's understanding of neuroanatomy but aid little in the solution of clinical problems. Only a very simple division of lesions into those above or below the clavicle is of practical value. Supraclavicular injuries include those of the nerve roots at the fourth cervical through first thoracic levels; the three trunks (upper, middle, and lower); the anterior and posterior divisions; and the three cords (lateral, posterior, and medial) (Fig. 5-6). Infraclavicular lesions are mainly those of the main nerve branches or combinations thereof.

The causes of plexus injuries are mainly missiles in war time and traction and fractures in civil practice. Most common is the motorcyclist who is projected from his vehicle and lands on his shoulder, with head and neck forced to one side, thus applying direct traction to the plexus. Fractures of the cervical spine are most often associated with nerve root injuries and clavicular fractures with supraclavicular damage to the trunks, divisions, and cords. However, shoulder fractures are more often associated with infraclavicular plexus and nerve trunk damage. Other signs of supraclavicular plexus injury are paralysis of muscles innervated from the proximal plexus, sensory loss and palpable swelling above the clavicle, and Horner's syndrome. The latter is a dire

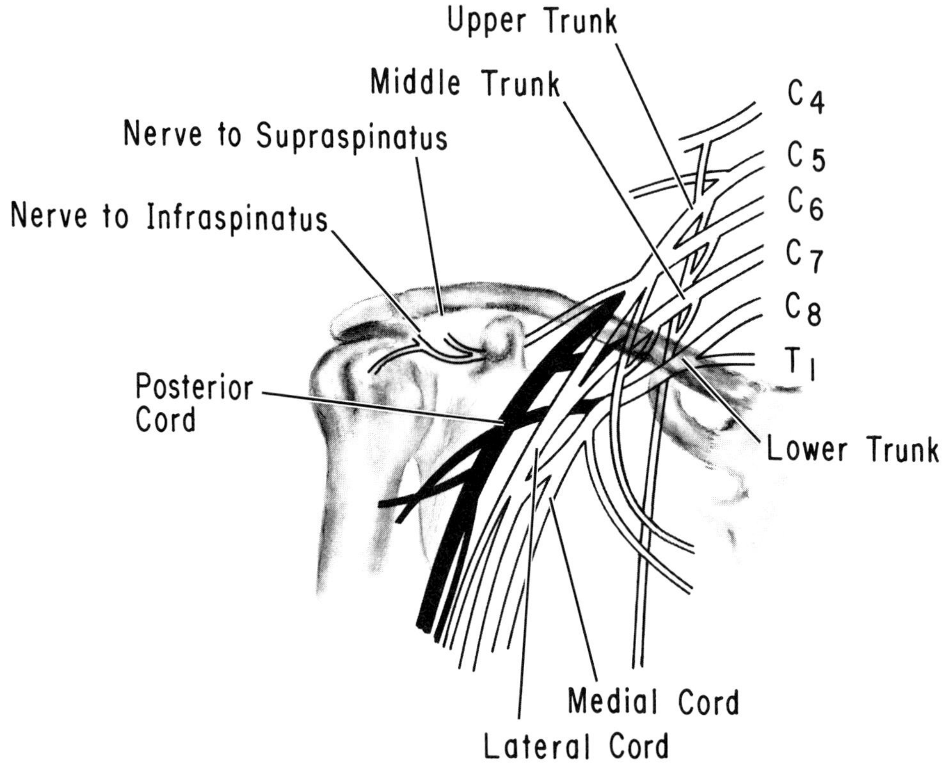

Fig. 5-6. Brachial plexus distribution. (Courtesy Richard Riggins.)

prognostic sign as it generally indicates an avulsion of the lower roots of the plexus. Roentgenographic evidence of vertebral, clavicular, scapular, or humeral fractures aids in the diagnosis. Cervical myelography may confirm nerve root avulsion.

The major motor nerves of the supraclavicular plexus are as follows: from the fifth cervical nerve root comes the *dorsal scapular* nerve to the rhomboid muscles which can be tested by having the erect patient place his hands behind his back, palms out, and push against the examiner's hand. From the fifth through seventh cervical roots, the *long thoracic* nerve supplies the serratus anterior, paralysis of which causes winging of the scapula when the patient pushes forward with his outstretched arm. (See Fig. 4-8 for an example of this condition.) From the upper trunk (and C-4, 5, and 6) comes the *suprascapular* nerve to the supraspinatus and infraspinatus muscles which initiate shoulder abduction. The *lateral and medial pectoral* (or *anterior thoracic*) nerves are united by a loop as they come off the medial (C-8, T-1) and lateral (C-5, 6, and 7) cords and supply the pectoralis major and minor muscles which are strong shoulder adductors. From the posterior cord come three separate motor nerves: the *upper subscapular* nerve (C-5 and 6) to the subscapularis muscle, the *thoracodorsal* nerve (middle subscapular nerve, C-7 and 8) to the latissimus dorsi muscle, and the *lower subscapular* (C-5 and 6) to the teres major. These latter muscles serve to rotate the arm internally and to adduct it from front to back.

Two sensory nerves originate from the medial cord and are the only significant sensory components of the supraclavicular brachial plexus. They are the *medial brachial cutaneous* nerve (T-1 and 2) to the medial surface of the arm and the *medial antebrachial cutaneous* nerve (C-8 and T-1) which supplies sensation to the medial aspect of the forearm. The former is the only upper extremity nerve with a contribution at the second thoracic level and is always spared in high brachial plexus injuries.

Only occasionally are the individual motor nerves of the plexus impaired. Injury more often involves areas or portions of the plexus and four basic types, based on the level of injury, can be recognized although one must bear in mind that many other combinations are possible.

Upper Trunk Paralysis (C-5 and 6) is marked by weakness or absence of abduction and external rotation of the shoulder and flexion of the elbow as in the Erb-Duchenne type of birth injury. Often there is only motor loss, but when sensation is also lost, it will only be on the lateral side of the arm and forearm and never distal to the wrist as many charts indicate.

Upper and Middle Trunks (C-5, 6, and 7). In addition to the above, there is also loss of shoulder adduction (pectoralis major, teres major, and latissimus dorsi), elbow extension (triceps), the extensor compartment muscles of the forearm, and sometimes the flexor carpi ulnaris. Sensory loss includes both sides of the thumb and index fingers.

Lower Trunk (C-8 and T-1). This is the same as a high combined median and ulnar paralysis except that the pronator teres and flexor carpi ulnaris (C-5 and 6) are spared. There is sensory loss of the anterior and posterior sides of the medial aspect of the forearm and hand as in a high ulnar palsy. Horner's syndrome, manifested by a small pupil, loss of sweating on that side of the face and neck, and narrowing of the palpebral fissure, is indicative of proximal damage to the eight cervical and first thoracic nerve roots.

Total Paralysis (C-5 to T-1). With this condition, all muscles distal to the shoulder girdle are paralyzed, and the upper extremity is totally insensitive except for a narrow strip from the axilla to the elbow which is supplied by the second thoracic nerve root (medial brachial cutaneous nerve). Horner's syndrome is common, as is edema of extremity.

Axillary Nerve (C-5 and 6)

The axillary or circumflex nerve derives from the posterior cords and winds about the posterior aspect of the neck of the humerus to supply the deltoid and teres minor muscles and, through the lateral brachial cutaneous nerve, an area of skin a few centimeters in diameter on the lateral aspect of the shoulder. Anesthesia in this area is an important diagnostic indicator of axillary nerve damage.

Injury to the axillary nerve is usually due to fracture of the proximal end of the humerus or to dislocation of the shoulder. The next most common cause is traction, in which case the nerve is rarely injured alone but in combination with other brachial plexus components. Although it is the supraspinatus which initiates the first 30 degrees of abduction of the humerus, beyond this the deltoid becomes the main abductor. It is best tested first by abduction against gravity alone, then against resistance. If the muscle is palpated as the patient attempts abduction, a clearer appreciation of the state of the muscle can be obtained.

Musculocutaneous Nerve (C-5 and 6)

This nerve arises from the lateral cord deep to the pectoralis major, pierces the coracobrachialis muscle which it supplies, and continues between the brachialis and biceps muscles which it also supplies. It terminates as the lateral antebrachial cutaneous nerve. It may be involved in brachial plexus injuries but may be injured alone by missile or stab wounds or by fractures of the humerus. Motor loss is confined to weakness or absence of elbow flexion, but in testing it is important to palpate the biceps and brachialis muscles as the brachioradialis and the forearm flexor group may be strong secondary elbow flexors.

Of the peripheral nerve injuries, surgical repair of the musculocutaneous nerve gives the best results; therefore, early recognition of severence is of particular importance.

Radial Nerve (C-6, 7, 8, and T-1)

The radial or musculospiral nerve is the direct continuation of the posterior cord of the brachial plexus. It passes posteriorly to the humerus in the musculospiral groove, pierces the lateral intramuscular septum, and passes to the anterior aspect of the distal brachium after giving off branches to the three heads of the triceps and the posterior brachial cutaneous nerve. Just proximal to the lateral epicondyle of the elbow it innervates the brachioradialis, the extensor carpi radialis longus, and the anconeus. At the level of the elbow joint, the nerve bifurcates into a deep motor branch and superficial sensory branches. Of the latter, one is the dorsal antebrachial cutaneous nerve and the other continues to supply the dorsal lateral aspect of the hand and dorsum of thumb as well as the middle and index fingers to about the level of the proximal interphalangeal joints. Due to overlapping sensory supply on the dorsum of the hand by both the median and ulnar nerves, the only area exclusively innervated by the radial nerve is an inconstant region 2 or 3 cm. in diameter on the dorsum of the area between the first and second metacarpals.

The deep motor branch at the elbow is called the posterior interosseous nerve and courses through the supinator muscle and supplies it as well as the extensor carpi radialis brevis, all extrinsic fingers and thumb extensors, as well as the abductor pollicis longus.

Radial nerve damage is most often incurred with fractures of the shaft of the humerus and next most often with open wounds, surgical damage, injections, and compression as in "Saturday night palsy." In complete radial palsy originating with nerve damage in the musculospiral groove, the triceps will generally be spared, but there will be a wrist-drop with loss of all wrist and finger extensors (Fig. 5-7). The wrist will be pronated due to loss of the supinator and brachioradialis which is also called the "long supinator." Extension will be possible of the middle and distal finger joints and in some cases of the distal thumb joint through action of the ulnar and median innervated intrinsic muscles of the hand.

When only the posterior interosseous nerve is affected, there will be no sensory loss, and as the extensor carpi radialis longus is spared, due to its higher branch, there will be wrist extension, although in some there will be radial deviation and loss of finger and thumb extension. Supplementary or trick movements may obscure the picture; occasionally finger extension may occur from forcible wrist flexion.

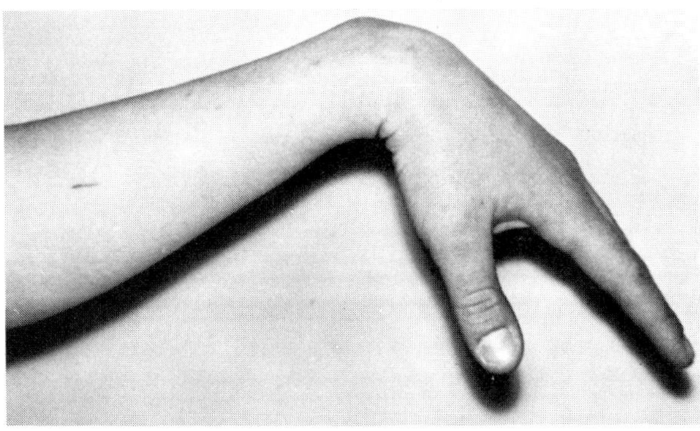

Fig. 5-7. The wrist-drop of a high radial nerve palsy. Not only are the wrist extensors out, but also those extensors of the fingers and thumb and the long abductor of the thumb. Extension of the interphalangeal joints of the fingers is still present through the interossei, which are ulnar-innervated.

Loss of sensation due to trauma of the superficial radial nerve on the dorsoradial aspect of the forearm and wrist causes no functional disability in the hand, but the nerve and its branches are particularly subject to the formation of painful neuromas which may be of great annoyance to the patient.

Median Nerve (C-6, 7, 8, and T-1)

The median nerve is formed by equal contributions from the lateral and median cords of the brachial plexus and courses with the brachial artery through the arm without branching. It can be readily palpated in the distal portion of the arm between the biceps and brachialis muscles.

Passing anterior to the elbow it gives off branches for the pronator teres, the flexor carpi radialis, the flexor digitorum sublimis, and the palmaris longus; continues on between the two heads of the pronator teres; gives off the anterior interosseous nerve to the flexor pollicis longus, the radial half of the flexor digitorum profundus, and the pronator quadratus; and continues to the carpal tunnel. It lies 4 or 5 cm. proximal to the transverse carpal ligament of the tunnel, it moves anterior to the flexor digitorum sublimis, gives off the palmar cutaneous branch, and lies beneath the antebrachial fascia to either side of, or under, the palmaris longus tendon. It then passes into the carpal tunnel formed by the carpal bones and roofed over volarly by the transverse carpal ligament. It is accompanied through the tunnel by the long, i.e., extrinsic, flexors of the thumb and fingers.

In the hand, the usual motor distribution is to the abductor pollicis brevis, the opponens pollicis, the superficial head of the flexor pollicis brevis, and to the lumbrical muscles of the index and middle fingers. There are many variations from this usual arrangement, and it is not uncommon for the ulnar nerve to give contributions to some or all of these thenar muscles.

At the distal end of the tunnel, as the ligament thins out, the main trunk of the median nerve gives off its motor recurrent branch or branches which run transversely to disappear into thenar muscles. The trunk then fans out into sensory branches supplying both sides of the thumb, the radial side of the index finger, and into two common digital branches which go to the second and third finger clefts where each common digital branch divides into individual nerves supplying the contiguous sides of the index, middle, and ring fingers.

The usual median sensory pattern is the palm, the thenar eminence, both radial and ulnar aspects of the volar (palmar or anterior) aspect of the thumb, index, and middle fingers, and the radial side of the ring finger and extending dorsally into each of these digits to include the thumb nail area and the distal two segments of the fingers. Except for the distal segments of the index and middle fingers, which are usually autonomous for the median nerve, any of these areas may have significant sensory contribution from the ulnar or radial sensory branches.

By far the most common median nerve lesion is its compression within the carpal tunnel. Transsection most commonly occurs with transverse lacerations at the wrist as a result of accidental or intentional knife or razor wounds. Fractures of the humerus or forearm bones and fractures about the elbow, as well as missile wounds, may injure the nerve. Colles' and other fractures of the distal part of the radius and ulna may cause traction, contusion, or compression injuries of the nerve just above or within the carpal tunnel. Transsection of the trunk within the carpal tunnel, or of the sensory branches just distal to it, commonly occurs in the child's hand as the result of a fall with the outstretched hand encountering a broken bottle or sharp piece of metal. Broken porcelain faucet handles, jars, and light bulbs may inflict similar injury. Some of these lacerations are deceptively small but may sever important nerves in the palm and fingers; a laceration in the palm warrants a careful sensory examination of the digits regardless of its size or seemingly innocuous appearance.

Motor examination for median nerve dysfunction is relatively simple and can be carried out in a few minutes with a cooperative patient. The lesion at, or proximal to, the elbow presents a rather typical resting hand position in which the thumb lies in the plane of the hand and the index finger is noticeably less flexed than the other fingers (Fig. 5-8). In the unconscious patient with an upper extremity injury, this resting position may be the only clue to median nerve damage. The high median lesion is characterized by loss of pronation, weak wrist flexion, and loss of flexion of the distal joints of the thumb and index finger. The median innervated muscles should be tested for individually. Pronator teres loss is apparent by loss of pronation of the wrist, but pronator quadratus paralysis can only be detected with the elbow in a position of acute flexion, thereby depriving the pronator teres of effective excursion. Flexor digitorum sublimis action is tested by voluntary flexion of the proximal interphalangeal joints of each digit while the adjacent fingers are held in extension by the examiner although some patients can demonstrate flexion of these joints even when the other fingers are not restrained. Thumb interphalangeal flexion by the flexor pollicis longus is easily tested as is the flexor digitorum profundus action on the distal interphalangeal joint of the index finger. Even though the median nerve classically innervates the flexor digitorum profundus of the middle finger, often this tendon works in conjunction with its counterpart to the ring finger or receives ulnar innervation; therefore, distal interphalangeal joint flexion of the middle finger is not a dependable sign of median function. Conversely, when the distal joint of the index finger flexes but not that of the other fingers, this may indicate an innervation variant in which the ulnar nerve supplies the ulnar-three flexor digitorum profundi and all of the flexor pollicis brevis, as well as the small and ring fingers and ulnar half of the middle finger.

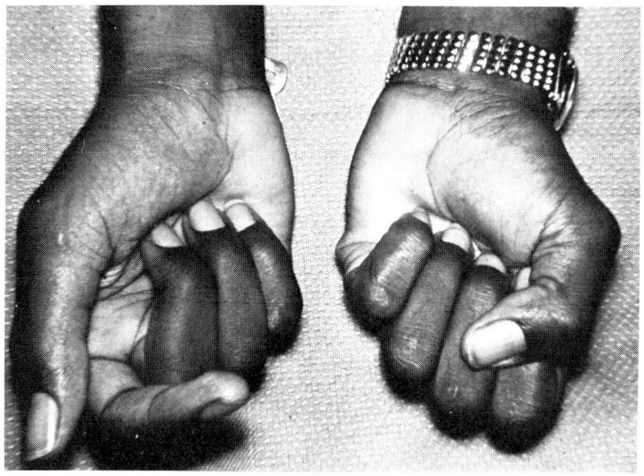

Fig. 5-8. High median nerve palsy on the right. Patient is unable to flex interphalangeal joints of the index finger or thumb. Note also the loss of mass in the thenar eminence and incomplete thumb metacarpophalangeal flexion.

Damage to the anterior interosseous nerve is demonstrated by loss of the flexor pollicis longus as well as the radial half of the flexor digitorum profundus and the pronator quadratus but with an intact pronator teres, flexor carpi radialis, flexor digitorum sublimis, palmaris longus, and thenar intrinsics. Isolated loss of anterior interosseous nerve function may be caused by compression of the nerve by various anomalies of the forearm musculature, fractures of the forearm or distal humerus, and by penetrating wounds.

Median intrinsic motor loss is usually reflected by a flattened thenar eminence but only when the paralysis has been present long enough for the palsied muscles to become atrophic and thereby lose noticeable bulk, a period of at least several weeks. The so-called "ape hand" results from paralysis of the abductor pollicis brevis, the opponens pollicis, and the superficial head of the flexor pollicis brevis (Fig. 5-9). Opposition of the thumb is lost, and the patient is unable to rotate the first metacarpal in an arc across the palm to bring the thumb into opposition with the fingers. Many variations are possible: in some median palsies there is great disability due to a complete loss of opposition, whereas in others the ulnar portion of the flexor pollicis brevis may act to give a fairly effective substitute for true opposition and may even result in hypertrophy with time and practice. In testing the thenar musculature, it is not enough to test the muscles against resistance; palpation of the thenar mass during abduction and rotation of the thumb will make the examination much more informative (Figs. 5-10, 5-11).

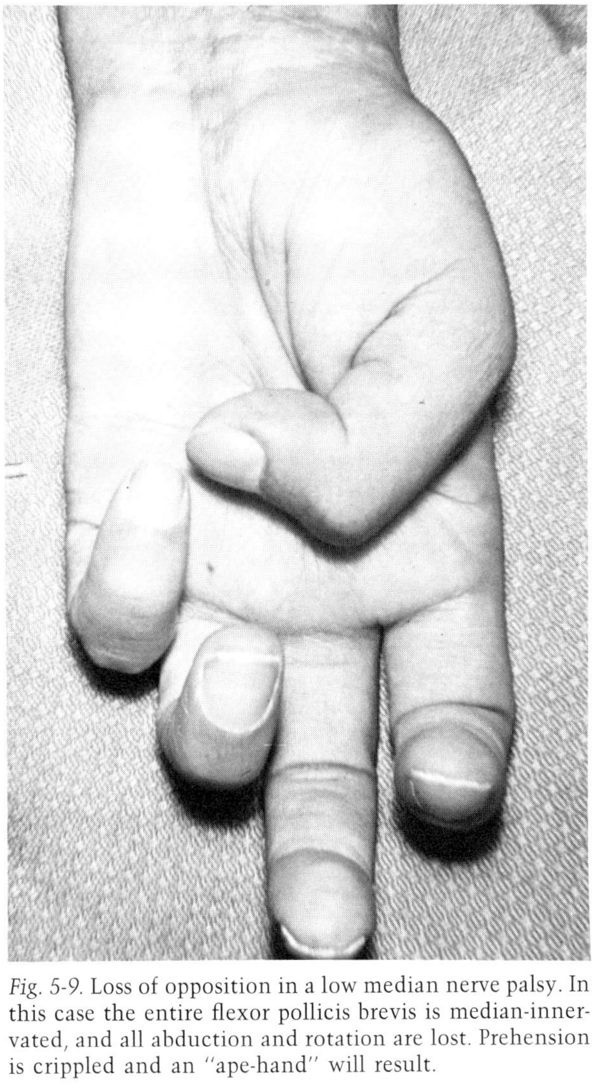

Fig. 5-9. Loss of opposition in a low median nerve palsy. In this case the entire flexor pollicis brevis is median-innervated, and all abduction and rotation are lost. Prehension is crippled and an "ape-hand" will result.

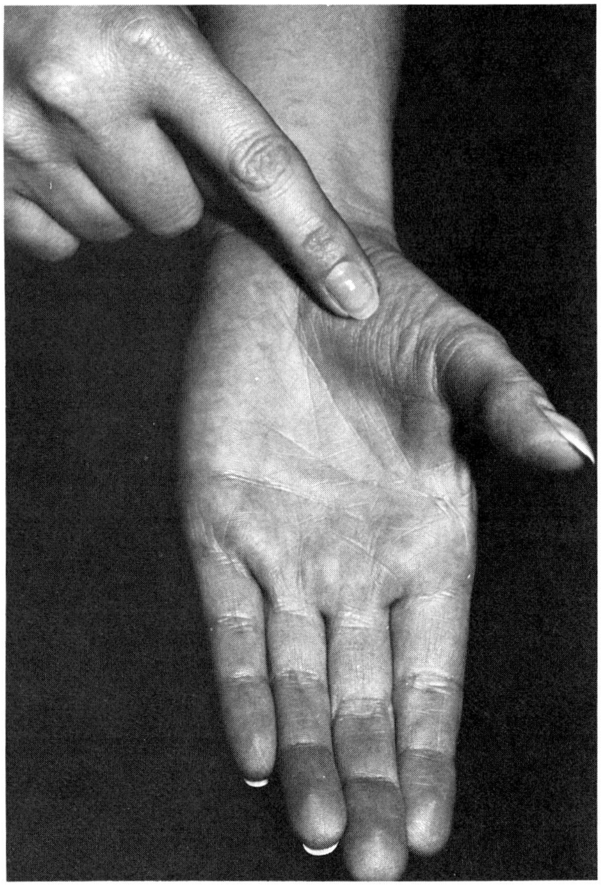

Fig. 5-10. Demonstrating the abductor pollicis brevis by observation and palpation. Its strength should also be tested against resistence.

Trophic and vasomotor changes in the index and middle fingers are common with median nerve lesions but are rarely seen in the thumb. The circumference of the fingers may be decreased, the skin dry and shiny and sometimes cyanotic, and the nails are often brittle or ridged. Stiffness of the index and middle fingers develops early in the median nerve paralysis of elderly patients.

Median paralysis is seen as part of the picture of Volkmann's ischemic contracture. This is usually due to ischemia which develops as the result of arterial injury which in turn may be secondary to fractures or dislocations about the elbow, open wounds, the development of massive edema and swelling in the flexor compartment of the forearm caused by snakebite, drug injection, or trauma. The median nerve injury in the Volkmann's contracture is due to ischemic changes within a long segment of the nerve, and these changes are extensive and irreversible once they are apparent. Early recognition of increasing swelling, or vascular insufficiency, is essential if early corrective action is to be taken.

Ulnar Nerve (C-8, T-1)

The ulnar nerve descends from the medial cord of the brachial plexus on the medial side of the arm, pierces the medial intermuscular septum, and continues in a groove behind the medial humeral epicondyle into the forearm. A branch or branches to the flexor carpi ulnaris is given off in the region of the elbow and distal to this, a branch to the medial half of the flexor digitorum profundus. The nerve trunk enters the forearm posteriorly between the two heads of the flexor carpi ulnaris where it may be constricted by a fibrous band between the muscle and the ulna; it is here that the nerve trunk is vulnerable to compression. The nerve lies to the medial side of the ulnar artery in the distal half of the forearm and just proximal to the wrist emerges from under the flexor carpi ulnaris to enter the canal of Guyon, the roof of which is the volar carpal ligament. From here, it passes between the pisiform and hamate bones, and at this point it divides into a deep motor branch to the ulnar innervated intrinsic muscles and a superficial sensory branch. The latter supplies both the dorsal and volar aspects of the ulnar side of the hand, all of the small fingers, and the ulnar half of the ring finger. The deep motor branch swings across the mid-palm dorsal to the flexor tendons giving off branches to the palmaris brevis and the three hypothenar muscles: the abductor, opponens, and flexor digiti quinti. It then supplies the four dorsal and three volar interossei, the lumbricals of the small and ring fingers, the adductor pollicis, and the deep head of the flexor pollicis brevis. Proximal to the wrist the palmar and dorsal cutaneous nerves of the hand are given off.

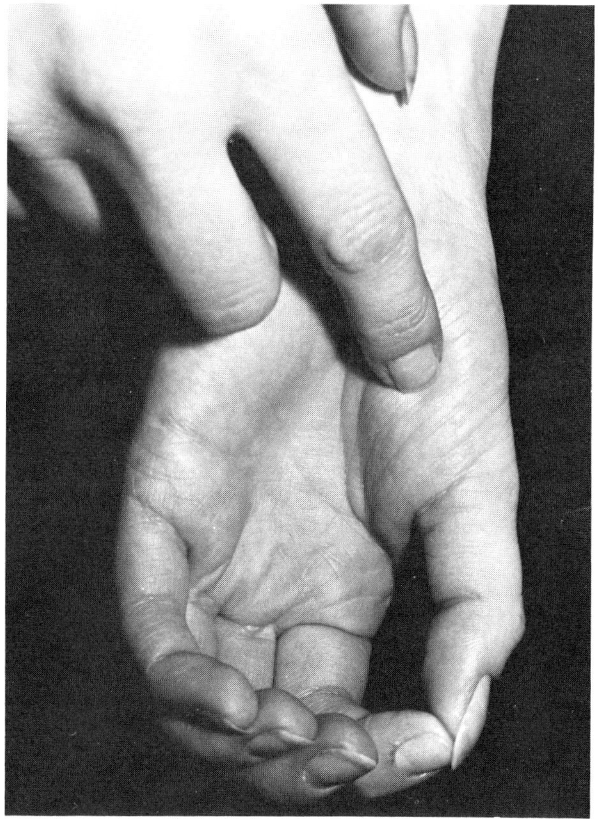

Fig. 5-11. Demonstrating the thenars during prehension. This is less specific than the test for the short abductor as all the thenars are contracted when pinching with force.

The ulnar nerve is the most commonly injured nerve of the upper extremity, and the results of surgical repair are the poorest. Open wounds, especially at the wrist, are the most common cause of injury, but compression or irritation of the nerve at either the wrist or elbow is not rare. Whereas the major functional loss in low median nerve palsy is sensory, loss of ulnar nerve function, as with radial nerve function, is predominantly a motor loss. Anesthesia in the ulnar distribution of the hand is, at worst, an inconvenience, but loss of all the interossei

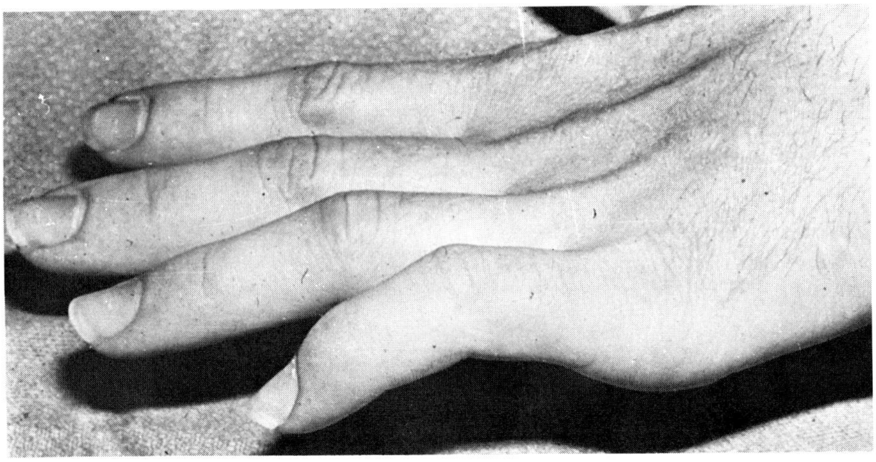

Fig. 5-12. Mild claw deformity. This may be due to an ulnar lesion proximal to the ulnar branch of the flexor digitorum profundus or may be due to a low ulnar lesion which has not yet led to stretching of the volar capsule of the metacarpophalangeal joints. Note the obvious interosseous atrophy between the extensor tendons indicating that the lesion must be at least several weeks old.

and the adductor pollicis interferes seriously with the strength and effectiveness of both grasp and prehension.

Ulnar clawhand, *main en griffe,* is primarily due to loss of the interossei, the major function of which is to flex the metacarpophalangeal joints. With their loss, the extensor action of the extrinsic finger extensors are unopposed, and a hyperextension deformity of the metacarpophalangeal joints begins. As the volar capsule of these joints stretches, the deformity, which may be barely apparent in the recently injured extremity, progresses. Lumbricals one and two are most commonly median-innervated; therefore, the index and middle fingers usually do not develop the deformity. The interossei and lumbricals also act as interphalangeal joint extensors, and with their paralysis these joints are held in flexion by the now unopposed flexor digitorum profundi and flexor digitorum sublimi which are at the same time overactive in their attempt to compensate for the lack of the interossei as metacarpophalangeal flexors. Thus, a vicious cycle is started, and the more the patient attempts to correct the deformity actively, the more it will become exaggerated. The degree of clawing is usually less apparent in the high ulnar palsy (Fig. 5-12) than when the ulnar half of the flexor digitorum profundus is spared, but the degree of clawing will also depend on other factors, such as the degree of ligamentous laxity in an individual patient's joints and on functions for which the hand is regularly used (Fig. 5-13).

Most obvious in the ulnar clawhand is the apparent deformity of clawing, a loss of the transverse arch of the hand, and visible atrophy of the interossei, particularly the first dorsal interosseous muscle mass, as well as hypothenar atrophy. Next most apparent is

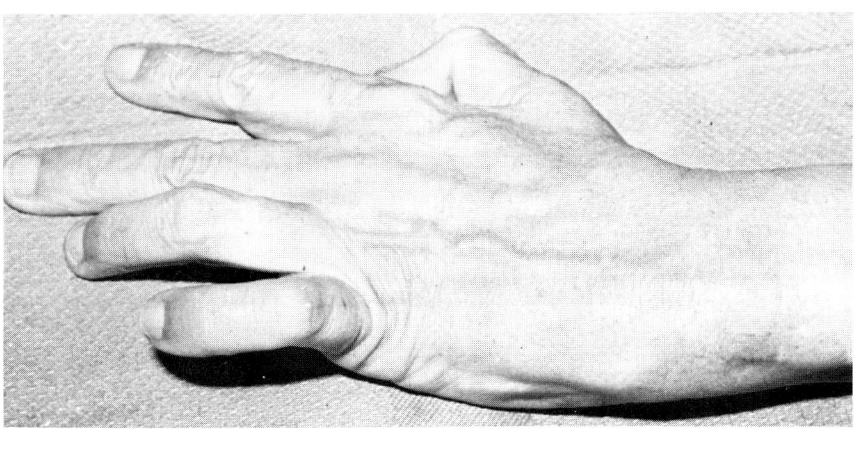

Fig. 5-13. Severe ulnar palsy due to a low lesion. Note wound on ulnar border of distal forearm.

the clumsy grip and the marked weakness of grasp. Normal grip strength in the adult male is approximately 90 pounds, and in the ulnar palsied hand the grip strength will only be one quarter to one third of that. It is this weakness which is most disabling for gross dysfunction of the hand, such as grasping a shovel or a suitcase handle.

More disabling for fine sophisticated use of the hand is the interference with normal pinch or prehension. The average strength of pinch in the adult male is 20 to 25 pounds, but with ulnar palsy, the strength is only 10 to 20 percent of that. This loss is due to paralysis of the adductor pollicis, half of the flexor pollicis brevis, and the first dorsal interosseous muscles. Their paralysis leads not only to weakness but also to gross deformity of pinch, manifested by hyperextension of the thumb metacarpophalangeal joint and hyperflexion of the thumb interphalangeal joint (Fig. 5-14). A good test of adductor pollicis and first dorsal interosseous function is to observe the position of pinch, test its strength, and palpate the first dorsal interosseous muscle on the radial side of the second metacarpal and the adductor pollicis deep in the thumb web while the patient attempts maximum strength of pinch. The extensor pollicis longus is an effective accessory thumb adductor, and the test in which a piece of paper is held by the thumb adducted to the index finger—incorrectly, but commonly, called Froment's sign—is not an accurate one.

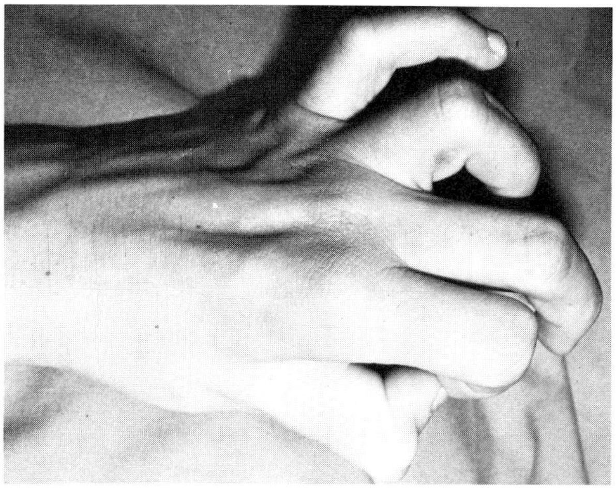

Fig. 5-15. Exaggerated claw hand and ulnar pinch deformity due to severance of the ulnar nerve at the wrist which occurred six months prior to the photograph.

The ulnar pinch deformity represents a reversal of the normal longitudinal arch of the first metacarpal and thumb, the integrity of which is dependent on the presence of the adductor pollicis and normal metacarpophalangeal flexion (Fig. 5-15). Many variations of the classic ulnar-palsied pinch are possible and are caused by variations in median and ulnar

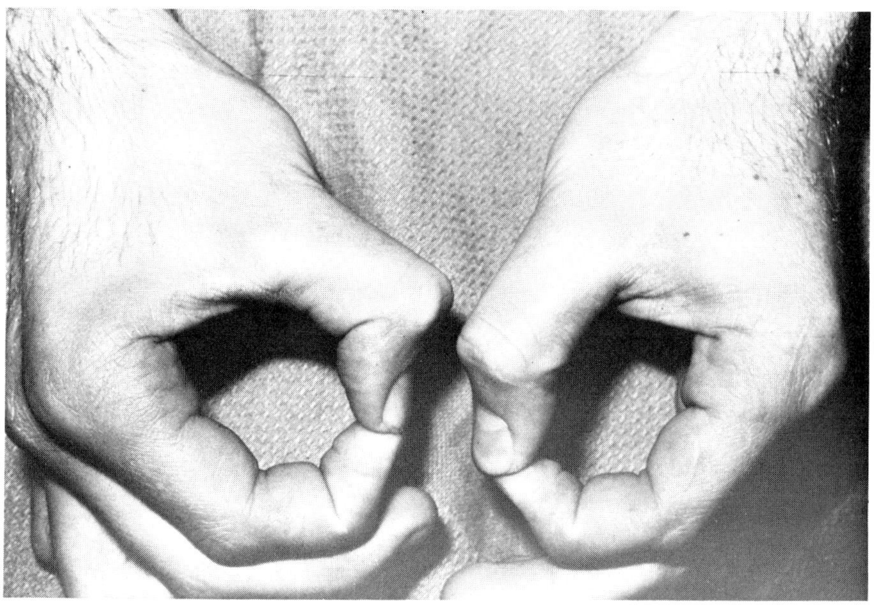

Fig. 5-14. Ulnar-palsied pinch of the right hand. Loss of the longitudinal arch of the thumb reflected by hyperextension of the metacarpophalangeal joint and hyperflexion of the interphalangeal joint. Note the flattening of the thumb web; palpation here will detect absence of the first dorsal interosseous and the adductor pollicis muscles. Pinch strength of involved hand is 3 pounds, as compared with 20 pounds for the normal hand.

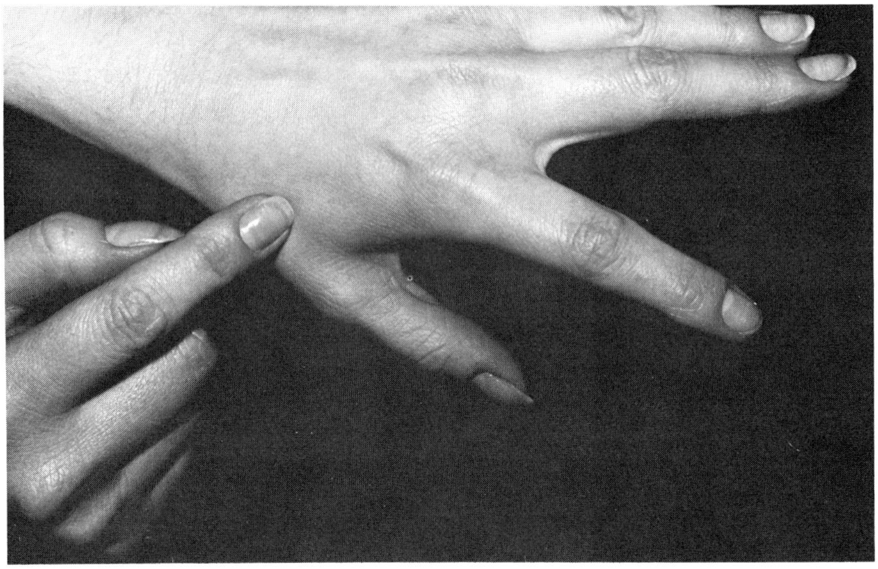

Fig. 5-16. First dorsal interosseous function. The muscle belly can be seen to contract, its action in abducting the index finger observed, and the muscle palpated as it contracts.

innervation of the intrinsics, whether or not the patient has "loose" or "tight" joints, and his occupation.

The ulnar-palsied hand in the recently injured patient will usually show only a suggestion of these deformities, and it is, therefore, most important to examine carefully the intrinsic muscles (Fig. 5-16) by visual observation of their action and by palpation of their muscle bellies while the patient attempts to contract them against resistance (Fig. 5-17). The flexor carpi ulnaris is easily examined as a flexor and ulnar deviator of the wrist; it may also be seen to contract in unison with the abductor digiti quinti as the patient attempts to abduct the small finger.

When possible, it is wise to measure (and record) the strength of grasp with a grip meter and that of pinch with a pinch meter. These instruments are seldom available in an emergency room, however, and a rough, but informative, estimate of strength can be made by having the patient grasp the examin-

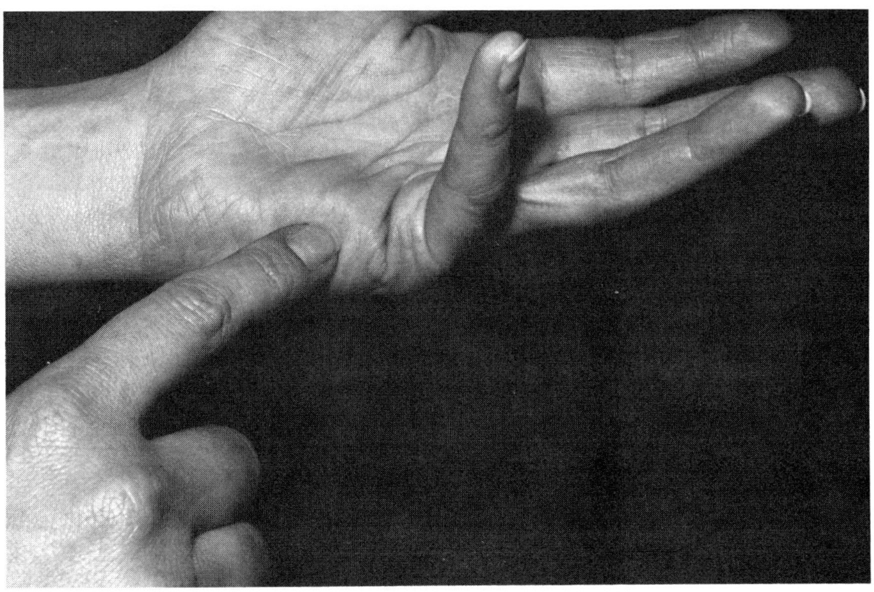

Fig. 5-17. Test for hypothenar muscles. With the hand palm up, the patient is asked to point the small finger to the ceiling without flexing the interphalangeal joints. The hypothenar mass is palpated during the test.

er's index and middle fingers with both hands simultaneously and then to pinch the examiner's index fingers in the same manner.

Referred pain in the distal ulnar distribution is common with subdeltoid bursitis and other painful shoulder conditions and occasionally in coronary artery disease but is not accompanied by objective findings. These same symptoms may occur with irritation of the ulnar nerve at the elbow and may progress to a tardy ulnar palsy with definite sensory and motor abnormalities.

Combined Nerve Lesions

Median and Ulnar Nerves. This is the most common combination and leaves the patient with a useless hand if the lesions are high enough to paralyze the extrinsic flexors of the wrist and digits. It is more common in the forearm and at the wrist in which case the hand is still badly crippled as it has then lost most of its useful sensation and all of its intrinsic muscles. The net result is a flat hand in which all five metacarpals are in the same plane, there is clawing of all four fingers, and loss of opposition of the thumb and any effective pinch (Fig. 5-18). A primitive pinch is still possible in the thumb cleft, activated by the flexor pollicis longus and the adductor power of the extensor pollicis longus. The insensitive fingertips are frequently burned or otherwise injured, and fingertip ulcerations and trophic changes of the entire hand are common. Intrinsic atrophy is obvious, and secondary finger joint contractures frequently occur.

Median and Radial Nerves. This combination usually occurs at or proximal to the elbow and affects the entire radial half of the hand with complete sensory and severe motor loss. Trophic changes in the thumb and index finger occur and opposition is impaired, but the overall picture is not as striking as in the combined median and ulnar lesion as most of the intrinsics are still functional although the wrist drop deformity is obvious.

Radial and Ulnar Nerves. Less serious than the preceding two, as median sensory function and some thumb motor activity is preserved, this combination is nonetheless crippling. Trophic changes are usually limited to the small finger, and there is a combination of radial wrist drop and ulnar clawhand deformity.

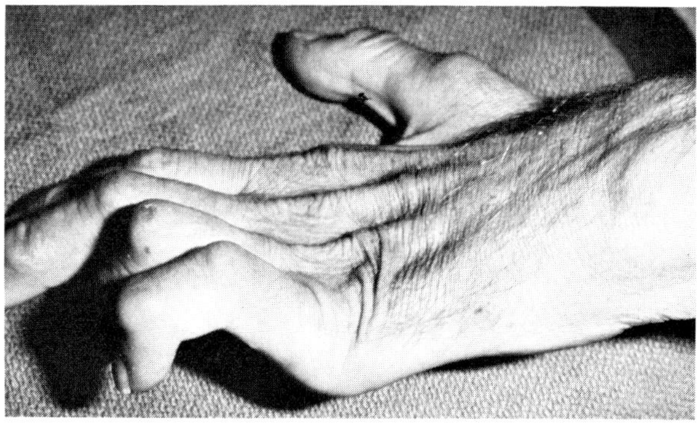

Fig. 5-18. Combined median and ulnar palsy due to a laceration on the volar aspect of the wrist which occurred several months prior to the photograph. The clawing is severe, the transverse arch of the hand is completely gone, and the thumb lies in the same plane as the remainder of the hand. Intrinsic atrophy is severe, and there is a burn on the dorsoulnar aspect of the ring finger proximal to the interphalangeal joint.

LOWER EXTREMITY NERVE LESIONS

Lumbar and Sacral Plexus

The lumbar portion originates from the first through fourth lumbar roots, and from its upper roots gives off the iliohypogastric, ilioinguinal, and the genitofemoral nerves. The second through fourth lumbar roots form an anterior and posterior division (Fig. 5-19); the anterior becomes the obturator nerve and the posterior division the femoral and lateral femoral cutaneous nerves. Similarly, the sacral plexus forms an anterior and posterior division, the anterior (from L-4, 5 and S-1, 2, and 3) forming the tibial portion of the sciatic nerve, the posterior (from L-4, 5, S-1 and 2) contributing the common peroneal portion of the sciatic nerve as well as the superior and inferior gluteal. In contrast to the brachial plexus, the lumbosacral plexus is rarely injured by traction and only occasionally by fractures but may be damaged by missiles or involved by cord or cauda equina lesions.

Femoral Nerve (L-2, 3, 4)

The femoral nerve (Fig. 5-20) emerges from the lateral border of the psoas muscle, descends below Poupart's ligament to enter the femoral triangle to the lateral side of the femoral artery, and then divides into its terminal branches. Above the inguinal ligament, it supplies the iliopsoas which is the major

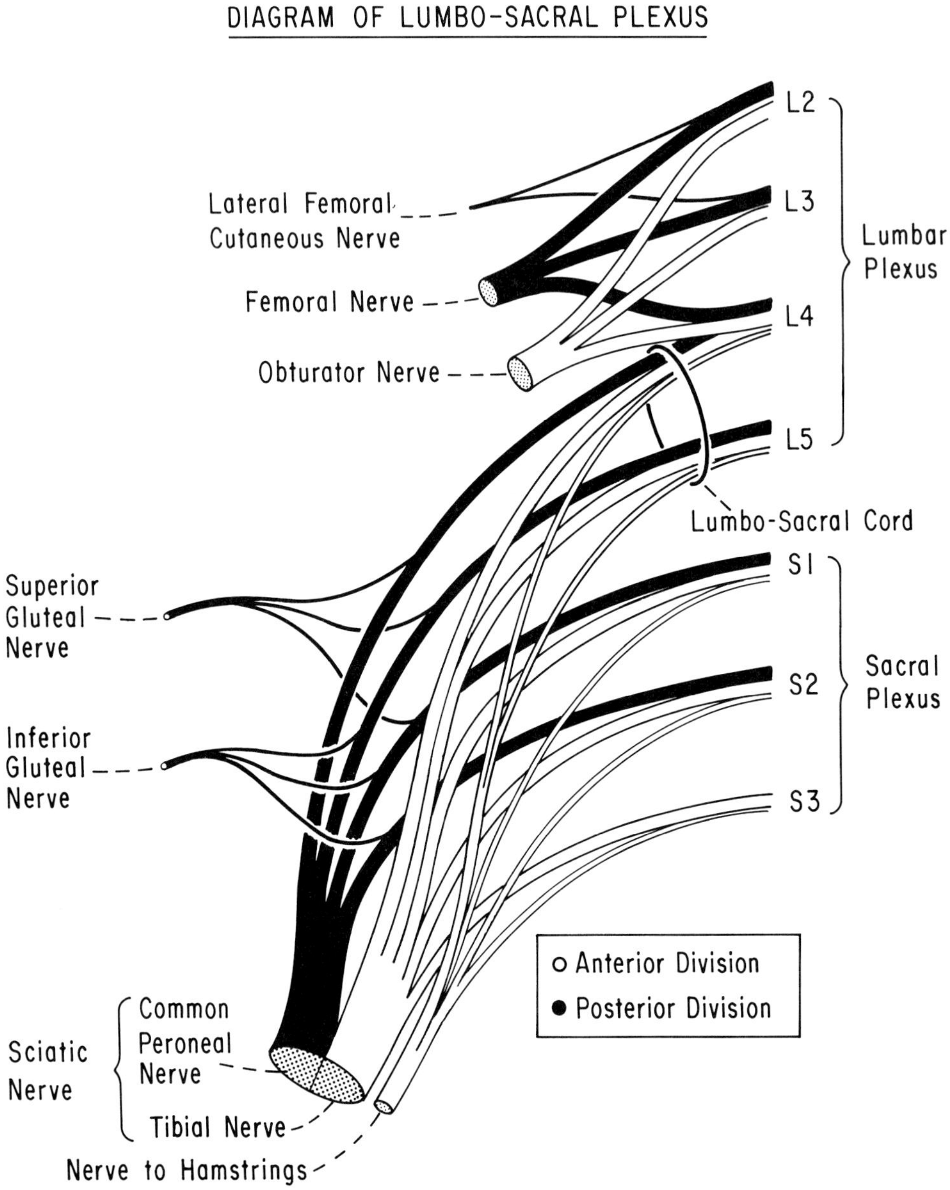

Fig. 5-19. Lumbosacral plexus. (From Seddon, H.: Surgical Disorders of the Peripheral Nerves, ed. 2. Edinburgh, Churchill, Livingstone, 1975.)

hip flexor. Below the ligament, it supplies the sartorius, pectineus, and the quadriceps femoris muscles. Its sensory branches supply the median and anterior aspect of the thigh and terminate as the saphenous nerve supplying the medial side of the leg and foot.

Quadriceps paralysis causes loss of active knee extension, and the patient walks with a type of steppage gait, lifting the knee high and using gravity and momentum to extend the knee passively as the hip is extended. He will usually assist this by pushing on the thigh with his hand. Atrophy develops quickly and is particularly apparent in the vastus medialis.

Peripheral injuries of the femoral nerve within the pelvis may be caused by tumors, fractures, or by psoas abscess. Within the femoral triangle, the nerve is vulnerable to damage by penetrating wounds and femoral artery aneurysms caused by shell fragment and bullet wounds. Small penetrating wounds below the inguinal ligament may be deceptive, just as in the palm, and the underlying nerve and artery must be carefully examined.

Obturator Nerve (L-2, 3, 4)

After leaving the medial side of the psoas near the pelvic brim, the obturator nerve passes lateral to the ureter and hypogastric vessels and enters the obturator canal in the upper part of the pelvic obturator foramen, splits into anterior and posterior branches entering the medial aspect of the thigh, and supplies the obturator externus, the adductor muscles, and gracilis. Except for a small area on the medial aspect of the thigh, its sensory contribution is negligible. Loss of the hip adductors and gracilis impairs adduction and external rotation of the hip and makes

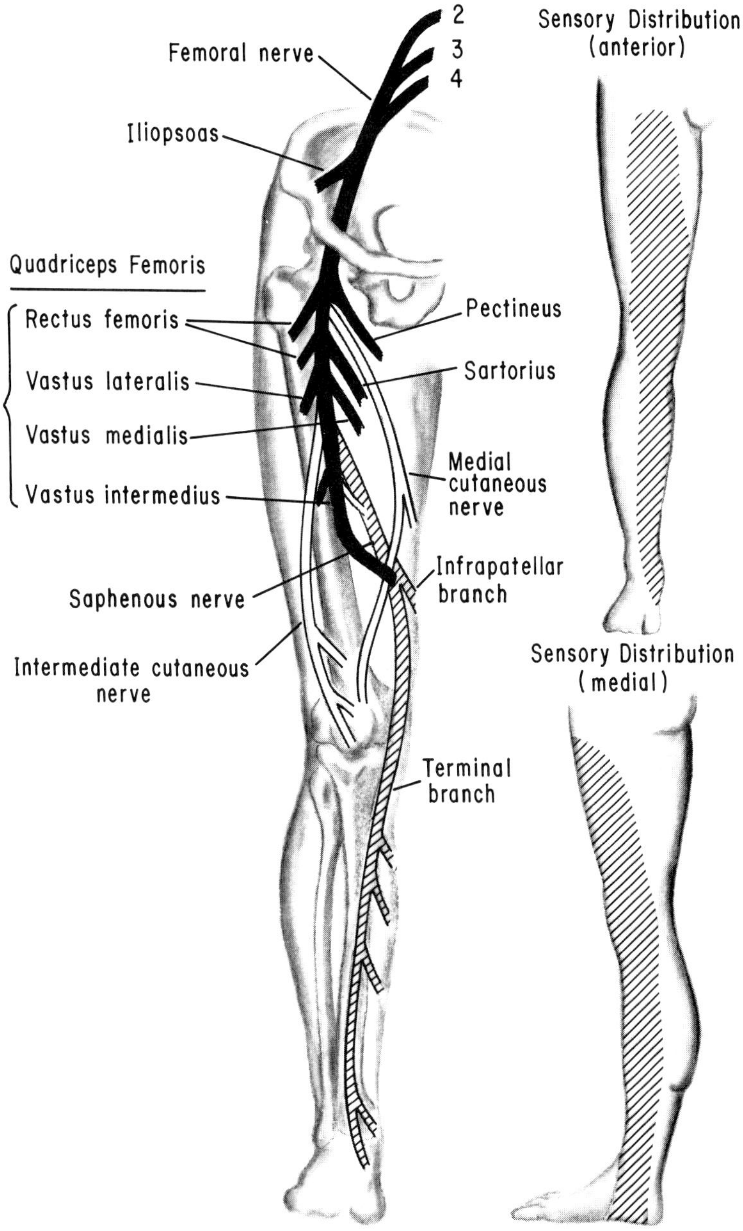

Fig. 5-20. Femoral nerve distribution. (Courtesy R. D. D'Ambrosia.)

crossing the legs difficult. The nerve may be injured by pelvic fractures or by trauma inflicted during a difficult delivery.

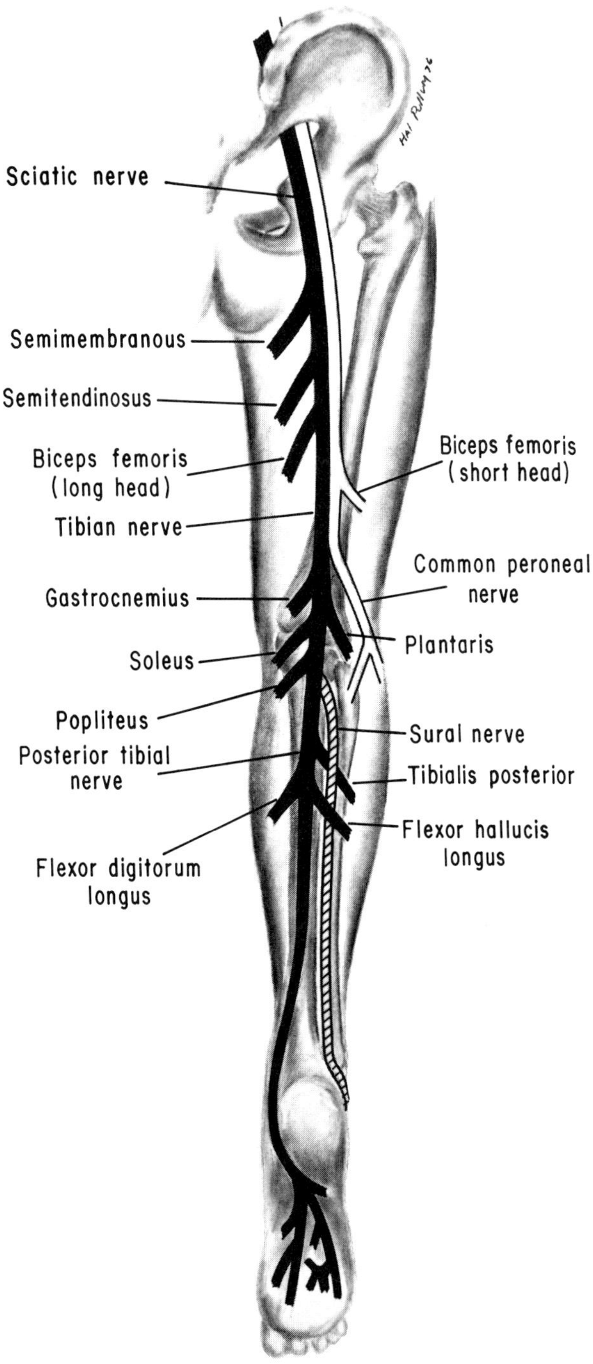

Fig. 5-21. Sciatic nerve distribution. (Courtesy R. D. D'Ambrosia.)

Sciatic Nerve (L-4, 5, S-1, 2, 3)

This is the largest nerve in the body and consists of the tibial and common peroneal nerves contained within a single sheath. It leaves the pelvis through the greater sciatic foramen below the pyriformis muscle, then along the posterior aspect of the thigh to the popliteal space where it divides into the two nerves, tibial and common peroneal (Fig. 5-21). From the tibial portion in the gluteal region, motor branches are given to the hamstrings, the semitendinosus, semimembranosus, and the long head of the biceps. The short head of the biceps is supplied by a branch from the common peroneal trunk.

In the gluteal region, the sciatic nerve is vulnerable to injury by drug injection. In the region of the hip, it may be damaged by fractures and posterior dislocation of the hip or by attempts to reduce them. It may also be injured in this region during hip operations. Femoral fractures of the neck, shaft, or supracondylar region may also injure the nerve. In wartime, missile injuries are the most common cause of injury.

Sciatic nerve loss is manifested by loss of knee flexion due to hamstring paralysis and by loss of all muscles of the leg and foot causing a steppage gait and inability to stand on toes or balance on heels. Sensation is preserved on the instep and medial malleolus but lost on the lateral side of the leg and the remainder of the foot. Incomplete injury may damage either component, or parts of each. Trophic and vasomotor changes and irritative phenomena are common with sciatic injury. The leg and foot are often edematous, and there may be ulcerations, discoloration, dryness, and hyperkeratosis.

Even with complete sciatic nerve loss, the functional picture may still be fairly good; the patient can still walk as the knee can be flexed by the gracilis which is supplied by the obturator nerve and the knee extensors supplied by the femoral nerve. The anesthetic foot is annoying, and pain at the nerve lesion may be severe but rarely is the patient prevented from walking.

Tibial Nerve (L-4, 5, S-1, 2, 3)

In the popliteal space the medial sural cutaneous nerve is given off to join with the lateral sural cutaneous from the common peroneal nerve to form the sural nerve which runs down the posterolateral aspect of the calf to the lateral aspect of the ankle and foot. Below the popliteal space, the tibial nerve (Fig. 5-21) supplies both heads of the gastrocnemius and the soleus (the triceps surae) and also the popliteus and plantaris muscles. It then gives off motor branches to the posterior tibial muscle, the flexor digitorum longus and the flexor hallucis longus and passes behind the medial malleolus to terminate as the medial and lateral plantar nerves. The medial plantar nerve is the counterpart of the median nerve of the hand and supplies most of the intrinsics acting on the great toe as well as sensation of the medial three-and-one-half toes. The lateral plantar nerve is the analog of the ulnar nerve and supplies the intrinsic musculature of the remainder (the major portion) of the foot and sensation to the outer one-and-one-half toes.

The tibial nerve may be injured by penetrating wounds of the popliteal fossa and in the leg, fractures and dislocations about the knee, inept knee operations, and the ischemia and compression from swel-

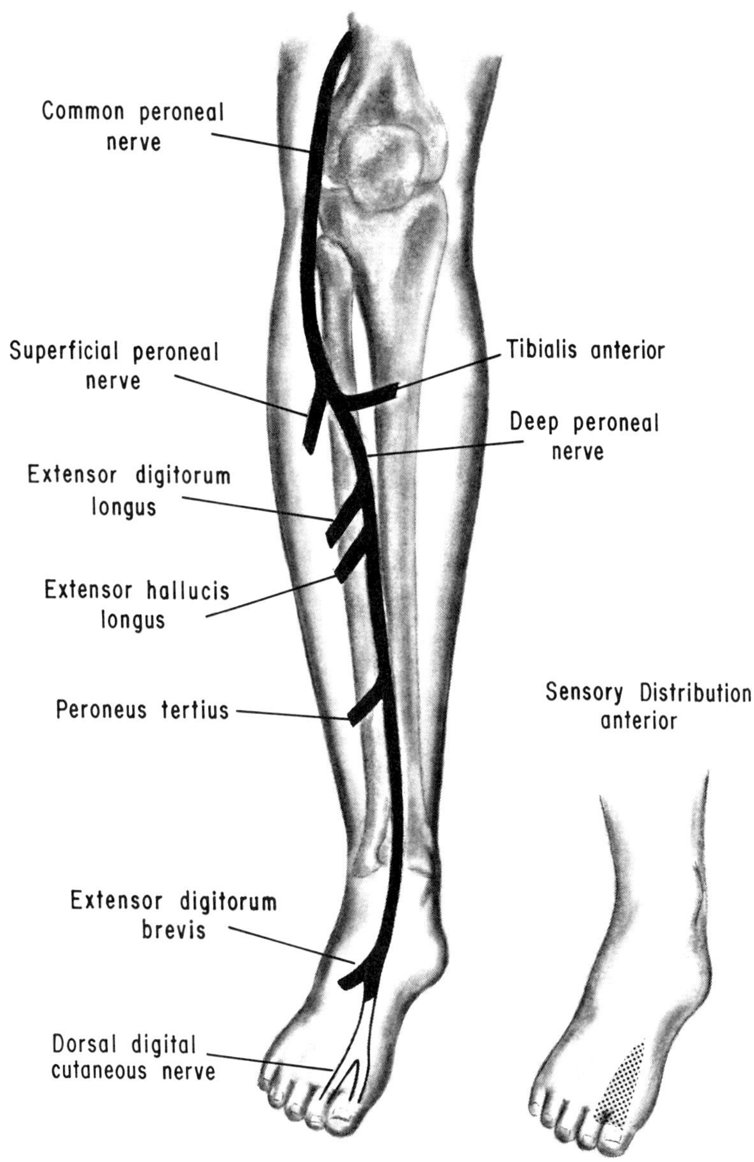

Fig. 5-22. Deep peroneal nerve distribution. (Courtesy R. D. D'Ambrosia.)

ling within the posterior muscle compartments. Volkmann's ischemic contracture of the leg and foot may be a part of the picture with severe ischemic injury.

Examination for tibial nerve damage in the recently injured patient is simple. If the wound or fracture is above the knee, it is enough to determine that there is sensation in the sole and that the calf muscles respond. If below the knee, check for sole sensation and toe flexion. With lesions of longstanding, the deformity is a clawing of the toes.

Common Peroneal Nerve (L-4, 5, S-1, 2)

After giving off the branch to the short head of the biceps while still a part of the sciatic nerve in the thigh, the common peroneal nerve leaves its tibial partner in the upper portion of the popliteal fossa, runs diagonally across the posterior aspect of the knee, where it gives off the lateral sural cutaneous branch to the sural nerve, continues around the head and neck of the fibula, and divides into three terminal branches: the recurrent articular nerve to the knee joint and the superficial and deep peroneal nerves.

The deep peroneal nerve (Fig. 5-22) descends in the anterior compartment of the leg to supply the tibialis anterior, the extensor hallucis longus, extensor digitorum longus, peroneus tertius, and the extensor digitorum brevis. It terminates as a sensory branch supplying the skin of the adjacent sides of the first two toes.

The superficial peroneal nerve (Fig. 5-23) descends along the intermuscular septum supplying the peroneus longus and brevis muscles and sensation to the

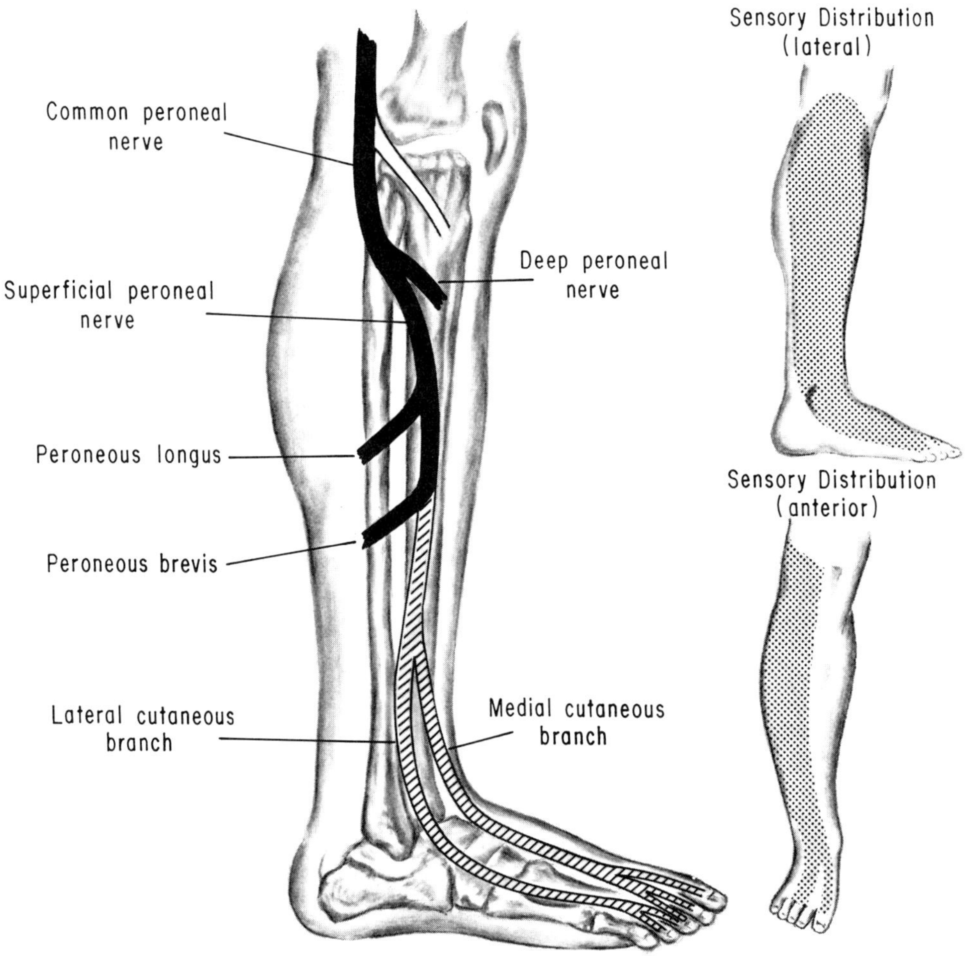

Fig. 5-23. Superficial peroneal nerve distribution. (Courtesy R. D. D'Ambrosia.)

front of the leg, the dorsum of the foot, and the proximal portions of the medial aspect of the great toe and the adjacent portions of toes two through five.

The common peroneal nerve is vulnerable to traction resulting from adduction injuries of the extended knee; the nerve may be injured with fractures and dislocations of the knee and may sometimes be entrapped in the lateral compartment of the knee. The traction or compression injury may be compounded by ischemia of the nerve secondary to the arterial damage which may be a part of either dislocation of the knee or open wounds in this area. The nerve is also susceptible to compression damage due to careless positioning of the anesthetized patient or by prolonged sitting with the legs crossed.

The anterior compartment syndrome, characterized by trauma to the leg, as in a tibial fracture, and swelling within the muscle compartment, causing nerve and muscle ischemia, may damage either peroneal nerve and lead to their paralysis and a Volkmann's ischemic contracture.

In the recently injured patient, active dorsiflexion and eversion of the ankle are generally enough to demonstrate an intact common peroneal nerve. In lesions of longstanding, foot drop is apparent and results in a steppage gait and a slapping of the foot on the ground. Vasomotor and trophic changes are not as commonly seen as they are with tibial nerve injury.

SUGGESTED READINGS

1. Bradley, W. G.: Disorders of Peripheral Nerves. Oxford, Blackwell Scientific Publications, 1974.
2. Chusid, J. G., and McDonald, J. J.: Correlative Neuroanatomy and Functional Neurology. ed. 14. Los Altos, Calif. Lange, 1970.
3. DeJong, R. N.: The Neurologic Examination Incorporating the Fundamentals of Neuroanatomy and Neurophysiology. ed. 3. New York, Harper & Row, 1967.
4. Haymaker, W., and Woodhall, B.: Peripheral Nerve Injuries, Principles of Diagnosis. ed. 2. Philadelphia, W. B. Saunders Co., 1953.
5. Mitchell, S. W.: Injuries of Nerves and Their Consequences. Philadelphia, J. B. Lippincott Co., 1972.
6. Seddon, H.: Surgical Disorders of the Peripheral Nerves. Baltimore, Williams & Wilkins, 1972.
7. Sunderland, S.: Nerves and Nerve Injuries. Baltimore, Williams & Wilkins, 1968.

6 The Neck

Henry H. Bohlman, M.D.

ANATOMY OF THE NECK

Topographical Anatomy

Knowledge of surface landmarks and regional areas, such as the cervical triangles in the neck, is extremely important. Anteriorly, the neck is divided into two major triangular areas by the sternocleidomastoid muscle: one triangle is anterior to the sternocleidomastoid muscle and the second is posterior to it (Fig. 6-1). The anterior triangle is bounded by the sternocleidomastoid muscle and inferior ramus of the mandible. It is subdivided by the digastric and omohyoid muscles and hyoid bone into the muscular, carotid, digastric, and submental triangles. The posterior triangle is bounded by the sternocleidomastoid and trapezius muscles and the clavicle. It is subdivided by the omohyoid muscle into the subclavian and occipital triangles.

Localization of deeper structures in the neck can be accomplished by palpation. Both the carotid sheath and pulsation of the common carotid artery deep to the sternocleidomastoid muscle can be identified by palpation. In the same area is an important bony landmark: the carotid, or Chassaignac's tubercle, the largest and most prominent tubercle on the lateral mass of C6. Also at the level of the 6th cervical vertebra is the cricoid cartilage. Above the 6th vertebra are the pharynx and larynx and below, the esophagus and trachea (Fig. 6-1).

The transverse process of C1 can be palpated halfway between the mastoid process and the angle of the mandible. The posterior ring of C1 is not palpable, but C2 is very prominent and just below the occiput. The anterior body of C2 can be palpated through the posterior pharyngeal mucosa if the latter is anesthetized. The most prominent spinous process is that of C7.

The jugular fossa is formed by the convergence of the two sternocleidomastoid muscles at the manubrium (Fig. 6-1). The supraclavicular fossa is a depression in the lower portion of the posterior triangle above the clavicle (Fig. 6-1). In this fossa one can palpate the subclavian artery and brachial plexus against the first rib.

Deep Anatomy

The major muscles and vessels are contained within well-defined fascial coverings. Anteriorly, the deep cervical fascial layers are divided into superficial, prevertebral, suprahyoid, infrahyoid, and visceral compartments. The superficial layer of investing fascia splits to encircle the sternocleidomastoid muscles anteriorly and the trapezius muscles posteriorly. The prevertebral fascia is cylindrical in form encircling the vertebral bodies, longus coli, scalene muscles, and posterior (extensor) muscles of the neck. The suprahyoid fascia encircles the digastric and stylohyoid muscles and extends up to the mandible. The infrahyoid fascia encloses the strap muscles (flexors) in two layers. The visceral fascia is composed of two parts: the pretracheal fascia circles the trachea, larynx, and thyroid gland, whereas the buccopharyngeal fascia is continuous posteriorly covering the esophagus, blending with the pretracheal fascia. The carotid sheath is bounded by its own layer of fascia. There is a separate plane in the retropharyngeal space formed by the alar fascia, which is just anterior to the prevertebral fascia (Fig. 6-2).

Posteriorly the erector spinae muscle group con-

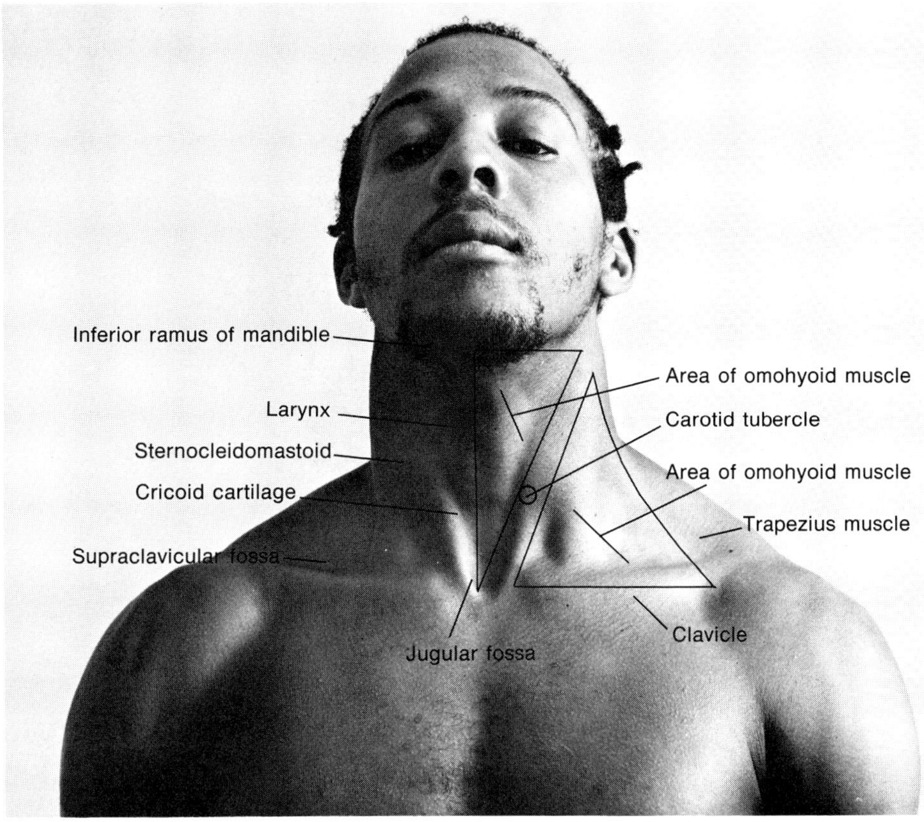

Fig. 6-1. Cervical triangles: (*left*) anterior triangle; (*right*) posterior triangle (Courtesy of Robert D'Ambrosia).

sists of the suboccipital muscles and minor deep cervical muscles, all of which serve to extend the skull and cervical spine. Superficially there are the longer semispinalis capitis and splenius capitis muscles. The deeper rectus capitis and oblique capitis muscles form boundaries of the suboccipital triangle, the floor being the posterior atlanto-occipital membrane. Through the suboccipital triangle the vertebral artery, suboccipital nerve, greater occipital nerve and occipital artery all pass (Figs. 6-3, 6-4).

Neuroanatomy

In the cervical region, the spinal cord comprises one-half of the spinal canal space. There are 7 cervical vertebrae and 8 cervical nerve roots. Each nerve root is formed from a ventral motor and a dorsal sensory rootlet. The nerve roots exit from the spinal canal through neural foramen. The first cervical root exits between the occiput and C1 vertebra; C2 exits above the C2 vertebra. Each nerve root exits above its numbered cervical vertebra, except C8, which passes out below C7 vertebra and above T1. The spinal cord and proximal portions of the nerve roots are covered with a fibrous layer of dura mater. Beneath the dural covering is another layer of thin tissue called the arachnoidea, through which the spinal fluid circulates. Directly adherent to the spinal cord is the pia mater, which covers the delicate nutrient vessels of the spinal cord. The spinal cord is surrounded by a protective layer of fatty tissue between the bone and dura mater. Thin epidural fat contains the plexus of veins and arteries (Fig. 6-5).

The internal structure of the spinal cord consists of central gray matter containing the anterior horn motor cells which innervate the muscles of the neck and upper extremities. The dorsal horn cells of the gray matter receive sensory impulses from the dorsal roots. Within the central gray matter are internuncial fibers which aid in transmission of impulses from sensory roots and long tracts to the

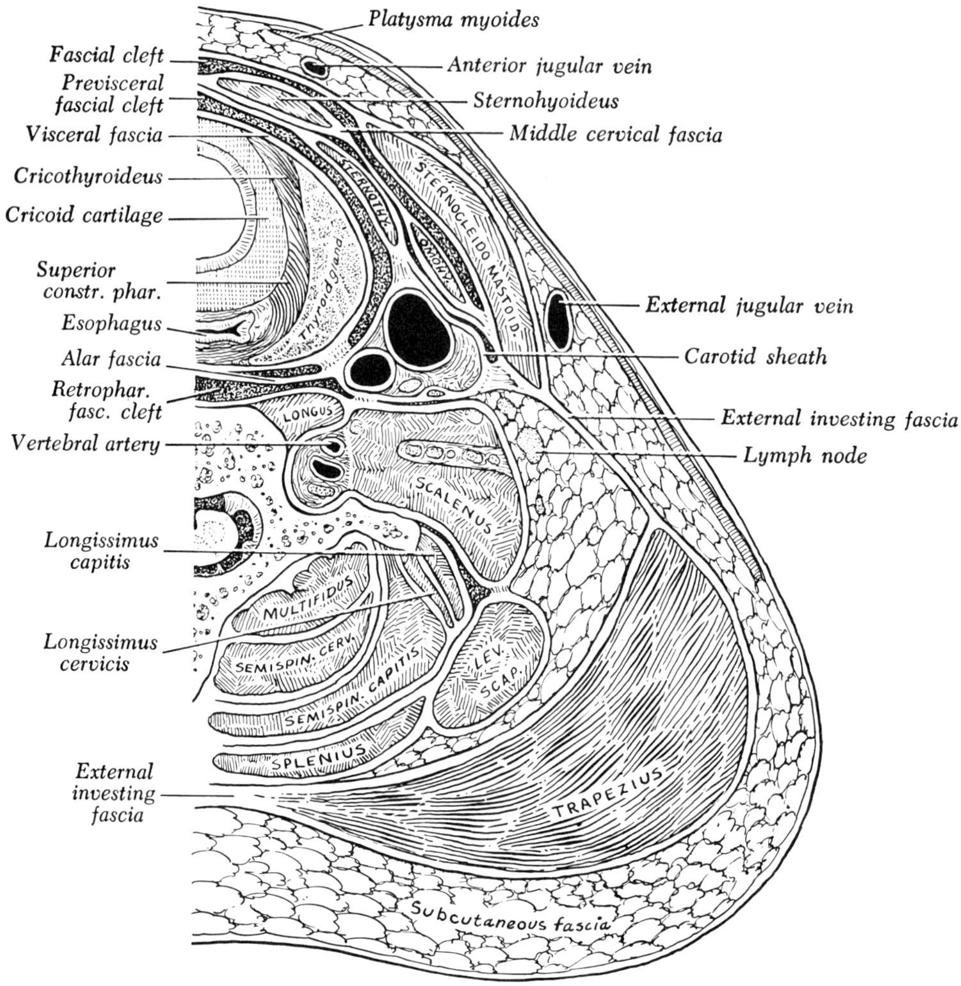

Fig. 6-2. Section of the neck at about the level of the sixth cervical vertebra (Goss, C. M. [ed.]: Anatomy of the Human Body by Henry Gray, F.R.S. ed. 29. Philadelphia, Lea and Febiger, 1973).

thalamus.The more peripheral white matter contains the long tracts for sensation and motor impulses to and from the trunk and extremities. In the cervical cord region are the lower motor neuron fibers for the arms and upper motor neuron fibers to the legs (Figs. 6-6, 6-7, 6-8, 6-9).

Osseous Cervical Spine

In general, the cervical spine has greater mobility than the thoracic or lumbar spine. There are seven cervical vertebrae; the first two are unique in structure and are responsible for major motion in flexion, extension, and rotation.

The first cervical vertebra or atlas is shaped like a ring and articulates with the occipital condyles of the skull with its large lateral masses. The caudal side of the lateral masses of the atlas articulate with the axis or C2. Approximately one-half of the flexion extension motion of the cervical spine occurs at the atlanto-occipital joints (Fig. 6-10).

The second cervical vertebra or axis has a very large vertebral body and a cephalic projection called the odontoid process. The odontoid process is stabilized to the ring of the atlas anteriorly by the strong transverse ligament. Anterior subluxation of C1 or C2 is limited by the transverse ligament. One-half of the cervical spine rotation occurs at the atlantoaxial joint and is stabilized by the alar, check-reign ligaments which attach the odontoid to the occipital

(Text continues on page 184.)

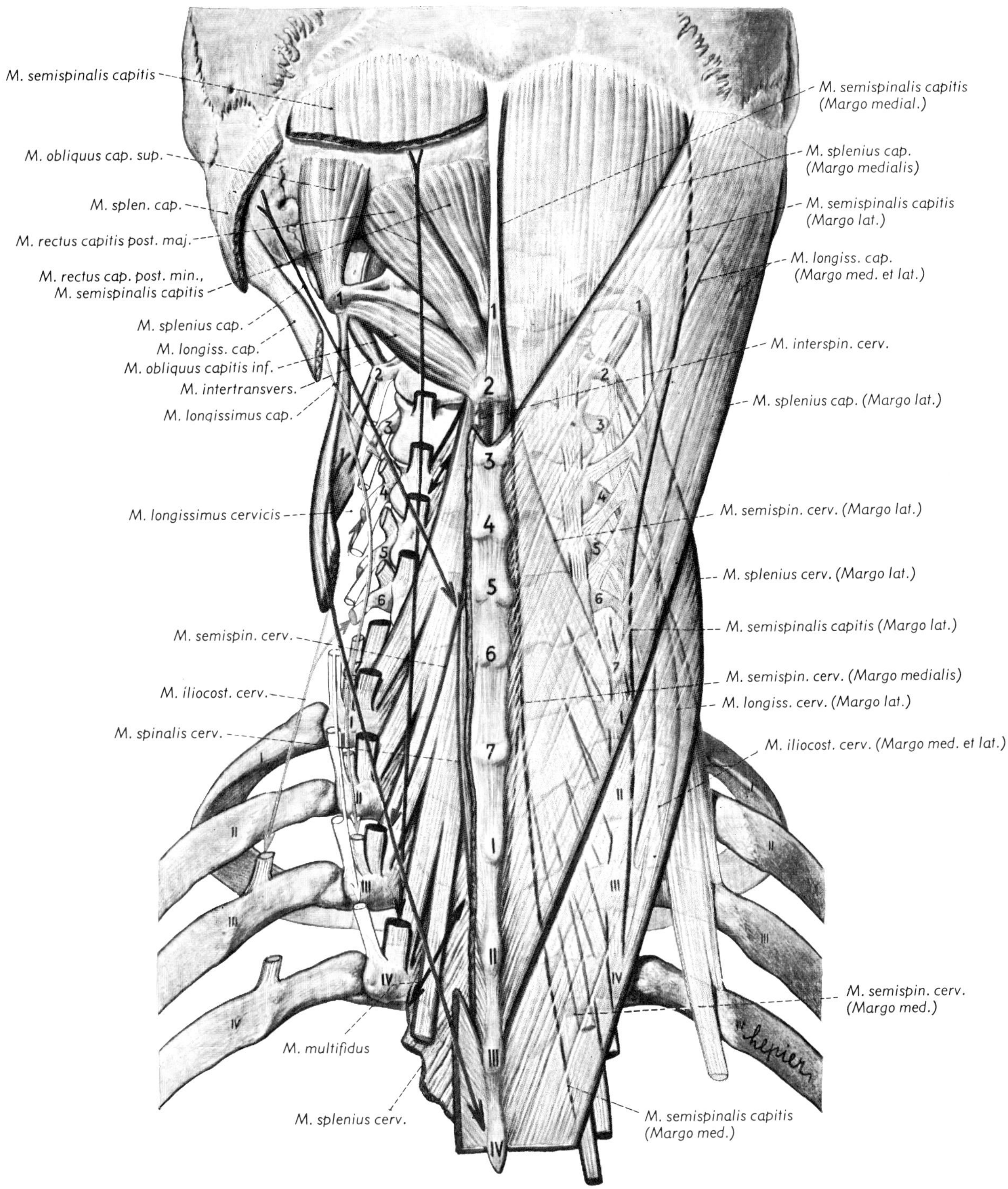

Fig. 6-3. The intrinsic muscles of the posterior neck region. The superficial muscles on the right side have been drawn translucent; on the left side only the origins and insertions have been indicated in order to bring into view the underlying muscles. The directions of contraction of the fibers of the muscles on the left side are indicated by arrows. (Pernkopf, E.: Atlas of Topographical and Applied Human Anatomy. Philadelphia, W. B. Saunders, 1963.)

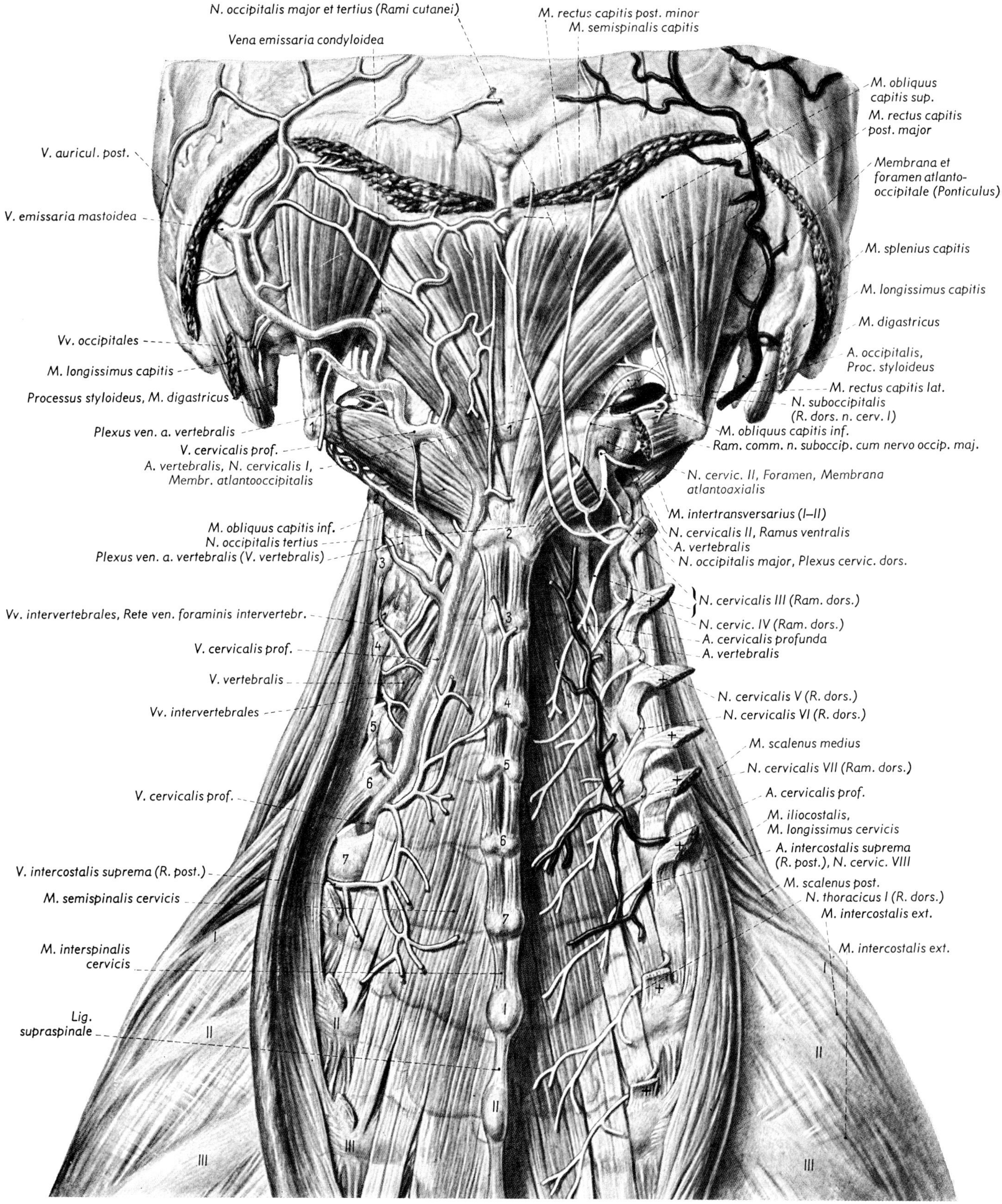

Fig. 6-4. The deep muscles, blood vessels, and nerves of the back of the neck. The arteries and nerves are shown on the right side, and the veins on the left side. The shoulder girdle with its muscles as well as m. splenius, m. semispinalis capitis, and m. longissimus colli have been removed. (Pernkopf, E.: Atlas of Topographical and Applied Human Anatomy. Philadelphia, W. B. Saunders, 1963).

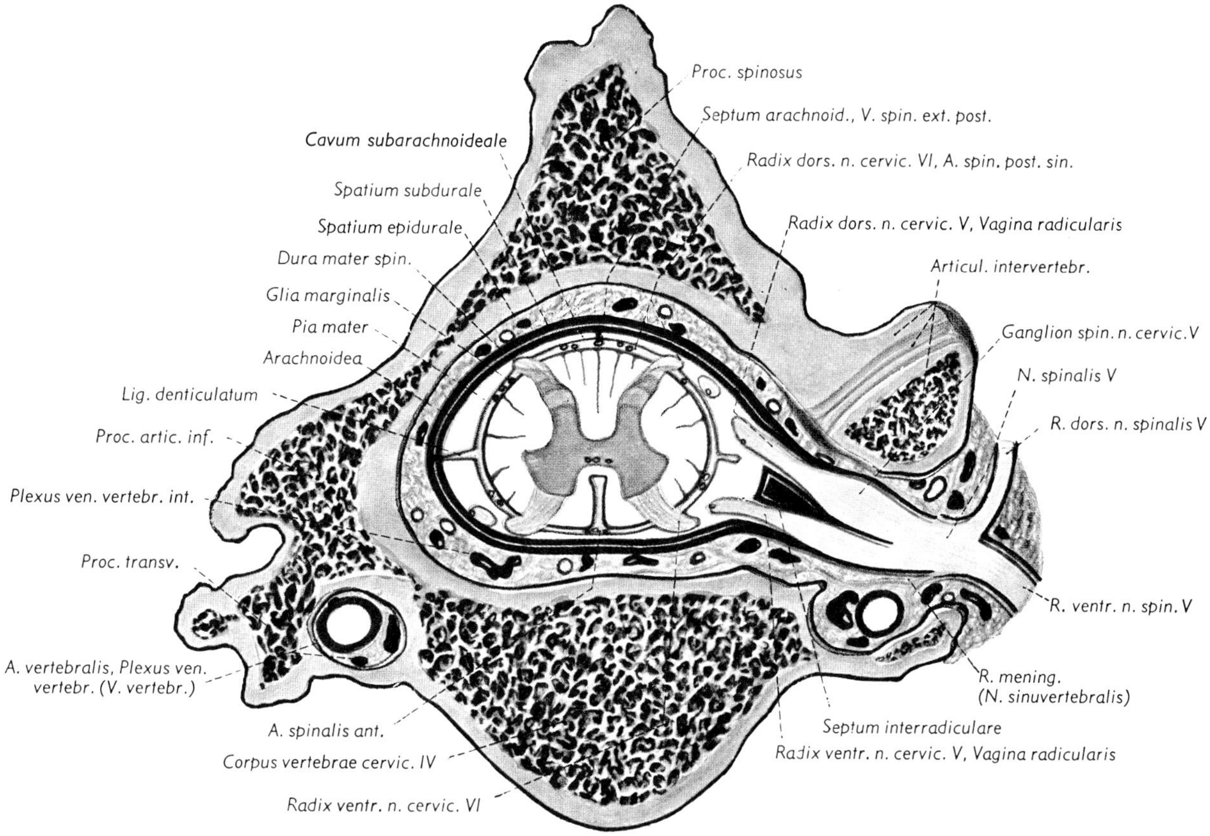

Fig. 6-5. Transverse section through the vertebral column of the neck and the contents of the vertebral canal: the spinal cord and its investing membranes in cross section. Section at the level of the 4th cervical vertebra; plane of sectioning is somewhat higher on the right side and lower on the left. A. and v. vertebralis lie in the enclosed right foramen transversarium. (Pernkopf, E.: Atlas of Topographical and Applied Human Anatomy. Philadelphia, W. B. Saunders, 1963.)

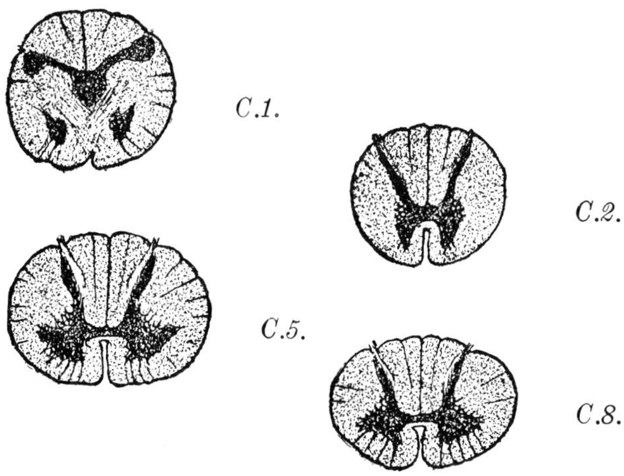

Fig. 6-6. Transverse sections of the spinal cord at C1, C2, C5, and C8 (Goss, C. M. [ed.]: Anatomy of the Human Body by Henry Gray, F.R.S. ed. 29. Philadelphia, Lea and Febiger, 1973).

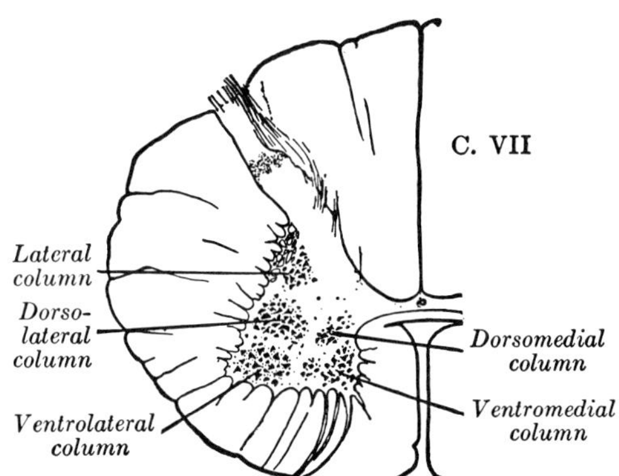

Fig. 6-7. Transverse section of the spinal cord at C7 showing the arrangement of the principal cell columns (Goss, C. M. [ed.]: Anatomy of the Human Body by Henry Gray, F.R.S. ed. 29. Philadelphia, Lea and Febiger, 1973).

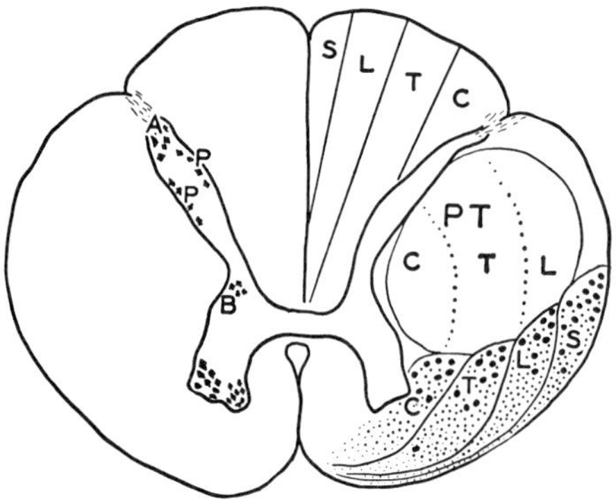

Fig. 6-8. Semi-schematic drawing to show on the left side the cell groups of the posterior horn, and on the right side the arrangement of the spinothalamic and other tracts in the lower cervical region. The heavy dots represent fibers concerned with temperature; the medium-sized dots, fibers mediating pain, and the fine dots, fibers carrying touch and pressure impulses. Note the overlapping and topical arrangement of the fibers. *A*, apical group of large ganglion cells of the posterior horn; *B*, basal group of large ganglion cells of the posterior horn; *C*, fibers from the cervical segment of the spinal cord; *L*, fibers from the lumbar segment of the spinal cord; *P*, pericornual groups of large ganglion cells of the posterior horn; *PT*, tractus pyramidalis; *S*, fibers from the sacral segment of the spinal cord, and *T*, fibers from the thoracic segment of the spinal cord. (Walker, courtesy of Arch. Neur. and Psych. *In* Goss, C. M. [ed.]: Anatomy of the Human Body by Henry Gray, F.R.S. ed. 29. Philadelphia, Lea and Febiger, 1973).

condyles at the lateral edges of the foramen magnum. A small apical ligament passes from the tip of the odontoid process to the occiput at the anterior aspect of the foramen magnum (clivus) (Figs. 6-11, 6-12).

The vertebrae between C3 and C7 are similar in structure to each other. They provide limited flexion and extension with a small amount of tilt and lateral rotation. The bodies of the vertebrae are concave superiorly and convex inferiorly. The intervertebral disks are composed of a soft nucleus pulposus centrally with a surrounding anulus fibrosis. The disks allow articulation of adjacent vertebrae. The transverse processes of the vertebrae provide the vertebral foramen through which the vertebral artery passes from C6 to C1. The superior and inferior articular surfaces of the lateral masses comprise facet joints.

These joints are angled 45 degrees from horizontal in a coronal plane and allow for flexion and extension but little rotation. Nerve roots exit the spinal canal in a groove between the vertebral artery anteriorly and the facet joint posteriorly. This groove lies on the superior surface of the vertebral pedicles (Fig. 6-13).

The laminae of the vertebrae arise from the lateral masses and complete the dorsal closure of the spinal canal to cover the spinal cord, and the spinous processes project posteriorly (Fig. 6-14).

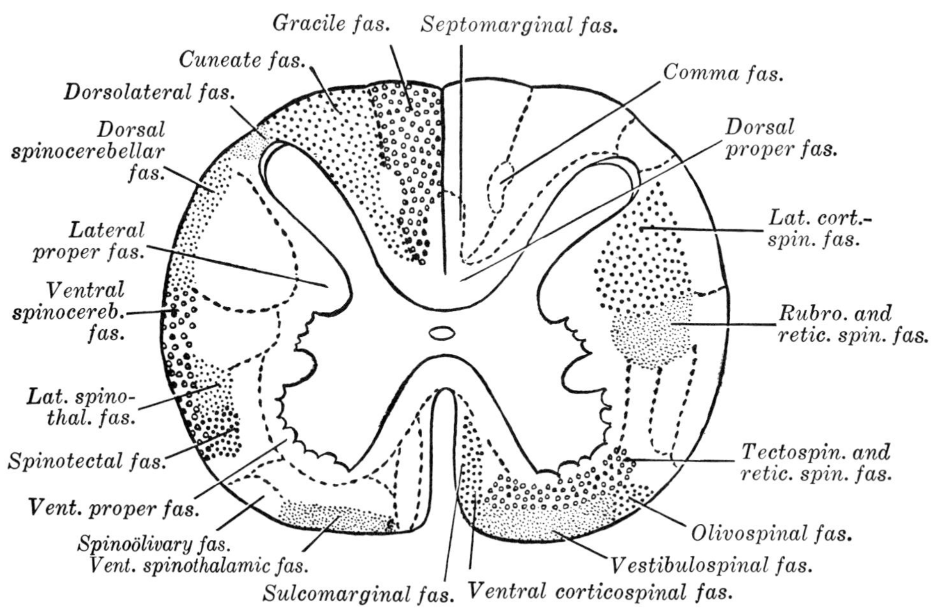

Fig. 6-9. Diagram of the principal fasciculi of the spinal cord (Goss, C. M. [ed.]: Anatomy of the Human Body by Henry Gray, F.R.S. ed. 29. Philadelphia, Lea and Febiger, 1973).

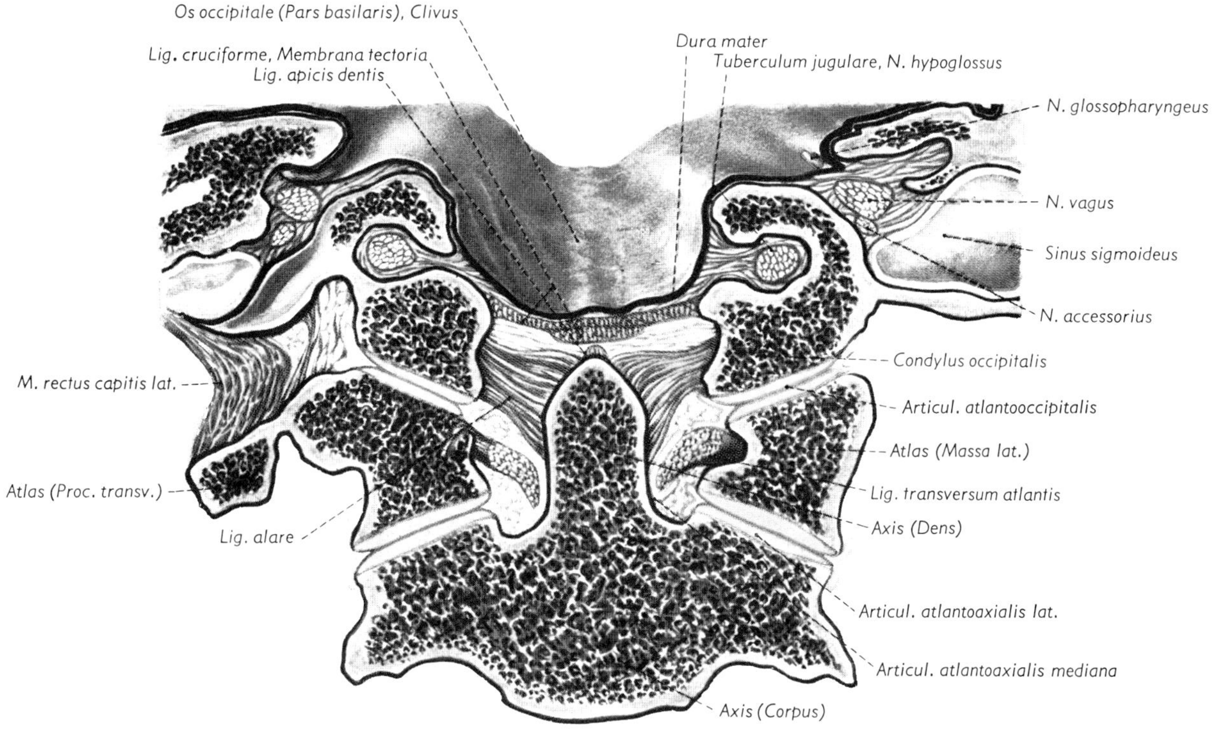

Fig. 6-10. Frontal section through the region of the craniovertebral joints. Dorsal view of the cut surface. (Pernkopf, E.: Atlas of Topographical and Applied Human Anatomy. Philadelphia, W. B. Saunders, 1963.)

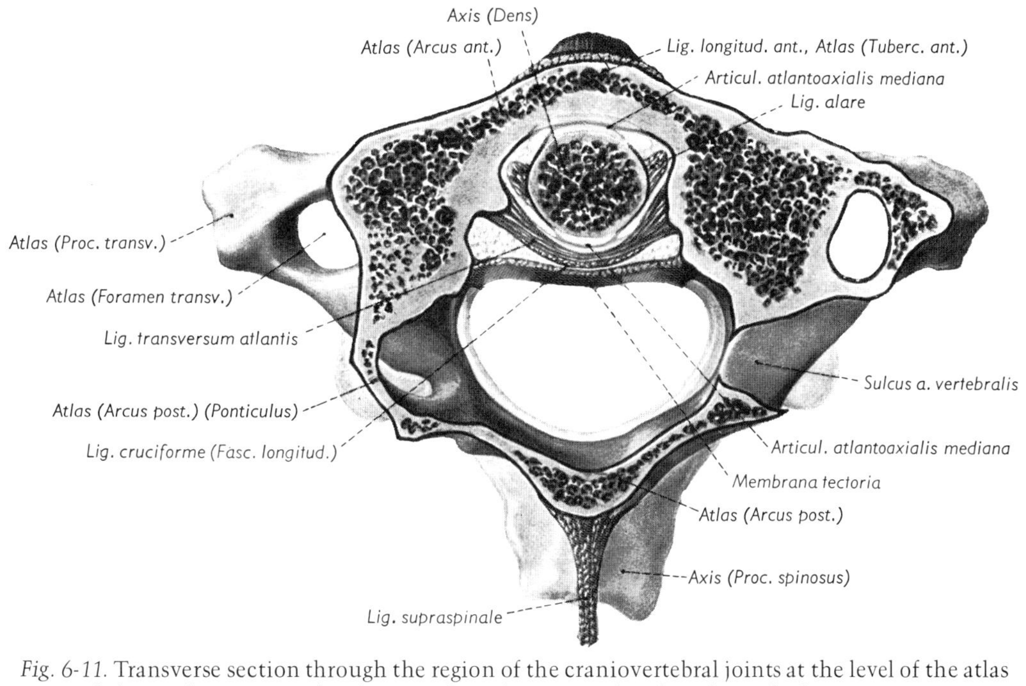

Fig. 6-11. Transverse section through the region of the craniovertebral joints at the level of the atlas (viewed from above). (Pernkopf, E.: Atlas of Topographical and Applied Human Anatomy. Philadelphia, W. B. Saunders, 1963.)

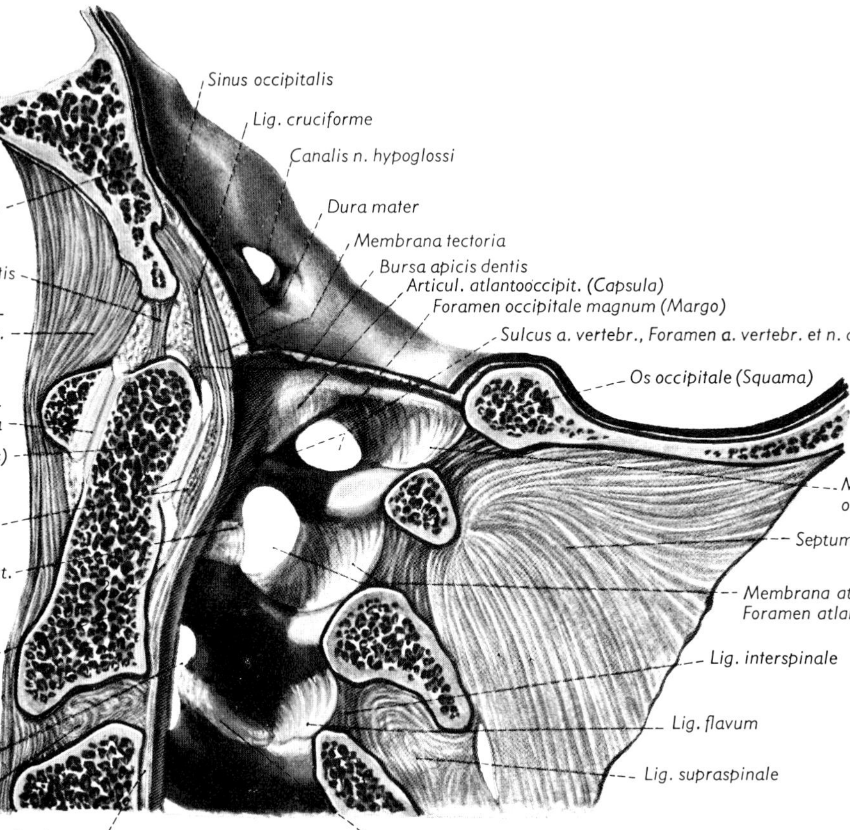

Fig. 6-12. Midsagittal section through the region of the craniovertebral joints (right half). (Pernkopf, E.: Atlas of Topographical and Applied Human Anatomy. Philadelphia, W. B. Saunders, 1963.)

The vertebral artery enters the 6th vertebral foramen, excluding the 7th, and passes cephalad through all vertebrae above and then loops posteriorly after passing through C1. The artery continues medially over a groove in the atlas lamina posterior to the lateral mass and passes cephalad where it joins its counterpart from the opposite side to form the basilar artery (Fig. 6-15).

The ligamentous structures of the lower cervical spine include a strong anterior longitudinal ligament covering the anterior surface of vertebral bodies and disks, continuing cephalad to form the anterior atlanto-occipital membrane. The posterior longitudinal ligament extends cephalad at C1 as the tectorial membrane. Between the facet joints posteriorly are found the capsular ligaments, and the laminae are held together by the thick ligamentum flavum.

REGIONAL EXAMINATION

Introduction

Examination of the patient with suspected cervical orthopaedic disease must begin with a *general observation* of the patient while taking a detailed history of the chief complaint, present illness, review of systems, and history of previous illness. The examiner questions the patient with regard to the general disease categories of trauma, tumors, infections, inflammatory disease, congenital anomalies, and the acute herniated disk. Details of the various categories depend on the age of the patient. General observation of the patient should include the position of the head in relation to the neck, facial expression of pain, general health of the patient, peculiar mannerisms, gait, and response to questioning.

(*Text continues on page 189.*)

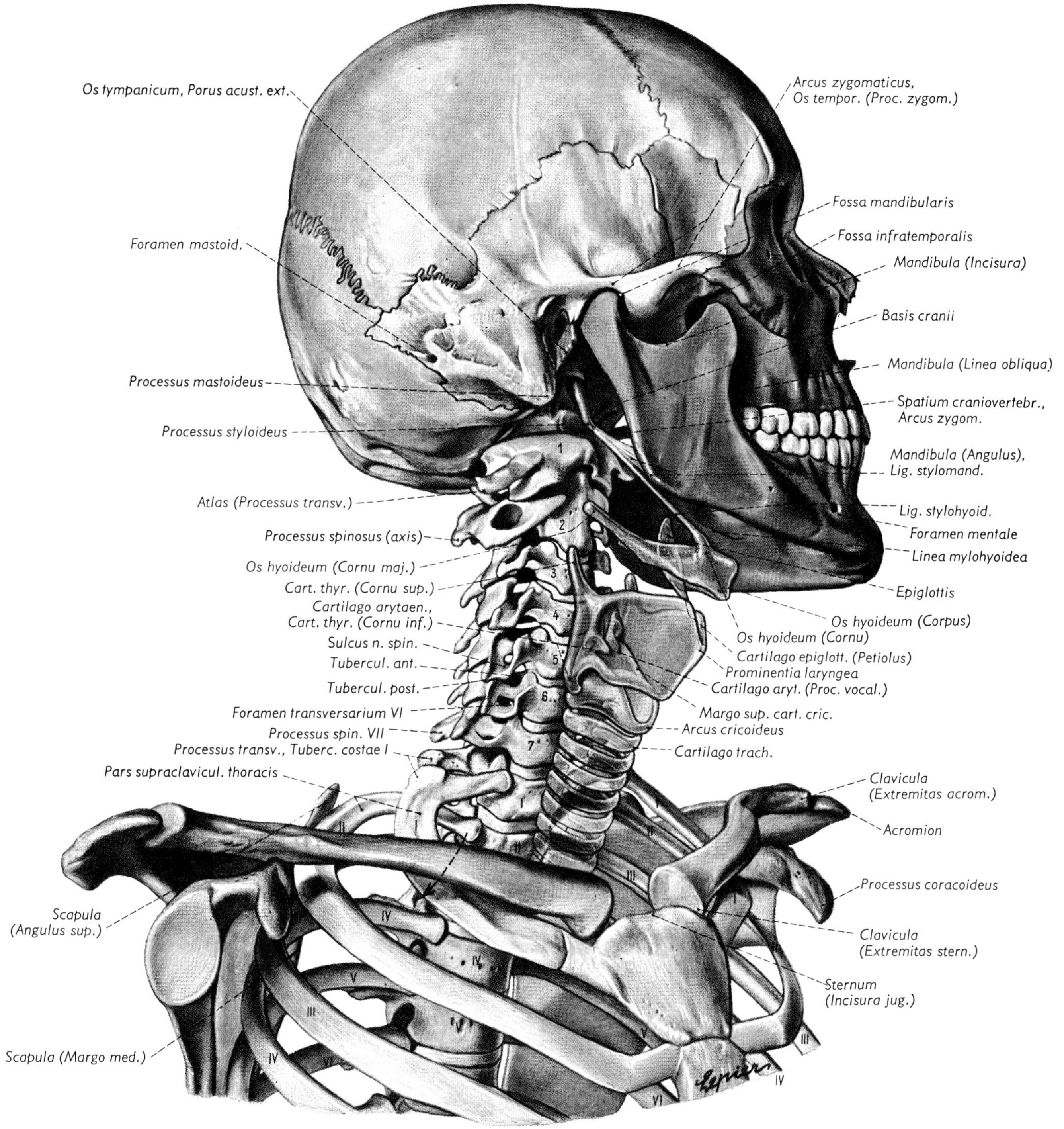

Fig. 6-13. Skeleton of the head and neck, viewed from the side with the head turned somewhat to the left. (Pernkopf, E.: Atlas of Topographical and Applied Human Anatomy. Philadelphia, W. B. Saunders, 1963.)

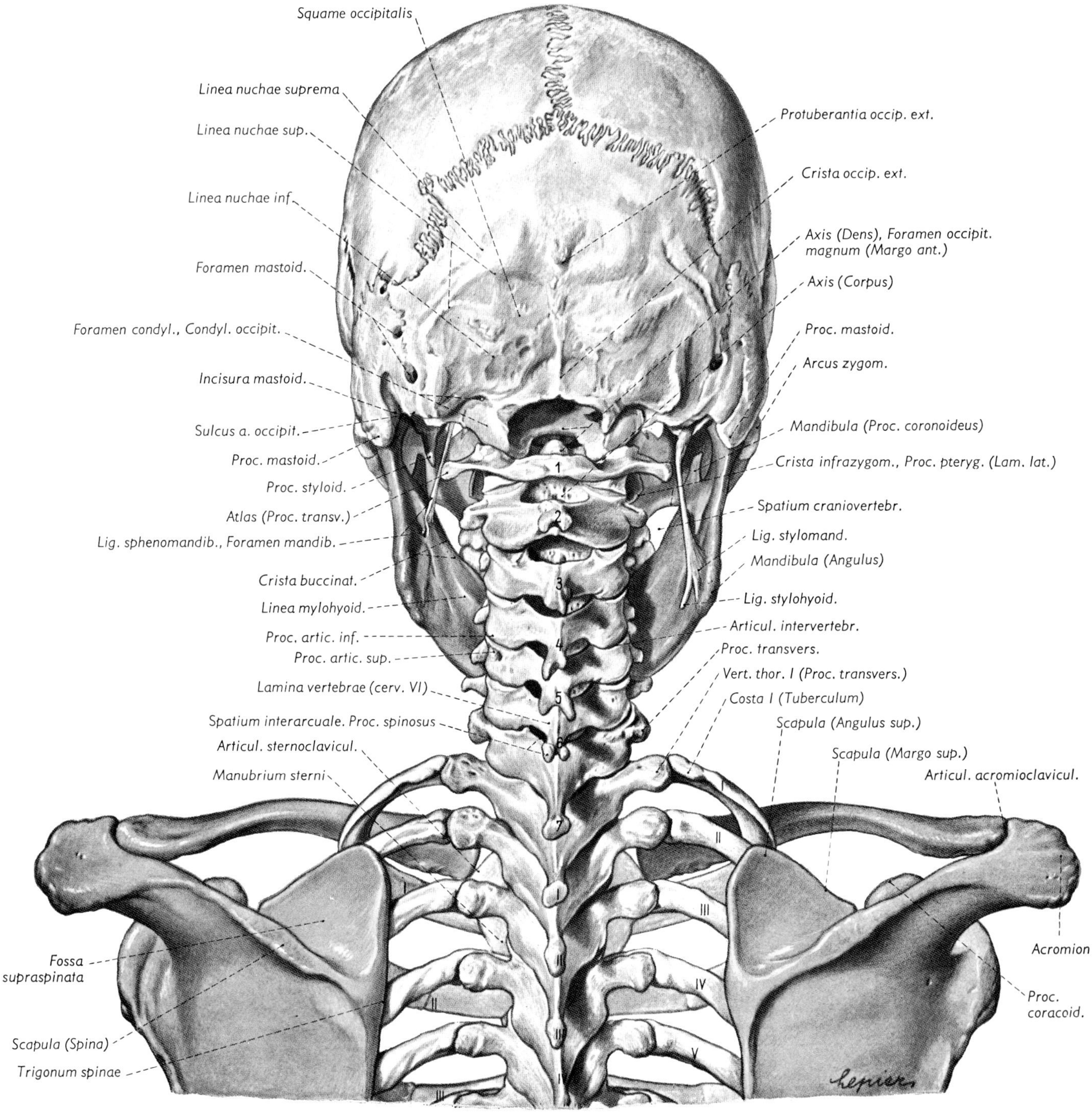

Fig. 6-14. Skeleton of the neck and associated parts, particularly the head. Dorsal view with the head bent slightly forward. (Pernkopf, E.: Atlas of Topographical and Applied Human Anatomy. Philadelphia, W. B. Saunders, 1963.)

Fig. 6-15. The internal carotid and vertebral arteries. Right side. (Goss, C. M. [ed.]: Anatomy of the Human Body by Henry Gray, F.R.S. ed. 29. Philadelphia, Lea and Febiger, 1973.)

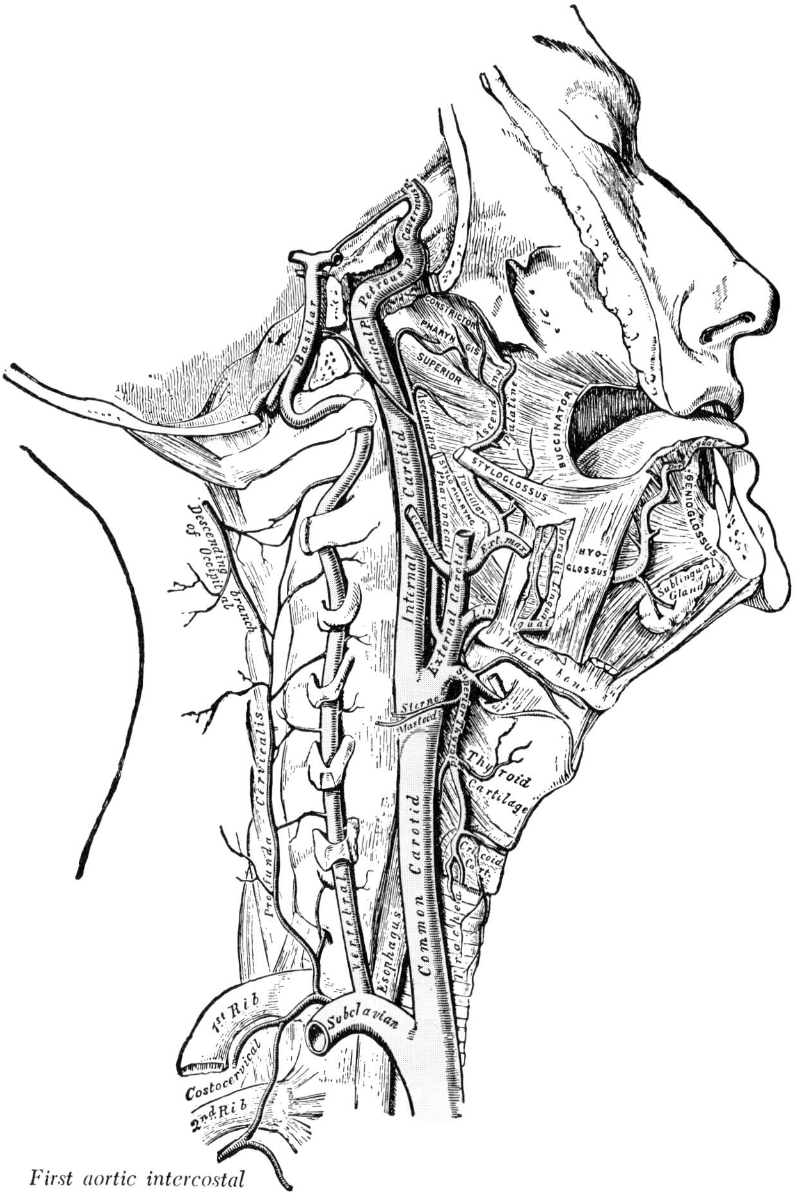

Neck Pain

Invariably, the chief complaint is of neck pain; therefore, diagnosis of the present illness evolves from detailed questions with reference to the pain. What was the date of onset of the pain? Was it recent, associated with trauma, or chronic for many months? What time of day does the pain occur? Is it at night? Is the pain intermittent or constant? Is it related to particular activities such as coughing or sneezing, and is it relieved by rest and lying down? One should ask if the pain is related to head and neck position. The pain should be characterized as a sharp or dull ache and whether it radiates to the head, shoulders, or extremities. Most important, the patient should point to the site of the pain and describe its distribution. Does the pain radiate to the arms, forearms, or fingers? Is the pain interscapular in association with the neck or in the chest region? A description of pain is found in Table 6-1.

Table 6-1. Description of Pain

Date of onset: acute or chronic duration: intermittent or constant?
Relation to trauma, fever, weight loss, disease
Character: sharp, dull, lancinating
Site and distribution
Chronology: day or night
Relation to position of head and neck
Associated neurologic problems

Once the pain syndrome has been elucidated, it must be related to other general disease categories. For instance, in the case of trauma (i.e., car accident, sports injury, or fall), care must be taken to have the patient describe the mechanism of injury. Did he strike his head? If so, at what site? Was a facial laceration present? Sites of head trauma are clues to the mechanism of injury (i.e., flexion, extension, lateral rotation, or a combination of forces). The mechanism of injury will be related to the type of soft tissue involved. The magnitude of the traumatic episode will determine the degree of injury. That is to say, the patient may have a simple cervical sprain with stretching and disruption of the soft tissue structure about the cervical spine, or a more severe injury, such as a fracture or dislocation of the cervical spine may be present. Was there a loss of consciousness? Was there associated extremity weakness, paresthesias, or loss of bowel and bladder control?

The patient who presents with neck pain associated with trauma must be questioned regarding previous degenerative disk disease, tumor, infections, herniated disk, and congenital anomalies. Here, past history and review of systems are most important. Not infrequently, however, it is a traumatic episode that brings the patient to the physician and the above traumatic entities are incidently discovered by roentgenogram. Chiropractic manipulation may induce collapse of a tumorous vertebra or dislocation of a previously unstable spine.

Tumors of the cervical spine are most frequently secondary to metastatic disease so that history of the present illness must include a review of systems with regard to a primary malignancy. Similarly, infections of the spine are usually blood-borne and originate at sites remote from the cervical spine, as in pulmonary tuberculosis or urinary tract and joint infections.

Cervical spondylosis or degenerative disk disease may be present for years without major symptoms and then may become painful after stress or injury. Unlike the lumbar spine region, herniated cervical nucleus pulposus is not usually associated with trauma. The patient most frequently has slept in an awkward position and awakens with neck and arm pain. Cervical spondylosis as well as a herniated disk may be associated with nerve root or spinal cord compression. Therefore, a proper history must include questions regarding weakness of extremities, paresthesias, bladder and bowel paralysis, and gait difficulties.

Congenital anomalies may be present and asymptomatic for years. Only in later life do patients with congenitally fused vertebrae develop degenerative disk disease and pain with added stress above the fusion. Dysplasia or absence of the odontoid process may result in dislocation of the atlas on the axis with pain and syncopal episodes in teenage or adult life. Finally, the patient with a congenitally narrowed spinal canal may not develop spinal cord compression until the cervical spine becomes severely arthritic and further compromises the diameter of the spinal canal.

Past History

The history is extremely important with reference to previous similar episodes of pain, herniated disks, types of treatment, and injuries in years past which may have predisposed to degenerative disk disease. The mere fact that a patient has diagnosed rheumatoid arthritis and has been treated with steroids should alert one to the fact that subluxation or dislocation of vertebrae may be present. In contrast, juvenile rheumatoid arthritis results in spontaneous fusions of the cervical vertebrae as does ankylosing spondylitis. Previous traumatic episodes may produce dislocated vertebrae which go undiagnosed for months or years.

Physical Examination

Following a detailed history of the present illness and review of systems, a thorough physical examination is performed. The patient's active as well as passive range of motion is tested. Extension is tested by asking the patient to move his head backward as far as possible and flexion is tested by touching the chin on the chest (Fig. 6-16). Lateral bend to either side is tested by asking the patient to touch his chin on either shoulder (Fig. 6-17). Rotation is tested both

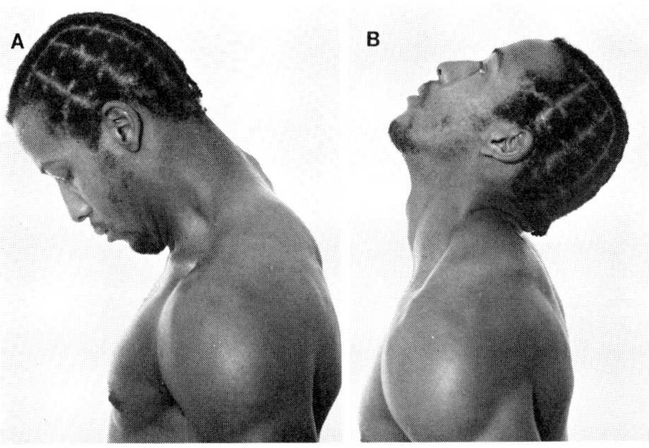

Fig. 6-16. Extension (*A*) and flexion (*B*) of the cervical spine. It may be indicated by degrees from neutral or the distance in inches from the chin to the chest. (Courtesy of Robert D'Ambrosia.)

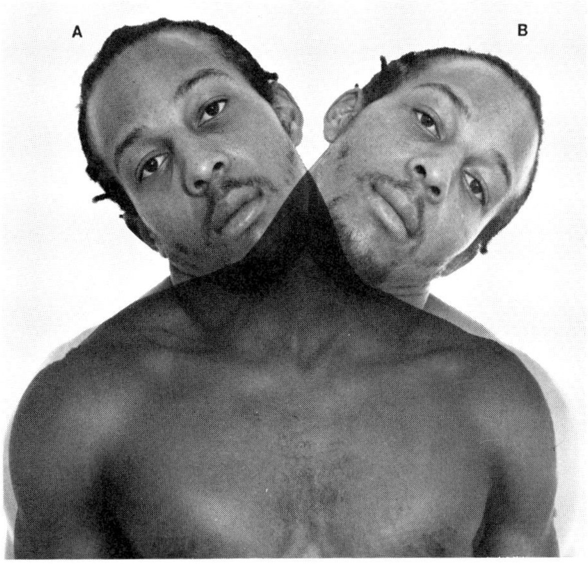

Fig. 6-17. Right (*A*) and left (*B*) lateral bend can be measured in degrees or the distance in inches from the ear to the shoulder. (Courtesy of Robert D'Ambrosia.)

to the right and left from the neutral position (Fig. 6-18). Muscle spasm, arthritis, or guarding a painful neck will prevent full range of active motion. Passive range of motion is tested by gently grasping the patient's forehead, extending the head backward as far as possible, then rotating the head in neutral position to either side. Forward flexion is tested by grasping the occiput and moving the head and chin toward the chest. All ranges of motion should be recorded in degrees from neutral position to most complete motion in each direction. Any crepitus or cracking of the neck is noted.

Topographical anatomy and landmarks are quite important in the next step of physical examination: palpation of the neck. First, the posterior spinous processes are palpated, the second cervical being most prominent in the upper part of the spine and the seventh cervical, in the lower region of the neck. If a particular vertebra is tender, this should be recorded. The transverse processes of the atlas may be felt halfway between the mastoid process of the skull and angle of the mandible. Anteriorly, the vertebral bodies may be palpated by pressing the index and middle fingers through an imaginary anterior surgical approach to the neck; that is, between the carotid sheath and sternocleidomastoid muscle laterally, and the trachea, esophagus, and thyroid gland medially. Patients with acute sprains exhibit tenderness over the longus colli muscles as well as posterior extensor neck muscle groups. The latter may be taut with muscle spasm secondary to injury.

An important specific compression test for suspected ruptured cervical disks is the Spurling test, which is performed by hyperextension, lateral rotation, and compression on the forehead with the hands. It produces a shocklike sensation of pares-

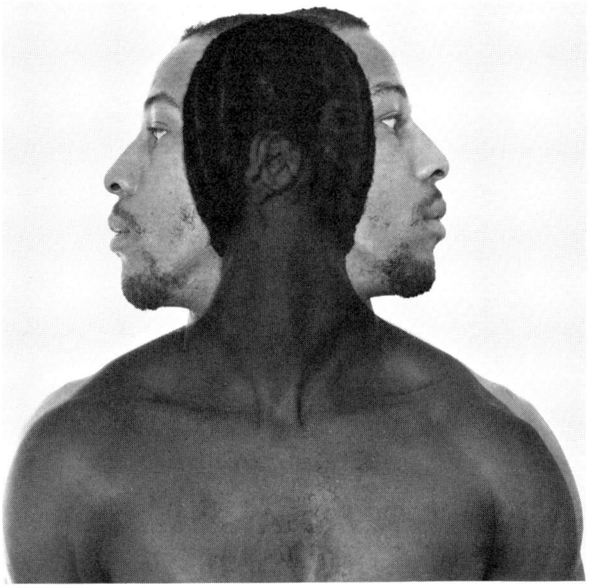

Fig. 6-18. Rotation is measured in degrees from the neutral position. (Courtesy of Robert D'Ambrosia.)

thesias in the nerve root distribution of the particular cervical root compressed. One may also reproduce pain and paresthesias by percussing directly over the lesion posteriorly with a rubber hammer.[5] Also, applying upward traction by grasping the chin and occiput may produce enough traction on the neck to relieve the pain of a ruptured disk.

Palpation of the specific anterior and posterior muscle groups must be carried out to determine the degree of muscle spasm present. At the same time, soft tissue masses should be noted (i.e., enlarged thyroid, lymph nodes, or a sternocleidomastoid mass in the infant with congenital torticollis).

A complete neurologic examination should then be performed. This must include gait patterns to rule out myelopathy associated with cervical spondylosis, acute central disk herniation, or dislocation of the atlas and axis in certain nontraumatic diseases. Complete muscle testing is performed for motor weakness with special reference to upper extremity nerve root distribution. Any atrophy or fasciculations are recorded as evidence of peripheral nerve disease or compression. Muscle weakness is graded and recorded for future comparison and reference. The sensory examination must include pinprick sensation and recording of various dermatome sensory loss. Position, vibratory, and touch sense in upper and lower limbs are tested for documentation of any posterior column impairment which may occur late in cervical spondylosis. Reflex examination is extremely important in regard to ruptured cervical disks as well as cervical spondylosis with spinal cord compression. In the former, the deep tendon reflexes are decreased or absent, and in the latter reflexes are exaggerated. Notation must be made of any pathologic reflexes, such as positive Hoffmann or Babinski reflexes and clonus.

Roentgenography

Proper radiologic studies must be ordered, including anteroposterior, lateral, oblique, and odontoid views. Special views may be requested depending on the explicit area of the cervical spine that is suspect. Often flexion-extension lateral views are helpful in differentiating certain diseases.

Table 6-2. Congenital Anomalies of Infancy

Basilar invagination or impression
Occipitalization of the atlas
Dysplasia of the odontoid process
Fusion of cervical vertebrae
Spinal dysraphism

DIFFERENTIAL DIAGNOSIS

CERVICAL DISORDERS PRESENTING IN INFANCY AND USUALLY PAINLESS

In contrast to cervical spine disorders in the adult, the infant presents with a deformity and rarely manifests pain as a presenting symptom.

Congenital Torticollis

Torticollis is a rotational deformity of the head and neck in which the sternocleidomastoid muscle is contracted or spastic; the head tilts toward the latter muscle, and the chin is rotated away to the opposite side. In the infant, there is usually a palpable fibrous tissue mass in the midportion of the affected muscle. As the affected, untreated infant grows older, there may be gross asymmetry of the external facial features. Radiologic examination should be performed to rule out congenital bony abnormalities of the cervical spine.

Congenital Anomalies of the Cervical Spine

Congenital bony anomalies of the cervical spine in the infant are believed to originate during the six and seventh weeks of embryonic life. The adage that congenital anomalies of one organ system are often associated with anomalies of other systems is quite true in the cervical region. For instance, intramedullary cavitation (syringomyelia) is often associated with anomalies of the craniovertebral junction. One-third of the patients with Klippel-Feil syndrome (fusion of cervical vertebrae) have genitourinary tract anomalies.

Usually these malformations remain asymptomatic until adolescence or adulthood when neurologic signs develop. The various congenital anomalies of infancy are listed in Table 6-2.

Basilar Invagination (Impression). Basilar invagination occurs when the margins of the foramen magnum are turned upward. This is frequently associated with anomalies of the atlas and axis. Signs of syringomyelia are often associated with sensory loss to pain and temperatures over the neck, shoulders, and upper extremities. There may also be weakness and atrophy of the arms and hands. Roentgenologic signs of basilar invagination are displacement of the rim of the foramen magnum above McGregor's line (drawn from hard palate to external squamous occipital cortex). Chamberlain's line is drawn from the hard palate to the internal squamous occipital cortex. McRae's line lies along the plane of the clivus. When McGregor's line subtends an angle with McRae's line of more than 145 degrees, there is platybasia or flattening of the base of the skull which is often associated with basilar impression.

Symptoms occur later in life if the odontoid process protrudes into the foramen magnum, compressing the medulla oblongata.

Occipitalization of the Atlas (Atlanto-occipital Fusion). Occipitalization of the atlas implies fusion of all or portions of the atlas to the base of the skull. This entity may be associated with basilar impression or dysplasia of the odontoid process. The diagnosis of this entity cannot be made clinically but must be elucidated radiologically with laminagrams and flexion-extension lateral roentgenograms demonstrating no motion between the atlanto-occipital joint. Symptoms are neurologic in origin and usually do not affect the infant but become manifest later in adolescence or adult life. In about one-half of the cases of occipitalization of the atlas there is fusion of C2 and C3.

Dysplasia of the Odontoid Process and Atlantoaxial Instability. Dysplasia or malformation of the odontoid process may be congenital or associated with various forms of dwarfism and Down's syndrome. The odontoid process may be completely absent or aplastic; it may be partially formed or dysplastic. Dislocation of the atlas on the axis anteriorly is frequently associated. The infant may have a torticollis, but symptoms or signs usually occur later in childhood. Chronic dislocation of the atlas on the axis may produce spinal cord compression with neurologic symptoms. Diagnosis can only be made by lateral flexion-extension roentgenograms and laminagrams.

Fusion of Cervical Vertebrae. The Klippel-Feil syndrome consists of three signs: short neck, low hairline, and restricted neck movement with unusual posture of the head. This syndrome consists of fusion of two or more cervical vertebrae because of failure in segmentation between the vertebrae. The diagnosis may seem obvious from the clinical appearance of the infant, but roentgenograms must be taken. Disk spaces are small or nonexistent in the fused segments. Anomalies of the central nervous system are often associated (i.e., cervical meningocele or Arnold-Chiari malformation). Hypermobility in the unfused segments may predispose to disk degeneration later in life.

Spinal dysraphism is a condition related to failure of formation of the dorsal elements during embryonic development. It includes spina bifida, meningomyelocele, diastematomyelia, and dermal cysts. In the cervical region, the more severe anomalies are fatal whereas the lesser ones produce only a hairy nevus or radiologic bony anomalies.

Birth Injuries

Injuries to the cervical spine at birth or during infancy are rare but still occur. The infant spine is hypermobile, and the spinal cord at birth has immature myelin development in the white matter for protection against shear or stretching forces. The breech or difficult delivery can require manipulation of the baby's head and neck to a degree which produces damage to the spinal cord without dislocating the cervical spine itself. Complete transection of the spinal cord can occur during a breech delivery, with a resultant quadriplegic (Fig. 6-19).

Massive epidural hemorrhages have been seen in infants sustaining birth trauma.

The neurologic examination revealing partial or complete quadriplegia should alert the physician to the possibility of cervical trauma.

Infants who have been dropped or injured in auto accidents can sustain cervical spine injuries as well, usually associated with cerebral trauma.

An increasingly common incidence of cervical trauma is the battered child. The infant who holds his neck rigidly should alert the physician with a high level of suspicion. Appropriate radiologic studies may reveal a fracture, dislocation, or callus formation with partial healing.

CERVICAL DISORDERS PRESENTING IN CHILDHOOD OR ADOLESCENCE

Acquired Torticollis

Although congenital torticollis can be progressive (and manifest in later life), usually the torticollis seen in childhood and adolescence is acquired. This

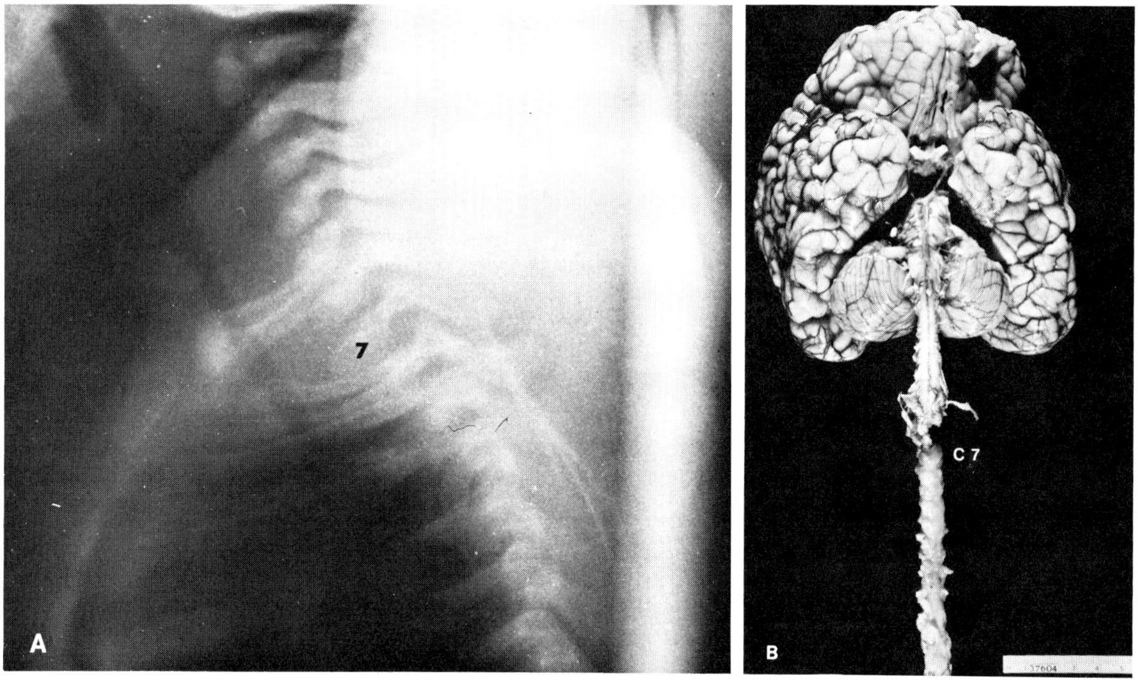

Fig. 6-19. (*A*) Normal cervical spine of quadriplegic birth injury secondary to breech delivery. (*B*) Transected spinal cord C7 level.

torticollis produces the same deformities as seen in infancy, with the head tilted to the side of the taut sternocleidomastoid muscle and the chin turned in the opposite direction. Frequently this condition follows an acute upper respiratory infection in the child presenting with a wry neck and acute cervical pain (Fig. 6-20A). Mild trauma may play a role also, with the child experiencing a "snap" when turning the neck. Roentgenograms usually reveal unilateral atlantoaxial rotatory subluxation with asymmetry of the lateral joints between the axis and atlas, secondary to the rotational deformity (Fig. 6-20B). The anteroposterior roentgenogram also shows tilting of the base of the skull in relation to the vertical axis of the cervical spine. Lateral view gives the appearance of atlantoaxial dislocation (Fig. 6-20C). Congenital anomalies of the upper cervical spine should be ruled out by roentgenograms. Occasionally a patient with a tumor of the upper part of the cervical cord or posterior fossa will present with acquired torticollis

Tumors of the Cervical Spine

Primary osseous tumors of the cervical spine are uncommon but do occur during childhood and adolescence. Metastatic tumors are extremely rare in this age group but are more common in adulthood. Primary tumors ordinarily present with neck pain and may be either benign or malignant. The most common benign tumors in this age group are aneurysmal bone cysts (Fig. 6-21), osteoblastoma, eosinophilic granuloma (Fig. 6-22), osteochondroma (Fig. 6-23), hemangioma, or histiocytosis (Fig. 6-24). Usually laboratory data are normal, and the diagnosis is made by roentgenographic studies. Laminagrams are helpful in determining the extent of tumor invasion in the anterior or posterior elements of the vertebra and the character of the tumorous bone (i.e., osteoblastic or osteolytic). The ultimate specific diagnosis must be made by open biopsy and pathologic study. Rarely primary tumors of the cervical cord present with neck pain, with or without paralysis. These tumors may be extramedullary or intramedullary in origin. Slow, insidious onset of pain without fever, abnormal gait, or arm pain may be clues to the lesion. Careful neurologic examination is critical. Cervical myelography is necessary to define the lesion.

Congenital Deformities

Various forms of Klippel-Feil deformity may present with neck pain during childhood or adolescence.

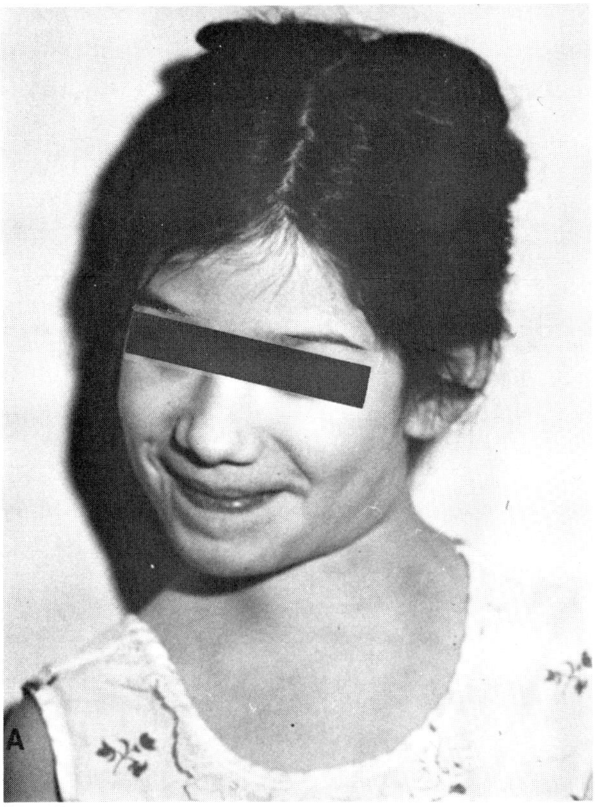

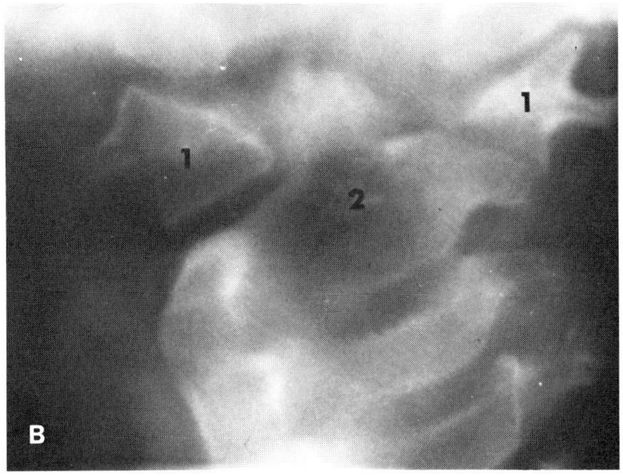

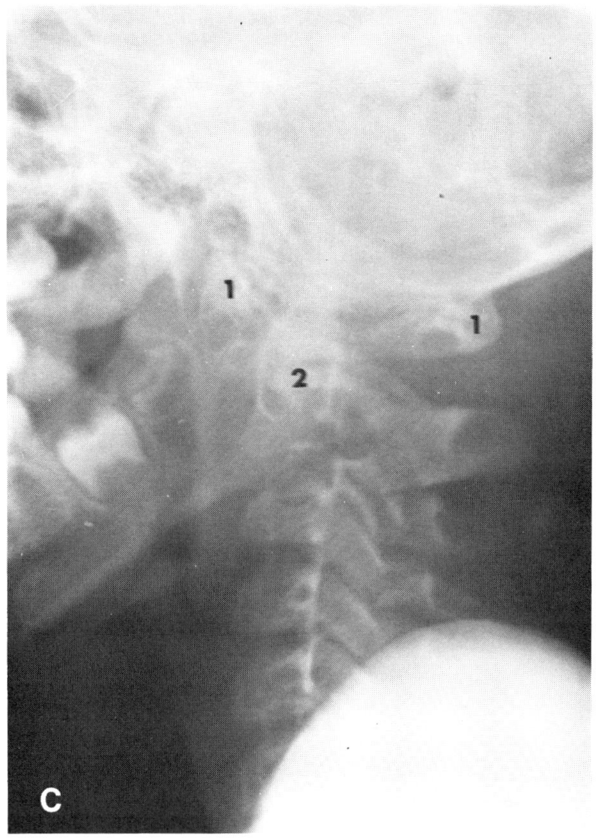

Fig. 6-20. Seven-year-old child with torticollis for four months following a febrile illness of chicken pox. (*A*) The head is tilted to the left and the chin rotated to the right. (*B*) Child with unilateral rotatory subluxation of C1-2. Note asymmetry of atlantoaxial joint spaces. (*C*) The atlas appears to be dislocated on the axis with a wide atlantodental interval.

As previously stated, degenerative disk disease and abnormal subluxations may occur in relation to the fused vertebrae. Diagnosis is initiated by the general appearance of the patient with a short neck, low hair line, and loss of motion when the bony deformities are extensive. When only two or three vertebrae are affected, diagnosis can only be made by appropriate radiologic examination. This should include flexion extension views to define abnormal motion segments (Fig. 6-25).

The dysplastic or malformed odontoid process at this age may present with neck pain or evidence of spinal cord compression (i.e., leg weakness at the end of the day, spasticity of the extremities, or fainting

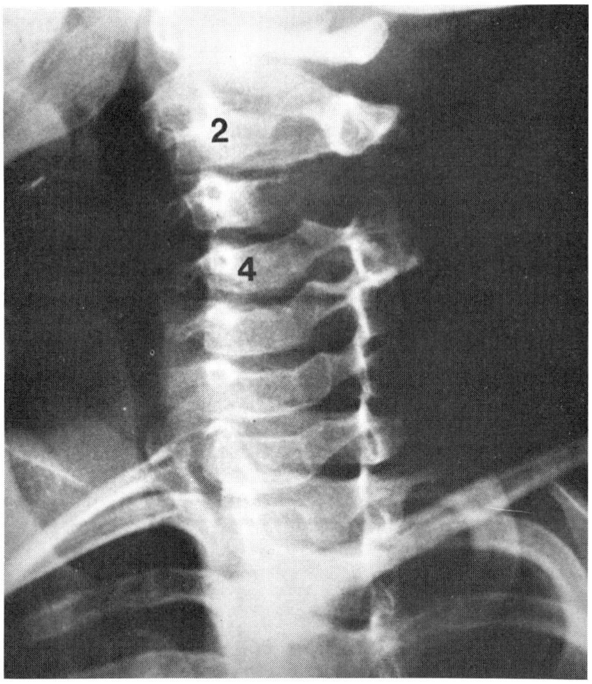

Fig. 6-21. Two-year-old child with purely lytic lesion of C3. The entire pedicle and posterior elements are destroyed. Excisional biopsy revealed aneurysmal bone cyst.

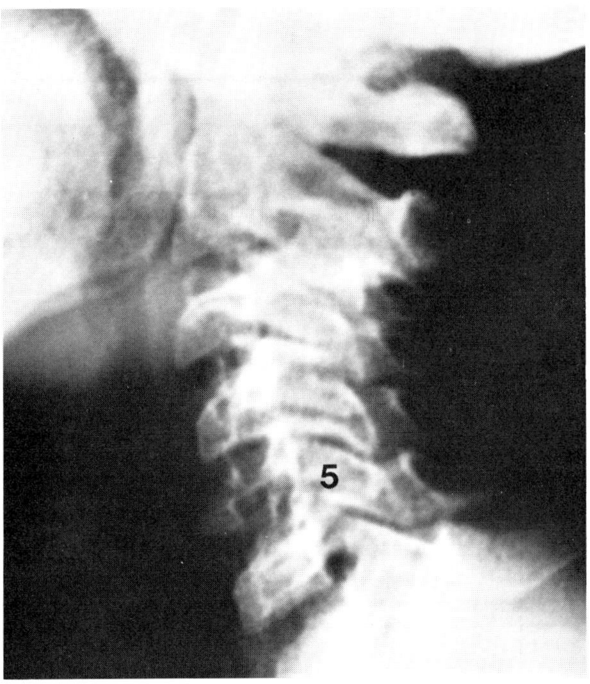

Fig. 6-22. Eosinophilic granuloma of the C5 vertebral body. Note lytic lesion.

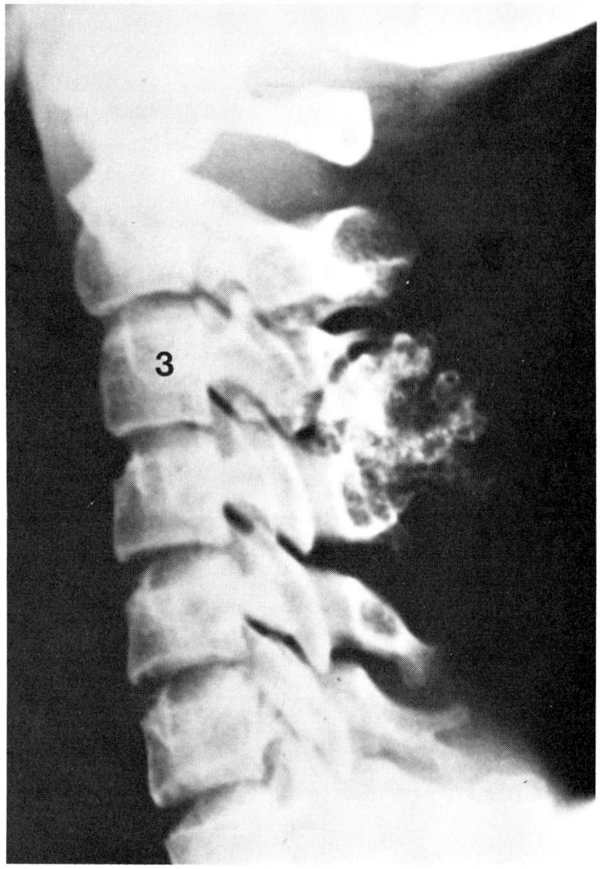

Fig. 6-23. Young child with osteochondroma of the posterior elements of C3. The lesion is osteoblastic.

episodes). Traumatic episodes may also aggravate this pre-existing condition. Radiologic examination may reveal entire absence of the odontoid process (aplasia), partial absence (dysplasia), or an extra ossicle at the apex of the process (os odontoideum).

Roentgenograms of the cervical spine must be obtained with flexion-extension laterals to determine the degree of instability. At this point, measurements are made of the distance between the anterior arch of the atlas and odontoid process. If this distance exceeds 4 mm. in childhood or 3 mm. in adults, it is considered abnormal. One must not be led into the trap of assuming excess motion in the second and third cervical segments or lower cervical spine is abnormal in the child. Catell and Filtzer have written about radiologic variations in the child's cervical spine.

Congenital anomalies of the vertebrae with kyphoscoliosis or curvature at the cervicothoracic junction may produce marked, progressive deformity in the child. Kyphosis refers to curvature in the anteroposterior direction, and scoliosis refers to curvature in the lateral direction. If a ventral segment of vertebra is congenitally fused, there may be overgrowth of a corresponding dorsal segment with resultant progressive kyphosis. Several anteroposterior and lateral roentgenograms are necessary over a long period of time to determine if there is progression of the deformity as the child is growing.

Arnold-Chiari malformation is a caudal elongation of the cerebellum and brainstem through the foramen magnum. The longitudinal growth of the spine does not keep up with that of the spinal cord. As a result, the cervical nerve roots may take an angular course cephalad then caudad after exiting from their foramina. Therefore, angulation of the nerve roots in this entity can produce symptoms similar to a herniated disk. Spinal cord as well as cerebellar compression may also occur. The entire clinical picture is characterized by headache, pain in the arms, paresthesias in a particular root distribution, difficult urination, and gait problems with weak legs and hyperreflexia. Following neurologic examination, appropriate roentgenograms must be taken and cervical myelography with contrast media performed.

Cervical ribs may be present in childhood but are usually asymptomatic.

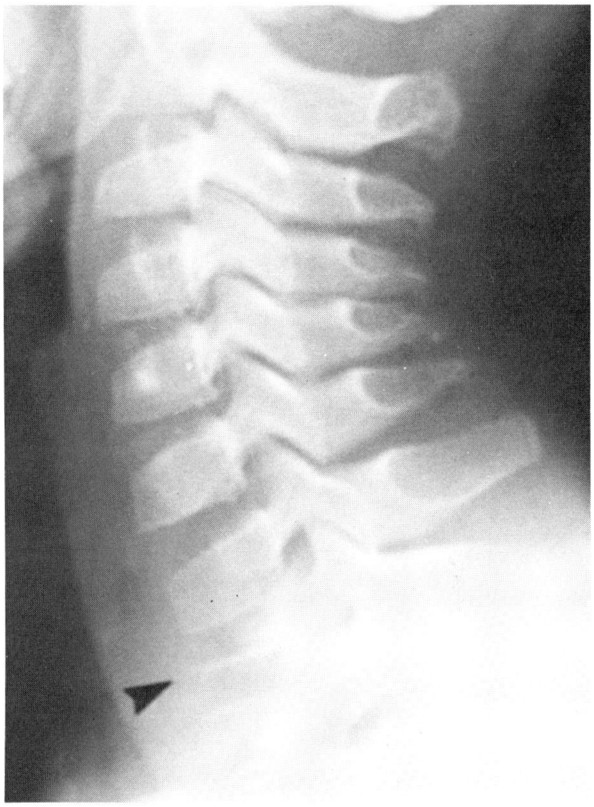

Fig. 6-24. Child with "vertebra plana" or flattening of vertebral body secondary to histiocytosis.

Metabolic Disease and Bone Dysplasias

Certain forms of dwarfism, such as Morquio's disease, spondyloepiphyseal dysplasia, or diastrophic dwarfism, may be associated with dysplasia of the odontoid process and atlantoaxial dislocation (Fig. 6-26). Subluxation of lower vertebrae may also occur. The signs and symptoms are similar to those previously mentioned, with congenital aplasia of the odontoid process. Morquio's disease is transmitted as an autosomal recessive trait, characterized by excessive urinary excretion of keratosulfate. There may be corneal opacities and dental abnormalities. The vertebrae are flattened on lateral roentgenograms, and there is a short neck with "chin on chest" deformity. Also, a thoracolumbar kyphosis occurs because of an upper lumbar wedge-shaped vertebra.

In spondyloepiphyseal dysplasia there is no abnormality of keratosulfate excretion and no corneal opacity. These patients also manifest flattened vertebrae, or platyspondylisis.

Neurologically, the patients are usually normal but may, on close questioning, be experiencing leg weakness and fatigue at the end of the day, with early spinal cord compression. Radiologically, there may be a separate or dysplastic odontoid process, with dislocation of the atlas on the axis in flexion-extension views. Air myelography may be the only method of demonstrating spinal cord compression in the upper cervical spine. Laminagrams are necessary to do this study, with the child sedated (Fig. 6-27).

Achondroplasia is a short-limbed dwarfism in which the signs are present at birth. It is transmitted as an autosomal dominant characteristic. There is prominence of the forehead and small face with flattening of the nose bridge. In these patients there is a decrease in the anteroposterior diameter of the spinal canal, leaving very little room for the spinal

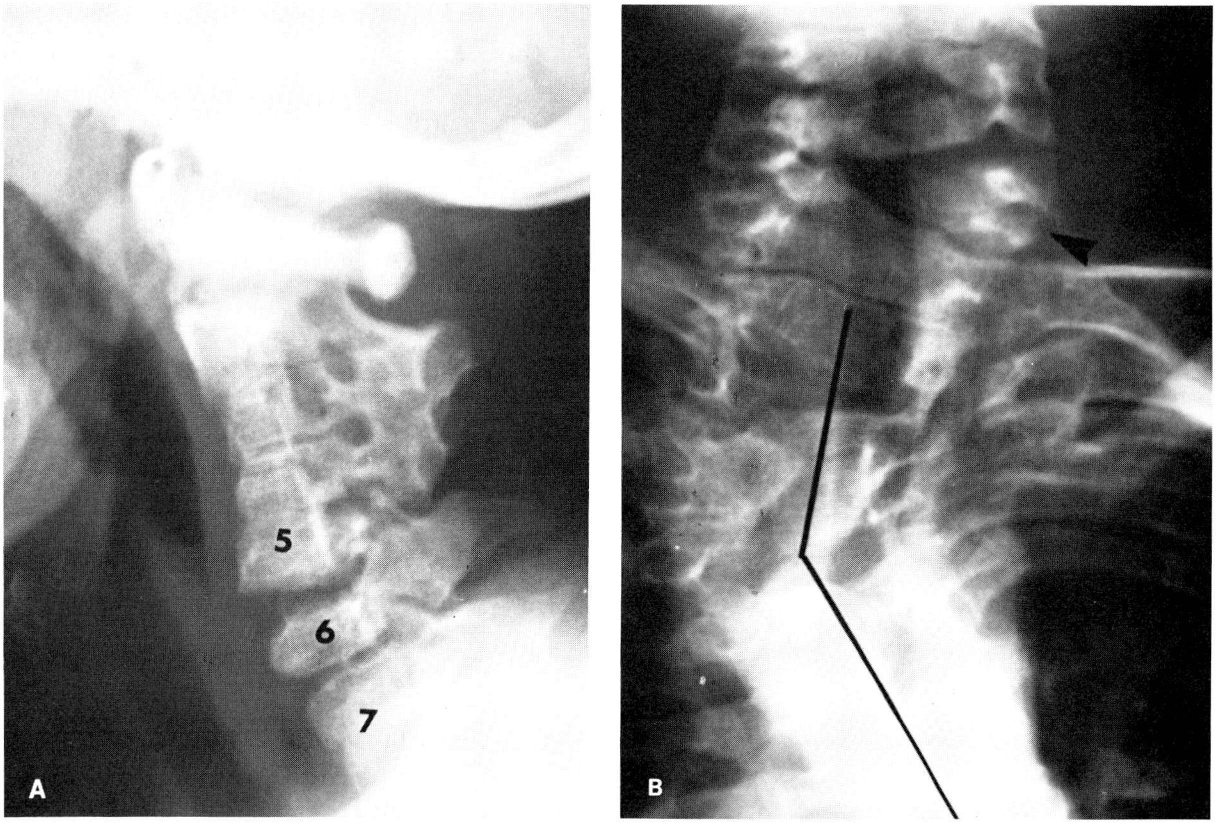

Fig. 6-25. (*A*) Lateral roentgenogram of four-year-old child with Klippel-Feil deformities. Note fusion of C2-3-4-5 vertebrae. (*B*) Anteroposterior roentgenogram of Klippel-Feil deformities. Note C6 hemivertebra and thoracic scoliosis.

cord. Small disk herniation can produce spinal cord compression.

All of the above patients are of normal intelligence. There are no abnormal routine laboratory findings in spondyloepiphyseal dysplasia or achondroplasia.

It should be mentioned that on rare occasions a metabolic change occurs in the child's cervical disk with calcification, which may present as neck pain. The etiology is unknown, and the process is manifest by central opacification of the disk on roentgenogram (Fig. 6-28).

Inflammatory Disease

Juvenile Rheumatoid Arthritis. In the childhood and adolescent age groups, certain inflammatory diseases of unknown cause may affect the cervical spine. Juvenile rheumatoid arthritis may begin as early as one year of age, and it manifests as monoarticular arthritis or polyarthritis and occasionally neck pain. Laboratory findings are similar to those of adults with an elevated sedimentation rate, except the rheumatoid factor is rarely positive, and the leukocyte count may be very high. As the disease progresses, the cervical spine may be affected by bony ankylosis of the apophyseal joints, especially in the upper cervical spine (Fig. 6-29). Loss of neck motion occurs and is permanent. Spontaneous fusion begins posteriorly and over the years becomes anterior as well in many cases. Radiologic examination as well as physical demonstration of decreased motion of the cervical spine is necessary for diagnosis of fusion. The posterior facet joints will be ossified as well as the interspinous ligaments between the spinous processes.

Ankylosing spondylitis is an arthritis of adolescence with progressive inflammatory disease of the spine and large joints producing ankylosis and deformity. The etiology of the disease is unknown; it occurs predominantly in males. Early in the disease there is spinal pain, muscle spasm, and loss of chest expansion. The vertebral segments become rigid and eventually ankylosed with ossification of the longitudinal ligaments and para-articular structures. The erythrocyte sedimentation rate is usually elevated throughout the course of the active disease. Usually symptoms begin in the lower lumbar and sacroiliac region, but the cervical spine may be affected with pain. Occasionally there may be ligament laxity above a rigid segment, and atlantoaxial dislocation occurs.

Radiologic studies of the cervical spine demonstrate progressive loss of motion between vertebrae with ossification of the ligaments and disk spaces. As opposed to degenerative disk disease, the disk spaces are not narrowed. Congenital fusion of the vertebrae can be differentiated by the narrowing of the vertebral bodies in the anteroposterior diameter on lateral roentgenogram as well as the little or no disk formation between affected vertebrae.

Infectious diseases of the cervical spine or disk spaces are unusual in childhood and adolescence but do occur. Etiologically, they may be divided into pyogenic and tuberculous infections. The route of introduction is usually hematogenous but may be postsurgical, by contiguous infection, or from diagnostic procedures. Acute osteomyelitis is usually blood-borne and originates at distal sites. Urinary tract, dermatologic, and pulmonary infections may create the bacteria carried via the blood stream to the highly vascular vertebrae. The most common organisms of pyogenic osteomyelitis are *Staphylococcus aureus,* streptococcus, klebsiella, or pseudomonas. Tuberculous osteomyelitis of the spine usually originates from active pulmonary disease. The earliest clinical symptoms are pain and rigidity of the neck. These precede the roentgenographic findings. The patient is very protective of any neck motion and may hold the neck in a torticollis position. There is tenderness to percussion posteriorly as well as to palpation anteriorly, where an abscess may be felt.

Neck pain is constant, both night and day, but may be somewhat relieved by recumbancy. The pain may radiate to the occiput or shoulders. If the abscess is quite painful, the child will support the head in his hands. The patient can develop quadriplegia or arm paralysis if the abscess expands into the spinal canal, causing extrinsic pressure on the anterior spinal cord. The paralysis is usually spastic with hyperactive reflexes, positive Babinski sign, sustained clonus, and inability to void. Pathologically, the tuberculous infection involves the vertebral body, where it may be central, anterior, or epiphyseal in location (Fig. 6-30). Osteoporosis occurs following exudative inflammation with hyperemia. As the infection advances, it involves the end plate of the bone and eventually breaks into the disk space. The vertebra may collapse secondary to bone destruction and form a wedge shape with increased density compared to decreased density in other areas of destruction by roentgenography. The abscess may progress to lie anterior to the posterior longitudinal ligament and protrude into the spinal canal. By the same process the abscess may lie under the anterior longitudinal ligament or break out into the retroesophageal space. A paravertebral abscess may also

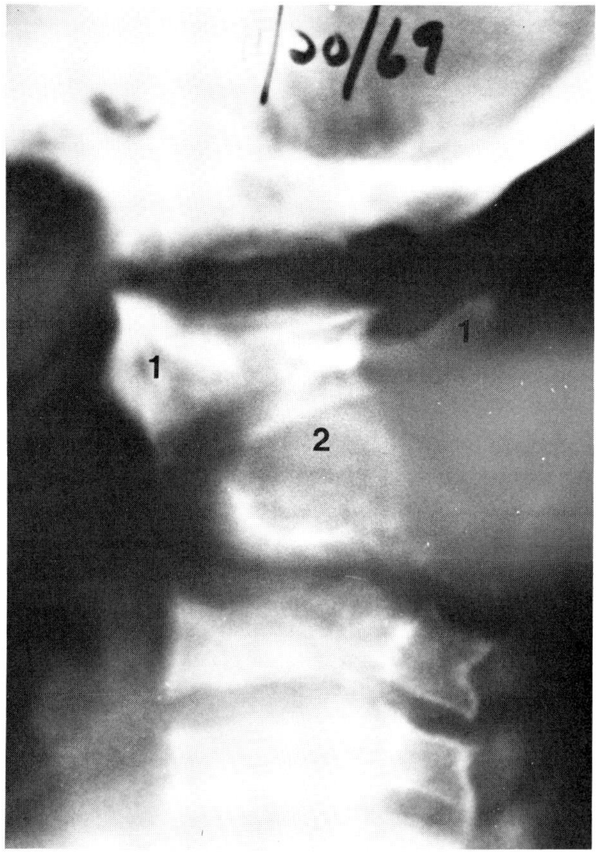

Fig. 6-26. Achondroplastic dwarf with dysplasia of the odontoid and atlantoaxial dislocation. Lateral tomogram.

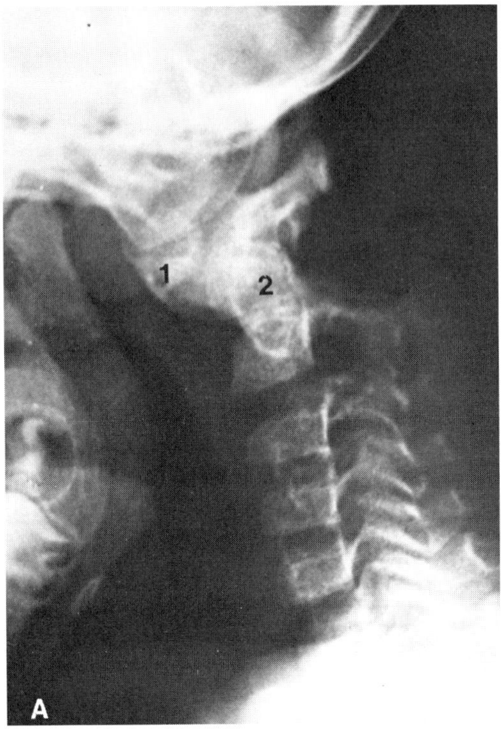

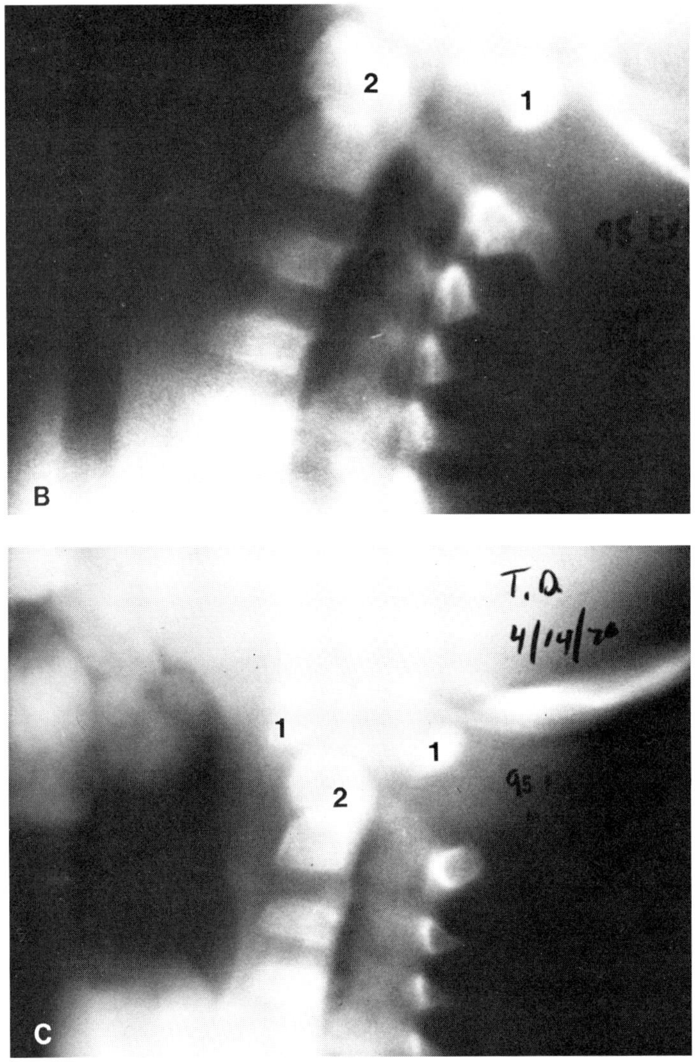

Fig. 6-27. Dwarfed child with Scott's syndrome. (*A*) Dysplastic odontoid and atlantoaxial dislocation. Air myelogram in extension. (*B*) Lateral tomography used to define details of air column within canal. (*C*) Flexion during air myelography. Note pinch-off of air column at C2.

extend into the thorax or vice versa. Pyogenic osteomyelitis may involve the disk space earlier, and there may be sclerosis or increased density of the vertebra with reactive bone formation. Consequently a radiologic picture of osteomyelitis demonstrates an enlarged retroesophageal space on the lateral view greater than 3 to 4 mm. anterior to the 3rd cervical vertebra, destruction or lysis of the vertebral body, or generalized osteoporosis. The vertebral body often collapses into a wedge-shaped mass. In pyogenic osteomyelitis there is usually greater disk space destruction with more reactive bone formation and sclerosis. Laminography helps to delineate bone detail to differentiate the lesion from tumor. Cervical myelogram may be necessary in patients with paralysis to determine the exact level of the spinal abscess. Less severe infections occur with pyogenic organisms and may only involve the disk space and adjacent bony end plates. In children, primary retroesophageal abscesses can occur in association with such regional infections as lymphadenitis, tonsillitis, and oral abscesses. In these cases there may be large increases in the retroesophageal space on lateral roentgenogram and they may be unrelated to the vertebrae. Normally, inspiration increases the space if the child is crying.

Laboratory data indicates acute infection when the patient is clinically ill. That is to say, the white blood count is quite high, with increased mononuclear cells in tuberculosis and polymorpholeukocytes in pyogenic infection. The erythrocyte sedimentation rate is elevated as well as the temperature. Blood cultures should be performed, and eventually surgical drainage usually confirms the diagnosis with appropriate cultures and sensitivities. Skin tests may be necessary to rule out tuberculosis or fungal infections. It can be difficult to differentiate osteomyelitis from tumors of the cervical spine because active destruction of bone is present in both diseases.

Trauma

During childhood and adolescence, trauma to the cervical spine is usually related to sporting injuries or vehicular accidents by the very nature of the child's activities. In early childhood, the cervical spine growth is incomplete, and the epiphyseal or apophyseal centers may be immature. Cartilage end plates are thick between the disk and vertebral bodies, and the mobility of the spine is great.

Cervical spine injuries may only involve the soft tissues (i.e., the ligaments and disks), or bony fracture and dislocation may occur. With either of the above there may be an associated neurologic injury.

Acquired torticollis may occur in children as a result of mild trauma. The etiology is rotatory subluxation of the atlas on the axis, probably secondary to laxity of the capsular ligaments of those joints. The position of the head and neck is with the head tilted to the side of subluxation with the chin rotated in the opposite directon. The characteristic wry neck is easily recognized clinically and the patient presents with upper cervical pain. Lateral and open-mouth odontoid views must be taken to demonstrate asymmetry of the atlantoaxial joints. It is important

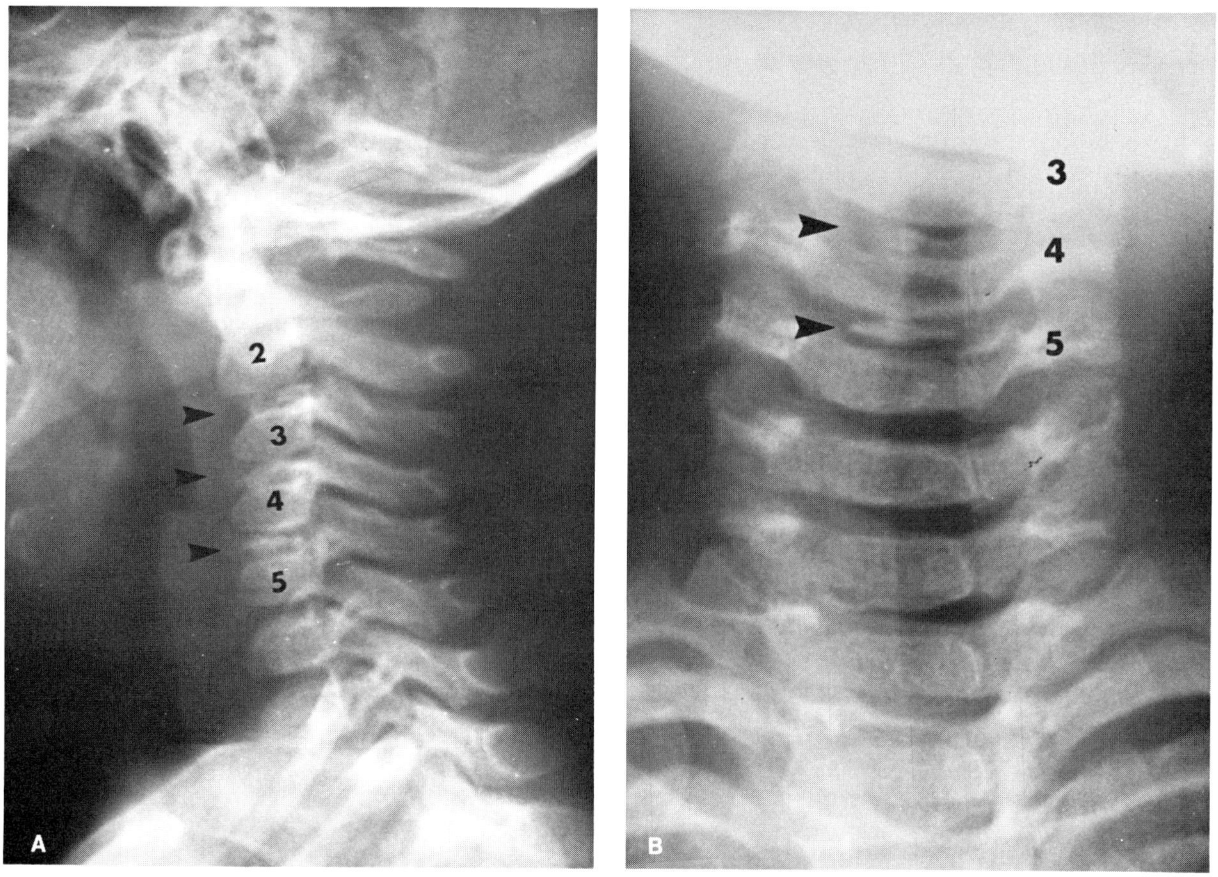

Fig. 6-28. (*A*) Lateral roentgenogram of child two years of age with neck pain and calcification of three cervical disks. (*B*) Anteroposterior roentgenogram of calcified disk nuclei.

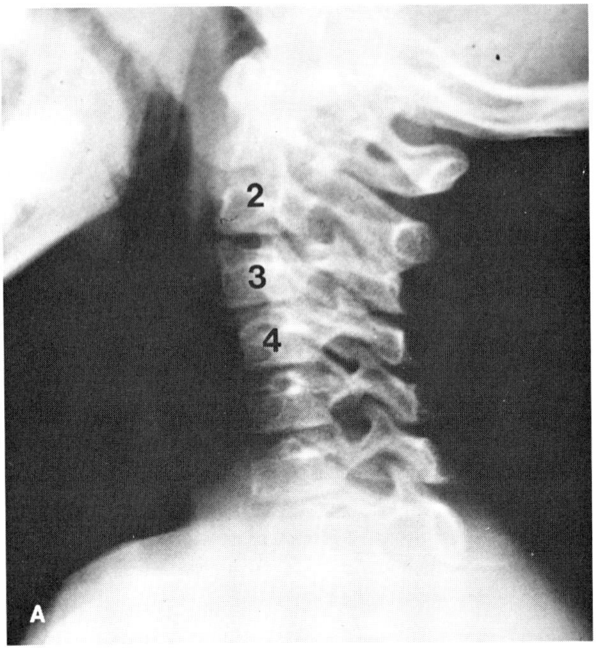

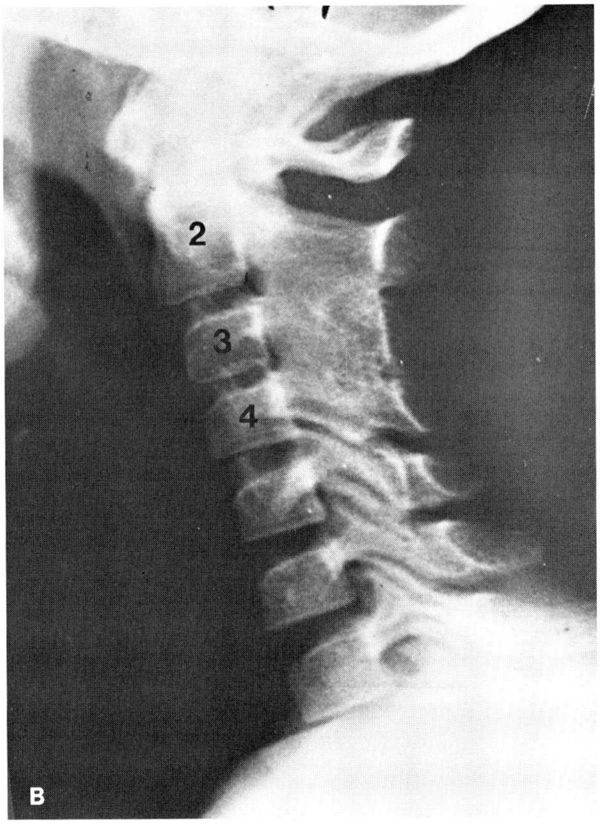

Fig. 6-29. (*A*) Juvenile rheumatoid arthritic child with normal appearing cervical vertebrae in 1966. (*B*) Spontaneous posterior element fusion of C2-3-4 has occurred over a 4-year period.

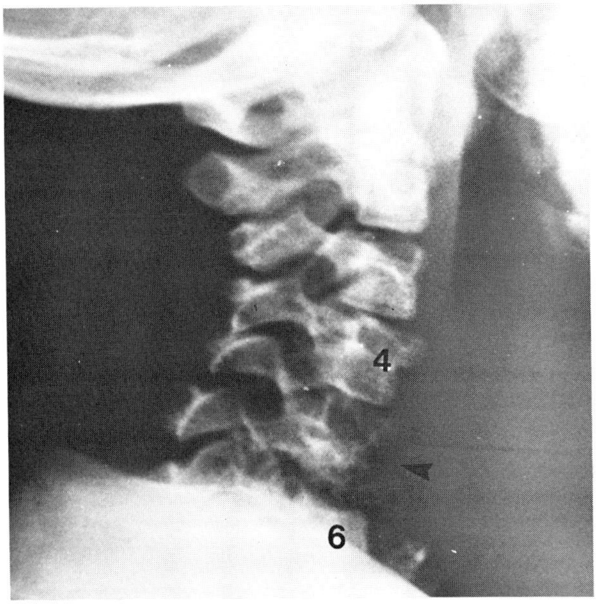

Fig. 6-30. Two-year-old child with destructive tuberculous lesion of C5 vertebral body.

to note that the lateral bodies of the atlas and axis remain parallel, and only the horizontal atlantoaxial joint spaces are asymmetric. In a Jefferson or "blow-out" fracture of the atlas, the lateral masses of the atlas are both displaced beyond the lateral borders of the axis. Mere rotation or tilting of the head on the neck can produce differences in the distance between the odontoid process and medial borders of the lateral masses. The latter is a normal variation.

Cervical sprain in a child is not as common as in the adult whose tissues are more inelastic. The term *sprain* implies microscopic tearing of tissues which have been stretched beyond their elastic limit. When a ligament or muscle is grossly torn, it is termed a *rupture*. Etiologically, soft tissue injuries of the cervical region occur by flexion, extension, and/or rotation forces. More severe injuries tear the deep structures, such as facet joint capsules or longitudinal ligaments, and disrupt the disks. Physical examination of the child with an acute neck sprain reveals that the head is held rigidly in one position and there is considerable muscle spasm, which can be palpated as hardened contractions of the posterior erector spinae groups. The patient guards against any attempt at moving the neck in flexion or extension. Pain is generalized and not usually referred beyond the shoulder or scapular levels. Only if the brachial plexus is stretched will there be subjective paresthesias of the arms or hands. There may be an occipital headache. Neurologically the child should be normal. Neck discomfort may last for days or weeks but usually subsides with rest and immobilization in a collar.

Epiphyseal injuries of the axis can occur in the young child before fusion through the epiphyseal plate has occurred. This injury may be associated with significant cranial trauma (Fig. 6-31).

On rare occasions, avulsion of the anterior apophyses of the vertebrae occurs in children with hyperextension injuries. Appropriate anteroposterior as well as lateral roentgenograms are required to outline the specific injury.

In young children with severe trauma to the cervical spine, the cartilage end plates of the vertebral body break away from the bony end plates. This lesion can only be demonstrated at autopsy.

Dysplasia or aplasia of the odontoid process may predispose a child to atlantoaxial dislocation in association with a traumatic episode, such as an auto accident or football injury.

One must be very cautious in the emergency room situation that the child with a head injury and decreased level of consciousness has had a cervical spine roentgenogram to rule out fracture or dislocation.

The more common osseous and neurologic patterns of cervical fracture-dislocations will be discussed in the section on adult trauma.

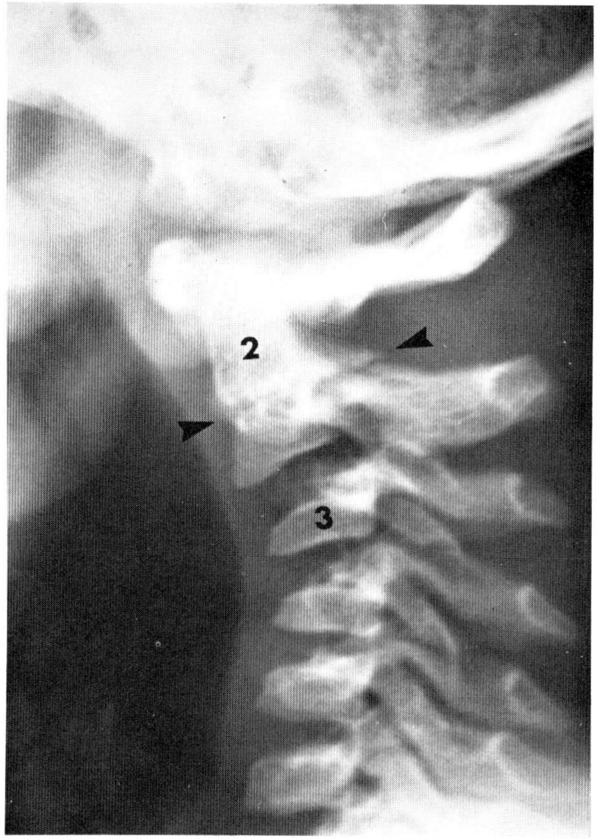

Fig. 6-31. Four-year-old child with fracture through the epiphyseal plate of the axis, extending through the pedicles of C2.

CERVICAL DISORDERS PRESENTING IN ADULTHOOD AND USUALLY PAINFUL

Congenital Anomalies

The basic forms of congenital anomalies have already been described, so only the adult clinical manifestations and differential diagnosis will be stressed here. One should be aware of the predisposition to problems in adult life that congenital anomalies pose.

Anomalies of the craniovertebral area include the previously mentioned basilar invagination, occipitalization of the atlas to the occiput, and Arnold-Chiari malformation anomalies of the atlantoaxial vertebrae, with or without dislocations. There is a high association of vascular as well as neurologic anomalies with the osseous abnormalities. There may be aplasia of one vertebral artery, producing cerebral ischemia or associated central nervous system anomalies.

Frequently, congenital cervical anomalies are not diagnosed until adulthood, when, after trauma, the patient is symptomatic and roentgenograms are taken (Fig. 6-32).

McRae and DeBanos described in detail the symptoms of congenital anomalies of the cervico-occipital

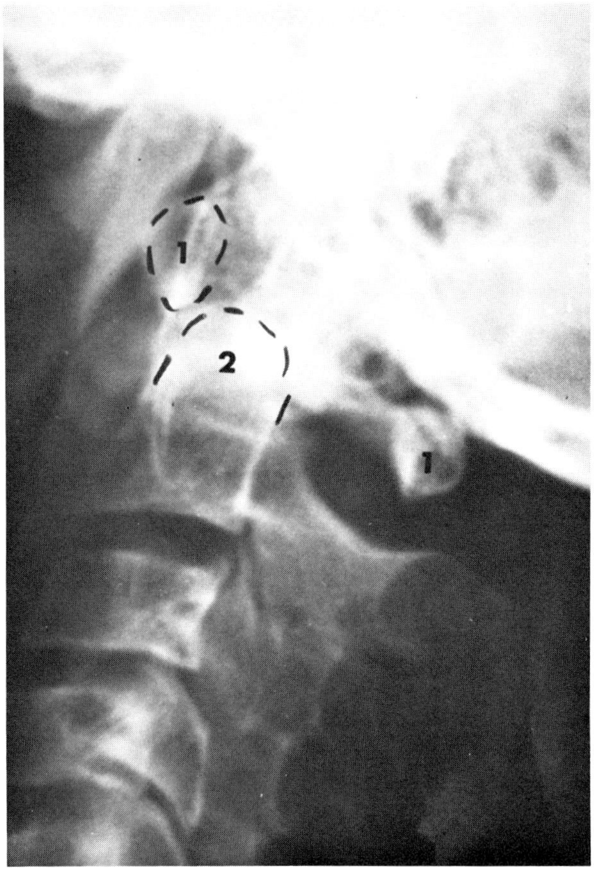

Fig. 6-32. Hypoplastic odontoid process in adult, recognized by roentgenogram after traumatic episode.

junction. These include cervical-occipital pain and headaches, weakness and paresthesias of the upper extremities, as well as weakness and ataxia of the lower extremities. Long tract signs may occur in the arms as well as legs. Mild trauma may aggravate the symptoms.

Results of examination of the patient with cervical spine anomalies may be completely normal or there may be limited neck motion, with or without neurologic signs of the spinal cord compression or vertebral artery compression. Chronic atlantoaxial dislocation may produce syncopal episodes in flexion; pain, especially occipital; limited neck motion with guarding; and evidence of spinal cord compression. Early neurologic signs may be quite subtle, and only manifest by fatigability of the legs, difficulty with balance on ambulation, or occasionally a shocklike sensation down the torso and legs on hyperflexion of the neck. Careful neurological examination is important.

Diagnosis of the particular anomaly may require dynamic lateral flexion-extension roentgenograms of the cervical spine, laminagrams, both air and contrast myelography, as well as arteriography to rule out associated vascular anomalies.

Congenital stenosis or narrowing of the cervical spinal canal is extremely important to recognize because it predisposes the patient to spinal cord injury during sporting activities and other trauma (Fig. 6-33). The cervical spinal cord becomes endangered later in life also with progressively severe cervical spondylosis and disk protrusions which further compromise the spinal canal. A congenitally narrow spi-

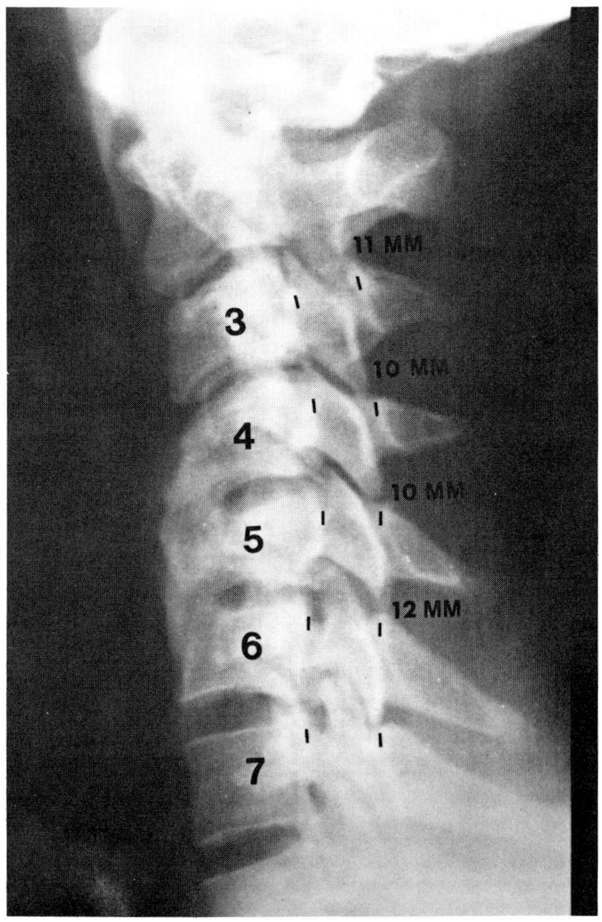

Fig. 6-33. A trampoline injury resulted in a compression fracture of C5 and anterior cervical fusion C4-C6 and quadriplegia. Note congenitally narrow spinal canal which predisposes to severe spinal cord injury.

nal canal complicated by progressive cervical degenerative disk disease, when producing early spinal cord compression, is manifested by ataxia, spasticity, or weakness of the extremities. Following trauma the patient may note subjective weakness of the legs or paresthesias with some difficulty in gait. Neck pain may be present and the patient may state "my legs just don't feel right." This is a manifestation of spinal cord concussion, and no positive neurologic signs may be present unless the injury is more severe.

At the upper cervical level, the anteroposterior diameter of C1 between the odontoid process and inner arch of the atlas must be less than 18 mm. before neurologic signs appear. Hinck et al. have written monographs on the normal and abnormal sagittal diameter of the cervical spinal canal in adults and children. Payne and Spillane were first to recognize that development of spinal cord myelopathy was related to the initial size of the spinal canal. It is, therefore, important in the patient having gait difficulties, with or without neck pain, to focus on the cervical spine. Appropriate lateral roentgenograms must be taken at the standard 6-foot distance as well as other routine views. Physical examination of the cervical spine in older patients only reveals decreased motion, particularly in extension. Neurologic examination of the patient with a narrow spinal canal and cord compression usually reveals hyperactive reflexes, pathologic reflexes, and difficulty with their gait to the point of being unable to walk without aid. There may be no gross weakness or sensory loss. The anteroposterior diameter is measured from the posterior aspect of the vertebra to the corresponding inner cortex of the lamina. In adults, less than 13 to 15 mm. between C4 and C7 is an ominous sign and warns one of the possibility of spinal cord compromise by trauma or spondylosis.

Klippel-Feil syndrome with multiple fusions may not be symptomatic until adulthood. Over many years, the normal disks are stressed by the fused segments. A person with congenital fusion of C3-4 and C4-5, for instance, may develop a degenerative disk with protrusion at C5-6. This may result in rather severe neck pain. Severe problems only occur when all vertebrae are fused except one at the midcervical level (Fig. 6-34). These patients are more apt to develop disk degeneration, protrusion, and neurologic deficit. Physical findings are those of decreased neck motion and pain on extremes of motion or on palpation of the spinous processes where there is a mobile segment.

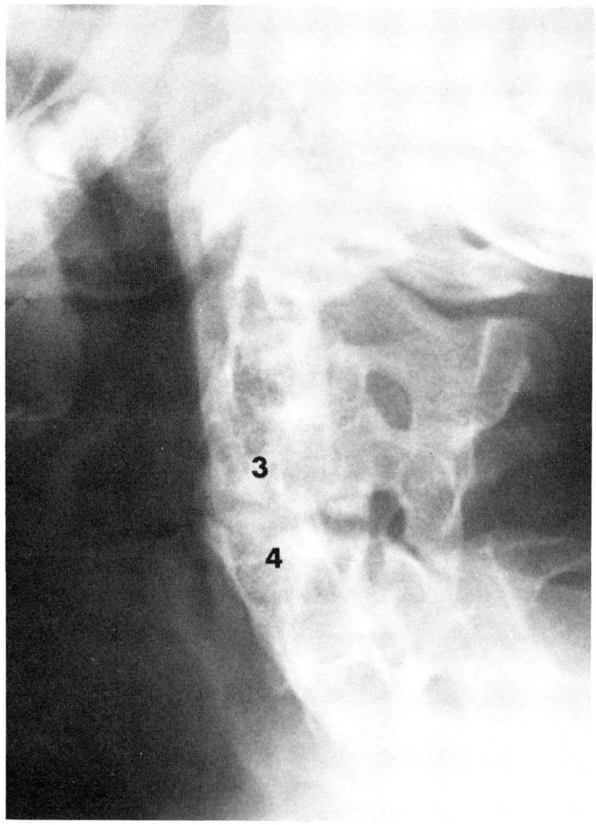

Fig. 6-34. This roentgenogram of a patient with Klippel-Feil syndrome reveals a rigidly fused cervical spine with a mobile segment at C3-4.

Radiologically, lateral views demonstrate poorly developed or totally absent disk spaces, fused posterior articulations on the obliques, and inadequate neural foramina. There may be spina bifida and reduced numbers of vertebrae.

Arnold-Chiari malformation has been discussed under childhood congenital anomalies. It should be remembered that this entity can simulate a herniated cervical disk without trauma, causing neck and occipital pain as well as spastic paresis. Myelography must be used to delineate the anomaly.

Cervical ribs may occur at the 7th cervical level. Embryologically they have the same origin as the costal processes and may be differentiated from the latter by their downward course. Cervical ribs are supernumerary structures and may be associated with fibrous bands attaching to the first thoracic rib.

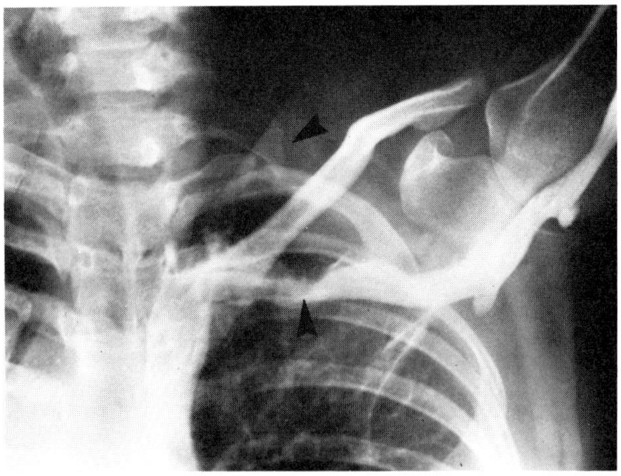

Fig. 6-35. Seventh cervical rib with fibrous band producing compression of the subclavious vein when the shoulder is abducted.

This extra rib may compress the lower cord of the brachial plexus and subclavian vessels. Ordinarily, the symptoms are paresthesias and pain in the ulnar distribution. Radiologic examination will demonstrate the cervical rib which may be bilateral (Fig. 6-35). The mere presence of a cervical rib, however, does not mean that it is symptomatic or causing neurovascular compression. On physical examination, it may be possible to palpate the extra rib in the supraclavicular fossa, at the base of the neck. The Adson sign is positive with reproduction of symptoms when the head is rotated toward the opposite side with hyperextension of the neck (see Fig. 8-43). This maneuver often obliterates the radial pulse. It may be necessary to do radiologic vascular contrast studies to determine the level of compression.

When there are similar signs and symptoms of a cervical rib but the rib is absent on roentgenogram, the scalenus anticus syndrome must be considered. Similar compression of the neurovascular structures may occur between the insertion of the anterior scalene and middle scalene muscles.

Tumors

Tumors of the adult cervical spine may be primary, arising from the bone, or secondary, that is, metastatic from a distant primary site. The most common sites of origin of metastatic tumors are prostate gland and lung in men, breast in women, followed by gastrointestinal tract, kidney, and undifferentiated tumors of unknown etiology.

The presenting symptom of metastatic tumor to the cervical spine is pain which is constant, persistent through the night, and usually not relieved by rest. Physical examination may reveal an external mass, pain on palpation of the spine, and pain on motion of the spine. Pain may be aggravated by manipulation and with progressive vertebral body collapse, bone may protrude into the spinal canal, compressing the anterior spinal cord surface and producing paralysis (Fig. 6-36). Positive diagnosis must be made by open biopsy and appropriate treatment instituted.

Primary tumors of the cervical spine may be benign or malignant. *The most common benign tumors of adults* are osteochondromas, osteoblastomas (Fig. 6-37), aneurysmal bone cysts, chondromas, osteoid osteoma, and hemangiomas (Fig. 6-38). *The most common malignant tumors* are osteogenic sarcoma, giant cell tumor, and chordoma (Fig. 6-39). Location of the tumors is significant in relation to chordomas which are usually found in the upper cervical spine. Certain tumors have predilection for the posterior elements and pedicles, such as osteoid osteomas, aneurysmal bone cysts, and osteochondromas. Other tumors most commonly affect the vertebral bodies, such as metastatic tumors, giant cell tumors, hemangiomas, and osteogenic sarcomas.

Most tumors of the cervical spine, whether primary or secondary, produce bone destruction or radiolucency on radiologic examination. Some tumors will also be osteoblastic in nature—with some areas of increased density. The latter include prostatic carcinoma, osteogenic sarcoma, and some giant cell tumors. Tomography is extremely helpful in diagnosing the extent of the tumor invasion and planning the type of surgical approach, that is, anterior and/or posterior. Myelography is used to determine the amount of cord compression. Arteriography is performed when the tumor involves the lateral aspect of the vertebra near the vertebral foramina.

Tumors may be differentiated from infection by appropriate laboratory studies (i.e., sedimentation rate, skin testing, temperature charting, white blood count with differential, and biopsy). Adequate history is also very important to relate previous episodes of infection, primary tumors at a remote site, and duration of the present illness.

Tumors of the cervical cord must be considered in diagnosing the cause of neck pain. These tumors can be primary, metastatic, extramedullary, or intramedullary. Pain of insidious onset, with or without neurologic symptoms and signs, may occur. Neurologic signs may be slow to develop with progressive leg weakness, bladder paralysis, and with sensory loss. The type of paralysis may be upper motor neuron and spastic, or lower motor neuron with root pain

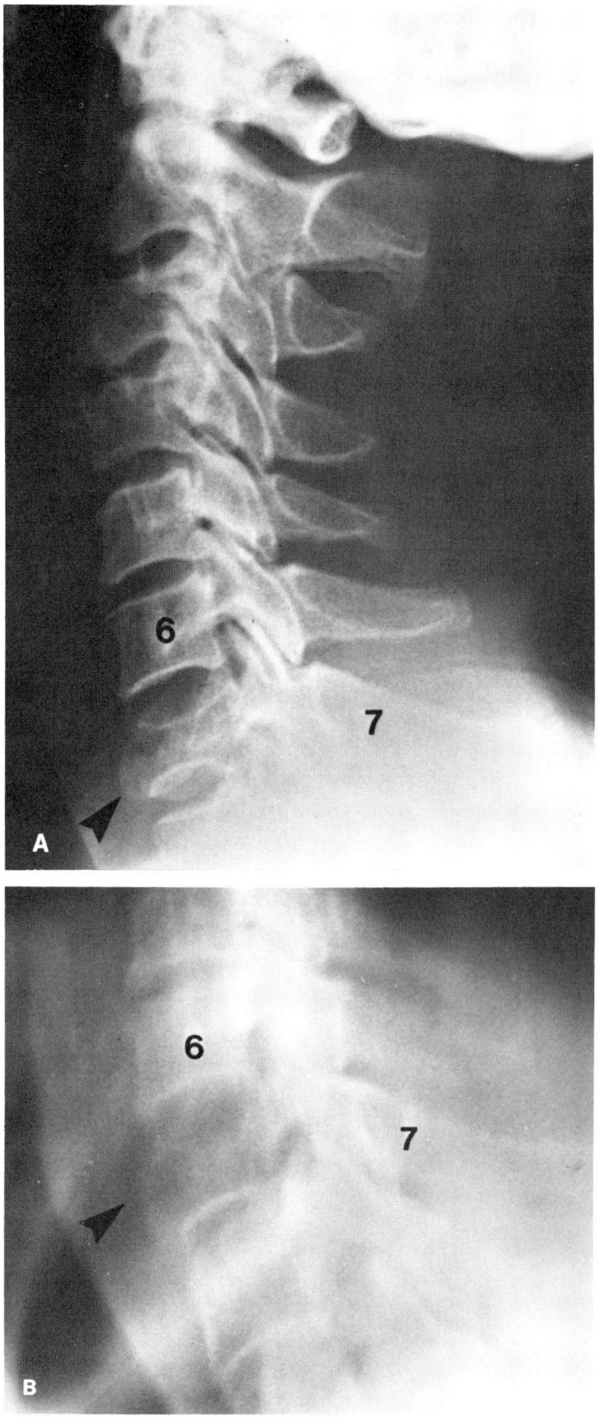

Fig. 6-36. (*A*) C7 vertebra with metastatic carcinoma was crushed by chiropractic manipulation, producing paralysis of the left arm. (*B*) Tomogram of C7 revealing lytic destruction of the vertebral body.

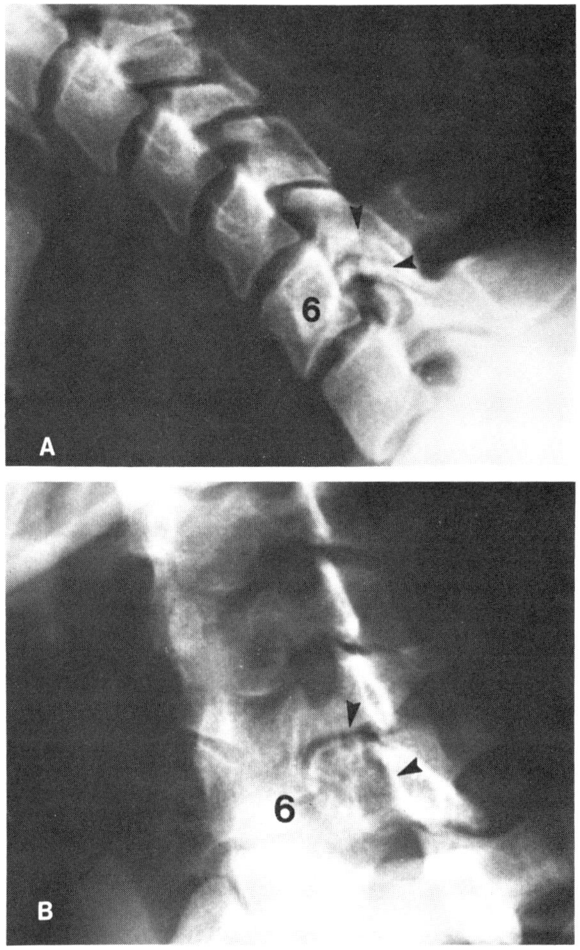

Fig. 6-37. (*A*) Lateral roentgenogram of osteoblastoma of C6 lateral vertebral elements. Note irregularity of the facet joint with increased density. (*B*) Oblique roentgenogram of an osteoblastoma C6 showing obliteration of the foramina. The tumor had also encircled the vertebral artery.

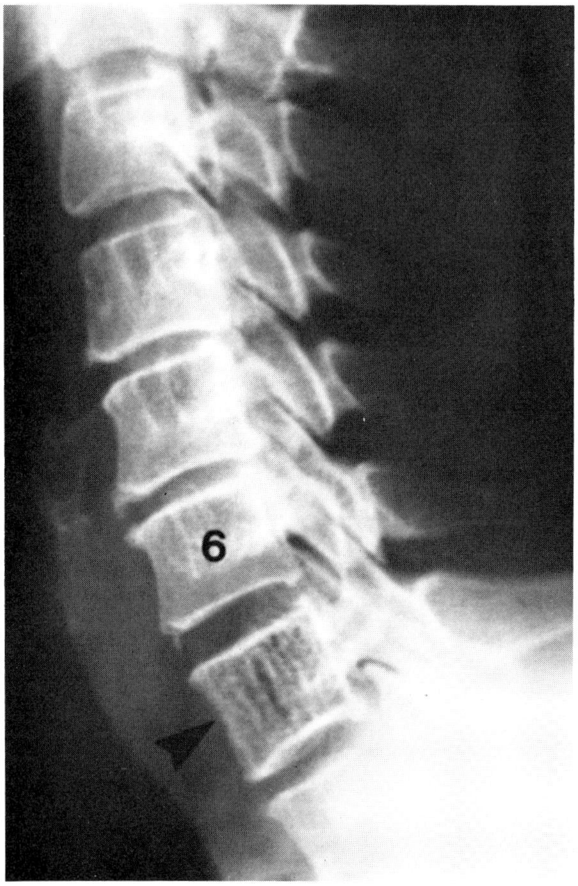

Fig. 6-38. Roentgenogram from an adult with hemangioma of C7 vertebra. Note the vertical trabecular pattern.

and paralysis. Extramedullary tumors present with early, radicular pain and contralateral loss of pain and temperature, most marked at the level of the lesion. Pyramidal tract involvement is prominent early. Intramedullary tumors, on the other hand, present with poorly localized burning pain, variable sensory changes, late pyramidal tract signs, and marked atrophy and fasciculation of the lower motor neuron or anterior horn cell involvement.

Tumors of the cervical spinal cord and roots cause bone destruction by direct bone compression (Fig. 6-40).

Diagnosis of spinal cord tumors is by roentgenography as well as neurologic examination. Analysis of the spinal fluid, protein dynamics, and cell count are important. Myelography may differentiate intra- from extra-medullary tumors as well as the level of the lesion.

One must remember that a large central herniated cervical disk may simulate a spinal cord tumor.

Inflammatory Diseases

The two major inflammatory diseases affecting the cervical spine are ankylosing spondylitis and rheumatoid arthritis. Both of these entities have been mentioned in the discussion of adolescent cervical spine afflictions.

Ankylosing Spondylitis. The major problem with ankylosing spondylitis in adulthood is total loss of motion. There may be some motion at the upper cervical spine between the occiput, atlas, and axis, but this frequently is also lost (Fig. 6-41). Simple observation of the individual reveals rotation of the eyes, torso, head, and shoulders as a unit. The patient is pain-free. Occasionally, either spontaneously or because of mild trauma, the patient develops a fracture through an ossified disk space with motion and pseudarthrosis. This is clinically manifest by a "chin-on-chest" deformity. The level of the lesion is usually lower cervical. This produces great disability. It may be corrected with a halo-cast and/or surgery. Traumatic episodes may cause fracture through a disk space resulting in vertebral dislocation with or without major paralysis. Rarely, progressive quadriparesis may develop secondary to massive epidural hemorrhage. One must be aware of this entity in ankylosing spondylitis and do repeated neurologic examinations. Massive epidural hemorrhage does not occur in other fracture-dislocations of the cervical spine.

Radiologically it is of interest that patients with totally ankylosed cervical spines have no osteophyte formation in the foramina on oblique views because of bone remodeling and complete loss of motion at the fixed segments. This is in contrast to cervical spondylosis in which abnormal motion and reactive bone formation is produced until spontaneous or surgical fusion occurs.

Rheumatoid Arthritis. In the adult patient with rheumatoid arthritis, a number of pathologic changes affect the cervical spine. Synovial tissue invasion destroys joint surfaces and produces ligamentous laxity, as it does in other sites of the body. Neck pain is exacerbated by flareups of the disease. Osteoporosis affects the osseous structures in the cervical spine. All of these problems may be complicated by the administration of steroids for the gen-

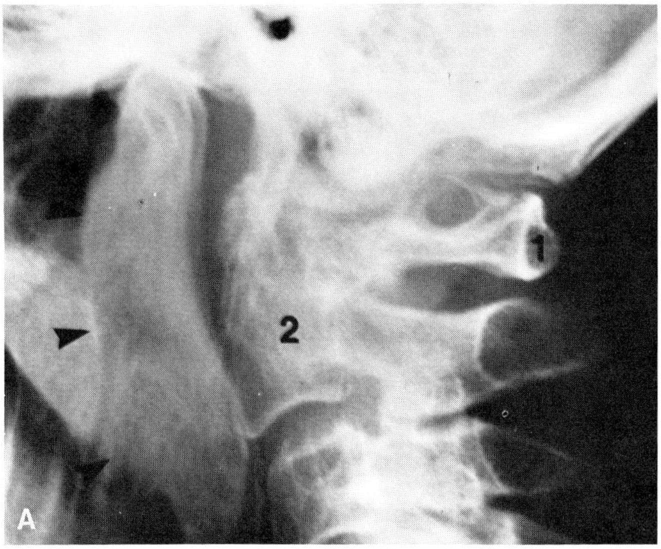

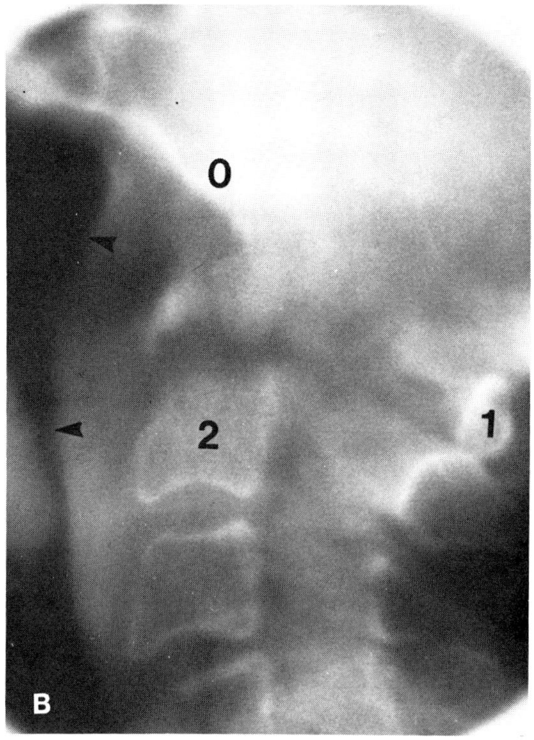

Fig. 6-39. (*A*) Chordoma involving vertebral body and odontoid process of C2. Note large prevertebral mass anterior to C2. (*B*) Tomogram of chordoma. Note destruction, purely lytic lesion of C2.

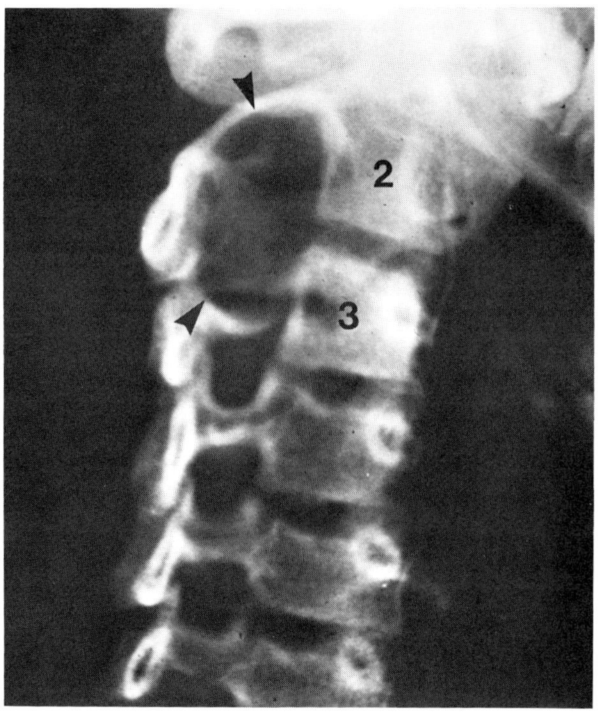

Fig. 6-40. Neurofibroma involving C2 and C3 pedicles. Expansile lesion causing erosion of bone by direct pressure, and enlarged foramina.

eral disease. Increased ligamentous laxity at the lower as well as upper cervical spine occurs with subluxations as well as dislocations of the vertebrae (Fig. 6-42). Particularly susceptible and dangerous is lysis of the transverse ligament of the atlas producing atlantoaxial dislocation (Fig. 6-43). All rheumatoid patients should have roentgenograms of the cervical spine to document such lesions. Dislocations of the cervical spine in rheumatoid patients may be totally asymptomatic or may be manifested by progressive pain and myelopathy. In patients with myelopathy, the neurologic manifestation may be quite subtle (i.e., easy fatigability or difficulty in walking, without sensory loss or gross paralysis). This clinical picture may be mistaken for exacerbation of the rheumatoid disease.

Dynamic flexion-extension views of the cervical spine must be carried out for accurate diagnosis. A gap of 3 mm. or greater between the anterior atlas and odontoid process is significant and indicates a pathologic condition. Forward subluxation of 4 to 5 mm. of the lower vertebral bodies is also significant. Both should be treated by immobilization initially and the question of surgical stabilization re-

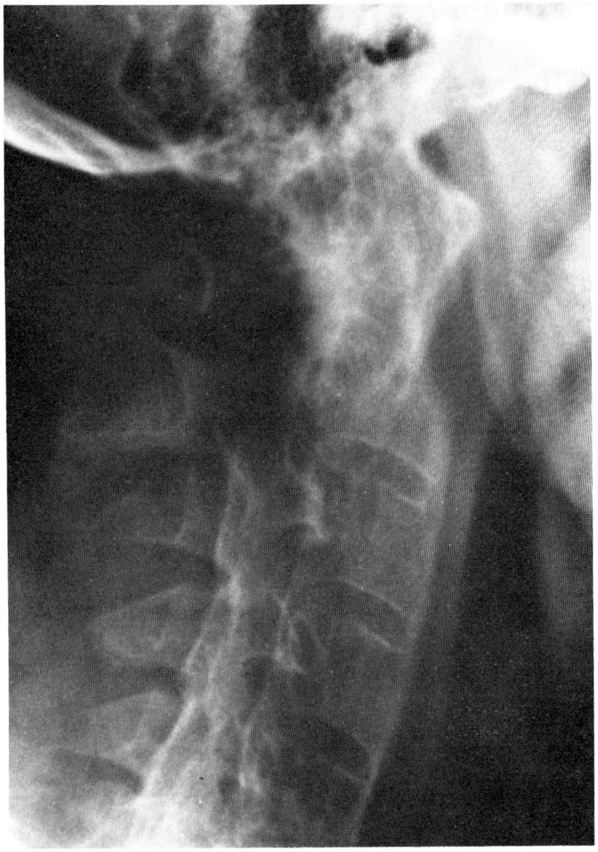

Fig. 6-41. Note fusion of occiput to lower cervical spine in this roentgenogram from a patient with ankylosing spondylitis of long standing.

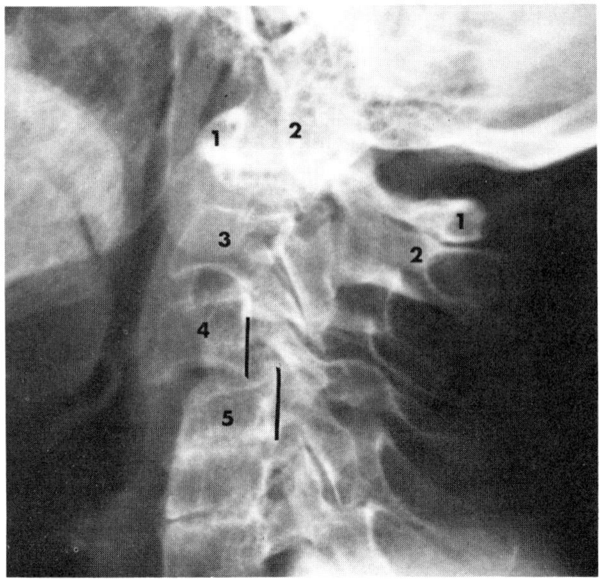

Fig. 6-42. Rheumatoid arthritic patient demonstrating anterior subluxation of C4 and C5 and basilar invagination of the odontoid process through the arch of C1.

solved later. Cervical myelography either by air or contrast material is indicated when neural signs appear.

Late in the disease and especially after long treatment with steroids, the odontoid process may migrate proximally into the foramen magnum, producing basilar invagination and medullary compression. This can be especially severe if associated with atlantoaxial dislocation (Fig. 6-44). Clinical signs include respiratory distress, cardiac abnormalities, intermittent quadriparesis without sensory loss, and occipital pain. Radiologic diagnosis and accurate delineation of the bony structures can best be carried out by anteroposterior and lateral tomography. Sudden death may result if this lesion is not stabilized surgically by fusion.

Infections of the cervical spine and disks are uncommon and usually caused by tuberculosis or pyogenic organisms. The peak ages of occurrence are in the second and fifth decades. Diagnosis and early treatment are important because of the disastrous effects of infection extending into the spinal canal with resultant paralysis.

Etiologically, the mode of introduction of the organism may be by hematogenous route, contiguous spread, postsurgical or by direct introduction via

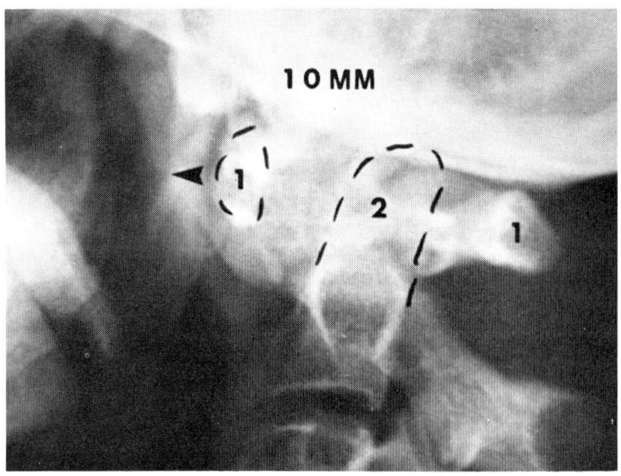

Fig. 6-43. This roentgenogram was taken from a rheumatoid arthritic patient treated with steroids; there is marked atlantoaxial dislocation. The patient was quadriparetic. Note the small amount of room for the spinal cord between the posterior arch of C1 and the odontoid process.

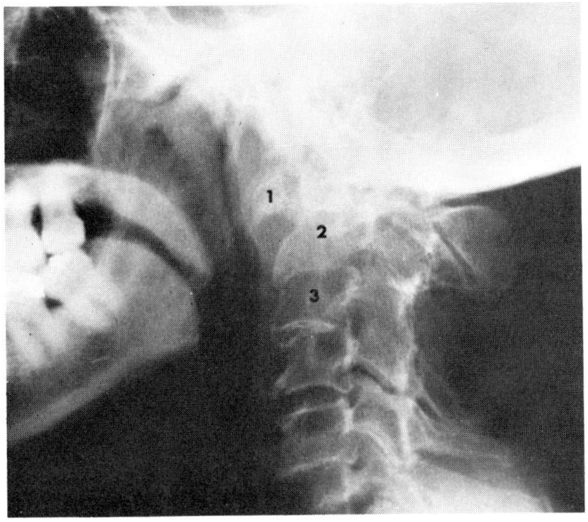

Fig. 6-44. Roentgenogram of the cervical spine of a patient with long-standing rheumatoid arthritis treated with steroids. Note basilar invagination with C1-2 dislocation. The patient was quadriparetic.

diagnostic procedures. In the younger patient infections or abscesses at a distant site are usually the cause. Middle-aged patients may develop osteomyelitis of the cervical spine secondary to genitourinary tract procedures, direct introduction by diskography, postoperative infection, or from other distant sources, such as pulmonary tuberculosis. Staphylococcus is the most common pyogenic organism in adults, but gram-negative bacteria are becoming manifest more frequently. Streptococcus is predominant in children.

Pathologically the organism which is blood-borne lodges in the vertebral body capillary loop, sludging the blood and setting up an inflammatory reaction. Necrosis of bone occurs, and the infection extends out of the vertebra under the anterior or posterior longitudinal ligaments. A paravertebral abscess may form or the adjacent disk space may be involved.

If the abscess extends into the spinal canal, direct pressure on the neural structures creates anterior cord compression, manifested by spasticity and extremity weakness, with relative sparing of posterior column modalities (i.e., position and vibratory sense).

Diagnosis must begin with an accurate history and physical examination. The earliest sign and symptoms are neck pain and fever. Neck pain may be present prior to any bone destruction seen on roentgenogram. Usually there will be very guarded motion of the neck, muscle spasticity, and occasionally dysphagia if the anterior abscess is large. Palpation of the neck may reveal an abscess mass anteriorly, or tenderness. Neck pain may be referred to the inner scapula region or shoulder.

Associated diseases are quite important to analyze. Subacute bacterial endocarditis may produce blood-borne infections of the cervical spine (Fig. 6-45).

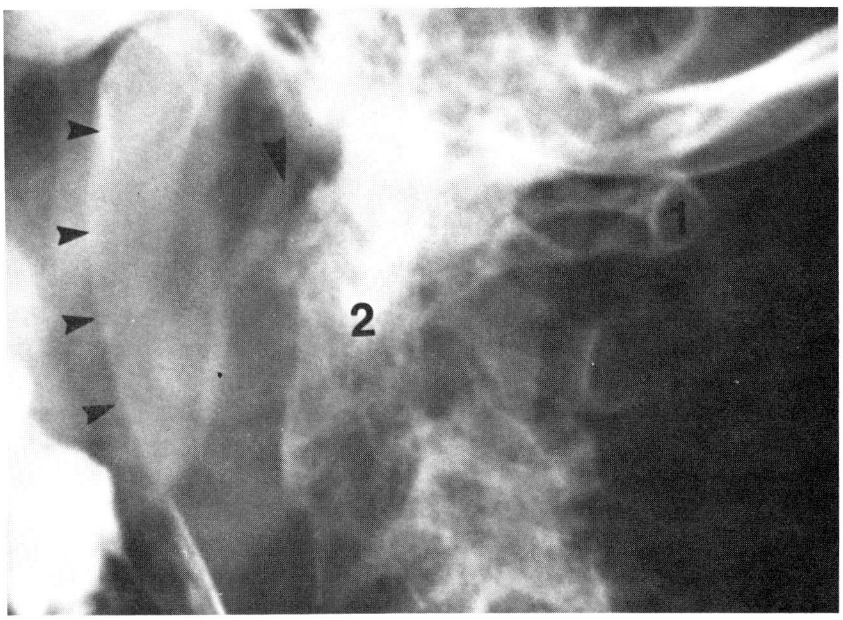

Fig. 6-45. Note prevertebral abscess, and destruction of odontoid as well as the anterior arch of C1. Patient had high fever, known subacute bacterial endocarditis and two-month history of upper neck pain.

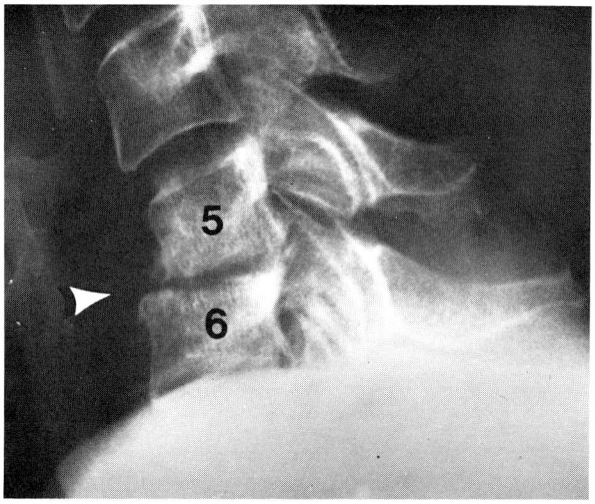

Fig. 6-46. A patient with rheumatoid arthritis, treated with steroids, presented in staphylococcal septicemia, with central cord quadriparesis, and destruction of C5-6 disk space. Note osseous end-plate destruction, and narrowed disk space.

Patients with rheumatoid arthritis have frequently been treated with steroids for years and are especially susceptible to blood-borne infections (Fig. 6-46). Diabetics are well known to have low resistance to infections. The patient may present with the other usual manifestations of infection (i.e., anorexia, chills, fever, and malaise).

Laboratory tests should include white blood count, sedimentation rate, blood cultures, and skin testing to rule out tuberculosis or fungal infections.

Radiologically the findings of pyogenic infection include early rarefaction of bone, disk space destruction and narrowing with erosion of the bony end plates. Soft-tissue swelling occurs anteriorly on lateral roentgenogram as well as paraspinous enlargement on the anteroposterior view. Clinical symptoms precede radiologic changes in pyogenic infections, whereas the opposite is true in tuberculous infections. Radiologically there may be much more sclerotic reaction of bone in pyogenic infections, as well as disk space destruction.Tuberculous infection of the spine produces a more central bony destruction of the vertebral body and later disk space narrowing (Fig. 6-47).

If a patient presents with neck pain and fever, and the physician suspects that there is infection, the burden of proof is on the physician to search diligently for radiologic clues. Bone scan and laminagrams are of great benefit early in the course of osteomyelitis as they delineate early bone destruction and disk space narrowing.

Differential diagnosis must include tumors of primary osseous origin or metastatic carcinoma. Tumors generally do not affect the disk space first. Infection usually is confined to the anterior vertebral body elements of the spine. Ultimately the diagnosis is made by direct open biopsy via the anterior approach and is usually necessary to prove the exact nature of the organism.

DEGENERATIVE DISK DISEASE

The etiology of degenerative disk and joint disease of the cervical spine is uncertain. Many factors may be related: trauma, congenital anomalies, and the aging process. The cervical spine is quite mobile and subject to greater stresses than the lower spine. With aging, the cervical disk loses its water content and the disk space narrows. The pathophysiology of cervical degenerative joint disease is the same as other joints in the body. Initially there is narrowing of the disk, abnormal motion follows at the affected segment with synovial tissue proliferation and reactive bone formation, especially at the joints of Luschka posterolaterally. Vertebral body spurs form anteriorly as well as posteriorly. Degenerative changes are more common anteriorly in the lower cervical spine and in the posterior apophyseal joints of the upper cervical spine.

Degenerative changes in the cervical spine are present in 40 percent of the population in the fourth decade of life, and 70 per cent of men and women by age 65. Not all of these people are symptomatic. Frequently the pre-existing degenerative disk becomes symptomatic following a flexion-extension injury.

The etiology of neck pain secondary to degenerative disk disease is uncertain. It is known, however, that the outer layers of the anulus fibrosus, facet joint capsules, and anterior and posterior longitudinal ligaments have all been shown to be innervated by gamma or C nerve fibers with simple termination in these structures. Human and dog bone is thoroughly innervated. Robinson demonstrated pain patterns by injecting cervical structures with local anesthetics. He postulated that a mechanical defect at a

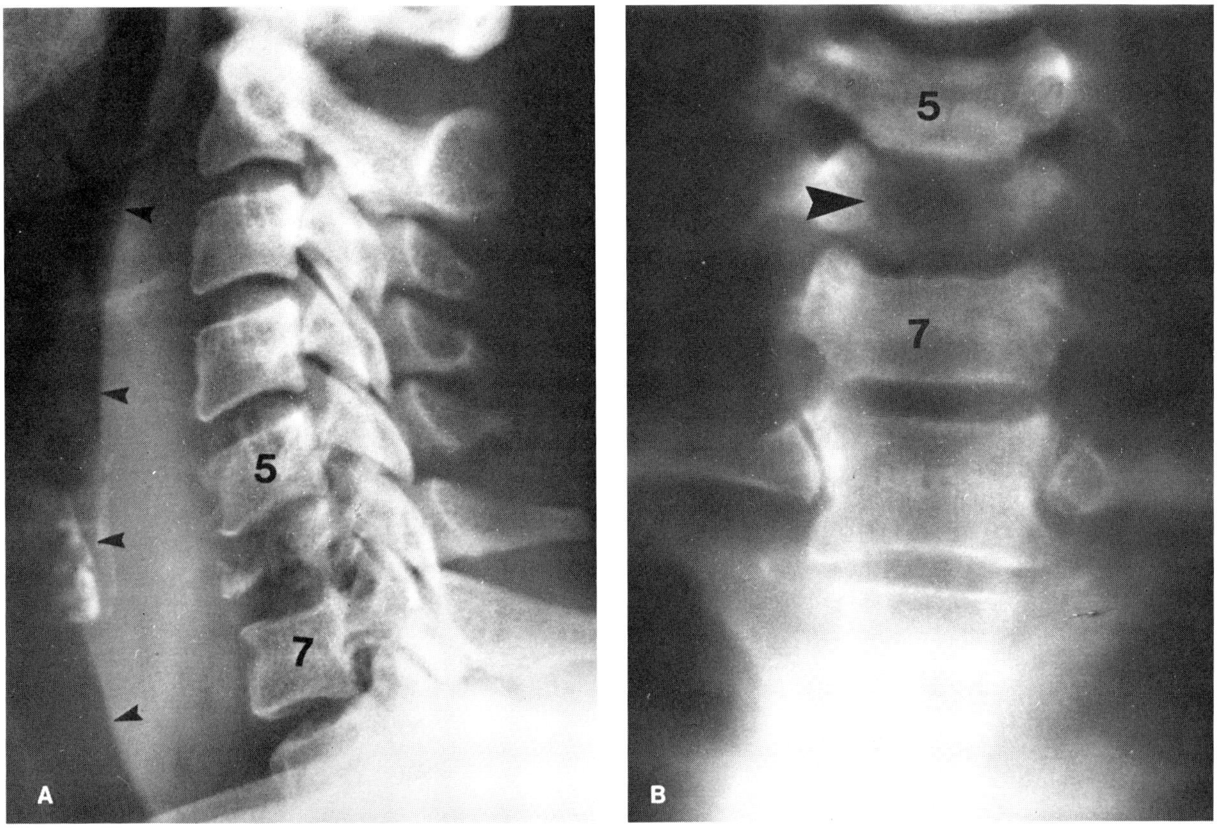

Fig. 6-47. Tuberculous prevertebral abscess with destruction of the C6 vertebral body. (*A*) Note relative preservation of the disk spaces. (*B*) Anteroposterior tomogram of tuberculous destruction of C6 vertebra.

motion segment of the cervical spine distorts the soft tissue or produces a disk bulge against the posterior longitudinal ligament and anulus. This in turn overstimulates the C fibers and produces cortical perception of those stimuli as pain. This pain may not be well localized. It can be called "diskogenic pain."

The clinical picture of the patient with symptomatic degenerative disk disease is that of neck, interscapular, occipital, and shoulder pain. There may be referred pain to the arm and forearm in lower cervical lesions. Subjective paresthesias occur, which are vague in distribution and unlike those of specific nerve root compression. Neck stiffness with muscle spasms and limited motion is present. The pain is frequently relieved by lying down or immobilization with a cervical collar. Tenderness is present over the spinous processes of the affected cervical segments. Cervical motion may be very limited in flexion and extension.

Laboratory studies may be of no help. Radiologic studies, however, may point to one particular degenerative segment with a narrowed disk, spur formation, and partial obliteration of the foramina on the oblique views. Posterior lipping of the vertebrae is observed on lateral roentgenograms, and there is sclerosis of the vertebral body end plates. It is important to note the width of the spinal canal on the lateral roentgenogram.

Rarely does cervical degenerative disk disease present with radicular symptoms, unless there is a superimposed herniated disk with root compression.

CERVICAL SPONDYLOSIS AND ACUTE HERNIATED DISK

Cervical spondylosis encompasses a more severe degenerative process involving all parts of the cervical spine, including disks, joints of Luschka, apophyseal joints, vertebrae, and foramina. Cervical spondylosis may cause nerve root compression producing a radiculopathy, spinal cord compression resulting in myelopathy, or both in combination, which complicates the diagnostic problem.

An important consideration in cervical spondylosis is that of a pre-existing congenital spinal stenosis (i.e., a lower cervical canal that is 13 mm. or less to begin with and has superimposed upon it a herniated disk, large spur formation, and thick ligamentum flavum). This may easily produce neural compression anteriorly or laterally.

Brain's monograph on cervical spondylosis describes the pathophysiology and symptoms of cervical spondylosis. Basically, the patient presenting with cervical radiculopathy is usually middle-aged, with insidious onset of neck and arm pain with paresthesias. The pain distribution varies with the level of nerve root compression. The presentation of *acute radiculopathy* in cervical spondylosis is not just secondary to spurs present in the foramen but ordinarily a result of acute superimposed *herniated cervical disk*. Usually no trauma is associated, but the patient awakens in the night with acute pain after sleeping in a stressful position. The pain may begin during the day without any episode of lifting or injury. Past history is frequently associated with old remote trauma, such as an auto accident or fall. The pain may be aggravated by sneezing or coughing. Physical examination reveals a patient in acute distress with limited motion in all directions, but especially lateral rotation to the side of the lesion with extension. The Spurling test may be positive. Pressure on the top of the head accentuates the symptoms. There will be marked muscle spasms. Traction by the examiner, pulling gently upward simultaneously on the chin and occiput, relieves the symptoms. Weakness of certain muscles may be subjective with complaints of dropping objects from the hands. There may be objective weakness, atrophy, or fasciculations, depending on the nerve root involved. There are eight cervical nerve roots; the first leaves the spinal canal above the atlas and the remaining roots exit above the numbered vertebrae. That is, the 6th root exits between the 5th and 6th cervical vertebrae. The 8th root exits below the 7th vertebra. Therefore, a laterally ruptured disk between the 5th and 6th vertebrae produces compression of the 6th nerve root. If a disk is herniated centrally it may compress the spinal cord anteriorly and may affect more than one level of root function. Centrally herniated disks produce central neck pain whereas laterally herniated disks produce lateralized pain from the neck to shoulder and referred down the arm. Rupture of the 4th cervical disk (C4-5) produces pain and paresthesias of the shoulder and arm region, with hypesthesia of the 5th root distribution, and weakness of the deltoid or biceps (see Fig. 5-1B). A ruptured 5th cervical disk (C5-6) produces 6th nerve root compression, with hypesthesia of the lateral aspect of the forearm and thumb with biceps and supinator weakness (Fig. 6-48) (see Fig. 5-1B). A ruptured 6th cervical disk (C6-7) (Fig. 6-49) compresses the 7th root, producing hypesthesia of the index and middle fingers, triceps, and grip weakness (see Fig. 5-1B). The less common 7th disk herniation (C7-T1) compresses the 8th cervical root and causes intrinsic weakness and ulnar hypesthesia in the hand (see Fig. 5-1B). At each particular level of nerve root compression, the deep tendon reflexes are depressed or absent and should be noted. Atrophy and fasciculations may be present in the affected muscles.

Interestingly, an acute herniated cervical disk usually occurs at a cervical segment where there has been mild degeneration of the disk, and rarely occurs with severe spondylitic change in association with foraminal spurs or large posterior osteophytes. One should not be misled by roentgenograms showing marked degenerative disk disease at a particular level. Myelography must always be carried out to localize the lesion. As Brain pointed out, the clinical neurologic level does not always correlate with the myelographic defect level. Frequently the acute disk herniation is above or below the degenerate level indicated on the roentgenogram. Electromyography may be very helpful in localizing the lesion to a specific nerve root and differentiating from peripheral neuropathy or entrapment. Nerve conduction delay at the first rib, elbow, or wrist may focus the attention on entrapment of a peripheral nerve distal to the cervical spine. Differential diagnosis must include the Pancoast's tumor (Fig. 6-50A), cervical rib (Fig. 6-50B), or scalenus anticus syndrome, primary shoulder lesions, and osseous tumors of the cervical spine. The previously mentioned Arnold-Chiari malformation may reproduce symptoms of spastic paresis or nerve root compression.

Severe cervical spondylosis occurs at multiple lev-

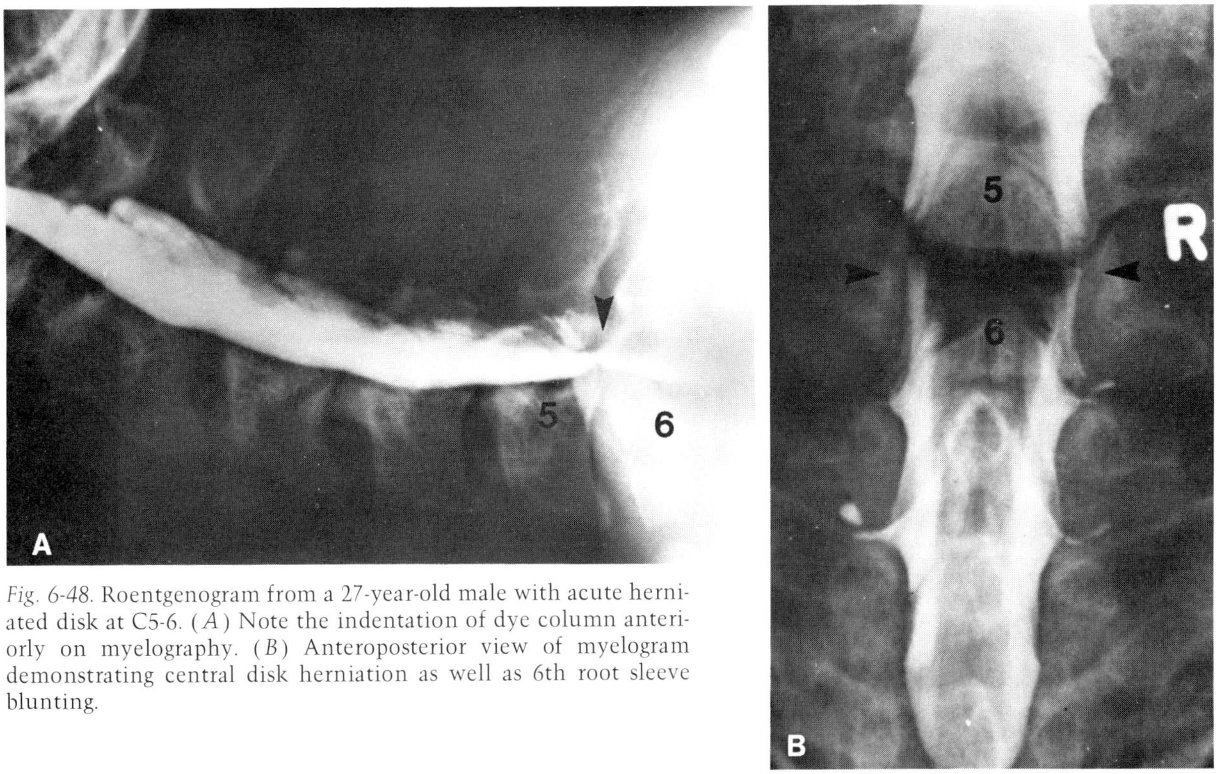

Fig. 6-48. Roentgenogram from a 27-year-old male with acute herniated disk at C5-6. (*A*) Note the indentation of dye column anteriorly on myelography. (*B*) Anteroposterior view of myelogram demonstrating central disk herniation as well as 6th root sleeve blunting.

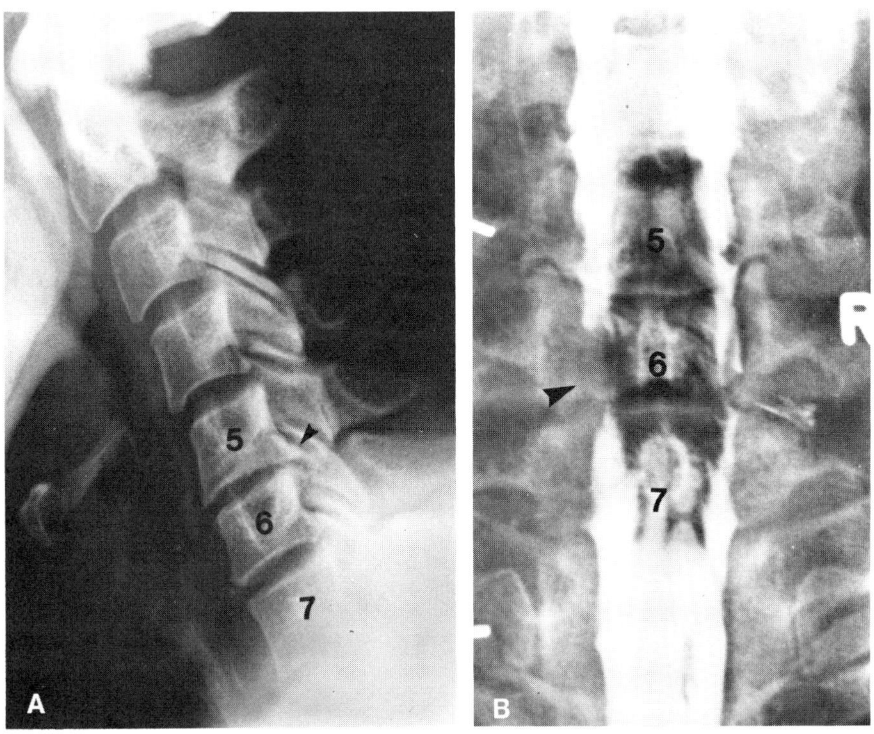

Fig. 6-49. Roentgenogram depicting posterior osteophytes in a patient with degenerative disk disease at the C5-6 level. (*A*) Acute herniated disk occurred at the less degenerated C6-7 level. (*B*) Anteroposterior myelogram demonstrated on the left, C6-7 disk herniation and compression of the 7th root.

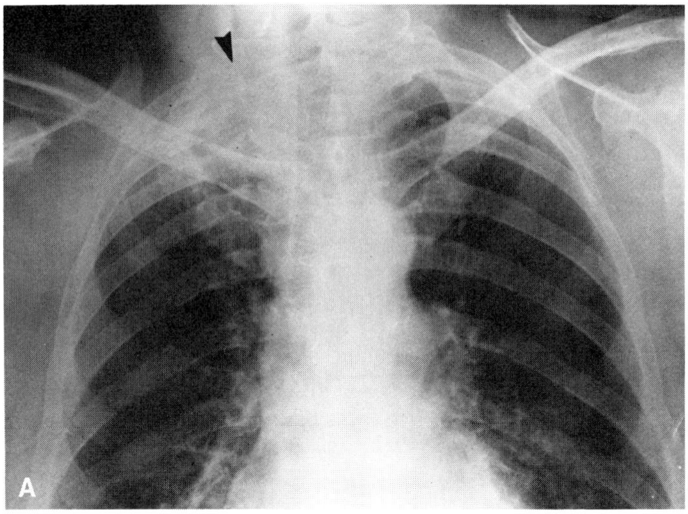

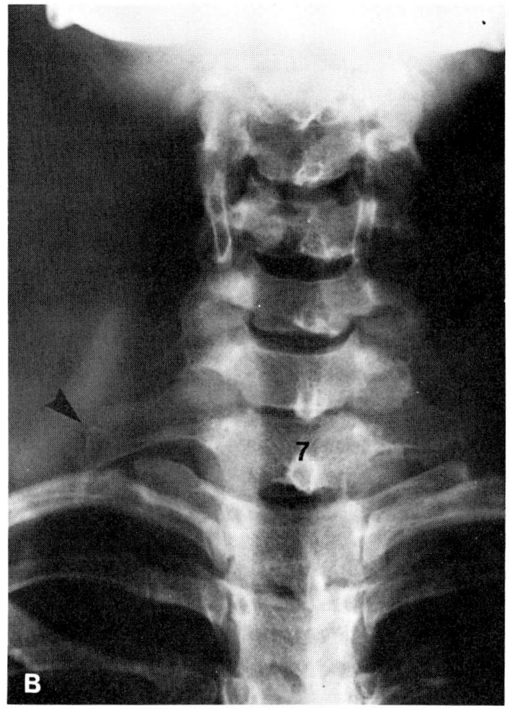

Fig. 6-50. (*A*) Pancoast tumor, producing neck, right shoulder, and arm pain. (*B*) Elongated right transverse process of C7, producing right arm pain and paresthesias.

els and increases with the aging process but usually is asymptomatic unless associated with a congenitally narrow spinal canal. Pain is not always a presenting symptom. Spurs and osteophytes may be present for decades and not produce any problem except decreased range of motion of the cervical spine. Cervical spondylosis in the presence of congenital spinal stenosis may produce radiculopathy, myelopathy, or a combination of upper and lower motor neuron signs. Another predisposing factor in severe spondylosis is that of spontaneous fusions, usually at lower cervical segments, producing more stress at the upper, more mobile, segments and resulting in hypermobility, stretched ligaments, and abnormal subluxations. The latter may cause spinal cord or nerve root compression with pain (Fig. 6-51). Flexion-extension lateral roentgenograms may be the only way to demonstrate this problem. Myelography is done to localize the pathologic condition.

In the patient with severe spondylosis and *insidious onset of peripheral root signs,* the etiology is thought to be a combination of increased spur size in the foramen, increase in soft disk protrusion, and scarring around the root. These are gradual problems which occur over a long period of time unless there is a superimposed herniated disk as has been described. The neuropathy may involve more than one level. Pathologically a large soft disk protrusion and posterior vertebral body osteophyte may cause direct compression of the anterior horn cells. It may also cause ischemia by compression of the anterior spinal artery and the resultant peripheral root signs of atrophy, fasciculation, and radicular pain with paresthesias. The physical signs on examination will be similar to those of an acute herniated disk. Routine roentgenograms, including anteroposterior, lateral, and oblique views are necessary to visualize the foraminal encroachment by osteophytes. Myelography is used to delineate the level of the lesion. One must be careful not to implicate the commonly seen arthritic cervical spine until other causes of peripheral neuropathy have been ruled out (i.e., diabetes, entrapment syndromes, and chronic alcoholism).

Not infrequently, a patient with severe cervical spondylosis may develop signs of *cervical spinal cord myelopathy.* This is highly associated with a congenitally narrowed spinal canal. These patients may live for many years with large osteophytes, narrowed disks, and narrow canals, then insidiously over 3 to 6 months they experience difficulty in walking, stumbling, clumsiness with their hands, and, rarely, neck pain. It is my belief that the acute pathologic condition is caused by a few more millimeters of soft disk protrusion beyond their osteophytes; this produces anterior spinal cord compresson and ischemia. Only late do patients exhibit signs of loss of position and vibratory sense of the posterior column. It is in the latter case that irreversible scarring, anterior horn cell loss, and intraneural fibrosis has occurred. Clinical complaints in the spondylitic patient with myelopathy include difficulty in walking, weakness of the hands and legs, and later difficulty in controlling urination. History may include frequent falls, stumbling, and loss of balance. On examination, hyperextension of the neck is very limited or guarded and may even produce a shocklike sensation down the back or legs, a positive Lhermitte's sign. Lateral rotation of the neck is limited also by severe arthritic change. There is usually no pain on palpation of the cervical spine. Neurologic examination may reveal evidence of lower motor neuron signs in the upper extremities, that is, atrophy, fasciculations, and sensory loss. Upper motor neuron signs are also present with positive Hoffmann and Babinski, ataxia, hyperreflexia of the extremities, and clonus of the ankles. There may be various gradations and combinations of upper and lower motor neuron signs.

Proof of the particular cervical levels at risk is by plain roentgenograms, measurement of the anteroposterior canal diameter, and cervical myelography (Fig. 6-52). There may be one or more cervical segments compromising the spinal canal. Occasionally lateral tomography is helpful in delineating the narrow canal. Bed rest and cervical immobilization may relieve the symptoms of myelopathy, but usually anterior cervical diskectomy and eventual spur remodeling following fusion is required to arrest the problem (Fig. 6-53).

Differential diagnosis must include other neurologic diseases, such as amyotrophic lateral sclerosis, muscular dystrophies, multiple sclerosis, and tumors of the spinal cord and cervical spine.

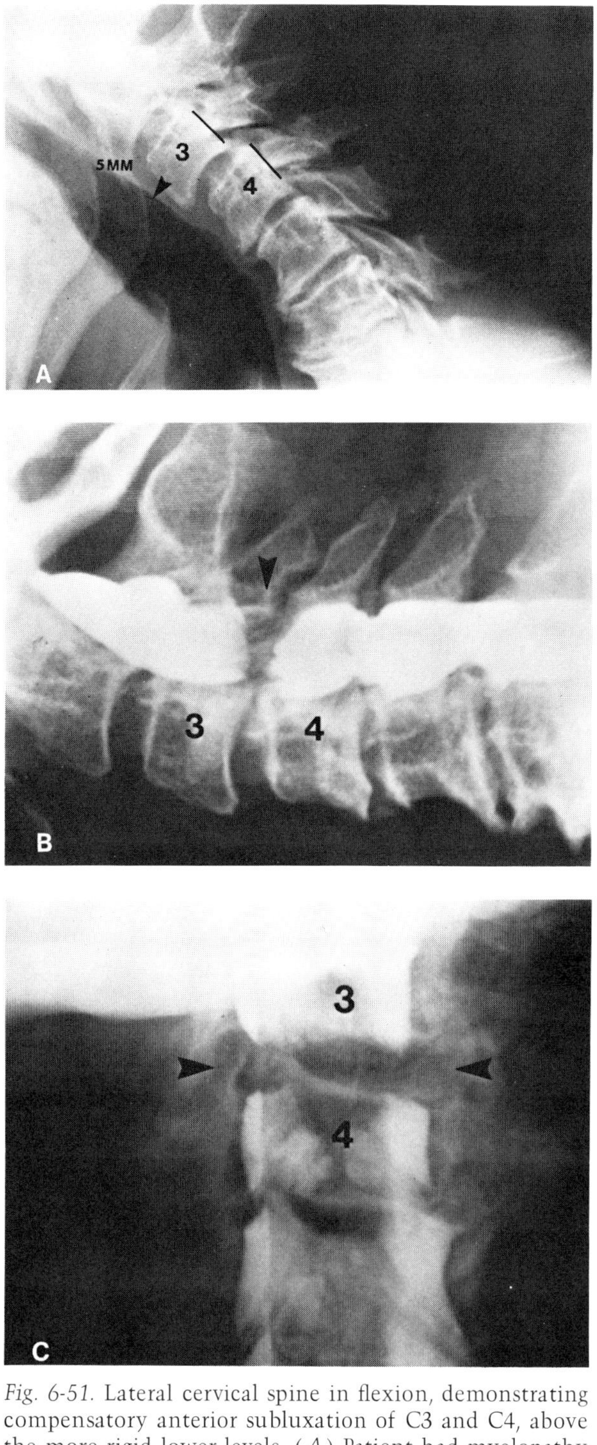

Fig. 6-51. Lateral cervical spine in flexion, demonstrating compensatory anterior subluxation of C3 and C4, above the more rigid lower levels. (*A*) Patient had myelopathy with cord compression signs, gross weakness of all muscles of the upper extremities and inability to walk with spastic legs. (*B*) Cervical myelogram (lateral view) revealing obstruction at the C3-4 disk space. (*C*) Anteroposterior myelogram demonstrating compressive bar at C3-4.

TRAUMATIC INJURIES OF THE CERVICAL SPINE AND SPINAL CORD

Cervical spine injuries may be very mild, involving just the soft tissues, or more severe with associ-

(*Text continues on page 220.*)

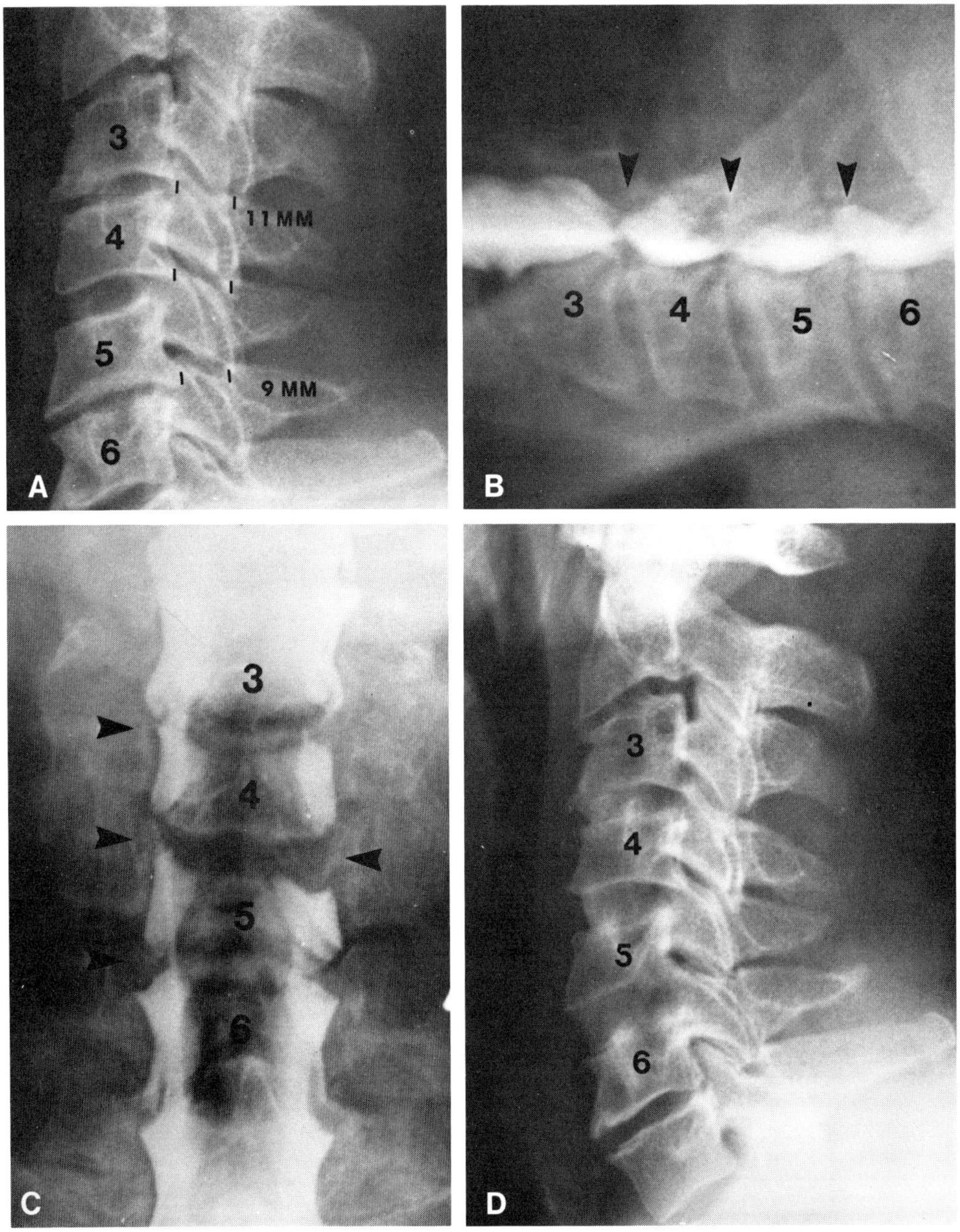

Fig. 6-52. Roentgenograms from a patient who presented with difficulty walking, spastic gait, and weakness of the upper extremities and hands. (*A*) Note the degenerative disk disease and narrow spinal canal, measuring from 9 to 11 mm. (*B*) Lateral myelogram demonstrating disk protrusions at C3-4, C4-5 and narrow spinal canal between C3 and C6. (*C*) Anteroposterior myelogram revealing disk protrusion at C3-4, C4-5, with nerve root sleeve blunting at multiple levels. (*C*) Note the predominant dye column interruption at C4-5 with a horizontal bar defect. (*D*) Lateral cervical spine roentgenogram of same patient following Robinson anterior diskectomies and block fusions at C3-4, C4-5, and C5-6 levels. Patient regained his muscle strength and walking ability 6 months postoperatively.

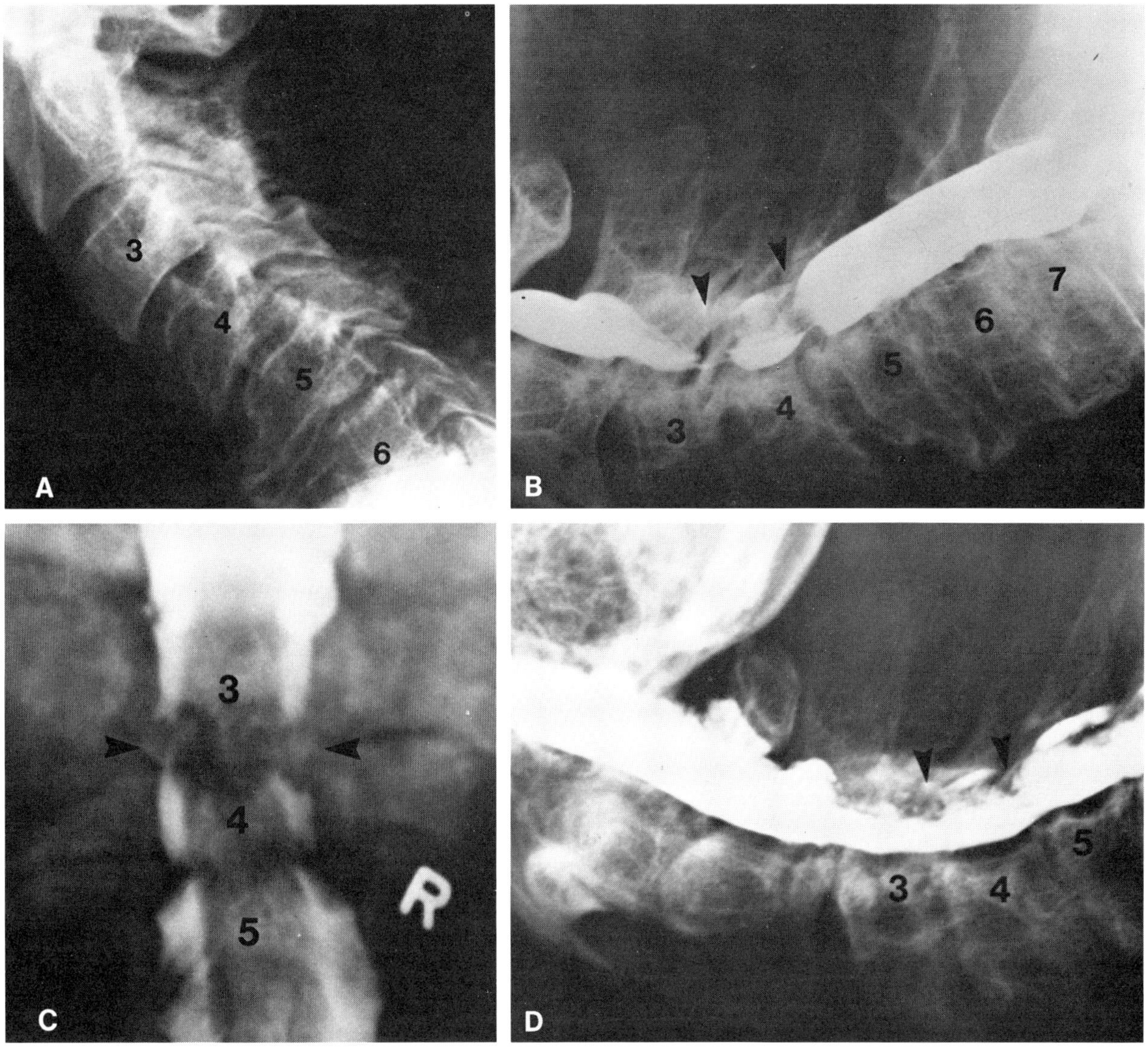

Fig. 6-53. (*A*) Myelogram from a patient with cervical spondylitis, with multiple levels involved, and slight anterior subluxation of C3 and C4. (*B*) Lateral myelogram showing disk protrusion at C3-4 and C4-5. Note complete filling of dye column at C5-6 and C6-7, where there are spontaneous anterior fusions. (*C*) Cervical myelogram showing a large horizontal bar at C3-4, smaller bar at C4-5, as well as nerve root sleeve blunting at both levels. (*D*) Same patient seven months following Robinson anterior cervical diskectomies and fusion at C3-4, and C4-5. No attempt was made to remove posterior osteophytes. The dye column is quite smooth now.

Table 6-3. Cervical Trauma

I. Soft tissue injury, disk injury or both
  A. Without neural deficit
  B. With neural deficit
    1. Root signs
    2. Cord signs
II. Bony fracture or dislocation without neural deficit
  A. Stable
  B. Unstable
III. Bony fracture with neural deficit
  A. Complete quadriplegia
  B. Incomplete quadriplegia
    1. Anterior cord syndrome
    2. Central cord syndrome
    3. Brown-Séquard syndrome
  C. Nerve root injury

ated fractures and dislocations resulting in neurologic damage.

Cervical trauma may be classified for clinical purposes as in Table 6-3.

CERVICAL SPRAIN

The most common mildest form of neck injury is the cervical sprain. Flexion, extension, and rotational forces may stretch the soft tissues beyond their elastic limit. Tearing of the cervical musculature, ligamentous complexes, and facet joint capsules occurs. These injuries cannot be demonstrated radiologically unless they are severe enough to tear many structures at once, causing separation of the vertebral bodies and damage to the disk itself.

The mechanisms of injury include: flexion, flexion-rotation, axial load, compression, extension, lateral flexion, missile wounds, or direct blows to the neck.

History taking from the patient with cervical trauma should include definition of mechanisms of injury, whether the patient struck his head, and if so, at what site. Was the patient thrown from a vehicle? Most commonly a patient will have sustained an acceleration or deceleration force during a rear-end auto accident. Inquiries must be made as to whether the patient had a head rest in the car preventing hyperextension. Did he strike the car in front after rear impact? Occasionally patients describe blurred vision and difficulty in thinking after the accident which may be secondary to transient vertebral muscle spasms. Frequently the cervical pain has a delayed onset, from one day to a week later.

The cause of most sports injuries is usually a flexion or flexion rotation force, regardless of the type of sport.

The patient with a cervical sprain presents with pain and stiffness of the neck. The neck is usually held rigidly and the lower torso is used to rotate the head. Physical examination of the patient with an acute injury usually reveals muscle spasm of the erector spinae muscle group as well as sternocleidomastoid muscles. Particular levels of spinous processes may be painful and give a clue to the level of injury. Pain is often generalized, involving the neck and shoulders, and may radiate to the occiput with a headache. Arm pain is usually not present unless nerve roots have been injured. Motion of the cervical spine is limited.

Specific radiologic views should include anteroposterior, lateral, and oblique projections. Open-mouth odontoid views should be obtained. Usually the only positive sign is decrease or reversal of the normal lordotic curve, which may be indicative of acute muscle spasm. Careful neurologic examination is important to rule out nerve root or spinal cord injury or compression.

CERVICAL DISK DISRUPTION

The pathology of 50 fatal craniospinal injuries has been studied in detail by the author. In these patients disk disruption without protrusion was common. This cannot be demonstrated radiologically by the routine examination. Disk disruption in milder cervical trauma may be the cause of acute as well as a chronic pain syndrome. Pain arising from a disrupted disk may be called diskogenic pain, as described in the previous section on degenerative disease. This type of pain pattern can become chronic over many years without resolving. The areas affected by pain include the neck, inner part of the scapula, shoulder, and arm. This pain is relieved by rest, immobilization, and traction. The pain recurs when the patient becomes active again. Although the patients complain of subjective, ill-defined paresthesias of the arms and hands, there is no neurologic deficit. They complain of the unintentional dropping of objects from their hands. Occipital headaches are common.

Radiologic diagnosis is difficult. The cervical spine films may be completely normal with the exception

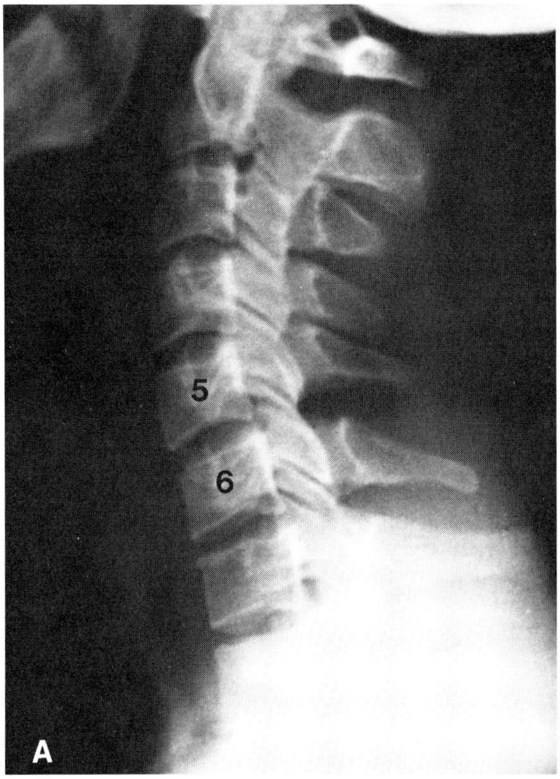

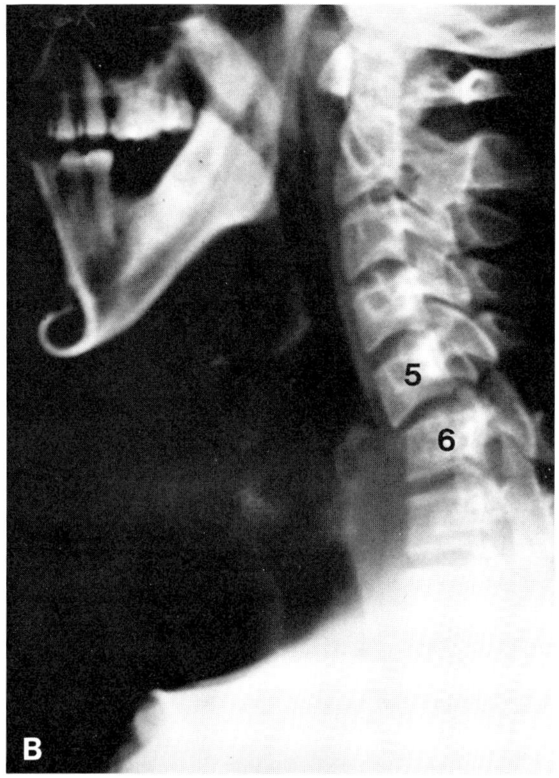

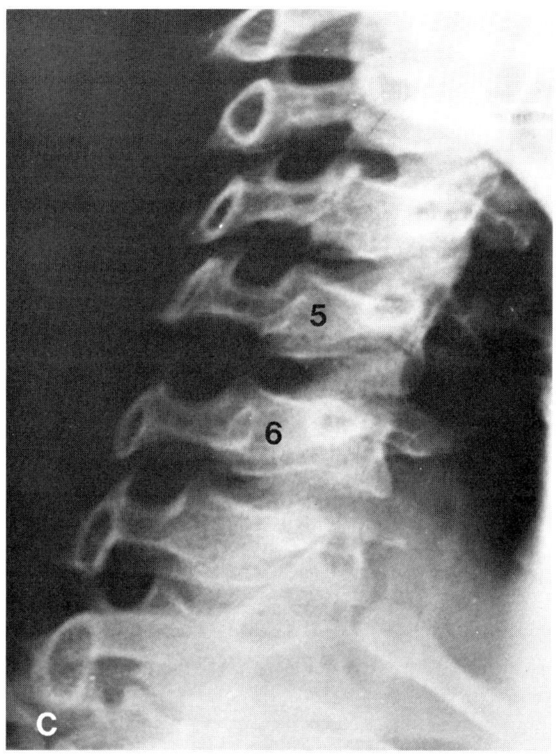

Fig. 6-54. Roentgenograms of the lateral cervical spine of a young adult who rolled over in his car; came to the emergency room complaining of cervical pain. No diagnosis of neck injury was made and the patient was discharged. (*A*) Note the slightly widened interspinous space between C5 and C6 posteriorly. (*B*) Lateral cervical spine film of same patient 10 days later in an orthopedist's office. Neck pain continued and this roentgenogram reveals subluxation of C5 anteriorly on C6. (*C*) Oblique roentgenogram showing "perched" facets of C5-6.

of slight disk space narrowing, or slight anterior subluxation of one vertebra upon another. Occasionally there will be slight widening of the posterior interspinous space indicating ligament disruption (Fig. 6-54).

Positive diagnosis is only possible by operative cervical diskograms in which the anterior surgical approach is utilized. The various levels of disks are then tested by injecting a water-soluble radiopaque dye into the nucleus pulposus. If more than 4 mm. of dye is accepted, disruption of the anulus fibrosus and posterior longitudinal ligament is indicated. Dye will be seen extravasating laterally along the nerve root sleeves on the anteroposterior view and pool along the anterior border of the posterior longitudinal ligament on the lateral view. Operative cervical diskography is only carried out in those patients in whom one to two years of conservative therapy has failed and the roentgenograms of the cervical spine are normal (Fig. 6-55). Anterior cervical diskectomy and fusion alleviates the problem.

CERVICAL FRACTURES AND DISLOCATIONS

Introduction

More severe cervical trauma may produce total disruptions of the ligament complexes, fractures, and dislocations. The common causes of severe cervical trauma are vehicular accidents, falls, such sporting injuries as diving into shallow water, and gunshot wounds.

Diagnosis by history and physical examination is all-important. The author has carried out a detailed review of over 300 injuries of the cervical spine, with and without neurologic deficit. Delay in diagnosis in various emergency rooms was common. One hundred of 300 severe cervical spine injuries were initially missed at various hospitals. This included patients with neurologic deficit. Delay in diagnosis ranged from one day to over a year. The most common causes for missed diagnoses were associated head trauma, acute alcoholic intoxication, and multiple injuries. Patients with decreased levels of con-

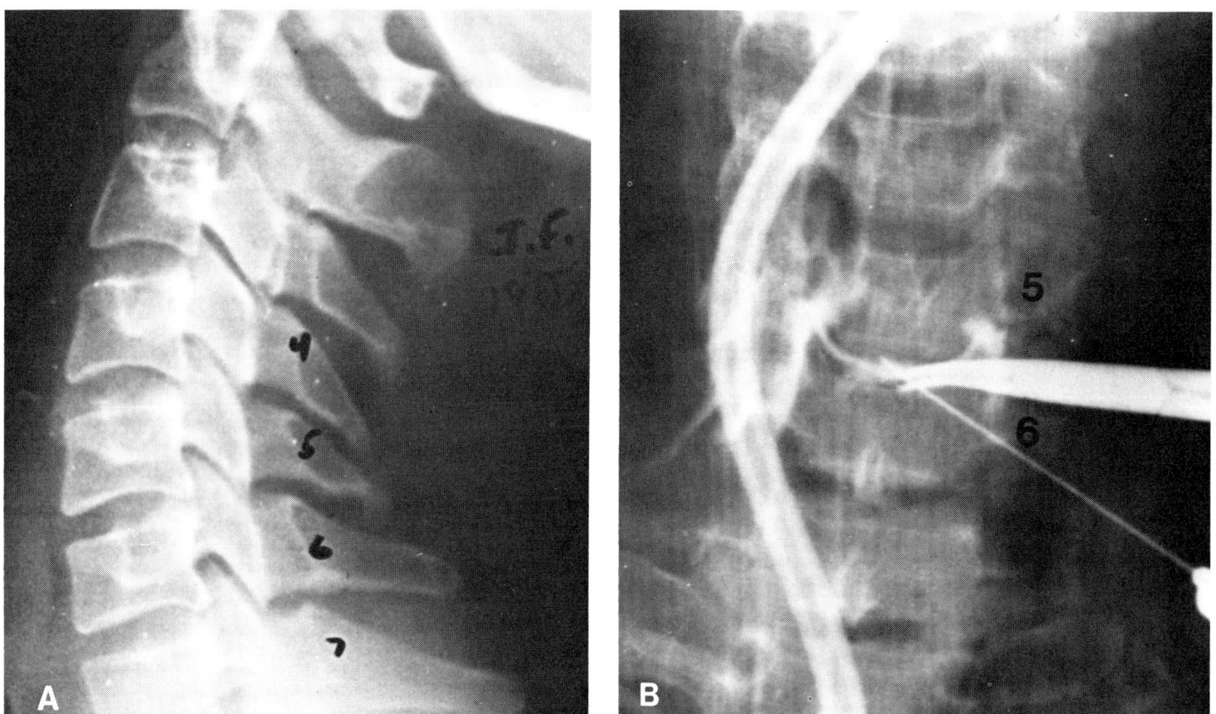

Fig. 6-55. (*A*) Normal lateral cervical spine roentgenogram on patient with a 6-year history of neck, inner scapular, and shoulder pain. (*B*) Positive operative diskogram at C5-6. Note cleft in the disk space and dye extravasating out the nerve root sleeves. Patient was relieved of pain by anterior cervical diskectomy and fusion.

sciousness (Fig. 6-56) or comatose patients do not complain of neck pain (Fig. 6-57). Also, patients who have sustained severe facial or scalp lacerations bleed profusely and distract attention from the cervical spine problem (Fig. 6-58). The intoxicated patient does not complain of pain either (Fig. 6-59). Also, the patient with multiple injuries may be in a state of shock, and may not complain of pain, and many of the ancillary injuries distract attention from his cervical spine (Fig. 6-60). Occasionally, a patient will have a Brown-Sequard type of hemiparesis which is mistaken for a stroke (Fig. 6-61).

A very high correlation of head and neck pathology has been demonstrated in a study of fatal cranio-

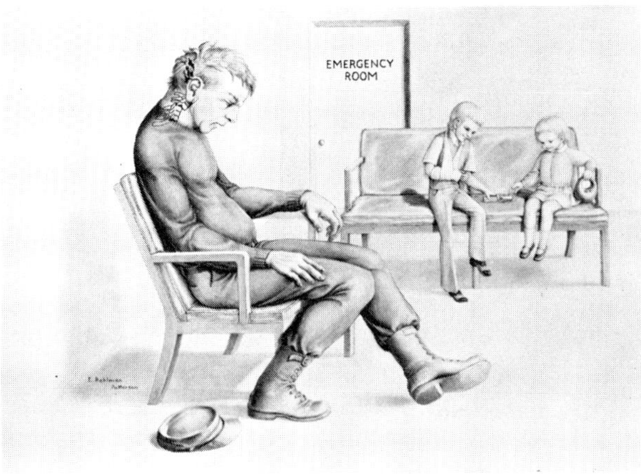

Fig. 6-56. Patient sitting in emergency room with head and neck injury and associated lethargic level of consciousness.

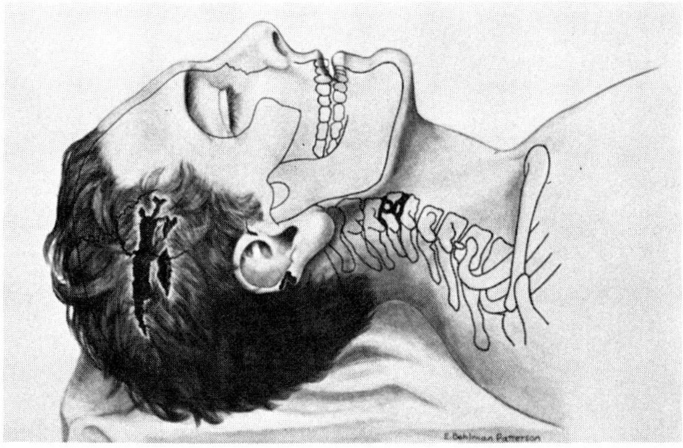

Fig. 6-57. A patient in comatose level of consciousness with cervical fracture and scalp laceration. Since this patient will not complain of pain, cervical spine roentgenograms must be taken for diagnosis of neck injury.

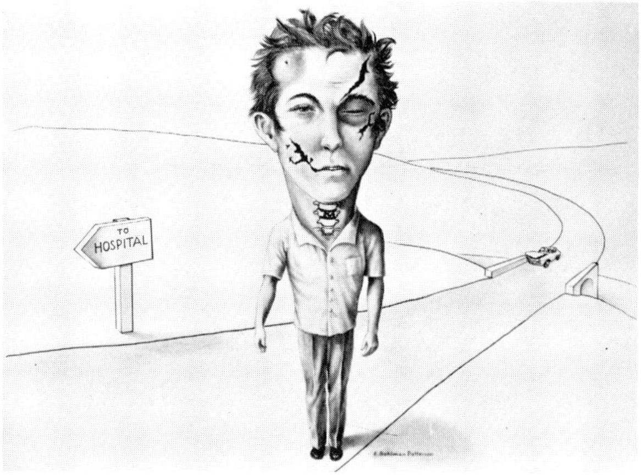

Fig. 6-58. A patient with severe scalp lacerations which distract attention from cervical fracture.

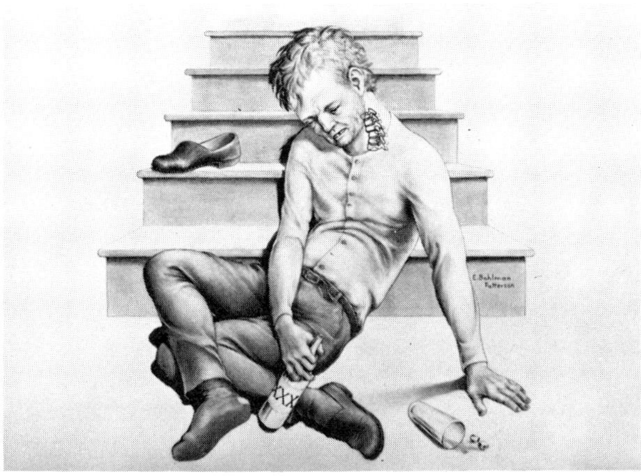

Fig. 6-59. The acutely intoxicated patient usually sustains a cervical spine fracture by falling down the stairs. The obtunded patient will not complain of pain. Cervical spine roentgenograms must be taken for diagnosis.

spinal injuries. The same is true of the injuries in the author's clinical review series. It is evident from these studies that the head and neck should be treated as a unit. In the clinical setting, one should always obtain roentgenograms of the cervical spine when there is any evidence of head injury. In severe cervical trauma, a detailed *history* as to the mechanism of injury is critical. One must ask if the patient was unconscious, transiently numb or paralyzed in the arms or legs, or struck his head. Past history is important from the standpoint of pre-existing problems, such as cervical spondylosis, ruptured disks, or

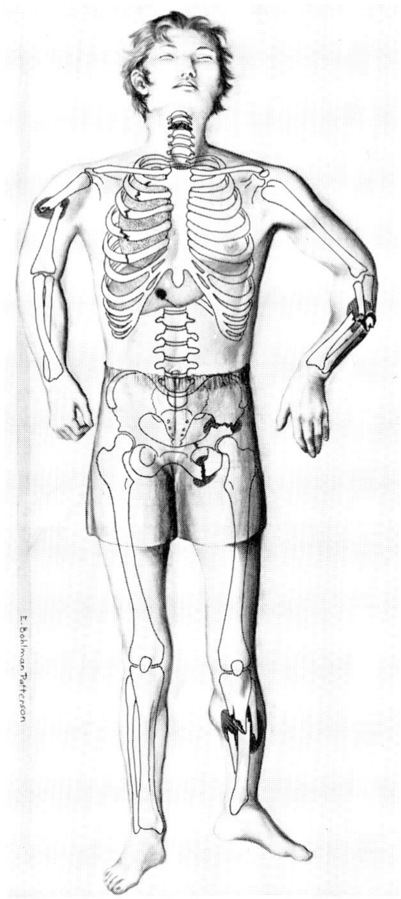

Fig. 6-60. The patient with multiple trauma is frequently in shock and will not complain of neck pain. Paralysis, if incomplete, may also be difficult to evaluate.

other injuries and neurologic diseases. The examining physician must ask the patient if he has neck pain. Intoxicated patients or those with head injury will not volunteer this information. Any patient complaining of neck pain or weakness of the arms or legs, with or without numbness, should be immediately suspected of having cervical spine or cord trauma and be immobilized with sand bags or head halter traction.

General *physical examination* is carried out with the patient in the supine position. One must examine the head for evidence of lacerations, bruises, and facial fractures. Ear canals are examined with an otoscope to rule out basilar skull fractures characterized by leaking spinal fluid. Gentle palpation of the posterior cervical spine reveals reaction to pain on the patient's part when a painful spinous process is touched. This may be very reliable in the face of alcoholic intoxication and decreased level of consciousness. It may also reveal a dislocation. The anterior cervical spine may be palpated via the "imaginary" anterior surgical approach.

Gentle rotation of the head occasionally elicits pain. The general attitude of the upper extremities may reveal flexed position of the elbows if there is loss of function below the biceps or extension of the elbows if the paralysis is at a higher level. Penile erection and incontinence of bladder or bowel all indicate severe spinal cord damage or compression.

Quadriplegia is usually quite obvious when one observes flaccid paralysis of the lower as well as some

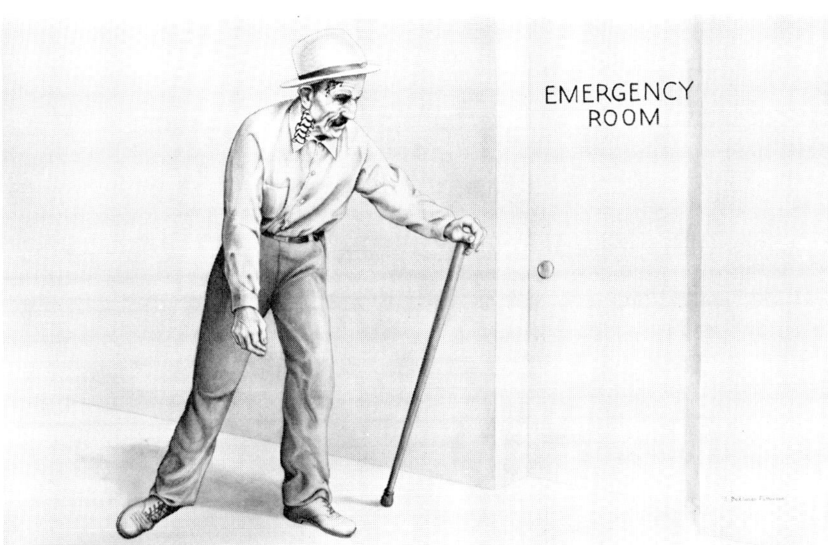

Fig. 6-61. Elderly patient with scalp laceration and unilateral facet dislocation may consequently have hemiparesis. This clinical pattern may be mistaken for a cerebrovascular episode.

weakness of the upper extremities. Vital signs initially may reveal a decreased blood pressure because of spinal cord shock. The pulse is not rapid as it is in hypovolemic shock from the blood loss, unless there is associated major trauma. The chest, abdomen, and extremities must be carefully examined for evidence of other injuries.

It should be strongly emphasized that initial physical and neurologic examination in the emergency room is the most crucial factor in a series of events that will comprise the acute as well as long-term treatment of patients with spinal cord injuries and, therefore, determine the prognosis.

Neurologic examination must be meticulous. The physician must look for any evidence of sensory or motor function sparing below the level of obvious quadriplegia.

Sensory examination is first carried out with a pin, beginning at the occiput, face, and neck, and working distally to examine particular dermatome distribution. Sensation may be normally sharp, oversensitive (hyperesthetic), decreased (hypesthetic), or dull (anesthetic) without any perception of a pin. Pinprick should be tested slowly with gentle pressure to avoid summation of impulses. The nipple line is T4 with T3 just above, and T2 extends across the chest to the axillae. First thoracic is along the inner forearm and arm. The next level above T2 is C4, beneath the clavicles. In quadriplegic patients there is usually a band of hypesthesia above the anesthetic level. Once a sensory level is established one must examine carefully the trunk, perineal areas, and distal extremities. It is of particular importance to look for any evidence of sacral sensory sparing in which case the diagnosis of an incomplete spinal cord injury is established. The only sparing of sensation distal to the obvious cervical level in a quadriplegic patient may be in the perianal region. Documentation of this fact may mean potential recovery of motor as well as sensory function. The skin is marked where sensation is present and then the examiner should proceed to the motor examination.

The physician must differentiate between complete versus incomplete quadriplegia and a pure nerve root lesion. A single herniated cervical disk or unilaterally dislocated facet may produce an isolated nerve root paralysis. There will be specific paralysis of biceps in the case of C5-6 disk protrusion or triceps paralysis with C6-7 protrusion.

Quadriplegia at the C3 level or above is infrequently seen because of immediate paralysis of the diaphragm and inability to breath independently. Active diaphragm, sternocleidomastoid, and trapezius muscles indicate C4 level of function. Deltoid and biceps function can occur if C5 level is intact. Active supination and wrist extension indicate that the C6 nerve root level is intact. Functioning pronator teres, flexor carpi radialis, triceps, and finger extensors, all document C7 level function. Flexor digitorum sublimi or profundi function are evidence of C8 level, and intrinsic function is T1 level.

Following examination of the upper extremities, the torso and lower extremities should be tested for any voluntary contractions. It is very important to look for evidence of sacral motor sparing, which consists of voluntary, rectal sphincter, or toe flexor contractions. If present, this indicates sparing of corticospinal tract function, and the prognosis is good for recovery of motor function.

Rectal examination is important to verify complete versus incomplete spinal cord injury. If a patient can feel a gloved finger on rectal examination or perianal pinprick, then an incomplete cord lesion can be documented. Also if voluntary contraction of the rectal sphincter is present, this adds proof of incomplete paralysis.

Reflexes must be documented in the patient with an acute spinal cord injury. Flexion withdrawal of the legs following pinprick stimulation does not indicate voluntary motion. Usually the paralyzed patient is areflexic when initially testing deep tendon reflexes. This is the period of spinal cord shock. If clonus or a positive Babinski reflex is present in an incomplete cord injury, this may indicate spinal cord compression from dislocation or disk protrusion. Spinal cord shock rarely lasts more than 24 hours. A patient must be tested for the bulbocavernosus reflex. This is elicited by tugging on the urethral catheter, squeezing the glans penis, or applying pressure on the clitoris, which will in turn cause contraction of the rectal sphincter. A positive bulbocavernosus reflex indicates that the spinal shock is over. If at that time there has been no documentation of motor or sensory function below the cervical paralytic level, then the patient can be diagnosed as having a complete spinal cord injury, and no recovery in the trunk or lower extremities is expected.

Spinal Cord Lesions

Determination of whether a patient has complete or incomplete cord injury is important in the overall prognosis of the patient and cannot be overemphasized. This should be determined with few exceptions within the first 48 hours by the previously mentioned criteria.

By definition an incomplete spinal cord injury is one in which there is sparing of some motor or sensory function distal to the level of cord injury. Incomplete spinal cord injuries may be a Brown-Sequard syndrome, central cord syndrome, anterior cord syndrome, or rarely, a monoparesis of the upper extremity.

The Brown-Sequard syndrome is an injury to either half of the spinal cord producing ipsilateral motor paralysis, and contralateral hypesthesia to pain and temperature. This offers good prognosis for recovery of motor and sensory function.

The central cord syndrome is an injury to the central area of the spinal cord, both gray and white matter, affecting most severely the centrally located arm tracts in the corticospinal area and to a lesser extent the leg tracts. The patient presents with a quadriparesis involving upper extremities to a greater degree than the lower. The sensory sparing may be variable, but usually there is sacral pinprick preservation (Fig. 6-62). These patients may show immediate partial recovery after being placed in skull traction. Depending on the amount of edema centrally versus the amount of cord contusion, the prognosis is good for recovery of leg, bladder, and bowel function. Arms and hands recover to varying degrees. There are two mechanisms of injury that produce central cord quadriparesis. First, the older spondylitic patient sustains a blow to the face or forehead, hyperextending the neck. This buckles the posterior ligamentum flavum posteriorly and pinches the cord

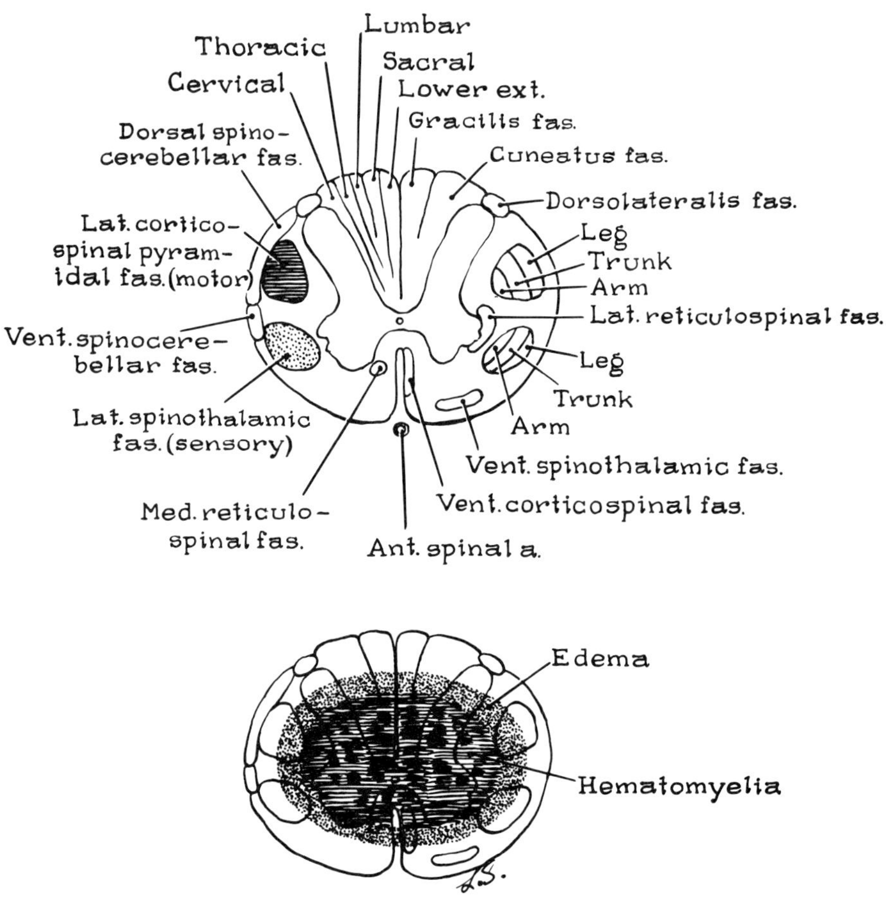

Fig. 6-62. Diagram of the central cord syndrome. Centrally placed tracts are affected by central edema or necrosis. Note the most medial portion of the pyramidal tract is for arm function. The upper extremity paralysis is therefore greater than the lower extremity.

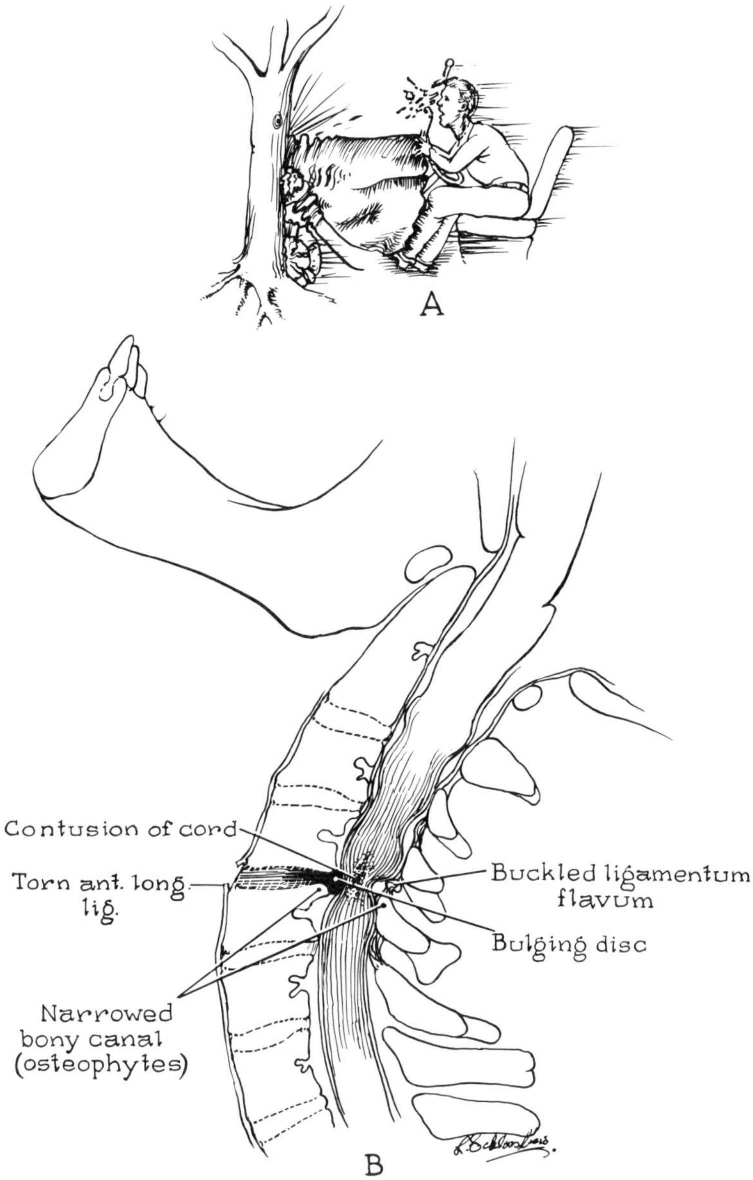

Fig. 6-63. (*A*) Frontal head injury, producing hyperextension with cervical spondylosis. (*B*) Note the ligamentum flavum buckles inwardly against the posterior spinal cord while the bulging disk compresses the cord anteriorly. The combined forces contuse the cord. The disk is also disrupted.

against the posterior vertebral osteophytes anteriorly (Fig. 6-63). The second mechanism is the younger patient with a flexion injury.

The anterior cord syndrome is an injury or ischemia of the anterior two-thirds of the spinal cord indicated by a quadriplegia with the lower extremities completely paralyzed with lesser weakness of the arms. The posterior columns are spared to varying degrees. There is preservation of proprioception, touch, deep pressure, and sacral sparing. Prognosis is good for recovery if after the first 24 hours there is toe function, good preservation of posterior columns, and sacral sparing. The mechanism of injury here is a flexion injury with bone or disk fragments compressing the anterior spinal artery and cord (Fig. 6-64).

The complete cord syndrome is manifested by total motor and sensory loss distal to the level of injury. If after 24 hours the patient has had no return of sacral sensation or motor function and the bulbocavernosus reflex is positive, then the patient will be permanently and completely paralyzed. The positive bulbocavernosus reflex indicates cessation of spinal

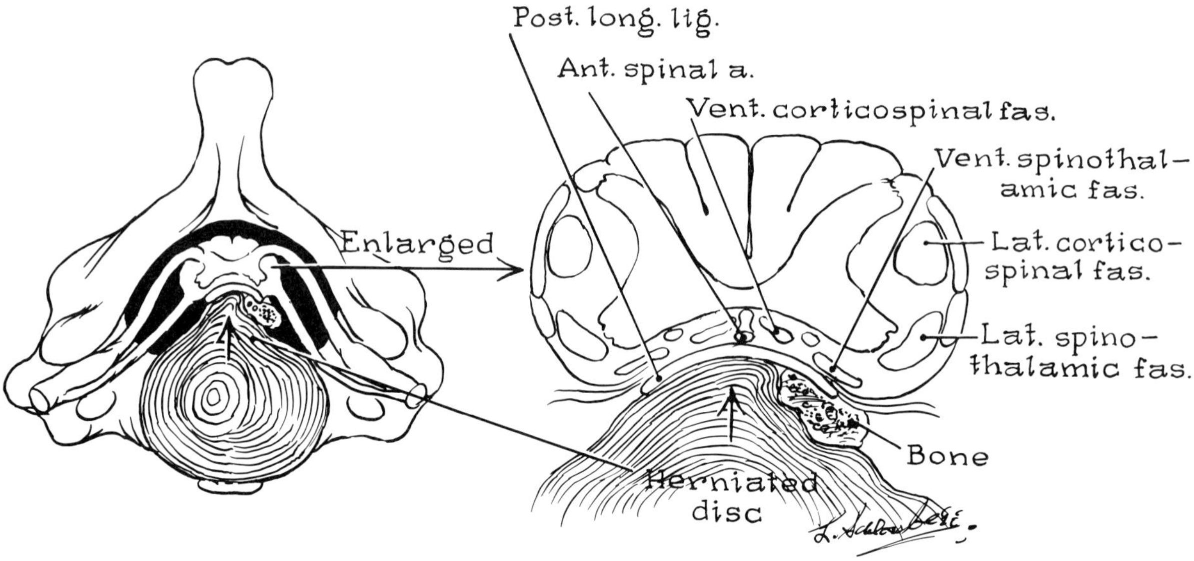

Fig. 6-64. Diagram of the anterior cord syndrome. A herniated disk or bone fragment compresses the anterior spinal artery and cord. This may produce ischemia of the anterior two-thirds of the cord, sparing posterior column function (touch, position, and vibratory senses).

shock and return of local spinal cord reflex activity. This patient will only regain root function in the upper extremities but no leg function. It should be mentioned here that a patient may have complete quadriplegia without fracture dislocation or disk herniation especially if there is a congenitally narrowed spinal canal.

The spinal fluid dynamics can be tested in the patient with an acute spinal cord injury, but do not relate to the prognosis and should not be the criteria for surgery. Complete block versus incomplete block on the Queckenstedt test does not give any indication of the potential for recovery of function. Only in a general way does the positive Queckenstedt test relate more commonly to a complete cord injury and the negative test to the incomplete cord lesion. The test is performed by doing a puncture of the lumbar spine and when pressure is applied to both jugular veins in the neck, spinal fluid in the manometer should rise and fall freely. If the spinal fluid level does not rise rapidly or fall, this indicates obstruction to flow of spinal fluid in the subarachnoid space and a positive Queckenstedt test.

Once a cervical spine injury is suspected in the emergency room, the patient is immediately placed in head halter traction and appropriate radiologic studies performed. The initial neurologic examination may give a clue to the expected level of spinal trauma. The entire cervical spine and first thoracic vertebra must be visualized by various roentgenographic studies. The most frequently missed significant fractures on roentgenograms are those of the odontoid process and at the C7 or T1 levels. Initially, anteroposterior and lateral films are made. Then, if C7 is not visualized, the arms are pulled down by the physician, and at the same time the patient is asked to relax his shoulders. A swimmer's view can be obtained to adequately visualize the C7-T1 levels. This is carried out by abducting one arm 180 degrees, with the other held down at the patient's side. The roentgen cassette is held against the abducted side, and the beam is directed laterally at the C7 level. Distorted oblique films are taken without turning the patient. This is done by placing the cassette under the patient's neck and shoulder, slightly to the side of the facets. The roentgen beam is then directed at a 45 degree angle laterally and 10 degrees cephalad to visualize the foramina. This procedure is repeated from the other side. Oblique films are necessary to determine the nature of the pathology in the posterior elements. The anteroposterior view should be angled cephalad 20 degrees to visualize the vertebral bodies and joints of Luschka for compression fractures. Lateral displacement of one spinous process on another in the anteroposterior view indicates rotation of one vertebra on another, such as a unilateral facet dislocation. An open-mouth odontoid view should also be obtained.

Usually a single lateral roentgenogram of the cervical spine is sufficient to initiate the diagnosis of fracture or dislocation. One of the following conditions will be evident: slight 1 to 3 mm. posterior subluxation of the upper vertebra on the lower one (Fig. 6-65); moderate 3 to 5 mm. anterior subluxation of the upper vertebra on the lower one (Fig. 6-66); or 5 mm. or greater maximal anterior dislocation (Fig. 6-67). Slight posterior subluxation usually occurs with extension injuries in cervical spondylosis where there is a crack through the disk space. This may be very subtle. Moderate anterior subluxation on the lateral roentgenogram indicates a unilateral facet dislocation, a unilateral facet fracture, or bilaterally "perched" facets (Fig. 6-68). These entities may cause incomplete quadriparesis or nerve root compression.

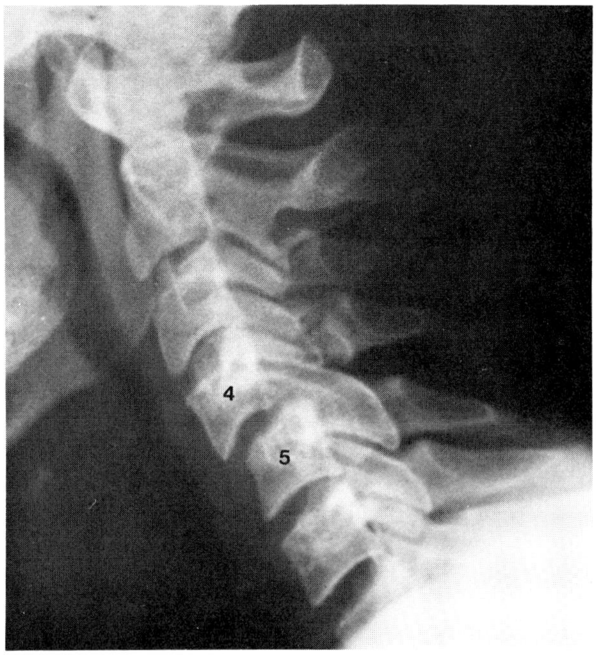

Fig. 6-66. Lateral roentgenogram from a patient with moderate (5 mm. or greater) anterior subluxation of C4 or C5. Oblique views must be taken to determine the exact posterior element pathology.

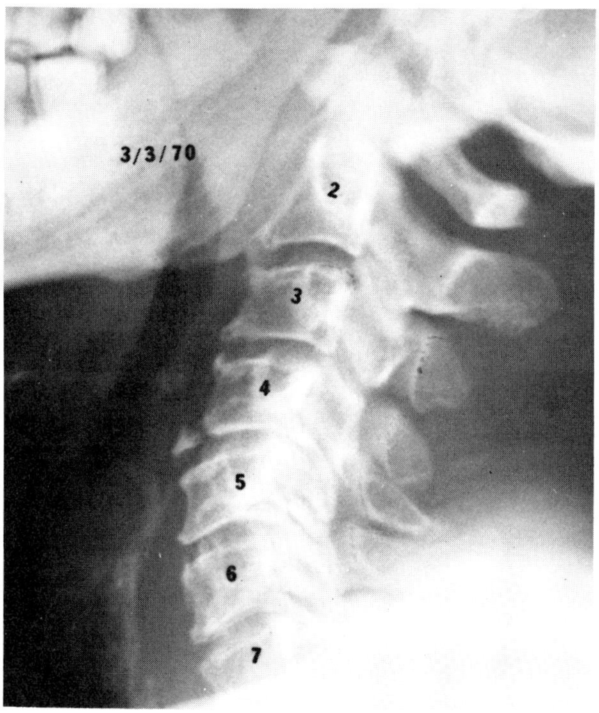

Fig. 6-65. Lateral cervical spine roentgenogram in a totally quadriplegic patient at the C5 level. Note the slight posterior subluxation of C4 on C5. Avulsion fracture of the anterior, inferior body of C4 indicates a hyperextension injury. This corresponds to the diagram in Fig. 6-63.

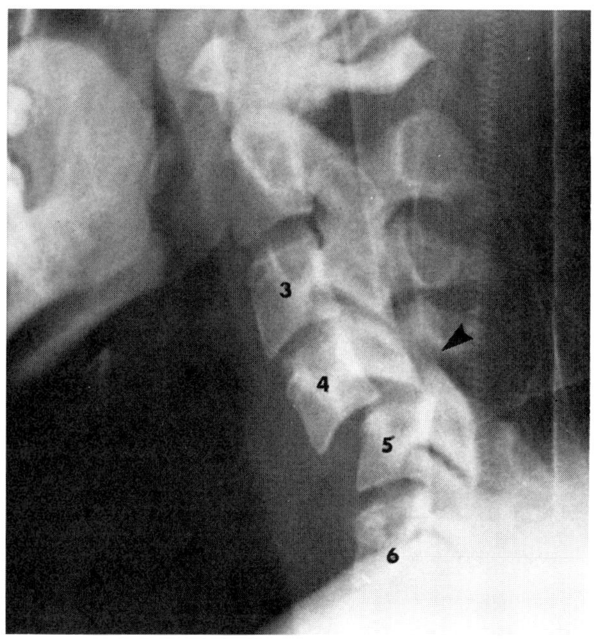

Fig. 6-67. Roentgenogram from a patient with maximal anterior dislocation. There is complete bilateral facet dislocation of C4 on C5 with complete quadriplegia.

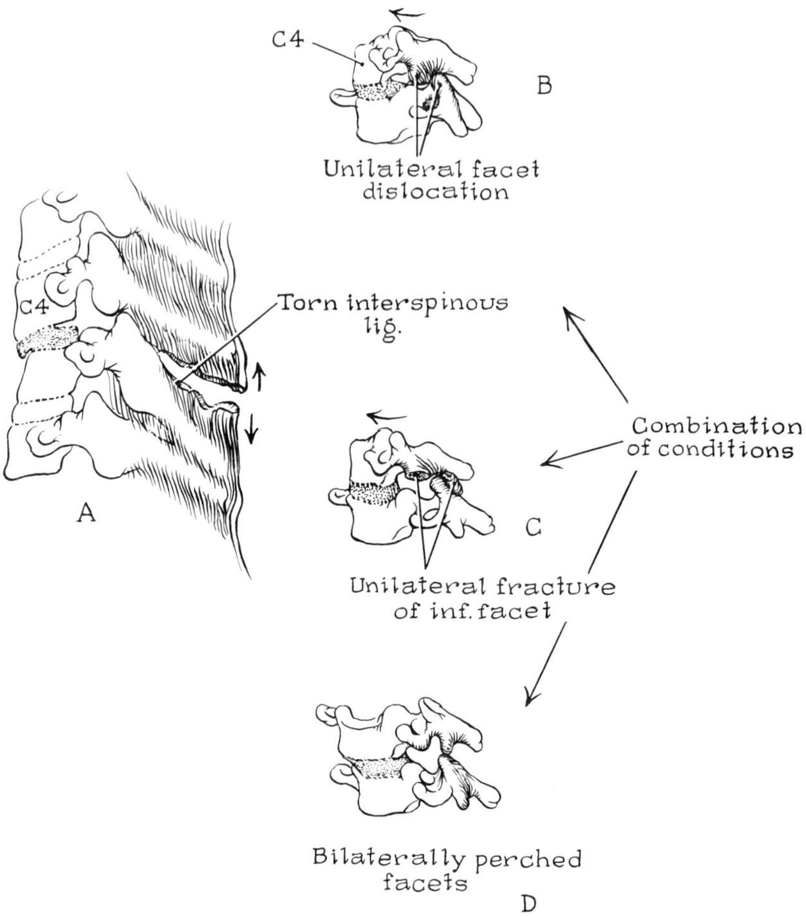

Fig. 6-68. Diagram of moderate anterior subluxation (*A*). The causes are (*B*) unilateral facet dislocation, (*C*) unilaterally fractured facet, and (*D*) bilaterally "perched" facets.

Maximal anterior dislocation indicates complete bilaterally dislocated facets and usually is associated with complete quadriplegia. The above radiologic interpretation is important in determining the type of fracture, and, therefore, the treatment approach.

Fractures of the laminae are frequently missed because they are not visualized well on routine views. The Abel view, performed in the anteroposterior plane angling the beam 30 degrees caudad, is very difficult to do in the acute situation. Also, fractures of the laminae are not important clinically because they do not compress the spinal cord. Pillar views can be taken to rule out lateral mass fractures.

Laminography may be helpful in determining lateral mass atlas fractures as well as odontoid and pedicle fractures. If the patient demonstrates no fractures or dislocations on routine roentgenograms, then gentle, controlled flexion-extension views may be obtained with the patient in cervical traction. These may demonstrate slight subluxation of the vertebrae or spreading of the interspinous space posteriorly, indicating the level of injury.

Air or panopaque myelography may be of benefit in acute spinal cord injury or later in the course of the patient's treatment to determine the possibility of herniated disk or protruding bone fragments which may be compressing the anterior cord surface. The patient must be protected from untoward manipulation by cervical traction if it is to be done in the acute situation. The finding of complete block is no indication to do surgery and may only be a result of spinal cord edema. More important is the demonstration of an incomplete block, with a protruding bone or disk fragment in a patient with an incomplete spinal cord injury. In this situation early anterior decompression may be of great benefit, in the author's opinion. Myelography should not be performed if the spinal fluid is grossly bloody or the patient has a complete cord injury. In younger patients sustaining flexion injuries, the causes of cord damage are protruding disk or bone fragments against the anterior cord surface secondary to compression fractures.

Fractures and dislocations of the cervical spine may be classified according to spinal levels as listed in Table 6-4. An understanding of cervical spine trauma must involve knowledge of the mechanisms of injury as well as the radiologic appearances of various fractures, dislocations, or subluxations. One must be specific in description to be accurate in diagnosis. Subluxation of a joint indicates abnormal position or motion, and dislocation indicates total incongruity of the articular surfaces, without bony apposition.

Table 6-4. Fracture-Dislocations of the Cervical Spine

I. Atlanto-occipital dislocations
   - Anterior
   - Posterior

II. Isolated fractures of the atlas
   - Posterior arch
   - Anterior arch
   - Both (Jefferson fracture)
   - Lateral mass compression fracture

III. Atlantoaxial dislocations without fracture
   - Anterior
   - Posterior
   - Rotary

IV. Atlantoaxial fractures and dislocations
   - Anterior with odontoid fracture
   - Posterior with odontoid fracture
   - Pedicle fracture of axis

V. Lower cervical spine fractures and dislocations (C3-C7)
   - A. Posterior elements
     - Unilateral facet dislocation
     - Bilateral facet dislocations
     - Bilateral perched facets
     - Fractured facets
     - Spinous process fracture (clay shoveler's fracture)
     - Laminae fractures
   - B. Anterior elements
     - Compression fracture of vertebral body without displacement
     - Compression fracture of vertebral body with displacement
     - Avulsion fracture
     - Fracture through disk space (spondylitic)
   - C. Lateral elements
     - Lateral mass fracture

VI. Gunshot wounds

Atlanto-occipital Dislocations

It is rare that a person sustains severe enough trauma to have an atlanto-occipital dislocation and survive. There are three reported cases in the literature of anterior dislocation, (Fig. 6-69) and the author has seen and treated one case of posterior atlanto-occipital dislocation with survival (Fig. 6-70). In a study of fatal craniospinal pathology by the author and Davis, a major portion of the spinal injuries were between the occiput and C3. Major ligamentous tearing must occur to produce these injuries. This includes disruption of the alar and apical ligaments, the tectorial membrane, and posterior

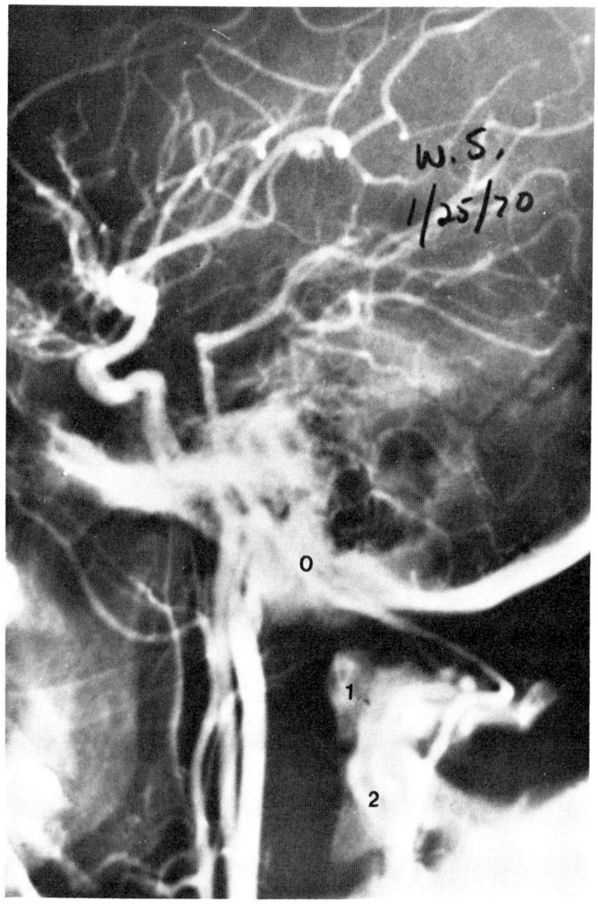

Fig. 6-69. Arteriogram from a pedestrian who was struck by an automobile, sustaining an anterior dislocation of the occiput on the atlas. Arteriography was performed because the patient was comatose. Note forward displacement of the occipital condyles on the C1-2 complex. The patient died 48 hours after injury.

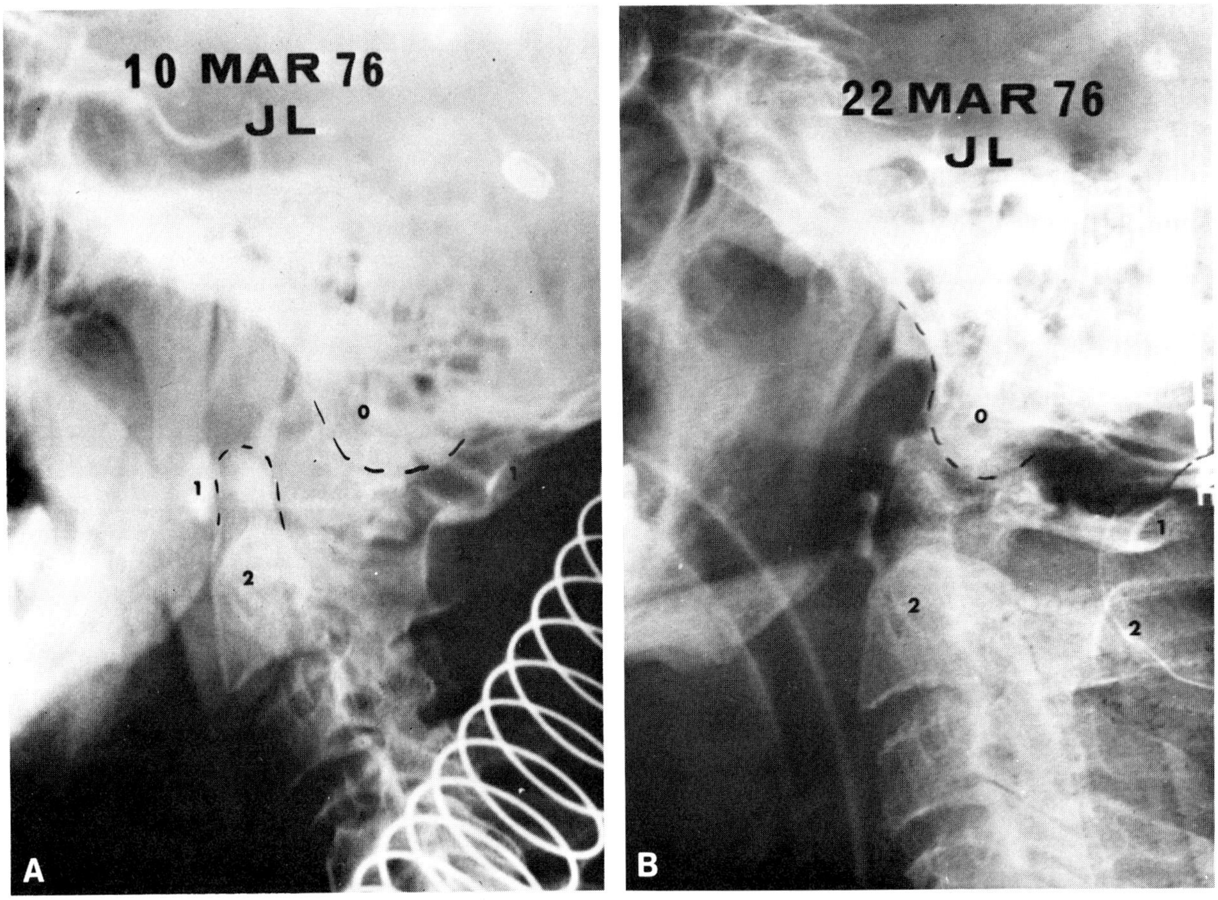

Fig. 6-70. Posterior dislocation of the occiput on the atlas, with survival. (*A*) Note the occipital condyles being displaced with a fractured posterior arch of C1. Patient had episodes of respiratory distress and was on a respirator. (*B*) Atlanto-occipital dislocation reduced with gentle tong traction in flexion. Patient was later placed in a halo cast and posterior occiput to C3 fusion performed.

atlanto-occipital ligaments. The mechanism of injury can be flexion or extension. There may be vertebral artery compression as well as spinal cord compression above the level of decussation of the arm pyramidal tracts producing the so called "cruciate paralysis" described by Bell. This involves upper extremity weakness and various cranial nerve palsies without sensory loss.

Isolated Fractures of the Atlas

Fractures of the atlas may occur by vertical force applied to the head, with or without flexion-extension. Fractures may occur as isolated entities at the thinnest aspects of both the anterior and posterior arch. Fracture of the posterior arch requires an extension force applied to the head, and anterior arch fractures are usually associated with axial load as well as flexion. When there is a severe blow to the head, such as in falling or being struck on the head in an auto accident, the axial force is transmitted to the occipital condyles, down to the articulation of the atlas at the lateral masses. The centrifugal force applied to the wedge-shaped lateral masses forces expansion, and the atlas fractures anteriorly at two points as well as posteriorly at two weaker points near the grooves for the vertebral arteries. This "blow-out" fracture is also called the *Jefferson fracture.* There is usually no neurologic deficit associated because there is no neural tissue compression. Diagnosis of the Jefferson fracture is made by open

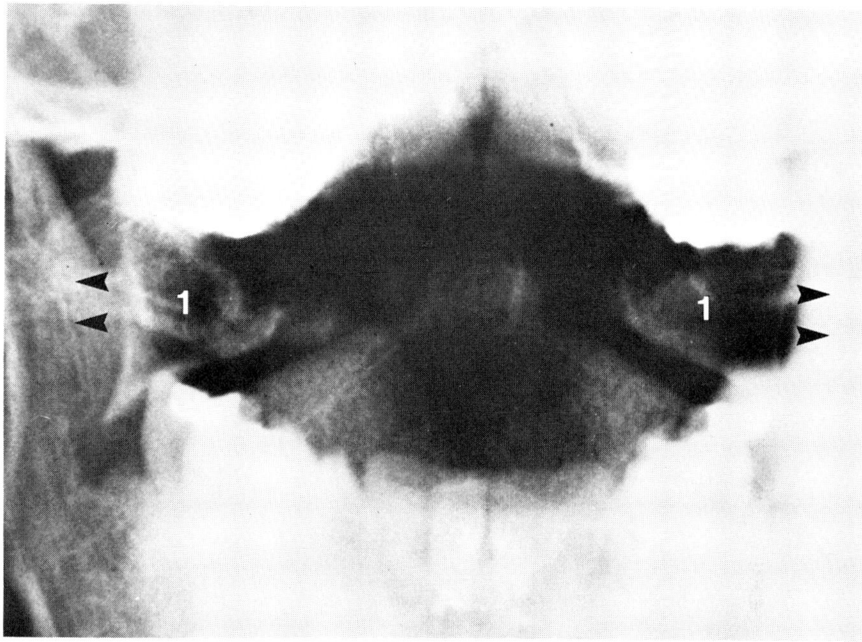

Fig. 6-71. Jefferson fracture of the atlas with bilateral lateral displacement of the lateral masses of the atlas in relationship to the odontoid process.

mouth odontoid view, when the lateral masses are both symmetrically displaced laterally beyond the borders of the vertebral body of the axis (Fig. 6-71). Fractures of either arch of the atlas are recognized by the same view or by lateral roentgenograms and tomography if necessary. Occasionally the axial force applied to the head will not be severe enough to cause a Jefferson fracture but will compress the lateral masses (Fig. 6-72). These patients complain of pain on lateral rotation of the head as well as crepitus and "cracking" with rotation. Anteroposterior tomography may be necessary to confirm the diagnosis on routine roentgenograms.

Atlantoaxial Dislocations

Atlantoaxial dislocations may occur without fractures. Anterior dislocation is a result of rupturing the strong transverse ligament by a flexion injury (Fig. 6-73). Dislocation may occur with congenitally dysplastic or small odontoid processes following trauma (Fig. 6-74.) Posterior dislocation of the atlas on the odontoid process can occur but is rare and usually does not rupture the transverse ligament. Instead, the alar ligaments are avulsed from the occipital condyles (Fig. 6-75). Atlantoaxial dislocations may produce neural compression with paralysis or sudden death. The fixed odontoid process produces anterior cord compression and the posterior arch of the atlas, posterior spinal cord compression. Chronic dislocations may produce signs of progressive myelopathy with spasticity, ataxia, and extremity weakness (Fig. 6-76).

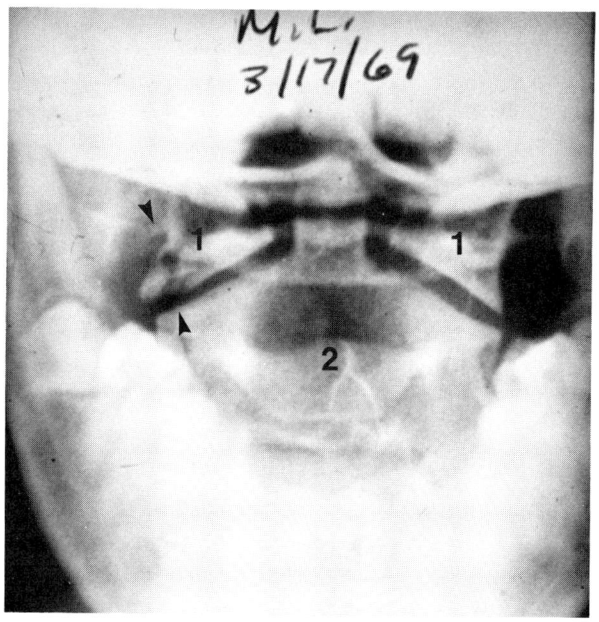

Fig. 6-72. Fractured lateral mass of the atlas.

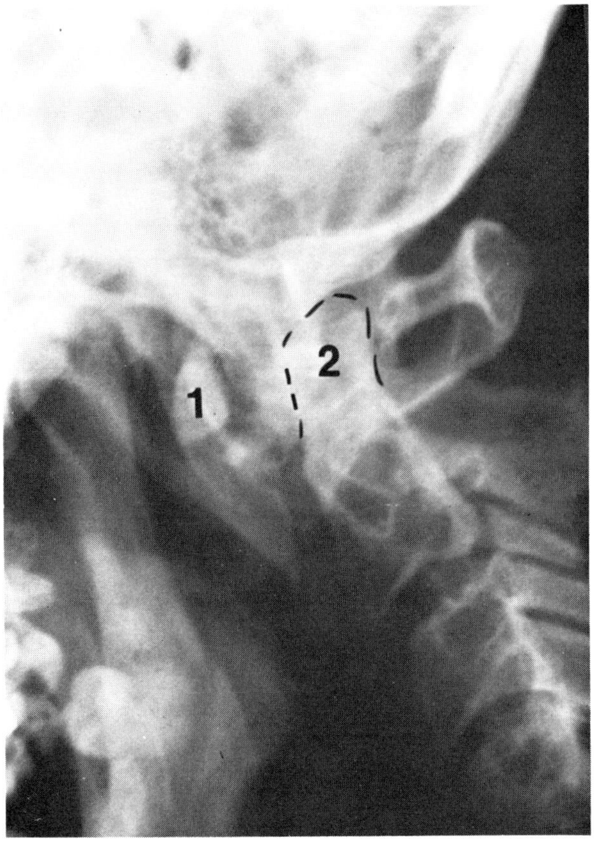

Fig. 6-73. Roentgenogram from the driver of a milk truck which was struck by a train. Anterior dislocation of the axis on the atlas without fracture. This is evidence of a ruptured transverse ligament.

Rotary dislocations of the atlas on the axis may occur with trauma but are usually associated with cervical inflammatory disease in children.

Atlantoaxial Fractures and Dislocations

Atlantoaxial dislocations may occur with a fractured odontoid process which is anteriorly displaced, most commonly (Fig. 6-77). The mechanism of injury is severe flexion or a posterior force applied to the head. Much rarer is the posterior fracture dislocation of C1-2 (Fig. 6-78). In both instances the transverse ligament remains intact and carries the fractured odontoid process with the atlas dislocation. Neural compression is less apt to occur when the odontoid process is fractured than when it is fixed.

Fractures of the odontoid process in adults occur in two different planes. They may occur through the

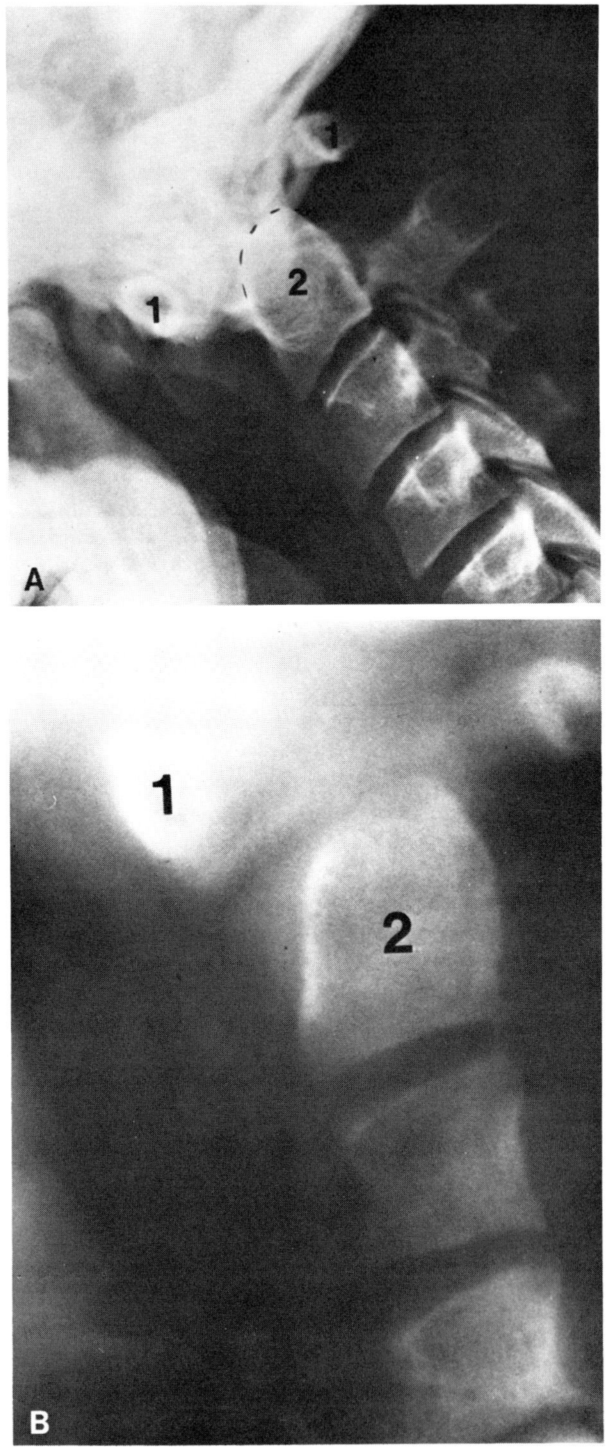

Fig. 6-74. Atlantoaxial dislocation diagnosed by roentgenogram taken following an auto accident. (*A*) Note hypoplastic odontoid process. (*B*) Lateral tomogram demonstrating hypoplastic odontoid process.

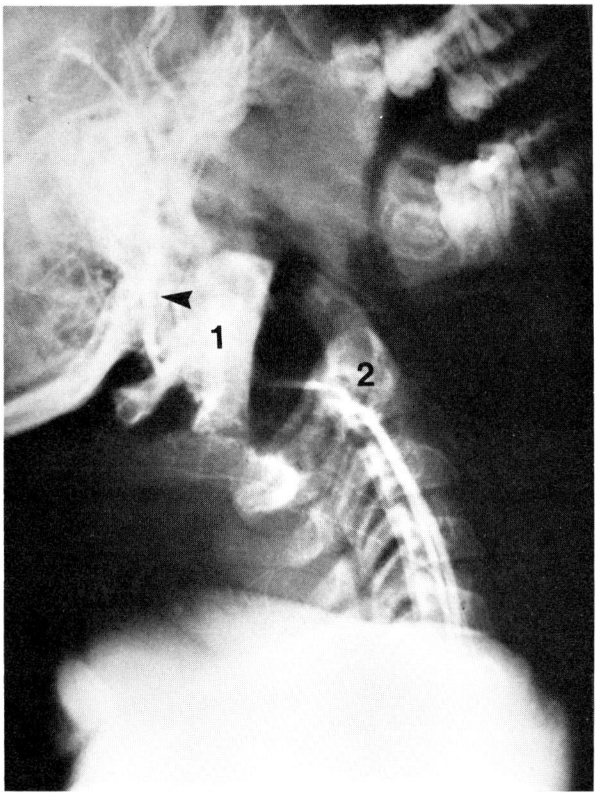

Fig. 6-75. Autopsy roentgenogram of child struck by a car, resulting in secondary posterior atlantoaxial dislocation.

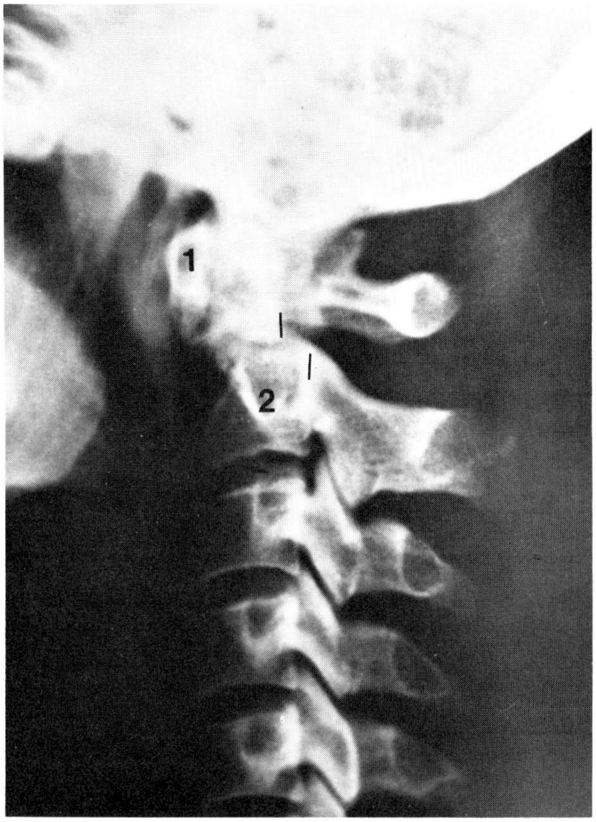

Fig. 6-77. Fractured odontoid process with anterior displacement. The transverse ligament remains intact and carries the odontoid forward with the axis.

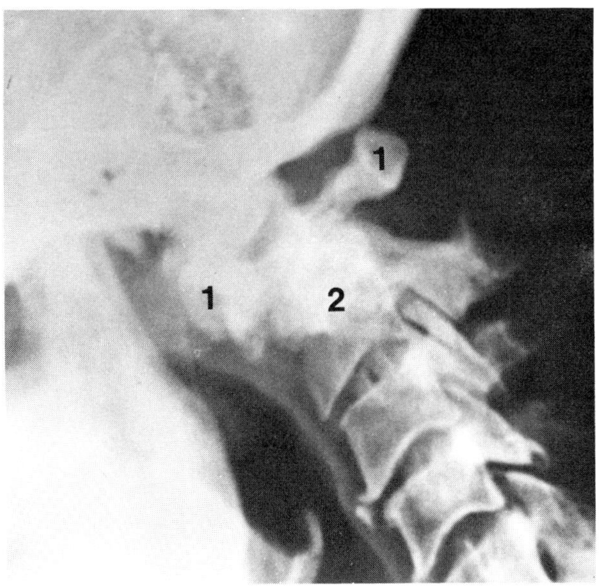

Fig. 6-76. Chronic, fixed anterior dislocation of the atlas on the axis with myelopathy following trauma.

waist of the odontoid process in which case healing is difficult (Fig. 6-79), or the odontoid may also fracture obliquely down into the body of the axis where medullary bone heals well with proper immobilization.

Pedicle fractures of the axis occur as a result of hyperextension of the head on the neck. The occiput is forced down against the posterior arch of the atlas, which in turn is forced against the pedicle of C2. With a flexion component added there may be disruption of the disk and ligaments between C2 and C3 with forward subluxation of these vertebral bodies. Because of the relatively great amount of room in the spinal canal at this level, there rarely are neurologic signs with this fracture. The fracture of the pedicles of C2 has been called the "hangman's fracture" (Fig. 6-80). Lateral tomography of the axis may be of benefit in diagnosing nondisplaced pedicle fractures.

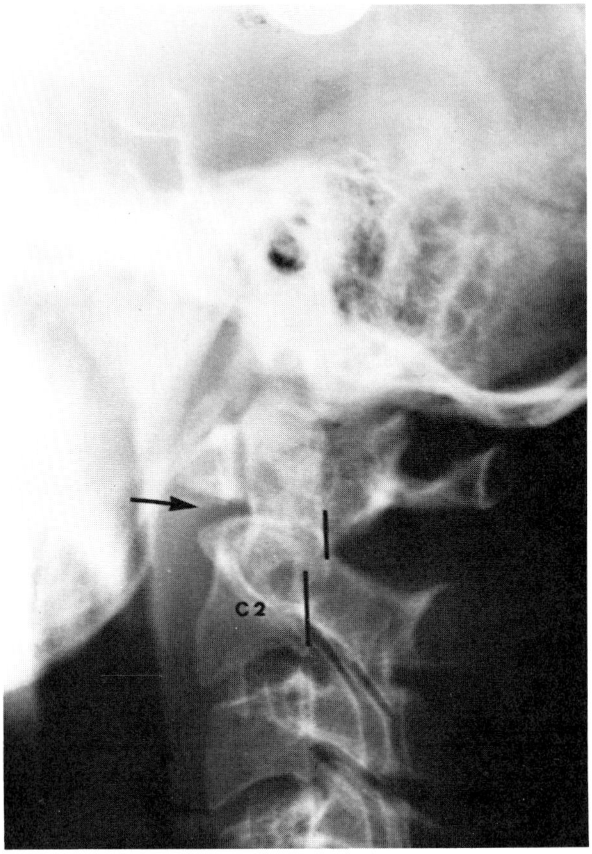

Fig. 6-78. Fractured odontoid process with posterior displacement. The transverse ligament remains intact.

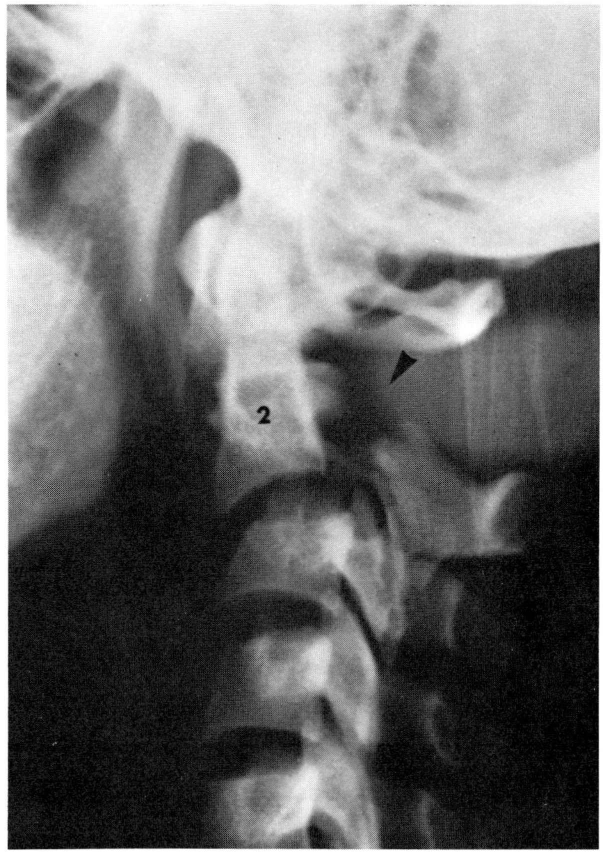

Fig. 6-80. Lateral roentgenogram of bilateral pedicle fracture of the axis. Note subluxation of C2 on C3 with probable disk and ligament disruption.

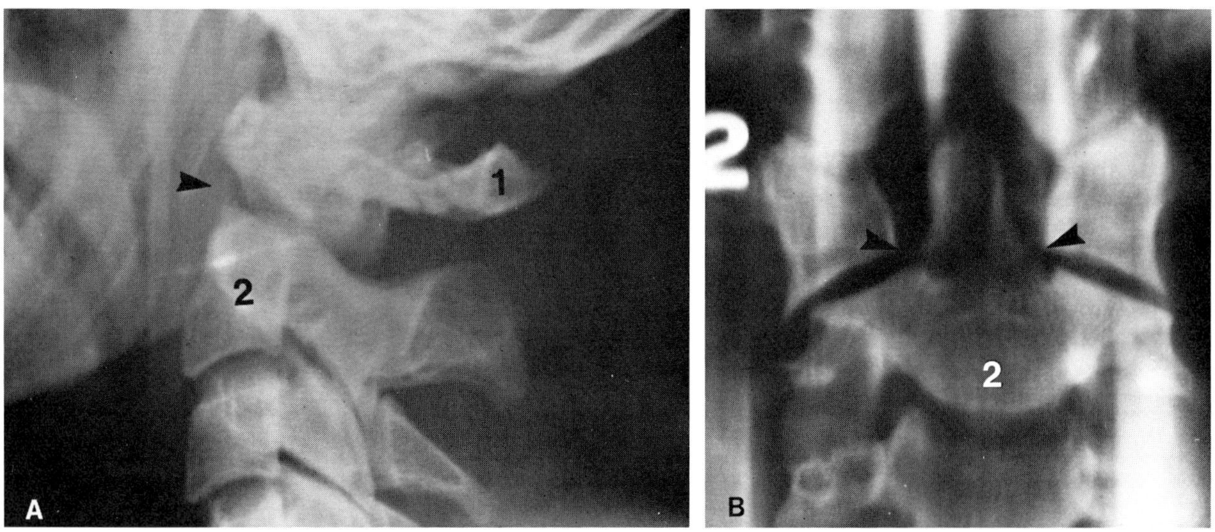

Fig. 6-79. (*A*) Lateral view of fracture through the waist of the odontoid. (*B*) Anteroposterior tomogram of odontoid fracture through the waist of C2.

Lower Cervical Spine Fractures and Dislocations

Posterior Elements. *Unilateral facet dislocations* result from flexion-rotation forces applied to the neck. Tearing of the facet joint capsule and posterior ligament complex occurs. These fractures are stable but may compress the nerve roots, creating an isolated upper extremity muscle paralysis, or produce a unilateral spinal cord compression with a Brown-Sequard syndrome. On the anteroposterior roentgenogram, the spinous processes are displaced laterally to midline above the dislocation. Oblique views confirm the diagnosis. Lateral views reveal moderate anterior subluxation of the vertebral bodies.

Bilateral facet dislocations are a result of severe flexion forces and usually are associated with severe neurologic deficit or complete quadriplegia secondary to spinal cord damage. The facet capsules are torn as well as the posterior ligament complex. The intervertebral disk is disrupted, and the anterior longitudinal ligament usually remains intact. Lateral roentgenogram reveals marked displacement of the vertebral bodies one-half their width or greater. Oblique views reveal the dislocated facets. Dislocated facets may also be associated with fractured facets (Fig. 6-81).

Bilateral "perched" facets (tip-to-tip) occur as a result of pure flexion force where the posterior liga-

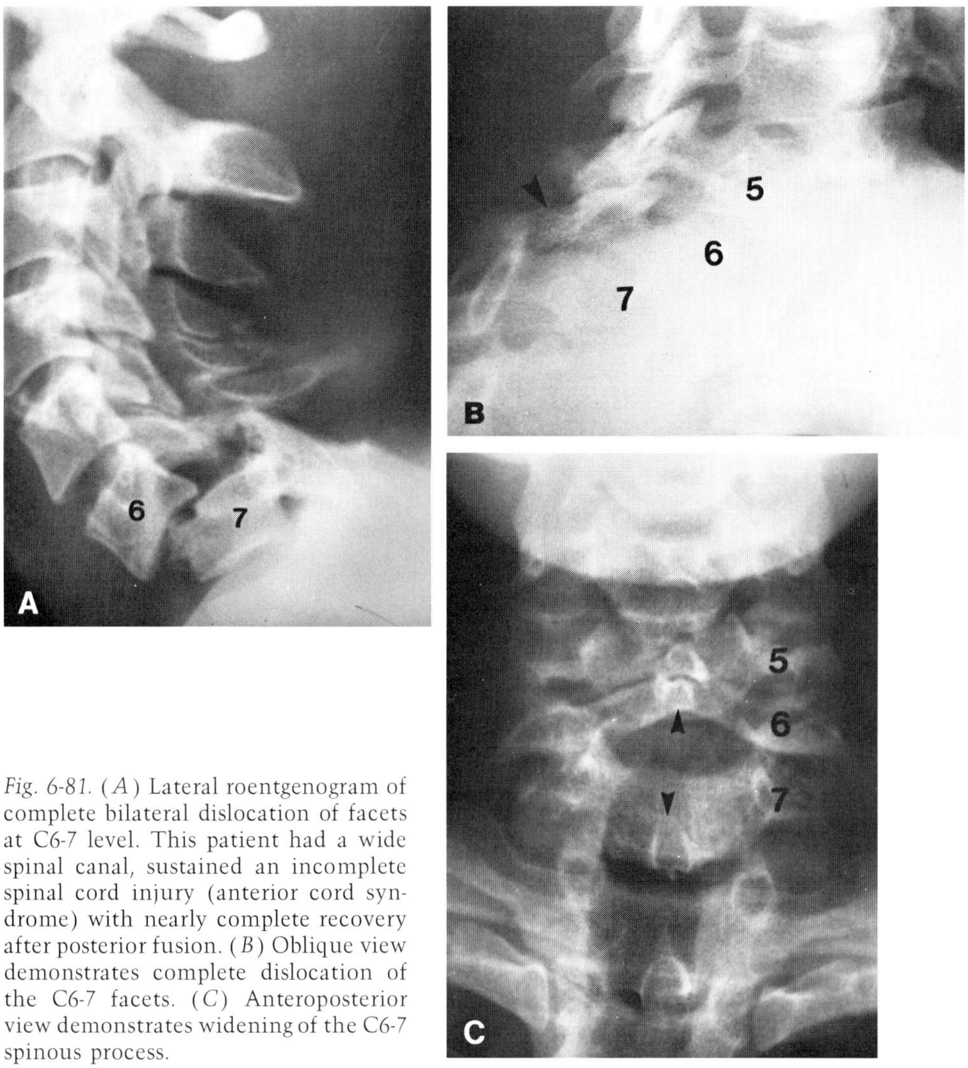

Fig. 6-81. (*A*) Lateral roentgenogram of complete bilateral dislocation of facets at C6-7 level. This patient had a wide spinal canal, sustained an incomplete spinal cord injury (anterior cord syndrome) with nearly complete recovery after posterior fusion. (*B*) Oblique view demonstrates complete dislocation of the C6-7 facets. (*C*) Anteroposterior view demonstrates widening of the C6-7 spinous process.

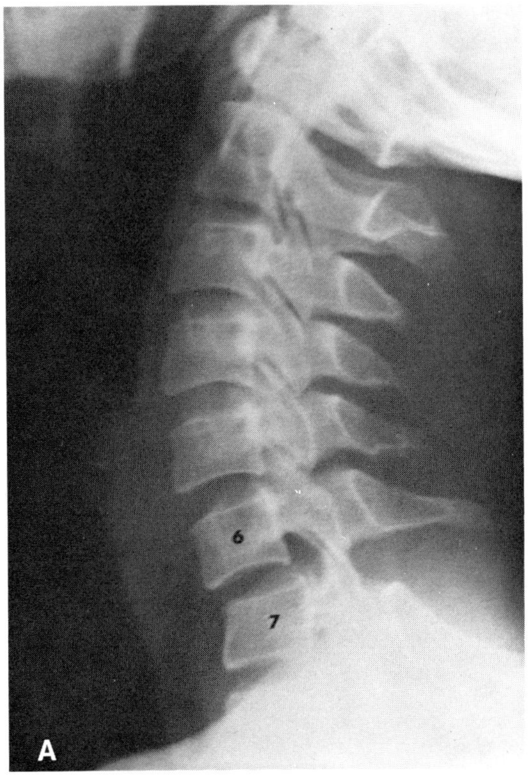

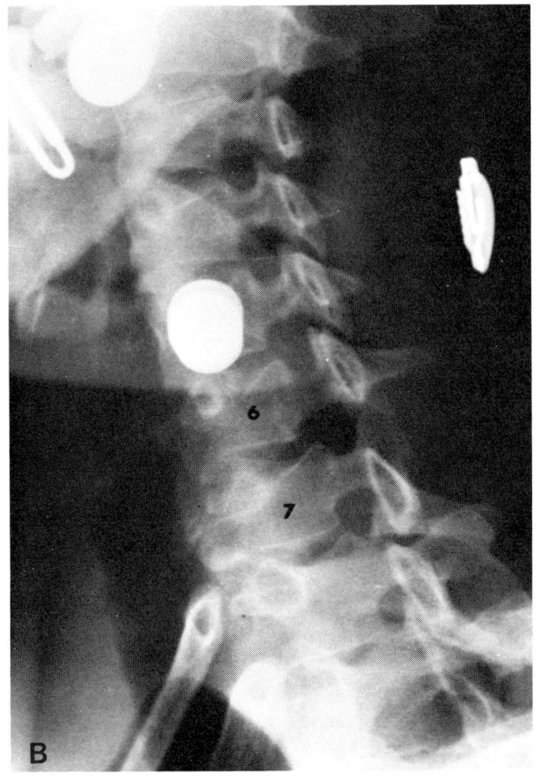

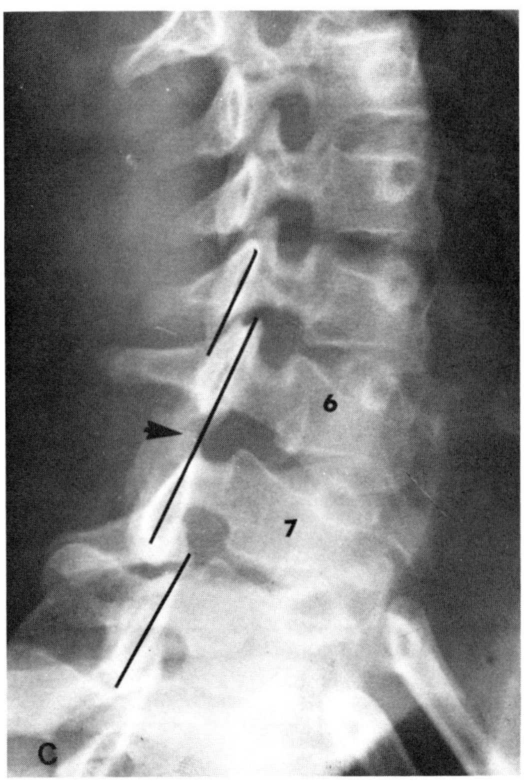

Fig. 6-82. (*A*) Lateral roentgenogram of subluxation of C6 on C7. Note slight anterior displacement of C6 vertebra. There is widening of the interspinous space posteriorly indicating a torn interspinous ligament. (*B*) Oblique view revealing "perched" C6-7 facets. The tips of the laminar cortices oppose each other instead of overlapping. (*C*) Diagnosis of "perched" facets is made by drawing lines through the laminar cortices. Normally these lines overlap (C5-6) (C7-T1), but at C6-7 they intersect.

ment complex tears. Usually there is no associated neurologic deficit except for a possible single root paralysis. Lateral roentgenograms reveal spreading of the interspinous space and angular anterior subluxation of the upper vertebra on the lower one. Oblique views confirm the tip-to-tip position of the laminar cortices and facets. Ordinarily, parallel lines drawn through the laminar cortices on the oblique views will overlap like shingles on a roof. If they intersect at one level, the facets are "perched" (Fig. 6-82).

Fractured facets may occur as an isolated entity with flexion-rotation forces applied to the cervical spine. This fracture may compress the nerve root in the foramina and produce a single muscle paralysis. Lateral roentgenograms reveal slight forward subluxation of the vertebral bodies, and oblique views confirm the diagnosis (Fig. 6-83).

Fractures of the spinous processes may result from strenuous muscle exertion which avulses a portion of the spinous process. This is the "clay shoveler's fracture." These may be identified by lateral roentgenograms of the cervical spine.

Fractures of the laminae are commonly missed on routine films of the cervical spine because of the 30 degree angle of their inclination. These fractures do not compress the neural structures but remain free-floating in an acute injury.

Anterior Elements. *Anterior element fractures* between C3 and C7 are usually caused by flexion forces. The vertebral body may be mildly compressed without posterior displacement following a flexion injury. These fractures may be associated with disk disruption or protrusion causing diskogenic pain or nerve root compression by a disk fragment. Tomography may be necessary to identify compression fractures of the vertebrae with depression of the bony end plates (Fig. 6-84). A *flexion injury* may result in an isolated posteriorly herniated disk with anterior spinal cord compression (Fig. 6-85).

Axial loading with flexion produces the more se-

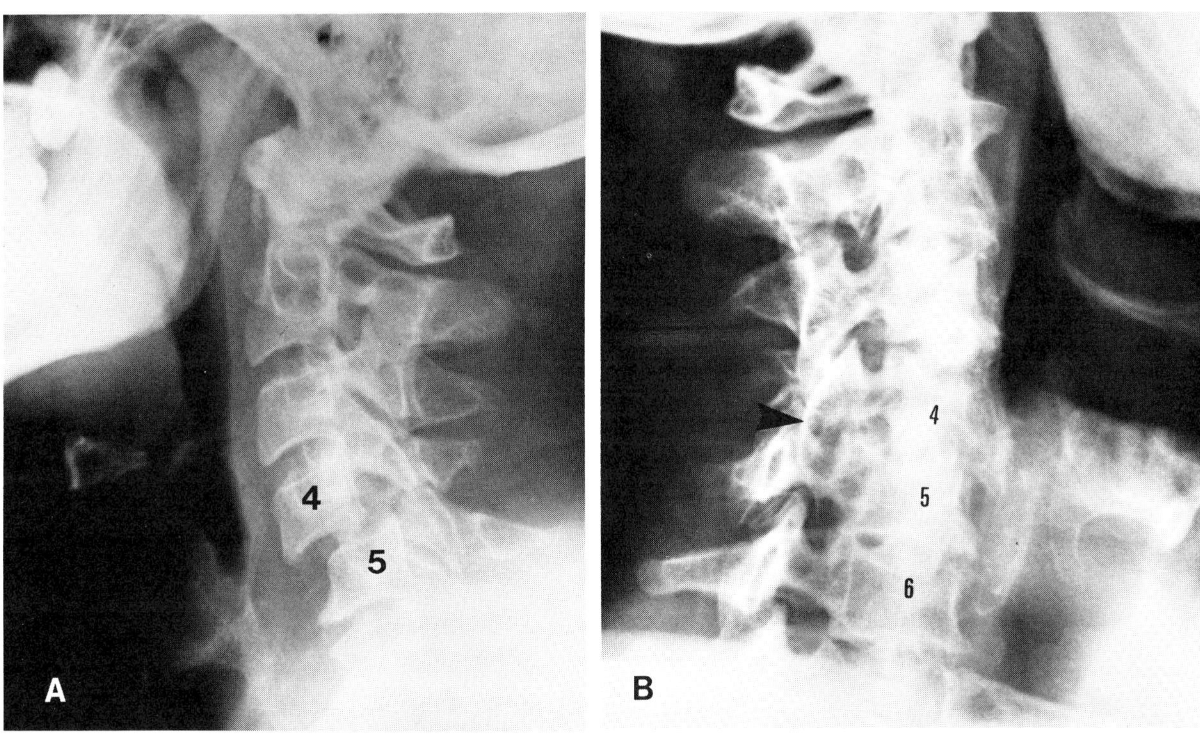

Fig. 6-83. (*A*) Roentgenogram from a patient with anterior dislocation of C4 on C5 vertebrae. Marked deltoid and mild biceps weakness was present on the right. Dislocation was missed for 6 weeks because patient was initially intoxicated and did not complain of neck pain. (*B*) Right oblique roentgenogram demonstrates a dislocated C4 facet and a fractured facet occluding the C4-5 foramina. The latter pathology caused compression of the right 5th nerve root.

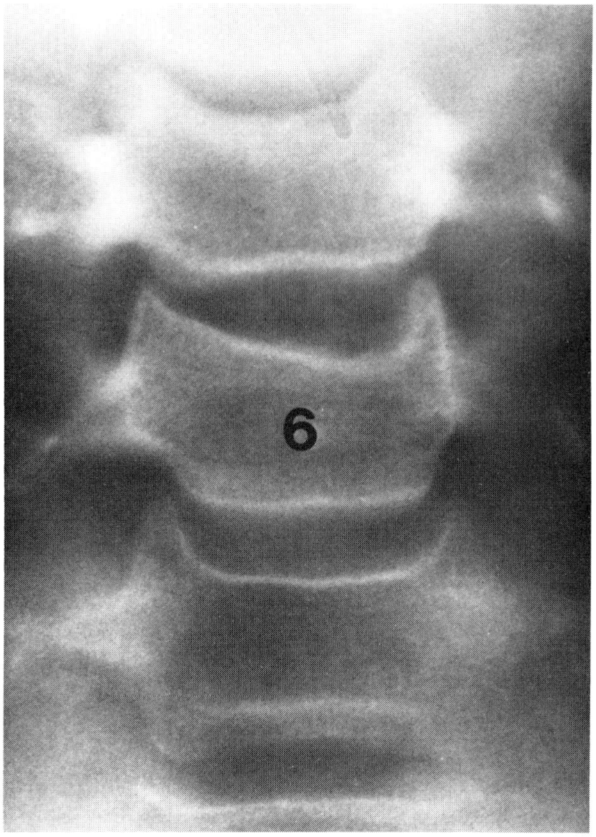

Fig. 6-84. Compression fracture of the superior end plate of C6 vertebra demonstrated only by tomography. Patient had continued neck pain following injury with a normal lateral cervical spine roentgenogram.

vere compression fracture of the vertebral body with posterior displacement of fragments into the spinal canal (Fig. 6-86). These injuries occur as a result of the patient's diving into shallow pools or lakes and striking his head on a stationary object. A portion of the vertebral body is displaced anteriorly while usually a larger fragment is pushed posteriorly into the spinal canal. Most bone and disk fragments lie anterior to the posterior longitudinal ligament and not free in the spinal canal. This is an important consideration in support of the anterior approach for decompression of the canal.

Occasionally a hyperextension injury avulses a fragment of bone from the anterior superior vertebral body. Severe extension may produce a spinal cord injury, with very little evidence of bony damage (Fig. 6-87). The degenerate intervertebral disk is disrupted

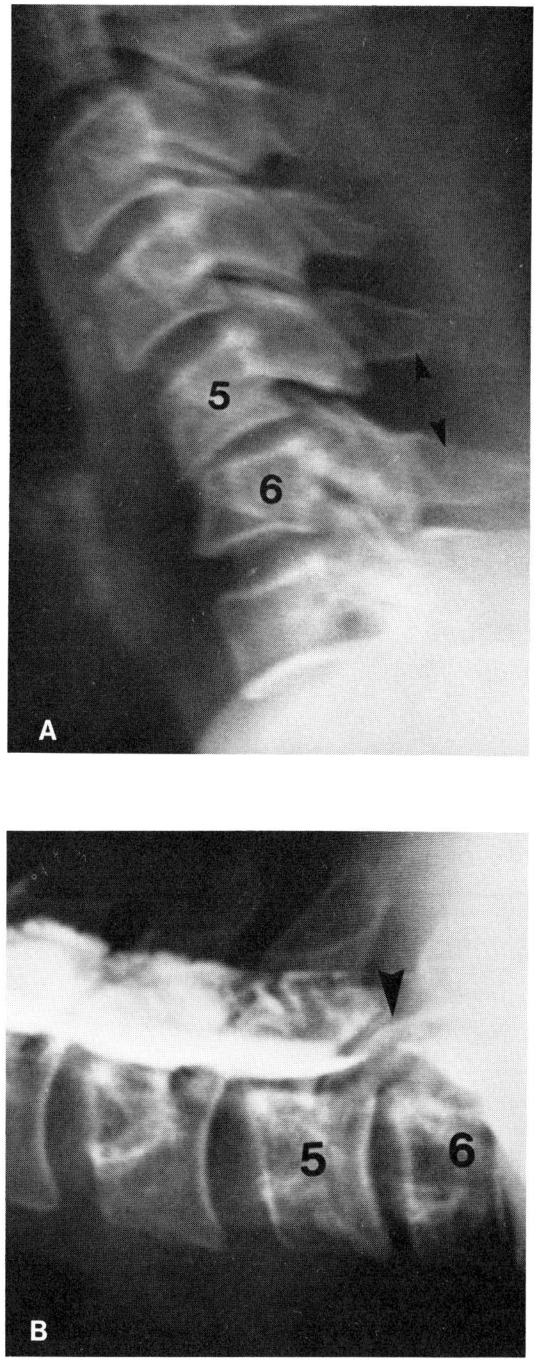

Fig. 6-85. (*A*) Flexion injury with anterior subluxation of C5 on C6 and tearing of the interspinous ligaments. The patient was quadriparetic with an anterior cord syndrome. (*B*) Cervical myelogram on same patient demonstrating a large herniated disk at C5-6 compressing the anterior spinal cord. Anterior diskectomy and fusion resulted in recovery of paralysis.

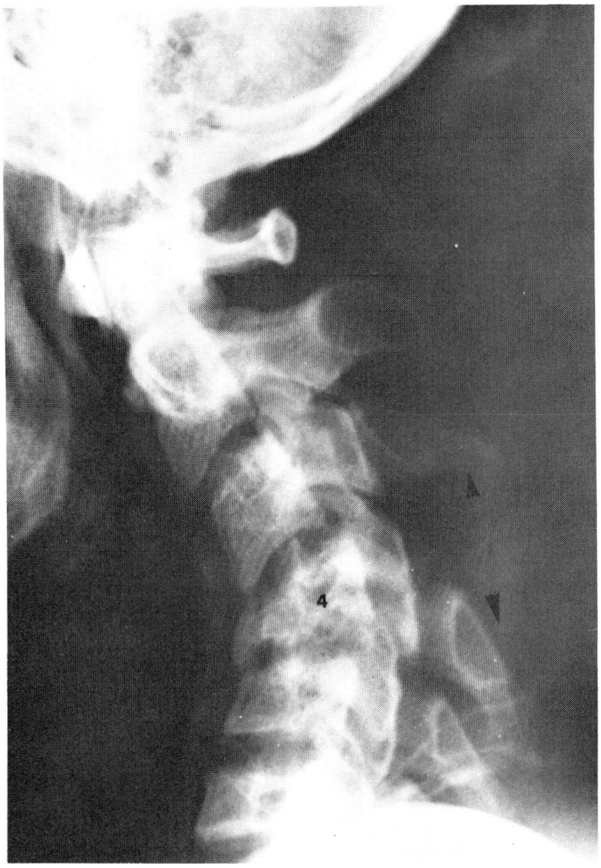

Fig. 6-86. Roentgenogram from a patient who sustained a diving injury producing a severe compression fracture of C4 vertebra with kyphotic deformity and bony fragment protrusion into the spinal canal. This patient was quadriparetic with a central cord syndrome.

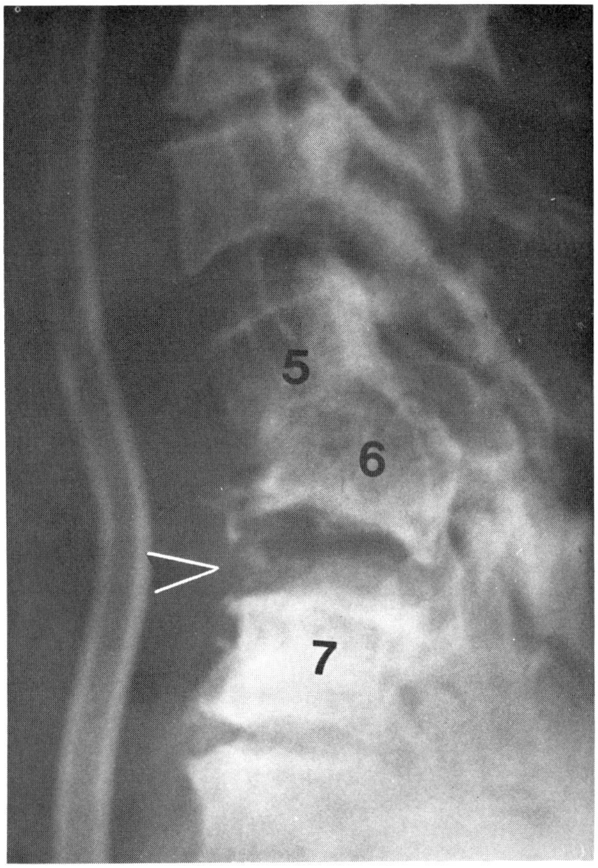

Fig. 6-87. Lateral roentgenogram of hyperextension injury in a complete quadriplegic. Picture taken in traction. Note the old fracture of C6 with spontaneous C5-6 fusion. The new injury is total disruption of the C6-7 disk space and longitudinal ligaments.

as well as longitudinal ligaments, producing a posterior or reverse subluxation of the vertebrae.

Lateral flexion forces produce fractures of the pedicles, lateral masses, or facet joints. These injuries are rarely associated with neural damage (Fig. 6-88).

Gunshot Wounds

Direct missile wounds may damage the spine or spinal cord to varying degrees. Obviously, low velocity civilian wounds cause less osseous damage. However, complete quadriplegia can result without evidence of osseous injury by roentgenogram (Fig. 6-89).

Nerve Root Lesions

A nerve root may be damaged or compressed as an isolated lesion with cervical trauma. This can be caused by a fractured facet, unilateral facet dislocation posteriorly, or a herniated disk fragment anteriorly. These are peripheral nerve injuries, and recovery may follow reduction of the dislocation of proper surgical decompression and fusion. Root avulsion can occur in conjunction with cervical spine injury.

SYSTEMIC DISEASE CAUSING ALTERATIONS IN BONE TEXTURE OF THE CERVICAL SPINE

Certain systemic diseases which affect osseous tissues of the body in general can specifically cause alterations in the cervical spine. They are anemias, leukemias, Hodgkin's disease, Paget's disease, and

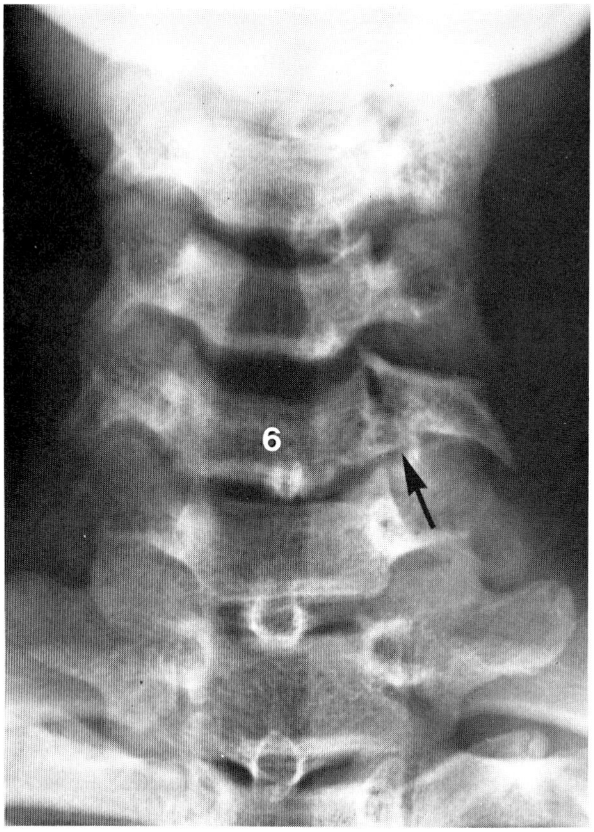

Fig. 6-88. Anteroposterior roentgenogram demonstrating a lateral mass fracture of C6.

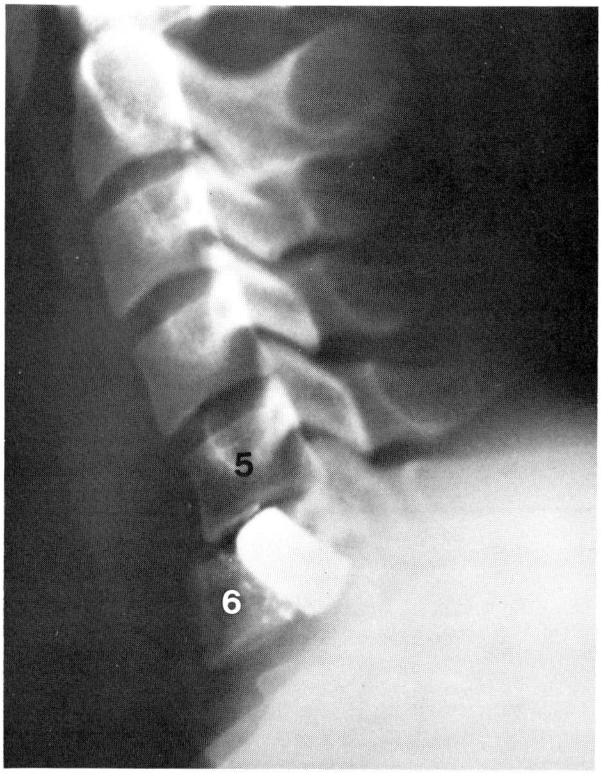

Fig. 6-89. Roentgenogram of a civilian gunshot wound of C6 that resulted in complete quadriplegia. The patient died of ascending necrosis of the spinal cord, a rare occurrence.

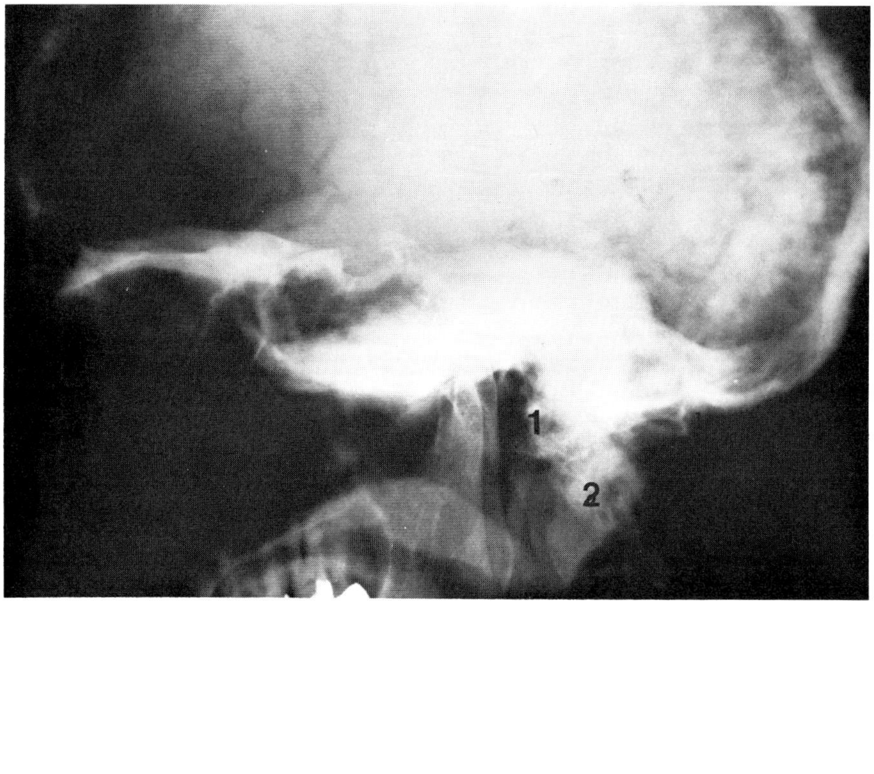

Fig. 6-90. Roentgenogram of Paget's disease of the skull with acquired basilar invagination. Note flattening of the base of the skull. (Courtesy Dr. Benjamin Kaufman, Department Radiology, University Hospitals, Cleveland.)

osteoporosis. The anemias and leukemias may produce osteolysis locally or generally. Bone density decreases, and in the vertebral bodies there is an accentuation of the trabecular pattern. Pathologic compression fractures may occur. The presenting symptom is usually neck pain which is rather constant.

Hodgkin's disease may cause lysis of the bone or a very dense sclerosis of the vertebra much like Paget's disease. Neural compression occurs following collapse of the vertebral body with protrusion of bone and tumor into the spinal canal. In Hodgkin's disease there may be direct invasion of the neural structures without major bony involvement.

Paget's disease may produce osteoclastic destruction and fibrous replacement of bone at any site in the body. There may be a reparative process at the same time, producing irregular new dense bone. The new dense mosaic bone may be very sclerotic, producing the so-called "ivory vertebra." There is always the danger of malignant degeneration of the pagetoid bone. Another life-threatening situation occurring in Paget's disease is progressive basilar invagination of the odontoid process with platybasia. This may result in medullary neural compression (Fig. 6-90).

Generalized osteoporosis, whether primary or secondary to steroid administration, may affect the cervical spine. Compression fractures occur, and ligamentous laxity with spontaneous dislocations are a danger. The latter has been mentioned in conjunction with rheumatoid arthritis.

I should like to thank the Medical Media Production Service, Veterans Administration Hospital, Cleveland, Ohio, for preparing the radiologic photographs in this chapter.

SUGGESTED READINGS

Anatomy of the Neck

Gatz, J. T.: Manter's Essentials of Neuroanatomy and Neurophysiology, ed. 4, Philadelphia, F. A. Davis, 1970.
Goss, C. M. (ed.): Gray's Anatomy of the Human Body. ed. 29. Philadelphia, Lea and Febiger, 1973.
McKusick, V. A.: Heritable Disorders of Connective Tissue. ed. 4. St. Louis, C. V. Mosby, 1972.
Pernkopf, E.: Atlas of Topographical and Applied Human Anatomy, vol. 1 Head and Neck. Philadelphia, W. B. Saunders, 1963.

Regional Examination

Spurling, R. G., and Scoville, W. B.: Lateral rupture of the cervical intervertebral discs. Surg. Gynecol. Obstet., **78:**350, 1944.
Turek, S. L.: Orthopaedics: Principles and Their Application. Philadelphia, J. B. Lippincott, 1967.

Differential Diagnosis of Cervical Disorders Presenting in Infancy and Usually Painless

Hinck, V. C., Hopkins, C. E. and Savara, B. S.: Diagnostic criteria of basilar impression. Radiology, *76:*572, 1961.
McGregor, M.: The significance of certain measurements of the skull in the diagnosis of basilar impression. Br. J. Radiol., *21:*171, 1948.
McRae, D. L., and Barnum, A. S.: Occipitalization of the atlas. Am. J. Roentgenol., *70:*23, 1953.
McRae, D. L.: The significance of abnormalities of the cervical spine. Am. J. Roentgenol., *84:*3, 1960.

Cervical Disorders Presenting in Childhood or Adolesence

Bailey, J. A., II: Orthopaedic aspects of achondroplasia. J. Bone Joint Surg., *52A:*1285, 1970.
Catell, H. S., and Filtzer, D. L.: Pseudo subluxation and other normal variations in the cervical spine in children. J. Bone Joint Surg., *47A:*1295, 1965.
Davis, D. E., et al.: The pathological findings in fatal craniospinal injuries. J. Neurosurg., *34:*603, 1971.
DeBarrows, M. C., et al.: Basilar impression an Arnold-Chiari malformation: a study of 66 cases. J. Neurol. Neurosurg. Psychiat., *31:*596, 1968.
Fielding, J. W.: Normal and selected abnormal motion of the cervical spine from the second cervical vertebrae to the seventh cervical vertebrae based on cineroentgenography. J. Bone Joint surg., *46A:*1779, 1964.
Greenberg, A. D.: Atlanto-axial dislocations. Brain, *91:*655, 1968.
Hinck, V. C., Hopkins, C. E., and Savara, B. S.: Saggital diameter of the cervical spinal canal in children. Radiol., *79:*97, 1962.
Hohl, M.: Normal motion of the upper portion of the cervical spine. J. Bone Joint Surg., *46A:*1777, 1964.
McRae, D. L.: The significance of abnormalities of the cervical spine. Caldwell Lecture, 1959. Am. J. Roentgen, *84:*3, 1960.
———: The cervical spine in neurologic disease. Radiol. Clin. North Am., *4:*145, 1966.
McRae, D. L., and Barnum, A. S.: Occipitalization of the atlas. Am. J. Roentgen., *70:*23, 1953.

Cervical Disorders Presenting in Adulthood and Usually Painful

Bell, H. S.: Paralysis of both arms from injury of upper portion of the pyramidal decussation: "Cruciate Paralysis." J. Neurosurg., *33:*376, 1970.
Bohlman, H. H.: Cervical spine injuries, a critical review of 300 cards. J. Bone Joint Surg., *54A:*1353, 1972.
———: Pathology and Curent Treatment Concepts of Cervical Spine Injuries. Instructional Course Lectures, Academy of Orthopaedic Surgeons, *21:*108, 1972.

Brain, L. and Wilkinson, M.: Cervical Spondylosis. Philadelphia, W. B. Saunders, 1967.

Dahlin, D. C.: Bone Tumors: General Aspects and Data on 3,987 Cases. ed. 2. Springfield, Ill., Charles C Thomas, 1967.

Davis, D. D. et al.: The pathological findings in fatal craniospinal injuries. J. Neurosurg., *34:603*, 1971.

Dejong, R. N.: The Neurological Examination. ed. 2. New York, Harper and Row, 1967.

Evarts, E. M.: Traumatic occipito-atlantal dislocation. J. Bone Joint Strg., *52A*:1653, 1970.

Feldman, F., and Seaman, W. B.: The neurologic complications of Paget's disease in the cervical spine. Am. J. Roentgenol; *105*:375, 1969.

Greenfield, G. B.: Radiology of Bone Diseases. ed. 2. Philadelphia, J. B. Lippincott, 1975.

Hinck, V. C. and Sachdev, N. S.: Developmental stenosis of the cervical spinal canal. Brain, *89*:27, 1966.

Jaffe, H. L.: Tumors and Tumorous Conditions of the Bone and Joints. Philadelphia, Lea and Febiger, 1964.

Kellgren, J. H., and Lawrence, J. S.: The relation of occupation to the incidence of degenerative joint disease. Br. J. Indust. Med., 9:197, 1952.

Lichenstein, L.: Bone Tumors. St. Louis, C. V. Mosby, 1965.

Payne, E. E. and Spillane, J. D.: The cervical spine and anatomical pathological study of 70 specimens with particular reference to the problem of cervical spondylosis. Brain, *80*:38, 1957.

Riley, L. H. Jr., et al: The results of anterior interbody fusion of the cervical spine. J. Neurosurg., *30*:127, 1969.

Robinson, R. A. and Smith, G. W.: Anterolateral cervical disc removal and interbody fusion for cervical disc syndrome. Bulletin, Johns Hopkins Hospital, *96*:223, 1955.

Schneider, R. C.: The syndrome of acute anterior spinal cord injury. J. Oeurosurg., *12*:95, 1955.

Schneider, R. C., Cherry, G., and Pantek, H.: The syndrome of acute central cervical cord injury with special reference to the mechanism involved in hyperextension injuries of the cervical spine. J. Neurosurg., *11*:546, 1954.

Stauffer, E. S. and Kaufer, H.: Fractures and dislocations of the spine. *In* Rockwood, C. A. and Green, D. P.: Fractures. Philadelphia, J. B. Lippincott, 1975.

Telford, E. D. and Mottershead, S.: Pressure at the cervical brachial junction, an operative and antomical study. J. Bone Joint Surg., *30B*:249, 1948.

Waldvogel, F. A., Medoff, G., and Schwartz, M. N.: Osteomyelitis: a review of clinical features, therapeutic considerations and unusual aspects. N. Engl. J. Med., *282*:198, 258, 314, 1970.

7 The Back: Thoracic and Lumbar Spine

Daniel R. Benson, M.D.

Back pain is probably the most common complaint heard by the practicing physician. Because the causes are so many and varied and because the modes of treatment are far from universal, the diagnosis and subsequent care of the spine has often been confusing.

On the other hand, the diagnosis and treatment can be a challenge if you have a basic understanding of the spine and intervertebral disks and their relationship to the spinal cord and its nerve roots. The multiple pathological processes, whether they be a fracture of spine, tumor of the spinal cord, herniation of a spinal disk, or whatever, fit into a definite organized pattern which will aid in making the diagnosis and selecting an appropriate treatment program.

ANATOMY

EMBRYOLOGY

The spine is a segmented structure, the precursor somites arising from the paraxial mesoderm as early as the 20th day of embryonic development. They form in a craniocaudal sequence over the next 10 days into 38 pairs of somites just behind the notochord. The somites then begin to show signs of specialization dividing into three distinct portions: the dermatome, the myotome, and the sclerotome. The dermatome gives rise to the integument, the myotome establishes the dorsal musculature, and the sclerotome forms connective tissue, cartilage, and bone. The development and subsequent migration of the sclerotome cells herald the formation of the membranous vertebral column which aligns along the long axis of the notochord. Eventually the notochord becomes surrounded by the somites which are each divided by an intersegmental artery.

The critical time of development is in the fifth to sixth embryonic week, the period of resegmentation. At this time, the somites resegmentate, the caudal half of one somite uniting with the cranial half of another. Thus, the intersegmental artery, formerly dividing the somites, ends up in the middle of vertebral bodies. Segmentation failures which show up as vertebral anomalies in the adult skeleton occur during this critical sixth embryonic week.

Shortly after resegmentation, the mesenchyme changes to chondroid, and the vertebrae become well formed in cartilage. During the seventh and eighth weeks, the anterior and posterior longitudinal ligaments are formed. Their relationship to the chondrous bodies is identical to that seen in the adult skeleton. During the process of cartilage formation, a thick ring of noncartilagenous cells, known as the anulus fibrosus, forms between the vertebral somites. The notochord becomes progressively less prominent and is gradually exuded into the intravertebral region. The anulus fibrosus surrounds the beads of notochord which remain as the anlage of the nucleus pulposus. The nucleus pulposus is what bulges or herniates thru the anulus fibrosus in the adult, causing the spinal disk syndrome.

Ossification centers appear in the cartilage about the eighth week. Each vertebra is derived from three primary centers: one for the centrum and two for the vertebral arch. The eventual fusion of the arches with the centrum occurs anterior to the pedicles, thus the terms "body" and "centrum" are not really interchangeable.

GROSS ANATOMY

Understanding back pain and its radicular patterns is impossible without a basic familiarity with the anatomic structure. This will be covered starting superficially with the back muscles and working down to the spinal cord and its nerve roots.

MUSCLES

When we view the back of a muscular individual, the muscles which stand out are the trapezius, latissimus dorsi, rhomboids, and erector spinae (Fig. 7-1).

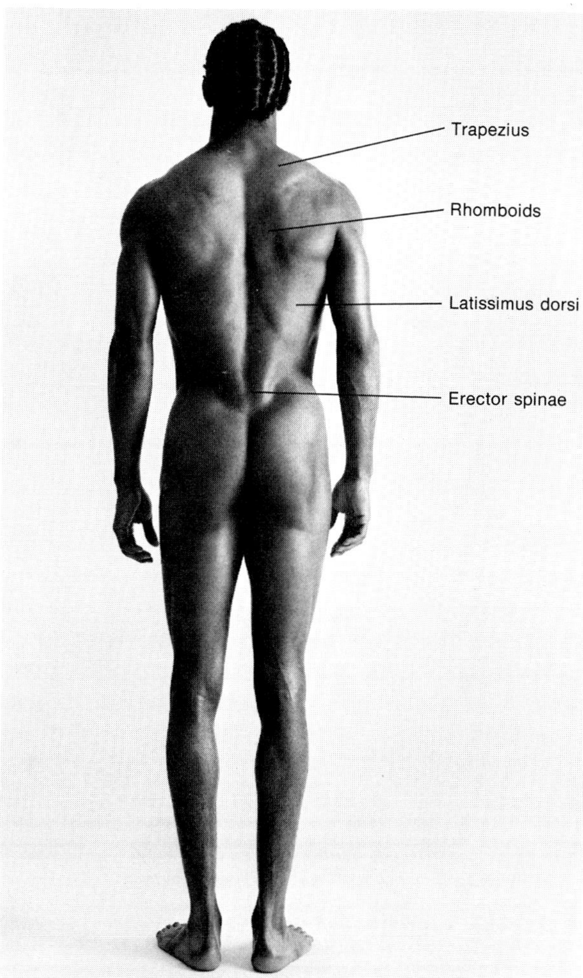

Fig. 7-1. A muscular individual demonstrating the outline of the trapezius, latissimus dorsi, rhomboids, and the erector spinae.

The trapezius originates from the external occipital protuberance, the ligamentum nuchae, and from the spinous processes of the seventh cervical through the twelfth thoracic vertabrae. The insertion begins superiorly on the lateral one third of the clavicle, the acromial process of the scapula, and along the spine of the scapula. Its action with the origin fixed is to adduct the scapula with the middle fibers, the upper and lower fibers providing stabilization; to rotate the scapula so the glenoid fossa faces cranially using the upper and lower fibers; and to elevate the scapula with the upper and depress the scapula with the lower fibers. With the insertion fixed and acting unilaterally, the upper fibers extend, laterally flex, and rotate the head and joints of cervical vertabrae so the head turns toward the opposite side. Acting bilaterally, the upper trapezius extends the head and neck. It is innervated by cranial nerve 11, the accessory, and the ventral rami of cervical nerves 2, 3, and 4.

The latissimus dorsi originates from the spinous processes of the last six thoracic vertabrae, last three or four ribs, through the thoracolumbar fascia from the lumbar and sacral vertabrae, and from the posterior one third of the iliac crest. It inserts into the intertubercular groove of the humerus. Its action with the origin fixed is to medially rotate, adduct, and extend the shoulder joint. Continued action causes depression of the shoulder joint and lateral flexion of the spine. With the insertion fixed, it assists in tilting the pelvis anteriorly and laterally. Acting bilaterally, this muscle assists in hyperextending the spine and anteriorly tilting the pelvis. This muscle is extremely important in relation to movements such as walking with crutches or parallel bars. Forceful arm muscles in swimming and rowing are dependent on this muscle. It is innervated by the thoracodorsal nerve.

The rhomboids are divided into minor and major divisions, the minor being most superior. Functionally, they can be considered as one muscle and are hard to separate anatomically. The origin is from the ligamentum nuchae and the spinous processes of the seventh cervical through the fifth thoracic vertabrae. They insert into the medial border of the scapula and act to adduct and elevate it in conjunction with the trapezius. The innervation of both muscles is the dorsal scapular nerve, which leaves the brachial plexus at root level. This is anatomically important because if the brachial plexus is injured and rhomboids are out, one can place the injury very close to the spinal cord. This is also true of the long thoracic nerve to the serratus anterior muscle, which is discussed next.

The serratus anterior originates from the outer surface and superior borders of the upper eight or nine ribs and inserts into the costal surface of the medial scapula. Its action is to abduct and rotate the scapula so that the glenoid fossa faces cranially. It also holds the scapula firmly against the thorax, and weakness of this muscle results in so-called "winging" of the scapula (see Fig. 8-15). Because of the long, superficial course of the long thoracic nerve, it is particularly susceptible to injury by either trauma to the lateral rib cage or viral infiltration.

The true back muscles present a rather complicated picture as they consist of numerous converging and diverging fascicles that are referred to as individual muscles. From a functional standpoint, it is useless to subdivide the back musculature as they generally all work together and are difficult to separate anatomically.

The main mass of back muscles can be most easily understood by starting in the lumbar region and following the muscles upward. The heavy musculotendinous band over the upper sacral and lower lumbar vertebrae represents the origin of a large segment of the spinal musculature, known collectively from its attachments as the sacrospinalis or as the erector spinae, as its action is to extend the spine. As the sacrospinalis continues cranially, it divides into three series of muscles. The most lateral division is the iliocostalis system which is broken down into lumborum, dorsi, and cervicis portions depending on the anatomical location. They all originate from midline musculature and insert into ribs. The next and more medial muscle is the longissimus system which is divided into dorsi, cervicis, and capitis portions. The most medial division is the spinalis muscle; it is usually poorly developed and has little function. Beneath the spinalis is the larger and more continuous semispinalis which is also divided into dorsi, cervicis, and capitis portions. This muscle consists of fibers which originate from transverse processes and insert medially into spinous processes of vertebrae four to five levels above. Deep to the semispinalis is the multifidus which resembles the semispinalis except the muscle fibers are shorter and traverse fewer vertebrae. Other muscles include the interspinales, intertransversarii, and the rotators, all small muscles which traverse only one or two vertebral levels.

The true back muscles are extensors, lateral flexors, and rotators of the vertebral column. The muscles of one side will act as a unit in carrying out these movements, and it is impossible to single out the individual muscles. Therefore, the entire sacrospinalis extends the spine. Unilaterally, this muscle will laterally flex the spine, the action especially being carried out by the iliocostalis since it is most lateral and has the greatest leverage. The innervation of all these muscles is via posterior branches of the local spinal nerves. The semispinalis and multifidus also aid in extension and lateral flexion. The intertransversarii presumably aid in lateral flexion, and the rotators are so named because it is believed that that is their function.

There are no muscles attached anteriorly to the thoracic vertebrae. In the lumbar region the psoas major, although primarily a lower limb muscle, has a direct action on the vertebral column. It takes its origin from the bodies and transverse processes of the lumbar vertebrae and aids in flexion of the lower spine. Most of the flexion, lateral flexion, and rotation of the spine is largely controlled by muscles which have little or no connection to the axial skeleton. The rectus abdominis is an excellent flexor, and the lateral abdominals flex and rotate the spine. Because the abdominal muscles create intra-abdominal pressure, it is believed that they provide approximately 30 percent of the lower spine support. This is why abdominal muscle strengthening is stressed in the rehabilitation of the patient with low-back pain.

Vertebral Column

In the adult, the spinal column is a segmented column of vertebrae intricately stacked one upon another. The vertebrae are held together by an exact system of ligaments and muscles which hold the spine erect yet allow flexibility. The spine supports the head and trunk and houses the delicate spinal cord and nerve roots.

The entire spinal cord contains 33 vertebrae. Seven cervical (included in Chap. 6), twelve thoracic, and five lumbar vertebrae compose the moveable portion of the spine. Five fused vertebrae make up the immobile sacrum which articulates with the pelvis as the sacroiliac joint. Caudal to the sacrum, four or five irregular ossicles make up the coccyx. In the fetus, the entire spine is in the shape of a long kyphotic curve. However, shortly after birth the normal cervical and lumbar lordosis are formed along with compensatory thoracic and sacral kyphosis.

The typical vertebra consists of a body and a vertebral arch (Fig. 7-2). These two enclose an area known as the spinal canal through which the spinal cord passes. The arch consists of two sides which are the pedicles and two laminas which form the roof. The spinous process projects from the roof and the transverse processes extend laterally from the junction between the pedicles and the laminas. Projecting cranially and caudally from the junction between pedicles and laminas are the superior and inferior articular processes. The meeting of an inferior process from one vertebra with a superior process from another constitutes the facet joint. This occurs bilaterally between each vertebra and accounts for the flexibility of the spine. Each of these articulations is a true diarthrodial joint, complete with a synovial lining and a joint capsule.

The lateral opening which is created between the pedicles and the articular facets of two adjacent vertebrals provides an exit for spinal nerves and is called the intervertebral foramen (Fig. 7-2). Within the foramen, the spinal nerves have limited room and are susceptible to compression by bony spurs, tumors, or protruding disks. This is particularly true in the cervical region where the foramina are small and nerve roots virtually fill up the entire anteroposterior diameter of the canal. In the lumbar region the foramen is normally five to six times the diameter of the nerve root traversing it, thus allowing some maneuverability of the nerve. Between each of the vertebral bodies lies the intervertebral disk. This

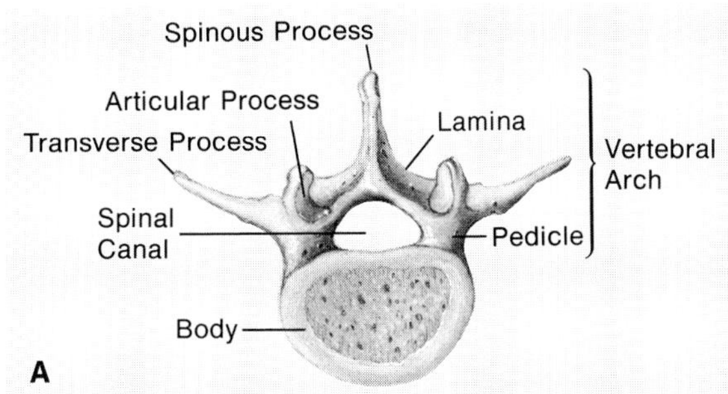

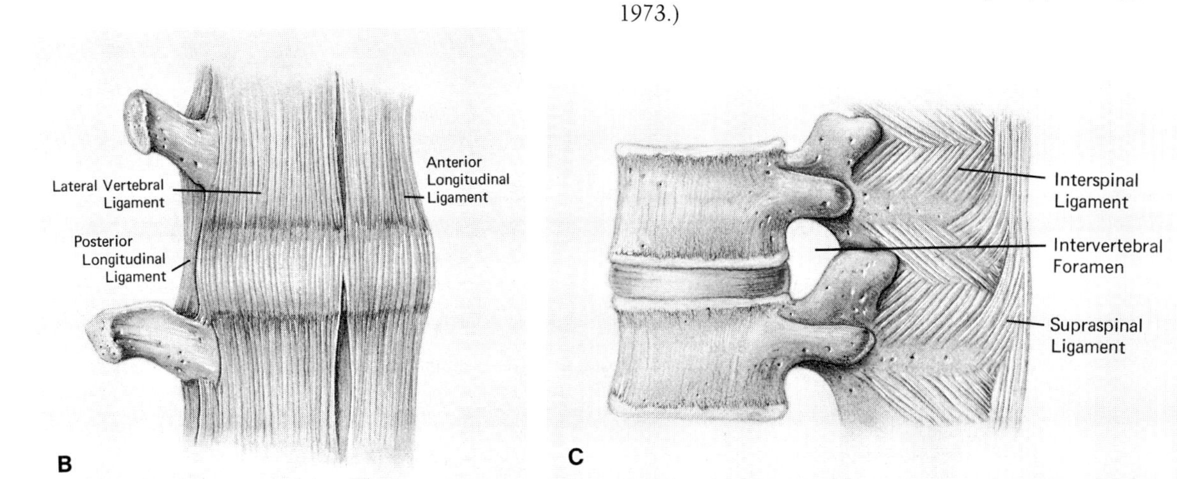

Fig. 7-2. (*A*) Typical lumbar vertebra. (*B*) Ligaments of the vertebra. The lateral vertebral ligaments consist of short fibers firmly adherent to the intervertebral disk and passing over the vertebral body to the adjacent vertebral disk. (*C*) Supraspinal and intraspinal ligaments. (Finneson, B. E.: Low Back Pain. Philadelphia, J. B. Lippincott, 1973.)

functions as an amphiarthrodial joint much like the symphysis pubis. It is composed of the strong, anulus fibrosus which is a concentric series of strong fibrous lamellae that encase the nucleus and hold the vertebrae firmly together. The lamellae insert into the vertebral body at its outer border as Sharpey's fibers. This area of insertion is known as the traction apophysis. The nucleus pulposus occupies an eccentric position within the anulus fibrosus. It is the definitive remnant of the embryonic notochord and is composed of fibrous strands dispersed in a spongy gelatinous matrix.

The intervertebral disk has the ability to convert vertical pressure to horizontal thrust extending energy out into the anulus fibrosus. The fluid behavior of the nucleus pulposus is essential in delivering this force and the anulus deforms with force. As the aging process occurs, less and less deformity is accepted, the anulus stiffens and rupture can occur. The more fluid nucleus then bulges or even escapes, causing nerve root or spinal cord compression. The disk can bulge either anteriorly or posteriorly, but most frequently it is seen in the posterior region where the ligament structure is slightly weaker. It is more significant if it ruptures posteriorly, as the spinal cord and nerve roots are more vulnerable than the structures which are anterior to the vertebral body.

A number of important ligaments hold the spine together (Fig. 7-2). The strongest is the anterior longitudinal ligament which runs along the anterior surface of the vertebral bodies, from cervical C-1 to the sacrum. The posterior longitudinal ligament runs along the posterior portion of the vertebral bodies just anterior to the spinal cord. The posterior longitudinal ligament is slightly weaker than its anterior counterpart, thus allowing for more frequent ruptures of the disk posteriorly.

In the posterior elements, the ligamentum flavum is the yellow ligament which bridges the space between adjacent laminas. It runs laterally out to the articular facets and is the ligament which is removed at laminectomy to provide access to the spinal canal. Between the spinous processes run intraspinous ligaments and superior to the spinous processes is the supraspinal ligament (Fig. 7-2C). Other ligaments include the intertransverse (between transverse processes), costotransverse (between ribs and transverse processes), and intercostal (between ribs) ligaments. The anatomical location of each of these ligaments, with the exception of the ligamentum flavum, is clearly indicated by its assigned name.

The facet joint alignment at various vertebral levels deserves discussion because of its anatomical significance. In the cervical region, the facets are arranged in a horizontal or transverse plane with only a small anteroposterior tilt. This allows for greater rotation in the cervical spine and also accounts for the frequency of dislocated facets without fracture. In the thoracic region, the facets slope inferiorly and can be compared to the arrangement of shingles on a roof. The lumbar facets range from a sagittal orientation at the first and second lumbar vertebrae to an almost coronal placement at the lower lumbar spine. This arrangement allows for flexion and extension but limits the rotation in the lumbar area. In contrast to the cervical region, the lumbar facets almost never dislocate without facet or body fracture.

Spinal Cord and Nerve Roots

The spinal cord lies in the spinal canal and is surrounded by the vertebral bodies, pedicles, and laminae (Fig. 7-3). The spinal nerves which arise from it then make their exit through the intervertebral foramina. A more definitive description of the spinal nerves and their clinical importance can be

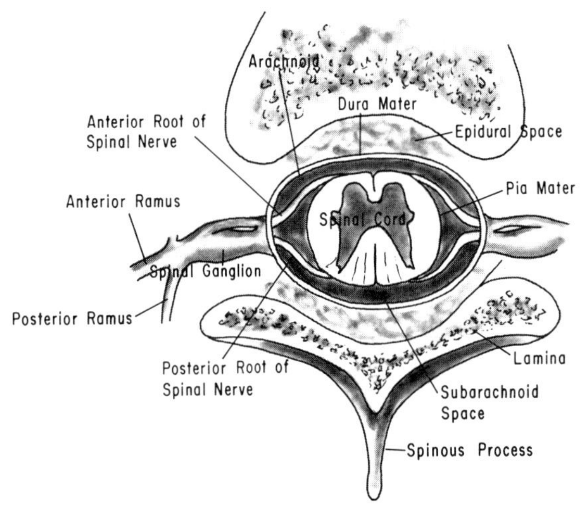

Fig. 7-3. Schematic drawing of the spinal cord and its nerve roots. The important anatomical landmarks are labeled.

found in the section on spinal disk herniations in this chapter.

The spinal cord is cushioned from the boney vertebral canal by a layer of epidural fat in which is embedded a rich venous plexus. There are three layers or coverings of the spinal cord, the first and most superficial being the tough dura mater. It extends from the foramen magnum where it is continuous with the dura mater of the brain to its attachment in the coccyx as a narrow fibrous cord. It surrounds the spinal cord and the exiting nerve roots much like a sac, the sac ending at the second sacral vertebra.

Just beneath the dura mater, separated by a thin fluid-filled space known as the subdural space, is the arachnoid membrane. Between the arachnoid and the pia mater is the large subarachnoid space. This is the area that is filled with cerebrospinal fluid and protects the cord from injury. The spinal cord is suspended within this fluid-filled space by bilaterally placed ligaments, known because of their tooth-like appearance, as the denticulate ligaments. The denticulate ligament on each side extends from the pia mater to the dura mater, in a series of processes, much like the teeth in a saw. These attach to the dura mater between the points of exit of the spinal nerves. Because their function is to support the cord and because the cord ends at lumbar 1, the denticulate ligaments are usually confined to the cervical and thoracic regions of the vertebral canal.

The pia mater is the third and the innermost covering of the cord and appears as the outer surface of the spinal cord to which it is firmly attached. The cord itself ends at lumbar 1 in the adult as the conus medullaris. The conus migrates to this level because skeletal growth is greater than neural growth. The conus is at the tip of the coccyx at the embryonic age of three months. By birth, it has risen to lumbar 3, and by age five it is at lumbar 1, its permanent position. Below this level, the cord is represented by a thin fibrous band called the filum terminale. Because of this shortening, the lumbar and sacral nerve roots slant considerably downward to make their exit at the appropriate level. This parallel group of nerve roots is collectively called the cauda equina or "horse's tail" because of their resemblance to the latter.

The area below lumbar 1 is occupied only by the filum terminale and the lumbar and sacral nerve roots. Thus, in the lumbar region the subarachnoid sac forms a cistern of good size into which a needle can be entered without damage to the cord itself. This is where spinal puncture can most safely be performed. Spinal fluid can be removed for diagnostic purposes, spinal fluid pressure can be measured, and medications or contrast agents injected. The nerve roots which are suspended in fluid tend to be pushed away from the needle; at a higher location, the fixed cord might suffer damage.

In the thoracic and lumbar regions, the nerve roots exit through the intervertebral foramen below their respective vertebrae. For example, the first thoracic nerve exits through the intervertebral foramen made up by the first and second thoracic vertebrae. Remember the cervical nerve roots exit above their respective vertebrae. There are eight cervical nerve roots and the last exits between cervical vertebra 7 and thoracic vertebra 1. This becomes important when describing spinal cord or nerve root injury. If this concept is understood, more exact localization of the problem can occur. This will be discussed further in the sections on spinal fractures (p. 264) and spinal disk herniations (p. 276).

The spinal cord itself varies in shape according to the level. There are cervical and lumbar enlargements at the areas where nerve roots exit to supply the arms and legs. The spinal nerves, 31 in all, arise at regular intervals along the length of the cord. Each is composed of two roots: a ventral (anterior) and a dorsal (posterior). Each of the dorsal roots exhibits a swelling or ganglion as it exits through the intervertebral foramen. Just lateral to the ganglion, the anterior and posterior roots join to form a spinal nerve. The subarachnoid space and, therefore, the pia mater, arachnoid, and dura mater all extend out along nerve roots to a point just beyond the ganglion. This area, when viewed on a myelogram (radiopaque dye in the subarachnoid space), is called the dural sheath or "nerve root sleeve." If it is absent or indented on the myelogram, compression of the nerve root should be suspected.

The fibers of the posterior roots arise from nerve cells in the posterior root ganglia and run centrally to the cord. The peripheral sensory fibers arise with the central ones, each posterior root ganglion cell giving off a single process which divides into a central and peripheral branch. Thus, sensory input from skin, muscle, intestine, or whatever, reaches the cord via the posterior root from throughout the distribution of each particular spinal nerve. The anterior roots arise from cells within the gray matter of the spinal cord. These fibers are strictly motor and, therefore, conduct impulses away from the spinal cord. When the anterior and dorsal spinal roots join, a mixed nerve (one containing both motor and sensory fibers) is formed. Shortly beyond this formation of the spinal nerve it branches into posterior and anterior rami, both of which are mixed nerves. The posterior rami or branches are distributed to innervate back muscles and supply sensation to a small area of skin over the back. These nerves tend to remain separate contrary to the anterior rami which may enter into plexus formation. The anterior rami of the second to fourth cervical nerves make up the cervical plexus; those of cervical 5 through thoracic 1 make up the brachial plexus; the upper lumbar nerves form the lumbar plexus; and the lower lumbar and sacral nerves enter into the formation of sacral and pudendal plexuses. The anterior rami of the thoracic nerves are kept apart by the innervation of the ribs and do not form plexuses. They are known, because of their course between ribs, as intercostal nerves. Each of these spinal nerves has a specific sensory distribution and motor innervation. By careful motor and sensory examination, injury to an individual nerve root can be almost exactly delineated. This will be expanded upon in the section on spinal disk herniations (p. 276).

REGIONAL EXAMINATION

Although the back may seem to be the most difficult region of the body to examine, it can be the easiest. The motion of the vertebral column is relatively simple in comparison to a joint such as the shoulder. The confusion arises because of the vertebral column's intimate relationship to the spinal cord. Both have to be considered together in analyzing pain and deformity of the back. In addition, back disease may be present as lower extremity weakness, pain or deformity, as bowel or bladder problems, or as abdominal distress. Therefore, a thorough assessment of the back includes rectal, pelvic, and abdominal examinations as well as complete examination of the lower extremities.

HISTORY

A careful history should be taken and chronologically recorded. It is important to have a set system so important areas will not be forgotten. The patient, whether young or old, should be the major contributor, as too frequently overzealous relatives or friends will cloud the picture by interjecting their feelings. If the patient can have his say, the orthopaedist will gain the needed insight into his feelings, hopes, and fears. The patient then leaves the office knowing the physician has talked to him or her. How important this must be to an adolescent or octogenarian who is beginning to doubt his own worth.

A spinal history should center around the chief complaint of what brings the individual to your office for examination. Pain or deformity are the two most common back complaints. Careful questioning as to exactly when and how these began is imperative. The course of the pain or deformity is recorded chronologically and previous operations or treatments listed in order.

The pain should be characterized in detail. What exacerbates the pain? For example, coughing, sneezing, or bowel movements may produce pain in an acute herniated disk. What makes the pain better? Lying with the knees flexed improves the disk syndrome but won't help if the problem is a spinal cord tumor. When does the pain occur? Pain and stiffness on arising may suggest one of the arthritis syndromes. Does the pain radiate? Pain into the lower extremities particularly with reflex changes, sensory loss, and weakness is a classic example of a herniated disk presentation.

Deformity is similarly pursued. When and by whom was it first noted? Has it changed or become worse in the interim? Is the deformity associated with pain? Idiopathic scoliosis invariably presents as a painless deformity. If pain is associated, the examiner is obligated to search for a cause—tumor, herniated disk, infection, or whatever. Back deformity with lower extremity weakness or deformity, bowel or bladder incontinence, or sensory disturbances may suggest an intraspinal tumor or bony anomaly.

If the problem is related to injury, try to find out the mechanism. Question the patient about lower extremity weakness or loss of sensation which occurred immediately after injury. Ask about bowel or bladder control. Find out if the pain or deformity occurred at the time of injury or has developed subsequently.

Some of the spinal deformities, particularly the nonpainful ones, require a thorough family history as many are inherited. Similar deformities may be present in the younger sibling of your patient and because of your persistence might be picked up earlier and treated. Idiopathic scoliosis, muscular dystrophy, and neurofibromatosis are only a few examples of this.

The congenital or developmental deformities require a history going back to the early months of gestation. As was discussed in embryology of the spine, its precursor is noted at the twentieth day of embryonic development. Defects, such as spina bifida, probably occur as early as the third embryonic week and other congenital vertebral anomalies at the fifth to sixth embryonic week, the period of resegmentation.

The nature of the process that causes abnormalities in humans is not known. In animals, various drugs, roentgenograms, vitamin deficiencies, anoxia, and viral infiltration have all been implicated. Any information regarding trauma, drug usage, illness, or radiation during the first trimester should be gathered.

In problems such as cerebral palsy, information such as the length of labor, the delivery presentation, the birth weight, and Apgar score *may* be important. Developmental history should be compared to standards so the examiner has an idea where the patient stands among his peers.

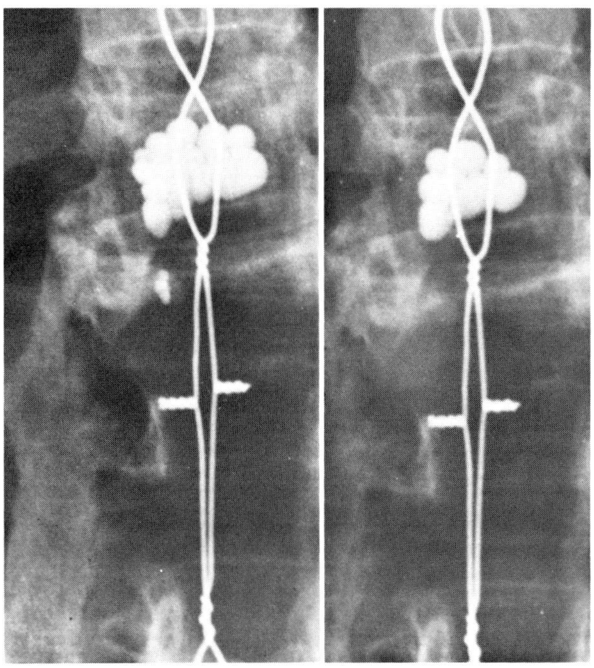

Fig. 7-4. Roentgenogram demonstrating an old compression fracture at lumbar 2. The wire from a previous posterior fusion is present, as is the myelographic dye which is blocked at the level of the compression fracture.

Past history is important in back examinations in diseases such as poliomyelitis, when an early febrile illness may be the cause of a severe spinal curvature. Past history is also helpful in evaluating progressive diseases, such as muscular dystrophy, Marfan's disease, or amyotrophic lateral sclerosis.

Multiple system questioning may reveal other already diagnosed or treated problems that may be helpful in your prognosis. These might include hydrocephalus in association with myelomeningocele, kidney or heart anomalies with congenital scoliosis, or aortic regurgitation in Marfan's syndrome; these few examples serve to remind us of the frequency of multiple system disease.

The social history is necessary to help understand the patient's feeling about himself and his desire to get well. This is where malingering and hysterical patients may be detected. The hysterical patient actually does have pain but it is the product of anxiety and inadequate psychological defenses rather than organic disease. Generally, the patient presents with the symptoms dramatically and reacts to examination in a bizarre manner. Because these patients can fool even the most astute, the examination must be extremely thorough.

Recently, a patient presented with a compression fracture of the second lumbar vertebra with impending paraplegia which was secondary to an automobile accident. Twice before the same symptoms of stocking glove anesthesia and weakness of the legs, bowel and bladder difficulties, and pain had prompted posterior surgical exploration and fusion of the spine. Each time, she had almost complete return of function, but this was short lived. She arrived by airplane for consideration of anterior decompression and fusion of lumbar 2. She demonstrated complete anesthesia to pinprick, almost absolute weakness of the lower extremity muscles, and a history that indicated progressive deterioration. On myelogram, a complete block was demonstrated at the old compression fracture site (Fig. 7-4). A difficult anterior approach to the spine was all but scheduled when careful questioning suggested some psychogenic overlay. Her affect toward this dangerous surgery was very flat—"la belle indifference." When her weak muscles were tested again slightly different results were obtained, and there was a suggestion of "cogwheel" rigidity. Her history revealed thirteen marriages with seven of these to the same man. Nothing really specific but enough to delay surgery. A repeat myelogram in the prone position revealed flow past the fracture, a frequently overlooked phenomena in this kind of fracture deformity (Fig. 7-5). Muscle testing under sodium pentothal revealed very little weakness, and the patient had a normal electromyelogram. Psychiatric consultation was obtained and the diagnosis of hysteria confirmed. Two weeks later, the patient walked out of the hospital without an operation. At last word, she had married for the fourteenth time. This is a graphic example of a patient whose psychological problem was so complex that she would submit to a life-threatening operation.

The malingerer with low back pain has some secondary gain in mind. It does not necessarily have to be financial in nature. Frequently, the malingerer is simply directing his frustration toward his job or family. This is his way of bringing attention to himself. Without a good history and understanding of basic psychology, these patients will plague the physician with doubt because they never get better. Psychological testing is very helpful in this type of patient.

The patient who is only seeking financial remuneration for his back pain is the easiest to detect. Most likely he will have a law suit pending or start the interview by asking you to fill out disability papers. Some will openly admit they don't want to get better until the suit is settled or disability runs out. It is important to remember that they, too, deserve the best you have to offer.

Questioning should also include an occupational history. The significance of a severe low back syndrome is less for a bookkeeper who sits all day than for a heavy laborer who relies on his back for his livelihood. In 1965, the United States Department of Labor and Industry collected some interesting statistics. Twenty-four percent of lost work days were due to back pain. Of the patients out with back pain longer than six months, only 50 percent ever returned to work. Of those off longer than one year, only 25 percent returned to work. In Sweden, where statistics are easy to obtain because of their health care system, 53 percent of light workers and 64 percent of heavy laborers are plagued with some back pain.

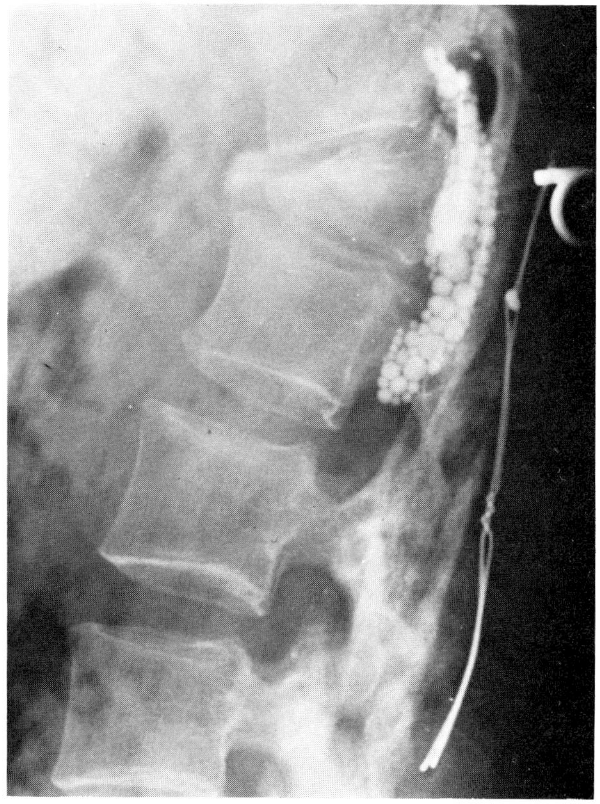

Fig. 7-5. Lateral roentgenogram of the same compression fracture at lumbar 2 with the patient in the prone position. The dye now flows past the fracture by changing the position of the patient. This is a frequently overlooked phenomenon in a patient with a kyphotic deformity.

Emotions can play a role in your diagnosis. Certain ethnic groups, such as the Chinese or American Indian, are so stoic that the degree of pain is underestimated. Other ethnic groups will overemphasize their pain. And finally, the same amount of pain to individuals of the same sex, race, and age is interpreted differently by each. The myriad number of reasons that makes this true are too complex to even attempt rational explanation.

PHYSICAL EXAMINATION

EXAMINATION OF THE BACK

Examination of the back follows exactly the same guidelines as examination of the rest of the body.

Observation is followed by *palpation, percussion,* and, if indicated, *auscultation.* The lower extremities, as part of the back examination, are similarly examined. Range of motion of the spine, hips, knees, and ankles is evaluated. Careful neurological examination of the lower extremities is performed, along with sensory examination of the torso. Rectal and pelvic examination are essential to a complete examination. These, along with breast, thyroid, or abdominal examination might prove to be diagnostic in patients who have metastatic tumors of the spine.

Observation

The patient should be observed as he walks into the office. The gait pattern may suggest a shortened extremity, antalgic gait, or restricted motion. The body build, general posture, and presence or absence of deformities is noted. Their rapport in dealing with your secretary, nurse, or their own relatives might provide insight into the personality of the patient. Thus, before you ask the first question you have some feeling for the patient's problem.

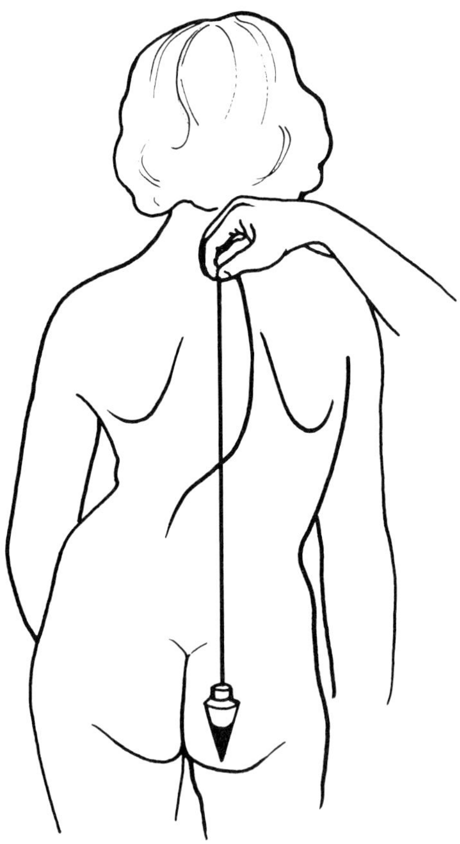

Fig. 7-6. Plumb bob being dropped from the vertebra prominens inferiorly. The patient has a right thoracic scoliosis shifting her in that direction. Therefore, the line of the plumb bob is slightly to the right side of the gluteal cleft.

The patient should be allowed to tell his history while fully clothed. This gives the examiner the additional opportunity to observe the patient undressing and mounting the examination table. With experience, the physician is able to estimate the quality and quantity of pain the patient is really having by this simple method.

Females should be examined in undergarments and males in shorts alone. A gown may be used for discreetness. Shoes and socks must be removed. When the patient is seated on the table, he is asked to stand again for further examination. Standing behind the patient, the physician can evaluate the spine for any abnormal curvatures or deformities. Normally, the spine is straight, looking at it from this position. Lateral deviation indicates some abnormality in the spine or lower extremities. Similarly, the back is generally symmetrical and if one side protrudes more than the other, it is abnormal. Prominence of the right posterior thoracic chest is a common presenting finding in idiopathic scoliosis.

Standing to the side of the patient, the normal cervical and lumbar lordosis and thoracic and sacral kyphosis are noted. Any severe accentuation or loss of these curves is not normal. Increase in the normal thoracic kyphosis may indicate Scheuermann's kyphosis in the young or osteoporosis in the elderly. Increase in lumbar lordosis, particularly if a hollow is present at the base of the spine, may represent spondylolisthesis.

Pelvic obliquity is checked in both positions by placing the fingers on the iliac crests. Normally these are equal in height. If one is lower than the other, a shortened extremity, muscle contracture, or hypoplasia of the ilium is suggested.

The thorax and spine should be balanced so the head sits directly over the pelvis. In scoliosis, curvature of the spine, if uncompensated by another curve, may shift the body to one side. The balance should be checked by dropping a plum bob from the spinous process of the seventh cervical vertebra toward the floor (Fig. 7-6). Normally, the string should fall into the crease between the buttocks. If it deviates to the right or left, the distance should be measured as it indicates an abnormal shift of the body. This could be the result of fixed spinal curvature or muscle spasm. Muscle spasm is noted as a tautness particularly in the low back where the erector spinae stands in relief. One side may be tighter than the other with subsequent listing of the torso.

Observe the skin for any local swelling or cutaneous lesions such as cafe au lait spots, patches of hair, or dimples. Discoloration or ecchymosis might indicate areas of trauma. Record obvious chest deformities, such as pectus carinatum (pigeon breast) or pectus excavatum. Judge the extremity length in relation to the trunk. Increase in length particularly with arachnodactyly (long fingers) may represent Marfan's syndrome or homocystinuria. Shortened extremities associated with typical facial features and lumbar lordosis may represent achondroplasia.

Range of Motion

Thoracolumbar spinal motion is next tested and recorded for future reference. It is tested in flexion, extension, lateral bend, and rotation. Limitation in any of these directions may indicate pain, arthrodesis, or muscle spasm.

In evaluating spine motion, the zero starting position is standing as straight as possible, looking forward (Fig. 7-7A). *Flexion* is tested by having the patient lean forward attempting to touch the toes (Fig. 7-7B). Most flexion takes place in the hip joint, as demonstrated by the scoliosis patient with a fused spine. If these patients are supple, frequently they can touch their toes. Some flexion does occur in the thoracolumbar spine, and this is best known as a reversal of the normal lordosis and increase in the thoracic kyphosis. The most accurate way to measure this is to measure with a flexible tape from the spinous process of the seventh cervical vertebra to the spinous process of the first sacral vertebra. This is done first with the patient standing erect and then with the patient bending forward as far as possible. As the spine flexes and the spinous processes separate, this distance should normally increase. In a normal healthy adult, the difference is usually in the range of 4 inches. The method of recording the distance between fingertips and the floor can be misleading as some patients normally cannot touch their toes because of tight hamstrings and others with completely fused spines can.

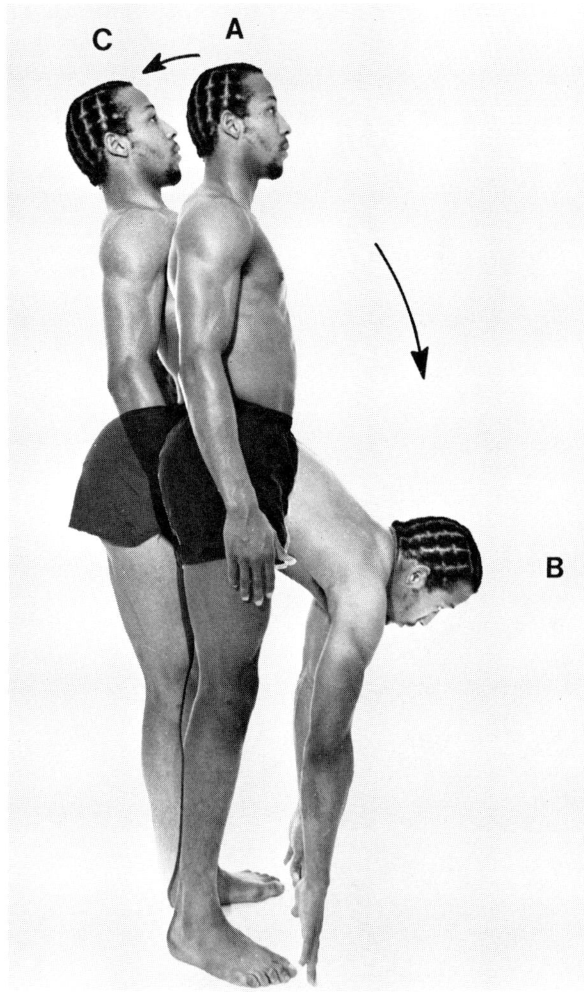

Fig. 7-7. (*A*) The straight neutral position is the zero starting position. (*B*) The patient is then instructed to flex forward, bending at the waist, attempting to touch the toes. (*C*) The patient is then instructed to hyperextend. Normally the spine extends from 20 to 30 degrees.

Another important sign to note is the increase in thoracic deformities as the spine flexes forward. As will be explained in the section on scoliosis, curvature of the spine is accompanied by rotation of the vertebrae. Because the ribs articulate with the thoracic spine, they become rotated and prominent unilaterally. As the patient bends forward, this deformity is accentuated. This is the standard test for screening children suspected of having spinal deformity. Extension or backward bending can be checked in either the erect or prone position (see Fig. 7-7C). The degree of extension is estimated by using a level pelvis and the spinous process of the seventh cervical vertebra as landmarks. Normally the spine extends from 20 to 30 degrees. This might be limited by a fixed dorsal kyphosis or ankylosing spondylitis.

Lateral flexion is measured in both right and left directions and should be symmetrical (Fig. 7-8). Here again, the pelvis is held fixed and level as the patient bends toward each side. The position of the spinous process of the seventh cervical vertebra is noted and lateral inclination estimated. Normally a patient laterally bends 30 to 35 degrees. In a patient with a painful herniated disk, this may be unilaterally limited and will be helpful in making the diagnosis. This motion is also valuable in evaluating scoliosis patients as the rigidity of the curves can be tested both clinically or by roentgenographic examination through side-bending.

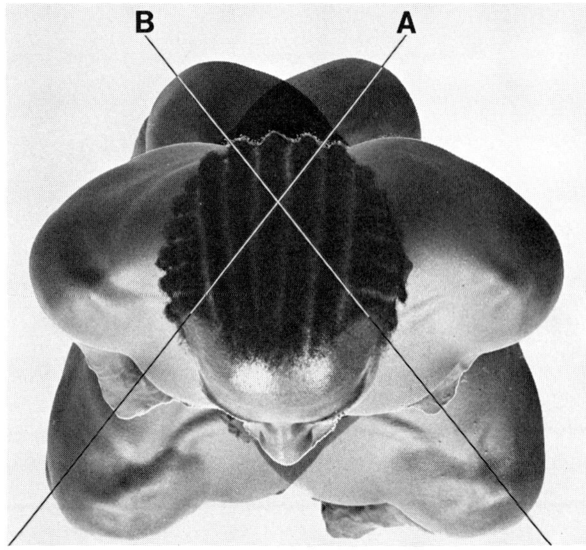

Fig. 7-9. With the examiner's hands placed firmly on the pelvic crests, the patient is instructed to rotate to the left (*A*) and to the right (*B*). This patient is viewed from above. Normally a patient can rotate 45 degrees to the left and right.

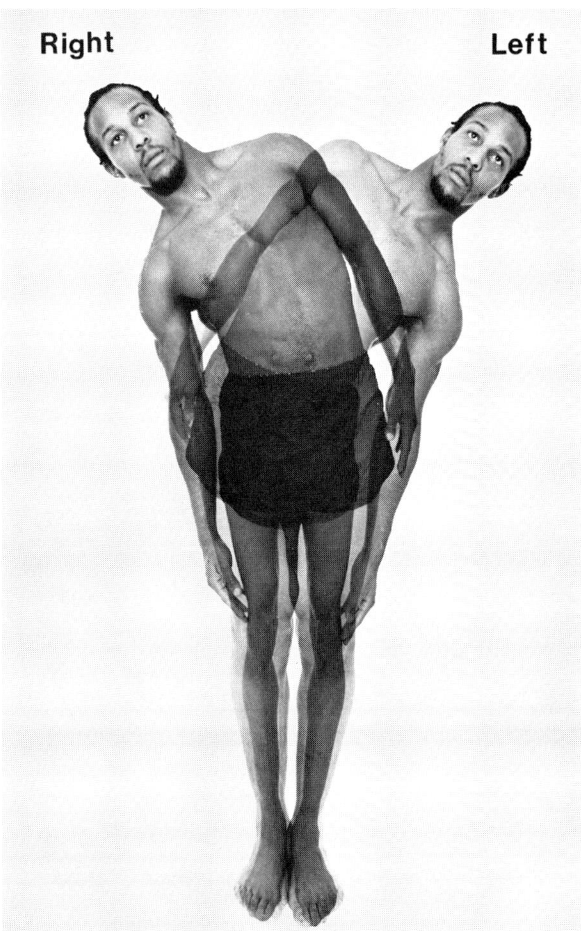

Fig. 7-8. Lateral bending to the left and the right. Normally a patient can laterally bend 30 to 35 degrees.

Rotation of the spine is tested in much the same manner (Fig. 7-9). With the examiner's hands firmly on the pelvic crests, the patient is instructed to rotate to the left and right. The rotation is estimated in degrees and normally is in the range of 45 degrees in each direction.

Chest expansion is measured using a flexible tape measure. This is done at the nipple line in maximum inspiration and expiration. A difference in the range of 3 inches indicates normal chest expansion. Limitation may reveal either chest disease (emphysema) or more likely in a back pain patient, ankylosing spondylitis. Limited chest excursion is secondary to ankylosis of the costovertebral joints.

Palpation

Any prominent masses or areas of swelling must be palpated. A mid-line mass which is cystic to palpation might represent a myelocele. Prominent muscle masses, particularly the erector spinae group, may show unilateral tenseness substantiating a diagnosis of acute muscular spasm. A fluctuant mass in the flank or iliac fossa could represent impending drainage of a tuberculous abscess. Asymmetry of the posterior chest, if bony, may indicate vertebral rotation with subsequent rib prominence or, if soft, may represent a soft tissue mass or hematoma.

The spinous processes are easily palpable in all but the most obese patient. Deviation of these processes laterally would suggest the diagnosis of scoliosis. Absence of spinous processes might suggest a congenital defect, such as spina bifida or an iatrogenic defect due to a prior laminectomy. The processes are generally equally spaced in the normal spine. After severe trauma, the ligaments can be torn posteriorly, and if associated with a compression of the vertebral body the spinous processes will separate. Palpation of the area of tenderness may suggest the true pathology of the fracture-dislocation even more clearly than by roentgenogram.

The defect of a severe spondylolisthesis where a vertebral body slips forward on the one below, can be palpated as a step off in the lumbar spine. This may be the presenting clinical finding. Kyphosis of congenital, tuberculous, or traumatic origin is palpated as a bony, hard, sharply angled mass, contiguous with the spine.

Palpation will also reveal areas of tenderness. For example, firm pressure over the sacroiliac joints may elicit pain in the patient with ankylosing spondylitis. When evaluating compression fractures in the aged, the only way to tell a fresh fracture from an old one is by palpation. If the area of compression seen on the roentgenogram is tender, it is assumed the fracture is a new one.

In a suspected herniated disk syndrome with radicular pain, tenderness can be elicited frequently in the sciatic notch. This is the area where the sciatic nerve trunk passes into the lower extremity. It is located midway between the ischial tuberosity and the greater trochanter, at the level of the gluteal fold.

Areas of local tenderness, such as the costovertebral articulations or the vertebral facet joints, if nonradicular and easily identified, can be located and treated with local anesthetic and steroid injections.

Percussion of the spine is also helpful in identifying more subtle spinal lesions. It will often differentiate the referred pain of a pyelonephritis from a true spinal problem. Tumors, infections, or neural impingement will almost always be tender on percussion of the spine. This, of course, should be done gently, but firmly, starting superiorly and working down to the base of the spine, then over the sacroiliac joints.

Auscultation

While this is a prominent feature in the cardiopulmonary patient, it is frequently overlooked in the examination of a back patient. Pulmonary tuberculosis with spinal spread is a classic example where auscultation might be helpful in the diagnosis. Congenital defects of the spine are associated with congenital heart disease, the scoliosis of Marfan's syndrome may be complicated by aortic regurgitation, and back pain in an elderly male which might really be an aortic aneurysm eroding the spine, all serve to remind us that the stethoscope may help to complete our examination.

Pelvic and Rectal Examination

As most orthopaedic clinics are not equipped for doing a pelvic examination, a gynecological consultation is often necessary to complete a back workup. A rectal examination should be done on most patients with back pain and certainly on all patients with back pain over the age of 30. In the male, the size and consistency of the prostate gland is evaluated to rule out carcinoma or prostatitis, either of which can present with back pain. In the female, the cervix can be palpated to reveal gross lesions or tenderness. Additionally, the pain of coccygeal origin can best be evaluated by rectal examination as the coccyx can be grasped between the index finger within the rectum and the thumb which is external.

In a patient with spinal cord injury or any patient in whom the bowel status is in question, anal sphincter tone requires evaluation. If the sphincter tone is absent, the presence of a bulbocavernosus reflex will indicate the completion of spinal shock and indicates a poor prognosis.

Examination of the Lower Extremities

Back problems are frequently reflected in abnormalities in the lower extremities because of the spinal column's close relationship to the spinal cord and its roots. Conversely, hip or knee disease can present as low back pain. The range of motion of ankles, knees, and hips should be evaluated when the patient has been placed in the supine position. An ankylosed or osteoarthritic hip or knee, because of the biomechanics involved, can create increased wear and tear on the lumbar spine and may be the primary source of back pain. Examination of the hip is covered in Chapter 10 and the knee in Chapter 11.

Leg length measurements are necessary to rule out a shortened extremity. Both true (from anterior iliac crests to medial malleoli) and apparent (from umbilicus to medial malleoli) lengths are important to differentiate a short extremity from a pelvic obliquity (Fig. 10-12). A difficult scoliosis problem may simply be a compensatory curve because of a short leg. To confirm the clinical diagnosis, the leg lengths can be compared by scanograms.

Measurements of the thigh and calf circumference are compared to the opposite extremity to rule out muscle atrophy secondary to disuse or denervation. The mechanics of these measurements will be discussed in the neurological examination.

The legs and feet should be evaluated for cutaneous lesions, deformities, vascularity, and neurological status. Cavus deformities of the feet, as discussed in Chapter 12, may be secondary to spinal cord impingement. Café au lait patches, lymphedema, or pseudoarthrosis of the tibia each could suggest the diagnosis of neurofibromatosis which manifests as scoliosis in half of the patients. Intermittent claudication of atherosclerotic origin may resemble the exercise claudication of spinal stenosis. A careful vascular and neurological examination can differentiate between the two.

Neurological Examination

The patient should stand facing away from the examiner. One can quickly scan for musclar weakness by having the patient stand on his toes, and then heels. This checks the gastrosoleus muscle complex (sacral 1-2) and the dorsiflexors of the feet (lumbar 4-5), respectively. The patient is then asked to squat like a baseball catcher, thus checking the quadriceps (lumbar 3-4). Any observable weakness or asymmetry is then checked more closely by individual muscle testing. Individual muscle testing will be discussed in the section on herniated nucleus pulposus.

The patient is then asked to sit on the edge of the examining table. More thorough muscle testing can be carried out at this point. Sensation of the legs is checked by comparing both extremities. The dermatomes of the human body are very specific so that a good sensory examination can localize a deficit of a particular nerve root (see Fig. 7-34).

The deep tendon reflexes are elicited and compared bilaterally. The ankle jerk can be obtained either in a sitting or kneeling position. If the reflexes are difficult to obtain, having the patient clinch his teeth or pull on his fingers may prove helpful. A change in the quality of a reflex or a difference between the two extremities is an important finding. Lower motor neurological damage, such as a herniated disk, will depress the reflexes and cause muscular flaccidity. Upper motor neuron disease, such as a cord tumor, produces hyperreflexia and spasticity.

The patient is then asked to assume a supine position, preferably with his head toward your left. Uniformity in performing the examination will aid in comparing the findings in each individual case. The calves are measured using a flexible tape at a measured distance from the anterior tibial tubercle. The point selected on the calf should be the area of largest circumference. They should measure within 0.5 inch bilaterally. The thigh is measured just above the patella, then at carefully measured 3, 6, and 9 inch intervals above the patella. Any difference greater than 0.5 inch would indicate atrophy of the smaller side.

The straight leg raising test followed by Laseque's test is accomplished to rule out sciatic irritation. If indicated, the femoral stretch, Kernig, or jugular compression test might be performed. If sacroiliitis is the suspected problem, then the described tests for irritation of the sacroiliac joint are done.

The superficial reflexes are checked, the abdominals, cremasteric, and the bulbocavernosus with rectal examination.

Special Diagnostic Tests

Tests for Sciatic Nerve Irritation

Straight Leg Raising Test (Fig. 7-10). With the patient in a supine position, the leg is slowly, passively elevated keeping the knee fully extended. Normally, the leg can be elevated to 90 degrees without too much discomfort. Pain, particularly of the electric type that radiates into the feet, the back, or to the opposite side, indicates nonspecific irritation of the sciatic nerve or root. If the knee is bent, the pain will be relieved. This is not true in afflictions of the hip joint where bending the knee has no effect.

Lasèque Test (Fig. 7-11). After the straight leg raising test has produced pain or hamstring spasm, further elevation of the leg is stopped and the foot is passively dorsiflexed. If there is sciatic irritation, dorsiflexion further aggravates the pain in the back and along the course of the nerve.

Femoral Stretch Test. In lumbar disk syndromes above the level of lumbar 4 to 5, the sciatic stretch is negative. By placing the patient prone and passively extending the thigh with the knee straight, pain will be produced due to stretch of the femoral nerve.

Tests for Meningeal Irritation

Kernig Test. With the patient lying in a supine position, the thigh and knee of one leg are flexed on the abdomen. When extension of the knee is attempted, resistance is met. A positive test is heralded by flexion of the opposite hip and knee when extension is attempted. A positive Kernig sign is indicative of meningeal irritation.

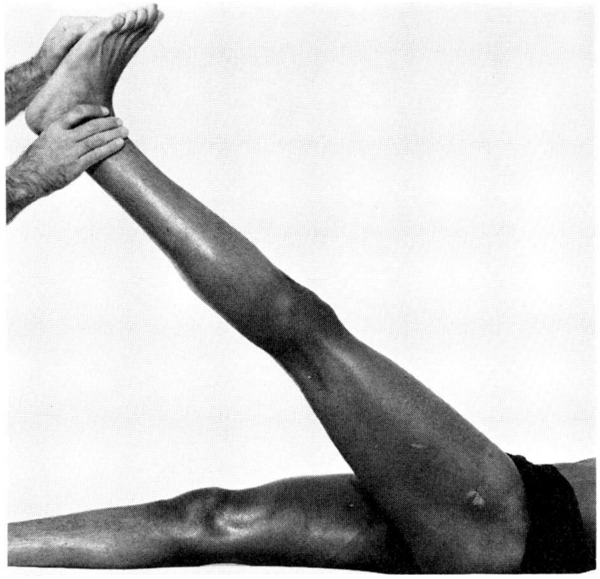

Fig. 7-11. Lasèque test. When straight leg raising has produced pain or hamstring spasm, further elevation of the leg is stopped and the foot is passively dorsiflexed. If there is sciatic irritation, further dorsiflexion aggravates the pain.

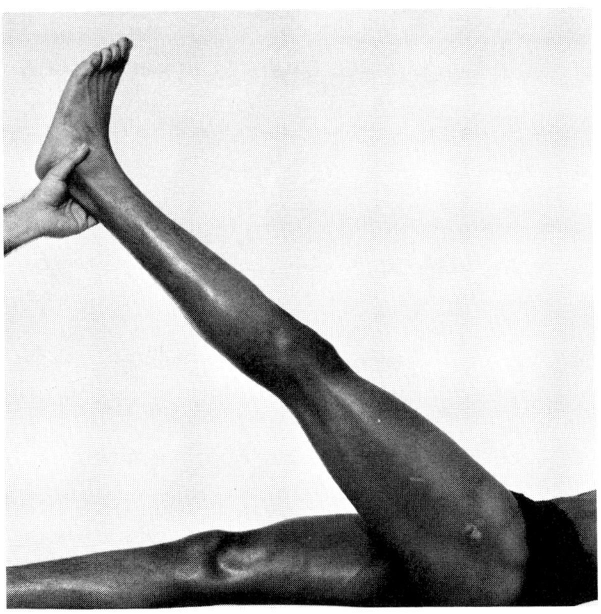

Fig. 7-10. Straight leg raising test. With the patient in the supine position, the leg is elevated keeping the knee fully extended. Normally the leg can be elevated to 90 degrees without discomfort.

Jugular Compression. When space occupying lesions, such as intraspinal tumors or intervertebral disk prolapse with nerve root impingement, are present, compression of the jugular vein may sufficiently increase the intraspinal pressure to cause pain. This pain may radiate down the course of the sciatic nerve. Coughing or sneezing will elicit the same response. This is also termed the Valsalva maneuver.

Vertebral Disease and Spinal Injury

Soto-Hall Test. With the patient in a supine position, the examiner passively raises the patient's head with one hand while controlling thoracic flexion by using the other hand to place pressure on the sternum. Because this tenses the intraspinous ligaments, pain is elicited at the site of the spinal lesions or recent fractures. This test should be done very carefully if a partial neurological deficit is present or suspected.

Sacroiliac Disease

FABERE Test or Patrick's Test. FABERE stands for flexion, abduction, external rotation, and extension. Such a maneuver places strain on the ipsilateral sacroiliac joint with pain, if arthritis or tumor are affecting it (see Fig. 10-25).

Gaenslen's Test. This test attempts to differentiate lumbosacral pain from sacroiliac pain. With the patient lying supine near the edge of the examining table, the inner hip and knee are flexed on the abdomen. The opposite thigh and leg are lowered over the edge of the table imposing sacroiliac strain and pain if that is the problem area.

Pelvic Compression. With the patient in a lateral position, firm compression over the iliac crest is applied. Pelvic compression by placing strain on the sacroiliac joints illicits pain if inflammation is present (see Fig. 10-23).

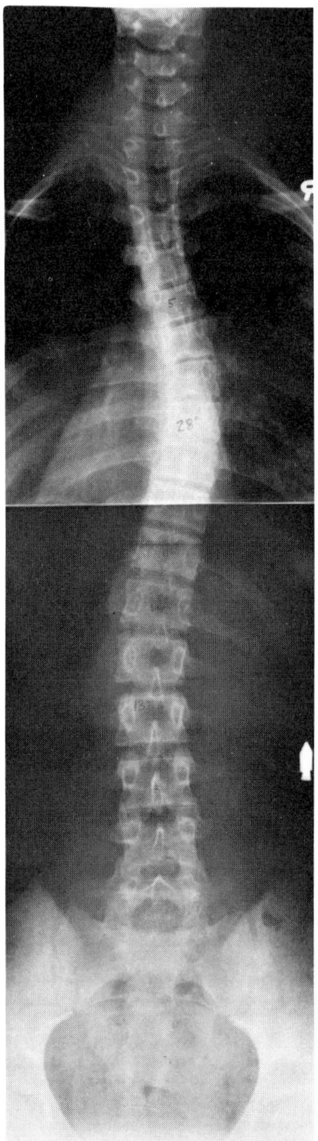

Fig. 7-12. A standard anteroposterior roentgenogram for a patient with spinal deformity. It is taken at a distance of 6 feet and includes the entire thoracolumbar spine. Note that the genital area is not covered by a lead sheet, which should be routine.

ROENTGENOGRAPHIC STUDIES

ROUTINE FILMS

If the deformity or pain is in the low back, certain routine films are necessary. These include anteroposterior, lateral, and oblique films of the lumbosacral spine. An anteroposterior view of the pelvis is added to view the sacroiliac joints if pain is centered in those areas. Generally, the hip joints are included on this view and can be evaluated for their contribution to the total picture.

Similar views can be taken of the thoracic spine if it is the area to be studied. For the scoliosis and kyphosis patients, special roentgenograms are necessary. The accepted view, according to the Scoliosis Research Society, is a 14 by 36 inch roentgenogram taken at a distance of 6 feet from where the patient is standing which includes the entire thoracolumbar spine (Fig. 7-12). If this larger film is not available, a standard large cassette is used.

STRESS FILMS

Stress films are helpful in several circumstances. Side-bending films are routinely used to evaluate the flexibility of scoliotic curves, and lateral hyperextension views are used to evaluate kyphotic deformities. Similarly, fusion masses in the spine can be checked for pseudoarthrosis by using stress views. A standing lateral view of the lumbosacral region, with weights on each shoulder, may demonstrate a spondylolisthesis that was not apparent on other views.

TOMOGRAMS—TOTAL BODY SCAN

Invaluable as the roentgenographic examination is, it suffers from one major shortcoming. On the film, structures overlap and are frequently difficult or impossible to distinguish from one another. This is particularly true when, as in the spine, the anterior and posterior structures are of the same density.

Every major hospital has the capacity to perform tomography. If a specific area of the spine is in question, as in congenital scoliosis, tomograms can more clearly delineate the abnormality. A series of progressive cuts are taken which, when looked at in sequence, offer a three dimensional view of the spine (Fig. 7-13). This kind of information has been greatly increased in the brain by the computer-operated EMI scanner and in the body by the total body scanner. These techniques have some major drawbacks; the units are costly and the detail produced is far poorer than standard roentgenograms. These are, however, the instruments of the future.

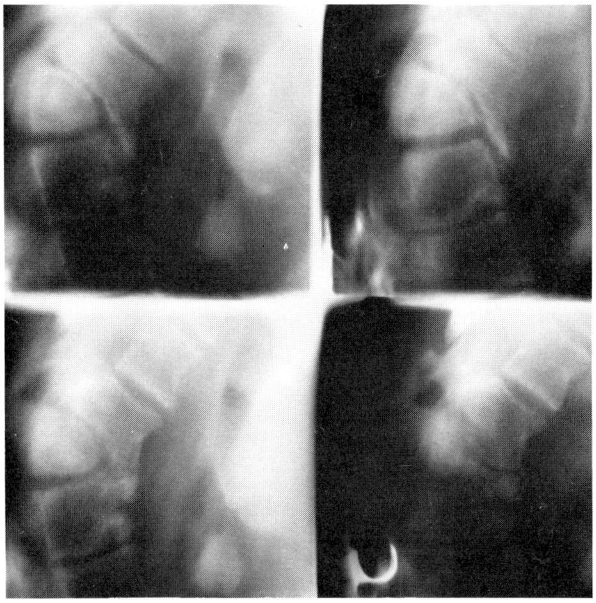

Fig. 7-13. Tomograms of the spine are helpful in delineating congenital anomalies, fractures, and infections. This figure demonstrates a healed fracture-dislocation of the thoracic spine which is clearly seen with the aid of tomography.

Oil Myelography

This is the most valuable roentgenographic examination in the diagnosis of lumbar disk disease. However, it is not a substitute for a thorough clinical examination but is requested to verify a suspected disk. It should probably be done before any intraspinal surgery, such as diskectomy, is performed. Additionally, it should be considered preoperatively in all congenital kyphosis and scoliosis correction and fusion.

The reasons for preoperative myelography are as follows: Tumors of the spinal canal that mimic disk disease will be revealed. More exact localization of the disk herniation and nerve root compression is offered. Double disk herniations which are unsuspected may be revealed. And finally, in congenital abnormalities, the bony or cartilagenous spurs frequently associated with diastematomyelia are outlined. These may tether the cord in such a way that straightening will cause paraplegia.

The technique is to perform routine spinal puncture in the lumbar spine and inject one of several oil base contrast media into the subarachnoid space. The sac and nerve root sleeves will be filled by the contrast medium and sharply outlined. Indentation of the dural sac or filling defects indicates abnormality which needs explanation (Fig. 7-14A, B).

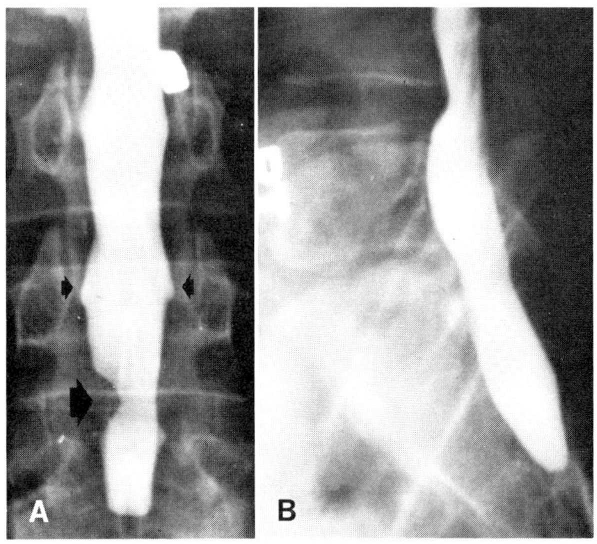

Fig. 7-14. (*A*) Anteroposterior myelogram of the lumbar spine indicating an indentation at the level of L5-S1 on the right. The nerve roots can be clearly seen at the level above, as indicated by the small arrows, and at L5-S1 a defect can be seen, as indicated by the large arrow. (*B*) Lateral view of the same patient demonstrating the disk indenting the myelographic dye column at the L5-S1 level. Note that the patient has an S1-S2 disk space, which can be a normal finding.

Because the needle usually remains in the back for removal of the dye, the study is done in the prone position. The examiner must be wary of a complete block of dye flow on myelogram. This may be seen in many conditions from tumor to trauma and prompts the neurosurgeon to recommend immediate decompression surgery. In the kyphotic patient, the flow of the dye is hindered by the kyphotic hump anteriorly. By removing the needle and placing the patient in the supine position, frequently the contrast agent will be seen to suddenly flow by the block. This may save the patient an unnecessary emergency operation which in the kyphotic may be detrimental to spinal stability.

The myelogram is only 80 to 90 percent accurate, with both false-positive and negative results. It should not be used in nonoperative candidates to prove or disprove legal claims and should not be used to decide whether a patient should undergo surgery. On the other hand, a patient who has a clear-cut neurological deficit, a positive straight leg raising test, and no improvement on conservative treatment should not be denied an operation because of a negative myelogram.

Complications of myelography have included meningitis, arachnoiditis, herniation of disk material, transection of a nerve filament, pulmonary embolism, and epidermoid formation.

Myelography with Water Soluble Contrast Medium

Radiopaque water soluble contrast has been used extensively in arteriography, intravenous pyelography, and several other roentgenographic tests to visualize internal organs. Because arachnoiditis and other bothersome complications have occurred after myelography using oil-based contrast media, attempts have been made to develop water soluble agents.

The difficulty with this material has been irritation of the nerve roots with pain and spasm. All agents developed thus far have been too irritating to allow contact with the spinal cord; therefore, the dye must be kept below lumbar 1. The incidence of transient headache and nausea is relatively high after examination. The quality of the myelogram produced is good. The density is less but the contrast agent tends to migrate further down the nerve root sleeves.

If a nontoxic, painless substance can be developed, this probably would be the agent of choice for myelography, as removal of the medium would not be necessary. This would save time and allow better positioning of the patient during the examination, as the needle could be removed.

Air Myelogram

This examination is rarely done in the United States although those centers that use the technique claim excellent results. Air as a medium of contrast is almost "ideal" in that it is quickly absorbed and is not toxic. A large amount of spinal fluid is removed so the injected air will float to the top when the patient is turned head-down. This technique, although difficult to interpret at first, is particularly effective in defining the spinal cord within the dural sac. This is important in the diagnosis of intradural lesions.

Diskography

Diskography is not a common procedure, although it has been done routinely prior to the injection of chymopapain into herniated disks. Diskography is performed by placing a 5-gauge spinal needle into the disk under radiographic control. Radiopaque dye is then injected into the interspace carefully recording the amount of dye accepted and the pressure required. This may be done with the patient awake in an attempt to reproduce pain. A normal diskogram can rule out degeneration, but abnormalities are so common that little reliability can be placed on abnormal diskograms.

Some other radiographic studies include intraosseous venography, selective arteriography of spinal arteries, and individual nerve root sleeve contrast studies. These studies are technically difficult to perform and interpret but offer additional help in diagnosis to those familiar with them. Texts specializing in treatment of the spine have a complete discussion of these studies.

OTHER STUDIES

Bone Scan

Scanning techniques have been developed in which bone-seeking isotopes are used. The radioisotopes most frequently used are technetium 99-M labeled diphosphonate derivative, fluoride 18, and strontium 85. They differ primarily in the half-life of the isotope and, when positive, are indicative of increased bone metabolic activity. It could represent infection, arthritis, malignant tumor, or fracture. Even the most astute nuclear medicine physician sometimes has difficulty differentiating these entities. It is, however, useful in locating a lesion which is symptomatic but not yet visible on roentgenogram.

EMG—Electromyogram

The electromyogram is extremely useful in evaluating nerve root denervation, muscular disease, and peripheral neuropathies. It is an essential tool in the evaluation of a herniated disk syndrome. It must be remembered that it takes 21 days before the EMG will record denervation potentials. The reader is referred to Chapter 2 for a complete discussion of this technique.

Cystometrogram

Incontinence and other disturbances of urinary bladder function occasionally will be the first manifestation of neurological disease. An associated rectal incontinence should suggest a common neurogenic cause of the disturbance. The cystometrogram is a quantitative measurement of the bladder tone. The differential diagnosis for motor and/or sensory deficit of the bladder and skin of the anogenital region is extensive. The roots involved are sacral 1, 2, and 3. The technique of performing this test is described in any urology text.

Needle Biopsy

When a definitive diagnosis is needed and all the clinical tests, short of surgical exploration, have been exhausted, needle biopsy is effective in obtaining pathological material from the spine. Ottolenghi, an Argentine surgeon, described techniques for obtaining needle biopsy material from all areas of the spine. Although biopsy above the level of lumbar 1 is dangerous because of spinal cord and lung proximity, it can be safely accomplished by following his technique under biplane image intensification. Thus, infectious lesions are biopsied and cultured and suspected tumors are pathologically studied.

DIFFERENTIAL DIAGNOSIS

Pain Syndromes of the Spine

Diskogenic Pain

Disk Space Infection

Disk space infection in children is probably different than pyogenic osteomyelitis of the spine and should probably be classified separately. This is exemplified by the poorer prognosis and more extensive vertebral destruction seen with pyogenic osteomyelitis in the late adolescent and adult. Most patients are less than 20 years of age, mean of 11 years, with no sex predilection.

An infectious cause is assumed by most authors although this is not universally accepted. Speigal and associates reported a series of 48 cases and concluded that objective data for an infectious cause, although not conclusive, cannot be disregarded. In 15 biopsy specimens, they obtained four positive cultures and eight specimens which showed inflammation. Boston and coworkers obtained specimens for culture in 11 patients with positive results in nine. Seven of the nine grew Staphylococcus aureus. The spread of the organisms is thought to be hematogenous. Vascular channels usually cannot be found in the intervertebral disk in those over the age of 30.

The patient usually presents with severe backache and progressive limp. The most useful symptom in the younger child is a refusal to ambulate because of pain. Night pain is usually a prominent part of the pattern. There may be an antecedent history of trauma although this is not usual. Temperature elevations in the range of 102 to 105 degrees F can be noted. This finding is frequently associated with an acute upper respiratory infection.

On examination, the patient makes every effort to guard or splint the spine. Usually, the involvement is lumbar, but it may be noted in the lower thoracic spine. The patient may present with a painful scoliosis.

Early in the course of the disease, the roentgenograms are negative, but by three weeks narrowing of the intervertebral disk space is usually noted. Progression leads to irregularity of the vertebral end plates on either side of the involved disk space (Fig. 7-15). The usual outcome is narrowing of the interspace with irregularity and sclerosis of the vertebral end plates (Fig. 7-16A, B). In some cases, the condition may progress to spontaneous fusion of the vertebrae.

The most consistent positive test is elevation of the erythrocyte sedimentation rate with levels approaching 100 being noted at one hour. The hemoglobin and leukocyte count are nearly always normal. Blood culture in the acutely ill patient may reveal a positive result. It may be necessary to perform a needle or open biopsy in adults, and if indicated, tomography, myelography, and appropriate skin tests.

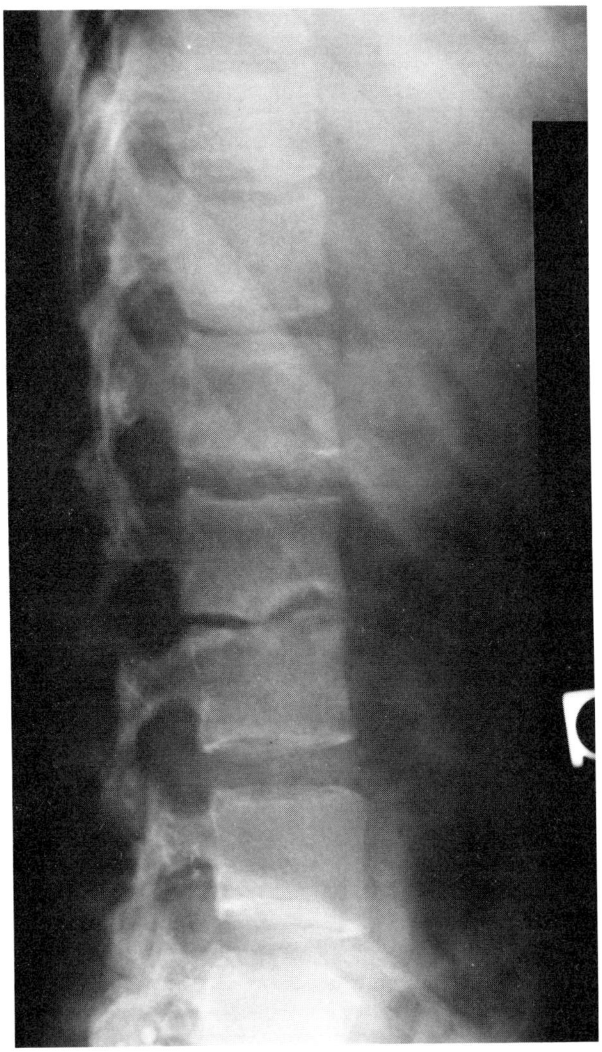

Fig. 7-15. Note the decreased disk space between lumbar 3 and 4 with irregularity of the vertebral end plates. Needle biopsy of this area produced a culture of *Staphylococcus aureus.*

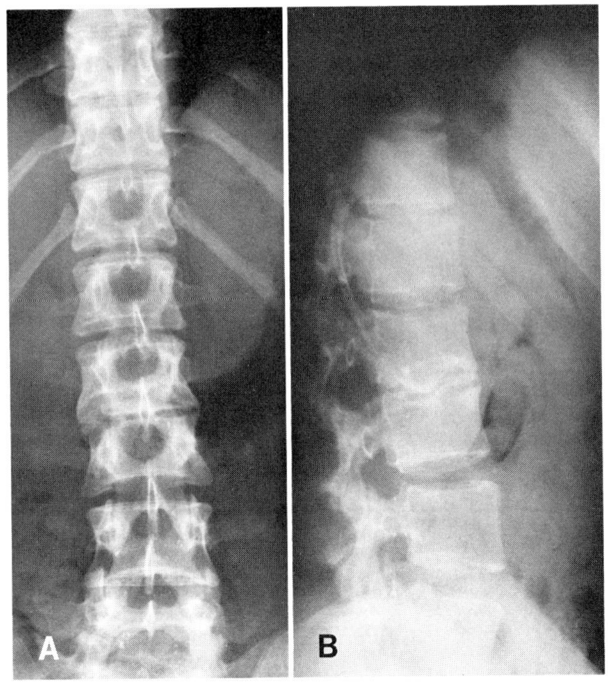

Fig. 7-16. (*A*) Anteroposterior roentgenogram one year later demonstrating the same patient in Figure 7-19 with almost complete loss of disk space and osteophytic formation about the vertebral body, indicating that spontaneous fusion may take place in the near future. (*B*) Lateral roentgenogram of the same spine showing loss of disk space and the potential for spontaneous fusion.

Vertebral osteomyelitis or paravertebral abscess must be differentiated so the appropriate treatment can be instituted. Antibiotics are not routinely used in disk space infection in children. Immobilization is the key to treatment and frequently is all that is needed.

Mechanical Insufficiency

Fracture-Dislocation of the Thoracolumbar Spine

In an accident, the spine is subjected to one of five types of stress: pure flexion, flexion and rotation, extension, vertical compression, or a direct shearing force.

With pure flexion stress, there is tension applied to the posterior ligament complex which does not rupture and compression applied to the body anteriorly. The result is a *simple wedge fracture* which remains stable (Figs. 7-17 and 7-18).

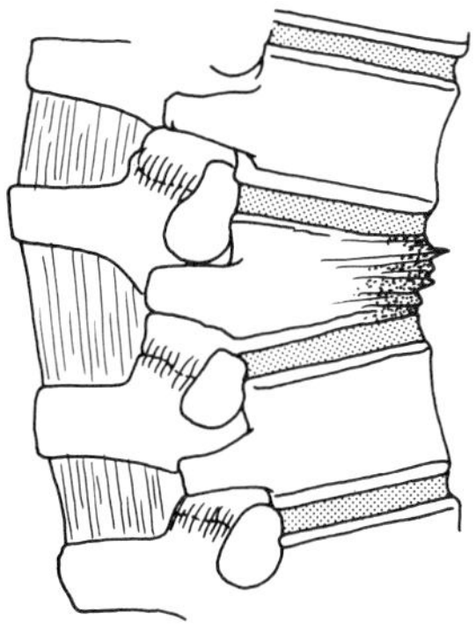

Fig. 7-17. Schematic drawing of a simple wedge fracture of a thoracic or lumbar vertebra.

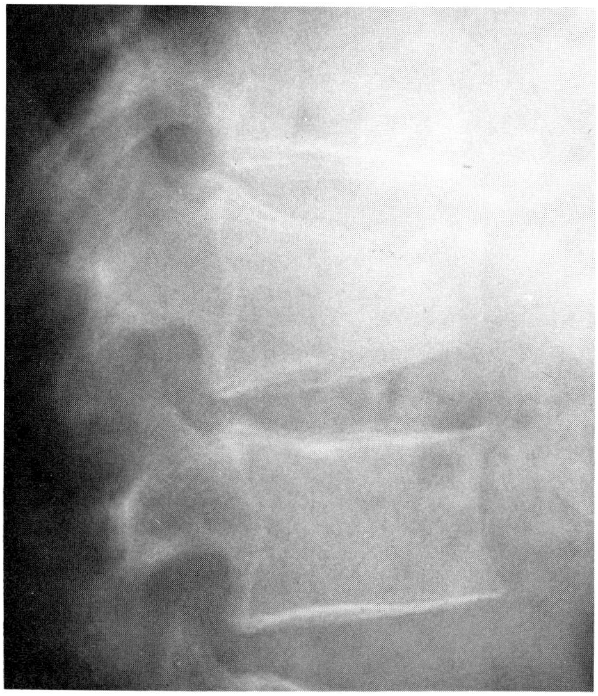

Fig. 7-18. Radiograph of a compression or wedge fracture of the first lumbar vertebra in a 45-year-old male. This is a stable injury.

With the flexion-rotation mechanism of injury, the posterior ligaments rupture and the upper vertebra rotates on the lower vertebra. In the lumbar region, because of large vertical facet joints, generally one or both of the articular processes fracture along with a slice fracture of the body of the lower vertebra (Fig. 7-19). The slice fracture is much more common than disruption of the disk. This is termed a *rotational fracture-dislocation;* it can occur anywhere in the thoracolumbar spine and is extremely unstable.

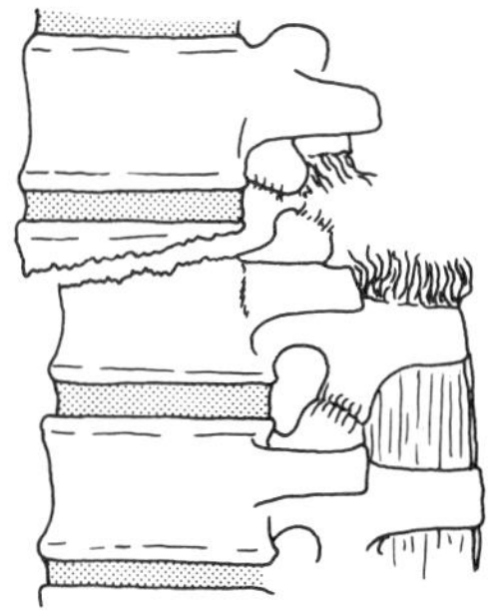

Fig. 7-19. A slice fracture, which is a rotational fracture-dislocation. This occurs in the lumbar region and one or both of the articular processes fracture along with a slice fracture of the body of the lower vertebra. This fracture is extremely unstable.

Pure *extension injuries* are limited to the cervical spine and will be discussed in the appropriate section.

Vertical compression injuries occur when severe force is applied to the buttocks, such as falling abruptly, and causes the applied force to be absorbed by the vertebral bodies. The vertebral end plate shatters, and the disk is forced into the body which explodes. This is commonly referred to as a *burst fracture* (Figs. 7-20 and 7-21A, B). The ligaments are not damaged, and the fracture is stable.

The *shearing type* of fracture occurs when a powerful force is applied directly to the back, particularly in the relatively fixed thoracic area. The upper vertebra is sheared off the lower vertebra with fracture of articular processes and rupture of all ligaments.

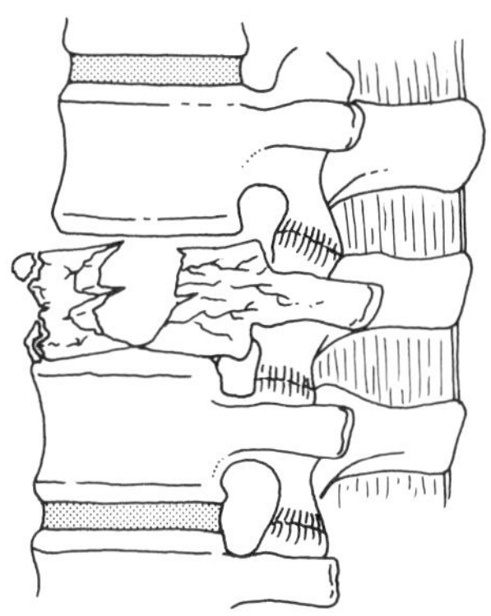

Fig. 7-20. Schematic demonstration of a burst fracture. In this case, the end plates shatter and the disk is forced into the body, which explodes.

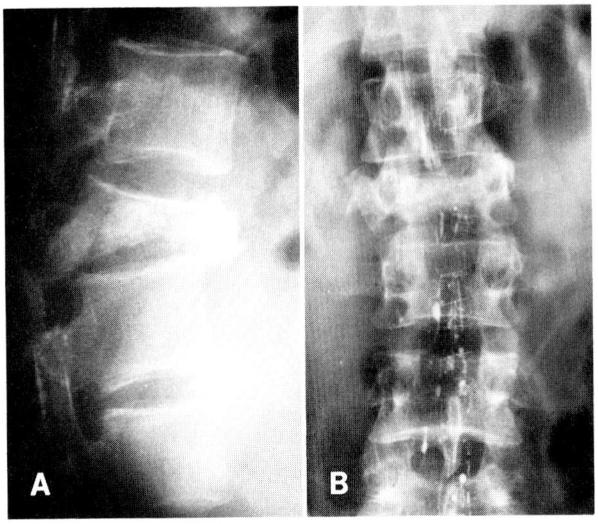

Fig. 7-21. (*A*) Lateral roentgenogram of a burst fracture of lumbar 2 in a 23-year-old male. These fractures frequently extend posteriorly compromising the spinal cord and its roots. (*B*) Anteroposterior roentgenogram of the same fracture. Note that the pedicles are slightly widened at the level of the fracture, indicating they have been exploded laterally.

These fractures frequently cause paraplegia because of displacement in the narrow thoracic vertebral canal but are stable due to the thoracic rib cage.

Other iniuries include fracture of the transverse processes. This occurs in the lumbar spine where the psoas muscle takes origin (Fig. 7-22).

A history of trauma associated with severe pain in the spine are the typical findings. It may be associated with varying degrees of transitory or permanent neurological deficit.

Inspection of the back can help determine the mechanism of injury. For example, abrasions over the shoulders would indicate a flexion-rotation injury. Palpation will reveal tenderness over the site of the fracture, and if the posterior ligaments are torn, a gap will be noted between the spinous processes. A palpable gap between the vertebral spines indicates instability according to Holdsworth.

The separation of the spinous processes can be confirmed on a lateral roentgenogram. Simple wedge fracture demonstrates compression of the vertebral body anteriorly, with intact end plates and no spinous process separation. Rotational fracture-dislocations frequently show a slice off the upper border of the lower vertebra and a lateral shift of the fractured articular processes. The burst fracture shows a fracture of the end plate with explosion of the body, and fragments frequently seen in the vertebral canal. The shear fracture is heralded by a forward displacement of one vertebra on another with fracture of the articular processes or pedicles or both.

The fractures are usually not a problem of diagnosis, but it is important to determine which are stable and which are unstable. Occasionally, an elderly patient will come to the emergency room with back

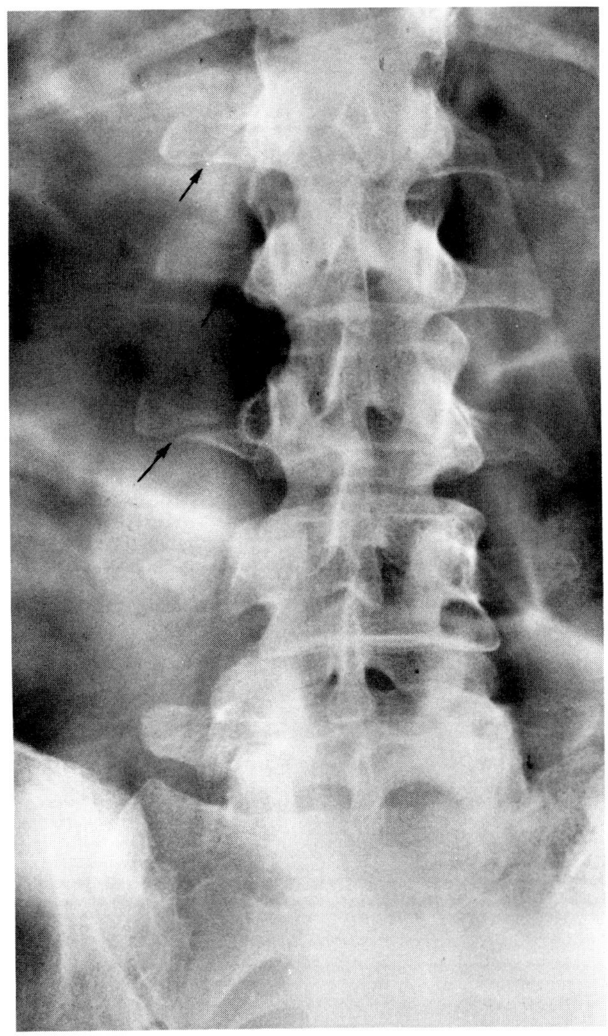

Fig. 7-22. Anteroposterior roentgenogram indicating fractures of the transverse processes of lumbar 1, 2, and 3 on the right side. Although this injury is not associated with any neurological problems, it can be quite painful and debilitating.

pain and roentgenogram reveals a compression fracture. Here the differential would include osteoporosis, tumor with pathological fracture, or an old fracture and new back pain.

In the paraplegic or paraparetic patient, an accurate diagnosis and prognosis of the neurological lesion depends on understanding the spinal cord anatomy and a careful, complete neurological examination on admission, combined with repeated examinations thereafter.

Spondylolisthesis and Spondylolysis

Spondylolisthesis is derived from the Greek "spondylo," meaning spine, and "listhesis," meaning to slide down a slippery path. Anatomically, this means one vertebra slides, usually forward or anterior, on another (Fig. 7-23). Spondylolysis pertains to a defect in the pars interarticularis, the "lysis" meaning to dissolve. Spondylolysis is usually requisite to slippage or spondylolisthesis. However, in some instances the pars interarticularis is stretched or traumatically fractured allowing the slip to occur.

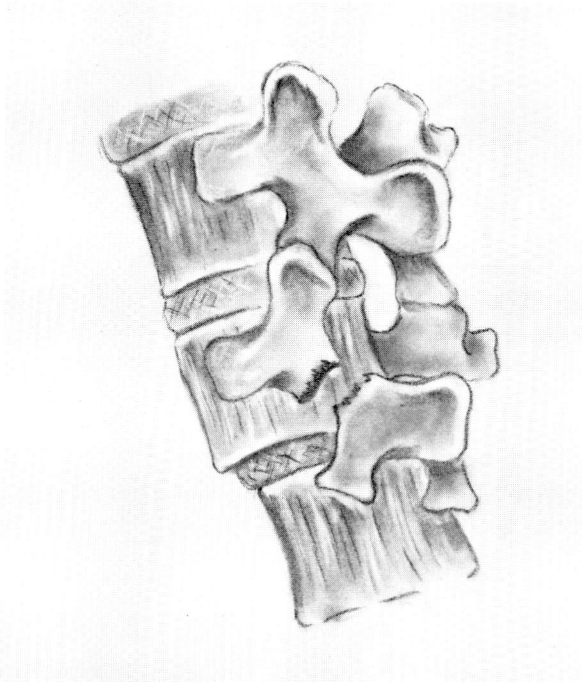

Fig. 7-23. Schematic drawing of spondylolithesis. Lysis of the pars interarticularis is demonstrated.

According to Wiltse about 50 percent of the cases having a defect in the pars interarticularis will not show appreciable slipping and are designated as spondylolysis without spondylolisthesis. In the younger patient these can usually be converted to a spondylolisthesis by the patient standing erect with weights on his shoulders allowing one vertebra to slide forward on another. This is usually the fifth lumbar sliding forward on the first sacral vertebra, but it can occur at any level.

Spondylolisthesis is most common in the lumbar spine but does occur in the cervical spine. There have been instances of pars interarticularis defects in the thoracic spine but spondylolisthesis only occurs secondary to fracture dislocation.

There are many causes of spondylolisthesis, the most common being simply a dissolution of the pars. This is the type seen in patients under the age of 50 and has been called "true spondylolisthesis." The cause of this condition has been extensively studied, with numerous theories being advanced as to its origin. Some of the interesting factors to be considered in determining the cause are discussed briefly in this chapter.

This disease only occurs in man who walks with a true upright stance and has lumbar lordosis. There is no evidence that this defect is ever present at birth, and it is not seen in patients who have never been ambulatory. The most common age of onset is between five and six years of age, but slipping can occur up until age 20. The period of most rapid slipping is between 10 and 15 years when the adolescent growth spurt is at its peak.

The overall incidence of this defect in the United States is around 5 percent. It is less common in blacks, being seen only half as often as in whites. The sex incidences show a predominance in males (2:1). Spina bifida is 13 times more frequent when associated with a defect of the pars interarticularis than in a normal spine. There is also a frequent association of scoliosis with spondylolisthesis. Finally, there is a familial tendency in the development of spondylolisthesis.

Wiltse's theory of etiology states that a defective pars is due to an inherited defect in the cartilage model of the vertebra. The defect appears when particular stresses and strains are placed on the pars interarticularis in the lumbar spine because of man's upright stance and lumbar curve. A stress fracture occurs which has diminished ability to repair itself.

Other types of spondylolisthesis include acute fractures of the pars interarticularis, elongation of the pedicles, degeneration of the facet joints with slipping, pathological fractures, and spondylolisthesis above or below a previous fusion. These are far less common clinically.

Although spondylolisthesis and spondylolysis usually occur during childhood and adolescence, symptoms during this period are uncommon. About 25 percent will have some back pain but only 10 percent will seek medical attention. More children will be seen for postural deformities and abnormalities of gait than pain. In the adult, pain is the usual presenting feature.

Symptoms are usually aggravated or initiated by some strenuous activity, and limitation of that activity or rest will usually decrease them. On occasion the patient will present with a radicular pattern of pain in the lower extremities but only a mild back problem. This suggests a more advanced spondylolisthesis with nerve root irritation.

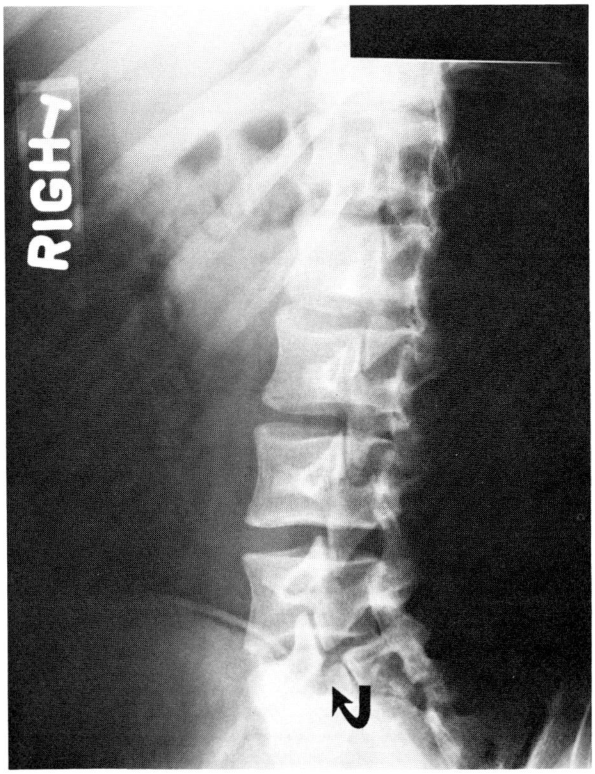

Fig. 7-24. Oblique roentgenogram demonstrating the defect in the pars interarticularis. Compare it with the schematic drawing in Fig. 7-23 to better visualize where the defect occurs in the spine.

Children, in contrast to adults, rarely show signs of objective nerve root compression (i.e., reflex changes, sensory loss, or motor weakness). However, careful testing for sacral anesthesia and bladder dysfunction should be carried out. Hamstring tightness is frequently associated with the symptomatic cases and is thought by some to be due to nerve root irritation. It can occur with either spondylolisthesis or spondylolysis. The exact mechanism which initiates this spasm is not known and nerve root irritation alone does not fully explain why it is so extensive and disappears after spinal fusion.

The hamstring spasm can be quite severe, the child being unable to flex the hips with the knees extended. The straight leg raising test may be positive at minimal degrees of leg elevation. This tightness is the cause of the peculiar gait which has been associated with spondylolisthesis in the child. The tight hamstrings keep the pelvis tilted backward and do not permit enough hip flexion for normal gait. The patient, therefore, walks stiff legged, severely rotating the pelvis. This has been described by Newman as a "pelvic waddle."

The physical examination can range from normal in the asymptomatic patient with a minor slip, to a myriad of anatomical and neurological findings in the severely affected. Lumbar lordosis can be severe and if the slip is advanced, a slip off or depression can be palpated in the lower lumbar area. Several types of scoliosis are frequently associated with spondylolisthesis, and they should be investigated together. The neurological findings can range from hamstring tightness to severe loss of reflex, bowel and bladder dysfunction, and motor weakness. The local pain in the adult can be incapacitating.

The radiolucent defect in spondylolysis of the pars interarticularis is visible on roentgenogram. If it is large, it can be seen on almost any view, but if smaller, may require special views, such as obliques, to place it in relief and make it stand out (Fig. 7-24). A visual aid is the "scotty dog" of LaChapele, the defect occurring at the dog's neck and is useful for those inexperienced in reading oblique views. The edges are typically smooth and rounded suggesting an old lesion rather than a fresh fracture.

Deficiency of the posterior elements is a common occurrence in spondylolisthesis. Malformed laminae have been observed in up to 40 percent of the patients with spondylolisthesis.

Forward subluxation of the vertebral body (spondylolisthesis) can best be visualized on the lateral roentgenogram (Fig. 7-25). Meyerding developed the simplest system for grading the amount of displacement. The top of the sacrum is divided into four equal sections, and the slips are given Grades of 1 to 4 depending on which quadrant the posterior portion of the superior vertebra falls. This should be judged on a standing roentgenogram, preferably with 10-pound sand bags on the shoulders, because the spondylolisthesis can reduce itself. In advanced slips the body develops a trapezoidal shape, the anterior portion being larger than the posterior. Flexion-extension views of the spine may be used to evaluate motion.

In less obvious cases tomography may better delineate the lesion. If neurological symptoms are present, myelography can be helpful. Typically, the spinal canal is indented anteriorly by the posterior aspect of the sacrum.

Spondylolisthesis presenting with low back pain and associated neurological signs can be confused with cauda equina tumors, diastematomyelia, tight filum terminale, and massively herniated disk syndrome. The radiographic features including myelography can help differentiate these diseases.

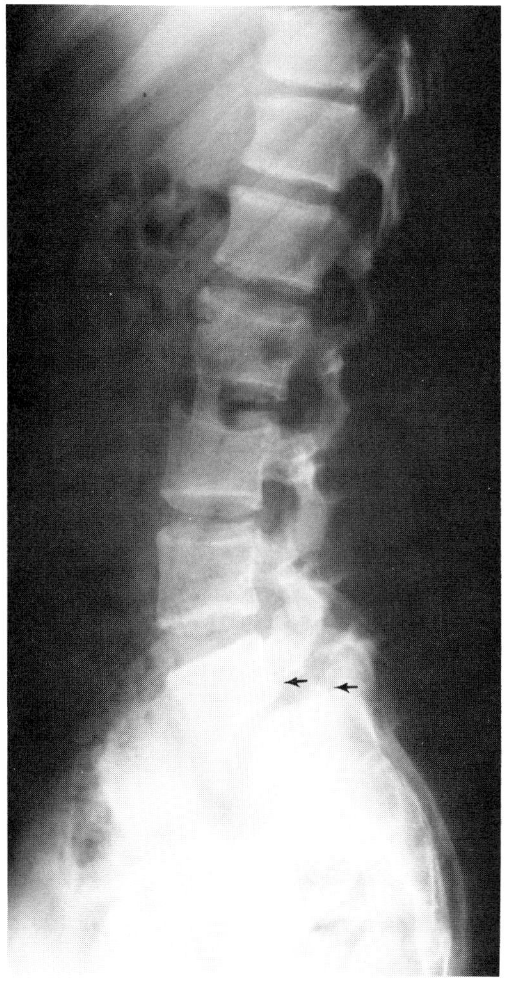

Fig. 7-25. Roentgenogram demonstrating a slip of L5 on S1. The arrows point to the posterior area of the fifth lumbar and first sacral vertebra respectively. Normally, these should line up. In this case, a second degree slip by Meyerding's system is noted.

Arthritis Pain Syndromes

Osteoarthritis

The most common of the arthritides to affect the spine is osteoarthritis. The cause is not known. Its development is closely related to the development and aging of the articular structures. The name primary osteoarthritis is used to designate those cases where there is no attributable cause. Secondary osteoarthritis results from abnormal stresses or trauma to the joints involved. In the back, these might be the abnormal stresses of a spinal deformity or simply obesity. Age remains the most important predisposing factor. It occurs almost exclusively in middle-aged and elderly people. No preference for sex is noted, but the occurrence of symptoms is particularly common in women approaching menopause. There is an element of inherited propensity and similar problems are seen in succeeding generations of families.

One of the interesting features of this disease is the striking lack of correlation between the symptoms and the degree of degenerative changes as evidenced on roentgenogram. A patient with advanced osteoarthritis of the spine may have little, if any, complaints, while those with only minor changes may be most uncomfortable.

Clinically, the most important symptom is an aching pain which occurs on exertion and is relieved by rest. Stiffness after sitting, particularly with the first few motions, is a common complaint. The stiffness is usually relatively short in duration resolving in minutes rather than hours as in the stiffness of rheumatoid arthritis.

Range of motion of the spine may reveal crepitus, creaking, or grating but these are uncommon findings. There may be localized tenderness particularly in the lumbar spine.

Associated disease is usually seen in the weight-bearing joints; hips, knees, and ankles. It is also associated with swelling in the distal interphalangeal joints of the fingers, with production of Heberden's nodes.

Degenerative arthritis is characterized histologically by degeneration and roentgenographically by hypertrophy of bone at the articular margins (Fig. 7-26). In the spine, the facet joints are more frequently involved. As the cartilage degenerates, the joint space narrows, and there may be erosion of the articular bone with alteration of the joint articulating surfaces (Fig. 7-27). This is best seen in the

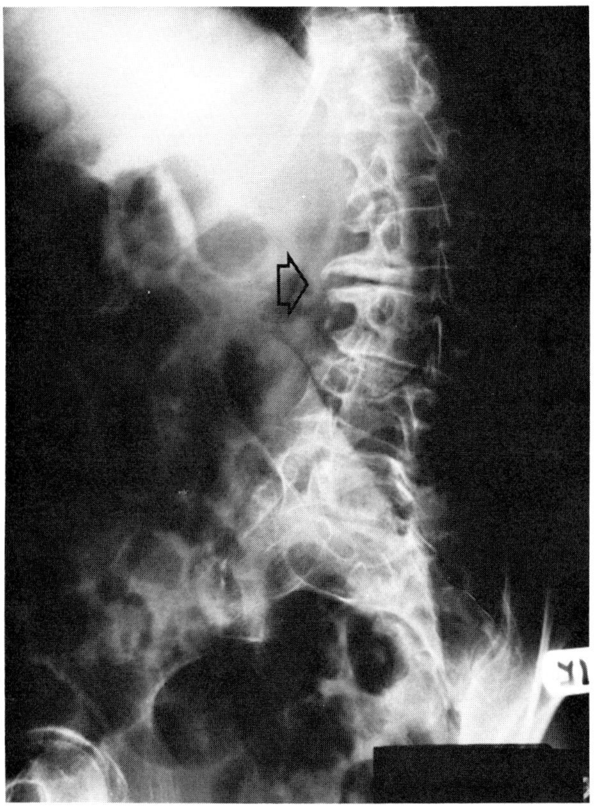

Fig. 7-26. Severe degenerative arthritis in the lumbar spine with horizontal osteophytes at almost every level. The arrow indicates several severe osteophytes at lumbar 3-4.

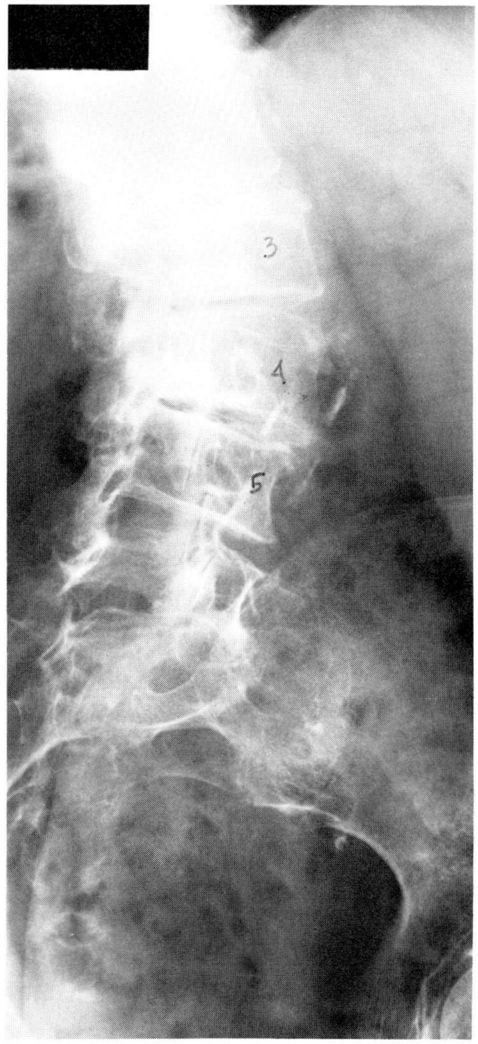

Fig. 7-27. Oblique roentgenogram of the lumbar spine clearly outlining the facet joints of the L4-L5 and L5-S1 levels. Joint space narrowing is present and the inferior facets have migrated cephalad. Also note that lumbar 4 has shifted slightly laterally on lumbar 5.

oblique projections which show the facet joints. Later, periarticular lipping becomes more conspicuous and is the predominant feature. These spurs can also occur about the vertebral disks particularly in osteoarthritis secondary to degenerative disk disease.

In the thoracolumbar spine, rheumatoid arthritis can usually be ruled out because of its preference for the cervical area, as well as the peripheral distribution of the disease. Gout, Charcot spine, and metastatic disease are more difficult pathological processes to rule out. Diffuse idiopathic skeletal hyperostosis (DISH) or Forestier's syndrome is similar in roentgenographic appearance to osteoarthritis and is probably part of the continuum.

Spondylitis of Rheumatoid Variants

Ankylosing spondylitis (formerly called "rheumatoid spondylitis"), Reiter's syndrome, psoriatic arthritis, and the arthritis of inflammatory bowel disease (ulcerative colitis and regional enteritis) were formerly considered "forme frustes" of rheumatoid arthritis but are now recognized as distinct entities. These arthritides are termed "rheumatoid variants" and may be distinguished from each other and from rheumatoid arthritis by clinical, laboratory, and roentgenographic characteristics, namely (1) the roentgenographic appearance of the spine when spondylitis is present, (2) the location of periosteal new bone formation and ligamentous calcification, (3) the joint distribution of the arthritis, (4) the presence of specific skin lesions, and (5) the HLA-W27 antigen. The diagnosis of spondylitis should not be a primary diagnosis unless it is idiopathic ankylosing spondylitis.

Ankylosing spondylitis is a systemic inflammatory disease with both intraarticular and extraarticular manifestations. It primarily affects the sacroiliac and apophyseal joints of the spine, but peripheral joints may also become involved. The extraarticular manifestations of primary concern are iritis which is potentially blinding and aortitis which may lead to the patient's demise. Less serious extraarticular manifestations include heel spurs and ligamentous calcification. The association between ankylosing spondylitis and Reiter's syndrome, JRA (juvenile rheumatoid arthritis), the spondylitis of IBD (inflammatory bowel disease), and psoriasis will be discussed under those disease entities.

Ankylosing spondylitis typically has its onset between 15 to 35 years, but it has been detected in some as young as age 7 and others in their 40s. It occurs nine times more frequently in males than in females, but the potential course of the disease is similar in both sexes.

The presenting complaint is usually low back pain of a nontraumatic and insidious onset. It may be constant but is more frequently intermittent, at least in the initial stages. About one fourth to one third of these patients present with peripheral joint complaints, usually in the large joints such as the hips or knees. Careful questioning usually elicits a history of back pain at an earlier date. And, finally, a very small number (about 2%) present initially with iridocyclitis. Whatever the onset, the symptoms are eventually accompanied by systemic manifestations which include fatigue, anemia, intermittent low grade fever, anorexia, and weight loss.

As the disease progresses, the spine slowly fuses in a caudad to cephalad fashion with back stiffness as the prominent feature. Diffuse costovertebral joint involvement is common, yet despite the decreased chest expansion (less than 2 cm.), those afflicted compensate with diaphragmatic breathing, and subsequent pulmonary compromise is minimal. One third of these patients are struck by acute uveitis at some point in the course of the disease, but chronic manifestations and blindness are rare. Aortic insufficiency and vertebral fracture are among the most serious complications and rarely may lead to death.

The sacroiliac joints are the first sites of spinal involvement (Fig. 7-28). Both are affected although initially one may be more involved than the other. The roentgenographic changes include irregularity

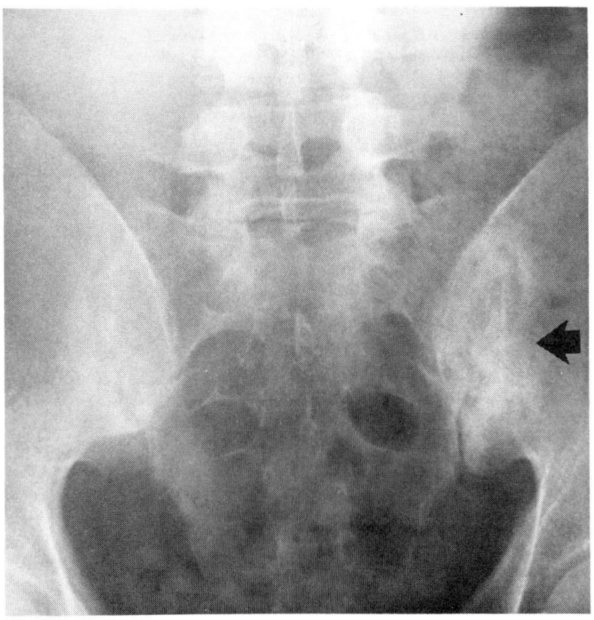

Fig. 7-28. An early case of ankylosing spondylitis with sacroiliac joint involvement. The arrow indicates the left sacroiliac joint where alternate areas of sclerosis and destruction can be seen.

and indistinctness of the subchondral bony margins with reactive sclerosis on both sides of the sacroiliac joint. The vertebrae and spinal joints are affected at the thoracolumbar and lumbosacral junctions. Cervical spondylitis may develop later. Vertebral erosions develop at the superior and inferior anterior aspect of the vertebral bodies, giving them a square appearance when viewed on the lateral projection (Fig. 7-29A). Syndesmophytes, paravertebral calcifications, develop near the above-mentioned erosions and bridge adjacent vertebrae. As they become generalized, the characteristic "bamboo spine" results (Fig. 7-29B). And finally, the apophyseal joints narrow and fuse. Extraspinal roentgenographic changes such as heel spurs, can also occur.

Mild anemia and an elevated ESR (in 80%) have been the only helpful laboratory data until recently, but they are nonspecific. The RA factor is no higher than in an age matched control population. In 1973 several reports linked the presence of ankylosing spondylitis with the HLA-W27 antigen. This antigen is present in 4 percent of the control population but is consistently present in greater than 80 percent with ankylosing spondylitis. Hence, the absence of this antigen does not rule out this disorder, but its presence, coupled with a strong clinical suspicion, is diagnostically helpful.

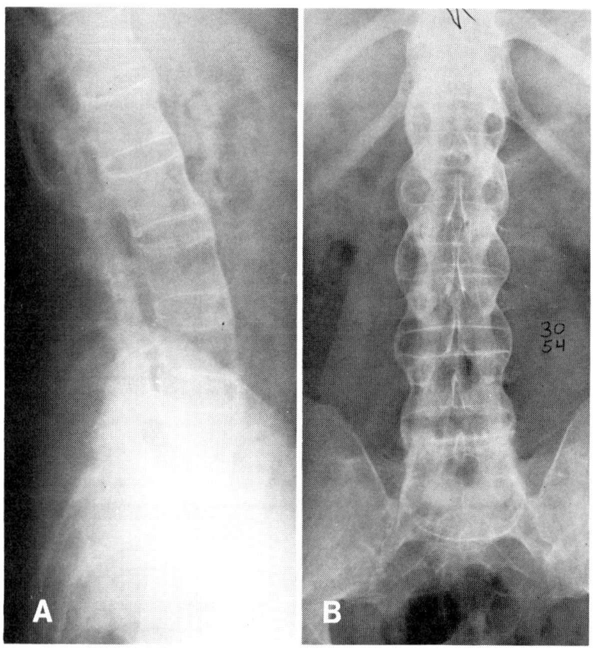

Fig. 7-29. Lumbar spine in a patient with ankylosing spondylitis. (*A*) The anterior longitudinal ligament is calcified. (*B*) Anteroposterior view of the same patient showing the characteristic "bamboo spine."

Reiter's Syndrome. The triad of nongonococcal urethritis, conjunctivitis, and arthritis (usually of the lower extremities) that has characteristically been used to describe Reiter's syndrome is too limiting. Keratodermia blennorrhagica, an exfoliative rash on the soles of the feet, and circinate balanitis, a rash on the glans, have been added to the unhappy trio.

The etiology remains unknown but it has certain associations. Shigella dysentery or nonspecific diarrhea have been known to precede it. More commonly, sexual exposure is antecedent. It should be noted that gonococcal urethritis may accompany this disorder. Generally this disease occurs in young males, but it may be seen in women and children.

The HLA-W27 antigen is present in at least 80 percent of patients with Reiter's and its inclusion is mandatory in an evaluation for this disorder. Cultures of urethral, prostatic, and conjunctival discharge are consistently negative.

The roentgenographic manifestations, when present, are axial and peripheral. We shall concentrate on the former. There may be a sacroiliitis indistinguishable from ankylosing spondylitis. However, in Reiter's syndrome the frequency of unilateral occurrence is higher. Paraspinal ossifications may bridge vertebral bodies, but unlike ankylosing spondylitis, they develop asymmetrically and are not generalized.

Psoriasis. The incidence of arthritis with psoriasis is probably in the neighborhood of 5 to 7 percent, and 20 to 30 percent of these have spinal involvement which is indistinguishable roentgenographically from Reiter's syndrome. It must be noted that often the skin lesions of Reiter's syndrome are indistinguishable from psoriasis. Laboratory tests for psoriasis are of no help. The HLA-W27 antigen is absent in psoriasis unless spinal involvement is present. The incidence then rises above 40 percent. Hence, the association is not as strong as in ankylosing spondylitis and Reiter's syndrome.

IBD—Inflammatory Bowel Disease. A seronegative arthropathy that is usually nonerosive and affects primarily the large joints has been described in association with inflammatory bowel disease. In addition, about 5 percent of the patients with regional enteritis and 20 percent of those with ulcerative colitis develop a spondylitis indistinguishable from ankylosing spondylitis. The spondylitis may antedate or postdate the appearance of the bowel disease. Moreover, the peripheral arthritis waxes and wanes with the activity of the bowel disease but once the spondylitis starts, it is progressive.

JRA—Juvenile Rheumatoid Arthritis. It is conceivable that juvenile rheumatoid arthritis and ankylosing spondylitis could occur simultaneously. However, the spondylitis of juvenile rheumatoid arthritis tends to affect the cervical spine, especially at C2-C3. Most occurrences of juvenile rheumatoid arthritis with ankylosing spondylitis are probably cases of ankylosing spondylitis, appearing in childhood, with the initial manifestations being inflammation of peripheral joints followed by spinal involvement. Roentgenographic changes of sacroiliitis without progression of spinal involvement is seen in patients with juvenile rheumatoid arthritis, but this is usually without symptoms.

Rheumatoid Arthritis. Seropositive RA does involve the spine, but this is predominantly in the cervical region and is discussed in Chapter 6. The thoracolumbar spine is conspicuously spared. Sacroiliitis is uncommon and clinically inconspicuous.

Diffuse Idiopathic Skeletal Hyperostosis

Ankylosing vertebral hyperostosis, described in 1950 by Forestier and Rotes Querol, has been recently more accurately called diffuse idiopathic skeletal hyperostosis (DISH). It occurs in those patients over the age of 50 and is characterized by ossification of the anterior and right lateral aspects of the vertebral column, usually in the middle and lower thoracic regions. This flowing ossification may also occur in the cervical region and produce osteophytes large enough to cause dysphagia.

The predominant symptoms of this disease are vertebral. Stiffness, back pain, and decreased range of motion are the most common findings. Cervical pain and dysphagia have been reported. Peripheral musculoskeletal complaints of pain and/or stiffness involving shoulders, knees, elbows, hips, and heels are present in less than one half.

Laboratory studies as of yet are no help in the diagnosis. The radiographic manifestations hold the key to recognition of this disease. The most common site of roentgenographic abnormality (and probably present in all) is the thoracic spine, usually T7 to T12, although involvement of the proximal and distal extensions is common. There is a distinct pattern of laminated new bone formation along the anterior and right lateral vertebral bodies (Fig. 7-30). Maintenance of disk space, absence of apophyseal changes, and absence of sacroiliac joint fusion distinguish this entity from degenerative disk disease and ankylosing spondylitis. In addition, osteoporosis is rare, and the vertebral bodies are not squared. C4-C7 is the most commonly involved ligament in the neck. Thick, flowing anterior osteophytes are present. It almost resembles a candle-wax dripping along the anterior cervical spine. Apophyseal joint involvement in this region is also absent.

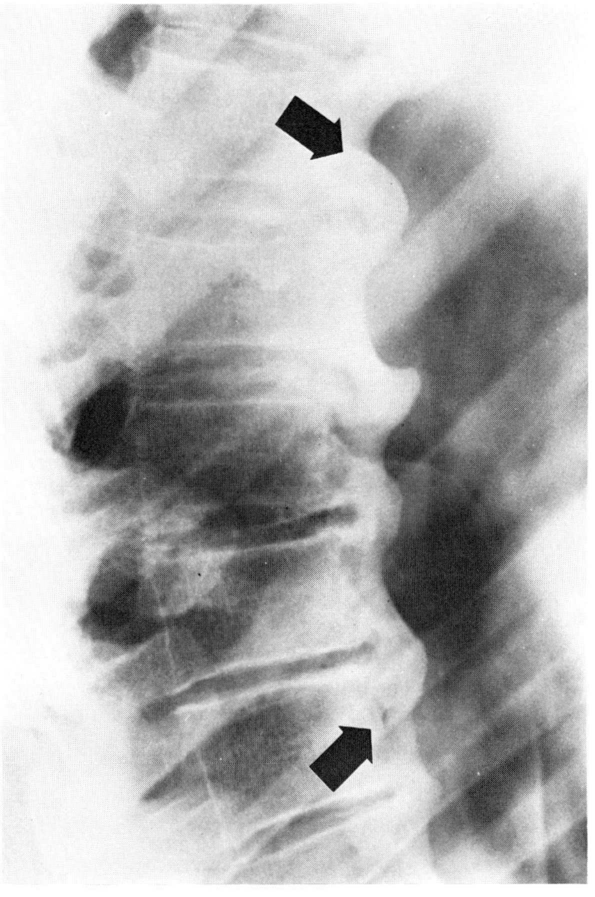

Fig. 7-30. Lateral roentgenogram of diffuse idiopathic skeletal hyperostosis. The arrows indicate laminated new bone formation along the anterior vertebral body. (Resnick, D., Shaul, S. R., and Robin, J. M.: Diffuse idiopathic skeletal hyperostosis [DISH]:Forestier's disease with extraspinal manifestations. Radiology, *115*:513, 1975.)

Ligamentous, tendinous, and paravertebral calcifications as well as heel spurs are the hallmarks of the peripheral manifestations (Fig. 7-31). These peripheral ossification sites have only recently been systematically studied as part of the disease process. Resnick feels that diffuse idiopathic skeletal hyperostosis represents an "ossifying diathesis" with resultant hyperostosis at tendon and ligament attachments. Initial involvement is predominantly axial but extra-axial skeletal involvement occurs. Roentgenographic recognition is important so that this disease entity will not be confused with diseases having entirely different prognoses, such as ankylosing spondylitis, acromegaly, fluorosis, hypertrophic osteoarthropathy, or pachydermoperiostosis.

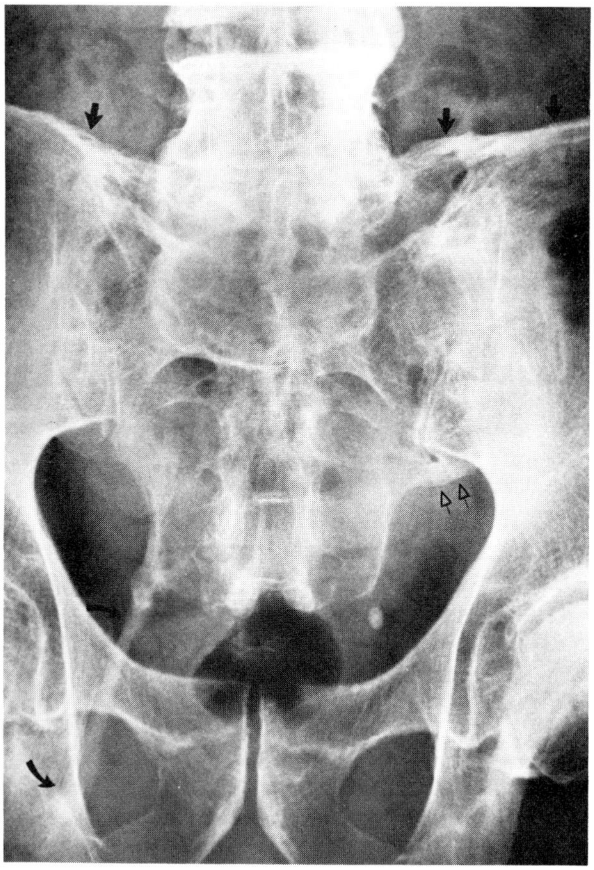

Fig. 7-31. Anteroposterior roentgenogram of the pelvis in diffuse idiopathic skeletal hyperostosis. The arrows indicate ligamentous calcifications which are hallmarks of the peripheral manifestations of this disease. (Resnick, D., Shaul, S. R., and Robin, J. M.: Diffuse idiopathic skeletal hyperostosis [DISH]: Forestier's disease with extraspinal manifestations. Radiology, *115*:513, 1975.)

Gout

Gout does involve the spine as evidenced from postmortem discovery of urate deposits in the intervertebral disks and articular joints. However, acute gout of the spine is only rarely described. The diagnosis is a clinical one based on a meticulous history and physical examination, hyperuricemia, and response to colchicine therapy. There will always be some doubt, however, as recovery of sodium urate crystals from the spine is virtually impossible. Roentgenographically, the findings are likewise nonspecific although Malawista and associates described sclerosis-rimmed cystic lesions adjacent to sacroiliac joints which they consider characteristic of gout.

Chondrocalcinosis (Pseudogout)

Pseudogout was first described by McCarty and Hollander, in 1961, as the deposition of calcium pyrophosphate crystals in the synovial fluid, producing an acute arthritis similar to gout. The arthritis and the accompanying radiographic picture was similar to the entity "chondrocalcinosis polyarticularis familiaris," described by Zitnan and Sit'aj in Czechoslovakia. We now know there are two distinct phases of the disease: the acute crystal-induced synovitis and a chronic degenerative arthropathy which is associated with deposition of crystals in cartilage. There is a definite association of chondrocalcinosis with other disease, such as gout, hemochromatosis and hyperparathyroidism. There is no known inheritance pattern, and involvement usually begins in the fifth to seventh decade.

As in gout, it is reasonable to assume that the pyrophosphate crystals may localize in the synovial lined joints in the spine. A diagnosis of acute pseudogout of the spine is indicated in a patient who has repeated episodes of acute spinal pain associated with crystal-diagnosed pseudogout in the peripheral joints. In chronic disease (chondrocalcinosis of the intervertebral disks), roentgenographic evidence of calcification of the disk does not necessarily mean the patient will have back pain.

Charcot Spine

Neurotropic arthropathy (Charcot joint) is a form of degenerative arthritis which develops as a result of impairment of normal pain or proprioceptive senses in the involved joint. Some of the known causes are tabes dorsalis (neurosyphilis), syringomyelia, paraplegia, congenital insensitivity to pain, and intraarticular corticosteroid therapy.

In the spine the defect is almost always limited to the lumbar area and is the result of tabes dorsalis. It can occur independently or in conjunction with peripheral joint involvement. The usual presenting complaint is pain in the low back, buttocks, and lower extremities. Weakness of the legs and deformity of the spine accompany the pain. The pain and deformity reflect the extreme spinal instability and subsequent cord and root compression. The degree of bony and neural involvement is clouded by the tabes dorsalis.

On examination the deformity and neurological findings greatly outweigh the symptoms. Roentgenographically, these patients demonstrate advanced spondylosis with compression fractures, large osteophytes, scoliosis, and extensive sclerosis.

Hemochromatosis

Hemochromatosis is a chronic disease in which excess iron is deposited causing fibrosis in many organs and tissues. The clinical manifestations are hepatomegalia, cirrhosis, skin pigmentation (due to increased melanin), diabetes, other endocrine dysfunction, and heart failure. Arthropathy occurs in 20 to 50 percent of the patients. Hemochromatosis is an idiopathic disease with a definite familial incidence. It may also be a result of alcoholic cirrhosis, excessive oral iron intake, chronic refractory anemia, or multiple blood transfusions. The symptoms occur between 40 and 60 years, with men being affected more frequently.

The most frequently affected joints are the hands, knees, and hips with the spine only being infrequently involved. Chondrocalcinosis is also seen in 30 to 60 percent of the patients with hemochromatosis. The most important laboratory tests are serum iron and serum iron binding capacity which are both greatly elevated. Liver biopsy is necessary to determine the extent of iron deposition and tissue fibrosis. Biopsy of the synovial tissue in the affected joints will show deposition of iron in the synovial lining cells.

Radiation Induced Pain

Chronic radium poisoning from iatrogenic administration or the ingestion of luminous paint by workers in watch factories has resulted in a toxic low back pain syndrome. These patients have developed aseptic necrosis of various bones, pathological fractures of vertebra, and radiation-induced sarcomas following long periods of ingestion. Because of the radiation effect on marrow, severe anemias have also been reported.

Similarly, radiation of certain benign tumors, such as aneurysmal bone cyst, has resulted in an increased incidence of osteogenic sarcoma 10 to 20 years later. In the young, radiation of the vertebral column for Wilm's tumor or neuroblastoma may cause cessation of epiphyseal growth unilaterally with subsequent spinal deformity, usually in the form of scoliosis.

Ochronosis (Alkaptonuria)

Ochronosis is a bluish-black discoloration of connective tissue which is associated with alkaptonuria. It is characterized by the presence of homogentisic acid in the urine. Homogentisic acid is an intermediate in tyrosine metabolism, and the patient's lack of the enzyme homogentisic acid oxidase allows excessive amounts of it to accumulate. It is inherited as an autosomal recessive trait and is frequently the result of consanguineous marriage.

Clinically the patients may have urine which turns black on exposure to oxygen. There may be blue pigmentation of ears, sclera, or skin. Back and peripheral joint pain may be noted early. The knees seem to be the most commonly affected peripheral joint. In the back, pain and stiffness are noted throughout the spine. There may be marked loss of range of motion in the dorsal and lumbar spine. The rate of progression varies but the entire spine may be involved in 10 to 15 years. The symptoms are similar to a herniated disk in a certain percentage because of weakening in the anulus fibrosus. Homogentisic acid can be positively identified in the urine utilizing a paper chromatography technique.

Roentgenographic findings occur as early as the second or third decade and include calcification and narrowing of numerous disks. This finding in a young patient is almost diagnostic of ochronosis. Osteoporosis of the vertebral bodies is also characteristic. In other patients, extensive osteophyte formation is the rule. The roentgenographic picture may resemble ankylosing spondylitis. However, fusion of the sacroiliac joints and bamboo spine are not features of ochronosis.

Osteitis Condensans Ilii

Osteitis condensans ilii is a lesion localized to the sacroiliac joints and is identified on roentgenograms. It should not be confused with the sacroiliitis of ankylosing spondylitis.

The etiology of osteitis condensans ilii is unknown. It is common in women and may be symptomatic during pregnancy. It is associated with increased stress, circulatory disturbance, urinary tract infection, and ankylosing spondylitis. It may be a source of low back pain.

Characteristically roentgenograms reveal bilateral or, rarely, unilateral triangular areas of sclerosis in the medial portion of the ilium. The base of the triangle is next to the sacroiliac joint, and the point extends laterally into the ilium. The size varies greatly. The sacrum is generally not affected.

Radicular Pain

Disk Herniation in Lumbar Spine

Low back pain with associated sciatic radiculopathy is most commonly due to a herniated nucleus pulposus (intervertebral disk) pressing on a nerve root. This occurs most frequently in the young adult (30 to 50 years of age), but can occur at any age. In the lumbar region the fourth and fifth "disks" are more frequently affected and produce rather characteristic syndromes. It should be remembered that disk degeneration can occur at any level from cervical 2 to the sacrum and depending on the amount of protrusion and level, produce a distinct pain and neurological picture.

As discussed in the anatomy section of this chapter, the intervertebral disk is composed of a gelatinous nucleus pulposus surrounded by an anulus fibrosus with high tensile strength. Normal function of the disk requires that the thick gel of the nucleus distribute forces evenly to the anulus fibrosus. With aging, certain biochemical changes lead to changes in gel behavior in the nucleus and loss of tensile strength in the anulus. When this occurs, nuclear pressure produces rupture or herniation of the weakened anulus fibrosus. Since the anulus is weakest posteriorly, the herniation most frequently occurs in that direction compromising the spinal cord and its roots. Because of this direct pressure, mechanical irritation occurs, with radiation of the pain along the dermatome of the affected nerve root. In addition, the motor fibers of the root are compressed leading to weakness and atrophy of the affected muscles.

The majority of the patients with lumbar disk degeneration initially present with low back pain. Most often the onset is insidious in nature, but occasionally a history of a lifting or a twisting episode accompanied by a "pop" with acute pain is elicited. The initial low back pain is usually not associated with leg pain or weakness. The pain is mechanical in nature, that is made worse by prolonged standing and improved by rest. The pain typically is intermittent, and the patient may complain of episodes which have progressively increased in severity and frequency. At this stage, "disk disease" cannot readily be separated from other mechanical causes of low back pain. These might include sacroiliac ligament strains, postural strain, neural arch defects, or spondylolysis.

Later there may be a pattern of pain referral. This can either be in the sclerotome or nerve root dermatome. The sclerotome is defined as the area that has the same embryonic origin as the mesodermal tissues being stimulated. When the ligaments, periosteum, joint capsules, and anulus fibrosus are stretched, a dull aching pain radiates into the sacroiliac area, buttocks, and posterior thighs. This is not nerve root compression pain and should not be confused with it.

When a herniated or ruptured anulus fibrosus compresses a nerve root, the irritation produces a syndrome of pain as well as motor and sensory loss of the lower extremities. As the nerve root becomes irritated, it becomes inflamed, and even more sensitive to pressures. The patient will note a sharp lancinating pain which begins in the thigh and progresses distally in a pattern typical of a dermatome. The onset may be gradual or extremely sudden and associated with a "popping" or "tearing" in the spine. This may represent the extrusion of disk material against a nerve root. When this occurs, the back pain will frequently resolve, and the patient is left with radicular symptoms.

Usually the disk rupture is lateral to the nerve root, and the patient lists or leans away from the side of the sciatica to release the pressure (Fig. 7-32). Occasionally the disk presents medially or in "the axilla" of the nerve root, and the patient will list toward the side of the sciatica (Fig. 7-33). The pain is

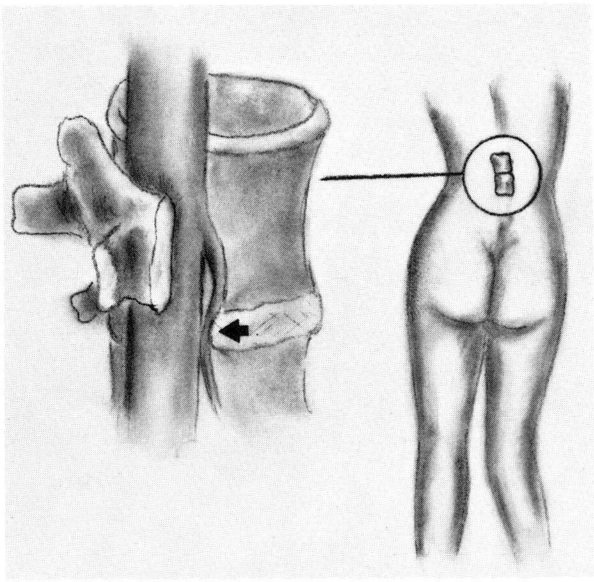

Fig. 7-32. In the usual case of herniated disk syndrome, the disk will protrude on the lateral side of the nerve root. In this instance, the patient will lean away from the side of the sciatica to release the pressure.

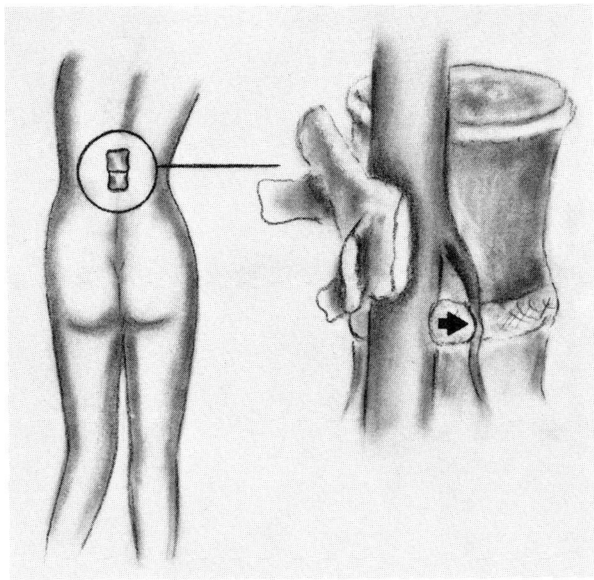

Fig. 7-33. On occasion, the disk will present medially or in (the axilla) of the nerve root. When this occurs the patient lists towards the side of the sciatica.

increased by any maneuver that suddenly increases intraspinal pressures such as a Valsalva maneuver (coughing, sneezing, or bearing down with defecation). The pain may be so severe as to "paralyze" the patient in a fixed position.

Rarely the major presenting symptom is motor weakness, particularly if the fourth or fifth lumbar nerve is affected. Weakness of the quadriceps with subsequent buckling of the knee (fourth lumbar) or a complete foot drop (fifth lumbar) without pain may be a confusing picture, challenging even the most astute examiner.

A large midline disk herniation can compress several roots of the cauda equina and mimic an intraspinal tumor. Usually low back and perineal symptoms predominate with radicular symptoms being masked. Difficulty with urination, consisting of frequency or overflow incontinence, may develop early. In male patients a recent history of sexual impotence may be elicited. The patients will experience pain down the posterior thighs to the soles of the feet with weakness of the legs and feet. When these findings are present a surgical emergency is indicated as only prompt relief of the cauda equina pressure will offer return of function.

Physical examination will reveal a patient listing away from or toward the sciatica depending on the presentation of the "disk." There commonly is limitation of movement in the lumbar spine but not necessarily so. The patient usually stands with the affected leg slightly flexed and is reluctant to place the foot on the ground. This presumably relaxes the sciatic nerve and relieves the root pressure. When the patient walks it is with an antalgic gait, with as little weight, for as short a time as possible, being placed on the affected leg.

The patients lose the normal lumbar lordosis and have unilateral or bilateral paravertebral muscle spasms. Palpation and percussion elicits pain at the level of the affected disk, sacroiliac joint, buttocks, and in the sciatic notch. This pain may either be local tenderness or more significantly radicular pain. There may be pain along the course of the sciatic nerve, for example in the popliteal region or calf.

The neurological examination is the most important part of the physical examination as it may yield objective evidence of nerve root involvement. The most common levels of disk herniation are L4-L5 and L5-S1 followed by L3-L4. In 10 percent of the cases two levels are involved. Because of the anatomical configuration of the cauda equina and lumbar spine, the herniated disk usually affects the nerve root exiting below the lesion. For example, a L4-L5 disk protrusion would compress the fifth lumbar and L5-S1, the first sacral nerve root. However, because of variations in the structure and size of the disk, any given disk can cause a variety of syndromes. Therefore, after clinical diagnosis of nerve root compression is made, the level is confirmed with myelographic and electromyographic examinations.

The neurological findings are threefold: motor weakness, sensory loss, and deep tendon reflex alteration. Compression of the motor fibers results in weakness or paralysis of those muscles innervated by that nerve root. Weakness is evaluated by muscle testing and atrophy of the lower extremity muscles. Atrophy is determined by comparative measurements of calf and thigh sizes. The muscle innervation at each root level and information as to how to muscle test is demonstrated in Chapter 4.

Sensory involvement usually follows the dermatome of the affected nerve root (Fig. 7-34). Typical patterns of motor and sensory involvement will be described at the end of this section for the most commonly involved levels.

The deep tendon reflexes are frequently changed by nerve root compression. The Achilles reflex is diminished or absent with involvement of the first sacral nerve root, and the knee jerk will be lost with involvement of the fourth lumbar nerve root. The

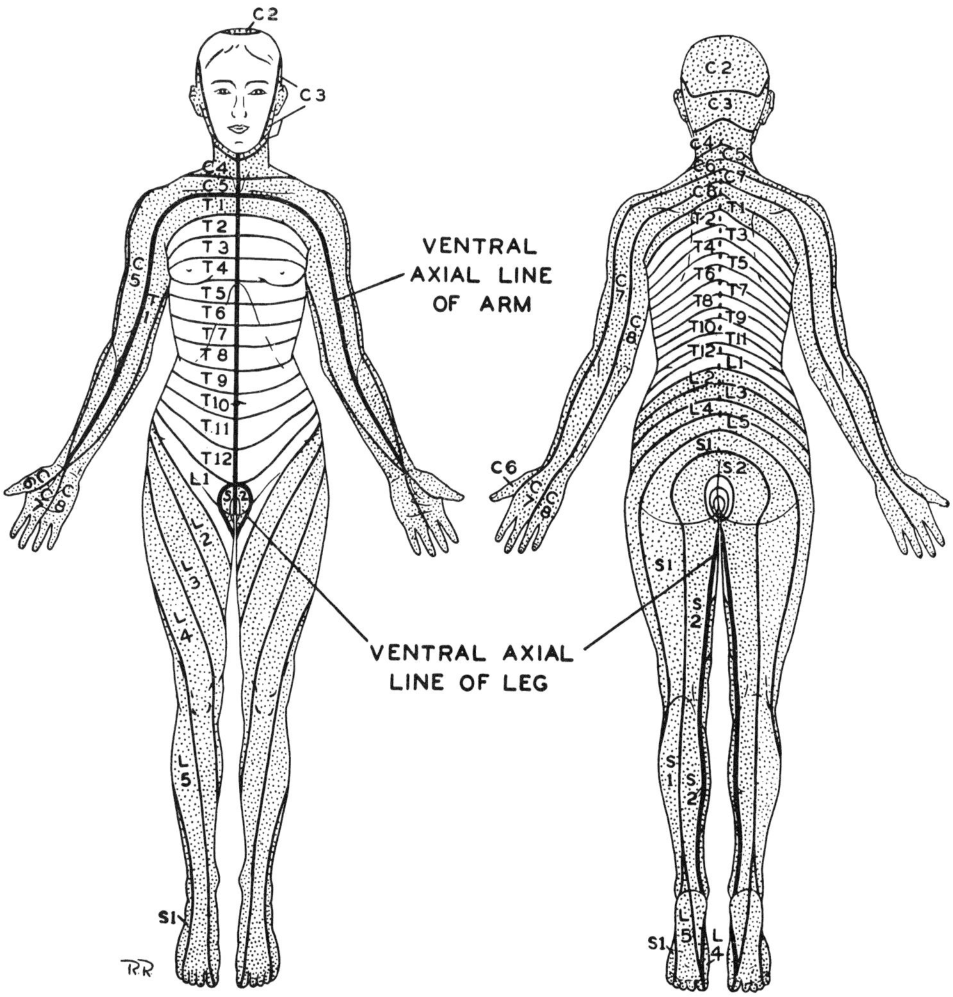

Fig. 7-34. Dermatome chart of the sensory level involvement of the lumbar sacral nerve roots. (Keegan, J. J., and Garrett, F. D.: Anat. Rec., *102*:411, 1948.)

fifth lumbar nerve root usually does not cause any reflex change, but on occasion a loss of the posterior tibial reflex will be noted. Absence of any of these reflexes has to be asymmetrical to be of significance. Increase or hyperreflexia is indicative of upper motor neuron lesions and indicates cord or conus medullaris pressure.

Several tests which tend to tighten the sciatic nerve and stretch it over the herniated disk were described in detail earlier in this chapter. The tests include straight leg raising with dorsiflexion of the foot and popliteal compression as adjuncts, contralateral straight leg raising, and reverse straight leg raising (for lesions of the fourth lumbar root).

Typical Lesions

Fourth lumbar nerve root (L3-L4 disk) demonstrates pain down the lower back, posterior lateral thigh, and anterior leg. Numbness is noted in the anterior medial thigh and knee. The quadriceps is weak and may be atrophied with decrease in the knee jerk reflex (see Fig. 1-5).

Fifth lumbar nerve root (L4-L5 disk) produces pain over the sacroiliac joint, hip, lateral thigh, and leg. Numbness will be noted on the anterior lateral leg and in the web dorsally between the great and second toe. There will be weakness of dorsiflexion of the great toe and foot (Fig. 7-35). Atrophy and reflex changes are minimal.

First sacral nerve root (L5-S1 disk) presents with pain over the sacroiliac joint, hip, posterior lateral thigh, and leg to the heel. Numbness is noted on the posterior calf, lateral heel, and small toe. There may be atrophy of the calf muscles, and the ankle jerk is diminished (see Fig. 1-5E).

Massive midline disk causes pain and numbness down the lower back, thighs, and perineum which may be bilateral. Variable amounts of weakness which may be profound are found in the lower extremities and are associated with bowel and bladder incontinence. All reflexes may be diminished.

Routine roentgenograms may be normal, but thinning or loss of disk height may be seen in disk degeneration. Sclerosis of the subchondral bone and the formation of peripheral osteophytes can be seen in chronic disk disease. The osteophytes are more common anteriorly and MacNab described them as having a unique horizontal appearance, 2 to 3 mm. from the disk space. He believes they are traction

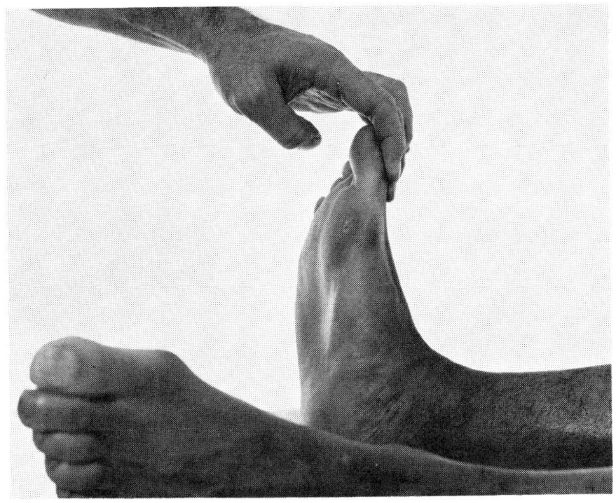

Fig. 7-35. This demonstrates a patient being examined for strength of dorsiflexion of the great toe. Since there is no reflex change for a lumbar 4-5 disk, this may be the only positive objective finding.

spurs which occur at the site of ligamentous insertion during the hypermobile stage of disk degeneration.

Herniation of disk material may occur into the vertebral body (Schmorl's nodules) and may or may not indicate disease. With degeneration of the disk, vertebrae may displace producing what has been called a "pseudo-retrospondylolisthesis." When this occurs, articular facets can encroach upon the intervertebral foramina with nerve root impingement. Calcification of the anulus fibrosus may occur.

Special tests for evaluation of the spinal column and its neurological elements were described in detail at the beginning of this chapter. They include oil myelography, water soluble myelography, air myelography, intraosseous venography, tomography, disk injection, and electromyography.

Thoracic Disk Herniation

Thoracic disk disease is discussed separately because of its unique, sometimes bizarre, presentation and the difficulties in making the diagnosis. Disk protrusion in the thoracic region was first recognized and described by Peet and Echols in 1932. It is not a common disease by any estimation. Of the total number of disk problems, thoracic presentation probably equals one to six cases per 1000. It appears predominantly in males, and the highest incidence is in the fifth decade. The interspace between T11 and T12 is the most commonly involved.

The patient's history and physical findings may vary greatly depending on the location, size, and duration of the herniation. The most common presenting complaint is pain. This may be unilateral or bilateral with girdle-like midline distribution. Patients with unilateral pain tend to have an extremely long history (years) while those with bilateral pain have a shorter history with more extensive spinal cord compression. In the low thoracic area, the pain can radiate into the abdomen, flank, or groin.

Sensory complaints are also common; they may either be sequential or in the presence of a large midline disk even cause paraparesis. The paraparesis will be spastic without sensory complaints. Bowel and bladder incontinence and sexual impotence can also present early or late in the disease process.

The only local sign is tenderness or percussion of the spine. In the lower extremities spastic paraparesis may be seen with increased deep tendon reflexes and a Babinski's sign. There may be sequential loss of the abdominal reflexes.

Plain roentgenograms of the thoracic spine are of little help in the diagnosis of thoracic disk disease. There may be narrowing of a disk space, calcification of the disk material, or local degenerative changes. These are late findings and usually not present in the acute disease. Positive contrast myelography is the most important diagnostic tool. Multiple projections, including oblique and decubitus views, will usually reveal the level of the offending disk. Selective angiography may be necessary to reveal the location of the "arteria radicularis anterior magna" of Adamkievich, which supplies the anterior two thirds of the spinal cord. This vessel is single, usually arising on the left side (80%) and entering with a nerve root between thoracic 9 and lumbar 2 (85%). If it is damaged, spinal cord infarction is possible; therefore, localization prior to surgery might circumvent this complication.

Thoracic disk protrusion is difficult to diagnose and, more often than not, will have a long puzzling history. It can be confused with ankylosing spondylitis, metastatic tumor, chronic duodenal ulcer disease, intercostal neuralgia, disk space infection, intramedullary spinal cord tumors, or neurofibromas.

NEUROGENIC PAIN

Intraspinal Neoplasms

Only a few cells within the spinal canal can become malignant. Distant metastasis to the cord is uncommon, the usual involvement being from extension of a vertebral lesion. Most remain extradural as the dura mater seems to provide a natural barrier against the malignant tumor. The extradural venous plexus is rarely invaded, but may be involved in the hematogenous spread of the tumor.

Extradural Tumors. These are the most common intraspinal tumors and comprise over 50 percent of the total. Virtually all are malignant. They are usually metastatic, entering from a contiguous space. Thoracic metastasis is very common, and this is explained by the proximity of the lung and breast to this area. The patients are generally over 50 and the sex predilection is dependent on the primary disease.

Pain, the hallmark of the disease, is usually unrelenting and severe. It is aggravated by activity but is not always relieved by rest. This is in direct contrast to most orthopaedic pain, including infections, herniated nucleus pulposus, and arthritis, which are relieved by lying down. The axial pain which is often accurately located by the patient is commonly the first complaint and overshadows the radicular symptoms.

Neurological symptoms usually occur rapidly as the tumor enlarges and cord or root compression is produced. Cord compression can cause a variety of neurological signs and symptoms. Lower extremity symptoms usually occur slightly before bowel and bladder difficulties. The root pressure produces radicular symptoms reminiscent of a disk syndrome.

Laboratory studies are usually not helpful except for a complete block when elevation of the spinal fluid protein does occur.

The bony changes are related to the type of tumor which is expanding into the epidural area. On myelogram, most epidural tumors will show a complete block which is described as "paint brush" in appearance. This is because the spinal cord is compressed between the dura on two sides which forms irregular edges. Air myelogram best demostrates the cord which is usually deviated to one side of the spinal canal.

Intradural-Extramedullary Tumors. Most tumors in this location are benign, over 50 percent being well encapsulated meningiomas and neurofibromas, and are primarily seen in the middle-aged female. These neoplasms tend to grow very slowly so neurological findings develop with less rapidity than in the extradural variety. However, the tumors grow in close relation to spinal roots, and radicular pain is common. For some reason, the pain may occur only at night with complete relief during the day.

With the neurofibromas a rather characteristic widening of the intervertebral foramen is seen on oblique spinal roentgenograms. This is due to the fact that neurofibromas tend to form along the nerve root as it leaves the spinal canal, widening the normal architecture. On myelogram, these tumors frequently present with a complete block. The margins of the block are smooth or lobulated rather than feathered as in the extradural tumors. The spinal cord can be pushed to one side of the spinal canal.

Intramedullary Tumors. Intramedullary tumors are the most uncommon of the three types discussed and most are gliomas. These tumors can progress insidiously and are often painless. The neurological findings are dependent on the anatomical location of the tumor. On myelogram, gliomas typically produce a fusiform swelling of the spinal cord shadow.

Syringomyelia is a fluid-filled intramedullary cavity and can be confused with a spinal cord glioma. It can either contain spinal fluid and communicate with the ventricular system or be associated with a glioma.

Spinal Epidural Abscess

Spinal epidural abscesses are separated into chronic and acute categories based on the length of symptoms as well as the surgical and pathological findings. The acute stage has the pathological finding of gross pus in the epidural space with a clinical symptom complex characterized by rapid progression of neurological symptoms. The principal findings in the chronic category are granulation tissue in the epidural space with a slower progression of neurological symptoms.

The infection may be secondary to a vertebral osteomyelitis, psoas abcess, decubitus ulcers (particularly in the sacral area), or from hematogenous seeding. One third of the patients have a history of prior back trauma. There is also an association with diabetes mellitus and intravenous drug use.

Spinal epidural abscesses can be seen at any age. In a study of 39 patients at the Massachusetts General Hospital, Baker and coworkers found a female to male ratio of 2:1 with an age range of 11 to 77 years. In this same series, the most common bacteria isolated was Staphylococcus aureus.

The most common location for epidural abscess is the thoracic or lumbar epidural space. The basis for destructive changes in the spinal cord itself are not entirely clear. The lesions in the cord are more extensive than can be accounted for by compression alone. The inflammatory mass probably causes vascular thrombosis with resultant impairment of the spinal cord's blood supply. Therefore, the neural damage is a result of both pressure and ischemic necrosis.

The clinical course of an epidural abscess can be subdivided into four phases: spinal ache, root pain, weakness, and paralysis. These occur within days of each other in the acute category while taking weeks to months in chronic cases. The spinal ache starts at the level of the affected spine and is excruciating. The patients usually seek physician consultation within 24 hours of the onset of pain. In the acute disease, root pain begins on the second or third day, the reflex changes are consistent with the level of the lesion. The reflexes are accentuated if the abscess lies over the cord and depressed if over the cauda equina. If untreated, motor weakness, ascending numbness, and impaired control of bowel and bladder develop until the patient becomes paraplegic. The patient may be febrile.

Patients in the acute category will usually have a serum leukocytosis in the 10,000 to 20,000 cells per cu. mm. range with an abnormal differential. The sedimentation rate can be elevated in both the acute and chronic categories. Spinal tap may yield evidence of pus in the epidural space if the needle is inserted at the area of spinal ache. Cerebrospinal fluid findings are typical of parameningeal infection.

Routine roentgenographic examination of the spine can be normal, show evidence of sciatic scoliosis, or be consistent with osteomyelitis of the spine. Myelograms are always abnormal showing evidence of either partial or complete block.

Major considerations in a differential diagnosis are meningitis, spinal subdural abscess, acute transverse myelopathy, disk space infection, and spinal cord tumors. Meningitis may present as a backache but headache is usually the major complaint. Spinal subdural abscess is much less common, but the signs are identical to those of an epidural abscess. The onset of acute transverse myelitis is more sudden, paralysis occurring within 72 hours. In osteomyelitis of the vertebral column, the spinal fluid examination is normal. The same is true of a herniated disk and epidural hematoma.

Syndromes Which Mimic Cord Pressure

Guillain-Barré Syndrome (acute postinfectious polyneuropathy, acute idiopathic polyneuritis) is a disease of unknown origin characterized by rapid onset of ascending weakness with associated sensory disturbance. All races, age groups, and both sexes are susceptible to this disease. The pathological picture is characterized by peripheral nerve demyelination and frequently by a mononuclear inflammatory reaction. There are numerous theories as to causation. One theory is that it results from an autoimmune reaction against peripheral nerve antigen, specifically myelin. Other theories postulate that it is secondary to a bacterial, viral, or neurotoxic substance. It is known that about one half of the cases will occur after an upper respiratory or gastrointestinal infection.

The typical history is of an acute upper respiratory illness followed in a few days by pins and needles paresthesia followed by weakness. Characteristically this is a symmetrical ascending motor weakness with minimal sensory changes and intact sphincter control. An aching pain or tenderness may be present but is not a prominent feature. A minority of patients exhibits profound sensory loss. Temporary bowel or bladder paralysis may occur but is always affected to a lesser degree than the lower extremities. The disease may ascend to involve the bulbar muscles, resulting in respiratory paralysis and death. The course of the disease ranges from several days to a week. If the patient survives the first two weeks, the prognosis is good. Motor power returns gradually over the course of a year.

Laboratory examination of the cerebral spinal fluid reveals a significant increase in the spinal fluid protein. Guillain stated that the protein should exceed 300 mg. per ml. to confirm the diagnosis. Although this is generally true, the diagnosis can be made with lower values. In subacute cases, the spinal fluid may be xanthochromic with protein in the range of 1000 mg. per ml. The spinal fluid pressure can be evaluated with papilledema. The white blood count in the spinal fluid is normal. There are no radiographic findings.

In a differential diagnosis of rapid motor paralysis of the lower extremities, it must be decided whether this is an acute disease of the peripheral nerves or the spinal cord. Poliomyelitis, acute postinfectious myelitis, and acute epidural abscess are spinal cord diseases which may be confused with this syndrome. Poliomyelitis can be differentiated by the meningitis, the asymmetry of the motor paralysis, and the complete absence of sensory changes. Acute disease of the spinal cord white matter as in postinfectious myelitis usually causes loss of sensation and motor function below a specific level. The bowel and bladder findings are pronounced and frequent. The same is true of the epidural abscess with the additional finding of severe back pain and fever.

Peripheral root diseases that should be included in the differential are acute porphyria, diphtheritic polyneuritis, and alcoholic neuropathy. Acute porphyria can be differentiated by a family history, abdominal pain, convulsions, and a darkly colored urine. The tempo of the disease in diphtheritic polyneuritis is much slower than in Guillain-Barré disease although spinal fluid protein is also elevated and the symptoms are similar. Alcoholic beri beri can look very similar, and the onset can be just as rapid; however, dietary insufficiencies are obvious, the paralysis less severe, and there is more pain and tenderness of the limbs. The spinal fluid protein is normal.

Acute Transverse Myelopathy (acute transverse myelitis, acute necrotic myelopathy). The syndrome of acute transverse myelopathy includes several entities which share a common clinical picture. Acute dysfunction of the spinal cord develops which can be either static or ascending, usually "transversely" involving both halves of the spinal cord. This can occur at any age, without prior history of neurological symptoms. The etiology in most cases remains unknown although it has been associated with previous viral and bacterial respiratory infections. It has been suggested that it develops as a result of direct viral invasion of the spinal cord or as a result of an allergic reaction to prior infection. Occlusion of the anterior spinal artery or a more proximal blockage of the spinal cord's blood supply (aortic occlusion, dissecting aortic aneurysm, or aortic clamping during surgery) is a cause in a certain percentage of cases. Some patients develop multiple sclerosis in the ensuing years.

The clinical course of patients with acute transverse myelopathy is variable, the incidence of the first neurological symptoms being evenly divided between muscle weakness, sensory loss or paresthesias, and back and root pain. The lapsed time from the onset of the first symptom to the greatest degree of neurological impairment can vary from minutes to weeks, the majority developing their complete deficit in the first 24 to 72 hours. About one third of the patients have a good recovery, in one third some recovery, and in one third there is no recovery. Death is a relative rarity unless the upper cervical cord is affected.

During the acute phase, spinal fluid examination may show cells or elevated protein. About one third of the patients will have serum leukocytosis. A myelogram is only indicated if the manometric examination reveals a subarachnoid block. Manometrics refer to the Queckenstedt maneuver of jugular compression. Routine roentgenographic examination is not helpful. Myelograms are usually normal but may show a partial block secondary to widening of the spinal cord.

It is important to differentiate this syndrome from treatable conditions, such as spinal epidural abscess, extramedullary tumors, or extradural hematomas. The syndrome of acute transverse myelopathy is eight times more frequent than acute spinal epidural abscess and they tend to mimic each other. Both acute spinal epidural abscess and extramedullary tumors tend to create a subarachnoid block, which is only occasionally seen in acute transverse myelopathy. There are no bony roentgenographic findings in acute transverse myelopathy, but there may be in the other two syndromes. Transverse myelopathy may be the presenting feature in multiple sclerosis but in the latter the onset is more insidious and the involvement less catastrophic than in the idiopathic syndrome.

Osteoporotic Pain

Osteoporosis is a condition in which the total volume of bone, both mineralized and unmineralized, is less than normal for age and sex matched control population. The etiologies are diverse and include dietary deficiencies, malabsorption syndromes, iatrogenic steroid administration, such endocrine disorders as acromegaly and hyperthyroidism, genetic abnormalities like osteogenesis imperfecta, and *idiopathic osteoporosis.* The latter usually develops in the elderly, and it is estimated that 20 percent of this population is affected. Females suffer more frequently than males; the difference is probably hormonal, but the details have not been delineated.

Osteoporosis is a generalized disorder, but it frequently manifests itself by vertebral compression fractures. They are most common at the thoracic 12 and lumbar 1 vertebral bodies initially and progress to involve other levels (Fig. 7-36). These fractures may be precipitated by minor, everyday trauma, sometimes the inciting event being so trivial that the

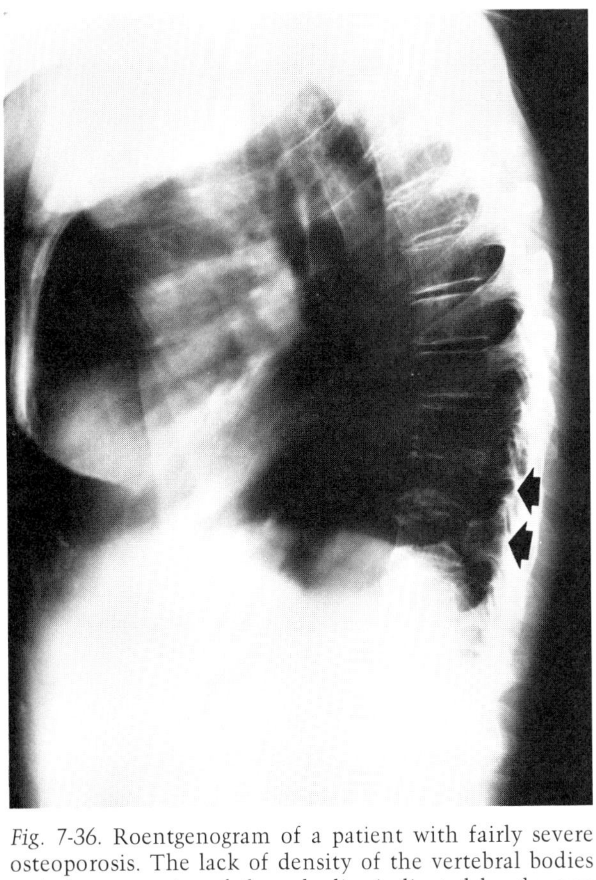

Fig. 7-36. Roentgenogram of a patient with fairly severe osteoporosis. The lack of density of the vertebral bodies and the concavity of those bodies indicated by the two arrows, are due to a loss of the total volume of bone, both mineralized and unmineralized.

patient cannot even recall exactly what it was. There is usually a sudden onset of pain which can last for months. If the fractures occur in the mid-thoracic region, the pain may be confused with myocardial ischemia. It must also be noted that compression fractures are sometimes asymptomatic.

As the fractures appear at multiple levels, the patient suffers a stepwise loss of height that may approach 4 inches in a single year. Kyphosis and sometimes scoliosis develop. Roentgenograms reveal porotic vertebrae that have collapsed into the characteristic codfish deformity (Fig. 7-37). Spinal cord involvement is rare with vertebral collapse unless a more severe underlying pathological process supervenes.

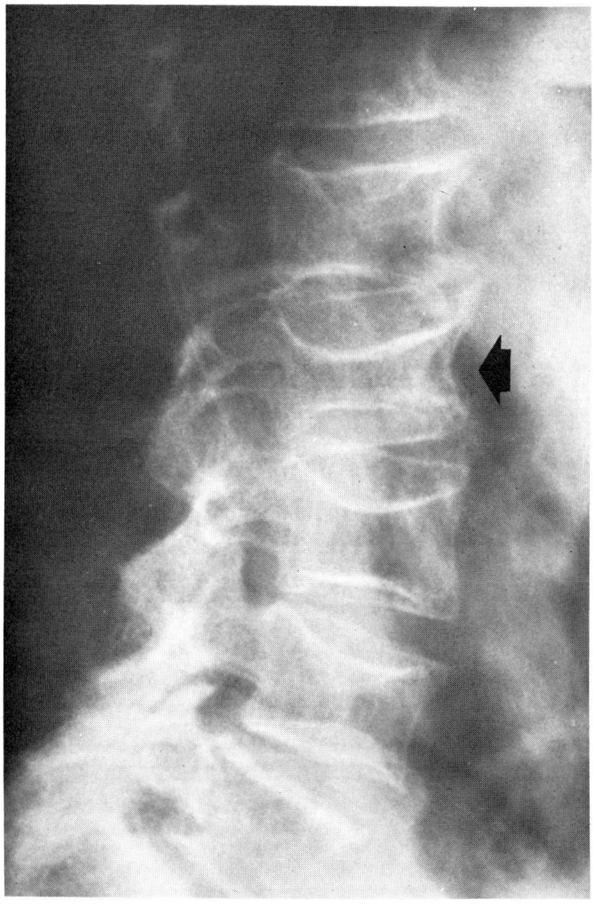

Fig. 7-37. Close-up of a lumbar vertebra in a patient with severe osteoporosis. The vertebra is porotic and collapsed into the typical codfish deformity. This is because a relatively normal disk has protruded into the abnormal vertebral body.

Osteogenesis imperfecta is a genetic disorder characterized by thin brittle bones which are easily fractured. Severely affected children are small with deformed extremities secondary to multiple fractures. They have blue scleras, lax ligaments, abnormal teeth (odontogenesis imperfecta), increased metabolism with excessive sweating, and tachycardia. These children are intelligent and many survive to adulthood with proper medical care. In the adult, deafness due to otosclerosis is seen.

Because of the weak bone, the vertebrae are affected as are the bones of the extremities. Severely affected children develop spinal deformity before age eight, and it is progressive. The deformity may be scoliosis and/or kyphosis. It is particularly difficult to treat because braces bend the soft ribs rather than hold the spine. Surgery is hampered by the soft bone and a bleeding tendency secondary to capillary abnormalities.

There are no specific laboratory tests for osteogenesis imperfecta but the family history and distinctive clinical appearance usually make the diagnosis easy. Radiographically the osteoporotic vertebrae show multiple areas of wedging, compression, or biconcavity (codfish vertebrae).

Homocystinuria is an inherited disorder of connective tissue similar to Marfan's syndrome. It is characterized by long extremities, ectopia lentis (dislocating lens which typically displace inferiorly whereas in Marfan's they displace superiorly), mental retardation, and multiple venous and arterial thromboses. Persons with homocystinuria often die early because of ischemic heart disease or massive thrombosis of the great vessels. The diagnosis is confirmed by the finding of homocystine in the urine.

Vertebral involvement includes osteoporotic wedging and biconcavity of vertebrae. An unusual finding is posterior wedging in the low lumbar spine. They may also have severe scoliotic deformities, probably because of weak ligamentous structure and vertebral wedging.

Both *male and female hypogonadism* during growth can lead to osteoporosis because of a failure to accumulate a normal complement of bone. The roentgenographic features are nonspecific. The diagnosis is made by chromosomal analysis and measurement of hormone levels.

Osteoporosis, compression fracture of the vertebrae, and kyphosis are well known features of

Cushing's syndrome (hyperadrenocorticism). It is differentiated from idiopathic osteoporosis by its preference for the axial skeleton and rib cage. Other features include moon facies, trunk obesity, purple striae, hirsutism, hypertension, and diabetes. Exogenous corticosteroid therapy can produce the same syndrome although the underlying disease may cloud the picture as it may also have an effect on the spine. The dose, type, and duration of steroid administered are all important in the degree of osteoporosis.

Hyperparathyroidism produces a high turnover osteoporosis, similar to that seen in hyperthyroidism. In most cases, the diagnosis is made on the other manifestations of the disease, the osteoporosis being an incidental finding. This usually, although not necessarily, is accompanied by high serum calcium levels.

Acromegaly produces a mild form of high turnover osteoporosis, with the compression fractures and other manifestations of symptomatic osteoporosis being conspicuously absent. The roentgenographic findings in the spine feature extensive osteophytic formation, disk space narrowing, and increased concavity of the vertebral bodies (Fig. 7-38).

Nutritional causes of osteoporosis include calcium deficiency, protein deficiency, scurvy, and intestinal malabsorption. These are complex problems usually affecting the growing child. Other causes of osteoporosis include chronic metabolic acidosis as a result of renal tubular disease or glycogen storage disease, large dose heparin administration, chronic anticonvulsant administration, methotrexate therapy, excessive alcoholic consumption, rheumatoid arthritis, and chronic disease or immobilization. In all cases the roentgenographic findings mimic those of idiopathic osteoporosis.

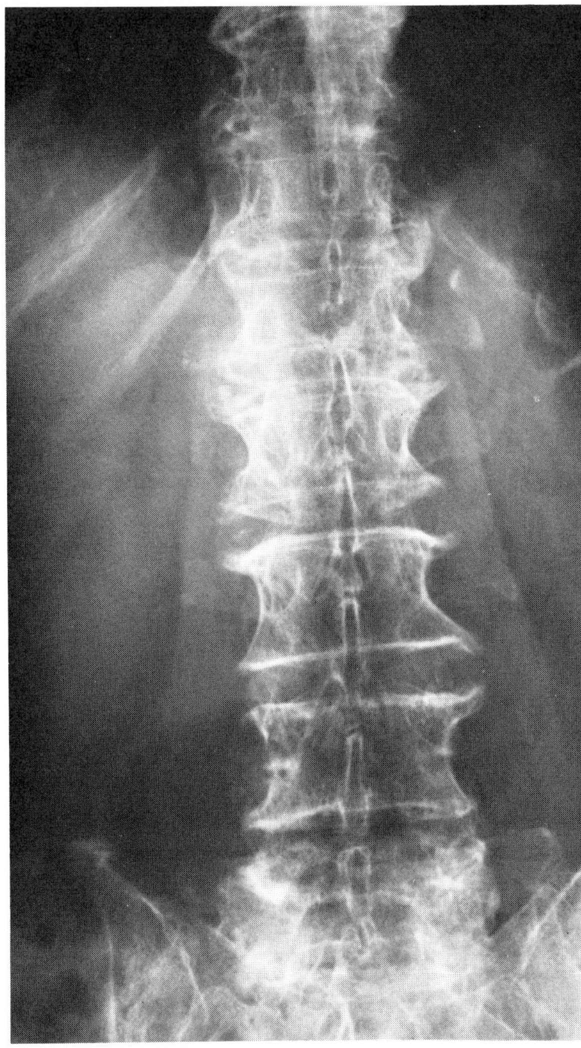

Fig. 7-38. Anteroposterior roentgenogram of a 53-year-old female with a diagnosis of acromegaly. The patient has extensive osteophytic formation and disk space narrowing. A lateral roentgenogram would reveal increased concavity of the vertebral bodies.

Stenosis of Lumbar Canal

The word stenosis is derived from the Greek "stenos" meaning narrow. Lumbar spinal stenosis is defined as any type of narrowing of the spinal canal, nerve root canals, or intervertebral foramina. It can be localized, segmental, or generalized. The etiology can range from bony encroachment, space occupying soft tissue lesions, such as disk inflammation or tumor, to a combination of any of the above. The signs and symptoms of the condition are based not only on cauda equina and nerve root pressure but also on vascular embarrassment of the nerve roots.

Verbiest in 1950 first drew attention to the association of lumbar spinal canal stenosis and intermittent cauda equina dysfunction. However, the abnormality of a shallow lumbar spinal canal was described 10 years before the related neurological deficits were recognized. This is exactly opposite that found in cervical canal stenosis where neurological symptoms were noted long before the narrowing.

There are three commonly recognized "claudication like" syndromes which may be caused by compression of the cauda equina. They are (1) herniated intervertebral disk or disks, (2) degenerative stenosis or hypertrophic ridging of the intervertebral canal, and (3) congenital narrowing of the spinal canal. These can occur singularly or in any combination.

Normally, the spinal canal space increases as the sacrum is approached. However, this is not the case in congenital stenosis of the spinal canal. While there is uniform narrowing at all levels, the fifth lumbar vertebra seems to be the narrowest. This is the kind of abnormality seen in achondroplasia, and rarely causes symptoms alone. However, when a small disk herniation or minor degrees of degenerative spondylosis are added, symptoms occur. Degenerative stenosis is one of the most common types of stenosis and is due to degenerative arthritis of the spine. The stenosis is most pronounced at the site of the articular facets, disks, and joints. The facets enlarge, laminae become dense, and the ligamentum flavum thickens. Central disks, particularly at multiple levels or any space-occupying lesion, can cause a relative stenosis.

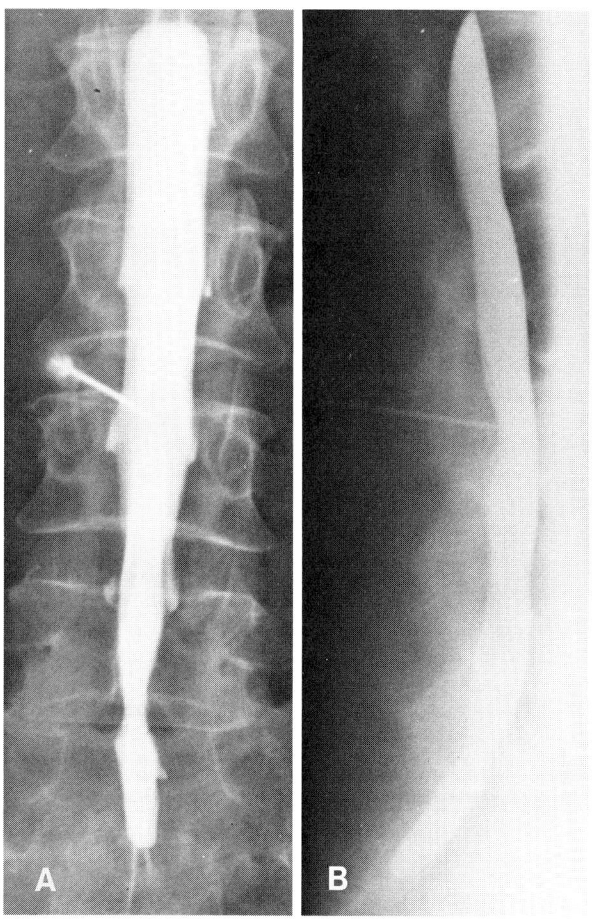

Fig. 7-39. Anteroposterior myelogram (*A*) of a 55-year-old male who carries a diagnosis of spinal stenosis. Note that the patient has narrowing at the lumbar 4-5 and lumbar 5–sacral 1 levels (*B*). Lateral myelogram in the same patient showing anteroposterior narrowing.

Males are affected more often than females, with the peak incidence in the fourth decade. The symptoms center around back and leg pain. The back pain is usually less acute than that seen in the patient with an acute herniated disk, but located similarly in the lumbosacral region. The radiating leg pain tends to simulate that seen in a herniated nucleus pulposus since the same nerve roots are involved in each. There may be "intermittent claudication" (periodic limping) but the rest-relief cycle which is seen in the arterial variety of this syndrome is not applicable. After activity the patient notes numbness or "tingling of the feet" and weakness or uncoordination of the lower extremities. The patient typically has a saddle-like distribution of these paresthesias and the signs of true sciatica, such as straight leg raising, are minimal. The manner of relief is also atypical with the patient having to sit or lie to obtain relief. It is also possible to lose deep tendon reflexes after exercise. The signs on examination mimic those seen in acute disk herniation, except they are not as pronounced. Spinal movement and straight leg raising are both restricted to some degree. There may be flattening of the normal lumbar lordosis or a sciatic scoliosis. The symptoms and signs are likely to be bilateral.

The normal depth of the lumbar spine canal on roentgenogram is 22 to 25 mm. in the anteroposterior diameter. This may be as small as 15 mm. and not be abnormal. Some patients, such as achondroplastic dwarfs, do not develop pedicles and have canals too small to support normal adult neurological function. They do not develop symptoms until middle age when further encroachment occurs.

The volume of the spinal canal can be estimated on anteroposterior (Fig. 7-39A) and lateral roentgenogram (Fig. 7-39B) of the lumbar spine. Myelography is frequently helpful in proving the diagnosis. The myelographic defects seen with spondylosis in a stenotic canal are large and often show huge defects or a complete block. If the panopaque is left a repeat roentgenogram in several days may show the dye to flow by the block. Multiple level defects with prominent root shadows and panopaque which will not move about is characteristic. It is most often confused roentgenographically with arachnoiditis.

The syndrome of cauda equina compression should be differentiated from disk herniation, arachnoiditis, intermittent claudication of arterial insufficiency, intraspinal tumors, and malingering. Disk herniation is usually unilateral and symptoms of sciatica are present. The symptoms of a stenotic vertebral canal are easily confused with arterial insufficiency because both have the intermittent claudication symptoms of periodic limping. However, in arterial insufficiency a constant exercise-pain, rest-relief cycle is seen. Other suggestive signs are absent pulses and a history of arterioiliac occlusive disease. The pain is genuine and a predominant feature. Pain relief is achieved in minutes with resting, while in the neurological variety it persists up to one hour. Reflex changes are not noted in arterial disease.

Scheuermann's Juvenile Kyphosis

A frequently unrecognized entity is round back deformity in the adolescent. The kyphosis is attributed to poor posture, and the teenager is unfairly asked to stand up straight by his parents and teachers. Because of the structural changes in the vertebrae and associated pain and rigidity, he is unable to accommodate their demands.

Juvenile kyphosis was first described in 1920 by Scheuermann, a Danish radiologist, as deformity caused by actual anterior wedging of the vertebrae. The etiology of Scheuermann's kyphosis has remained unknown; many have speculated as to the cause. The roentgenographic changes of Scheuermann's are rarely demonstrable before age 11. Bradford and associates reported a female to male ratio of 2:1, although in the literature the cases appear equally divided between the sexes. A familial incidence of this disease has been described, but it is not clear whether it is of genetic or environmental importance. The reported incidence in the general population has varied from 0.4 to 8.3 percent depending on whether the criteria for diagnosis are based on roentgenographic or clinical judgment.

The initial complaints are progressive pain and deformity at the apex of the deformity. Pain has been reported to be present in 20 to 60 percent of the patients. However, most patients present with simply a kyphotic deformity. On examination, a rigid thoracic kyphosis with an associated lumbar lordosis is noted. On attempted hyperextension of the thoracic spine, very little correction is obtained. Tenderness or muscle spasm may be present over the area of kyphosis. An associated scoliosis is found 30 to 40 percent of the time. In severe deformities, neurological testing may reveal spastic paraparesis secondary to spinal cord compression.

There are no laboratory examinations which are specific for Scheuermann's kyphosis.

Along with kyphosis, the characteristic finding, as seen on the lateral roentgenogram, is wedging of the vertebrae. Sorensen suggested that to make a correct diagnosis of Scheuermann's kyphosis it is necessary to have three adjacent vertebrae wedged 5 degrees or more. Most authors agree that this strict criterion is not necessary to make the diagnosis. There is also an increased incidence of Schmorl's nodules (invagination of disk tissue into the vertebral body) and irregularity of the vertebral end plates. Persistent vascular grooves may be present but are secondary to the vertebral immaturity rather than the disease itself. Scoliosis with rotation is frequently associated with the kyphosis. Late roentgenographic changes include concavity of the anterior vertebral border and anterior exostosis between vertebral bodies. Occasionally, tomography and myelography are indicated.

Traumatic injury such as a compression fracture to the spine may present a confusing picture in the differential diagnosis, but usually the trauma is limited to only one vertebra. Congenital anomalies of the spine resulting in kyphosis do occur and tomography is sometimes necessary for delineation of the abnormality. Kyphosis secondary to extensive laminectomy for tumor resection can be ruled out by clinical history and the presence of a scar.

Osteochondrodystrophies such as Morquio's and Hurler's disease must also be considered. These syndromes tend to have multiple joint involvement although not necessarily so. Mucopolysaccharide studies may be helpful.

Finally postural round back must be separated out. It is a supple deformity which corrects on hyperextension. Roentgenography does not reveal any vertebral wedging or end plate irregularity. Early in the course of the disease or in the preadolescent this differentiation may be very difficult.

BONY PAIN

Infections of the Spine

Pyogenic Infection. Pyogenic osteomyelitis may be difficult to diagnose clinically. However, the modern methods of diagnosis, including tomography as well as needle and open biopsy, have led to an increased frequency of accurate diagnosis. The causative organism is most commonly Staphylococcus aureus. Other common organisms include Streptococcus viridans and pyogenes, Escherichia coli, Clostridium perfringens, proteus, gonococcus, pneumococcus, pseudomonas, and the enteric group which includes Salmonella typhosa and paratyphi A and B. Actinomyces and brucellosis because of their uniqueness will be discussed separately. Common associations include sickle cell anemia with salmonella organisms, hard drug users with pseudomonas, and urinary tract procedures followed by infection with E. coli or proteus. Associated diseases include typhoid fever, pelvic and kidney infections, and diabetes.

The usual mode of spread is hematogenous from an infection elsewhere. Long bone osteomyelitis, impetigo, skin lesions, or thoracic infections may be the primary focus. However, osteomyelitis of the spine can occur after instrumentation of the bladder, catheterization, or any kidney, prostate, or pelvic infection. The spread in these cases is believed to be through the vertebral venous system known as Batson's plexus. Pyogenic osteomyelitis has been reported following removal of a herniated disk. Additionally, there may be local invasion from a focus of infection near the spine or secondary infection due to an open wound of the spinal column.

The site of involvement is the body of the vertebrae, rarely elsewhere. The lumbar spine is most frequently affected followed by thoracic involvement and last, the cervical and sacral spine are involved about equally.

The age of involvement has been increasing over the years. Studies prior to 1940 all showed large numbers of involvement in children. In the 1971 study of Griffith and Jones, there were fewer children and the most frequently affected patients were between 50 and 70 years of age.

Most studies in the past have indicated that pyogenic infections of the spine are slightly more common in males. The more recent study by Griffith and Jones has an equal ratio between men and women. Less than 5 percent of the cases of pyogenic osteomyelitis affect the spine. This is in striking contrast to the 50 percent involvement seen in tuberculous osteomyelitis.

The organisms reach the vertebral body through the blood stream and more than one bone at a time may be affected. The large sinusoidal veins or venous lakes of the vertebral body provide an excellent medium for multiplication of pathological bacteria. During the first two or three days pus is formed raising the intramedullary pressure. The perispinous ligaments and periosteum may then be raised by the expanding mass of necrotic tissue. A subperiosteal abscess if formed denudes the outer vertebral cortex of its blood supply. If the nutrient vertebral artery is also thrombosed by infection, then the entire vertebral body may be in jeopardy. The body then becomes a sequestrum, devoid of any blood supply. New bone is laid down subperiosteally forming an involucrum. This is similar to the sequence of events which occurs more commonly in the long bones. A paravertebral abscess may occur but is less extensive and common than those seen in tuberculosis. The spinal canal and its contents are involved in 15 percent of the cases of vertebral pyogenic osteomyelitis. This is termed an *epidural abscess* and is associated with a high mortality rate.

Clinically the symptoms are those of a generalized infection, with fever, chills, general malaise, and back pain being prominent. The onset may be rapid, the patient complaining of feeling ill within a matter of hours. The pain is severe, localized, and aggravated by motion. There may be muscle spasm or spinal rigidity. The child may refuse to walk because of pain. There may be referral to the hip joint with a limp due to spasm of the psoas muscle. There may be a history of prior infection but it is rare to find a primary source of infection. In adults there is a high incidence of associated urinary tract infections.

Examination reveals an elevated temperature with associated tachycardia. Local tenderness to palpation or percussion of the spine is a relatively constant finding early in the course of the disease. The range of motion of the spine may be severely limited. A hip flexion deformity may result from chronic irritation of the psoas muscle in the lumbar region. An accurate neurological examination should always be done to rule out cord involvement.

The erythrocyte sedimentation rate is invariably elevated. Classically it may rise to levels about 100 mm. Tuberculosis infections are never this high. Total white blood count may be normal early in the disease but not the differential which invariably is abnormal. Blood cultures are positive in about 50 percent of the cases. Ideally the cultures should be done when the fever spikes and before antibiotics are given. Serological tests used to identify staphylococcal infections are not particularly effective.

The only way to make an absolute diagnosis is to obtain pus for culture and sensitivities and this is best accomplished by needle biopsy using the technique of Ottolengi. It can be easily and safely done below lumbar 2, but above this biplane image intensification is necessary to avoid the spinal cord and lung. If needle biopsy proves unsuccessful or the infection is in an area difficult or dangerous to needle, then open biopsy may be indicated. This is accomplished through a transthoracic approach in the thoracic spine or through a retroperitoneal flank approach in the lumbar spine.

Roentgenograms are generally normal the first 10 to 14 days and remain so if the disease is promptly diagnosed and treated. The entire spine must be seen and as many views as necessary should be ordered. Early loss of the normal lumbar lordosis or thoracic kyphosis may be the only findings. The earliest roentgenographic signs are the presence of a paravertebral shadow or loss of the disk space. The first bony change is a small area of erosion, producing a lytic defect in the superior or inferior aspect of the vertebral body. It may not appear within the first months of symptoms. Tomograms are helpful in delineating these body changes more accurately than regular roentgenograms. The progressive erosion of the vertebral bodies results in its partial or complete destruction. A pyogenic paravertebral abscess is generally much smaller than those seen in tuberculous osteomyelitis.

Much later, there is a reactive sclerosis and an increase in density of the vertebral body resulting in a densely sclerotic or ivory vertebra. If two adjacent vertebrae are involved, spontaneous fusion may result.

Bone scan may localize the area of infection before the roentgenograms are positive because the increase in vascularity in the area enhances radioactive isotope uptake. In the presence of a sound clinical history with appropriate physical findings, a bone scan can localize the area of infection so needle biopsy can be accomplished.

If neurological symptoms are present, myelography may be indicated. Extreme caution must be used to avoid the area of infection when inserting the spinal needle.

The differential should include tuberculosis, brucellosis, and fungal diseases of the spine. Both primary and secondary malignant conditions appear radiographically similar to osteomyelitis because both have active destruction of bone. Needle or open biopsy is often required to provide material for a pathological diagnosis. Perinephric abscess, meningitis, suppurative arthritis of the hip, and arthritides of the spine can also present a confusing picture.

Tuberculosis. Hippocrates first described tuberculosis in 450 B.C., but it was identified in the spine of an Egyptian mummy dated 3000 B.C. Percivald Pott is credited with the first accurate description of tuberculosis and spinal involvement with a kyphotic deformity which still carries the name of Pott's disease.

The tuberculosis bacillus reaches the skeleton via the blood stream. There is a striking preference for the spine, with over 50 percent of the cases of bone and joint tuberculosis involving the vertebral column, compared to 2 to 7 percent of pyogenic osteomyelitis. Hodgson feels this may be because there is a different pathway of spread in spinal tuberculosis. Pyogenic bone infections secondary to postoperative sepsis in the pelvis almost invariably spread to the spine according to Henriques. He suggested that the spread was by way of Batson's plexus, the vertebral veins described first by Batson in 1940. Hodgson produced renal tuberculosis in monkeys and then followed the infection to the spine through the fourth venous plexus. The vertebra most commonly infected in tuberculosis is lumbar 1, which is at the level of the kidney. Therefore, the general belief is that tuberculosis of the spine spreads through the venous plexi rather than being seeded by arterial blood supply.

Tuberculosis can occur at any age but most often affects children and young adults. This is particularly true in undernourished areas. In the United States, the age of involvement tends to be higher. Males are affected slightly more often than females. It is rare in countries with adequate nutrition. The reduced incidence has been accomplished by a number of factors including improved housing, pasteurization of milk (eliminating bovine infection), and the use of specific antituberculosis drugs.

The tuberculosis bacilli reach the spine via the blood stream. The skeletal disease is a secondary local manifestation of disease elsewhere in the body, generally in the lungs or lymph nodes. When the infection starts in bone, a cavity filled with tuberculous granulation tissue and pus is formed. Eventually, a portion of the bone loses its blood supply and sequestration occurs. This is the start of the paraspinous abscess. The abscess contains pus with fragments of bone, the cartilagenous plate, and granulation tissue. The pressure strips the paravertebral tissues, may devascularize the vertebrae, and can eventually cause pathological fractures.

The disk does not become involved primarily because it is avascular. It may detach because of bony involvement, and if the bone on both sides becomes infiltrated, it may lose its end plate nutrition. At this point, the disk space may narrow.

Kyphosis occurs secondary to destruction of vertebral bodies, the worst deformities usually occurring at the dorsolumbar junction. Pott's paraplegia occurs because of cord pressure from the abscess or bony impingement. The dura mater may be penetrated by the tuberculous abscess and the cord involved. If the spinal cord has not been penetrated, the ensuing paraplegia can usually be reversed by rapid decompression. Once infiltration of the cord has occurred, the prognosis for recovery drops precipitously.

In addition to the systemic reaction, the most notable local symptom is pain which is aggravated by movement and is particularly severe at night. There may be a history of previous lymph or pulmonary infection or a positive family history for tuberculosis. If advanced, the kyphotic deformities associated with collapsed vertebrae are seen. If spinal cord pressure has occurred, some degree of mild spasticity will be present. If the cord has been penetrated, there will be marked spasticity with a withdrawal reflex.

Examination usually reveals one or more of the following signs: pallor, wasting, listlessness, and a low grade fever depending on the stage of the disease. There is tenderness with or without swelling about the spine. There may be areas of purulent drainage in the flank, buttock, or groin. These result from abscesses which have tracked along the course of least resistance and may burst, or have burst, as a chronic draining tuberculous abscess. Secondary infection with pyogenic organisms may occur secondarily once a sinus has formed. There may be muscle wasting and protective spasm, particularly in the spine or in joint involvement. Regional lymph nodes are sometimes enlarged and tender, and there may be pulmonary findings.

The erythrocyte sedimentation rate is usually raised when the disease is active, but extremely high readings are more suggestive of pyogenic arthritis. The hemoglobin is usually low in late untreated infections. A tuberculin reaction (Mantoux test) should always be positive at least in the 1/100 dilution. In active disease it is active in 1/1000, 1/10,000 dilutions. Generally one can be almost certain skeletal tuberculosis does not exist if the 1/100 dilution is negative. In disseminated tuberculosis, the skin test may be negative due to anergy.

Bacteriological diagnosis will confirm the suspected disease. Sputum specimens, early morning urine samples, and aspirated material from lymph nodes or the abscess itself are sent for culture, guinea pig inoculation, and pathological examination. The sensitivities of the cultured material are important particularly for patients who have previously received chemotherapy. As in pyogenic infections, fungal skin tests, serological tests, and blood cultures are useful in ruling out other disease entities.

A routine chest film should always be ordered as it may reveal the pulmonary lesion. The first roentgenographic sign is a generalized rarefaction of bone, particularly adjacent to the end plates. Later the disk space narrows from destruction of the end plate cartilage. This is often accompanied by destruction of the underlying bone. Bone lesions take the form of an irregular cavity with no surrounding sclerosis during the active phase of the disease.

The pus and sequestered vertebral material strip the paraspinous tissues and form the paravertebral abscess (Fig. 7-40). This is the mode of spread from vertebra to vertebra and the reason for multiple level involvement. According to Hodgson, 90 percent of

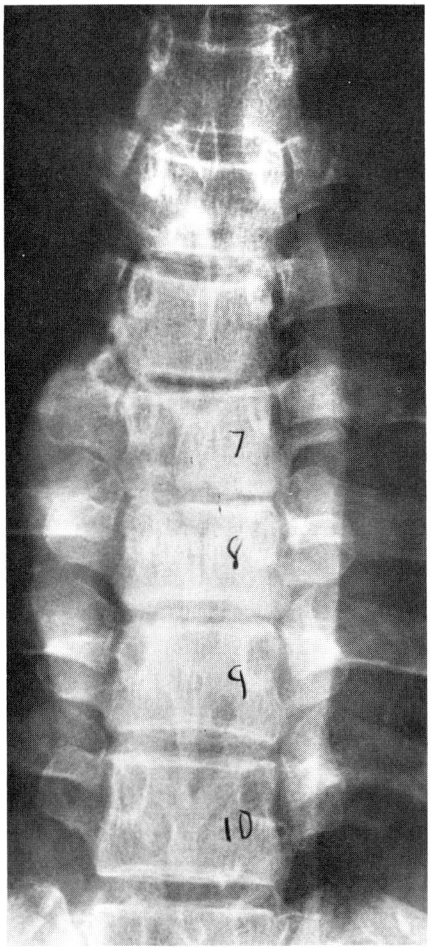

Fig. 7-40. Anteroposterior roentgenogram of a patient with a tuberculous abscess of the thoracic spine. This was created by the pus and sequestered vertebral material which stripped away the paraspinous tissues to form the abscess. This is the mode of spread from vertebra to vertebra and the reason for multiple level involvement.

the vertebral abcesses will be evident on roentgenograms. They are best seen in the thoracic region where the lung provides a sharp contrast.

Findings in advanced disease include the *aneurysmal syndrome* which is associated with long paravertebral abscesses in children. Hodgson believes this is due to a periosteal stripping process depriving the body of all vascularity allowing vertebral involvement and circumferential destruction. Concertina collapse (Fig. 7-41), unilateral collapse, or kyphosis (Fig. 7-42) are all due to vertebral destruction and collapse.

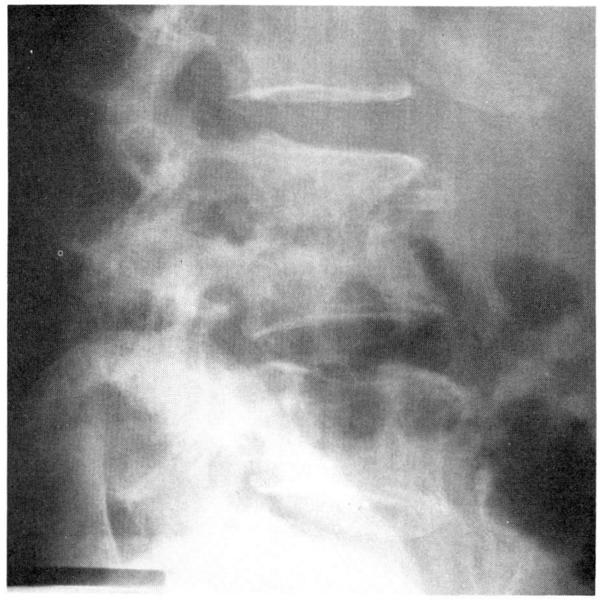

Fig. 7-41. Concertina collapse secondary to tuberculosis. The disk space is virtually destroyed and the superior vertebra is collapsing into the inferior vertebra.

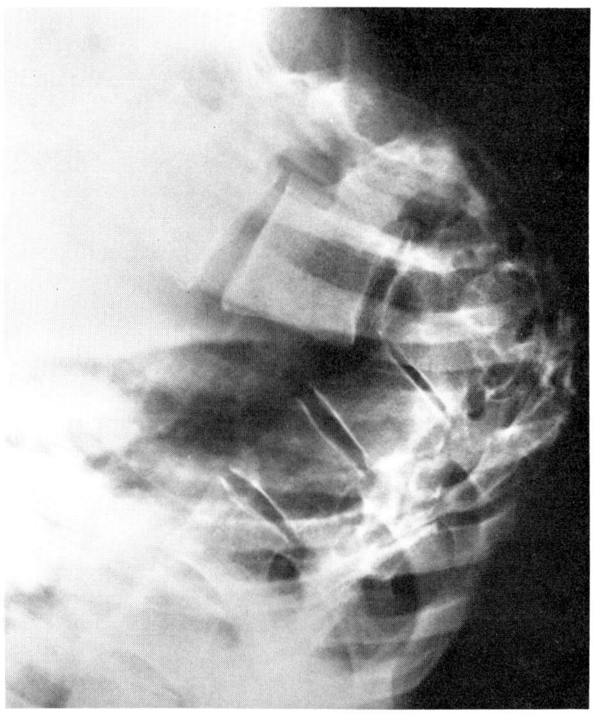

Fig. 7-42. Tuberculosis which occurred in infancy with destruction of vertebral bodies and a resultant severe kyphotic deformity. This patient had an impending paraplegia when seen in adulthood.

Later in the healing phase, revascularization occurs leading to a number of unusual roentgenographic findings which include *ivory vertebra* (a markedly white vertebra first described by Sougnes, Lafaurcade, and Terris in 1924), *vertebra within a vertebra* (new bone formation around an osteoporotic vertebra), and *bony bridging* (paravertebral ligament ossification).

The abscess may penetrate the surrounding organs. The lung is most frequently involved, and the sequence is as follows: the parietal pleura covering the abscess forms fibrin adhesions with the visceral pleura covering the lung. The lung collapses in the adhesion area, and pus escapes into the collapsed lung.

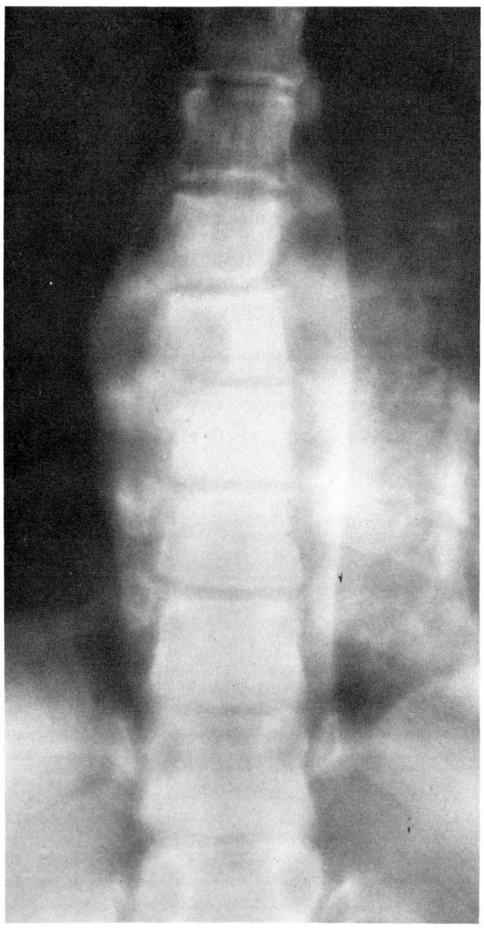

Fig. 7-43. Tomography is frequently helpful in visualizing a vertebral abscess if there is some question. A tomogram demonstrating a fusiform vertebral abscess involving over six levels.

Bone scan is helpful in delineating early lesions. The differential diagnosis should include low grade pyogenic infection, brucellosis, eosinophilic granuloma, typhoid fever, Scheuermann's disease, intervertebral disk disease, congenital anomalies (kyphosis), hemangioma, and neoplasms. Tomography, myelography, or vertebral biopsy may be helpful in arriving at the diagnosis and indicating prognosis (Fig. 7-43).

Brucellosis. The etiology in man is either of three species of brucella (B. melitensis, B. abortus, or B. suis). B. melitensis, the most invasive in man, is confined to the Mediterranean countries.

The spine is most commonly involved in the 40 to 60 year age group. There is no sex preference and the lumbar region is most commonly affected.

The organism enters by way of the lymphatics and passes into the blood stream, localizing in those organs abundant in reticuloendothelial cells. A granulation nodule is formed followed by abscess and caseation. A tissue hypersensitivity to brucellosis is produced.

The principal symptom is an irregular fever which lasts for many weeks and is accompanied by headaches, sweating, general weakness, and splenomegaly. Later rheumatic pains occur in all joints including the spine. Spine involvement is heralded by localized severe pain aggravated by any motion. About 12 percent of the patients have spinal cord compression.

A negative tuberculin test is helpful but blood cultures in the acute stage or biopsy from needle aspiration are most significant. However, a brucellosis agglutination reaction of 1/80 is regarded as diagnostic of the disease.

Once generalized symptoms occur, there is usually a period of several months before roentgenographic changes are seen in the spine. Changes may appear in the disk space, in the vertebral body, or at the margin of bone. An area of rarefaction at the upper anterior margin of the body is an early sign. The disk is involved early and becomes narrowed, but bony ankylosis is uncommon. There frequently are proliferative osteophytic outgrowths which may produce intervertebral bridging. This is similar to what is seen in tuberculosis except bone and disk destruction are less severe and a paravertebral abscess is not typical of brucellosis.

Actinomycosis. The infection is caused by Actinomyces israelii or Actinomyces bovis, and vertebral involvement is rare. It is more common in males by a ratio of 2:1, and there is no age preference.

The bones most commonly affected are the mandible, ribs, and vertebrae, the latter two by extension from pulmonary lesions. Essentially the lesion is a granuloma associated with suppuration and draining sinuses. The typical history and physical finding is that of a hard mass with discharging sinuses in the area of the spine or flank.

Diagnosis depends on isolation of the organism from the discharging sinus and the lesion must be cultured anaerobically. The disk spaces are usually spared, and vertebral collapse is uncommon. The vertebral body may show areas of destruction of a "honeycomb" appearance surrounded by reactive sclerosis.

Because of its atypical presentation, actinomycosis is relatively easy to differentiate from most diseases. The lack of vertebral collapse helps to separate it from tuberculosis and pyogenic infection.

Fungal Infections. *Coccidioidomycosis* is caused by Coccidioides immitis, the most infectious of all fungi capable of producing systemic disease. The localized form is usually benign but the disseminated form is progressive. Twenty percent of those with disseminated disease have osseous lesions. The fungus is endemic to southwestern United States, Central America, and parts of South America. It is particularly endemic to central California and carries the name of San Joaquin Valley fever.

Although the disease occurs in all ages, it is most prevalent in those 25 to 55 years of age, and dissemination is greater in males. The disseminated disease is ten times more common in blacks than whites and of even greater hazard to Filipinos.

If a patient in an endemic region comes down with respiratory symptoms and fever which last longer than one month, disseminated disease should be suspected. The organisms enter via the respiratory tract and are spread hematogenously.

In an endemic area, 50 to 84 percent of the population will have a positive coccidioidin skin test. It takes 3 to 6 weeks to become positive and due to anergy is unreliable when systemic disease is present. A serological complement fixation titer of $1/64$ or higher is thought to be diagnostic of disseminated disease.

Most lesions are lytic in nature and indiscriminantly involve the vertebral bones and other bone elements of the spine. Often multiple spinal lesions are found. Although the disks are spared, paraspinal masses are seen with contiguous rib involvement.

Blastomycosis (North American blastomycosis) is caused by Blastomyces dermatitidis, a chronic systemic fungus, respiratory in origin but capable of dissemination. It is endemic in the southeast and midwest United States. Males are affected nine times more frequently than females and all ages are affected, but there is a higher frequency in the third and fourth decade.

The disease usually begins as a mild respiratory infection but as the disease disseminates hematogenously generalized symptoms of fever, nightsweats, anorexia, and weight loss develop. Skin tests are frequently negative early in the disease but a culture of the skin or lesion reveals budding yeast cells. Serological tests may show a high titer only to Histoplasma capsulatum.

Osteomyelitis occurs frequently in disseminated blastomycosis and it has a greater tendency than coccidioidomycosis for fistula formation and erosion into joints. The disk cartilage is usually involved early, and large paravertebral masses involving ribs may be seen. There may be hilar adenopathy similar to tuberculosis on the chest roentgenogram.

Cryptococcosis is caused by Cryptococcus neoformans and is also a chronic systemic fungal disease originating in the respiratory tract. It affects all ages but is most prevalent between 40 and 60 years and is twice as common in males. This disease is commonly seen in patients with leukemia, Hodgkin's disease, or sarcoidosis who develop central nervous system findings. The pulmonary disease is rarely symptomatic. The spread is by a hematogenous route and frequently results in a cryptococcal meningitis, with 10 percent of the disseminated cases involving bone. The bony lesions are heralded by pain, swelling, and progressive loss of spine motion.

Blood, spinal fluid culture, or cultures from bony lesions may reveal the organism C. neoformans. The India ink preparation is helpful, especially in spinal fluid specimens.

Cryptococcus antibodies may be measured, and some authors believe their presence indicates a good prognosis. Roentgenographically the findings are indistinguishable from coccidioidomycosis.

Parasitic Disease. *Hydatid Cyst Disease (Echinococcosis).* While only 2 percent of hydatid cyst disease involves bone, the spine, sacrum, and pelvis are the bones most commonly involved. It is caused by the tapeworm Echinococcus granulosus when in the larval stage as hydatid cysts. The adult tapeworm is found in dogs and the cysts in man, sheep, swine, and cattle.

There are a number of special tests available including Casoni's test, complement fixation, and a precipitation test which are described in detail in Cecil and Loeb's *Textbook of Medicine.* The roentgenographic appearance is that of a multilocular cyst without cortical or periosteal reaction. The bone may be expanded and later the cortex is thinned with development of soft tissue lesions.

PAGET'S DISEASE (OSTEITIS DEFORMANS)

Paget's disease is a localized chronic disease which changes the size and shape of the involved bones. The basic process is creeping substitution of normal bone by new bone with abnormal architecture. The new bone is woven bone, which is gradually replaced by lamellar bone but the same disordered structure is preserved.

Paget's disease is seen in 3 to 4 percent of the population by roentgenographic examination. A great majority of these patients are asymptomatic. The disease rarely begins before age 40 with a slight preponderance of females.

The bone in Paget's disease goes through three basic phases: osteolytic, mixed, and sclerotic. The osteolytic stage is first and resorbs the normal bone much as a wave washes across the beach. Behind this resorption front, new woven bone is laid down in an irregular manner. This new bone is immature and structurally weak. It also has a rapid metabolic turnover and is rapidly divided into areas of resorption and proliferation. The roentgenographic appearance depends on the predominance of one phase over the other. Later as the disease becomes quiescent in a particular area, the woven bone is replaced by lamellar bone which is sclerotic and cannot be differentiated roentgenographically from the proliferative areas of the mixed phase. All three phases can occur in one bone at any given time.

Although any bone can be affected, the most common sites are the spine, pelvis, skull, femur, and tibia. Most patients are asymptomatic but complaints, if present, are usually related to weight-bearing, reflecting muscle action on the affected bone.

There is some involvement of the spine in almost all patients with the disease. In the spine, neurological complications may occur secondary to encroachment in the canal or intervertebral foraminae by abnormal bone. Collapsed vertebrae secondary to fracture of the weakened bone may initiate or compound the problem. In the thoracic vertebrae, cord compression can lead to paraplegia. However, neurological complications are rare, and when roentgenograms for back pain with neurological findings reveal Paget's disease, it is probably not the cause of the patient's problem. Other complications include deafness due to eighth nerve compression or involvement of the ossicles. The skin over an affected bone is usually warm and both skin and bone have increased blood flow. This is attributed to arteriovenous shunting and can lead to high output cardiac failure. Fractures through areas of woven bone are common, but they heal at a normal rate. Immobilization may occasionally lead to hypercalciuria and renal stones. The most severe complication is degeneration of Paget's disease bone into osteogenic sarcoma. Osteosarcoma is 30 times more common in patients with Paget's disease than in the normal populace and is particularly malignant. Fortunately, it is rare in the spine, accounting for only 3 percent of the total Paget sarcomas.

In the laboratory the most characteristic abnormality is elevation of the serum alkaline phosphatase, which grossly reflects the osteoblastic activity of the disease. The acid phosphatase is occasionally elevated but not nearly as high as in prostatic carcinoma. The total urinary hydroxyproline is also elevated.

Roentgenographically the findings vary with the stage of the disease. The osteolytic phase is best demonstrated in the skull (osteoporosis circumscripta) and is rarely seen in the spine. It is easily confused with metastatic disease. Once woven bone replacement begins in the vertebrae, the cortex is thickened and more dense, especially in the inferior and superior margins. Varying degrees of sclerosis can be seen, the most extreme being an "ivory vertebra," which may be an isolated finding. Roentgenographically, Paget's disease can be confused with metastatic carcinoma, particularly the sclerotic varieties, and bone biopsy is often required for differentiation.

TUMORS OF THE SPINE (Fig. 7-44)

Primary Tumors

Osteoid Osteoma

The osteoid osteoma is a small, solitary, painful lesion most commonly seen in the bones of lower extremities. It is of osteoblastic origin and is benign. It occurs at any age but is most prevalent in the second and third decades and is more common in males. In the spine, the lesion is usually seen in the vertebral arch or transverse process but can occur in the vertebral body.

The symptoms of osteoid osteoma are often unique and severe, but may be present for some time before the correct diagnosis is made. Characteristically the pain is more severe at night and is relieved by aspirin. The pain may radiate and in this way mimic other diseases. If a vertebra is involved, the pain may radiate in a manner similar to a herniated disk. Keim noted an associated scoliosis with osteoid osteoma in the spine in nine consecutive cases. The lesion is usually found at the apex of the curve, and is always on the concave side.

Roentgenographically the lesion usually presents in the posterior elements or transverse process as a dense sclerotic lesion with a central, usually radiolucent, nidus. They are usually less than 1 cm. in size. Tomography is usually effective in revealing a vertebral lesion that may otherwise elude detection.

Osteoblastoma

The osteoblastoma, an uncommon tumor, is also benign and of osteoblastic origin. It is a solitary tumor that often involves vertebrae and the long bones of the extremities. There is no sex predilection and it can occur at any age but the majority are between 10 and 35 years of age. Local pain is the chief symptom although spinal cord or root pressure may result in radicular pain. The pain is not more severe at night nor is it relieved by aspirin. These tumors have a tendency to be locally aggressive and may recur following resection.

The roentgenographic features can be variable, although the tumor is usually dense. The sclerosis is less than that noted with osteoid osteoma, and the lesions tend to be larger, in the range of 2 to 10 cm. The posterior arches, spinous processes, and bodies of vertebrae have been involved.

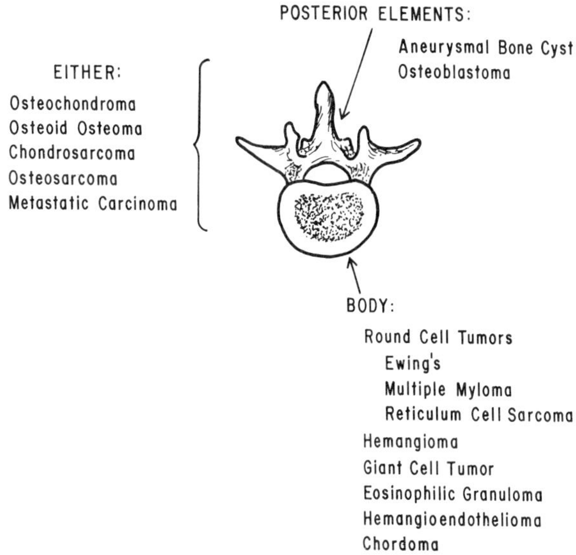

Fig. 7-44. The expected location of spinal column tumors. These are the usual locations in the spine. It should be emphasized that any given tumor can appear in either the posterior elements or the body. (Courtesy Dr. Alan Wolf.)

Osteosarcoma (Osteogenic Sarcoma)

Osteosarcoma is a rare neoplasm also of osteoblastic origin but malignant. It represents in Dahlin's series, 21 percent of malignant tumors of bone. Although the majority of these lesions affect the metaphyseal ends of long bones, the vertebral column is also affected. This is particularly true in patients who have had previous radiation to or preexisting Paget's disease of the spine. It is known that osteosarcoma may develop in these predisposed areas. In Paget's disease, the osteosarcoma that does develop tends to be more malignant, and the prognosis is quite poor. It occurs at any age but the peak is in the second decade with a steady decline thereafter. However the post-irradiation and Paget's sarcomas occur later in life. There is a slight male preference and distant spread takes place hematogenously with metastasis most commonly going to lung.

Pain and swelling are the most common symptoms. Because of the aggressive nature of this tumor, patients usually seek medical treatment within a few months of onset of symptoms. There may be a soft tissue mass with swelling and increased warmth over the lesion. The lesions are usually extremely aggressive and compression of the spinal cord and nerve roots can occur early, producing positive neurological findings (Fig. 7-45). The diagnosis is proven by biopsy. The alkaline phosphatase is elevated in approximately one half the cases and indicates osteoblastic activity.

An area of the spine can show roentgenographic evidence of both bone destruction and bone formation. Generally there is destruction of the bony cortex with subperiosteal bone formation. The classic signs of osteogenic sarcoma seen in the long bones, such as Codman's triangle and a sunburst appearance, are not as readily seen in the spine.

Plasma Cell Myeloma (Multiple Myeloma)

Multiple myeloma is of marrow origin and is the most common primary malignant tumor of bone. It originates from bone marrow and invades and destroys the skeleton. The vertebral bodies are frequently the site of skeletal involvement. It occurs between 20 and 80 years of age with the average age being 64 years. There is a sex predilection in men, 2:1.

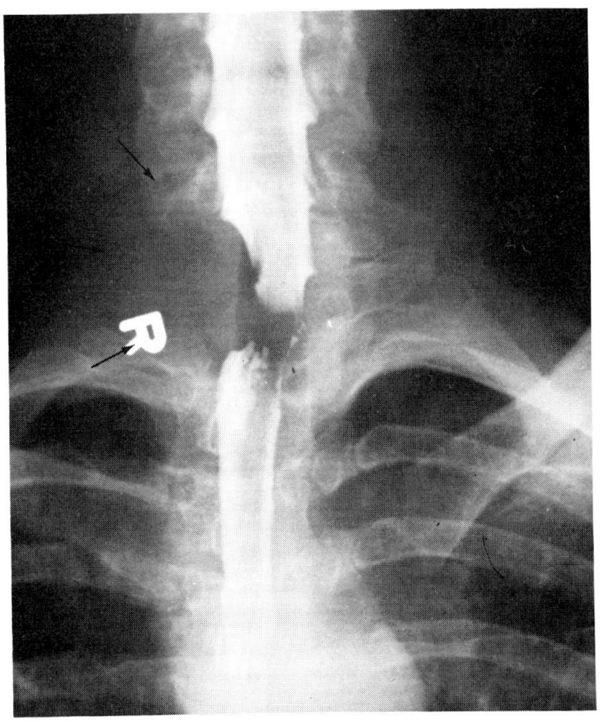

Fig. 7-45. Anteroposterior roentgenogram of a lytic osteogenic sarcoma in a 25-year-old female. The tumor has destroyed the body and lateral processes of the cervical 7 and thoracic 1 vertebrae. There is a block of the dye column. This patient became quadriplegic before suffering an untimely death.

Plasma cell myeloma is a neoplastic proliferation of the plasma cells of the bone marrow and may present as a solitary bone lesion or as a systemic disease. Clinical manifestations can be related to the excessive production of abnormal plasma cells and immunoglobulins with resultant decrease in ability to ward off infection.

The symptoms include bone pain, anemia, spinal deformities, pathological fractures, neurological involvement, hypercalcemia, and kidney failure. Pain is the initial symptom and is rather characteristic in nature. It is deep and persistent, never completely disappearing. The spine including the cervical, thoracic, and lumbar regions, frequently is the area first involved. The neurological problems are related to the associated compression fractures of the vertebral column. Carson and co-workers reported an incidence of 66 percent with fracture in those patients with vertebral involvement.

In the disseminated disease, anemia is usually present. The leukocyte count is generally normal or slightly elevated. Hypercalcemia is seen in one third to one half of the patients, and hyperuricemia may also be noted. The total serum protein is usually elevated, practically always in the globulin fraction. Abnormalities of the globulin fragment are detected by serum electrophoresis and are noted in 90 percent of those with disseminated disease. The urine electrophoresis may show an abnormal pattern even when the serum is normal. Bence Jones protein can be demonstrated in the urine in one half of the patients with disseminated disease.

Plasma cell myeloma is almost always destructive of bone, but as in any tumor, it may appear sclerotic. The vertebral body may demonstrate a compression fracture as a result of massive bony involvement (Fig. 7-46). The disk space is usually preserved. Occasionally, the only roentgenographic finding is generalized osteoporosis.

Since myeloma is generally a disseminated disease and by the time the orthopaedist is involved lesions are found in other bones, a bone survey should be ordered routinely. The skull in particular is prone to show punched out lesions.

Bone marrow biopsy of the sternum or iliac crest

marrow may be necessary to demonstrate the abnormal plasma cells. Open or needle biopsy of the lesion is often necessary to pathologically prove the diagnosis.

Eosinophilic Granuloma

The eosinophilic granuloma is also of marrow origin but unlike myeloma is benign. It is usually classified as a member of the reticuloendothelial proliferative diseases that include Letterer-Siwe and Hand-Schüller-Christian diseases. They may or may not be of common origin. Liebermann and associates tend to favor the latter, after a review of 82 cases of the three diseases. The lesions of eosinophilic granuloma are usually multiple but may be solitary. In the spine, the body is usually involved, and collapse causes a typical flattening termed vertebra plana or Calve's disease.

It can occur from birth to the sixth decade, but the peak incidence is between 5 and 10 years of age with a slight predominance in males. Local symptoms include pain and swelling in the younger child who refuses to walk because of pain. The vertebral involvement may lead to pathological fracture and collapse.

The lesion usually appears as a lytic defect until fracture when the body flattens. Later the vertebral body may reconstitute itself and appear absolutely normal. The disk spaces are almost invariably spared. Lesions should be searched for roentgenographically elsewhere, particularly in the skull and long bones.

Giant Cell Tumor (Osteoclastoma)

This tumor is of uncertain origin and rarely involves the spine but when it does, it nearly always involves the vertebral body with a high incidence in the sacrum. It occurs between 20 and 50 years of age, predominantly in women, and pain is the presenting symptom. The lesions are totally destructive and practically always involve the entire vertebral body. There is little, if any, periosteal reaction.

Hemangioma

This rare benign tumor is of vascular origin and may occur within the vertebral body and produce mild symptoms. Most are asymptomatic and need no treatment. It is common in the middle decades with no sex predilection. The main symptom is pain, particularly when the lesion is associated with a

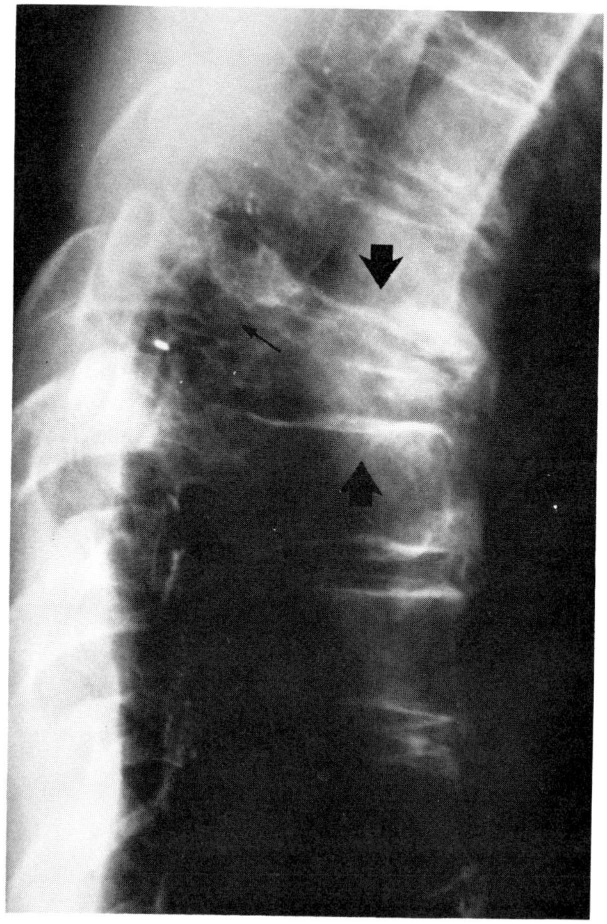

Fig. 7-46. Lateral roentgenogram of a plasma cell myeloma which has created a severe compression fracture as a result of massive bony involvement. The plasma cell myeloma is very destructive of bone and frequently presents as vertebral collapse.

pathological fracture. Neurological symptoms may be produced by the resultant fracture and swelling. Roentgenographically, the characteristic features in the vertebral body include decreased density of bone associated with parallel vertical linear streaks (Fig. 7-47).

The body may be enlarged or collapsed. The lesion is often mistaken for myeloma, metastatic carcinoma, or Paget's disease.

Aneurysmal Bone Cyst

Aneurysmal bone cyst is a benign tumor of bone of vascular origin. It may involve the spine and typically is seen in the posterior elements. It is more

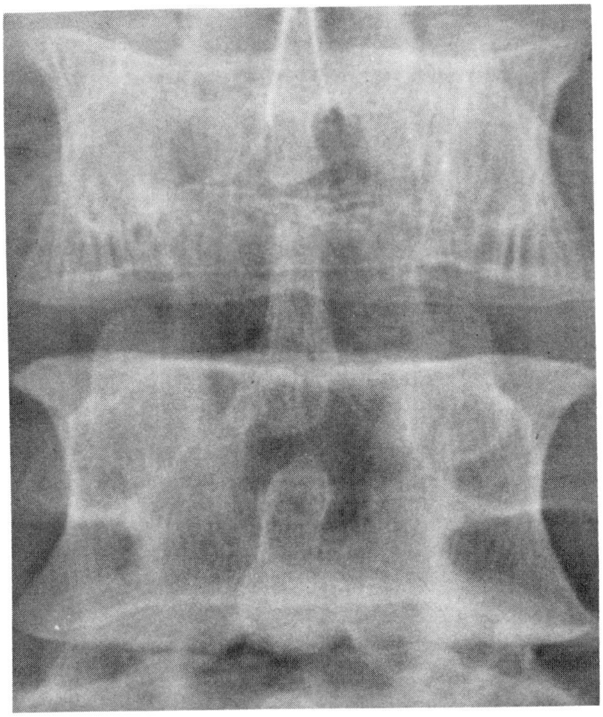

Fig. 7-47. Anteroposterior roentgenogram of a lumbar vertebra with a hemangioma. The characteristic features include decreased density of bone associated with parallel vertical-linear streaks.

common in females in their second or third decade of life.

Swelling, pain, and tenderness are the typical symptoms of an aneurysmal bone cyst. In the vertebral column, expansion of the mass may compress the spinal cord producing a myriad of neurological signs and symptoms.

The lesion is destructive and expansible with an expanded cortex that is thin but intact and produces the roentgenographic feature that gives the disease its name (Fig. 7-48). It is the only benign lesion that may extend from one vertebra to another. This may be helpful in distinguishing an aneurysmal bone cyst from other tumors of the spine.

Ewing's Sarcoma

This tumor occasionally occurs in the spine and is extremely malignant. The vertebral bodies are most frequently involved with extension into the pedicles. Ewing's sarcoma is a disease of childhood and adolescence and is more common in males by 2:1. The main symptom is severe, unrelenting pain not responding to the usual modalities of treatment. On roentgenogram Ewing's sarcoma is a moth-eaten destructive lesion involving the vertebral bodies and it may be associated with compression fracture of the vertebra. Surgical biopsy establishes the diagnosis as eosinophilic granuloma, aneurysmal bone cysts, osteogenic sarcoma, and bone infections which all can look alike.

Chondrosarcoma

Chondrosarcoma is a malignant tumor of cartilagenous origin which may arise de nova in a vertebral body or be superimposed on a preexisting cartilagenous lesion. Patients might include those with hereditary multiple exostosis or enchondromatosis

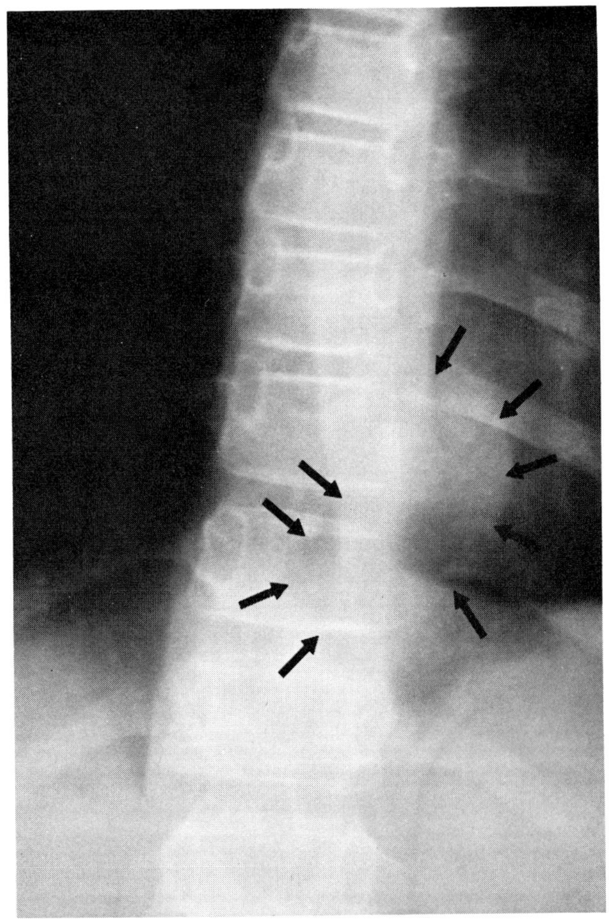

Fig. 7-48. Anteroposterior roentgenogram demonstrating an aneurysmal cyst involving the 11th thoracic vertebra. Note the disappearance of the pedicle shadow and the associated soft tissue mass.

(Ollier's disease) as both are highly susceptible to the development of chondrosarcoma.

It is common in children and adolescents and generally occurs in males (2:1) in their fourth or fifth decade of life. The majority of the patients present some degree of pain and swelling which has been present for a long period of time.

On roentgenogram the vertebral chondrosarcoma is mainly destructive involving any area of the spine but can extend from the bone as a lobulated mass. Frequently the tumor is speckled with calcifications. This may be a prognostic as well as diagnostic sign as the more calcification present, the more differentiated the tumor.

Laboratory studies are not helpful in these lesions and the only way to make a diagnosis is by surgical biopsy.

Chordoma

Although chordoma is an uncommon tumor of notochord origin, it has a predilection for the axial skeleton, most commonly being found in the sphenoid and sacrococcygeal areas. The lesion is almost always solitary and usually slow growing. It is only infrequently seen before the age of 30 and is more common in males (2:1). The symptoms are those of a space-occupying lesion rather than bony destruction. Pain is the most frequent presenting symptom but it may be mild. When the tumors arise in the sacrum, the symptoms may include compression of the sacral roots with bowel and bladder incontinence. A frequent physical finding is a presacral mass discovered on rectal examination.

Roentgenographically chordomas present as lytic destruction of the sacrum or, if higher, the vertebral body. These findings may be only a small part of the total picture as minimal roentgenographic changes can be associated with a massive soft tissue lesion (Fig. 7-49).

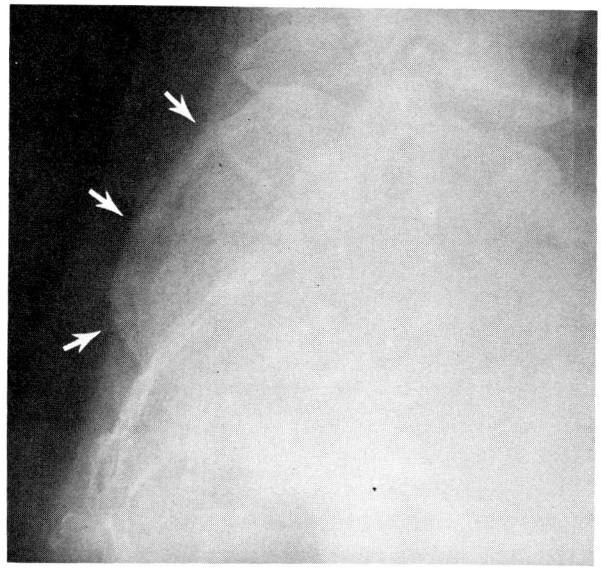

Fig. 7-49. Chordoma of the sacral area. A large posterior mass to the sacrum is indicated by the arrows. This patient had metastasis of the chordoma to the lung when first seen.

Metastatic Carcinoma

Any malignant tumor can metastasize to bone but some occur more commonly than others. Most common are those of the breast, prostate gland, kidney, thyroid, and lung. While malignant primary tumors, except for multiple myeloma, are relatively rare in the spine, metastatic tumors are not. This is particularly true in the patient over 50 years of age. In fact, metastatic bone cancer is the most common malignant tumor of bone. Abrams and coworkers et al. found metastatic bone disease in 27 percent of patients who died of carcinoma. In patients with breast carcinoma, the percentage was 73 percent. Jaffe feels that with more extensive sampling this figure could easily approximate 85 percent.

The two major pathways tumor cells reach the vertebral column are the venous and arterial systems. A third but less probable is through the lymphatic channels. Destruction of the bone occurs because of the proliferation of tumor cells, and bone production may be stimulated to combat the tumor's destructiveness. Therefore, both osteolytic and osteoblastic activity can be seen in any tumor. Most are osteolytic but some, particularly prostatic carcinoma, are predominantly osteoblastic.

Pain is the predominant complaint and in the spine it may mimic any of the other tumors, infection, or even a herniated nucleus pulposus. Pain is frequently present before roentgenographic signs develop. A thorough history and physical examination must be done as the orthopaedist may tend to gloss over examination of the thyroid, breasts, and prostate gland. Since metastatic disease of the spine can mimic arthritis, a high index of suspicion of the possibility of metastatic tumors, in patients over the age of 50, will encourage the examiner to inquire as to previous operations or diagnosed tumors.

The vertebrae are noted for having advanced metastatic disease in the absence of roentgenographic evidence. When signs are present, they may be osteolytic, osteoblastic, or both. The osteolytic lesions are destructive of bone and osteoblastic lesions are productive of bone. The large majority of metastatic lesions are lytic and include carcinoma of the kidney, thyroid, lung, and gastrointestinal tract. Breast carcinoma is usually destructive but may present as a mixed lesion. Carcinoma of the prostate gland almost invariably produces osteoblastic metastasis. Any segment of a vertebra may be involved including the lamina. Pathological fractures occur frequently, generally with preservation of the disk space. It is important to examine the pedicles of the vertebrae as in some cases absence of a pedicle may be the first roentgenographic finding.

There may be elevation of serum alkaline and acid phosphatase in prostatic carcinoma. The sedimentation rate can be elevated in any tumor. If a primary tumor cannot be found, then bone biopsy is necessary for diagnosis. Chest films, bone survey, mammograms, intravenous pyelogram, or upper or lower gastrointestinal series may help in the diagnosis of the primary tumor. Bone, thyroid, and liver scans may also be of assistance in the workup. However, it should be emphasized that nothing will be as helpful as a good history and physical examination in identifying the disease area.

REFERRED BACK PAIN

Extrinsic disorders can simulate spinal disease and should be carefully separated out. The pain of a *peptic ulcer* occasionally occurs only in the back between the eighth and tenth thoracic vertebrae. This localization may accompany penetration but is not pathognomonic of it. The diagnosis is usually made by obtaining a typical ulcer history with periodicity of symptoms and the relationship of pain to certain foods. Occult blood may be demonstrated in the feces and is often associated with an iron-deficiency anemia. The diagnosis is confirmed by barium studies of the stomach and duodenum supplemented with gastroscopy. If perforation has occurred, an upright view of the abdomen will reveal free air under the diaphragm.

Acute *pyelonephritis, perinephric abscess,* or a *carbuncle* of the kidney may all be confused with a back condition. In pyelonephritis an aching pain is noted in one or both costovertebral areas. The patient is usually febrile at 38 to 40 degrees C and has shaking chills. The flank areas will reveal tenderness to percussion. The laboratory studies reveal a polymorphonuclear leukocytosis, and the urine is loaded with leukocytes. Gram stain of the sediment reveals gram-negative bacilli, and culture will confirm this. An intravenous pyelogram may be helpful in confirming either perinephric abscess or a carbuncle.

Nephrolithiasis is the formation of stones within the kidney. These are subsequently passed via the ureters to the bladder and then through the urethra. These are usually due to the precipitation of calcium salts but can be urate salts, cystine, or rarely xanthine. The calcium-containing variety are seen most often in diseases associated with hypercalcemia. These include hyperparathyroidism, metastatic carcinoma, multiple myeloma, senile osteoporosis, specific renal tubular disease, hyperthyroidism, and Cushing's disease. Other conditions associated with calculus formation are infection, urinary stasis, dehydration, and excessive ingestion or absorption of calcium. Urate crystals are associated with gouty conditions and hyperuricemia.

The focal symptoms of nephrolithiasis are characterized by back pain radiating to the flank or iliac crest. *Ureteral colic* presents as an excruciating pain radiating down the course of the ureter into the urethra or groin area. These attacks are intermittent and can be accompanied by nausea, vomiting, sweating, and tachycardia. The diagnosis is made by history, physical examination, and examination of the urinary sediment. The urine usually contains red blood cells or is grossly bloody, and the sediment may reveal the type of stone. The diagnosis is confirmed by intravenous pyelogram.

The pain of *biliary colic* is usually recognized without difficulty. Occasionally the pain beneath the right costal margin may be confused with the girdle pain secondary to intracostal nerve compression.

The pain of *acute pancreatitis* may radiate into the back. Usually it originates in the epigastrium, is sudden, severe, and widespread. A diagnosis of acute pancreatitis can be made when a serum amylase exceeds 300 Somogyi units. The differential diagnosis usually centers around an abdominal catastrophe rather than spinal problems.

In *carcinoma of the pancreas*, the most frequent symptom is pain. It can be first noted as a paroxysmal or steady dull pain radiating from the epigastrium into the back. The pain is usually slowly progressive, worse at night, and unrelated to digestive activities. Other signs and symptoms include jaundice, weight loss, and gastrointestinal difficulties. This is predominantly a disease of males (2 or 3 to 1) and occurs in the sixth and seventh decades. If this disease is suspected, the patient should be given a full gastrointestinal workup.

On occasion an *abdominal aortic aneurysm* can cause severe back pain. Prompt diagnosis is imperative since rupture probably would result in death. The patients are usually males in the sixth or seventh decade of life who present with a deep, boring pain in the midlumbar region. Other stigmas of atherosclerosis, such as a history of coronary disease or intermittent claudication of the lower extremities, may be present. Physical findings may include a pulsating abdominal mass with a loud systolic bruit. The peripheral pulses may be diminished or absent. Routine roentgenograms of the spine may reveal a dilated abdominal aorta with calcification being noted in the atherosclerotic walls. The aneurysm may erode into the lumbar vertebrae.

Partial occlusion of the aorta or iliac arteries can be associated with ischemic muscle pain on exercise which may be confused with back or sciatic pain. The key to diagnosis is pain only with exercise; with rapid relief when exercise is stopped. The pulses may or may not be easily palpable. The diagnosis is made by arteriography.

The pain of an *acute myocardial infarction* may radiate into the thoracic spine area. Usually it is accompanied by a crushing compressing pain across the chest with an associated cold sweat, weak blood pressure, and thready pulse. There can be a pericardial friction rub or cardiac arrhythmia noted. The electrocardiogram, serum enzymes, and other laboratory data confirm the diagnosis.

Gonococcal prostatitis or prostatitis of unknown origin can present as a low backache. Rectal examination frequently reveals a swollen tender boggy prostate with urethral discharge after massage. Culture of the urethral discharge will reveal the etiology of the infection.

Gynecological disorders, such as retroversion of the uterus, uterine fibroids, endometriosis, and pelvic infections, can cause low back discomfort. The frequency of this being the source of many back problems is probably greatly overexaggerated. Diagnosis of pelvic disorders in the female is made by careful pelvic examination which should be included in all complete back workups.

Tumors, masses, and even endometriosis may involve the sacral plexus or its branches, causing severe pain which is sciatic in nature. Usually multiple roots are involved, and the pain is of a severe, burning nature. Diagnosis can frequently be made on rectal and/or pelvic examination.

Finally, the pain of a severely arthritic hip can radiate into the back and simulate sciatic pain. Characteristically hip pain is referred from the groin and anterior thigh to the knee. Irritation of the fourth lumbar nerve root simulates that pain. The hip joint should, therefore, be examined for range of motion and pain. A roentgenogram of the hip should confirm the arthritic findings suspected.

PSYCHOGENIC PAIN

When the workup for back pain leads to a dead end, psychogenic etiology should be considered. It is important to leave this to the last because each patient should have the benefit of a complete, unprejudiced examination. The examiner should try to put previous psychiatric illness, hysterical presentation, and pending law suits out of his mind during the initial evaluation. All persons should be examined for organic disease before assuming psychogenic overlay.

However, human behavior is such that both sociological and psychological factors influence our approach to problems. It is impossible to separate these factors from true organic pain, and this is particularly true in the low back pain syndrome. When the patient emphasizes what he cannot do because of the pain, rather than the pain itself, one must be suspect of some overlay. These patients may have years of experience in learning the appropriate painful behavior, and even the most astute physician can occasionally be fooled. An example is given in the history section of this chapter.

In the hysterical patient the cause of the pain is subconscious in origin, while in the malingerer there exists some conscious financial or social gain. The hysterical patient has severe pain as a product of inadequate defense mechanisms or severe anxiety. The anxiety leads to muscle tenseness, more anxiety, and then muscle spasm. The symptoms are usually exaggerated and not anatomical. These are the patients who develop "stocking glove" anesthesia with complete paraplegia.

The history is packed with anxiety symptomology and bizarre signs. The patient may be completely hysterical although this in itself should not rule out organic disease. Severe organic back pain can create the same state in an individual with low stress levels. Examination may reveal complete stocking glove anesthesia even to pin prick examination. Reflexes do not correspond to the symptoms. Cogwheel rigidity is present on straight leg raising testing with pain being completely out of proportion to the findings. Laboratory and roentgenographic examinations are necessarily completely negative.

The malingerer, on the other hand, has some secondary gain in mind. It may be financially based or directed at job or home difficulties. Many reports have shown that patients with compensable injuries who have had back surgery, remain in the hospital longer and have a subjectively poorer result than other control patient groups.

On examination, the patient may present symptoms as bizarre as the hysterical patient. On occasion they have been so well coached that the signs and symptoms closely parallel organic disease. The range of motion of the entire spine is usually diminished with increase in lumbar lordosis. Cogwheel rigidity of the back and legs suggests conscious protective guarding and is seen in these patients. Several good tests will help to weed out these exaggerated symptoms.

Extending the leg while the patient remains in a sitting position effects a straight leg raising test. If it can easily be done with the patient sitting but not when lying the patient probably is malingering. Another good test is to hold the heel of one leg in the palm of the hand and ask the patient to lift the opposite leg. If the patient has a true "back syndrome" he will press the heel into the palm while a malingerer will tend to lift it away. There is usually no objective neurological finding or muscle atrophy found. The laboratory and roentgenographic examinations do not reveal the source of the patient's extreme pain.

Wiltse and Rocchio have found it helpful to administer psychological examinations, specifically the Minnesota Multiphasic Personality Inventory, to help in predicting success of treatment. Patients who demonstrate high levels of hypochondriasis and hysteria have a statistically significant lower degree of success. This, along with the physician's preoperative rating as to the psychogenic origin of the disease, allows development of a prediction formula. It should be emphasized, however, that if objective signs justify surgery, the patient should, by all means, be operated on. It is helpful in the treatment of questionable cases with minimal signs and symptoms.

DEFORMITY OF THE SPINE WITHOUT PAIN

The history and clinical examination of patients with deformities of the spine have some special characteristics which will be discussed before presenting the disease processes.

Because progression of spinal deformities is most likely during the periods of rapid spinal growth, it is important to know the patients' age in years and months. This correlated with specific roentgen signs, the secondary sexual characteristics, and an estimation of the patients' expected height will usually give a fair idea of when growth is complete. Girls usually reach vertebral maturity at age 15 and boys at age 16. This can vary up to 2 years in either direction. The rapid growth period starts about age 9 and continues until vertebral growth is complete.

Information about the deformity should include how and when it was first noticed and whether it is accompanied by pain. A family history may reveal a similar deformity in a brother or sister. Muscular dystrophy, Marfan's disease, Ehlers-Danlos syndrome, and neurofibromatosis are familial diseases which are associated with spinal deformity. Significant past history might include a febrile illness, such as poliomyelitis, injury to the brain or spinal cord, or transverse myelitis. A previous thoracotomy with removal of ribs, radiation of the spine, or a severe thoracoabdominal burn can also cause vertebral deformity. Lower extremity problems can create unequal leg lengths resulting in a pelvic obliquity and scoliosis.

Any prior treatment is important, particularly if old reports and roentgenograms are available, allowing evaluation of the progression of the deformity. Previous bracing or surgical procedures should be examined in detail, as further recommendations may depend on their effectiveness or lack thereof. On physical examination, observation may reveal café au lait spots (neurofibromatosis) or a hairy nevus on the midline suggesting a diastematomyelia. Cutaneous nodules suggest neurofibromatosis, and hypermobility of joints associated with arachnodactyly raise the question of Marfan's syndrome. When the latter is associated with cutaneous elasticity, Ehlers-Danlos syndrome should be considered.

Roentgenography

In the anteroposterior roentgenogram of a normal spine, neither curvature nor vertebral rotation is seen. In each vertebra the transverse processes and pedicles are symmetric in relation to the sides of the bodies. The intervertebral spaces are parallel and the ribs symmetrical. When bending laterally, each vertebra leans toward the concavity of the curve, the intervertebral space narrowing on the concave and widening on the convex side. In scoliosis this balance or symmetry is lost.

With time, and as a result of the principles of the Hueter-Volkmann law, severe deformities develop in the vertebral bodies and arches, spinous processes, disks, ribs, and other structures attached to the spine. The vertebral bodies lose their rectangular shape and become wedged. The posterior elements and vertebral joints become hypoplastic on the concave side. As the vertebrae rotate the spinous processes, pedicle shadows move toward the concave side of the curvature. Simultaneously, because of their intimate relationship with the spine, the ribs are elevated posteriorly on the convex side and depressed on the concave side. This clinically produces the "rib hump" and thoracic valley which usually is the first sign of a scoliotic deformity.

At present there are two methods of measuring vertebral rotation on roentgenograms. Because three-dimensional rotation is taking place, neither is completely accurate but only gives an estimation of the amount of rotation. The Cobb method is based on the image of the spinous process and the lateral borders of the vertebral body. Frequently the spinous process is deviated or not clearly visible making this, at best, a gross estimate. The method of Nash and Moe is based on the relationship of the pedicle shadows and the edge of the vertebra (Fig. 7-50). This is based on an anteroposterior roentgenogram of the spine and is quantitated by dividing rotation into five grades. If the images are equidistant from the sides of the vertebral body, no rotation is present, and this is defined as Grade 0. Grade I indicates a shift of the convex pedicle toward the concave side

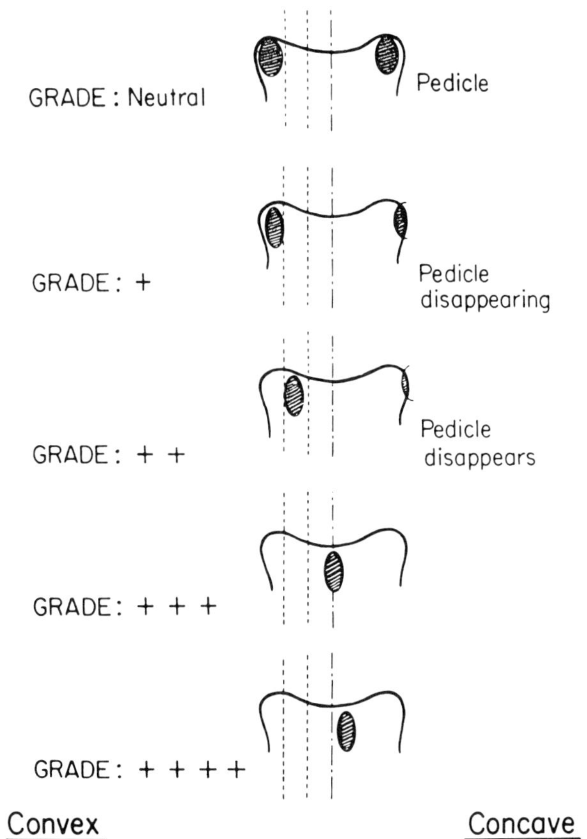

Fig. 7-50. Schematic drawing of the Nash-Moe method to estimate the rotation of a vertebra. On an anteroposterior roentgenogram of the spine, the images of the pedicles are evaluated for rotation. Grade I indicates a shift of a convex pedicle toward the concave side of the curve. When it approaches the midline it is defined as a Grade II, at the midline Grade III, and past the midline Grade IV. (Nash, C. L., and Moe, J. H.: A study of vertebral rotation. J. Bone Joint Surg., *51A*:224, 1969.)

of the curve. When it approaches the midline it is defined as Grade II, at the midline Grade III, and past the midline Grade IV. Mehter has shown it to be inaccurate if there is over 45 degrees of rotation because the pedicle shadow is lost. It also is dependent on the inclination of the vertebral body in the frontal and sagittal planes. However, it remains as the most reasonable estimate of rotation. It is important to recognize this rotation, as brace or surgical treatments are based on including the entire rotated portion of the curvature.

The normal physiological curves should be recognized on the lateral roentgenogram. Normally, thoracic kyphosis will be no greater than 35 degrees and lumbar lordosis no more than 50 degrees. These are measured by the Cobb-Lippman method which will be described next. The lumbosacral junction should be evaluated for spondylolisthesis as it and scoliosis are frequently associated.

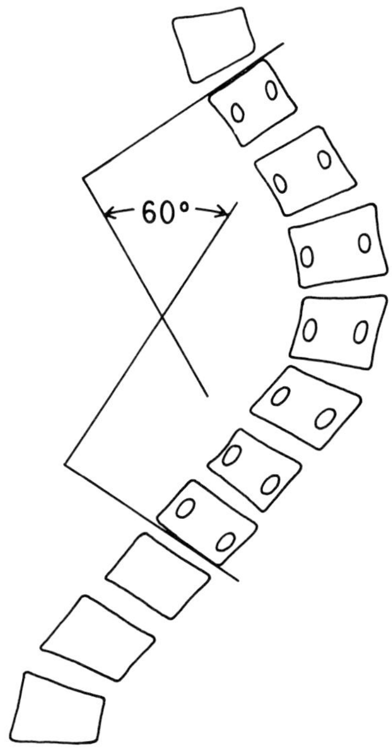

Fig. 7-51. Cobb-Lippman method of measurement of a lateral curve of the spine is characterized by measuring the curve through the angle formed by perpendiculars drawn on the tangents of the upper and lower margins of the limiting vertebral bodies of the curve. The limiting vertebral bodies are recognized as being the last vertebra tilting or rotating the same direction as the other vertebra in the curve.

Although there are several methods for measuring scoliotic curvature, the method of choice and that selected by the Scoliosis Research Society is the Cobb-Lippman method. The Cobb-Lippman method is characterized by measuring the curve through the angle formed by perpendiculars drawn on the tangents of the upper and lower margins of the limiting vertebral bodies of the curve (Fig. 7-51). The limiting vertebral bodies are recognized as being the last vertebra tilting or rotating the same direction as the other vertebrae in the curve. One problem with this measurement is that it concentrates on the ends of the curve rather than the apex. Because the curve is composed of independent vertebral segments, this can create a variety of discrepancies. Only experience in seeing many scoliosis films will conquer the need to strictly apply numbers and degrees to every curve. In time you begin to visualize them as "bad" or "not so bad," a subjective, but valid judgment.

The curves, when present, can be divided into structural and functional varieties. Curves are considered functional when the lateral tilt or bending of the trunk, toward the convexity of the curve, brings about complete correction. That is when the previously narrow intervertebral spaces on the concave become parallel or even widen. Generally when this occurs very little vertebral rotation will be present. Curves are considered to be structural when alterations in the anatomy of the spine limit its flexibility and complete correction is not possible. The apical vertebra (the centermost vertebra) usually is most rotated and is the last to alter its inclination.

In the roentgenographic examination of the spine for deformity, it is necessary to measure all of these variations of normal structure. Anteroposterior, lateral, and bending roentgenograms should be taken in the standing position. In this way the curvature will be maximized by the body weight and effects of gravity. If the patient cannot stand without crutches, a roentgenogram is taken in the sitting, unsupported position. This is because support of the arms on crutches or on the table can "straighten" the spine and lead to a false estimate of the extent of deformity. The study of vertebral flexibility in patients with pathological lordosis or kyphosis is done with the patient lying down. When the patient's torso is maximally flexed or extended to effect maximal correction, a roentgenogram is taken.

Special studies include wrist and hand films to estimate bone age and evaluation of the spine for

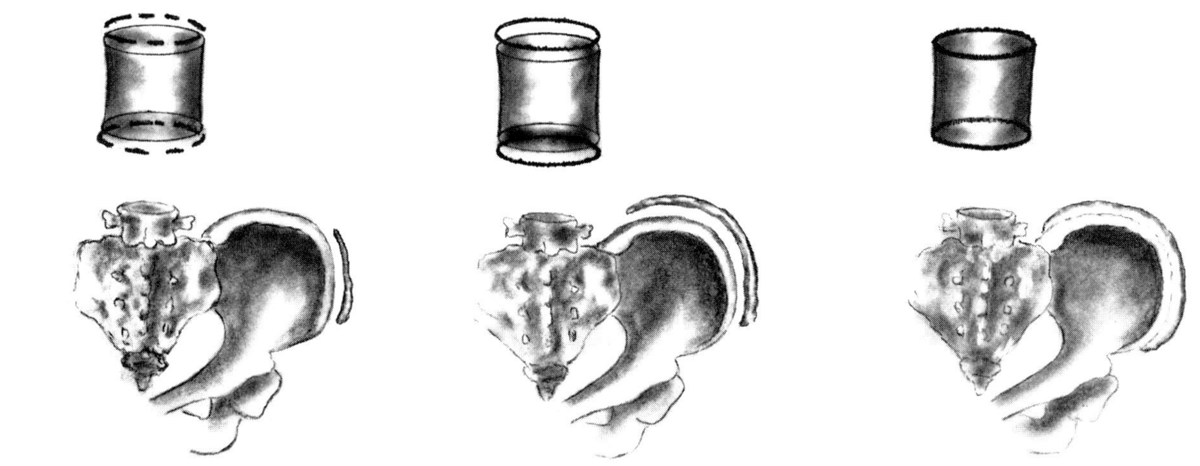
Risser Sign 2+
Open Incomplete Vertebral Ring Epiphysis.
Risser Sign 4+
Complete But Unfused Vertebral Epiphysis.
Risser Sign 5+
Vertebral Ring Epiphysis is Complete.

Fig. 7-52. Schematic illustration of ossification of the iliac crest epiphysis or Risser sign and the apophyseal centers of the vertebra. Both of these are indicators of vertebral maturity. Closure of the vertebral apophyses is particularly indicative of completion of spinal growth.

vertebral body ring and iliac crest epiphysis. The latter is termed the Risser sign. Anteroposterior roentgenograms of the spine usually show the whole extension of the iliac crest, allowing for evaluation of Risser's sign (Fig. 7-52). Because of its prognostic value in regard to the progression of the deformity, the study of Risser's sign is mandatory. According to Risser, the complete ossification of the iliac crest apophysis coincides with both the end of the vertebral growth and with the expected increase in deformity. The epiphyseal center of the iliac crest starts its ossification around the anterosuperior iliac spine and progresses along the upper border of the iliac crest until it reaches the posterior superior iliac spine. Risser's sign is referred to as degree 1 to 4 according to the extent of ossification. This corresponds to each of the 4 parts into which the distance between the iliac spine is divided. The average time span between a 1 degree Risser's sign to 4 is one year.

The ossifying center is often fragmented, but this does not rule out its significance. At other times, the images of the ilia are asymmetric, either when they appear or progress. In these cases, for prognosis of the curve, the image of later appearance or slower progression should be considered. Although Risser insists that degree 4 represents the end of the vertebral growth period and consequently the end of the deformity's progression phase, there are often exceptions to this rule. A definite sign of the end of the growth period is indicated by the image of apophyseal fusion to the iliac wing, referred to as Risser 5. The Risser 4 remains as indicative of the end of the peak growth period. Risser's sign 4 usually occurs at about 14 years of age in girls and 15 in boys. The figures vary if we consider their occurrence in patients from countries of different climate. Risser's 5 usually occurs in 16- to 17-year-old girls and in 17- to 18-year-old boys. The vertebral growth can also be assessed according to the degree of ossification in the apophyseal centers of the vertebra (See Fig. 7-52). Their fusion to the body of the vertebra means a definite stop in growth and coincides with a Risser 5.

Idiopathic Scoliosis

By far the most common type of scoliosis is the idiopathic or familial variety, accounting for at least 70 percent of the total. The etiology is unknown, but a strong familial tendency exists and, depending on the age, it primarily affects girls. It is divided into three groups, depending on the age of presentation.

Infantile familial scoliosis appears between birth and age 3. It is rare in the United States, but more common in Europe and England. Eighty to 90 percent of these curves resolve spontaneously and need no treatment, but a small percentage do progress and become extremely severe treatment problems. The rib angle difference measurement of Mehta is fairly reliable in recognizing those that will progress. The progressive curves are predominantly convex to the left and occur most frequently in males.

Juvenile familial scoliosis appears between the ages of 3 and 10. These curves are most commonly convex to the right, and the incidence is divided equally between males and females. They are usually recognized at age six and contrary to the infantile variety are never self-resolving and always need treatment.

Adolescent idiopathic scoliosis by definition starts after age 10 and is by far the most common variety of scoliosis seen in the United States. The right thoracic curve is so common (90%) that if a left thoracic curve is seen, other causes are suspected. This is generally reported as being eight times more common in girls although recent school surveys have shown more occult spinal curves in boys than had previously been suspected. Many of these curves are structural in type and tend to progress with growth. At the time of spinal growth (15 to 16 in females and 18 to 19 in males), the progression usually stops; although if the curve is severe (over 60 degrees) it can continue to worsen with age. The continued spinal curvature with the attendant vertebral rotation causes increasing deformity, pain, and cardiopulmonary compromise. Patients with severe thoracic curves tend to develop progressive pulmonary problems with the onset of severe respiratory infections and cor pulmonale in the fifth and sixth decades of life. The pulmonary function studies, particularly a low vital capacity, closely parallels the degree of cardiorespiratory disease. Nelsonne and Lundgren reported that the mortality rate for patients over 50 years of age with severe scoliosis is two times higher than what is seen in the normal population. Pulmonary disability with cardiac decompensation (cor pulmonale) was the cause of death in 60 percent of the scoliotic group.

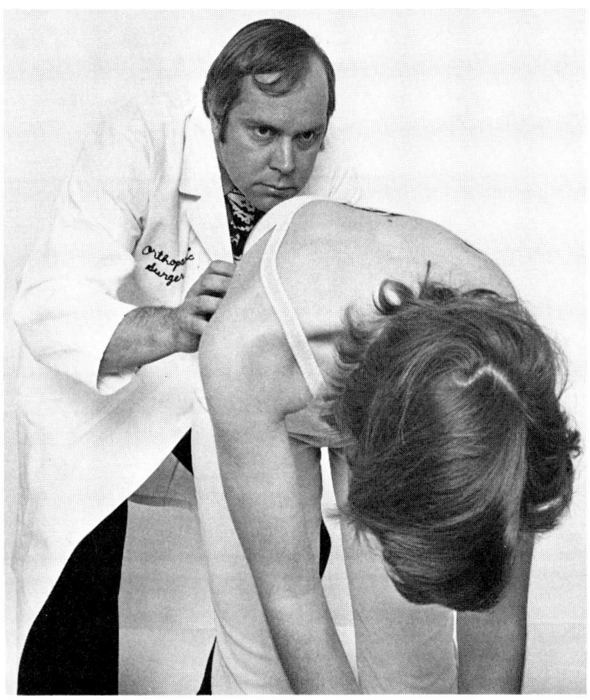

Fig. 7-53. Photograph of an examiner evaluating a suspected spinal curvature. The patient bends forward at the waist, dropping the hands with the palms together in front. Because of the scoliotic curve and subsequent vertebral rotation, a rib or flank hump may be present.

The scoliotic curve is best evaluated by having the patient bend forward at the waist (Fig. 7-53). Because of the scoliotic curve and subsequent vertebral rotation, a rib or flank hump may be present (Figs. 7-54 and 7-55). Bending forward accentuates the deformity and sets it in relief. This is the most reliable test and is used in school screening programs to diagnose early spinal curvature.

Neuromuscular Scoliosis

Scoliosis secondary to neuromuscular disorders can be the most deforming and difficult to treat of all the varieties. Neuromuscular scoliosis can be divided into *neuropathic* and *myopathic* types. The neuropathic type can further be divided into an upper motor neuron and/or lower motor neuron type. Spasticity or paraplegia is noted in the upper motor neuron disease. Examples are cerebral palsy, spinal cerebellar degeneration, syringomyelia, or spinal cord tumors. In cerebral palsy, spinal deformities are being recognized more and more frequently. It has been estimated that up to 25 percent of those afflicted will have some spinal deformity. Spinal cerebellar degeneration refers to a group of diseases which are not well understood and includes entities

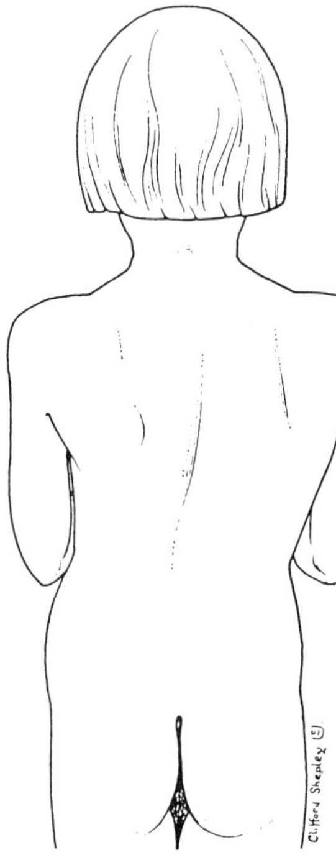

Fig. 7-54. Schematic drawing of the torso of a patient with scoliosis. (James, J. I. P.: Scoliosis. Edinburgh, Churchill-Livingstone, 1967.)

such as Friedreich's ataxia, Charcot-Marie-Tooth disease, and Roussy-Levy syndrome. These patients present in childhood with a clumsy gait, early muscle atrophy, cavus deformities of the feet, and spinal deformity. There is also loss of deep tendon reflexes, fever, proprioception, and tactile sensation. The disease is unpredictable and may progress to death or plateau without further progression.

The prototype of the lower motor neuron disease is *poliomyelitis.* Although the Sabin and Salk vaccines have virtually eliminated poliomyelitis in the United States, we still see the severe deformities in polio patients from other parts of the world. The anterior horn cell is affected leading to selected muscular weakness with subsequent imbalance. When this imbalance affects the spinal or abdominal musculature, vertebral column collapse and deformity will result. Another characteristic of poliomyelitis is the production of muscle and fascial contractures. The iliotibial band in the thigh and hip is a frequently affected area and its unilateral contracture can lead to pelvic obliquity and secondary spinal deformity. Additionally, the hip flexors, extensors, and adductors can be similarly affected creating a fixed deformity. The abdominal or spinal muscles can also become contracted and add to the pelvic obliquity. Examination of the patient with paralytic scoliosis secondary to poliomyelitis requires an accurate evaluation of the muscle weakness and contractures both above and below the pelvis. The pelvic deformity will need to be treated before the spinal problem.

Radiographically the curve of all paralytic diseases tends to be less acute and longer than that seen in idiopathic scoliosis. They are defined as long "C curves" and tend to be single rather than double. The ribs tend to "droop" toward the pelvis probably due to the muscular weakness.

Pulmonary and cardiac evaluation should be done preoperatively as patients with paralytic curves have the most severe cardiorespiratory problems. In a patient with advanced paralytic scoliosis, the vital capacity can be as low as 25 percent of the predicted amount. Many of these patients will die of cor pulmonale or respiratory insufficiency in the fifth and sixth decades.

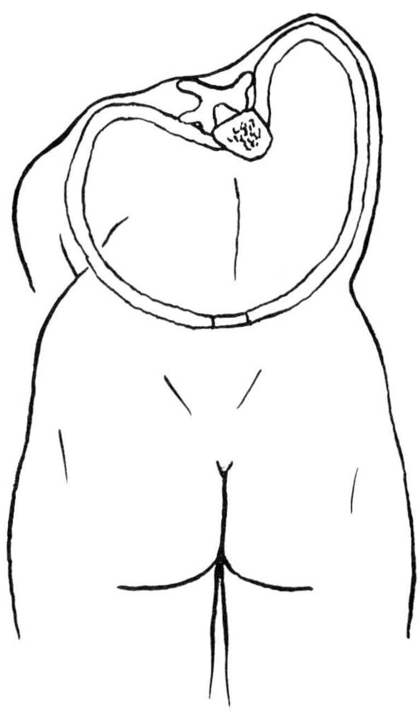

Fig. 7-55. Schematic drawing of a patient bending forward with a scoliotic curve. In this case, the curved rotated spine, because of its intimate attachment to the thoracic rib cage, has created a rib hump which is accentuated by the bending forward maneuver.

Progressive spinal atrophy of the Werdnig-Hoffmann type presents a rather poor prognosis. These are the children born with symmetrical paralysis of the trunk and limb muscles and are called "floppy babies." Most of these patients will die between the ages of three months and four years. Some, however, will survive to adolescence and will exhibit a profound paralytic scoliosis deformity.

In the child with an injured spinal cord, deformity will always develop if the injury is complete and above T12. This deformity is progressive during the growth years and needs to be treated. If a laminectomy has been performed after the injury, the deformity may be a kyphotic one. Otherwise, it usually presents as a long "C type" paralytic scoliosis.

Of the myopathic forms of neuromuscular scoliosis, progressive muscular dystrophy (Duchenne's) is best known. It is sex-linked recessive thereby occurring in boys. There is generalized wasting of muscles with replacement of the muscle fibers with large fat globules, causing what is called "pseudohypertrophy." The patient's calves may look quite developed when in fact they are weak. Life expectancy can extend into the twenties and thirties but severe spinal deformities further debilitate these chronically ill patients. The other forms of muscular dystrophy (limb-girdle, facioscapulohumeral) can cause deformity, but these tend to occur later and are less severe. In any muscular wasting disease, an important consideration is minimum recumbency. If these patients are kept in bed for long periods of time, they may never return to ambulation.

Neurofibromatosis (von Recklinghausen's Disease)

Kyphoscoliosis is seen in 25 percent of the patients with diagnosed von Recklinghausen's disease. These curves are particularly hard to treat as they are progressive even after spinal maturity and can lead to spinal cord compression with paraplegia. Those in whom neurological problems develop almost always have a kyphotic deformity associated with the scoliosis.

The patients will present with a fairly typical history and physical findings. Frequently there is a positive family history of neurofibromatosis. They may have been treated for pseudoarthrosis of the tibia (associated with neurofibromatosis in 50 percent of cases) or have had a positive biopsy of one of the multiple fibroma mollusca on the body. The skin exhibits café au lait patches or the bumps of molluscum fibrosum.

Roentgenographically, any curve pattern can exist but the classic presentation is with a short sharply angulated thoracic curve. The vertebrae are scalloped and wedged, and ribs leading away from the spine are "thinned" or "spindled."

Congenital Scoliosis and Kyphosis

It is important to review the embryologic development of the spine in the anatomy section of this chapter before considering congenital scoliosis. Each vertebra is well formed in primitive cartilage by the tenth embryonic week. Therefore, any failure of segmentation or formation must have occurred prior to that time. Experimental removal of the notochord results in growth only of the posterior elements but not the body. Removal of the spinal cord results in development of the body, but not the posterior elements. The latter may be important in patients with myelomeningocele.

Congenital scoliosis and kyphosis are, by definition, deformities caused by congenital anomalies of the spine. These are embryonic defects, not chromosomal or inherited in etiology. Although there have been a few isolated cases of familial occurrence, the defect is spontaneous and family histories are generally negative.

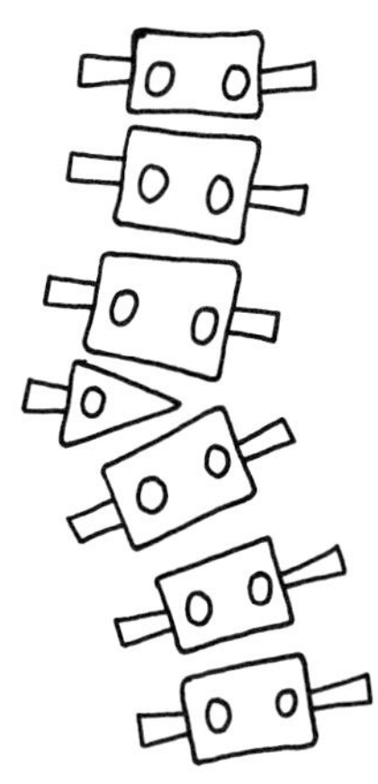

Fig. 7-56. Schematic drawing of a congenital scoliosis created by wedged or hemivertebra. This is a unilateral failure of formation.

The congenital spine deformities can be separated into "closed" and "open" varieties. The open varieties are associated with spina bifida or myelomeningocele with paralysis and will be discussed separately. In this section only the closed defects are considered and are divided into scoliosis and kyphosis. Congenital lordosis is possible but extremely rare.

The classification of congenital scoliosis most widely accepted was first proposed by MacEwan. In both scoliosis and kyphosis the anomalies are separated into three categories: failure of formation, failure of segmentation, and mixed varieties.

Unilateral failure of formation results in "wedged or hemivertebrae" (Figs. 7-56 and 7-57). Failure of segmentation unilaterally creates the most aggressive type of congenital scoliosis, a "unilateral bar" (Fig. 7-58). Because the growth potential is stopped on the bar side and normal on the opposite side, rapid, severe curves result. Bilateral failure of segmentation results in a "block vertebra or fusion." Failure of segmentation in the posterior elements creates the rare congenital lordosis mentioned earlier.

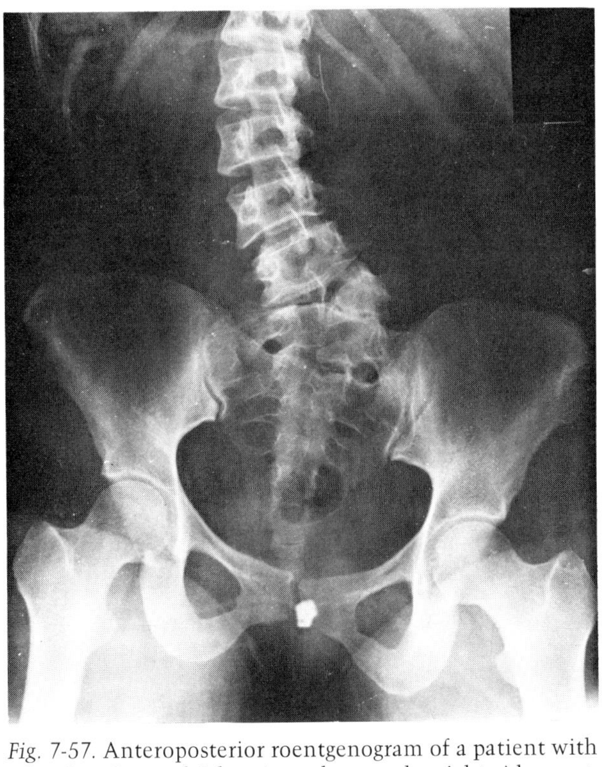

Fig. 7-57. Anteroposterior roentgenogram of a patient with a lumbar 5–sacral 1 hemivertebra on the right side creating a lumbosacral scoliosis.

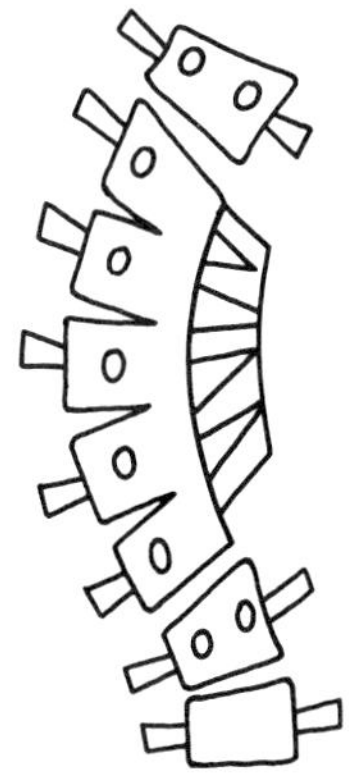

Fig. 7-58. Schematic drawing of a unilateral bar which is created by failure of segmentation. This is the most aggressive type of congenital scoliosis and usually needs to be treated early.

Congenital kyphosis can similarly be classified. Failure of formation of vertebral bodies results in an aggressive form of kyphosis which can rapidly progress causing paraplegia (Fig. 7-59). Failure of segmentation anteriorly produces an unsegmented bar which progresses less rapidly (Fig. 7-60).

The natural progression of congenital kyphosis tends to be more malignant than that of scoliosis. Although congenital kyphosis is approximately one fourth as common as scoliosis, it has approximately four times as many complications. However, in contrast to congenital scoliosis, where the unsegmented bar has the worse prognosis, an anterior unsegmented bar is usually associated with less deformity than failure of formation of vertebral bodies. The latter is commonly associated with a scoliotic component and needs to be treated aggressively and early. In the thoracic spine, progression often leads to paraparesis and finally paraplegia.

The above mentioned anomalies can occur singularly or in combination. When many anomalies are present in the same spine they are classified as a mixed type. These should be carefully distinguished from other curves occurring in infancy not caused by anomalous vertebrae (infantile idiopathic, neuromuscular, or the deformities of osteochondrodystrophy).

Other congenital anomalies which have an increased incidence with congenital vertebral anomalies include genitourinary tract (20%), diastematomyelia (5%), and anomalies of heart,

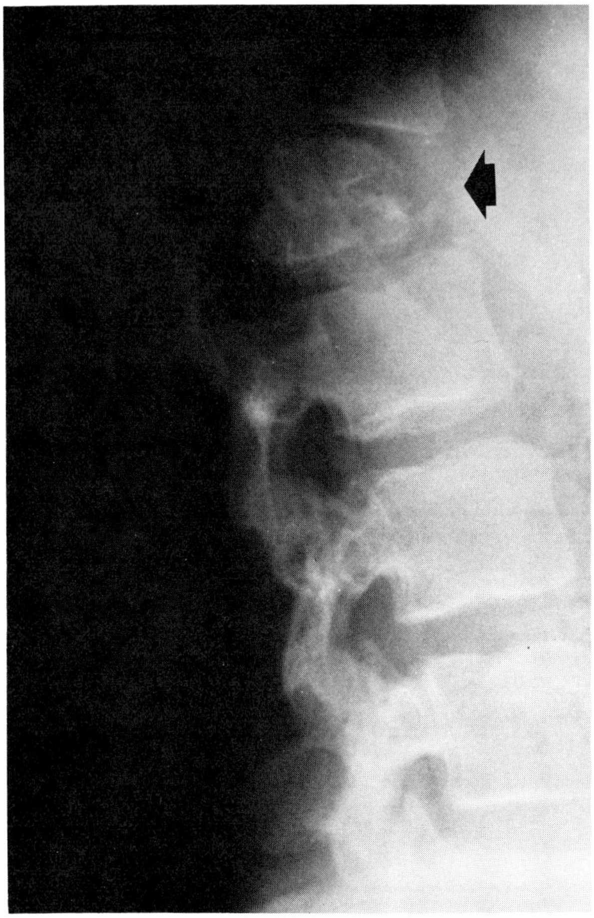

Fig. 7-59. Congenital kyphosis can be created by failure of formation, as demonstrated by this roentgenogram. This is the most aggressive type of congenital kyphosis and can progress rapidly to produce paraplegia.

chest wall, abdominal wall, and upper and lower extremities. The Klippel-Feil syndrome and Sprengel's deformity can be seen with congenital scoliosis.

In evaluating these problems it is best to think in terms of balance of growth. If one side has no potential of growth over three or four segments versus the other normal side, severe progression can be predicted. This is particularly true in the unilateral bar and when multiple hemivertebrae are seen on the same side. In both cases, progression is the rule. In all cases of congenital scoliosis reviewed by Winter and associates, progression occurred in 75 percent. The area of the spine affected has some relation to progression. The most common area involved is the thoracic spine, and this is where progression is most likely to take place. Curves with their apex at the thoracolumbar junction have an equal tendency to progress.

When performing the physical examination, it is important to look for hairy patches, cutaneous dimples, sinuses, or lipomas (Fig. 7-61). The lower extremities should be examined for leg length circumference, foot size, strength, and sensation. A positive finding should lead the examiner to suspect diastematomyelia which is tethering of the cord. A myelogram will be required to rule this out.

An intravenous pyelogram should routinely be

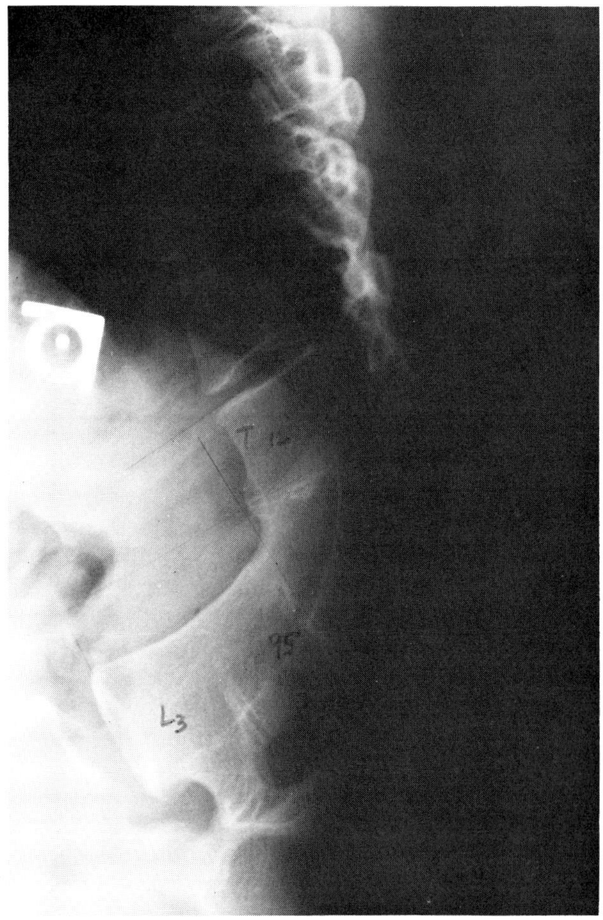

Fig. 7-60. A failure of segmentation anteriorly will produce an unsegmented bar as is demonstrated in this roentgenogram. This is an adult who has an unsegmented bar from thoracic 12 to lumbar 3 with a kyphotic curve of 95 degrees. She has had three children and now presents with low back pain.

obtained because of the frequency of genitourinary abnormalities which are potentially lethal (2.5 percent of cases). Hydronephrosis, hydroureter, and pelvic kidneys are a few of the problems seen. The uterus and vagina may be abnormally developed in the female and the penis and testicle may be abnormal in the male.

To make the diagnosis of congenital scoliosis, an anomaly of the vertebrae must be seen on the roentgenogram. These are alluded to in the discussion of the deformities. A frequent associated roentgenographic finding is fusion of adjacent ribs. Widening of the pedicle shadows would suggest diastematomyelia and should be confirmed with a myelogram. Other special radiographic studies include tomograms to clearly define the anomalies.

MYELODYSPLASIA

Spinal deformity in the myelodysplastic child has only recently begun to be appreciated as a serious problem. This is due to increased survival during the last 15 years which has allowed these children to reach adulthood. Early closure of the meningocele, antibiotics, and surgical control of the hydrocephalus have permitted these children to survive. Although alive, more than one half of these patients develop a significant spinal curve, the majority before age 10. The pattern of curvature can range from scoliosis, kyphosis, or lordosis individually to any combination of the three. Muscle weakness, vertebral structural imbalance (congenital scoliosis), and soft tissue contractures lead to progression of these curves. Once deformity starts it tends to progress rapidly.

The etiology of myelodysplasia has never been delineated although a number of exogenous factors have been investigated. Whatever the cause, its influence starts early in embryonic development before the nineteenth day when the neural folds meet to form the neural tube. The tube first closes in the thorax then proceeds cranially and caudally. The mesodermal somates arrange themselves around the neural tube as muscles and vertebrae. If the neural tube is dysrhaphic, the muscle and vertebrae fail to form properly and the vertebral laminae are left open posteriorly. Therefore, the vertebral level of deformity parallels the neurological level in most cases.

The extent of the lesion varies from a complete exposure of the neural elements to minor defects of the lamina with normal neurological findings. *Spina bifida occulta* refers to a bony defect of the laminae with no neurological deficit (Fig. 7-62). In the lumbar and sacral spine it is so common that it is frequently seen as an incidental finding on spinal films. It occurs in 5 to 10 percent of the population and generally has no clinical significance. It is frequently associated with spondylolisthesis and may be related to its pathogenesis.

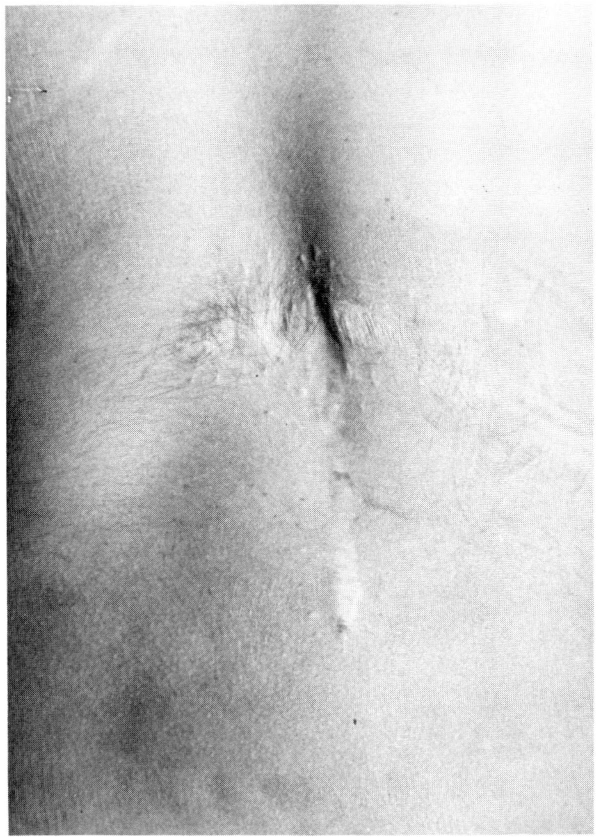

Fig. 7-61. In diastematomyelia it is important to look for hairy patches, cutaneous dimples, sinuses, or lypomas. Although only partially excised, this hairy patch indicated a diastematomyelia in an eight-year-old female.

A *dermal sinus* is a squamous epithelium-lined tube between the skin and dura mater of the spinal cord. It is most common in the lumbosacral area but can be located anywhere along the spinal column. It is commonly associated with laminar defects and may lead to the diagnosis of diastematomyelia. It may serve as an entrance for bacteria and lead to recurrent meningitis.

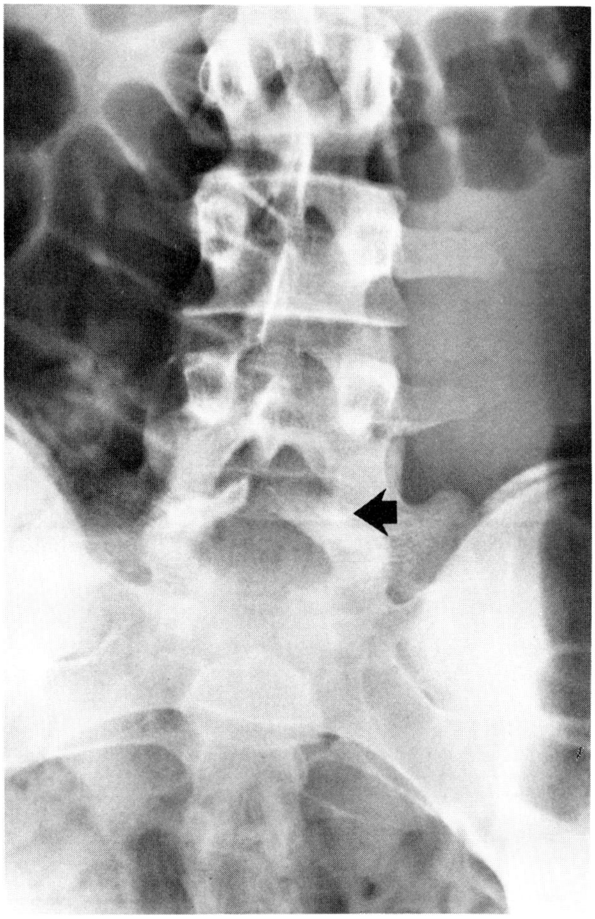

Fig. 7-62. Spina bifida occulta refers to a bony defect of the lamina with no neurological deficit. The bony defect in this situation is at the fifth lumbar level.

Pelvic obliquity is a common occurrence in myelodysplasia and can initiate or compound a scoliotic problem. A fixed pelvic obliquity is an elevation of one side of the pelvis when looking at the patient in the anteroposterior plane. It can result from contracture above, within, or below the pelvis due to the muscle imbalance seen in these patients. The obliquity must be corrected before the scoliosis can be treated successfully.

A *meningocele* is a herniation of the meninges through a posterior vertebral defect without inclusion of the spinal cord or roots (Fig. 7-63). The vertebral laminae are incompletely formed, and the canal is widened in the area of the meningocele. The meninges are only covered by a thin layer of skin, and the sac is filled with spinal fluid. Generally, there is no neurological dysfunction and sac closure offers a good result Fig. (7-64A, B).

A herniation of the neural elements through a posterior vertebral defect is termed a *myelomeningocele* (Fig. 7-65). It usually is not covered by skin but instead has only a thin tissue membrane (arachnoid) which is filled with spinal fluid. The dysplastic spinal cord and roots usually can be seen through the membrane. The vertebral bodies are widened in the transverse diameter with the rudimentary laminae and pedicles remaining as lateral ridges (Fig. 7-66). The neurological status depends on the vertebral level of involvement and the amount of associated hydrocephalus. Profound motor loss, absent or diminished sensation, bladder and bowel incontinence, and mental retardation are common.

Routine roentgenograms will usually reveal the level and amount of dysrhaphism. Once the spinal deformity begins, it should be followed closely with serial roentgenograms. As in any paralytic spinal deformity the amount of curve will be most appreciated in roentgenograms taken with the patient in the standing or unsupported sitting position. Unsupported means the child should not be allowed to support the torso with the upper extremities, as this may improve the spinal curve thus giving a false impression to the examiner and lead to inadequate treatment.

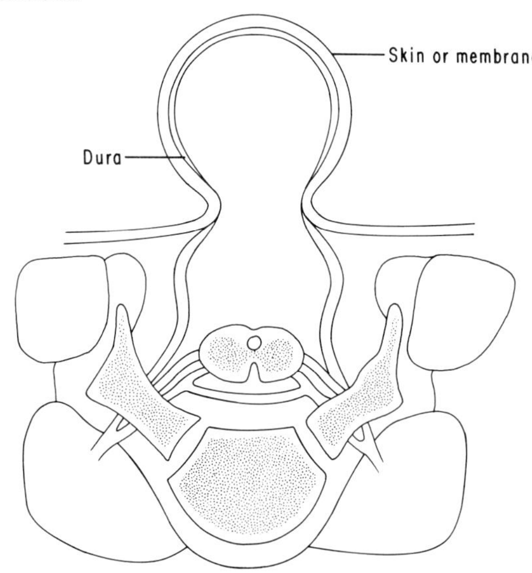

Fig. 7-63. A meningocele is a herniation of the meninges through the posterior vertebral defect without inclusion of the spinal cord or root. (Sharrard, W. J. W.: Paediatric Orthopedics and Fractures. Oxford, Blackwell, 1971.)

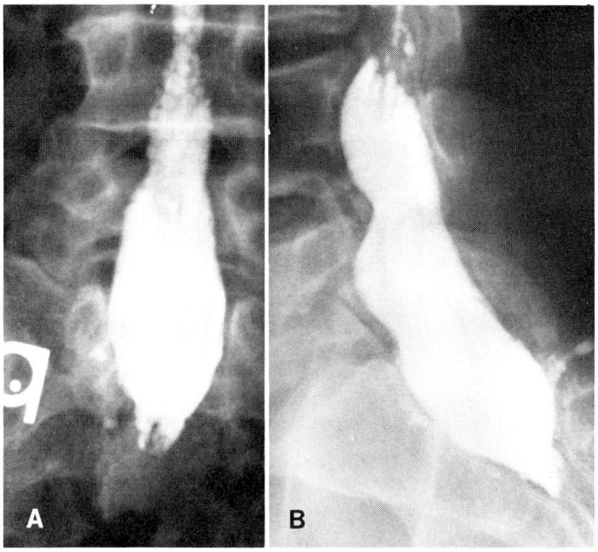

Fig. 7-64. (*A*) Anteroposterior myelogram of a patient with a meningocele in the sacral region. (*B*) Lateral myelogram of the same patient with intrasacral meningocele.

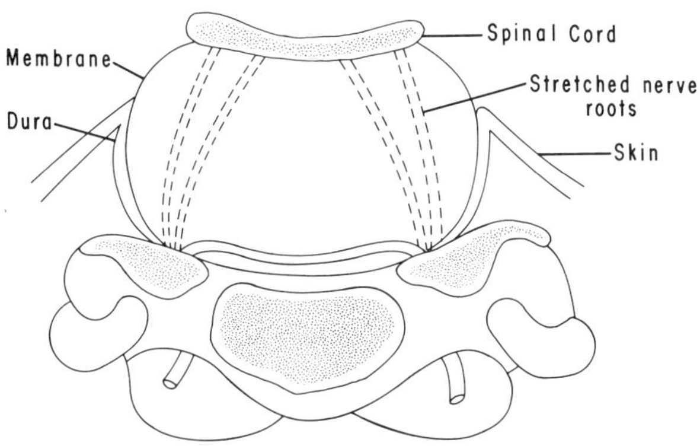

Fig. 7-65. Schematic drawing of a myelomeningocele. Herniation of the neural elements is covered only by a thin tissue membrane which is filled with spinal fluid. The dysplastic spinal cord and roots can usually be seen through this membrane. (Sharrard, W. J. W.: Paediatric Orthopedics and Fractures. Oxford, Blackwell, 1971.)

Lumbar and Sacral Agenesis

Lumbar and complete sacral agenesis can result in considerable neurological and bony deficit. Partial sacral agenesis may or may not have a detectable neurological lesion. Lesions above the twelfth thoracic level are usually incompatible with life but have been reported.

The deformity in humans is not completely understood, but can be compared to rumplessness in animals. This deformity can occur either by spontaneous mutation or by genetic transmission. Many noxious agents have been used to induce the condition in the embryo. The most interesting research to date has been that of Duraiswami, who produced rumplessness in chicks by injecting insulin into the eggs. Clinically, it has been noted that a significant percentage of children affected with distal vertebral anomalies have diabetic mothers or a strong family history of diabetes.

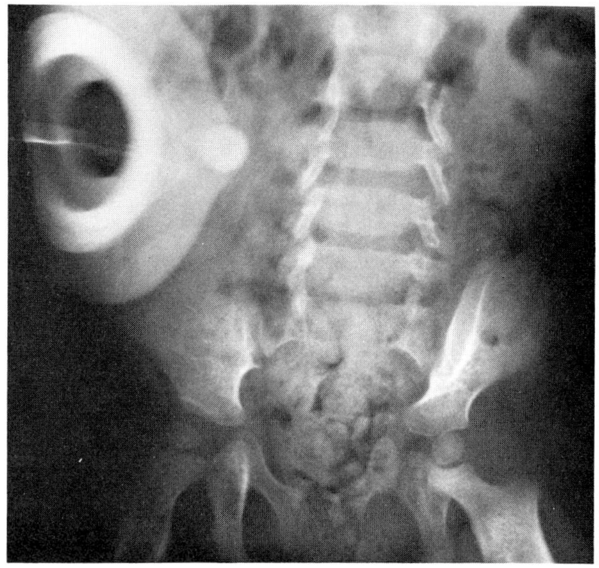

Fig. 7-66. Anteroposterior roentgenogram of the spine of a patient with a myelomeningocele with vertebral bodies which are widened in the transverse diameter with rudimentary laminae and pedicles remaining as lateral ridges. Note that this particular patient has an ileostomy sac in the right lower quadrant of the abdomen which is not uncommon for a patient with this problem.

The clinical appearance is dependent on the vertebral level of the lesion. Those with a partial sacral or a coccygeal agenesis may be entirely normal. On the other hand, the child with complete sacral or lumbar agenesis may be severely deformed with contractures of ankles, knees, and hips and an unsupported torso. The contractures of the lower extremities have been likened to a "sitting Buddha." The buttocks are narrowed because of an underdeveloped pelvis, with dimpling noted lateral to the gluteal cleft (Fig. 7-67). Inspection and palpation of the back may yield a bony mass representing the last vertebral segment,

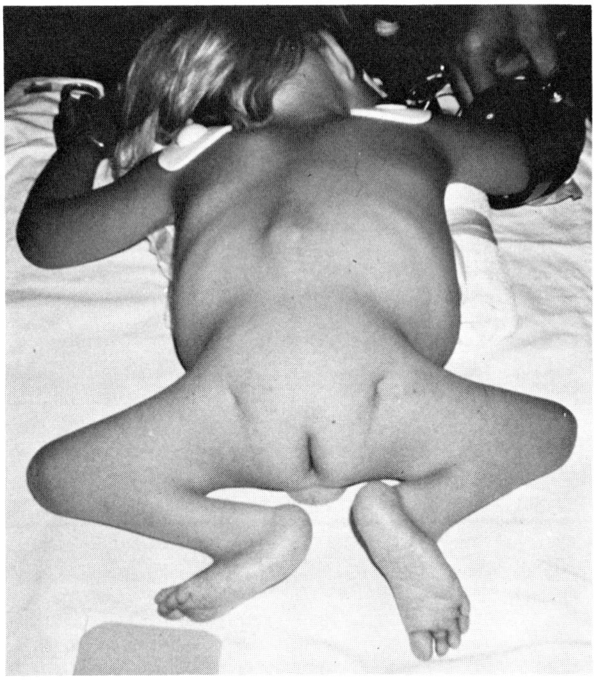

Fig. 7-67. Photograph of a patient with lumbosacral agenesis. Note that the buttocks are narrowed because of a underdeveloped pelvis with dimpling just lateral to the gluteal cleft. The last vertebral segment can be seen as a bony mass at the lower level of the rib cage.

generally with gross motion between it and the pelvis.

The paralysis is profound, and the legs are of no value to the patient. Ambulation is performed by hand walking, the pelvis and lower extremities swinging through. Sensation to the lower extremities does not necessarily parallel the motor loss and is usually present to some degree. Bladder and bowel incontinence, however, is a constant finding. The intelligence is not impaired, and the upper extremities are not involved. Commonly associated anomalies are scoliosis, hemivertebrae, spina bifida, and meningocele. Visceral anomalies have been reported in up to 35 percent of the cases, usually in the anogenital region or urinary tract.

Roentgenographic findings depend on the extent of the lesion and are readily seen on routine spine films (Fig. 7-68A, B). Because of the associated urological problems, an intravenous pyelogram should be performed on all patients.

The lower level lesions (i.e., coccygeal and sacral) may present with lower extremity deformities similar to arthrogryposis. The arthrogrypotic, however, has normal sensation and full control of bowel and bladder function. The arthrogrypotic patient will also have upper extremity involvement.

DIASTEMATOMYELIA

Diastematomyelia means a cleft of the spinal cord and is to be differentiated from diplomyelia, which is duplication of the spinal cord. In diastematomyelia the spinal cord or the spinal nerves are split in two by either a cartilagenous or bony mass attached anteriorly to the vertebral body and posteriorly to the dura mater. This may be localized to one vertebral level or extend over several segments. It is most commonly seen in the lumbar region but has been reported as high as the fifth thoracic vertebra.

The etiology of diastematomyelia is unknown but is in the realm of and is associated with the other congenital vertebral anomalies. The bony vertebral column and the spinal cord are of equal length until the third embryonic month when the vertebral col-

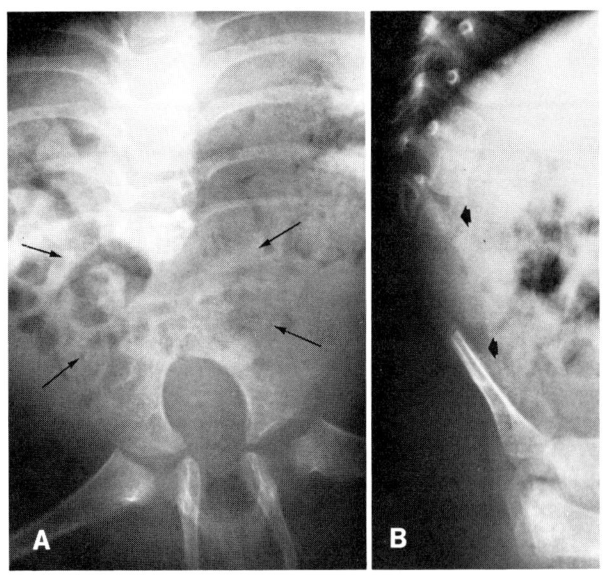

Fig. 7-68. (*A*) Anteroposterior roentgenogram of the spine of a patient with lumbosacral agenesis. The hypoplastic pelvis is seen inferior to the thoracic spine. The arrows surround the nonexistent lumbosacral spine. (*B*) Note the absence of the lumbosacral spine on lateral roentgenogram. The arrows point to the last thoracic vertebra and to the pelvic bone.

umn begins to accelerate. At birth the conus medullaris is at the second lumbar vertebra and continues to rise until age 5 when it terminates at the first lumbar vertebra. It is presumed that clinical consequences of diastematomyelia are due to the spur "tethering" the cord during its ascent.

Most patients have some cutaneous abnormality in the midline of the back, and this suggests the diagnosis (see Fig. 7-61). The form of the lesion is varied and may well be in an area distant to the diastematomyelia. The lesion may be a hairy patch, discrete pimple, fatty tumor, or hemangioma.

A majority will have a congenital deformity of one or both lower extremities, not recognized as being secondary to a neurological defect. As growth proceeds a progressing neurological deficit may be seen. The extremity may exhibit weakness, atrophy, sensory loss, or deformity. A frequent finding is a cavus foot with atrophy and skin ulcerations. Urinary and bowel incontinence may also be the presenting symptom. The level of the lesion obviously influences the neurological findings. If the cord or conus medullaris is involved, spasticity and pathological reflexes occur whereas low lumbar lesions result in weakness, reflex, and sensory loss.

The characteristic roentgenographic finding in diastematomyelia is a midline bony mass, projecting posteriorly from the vertebral body accompanied by a fusiform enlargement of the spinal canal (Fig. 7-69). If the spicule is cartilagenous it will not be seen on routine films and requires delineation by myelography. Tomography is also helpful in the less discrete lesions. The distance between the pedicle is usually widened at the level of the lesion and may be so over several vertebral segments. Occasionally the defect occurs in association with other vertebral anomalies.

Diastematomyelia is easily confused with spinal cord tumors of all types, congenital transverse bands, a taut filum terminale, arachnoid adhesions, and such progressive neurological diseases as Friedreich's ataxia or spinal muscular atrophy.

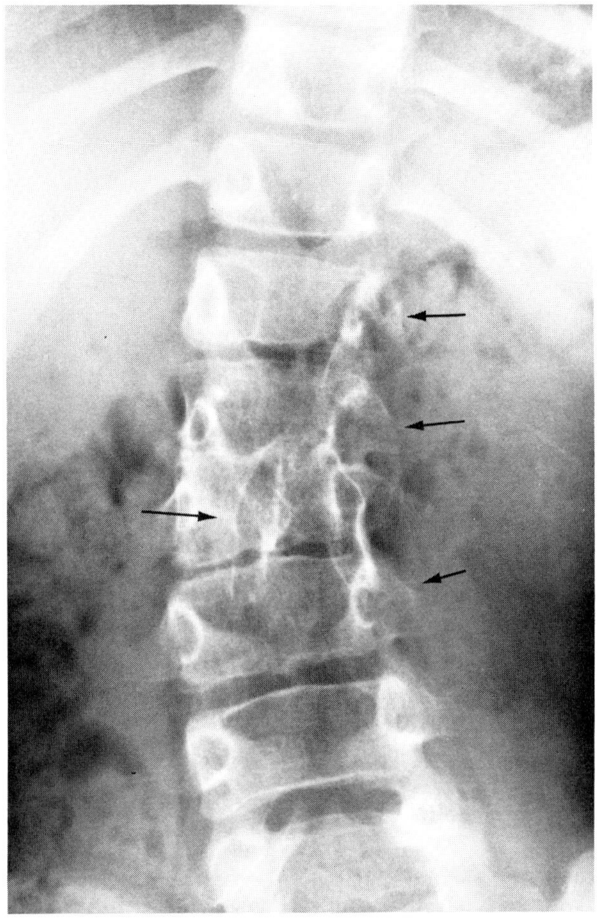

Fig. 7-69. Anteroposterior roentgenogram of the thoracolumbar spine in a patient with diastematomyelia. The arrow to the left demonstrates the bony midline mass which is splitting the spinal cord or, at this level, the spinal roots. A myelogram at this level would indicate the dye to flow past this lesion on both sides of it. Because of its tethering effect on the cord, it can cause a progressive neurological deficit. The arrows to the right indicate a unilateral bar which was an additional congenital anomaly present in this patient. The diastematomyelia was removed through a posterior approach and the spine fused in the area of the unilateral bar.

DYSPLASIAS

Achondroplasia

Achondroplasia is a common form of short limbed dwarfism. It is an autosomal dominant disease. However, 80 percent of the patients are new mutations. In general, the achondroplastic dwarf is intelligent with a normal life expectancy. The typical features include a large head, increased lumbar lordosis, and extremely short arms and legs.

In 1925 Donath and Voge first called attention to the vertebral anomalies which have become the hallmark of this disease. The normal spinal cord and cauda equina are housed in a spinal canal which is decreased in size in both the sagittal and transverse diameter. This "spinal stenosis" is a constant finding in all achondroplastic dwarfs and can lead to severe neurological problems in adulthood. A similar abnormal spinal configuration is seen in the animal prototype, the dachshund, which also has severe neurological problems.

The child is relatively free from lower extremity neurological problems; however, head enlargement with a mild dilatation of the ventricles is a common early finding in achondroplasia. If this progresses to a true hydrocephalus because of mechanical blockage, a high cervical compression with progressive quadriplegia can occur.

In the adult, neurological problems are usually due to further compression of the neural elements in the already compromised thoracic and lumbar spine. Any encroachment, such as a herniated disk or osteoarthritic spurring, can cause profound neurological symptoms in the achondroplastic patient. The same abnormality in a spinal column of normal dimensions would cause only a minor problem.

The onset of neurological symptoms is usually in the third or fourth decade but can occur at almost any age. The symptoms include low back pain, progressive motor and sensory loss in the lower extremities, and bowel and bladder problems. The neurological signs can be of either upper or lower motor neuron in nature. The signs and symptoms usually occur intermittently and are progressive. If sudden neurological symptoms occur, an acute herniated disk should be suspected.

Besides the hyperlordosis which is seen in 70 percent, about one third of the adults will have a scoliosis and another third kyphosis or kyphoscoliosis. Most of the patients who have neurological problems have some element of kyphosis.

The most consistent roentgenographic finding is a decrease in the interpediculate distance in the lumbar spine. Normally the distance between the pedicles increases from the first to the fifth lumbar vertebra. In achondroplastic dwarfs the interpediculate distance is least at the fifth lumbar vertebra. The pedicles tend to be thick and short, about one half the length of those in normal vertebrae. The disks are large and in the newborn can be as wide as the vertebral body. A mild thoracolumbar kyphosis is usual in the infant. As the child begins to ambulate this usually reverts to the typical hyperlordosis of the lumbar spine.

When neurological symptoms occur, myelography is helpful. Because of the lack of space in the lumbar region the contrast medium should be introduced suboccipitally and allowed to flow down. In the patient with a long history of symptoms, multiple areas of narrowing are usually seen. A single block should be carefully evaluated as it would be an unusual finding.

Patients with hypochondroplasia have similar skeletal changes but much milder in degree. In pseudoachondroplasia the skull is normal and epiphyseal ossification is severely disturbed.

Spondyloepiphyseal Dysplasia

Spondyloepiphyseal dysplasia is a congenital chondrodystrophy affecting the epiphyses of long bones and the spine. As a result epiphyseal ossification is irregular and multiple joint and spine incongruities occur.

There are three main divisions of this syndrome. *Spondyloepiphyseal dysplasia congenita* is the most severe and is recognized at birth. It is an autosomal dominant disease associated with myopia and/or retinal detachment in 50 percent of the cases, and clinically and roentgenographically, it can be confused with Morquio's syndrome. There are no known biochemical abnormalities associated with any of the spondyloepiphyseal dysplasias. *Pseudoachondroplasia* can occur as either a dominant or recessive form. The body habitus is similar to that of an achondroplastic dwarf except they have a normal head and deformities are rarely noted before age two. *Spondyloepiphyseal dysplasia tarda* is an x-linked recessive condition seen only in males, with the onset of findings occurring late in childhood. There is no mental retardation with spondyloepiphyseal dysplasia.

Except in the congenital variety, the clinical and radiological findings tend to occur during early childhood. These children look normal at birth but then develop progressive deformity with growth. A short trunk due to decreased vertebral height is common to all varieties of spondyloepiphyseal dysplasia. Spinal deformities, such as scoliosis, kyphosis, and lumbar lordosis, are to be expected. All peripheral joints, particularly the hips, can be involved with early degenerative arthritis.

Radiographically in all forms the vertebral changes are prominent and resemble those seen in Morquio's syndrome. Usually all vertebral bodies are involved and may range from anterior wedging to flattening (platyspondylia). There may be a "central tongue" appearance in the lumbar vertebrae. The vertebral end plates are irregular with multiple disk invaginations into the body. An important roentgenographic sign which may have clinical significance is dysplasia of the odontoid process. If this is unsuspected, serious neurological complications might occur during a minor accident or routine endotracheal intubation. The same vertebral abnormality is seen in Morquio's syndrome.

A source of confusion in the differential is Morquio's syndrome (mucopolysaccharidosis IV), but it can be separated on the basis of earlier, more severe involvement, corneal opacities, and urinary excretion of keratin sulfate. Occasionally the disks in the tarda variety can calcify and simulate ochronosis. The absence of homogentistic acid in the urine and the typical roentgenographic appearance can differentiate spondyloepiphyseal dysplasia from ochronosis.

Other dysplastic conditions which commonly have major vertebral manifestations include *diastrophic dwarfism* (progressive kyphoscoliosis in most cases), *metatrophic dwarfism* (progressive kyphoscoliosis with chest deformities), *Kniest disease* (dorsal kyphosis), spondylometaphyseal dysplasia of the Kozlowski type (kyphoscoliosis in adolescence), and *parastremmatic dwarfism* (severe kyphoscoliosis). The reader is referred to *Bone Dysplasias* by Spranger, Langer, and Wiedemann, W. B. Saunders, 1974 for further information about these dysplasias.

Mucopolysaccharidosis

The mucopolysaccharidoses (MPS) are inherited diseases of connective tissue. The skeletal manifestations in most types are qualitatively similar, the patients mainly differing in clinical severity and the specific type of mucopolysaccharide found. The afflicted individuals are unable to metabolize a specific mucopolysaccharide; therefore, it is allowed to build up in cells and is excreted in the urine. The three types that develop significant vertebral anomalies are MPS-I (Hurler's disease), MPS-IV (Morquio's syndrome), and MPS-VI (Maroteaux-Lamy disease). All three are autosomal recessive in inheritance pattern and characterized by dwarfism due to shortening of both spine and extremities. These children usually appear normal at birth but as the abnormal metabolite builds up, they develop the typical clinical features. The diagnosis usually is made at age 2 or 3 depending on the degree of involvement and the suspicion of the examiner. Hurler's disease (MPS-I) usually progresses rapidly and the children die before age 10. The prominent features are dwarfing, mental retardation, hepatosplenomegaly, and corneal clouding. The biochemical defect is a failure to break down heparin and dermatin sulfate.

Clinically the children have flexure contractions and limited motion of all peripheral joints. The neck is short due to decreased height of the cervical spine. They will typically have a gibbus at the thoracolumbar junction which can be quite severe. Roentgenographically, the vertebral bodies are ovoid with wedging of the vertebrae in the thoracolumbar area causing the acute kyphosis.

Morquio's syndrome (MPS-IV) is the most common of the mucopolysaccharidoses and is the prototype of dwarfism that occurs in later childhood. These patients have normal intelligence and survive well into adulthood. Morquio was an Argentinian physician who first described the clinical and roentgenographic findings in a family sired by parents who were first cousins. The defect in this case is believed to be in keratin sulfate and chondroitin-6-sulfate metabolism.

These children develop a typical clinical picture by the age of three or four. The neck is short and the facies characteristic. Corneal clouding and hearing defects are common. The patients have protrusion of the sterum with flaring of the rib cage and occasionally a dorsal kyphosis. There is laxity of ligaments and, therefore, hypermobility of the peripheral joints and the spine. Hypoplasia or aplasia of the odontoid is so common that fusion of the upper cervical spine is sometimes recommended routinely. If this instability is not carefully evaluated and treated, a spinal cord injury with quadriplegia and death is a possibility. Spinal cord compression secondary to the thoracolumbar gibbus can be a late complication.

Roentgenographically universal platyspondylia is characteristic with anterior wedging and beaking being seen at all levels. The majority will have an odontoid dysplasia, and this should be investigated with appropriate studies, such as tomography and/or cine radiograms.

This disease can be confused with any of the

dwarfisms. It can usually be separated from them by the keratosulfaturia and corneal opacities.

In Maroteaux-Lamy disease(MPS-VI) the patients have Hurler-like physical characteristics. However, they have normal intelligence and survive into adulthood. The metabolic error is in the metabolism of dermatin sulfate which is excreted in the urine. Clinically these patients have facies and joint contracture similar to Hurler's. Cardiac involvement with valvular deficiency is present, leading to failure and sometimes early death. The odontoid dysplasia seen in Morquio's syndrome is also seen in this disease. They also have corneal opacities. The vertebral findings on roentgenographic examination are similar to those seen in other mucopolysaccharidoses.

SUGGESTED READINGS

Disk Space Infections

1. Boston, H. C., Bianco, A. J., and Rhodes, K. H.: Disk space infections in children. Orthop. Clin. N. A. *6*:953, 1975.
2. Spiegal, P. G., Kengla, K. W., Isaacson, A. S., and Wilson, J. C., Jr.: Intervertebral disk space inflammation in children. J. Bone Joint Surg. *54A*:284, 1972.

Fracture Dislocation of the Thoracolumbar Spine

3. Holdsworth, Sir Frank M. B.: Fractures, dislocations, and fracture dislocations of the spine. J. Bone Joint Surg. *52A*:1534, 1970.

Spondylitis

4. Brewerton, D. A., Caffrey, M., Nicholls, A., et al.: The histocompatibility antigen (HL-A27) and its relation to disease. J. Rheum. *1*:249, 1974.
5. Calabro, J. J., and Maltz, B. A.: Ankylosing spondylitis. N. Engl. J. Med. *282*:606, 1970.
6. Calin, A., and Fries, J. F.: Striking prevalence of ankylosing spondylitis in "healthy" W-27 positive males and females. N. Engl. J. Med. *293*:835, 1975.
7. Engleman, E. P.: Psoriatic arthritis and Reiter's syndrome. Postgrad. Med. *51*:79, 1972.
8. Hollander, J. L., and McCarty, D. J.: Arthritis and Allied Conditions. ed. 8. Philadelphia, Lea & Febiger, 1972.
9. Ladd, J. R., Cassidy, J. T., and Martel, W.: Juvenile ankylosing spondylitis. Arthritis Rheum. *14*:579, 1971.
10. Moll, J. M. H., Haslock, I., MacRae, I. F., and Wright, V.: Associations between ankylosing spondylitis, psoriatic arthritis, Reiter's disease, the intestinal arthropathies, and Behcet's syndrome. Medicine *53*:343, 1974.
11. Morris, R. I., Metzger, A. L., Bluestone, R., et al.: HL-A-W-27: A useful discriminator in the arthropathies of inflammatory bowel disease. N. Engl. J. Med. *290*:1117, 1974.
12. Polley, H. F.: Anklyosing spondylitis. Postgrad. Med. *51*:71, 1972.
13. Primer on Rheumatic DB. Prepared by Committee of the American Rheumatism Association. Section of the Arthritis Foundation, 1973.
14. Reynolds, M. D., and Rankin, T. J.: Diagnosis of "Rheumatoid Variants." West. J. Med. *120*:441, 1974.
15. Rothman, R., and Simeone, F.: The Spine. Philadelphia, W. B. Saunders Co., 1975.
16. Schaller, J., and Wedgwood, R. J.: Juvenile rheumatoid arthritis. A review. Pediatrics *50*:940, 1972.
17. Schaller, J., Bitnum, S., and Wedgwood, R.: Ankylosing spondylitis with childhood onset. J. Pediatr. *74*:505, *1969*.
18. Schlosstein, L., Terasaki, P. I., and Bluestone, R., et al.: High association of an HLA antigen, W27, with ankylosing spondylitis. N. Eng. J. Med. *288*:704, 1973.

Diffuse Idiopathic Skeletal Hyperostosis

19. Forestier, J., and Lagier, R.: Ankylosing hyperostosis of the spine. Clin. Orthop. *74*:65, 1971.
20. Meeks, L. W., and Renshaw, T. S.: Vertebral osteophytosis and dysphagia. Two cases of the syndrome recently termed ankylosing hyperostosis. J. Bone Joint Surg. *55-A*:197, 1973.
21. Resnick, D., Shaul, S. R., and Robins, J. M.: Diffuse idiopathic skeletal hyperostosis (DISH): Forestier's disease with extraspinal manifestations. Radiology *115*:513, 1975.

Gout

22. Malawista, S. E., Seegmiller, J. E., Hathaway, B. E., and Sokoloff, L.: JAMA *194*:106, 1965.

Thoracic Disk Herniation

23. Benson, M. D. K., and Byrnes, D. P.: The clinical syndromes and surgical treatment of thoracic intervertebral disk prolapse. J. Bone Joint Surg. *57-B*:471, 1975.
24. Shaw, N. E.: The syndrome of the prolapsed thoracic intervertebral disk. J. Bone Joint Surg. *57B*:412, 1975.

Spinal Epidural Abcess

25. Baker, A. S., Ojemann, R. G., Swartz, M. N., and Richardson, E. P., Jr.: Spinal epidural abcess. N. Engl. J. Med. *293*:463, 1975.

Syndromes Which Mimic Cord Pressure

26. Birnbaum, G.: Guillain-Barré Syndrome, increased lymphoproliferative potential. Arch. Neurol. *28*:215, 1973.

Acute Transverse Myelopathy (Acute Transverse Myelitis, Acute Necrotic Myelopathy)

27. Altrocchi, P. H.: Acute transverse myelopathy, Arch. Neurol. *9*:111, 1963.
28. Altrocchi, P. H.: Acute spinal epidural abcess versus acute transverse myelopathy. Arch. Neurol. *9*:17, 1963.
29. Lipton, H. L., and Teasdall, R. D.: Acute transverse myelopathy in adults: A follow-up study. Arch. Neurol. *28*:252, 1973.

Stenosis of the Lumbar Canal

30. Blau, J. N., and Logue, V.: Intermittent claudication of the cauda equina. An unusual syndrome resulting from central protrusion of a lumbar intervertebral disk. Lancet *1*:1081, 1961.
31. Blau, J. N., and Rushworth, G.: Observations on the blood vessels of the spinal cord and their responses to motor activity. Brain *81*:354, 1958.
32. Cooke, T. D. V., and Lehmann, P. O.: Neurogenic origin of intermittent claudication. Can. J. Surg. *11*:151, 1968.
33. Ehni, G.: Significance of small lumbar spinal canal: Cauda equina compression syndromes due to stenosis. J. Neurosurg. *31*:490, 1969.
34. Evans, J. G.: Neurogenic intermittent claudication. Br. Med. J. *2*:985, 1964.
35. Joffe, R., Appleby, A., and Arjona, V.: Intermittent ischaemia of the cauda equina due to stenosis of the lumbar canal. J. Neurol. Neurosurg. Psychiat. *29*:315, 1966.
36. Kavanaugh, G. J., Svien, H. J., Holman, C. B., and Johnson, R. M.: "Pseudocaudication" syndrome produced by compression of the cauda equina. JAMA *206*:2477, 1968.
37. Kirkaldy-Willis, W. H., and McIvor, G. W. D.: Lumbar spinal stenosis. Clin. Orthop. *115*:2, 1976.
38. Moiel, R., and Ehni, G.: Cauda equina compression due to spondylolisthesis with intact neural arch. J. Neurosurg. *28*:262, 1968.
39. Paine, K. W. E.: Clinical features of lumbar spinal stenosis. Clin. Orthop. *115*:77, 1976.
40. Verbiest, H.: A radicular syndrome from developmental narrowing of the lumbar spinal canal. J. Bone Joint Surg. *36B*:230, 1954.
41. Verbiest, H.: Further experiences on the pathological influence of a developmental narrowness of the boney lumbar vertebral canal. J. Bone Joint Surg. *37B*:576, 1955.

Scheuermann's Juvenile Kyphosis

42. Bradford, D. S., Moe, J. H., and Winter, R. B.: Kyphosis and postural round back deformity in children and adolescents. Minn. Med. *56*:114, 1973.
43. Rothmann, R. H., and Simone, F. A.: The Spine. Philadelphia, W. B. Saunders Co., 1975.

Infections of the Spine

44. Cecil, R. L.: Cecil-Loeb Textbook of Medicine. pp. 332–334. Philadelphia, W. B. Saunders Co., 1963.
45. Cowan, N. J.: Cryptococcosis of bone. Case report and review of the literature. Clin. Orthop. *66*:174, 1969.
46. Dalinka, M. K., Dinnenberg, S., Greendyke, W. H., and Hopkins, R.: Roentgenogenic features of osseous coccidioidomycosis and differential diagnosis. J. Bone Joint Surg. *53-A*:1157, 1971.
47. Gehweiler, J. A., Capp, M. P., and Chick, E. W.: Observations on the roentgen patterns in blastomycosis of bone. Av. J. Roentgenol. *108*:497, 1970.
48. Ottolengi, C. E.: Aspiration Biopsy of the spine. J. Bone Joint Surg. *51-A*:1531, 1969.
49. Rob, C., and Smith, R.: Clinical Surgery Orthopedics. London, Butterworths, 1967.
50. Rothman, R. H., and Simeone, F. A.: The Spine. Philadelphia, W. B. Saunders Co., 1975.
51. Winter, W. G., Larson, R. K., Honeggar, M. M., Jacobsen, D. T., Pappagianis, D., and Huntington, R. W., Jr.: Coccidioidal arthritis and its treatment. J. Bone Joint Surg. *57-A*:1152, 1975.

Tumors of the Spine

52. Keim, H. A., and Reina, E. G.: Osteoid osteoma as a cause of scoliosis. J. Bone Joint Surg. *57-A*:159, 1975.
53. MacClellan, Donald I., and Wilson, Frank C., Jr.: Osteoid osteoma of the spine. A review of the literature and report of 6 new cases. J. Bone Joint Surg. *49-A*:111, 1967.
54. Prakash, B., Banerji, A. K., and Tandon, P. M.: Aneurysmal bone cyst of the spine. J. Neurol. Neurosurg. Psychiat. *36*:112, 1973.
55. Spjut, H. J., Dorfman, H. D., Fechner, R. E., and Ackerman, L. V.: Tumors of Bone and Cartilage. Bethesda, Md., Armed Forces Inst. Pathol., 1971.

Psychogenic Pain

56. Brown, M. D.: Diagnosis of pain syndromes of the spine. Orthop. Clin. N. Am. *6*:233, 1975.
57. Cecil and Loeb: Textbook of Medicine. Philadelphia, W. B. Saunders Co., 1963.
58. Keim, H. A.: Low back pain. CIBA Clinical Symposia *25*:2, 1973.
59. Wiltse, L. L., and Rocchio, P. D.: Preoperative psychological tests as predictors of success of chemonucleolysis in the low back syndrome. J. Bone Joint Surg., *57A*:478, 1975.

Congenital Scoliosis and Kyphosis

60. Mehta, M. H.: The rib vertebral angle in early diagnosis between resolving and progressive infantile idiopathic scoliosis. J. Bone Joint Surg. *54-B*:230, 1972.
61. Winter, R. B., Moe, J. H., and Eihlers, V. E.: Congenital scoliosis: A study of 234 patients treated and untreated. J. Bone Joint Surg. *50A*:1, 1968.
62. Winter, R. B., Moe, J. H., and Wang, J. F.: Congenital kyphosis: Its nature and treatment as observed in a study of 130 patients. J. Bone Joint Surg. *55-A*:223, 1973.

Dysplasias

63. Lloyd-Roberts, G. E.: Orthopedics Clinical Surgery—13. London, Butterworths, 1967.
64. McKusich, V. A.: Heritable Disorder of Connective Tissue, ed. 4. St. Louis, C. V. Mosby Co., 1972.
65. Rothmann, R. H., and Simeone, F. A.: The Spine. pp. 253–260. Philadelphia, W. B. Saunders, 1975.
66. Spranger, Langer and Wiedemann: Bone Dysplasia. pp. 55–62, 95–143. Philadelphia, W. B. Saunders Co., 1974.
67. Symposium on Myelomeningocele, American Academy of Orthopedic Surgeons, November 1970. St. Louis, C. V. Mosby Company, 1972.

8 The Shoulder

Richard S. Riggins, M.D.

When assessing a patient with complaints about the shoulder, the physician must first realize that the cause of the patient's symptoms may not be primarily in the shoulder mechanism. Dysfunction of the cervical spine, nerves, and vessels entering the upper extremity and even lesions in remote areas, such as the abdominal or thoracic viscera, may give rise to shoulder complaints. We will first deal with the anatomy, then the physical examination of the shoulder girdle and upper arm, and finally the differential diagnosis. The section on differential diagnosis will, by necessity, touch on material covered more completely in other chapters of this text.

ANATOMY

Shoulder Girdle

The shoulder girdle provides a mobile attachment of the upper extremity to the trunk. Actually, bony articulation with the trunk occurs only via the clavicle. Motions which occur about the shoulder include motion between the glenohumeral joint and motion between the scapula and the trunk, sometimes referred to as the scapulothoracic joint. The scapula moves in four directions: elevation (Fig. 8-1), in the cephalad direction; depression, in the caudad direction (Fig. 8-2); flexion (abduction) away from the midline (Fig. 8-3); and extension (adduction) toward the midline (Fig. 8-4). Combinations of these basic motions will cause a clockwise and counterclockwise rotation of the scapula with such movements as reaching above the head. Motion at the glenohumeral joint consists of flexion, extension, abduction (away from the trunk), and adduction (toward the trunk) (Figs. 8-5, 8-6, and 8-7). The humerus can also rotate in the glenohumeral joint. With the elbow flexed at 90 degrees, and the arm at the side, internal rotation brings the hand toward the trunk, and external rotation moves the hand away from the trunk (Fig. 8-8). These movements can also be carried out with the arm horizontal (Fig. 8-9). Motion at the glenohumeral joint, excluding rotational motions, occurs in concert with motions of the scapula on the trunk and through the acromioclavicular and sternoclavicular joints. Usually the first 30 degrees of motion occurs between the humerus and scapula, but from that point on for every 30 degrees of shoulder motion, 20 degrees occurs at the glenohumeral joint and 10 degrees between the scapula and the thorax.

Elevation of the scapula is performed chiefly by the upper fibers of the trapezius and the levator scapulae muscles (Fig. 8-10). Depression of the scapula occurs by the action of the lower fibers of the trapezius and by gravity. The trapezius is assisted in depression by the latissimus dorsi (Fig. 8-11) and pectoralis major (Fig. 8-12), acting through the glenohumeral joint. Adduction, or backward movement of the scapula, is performed by the rhomboids (Fig. 8-13) and the levator scapulae, again with some assistance from the trapezius. Abduction of the scapula is performed by the serratus anterior (Fig. 8-14), assisted by the pectoralis minor. The serratus anterior also steadies the scapula and holds it close to the chest wall. Paralysis of this muscle causes winging of the scapula when one attempts to push a heavy object with arms outstretched (Fig. 8-15). In movements about the glenohumeral joints, the supraspinatus (Fig. 8-16), infraspinatus (Fig. 8-17), teres minor, and subscapularis make up a group referred

(Text continues on p. 325.)

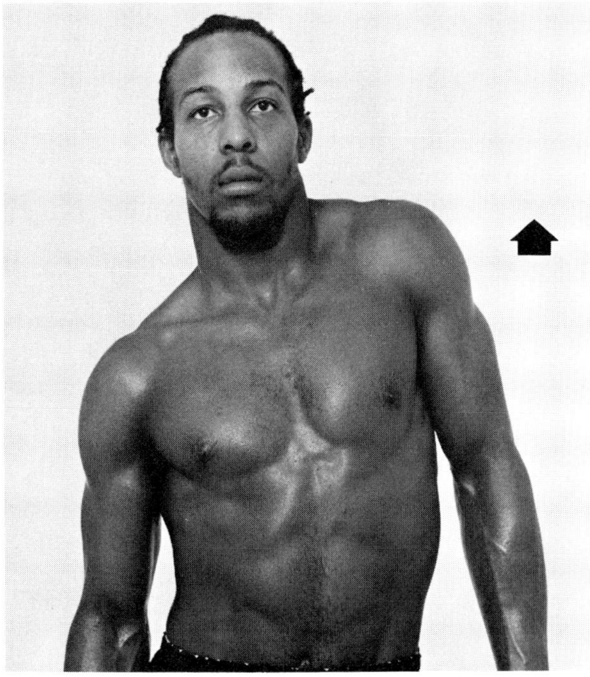

Fig. 8-1. Elevation of the scapula.

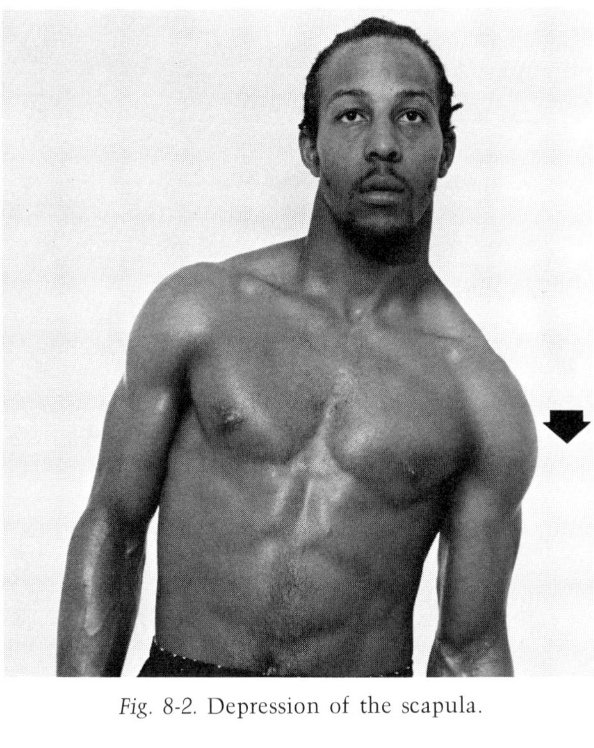

Fig. 8-2. Depression of the scapula.

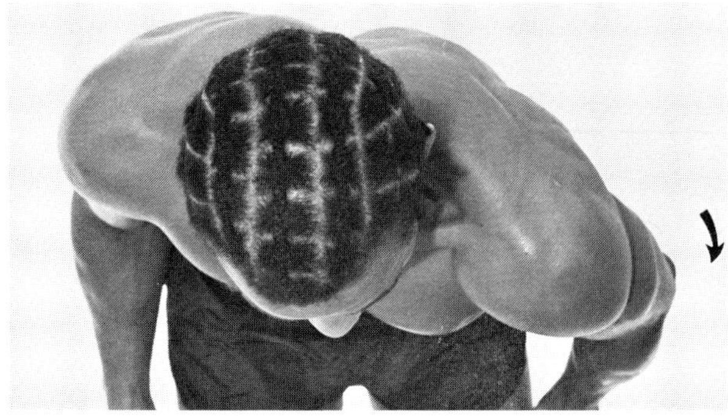

Fig. 8-3. Flexion (abduction) of the scapula.

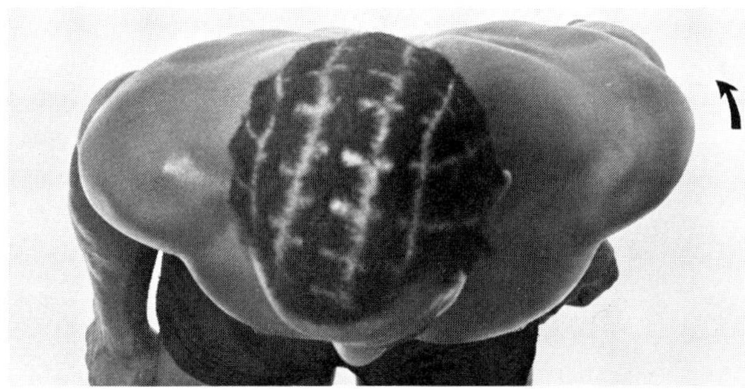

Fig. 8-4. Extension (adduction) of the scapula.

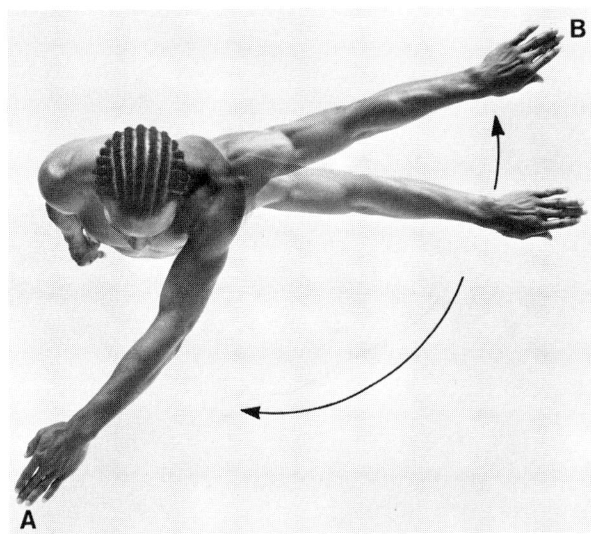

Fig. 8-5. Flexion (*A*) and extension (*B*) of the shoulder in the horizontal plane.

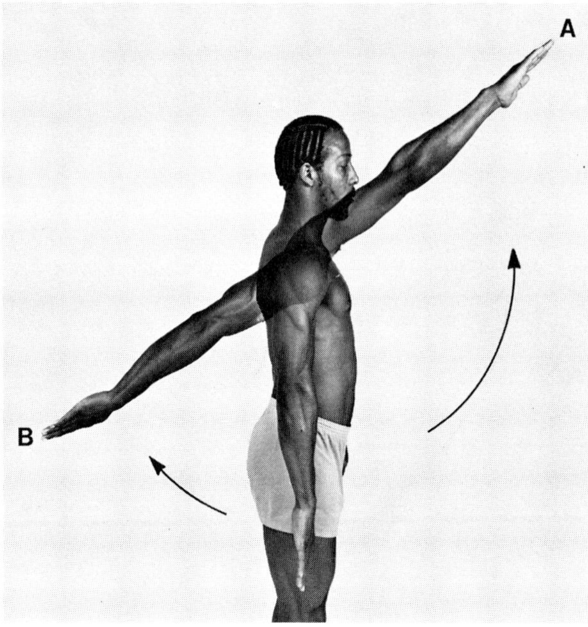

Fig. 8-6. Flexion (*A*) and extension (*B*) of the shoulder in the vertical plane.

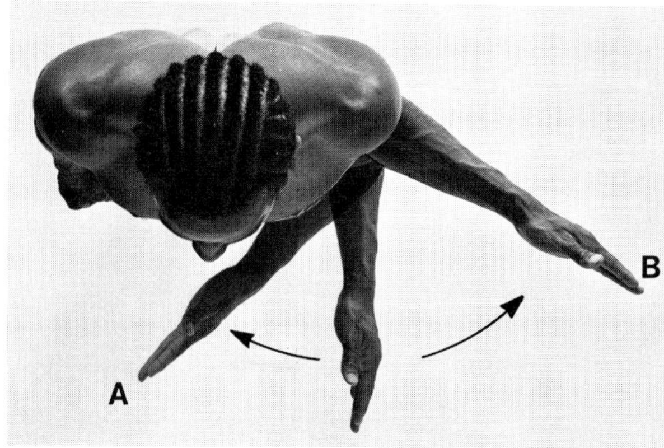

Fig. 8-8. Internal (*A*) and external (*B*) rotation of the humerus with the arm vertical.

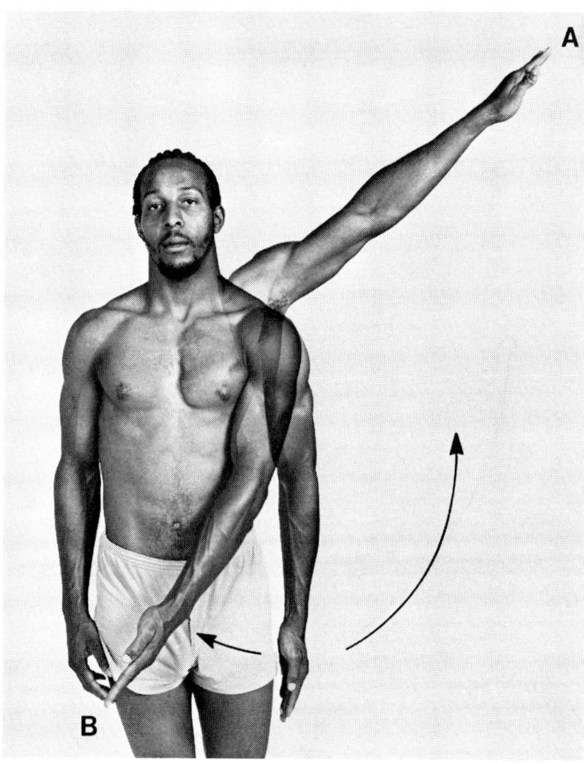

Fig. 8-7. Abduction (*A*) and adduction (*B*) of the shoulder joint.

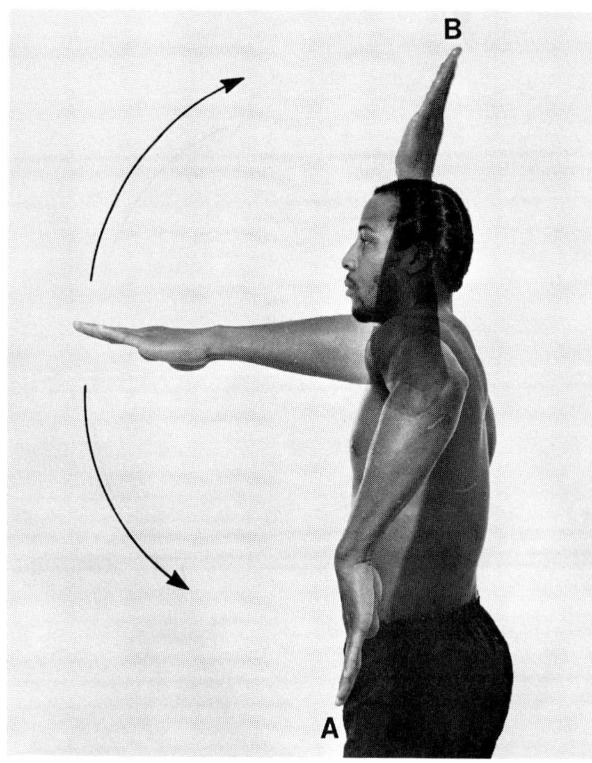

Fig. 8-9. Internal (*A*) and external (*B*) rotation of the humerus with the arm horizontal.

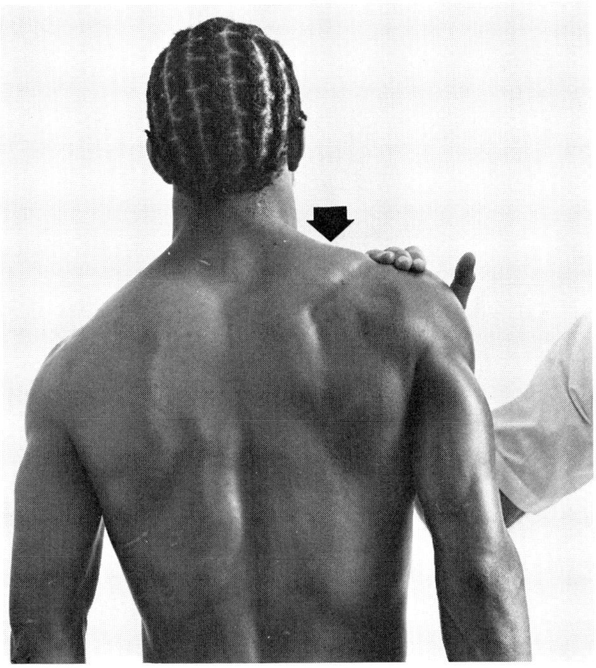

Fig. 8-10. Trapezius (spinal accessory nerve C3-C4). The patient elevates his scapula against resistance. The trapezius can be seen (*arrow*).

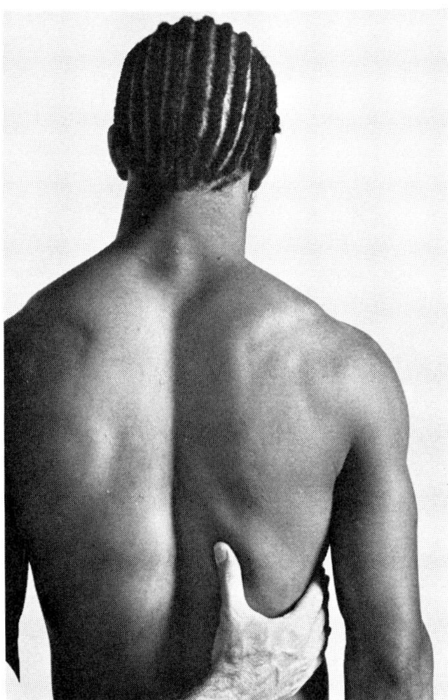

Fig. 8-11. Latissimus dorsi (thoracodorsal nerve C6-C7-C8). The muscle is firmly grasped and can be felt to contract when the patient coughs.

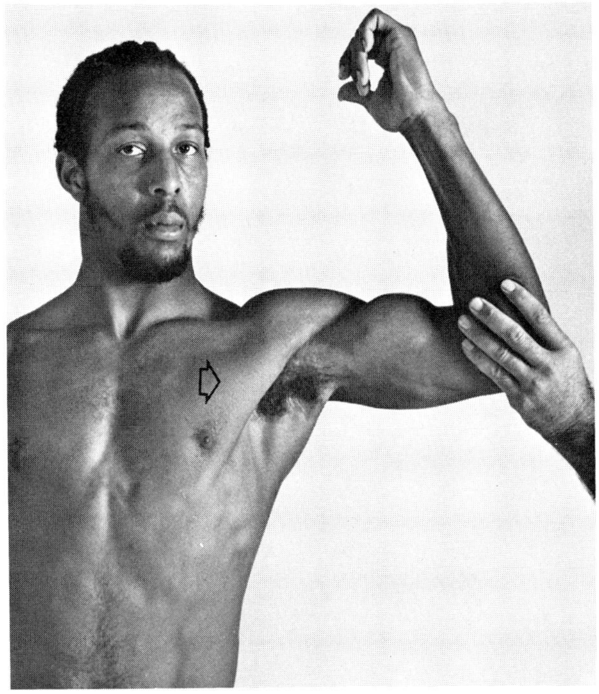

Fig. 8-12. Pectoralis major (lateral and medial pectoral nerves C5-C6-C7-C8). The arm is lowered and the elbow brought forward against resistance. The muscle can be seen (*arrow*).

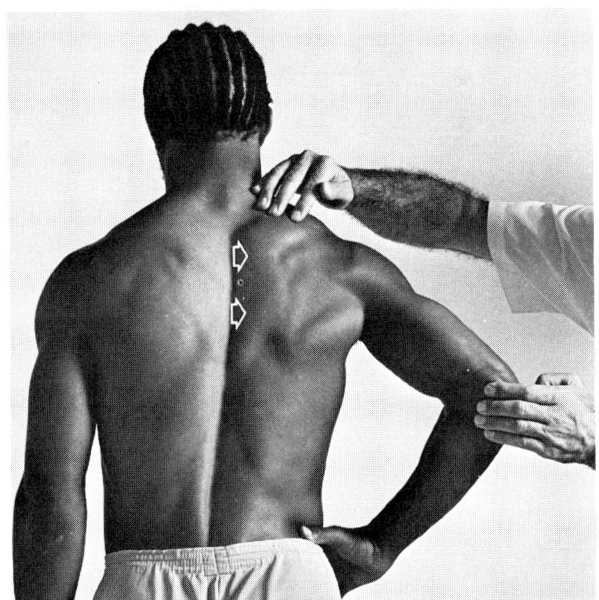

Fig. 8-13. Rhomboids (dorsal scapular nerve C4-C5). The scapula is extended against resistance. The rhomboids can be palpated deep to the trapezius (*arrows*).

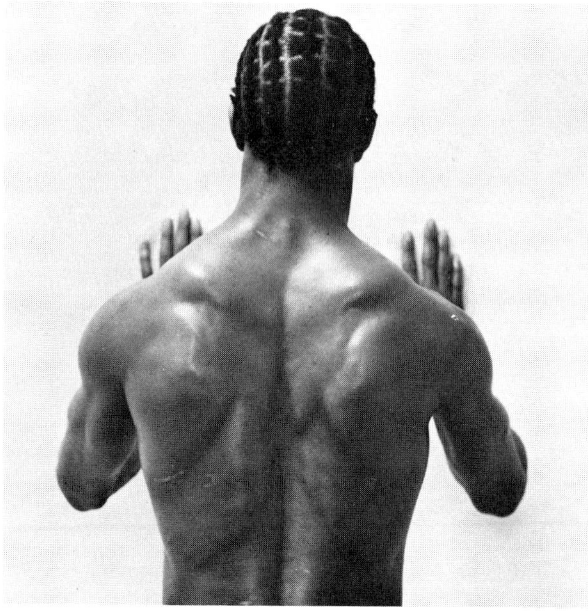

Fig. 8-14. Serratus anterior (long thoracic nerve C5-C6-C7). Attempts to push a stationary object will cause winging of the scapula if the serratus anterior is not functioning (see Fig. 8-15).

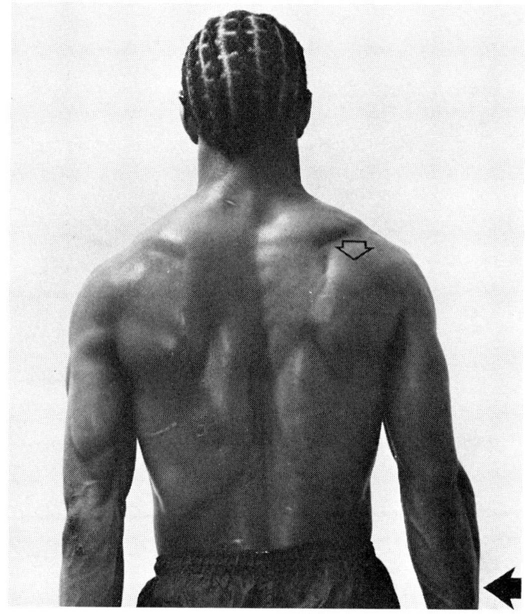

Fig. 8-16. Supraspinatus (suprascapular nerve C5). The subject attempts to elevate (abduct) the arm against resistance. The muscle can be seen (*arrow*) and palpated.

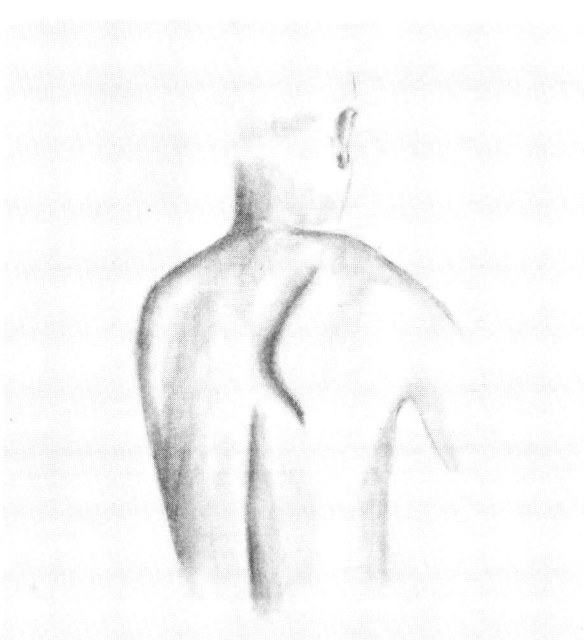

Fig. 8-15. Winging of the scapula secondary to paralysis of the right serratus anterior.

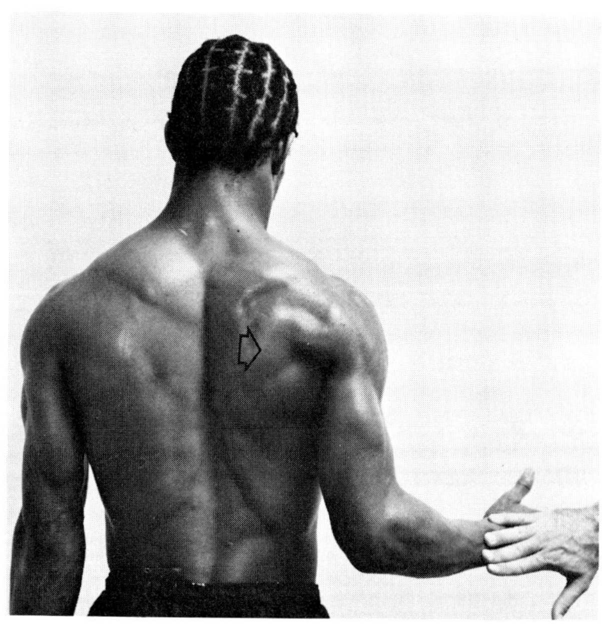

Fig. 8-17. Infraspinatus (suprascapular nerve C5-C6). With the elbow at the side attempts are made to externally rotate the arm against resistance. The infraspinatus can be seen (*arrow*) and palpated.

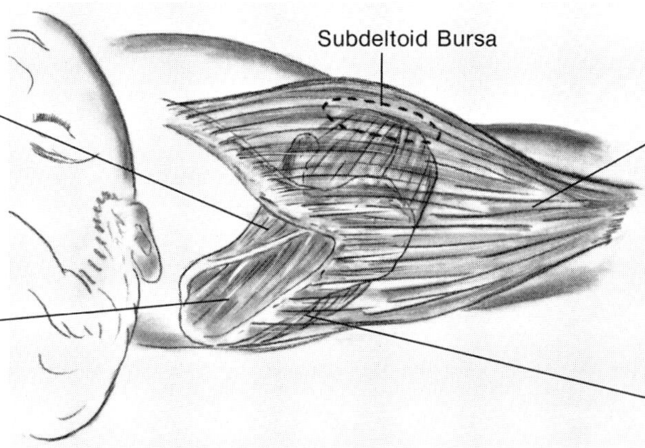

Fig. 8-18. The rotator cuff as seen from above and behind the shoulder. The subdeltoid bursa lies directly above the rotator cuff tendons which form its floor. The entire mechanism is covered by the deltoid muscle.

to as muscles of the rotary cuff (Fig. 8-18). They are mainly responsible for stability of the head of the humerus in the glenoid fossa. These muscles are not usually considered prime movers of the shoulder joint and serve instead as agonists assisting the larger muscles. Abduction of the shoulder joint is accomplished mainly by the deltoid muscle (Fig. 8-19) assisted by the biceps (Fig. 8-20) and the rotator cuff. Extension of the shoulder occurs by contraction of the latissimus dorsi, with some help from the posterior fibers of the deltoid muscle. Flexion of the glenohumeral joint is by the anterior fibers of the deltoid with some assistance by two muscles attached to the coracoid process, the biceps and coracobrachialis. Adduction of the arm occurs with contraction of the pectoralis major working synergistically with the latissimus dorsi. Medial rotation of the humerus

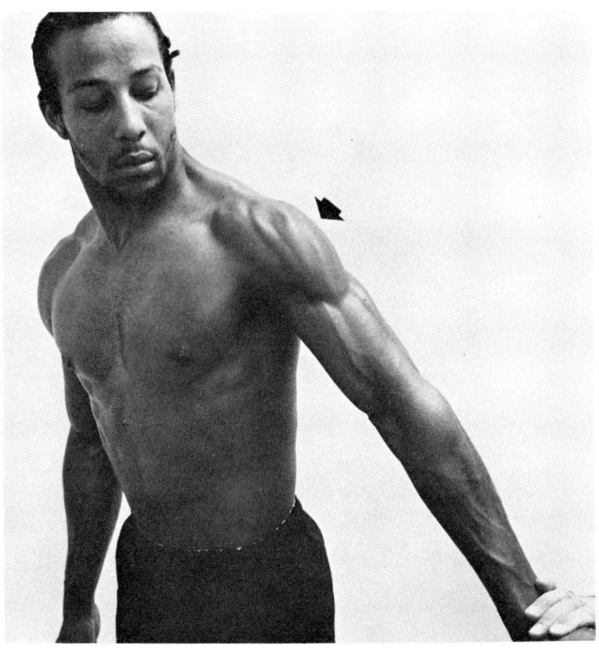

Fig. 8-19. Deltoid (axillary nerve C5-C6). The subject elevates the arm against resistance. The deltoid can be seen (*arrow*) and palpated.

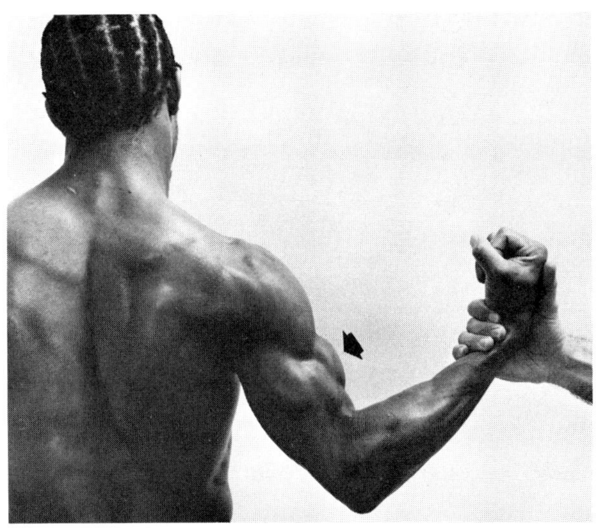

Fig. 8-20. Biceps (musculocutaneous nerve C5-C6). With the forearm supinated the elbow is flexed against resistance. The biceps and brachialis can be seen (*arrow*) and palpated.

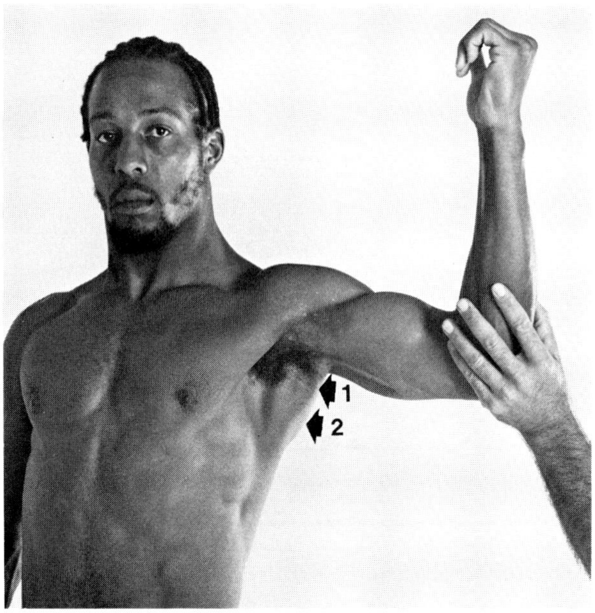

Fig. 8-21. Teres major (axillary nerve C5-C6). The arm is lowered and thrust laterally against resistance. The teres major (*arrow 1*) and latissimus dorsi (*arrow 2*) can be seen and palpated.

occurs by contractions of the pectoralis major and latissimus dorsi assisted by the teres major (Fig. 8-21) which is also an adductor of the humerus. Lateral rotation of the humerus is brought about chiefly by muscles of the rotary cuff, the infraspinatus, and teres minor. Muscles of the pectoralis region are all supplied by branches from the nerves of the brachial plexus, fifth cervical through first thoracic (see Fig. 5-6). The pectoral muscles are supplied by the lateral pectoral nerve from the lateral cord (C5, C6, and C7) and by the medial pectoral nerve which, in turn, is derived from the medial cord (C8 and T1). The serratus anterior is supplied on its superficial aspect by the long thoracic nerve (C5, C6, and C7). Because of its long, relatively unprotected course, this nerve may be paralyzed by direct trauma or viral infections, resulting in winging of the scapula (see Fig. 8-15). The latissimus dorsi is innervated by a single nerve, the thoracodorsal, which is a branch of the posterior cord of the brachial plexus (C5, C6, C7, and C8). The levator scapulae and rhomboids are both supplied from the anterior primary division of the cervical nerves (C4 and C5). The dorsal scapular nerve passes beneath the levator scapulae and the rhomboids, supplying all three muscles on their deep surface. The trapezius receives its nerve supply from the terminal fibers of the spinal portion of the spinal accessory nerve as well as from the cervical plexus (C3 and C4).

All muscles of the glenohumeral joint are supplied by anterior primary divisions of the fifth and sixth cervical nerves through branches of the brachial plexus. The supraspinatus and infraspinatus are supplied by the suprascapular nerve. The deltoid is supplied by branches of the axillary nerve (Fig. 8-22), which also supplies the teres minor, and terminates as a sensory nerve to the skin over the deltoid muscle. The subscapularis is supplied by the two subscapular nerves. The biceps receives its innervation from the musculocutaneous nerve (Fig. 8-23). The suprascapular nerve supplies 70 to 80 percent of the innervation to the shoulder joint (see Fig. 8-48). Blocking of this nerve can provide considerable symptomatic relief for patients with painful syndromes about the shoulder joint. A minor innervation to the shoulder joint also occurs from small articular branches of the axillary and lateral pectoral nerves.

The Arm

Anterior Aspect

The deltoid muscle is one of the prime movers of the shoulder joint (see Fig. 8-19). Its anterior fibers

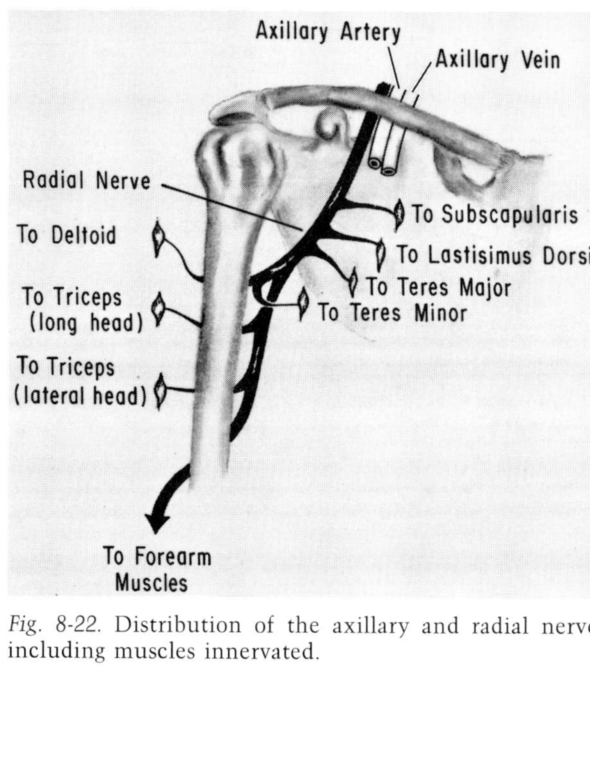

Fig. 8-22. Distribution of the axillary and radial nerve including muscles innervated.

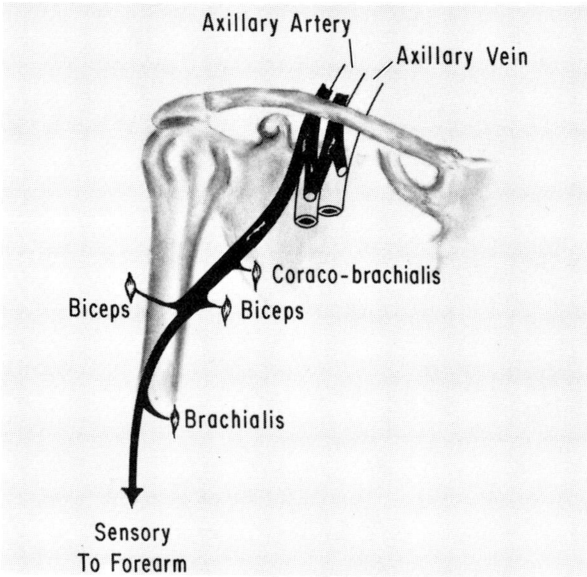

Fig. 8-23. Distribution of the musculocutaneous nerve and the muscles innervated. This nerve is responsible for elbow flexion.

assist in shoulder flexion, while its posterior fibers assist in shoulder extension. The lateral fibers are responsible for abduction of the shoulder. The muscles of the rotary cuff stabilize the shoulder joint and allow efficient action of the deltoid muscle (see Fig. 8-18). Without the stabilizing action of the rotary cuff, the deltoid can only maintain, not initiate, shoulder abduction (see Fig. 8-19). Loss of the deltoid muscle cannot be adequately replaced by function in any other muscle group in the shoulder, and shoulder fusion is usually recommended. The coracobrachialis flexes the shoulder and adducts it to the trunk. If the arm is externally rotated, the coracobrachialis can initiate internal rotation. The biceps and brachialis muscles are the main flexors of the elbow (see Fig. 8-20). The brachialis, by its insertion on the coronoid process of the ulna, can only flex the elbow, whereas the biceps, by virtue of its insertion on the tuberosity of the radius, can supinate the pronated forearm. The biceps can also act on the shoulder joint, creating flexion and some adduction. The long head of the biceps appears to stabilize the shoulder joint by passing through the joint to attach to the superior glenoid rim.

The deltoid muscle is innervated by the axillary nerve which comes through the quadrilateral space and winds beneath the muscle (see Fig. 8-22). The coracobrachialis, biceps, and brachialis are supplied by the musculocutaneous nerve containing branches from the fifth through seventh cervical nerves (see Fig. 8-23). The tendons of the muscles of the rotary cuff insert on the tuberosities of the humerus and are innervated by the fifth and sixth cervical nerves through the suprascapular and subscapular nerves (see Fig. 5-6).

Posterior Aspect

The posterior aspect of the humerus is covered in its entirety by the triceps muscle which is responsible for elbow extension (Fig. 8-24). The muscle arises from three heads: the glenoid rim, the scapula, and the back of the humerus. It extends to insert on the olecranon process of the ulna. The muscle is innervated by the radial nerve which rests in a spiral groove on the posterior aspect of the humerus (see Fig. 8-22). It is supplied by roots from the sixth and seventh cervical and first thoracic nerves. The major nerve supply is from the seventh cervical nerve, and the reflex arc of the triceps reflex is carried through the seventh cervical nerve root. Consequently, injuries to the seventh cervical nerve root will cause weakness of the triceps muscle and loss of the triceps reflex (see Fig. 1-4B).

Functionally, the triceps muscle is relatively unimportant in the normal individual. Gravity is sufficient for elbow extension, and triceps weakness

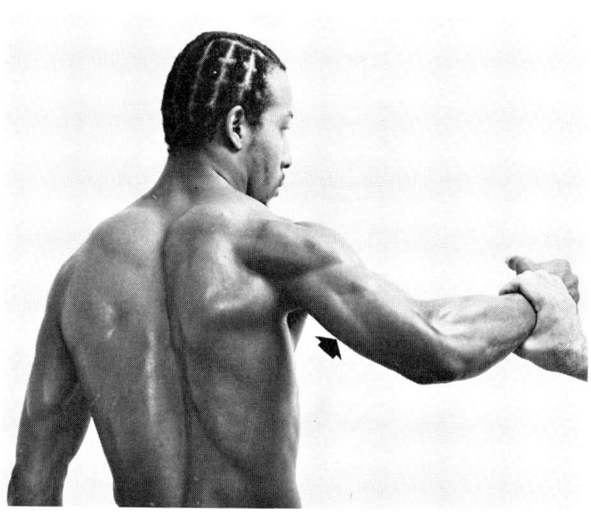

Fig. 8-24. Triceps (radial nerve C7-C8). The subject attempts to extend the elbow against resistance. The triceps can be seen (*arrow*) and palpated.

may go unrecognized. Patients who depend on crutches or a cane for ambulation require strong triceps musculature for the use of these implements. A strong triceps muscle is also required for active extension of the elbow against resistance, such as pushing away from the table or doing pushups.

Assignment of individual muscles to particular nerve roots is very difficult in the upper extremity. The biceps and deltoid are innervated chiefly by the fifth cervical nerve root. Also, the biceps reflex is carried through the fifth cervical nerve root so that injury to this nerve root will eliminate the biceps reflex (see Fig. 1-4A) and produce weakness of the biceps muscle. Usually, patients with cervical spine fractures which transect the cord at the sixth cervical level retain some shoulder abduction and elbow flexion. However, patients suffering with transection of the cervical cord at the fifth cervical level usually suffer complete loss of function in the upper extremity.

Ligaments

The coracoclavicular ligaments which attach the clavicle to the scapulas are the most important ligaments about the shoulder (Fig. 8-25). They are really two ligaments, the conoid and trapezoid, and complete separation of the acromioclavicular joint cannot occur until these ligaments rupture. The coracoacromial ligament (see Fig. 8-25) which forms

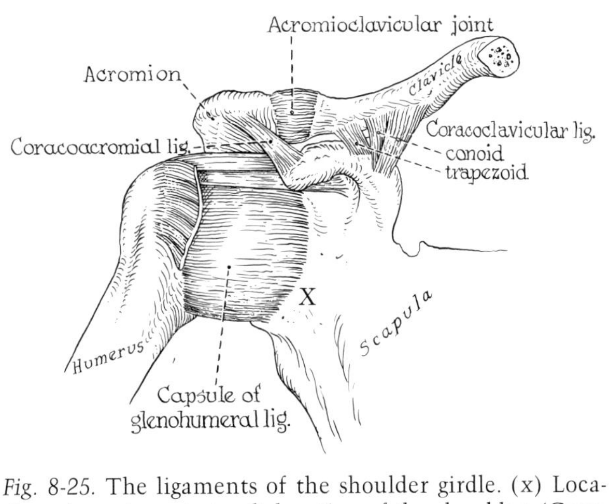

Fig. 8-25. The ligaments of the shoulder girdle. (x) Location of tear in anterior dislocation of the shoulder. (Courtesy R. D. D'Ambrosia.)

a protective roof above the supraspinatus tendon stretches across the anterior aspect of the glenohumeral joint and is sometimes implicated as a cause of painful shoulder syndromes. Lesions of the rotator cuff may impinge on this ligament with abduction and flexion of the shoulder, thus causing pain. The glenohumeral joint is stabilized mainly by its capsule and reinforced by surrounding muscles. This joint is deepened by a cartilagenous labrum attached to the glenoid rim which is at least functionally if not anatomically defective anteriorly and inferiorly. Tears at this level are the most common defects associated with shoulder dislocation. The shallow sternoclavicular joint is also dependent on the joint capsule for its stability, and tears of this structure usually result in some degree of permanent instability of the joint.

The most significant bursa about the shoulder is the subdeltoid bursa which lies between the tendon of the supraspinatus below and the deltoid and coracoacromial arch above. It separates the tendons of the rotator cuff from the deltoid muscle and serves as a lubricating mechanism. This bursa is frequently the site of calcific bursitis which begins in the tendons of the rotator cuff (see Fig. 8-18).

Nerves and Vessels

The entrances of the nerves and vessels into the upper extremity are important anatomical considerations because variation in their anatomy can be the cause of complaints about the shoulder and arm (Fig. 8-26). The anterior primary divisions of the lower cervical nerves (usually C5 through T1) pass through the scalenus muscles across the first rib and beneath the clavicle and coracoid process to enter the axilla. The subclavian artery joins the brachial plexus as it passes through the anterior and middle scalenus muscles. The subclavian vein passes anterior to the scalenus muscle so it does not join the neurovascular bundle until the nerves and the artery exit from the scalenus muscle. These structures are in close proximity until the individual nerves of the upper extremity separate from the vessels. Several neurovascular compression syndromes are associated with the anatomy of this area.

The functional anatomy of the nerves about the shoulder can be best understood by studying nerve injuries which occur at the various levels. Lesions of the upper cord of the brachial plexus (see Fig. 5-6) and root avulsions involving the fifth, sixth, and sometimes seventh spinal nerves produce weakness and loss of motion about the shoulder girdle and glenohumeral joint. There is sensory loss along the lateral and anterior aspects of the arm and forearm. The long thoracic nerve to the serratus anterior and the dorsal scapular nerve which supplies the rhomboids and levator scapulae emerge just distal to the spinal nerve roots. If function is lost in the rhomboids and levator scapulae which are supplied by these nerves, the injury probably has affected the spinal roots and is not repairable. Lesions in the lower portion of the brachial plexus, involving possibly the seventh cervical through first thoracic nerves, cause loss of function in the hand and wrist with sensory deficit over the posterior medial aspect of the arm and forearm. When motor or sensory deficit of the lower cord is noted one should look for a Horner's syndrome. It results from injury to the autonomic nervous system which accompanies the roots of the lower brachial plexus. The syndrome consists of ptosis of the eye, dilation of the pupil, and anhidrosis on the ipsilateral side of the face. The presence of a Horner's syndrome indicates an irreparable lesion of the lower roots of the plexus.

Injuries to the trunks of the brachial plexus (see Fig. 5-6) are extremely rare, but injuries to the cords of the brachial plexus which are more common produce a fairly regular pattern of functional loss. Injury to the lateral cord produces motor and sensory deficits in the distribution of the musculocutaneous nerve (paralysis of the biceps, coracobrachialis, brachialis: elbow flexors) and of the lateral root of the median nerve (paralysis of the flexor carpi radialis and pronator teres: forearm pronation and wrist flexion). Injury to the posterior cord causes motor and sensory deficit in the subscapular, thoracodorsal, axillary, and radial nerves. Clinically, the loss of the axillary nerve is denoted by the inability to abduct the arm, and the loss of the radial nerve is indicated by inability to extend the wrist and fingers and extension of elbow against resistance. Injuries of the medial cord produce a combined ulnar and median nerve deficit. This presents with loss of sensation over the hand and arm, plus complete paralysis of all intrinsic muscles of the hand and the extrinsic finger flexors.

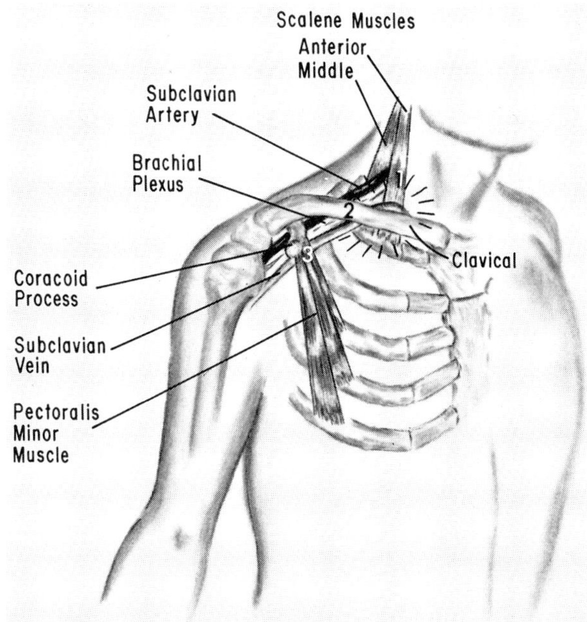

Fig. 8-26. Costoclavicular space and its relationship to the neurovascular bundle. (1) Brachial plexus and subclavian artery can be compressed between the scalene muscles. Compression by a cervical rib can also occur at this level (see Fig. 8-46). (2) Compression of the neurovascular bundle can occur between the first rib and clavicle. (3) Elevation of the arm may compress the neurovascular bundle against the coracoid process by the pectoralis minor.

Injuries can occur to individual major nerves from the brachial plexus. Interruption of the musculocutaneous nerve produces a loss of elbow flexion plus some weakness in shoulder flexion and abduction. Loss of the radial nerve in the upper part of the arm will result in inability to extend the elbow against resistance plus distal disturbances (see Chaps. 5 and 9).

There is extensive collateral circulation about the shoulder, and major vascular interruption about the shoulder is not always disastrous. Studies of major arterial injuries during World War II indicate gangrene of the upper extremity occurred with ligation of the subclavian artery in 29 percent of the cases, 43 percent in axillary artery ligations, 56 percent with ligation of the brachial artery in its proximal portion, and 26 percent with ligation of its distal portion. Quiring published an extensive study of the collateral circulation about the shoulder, and his text should be referred to for further details.

REGIONAL EXAMINATION

History

When eliciting a shoulder history the major areas to cover are the patterns of pain, losses of motion, symptoms of neurovascular dysfunction, and details of any past injuries. Because of potential litigation, circumstances of the injury should be well documented. The time, place, and the activity of the patient when the injury occurred are minimal requirements for an accurate history of any patient with shoulder complaints resulting from recent trauma.

Examination

Examination of the shoulder is best performed with the patient seated on a backless stool undressed to the waist. A halter is used to cover the breasts.

Inspection from the front and back should delinate any gross abnormalities such as an elevated scapula of a Sprengel's deformity (Fig. 8-27) or an absent clavicle as in cleidocranial dysostosis (Fig. 8-28). Careful inspection is made for atrophy, particularly the deltoid, supraspinatus, and infraspinatus muscles. In recent injuries, inspection alone frequently identifies fractures, dislocations, and, of course, any open injuries.

Palpation. It is unthinkable not to examine the neck when a patient is having shoulder difficulties because neck pain is often referred to the shoulder. Therefore, it is advisable to begin palpation in the area of the neck (see Chap. 6) before palpating the shoulder. Feel for tenderness over the spinous processes of the cervical vertebrae and the borders of the trapezius muscle. Look for masses in the supraclavicular area and thyroid gland on the anterior aspect of the neck. Evaluate the pulse of the carotid vessels. Special areas of concern about the shoulder are the intertubercular groove, through which the biceps tendon traverses, the rotator cuff and the acromioclavicular and sternoclavicular joints. The axillary artery and surrounding nerves are easily felt by abducting and externally rotating the shoulder. The

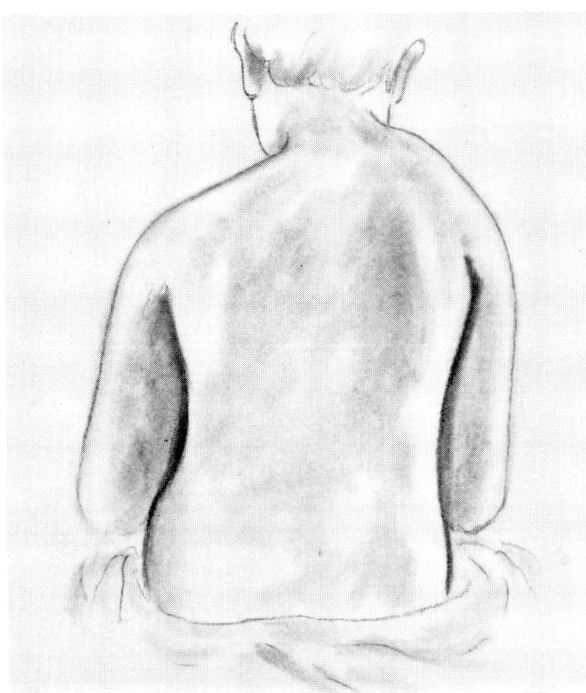

Fig. 8-27. Sprengel's deformity or congenitally undescended scapula. Embryonic connection with the cervical spine may persist as an omovertbral bone and anomalies of the cervical spine may also exist.

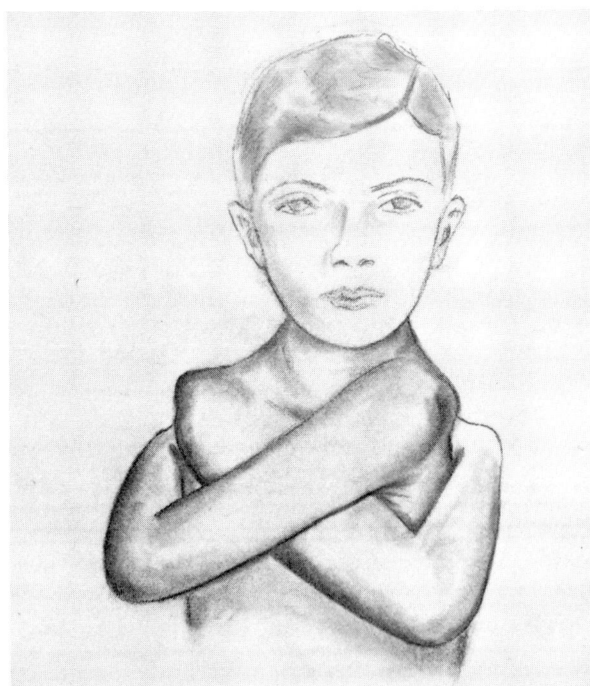

Fig. 8-28. Cleidocranial dysostosis. A congenital dysostosis involving multiple bones, most conspicuously the partial or complete absence of the clavicle allowing excessive flexion of the scapula.

artery is palpated just posterior to the pectoralis muscle in the anterior axillary fold (Fig. 8-29).

Range of motion, both active and passive, is evaluated. The neck and elbow are included to see if aggravation of the patient's symptoms occurs with their movement. Painful active abduction of the shoulder is present in tears of the rotator cuff, but passive abduction is relatively comfortable. The normal range of motions is described in the section on anatomy (Figs. 8-1 through 8-9).

Muscle testing is helpful in delineating tendonitis, tendon ruptures, and nerve lesions. The most common muscles tested and the methods used in examination are illustrated in Figures 8-10 through 8-17, 8-19, 8-20, 8-21, and 8-24. One must always be cognizant of both the segmental innervation and peripheral nerve innervation of each muscle tested as the location of a nerve injury is determined by the patterns of muscle weakness and sensory loss.

Sensory examination for light touch is performed noting both the dermatome distribution (see Fig. 5-1A, B) and the peripheral nerve distribution.

Reflexes. Examination of the three major reflexes, biceps (C5), brachioradialis (C6), and triceps (C7) can be helpful in localization of a particular nerve problem (see Fig. 1-4A, B, C).

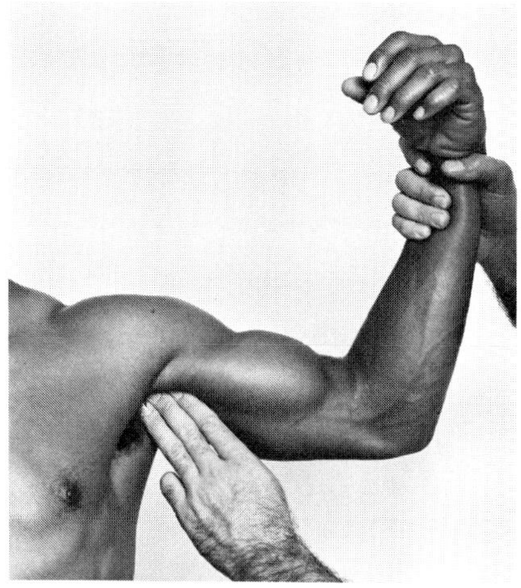

Fig. 8-29. The axillary artery and surrounding nerves can be palpated just beneath the pectoralis muscle in the axilla.

Roentgenography

Minimal roentgenographic examination of the shoulder includes an axillary lateral and anteroposterior view (see Fig. 8-34) in internal and external rotation. The differential diagnosis section can assist you in requesting specific roentgenograms for particular problems.

DIFFERENTIAL DIAGNOSIS

The various causes of pain in the shoulder are considered under three broad categories: lesions producing neck and shoulder pain; lesions producing only shoulder pain; and lesions producing shoulder pain with radiation into the upper extremity. These topics will be considered separately.

Lesions Producing Neck and Shoulder Pain

Cervical spondylosis is a term used which signifies degenerative disk disease of the cervical spine. The degenerative changes are usually found in the disk space between the fifth and sixth cervical and sixth and seventh cervical vertebrae. The disk spaces are narrowed and in the more advanced cases osteophytes develop at the margins of the vertebral bodies with occasional spontaneous interbody fusions. Malalignment of the facets is associated with advanced cervical spondylosis, and eventually degenerative changes are observed in these joints. The pain is described as aching, dull in nature, and poorly localized to the region of the trapezius muscle at the base of the neck and laterally over the posterior aspect of the shoulder. The pain is aggravated by movements of the neck and by holding the neck in one position for prolonged periods of time as occurs in driving or sitting at a desk. Roentgenograms of the cervical spine often reveal the degenerative changes (see Fig. 6-49A) although one must remember that patients past the age of 50 almost routinely show some degenerative changes of the disk and many of these patients are not symptomatic.

Postural disorders about the shoulder girdle produce pain and discomfort in the shoulder and neck. Those most subject to these symptoms are the typist or assembly line worker who perform repetitive work for long periods of time with little change in posture. The pain is described as a dull aching sensation about the shoulder and base of the neck and is frequently relieved by massage of the trapezius muscle or by change of position. Certain body types are also subject to postural disorders about the shoulder, such as individuals with long sloping shoulders which place the trapezius muscle at a mechanical disadvantage in operating the shoulder girdle (Fig. 8-30). Persons with a postural round back (Fig. 8-31) tip their scapula anteriorly which causes early impingement of the humerus on the coracoacromial ligaments making them particularly susceptible to postural shoulder pain.

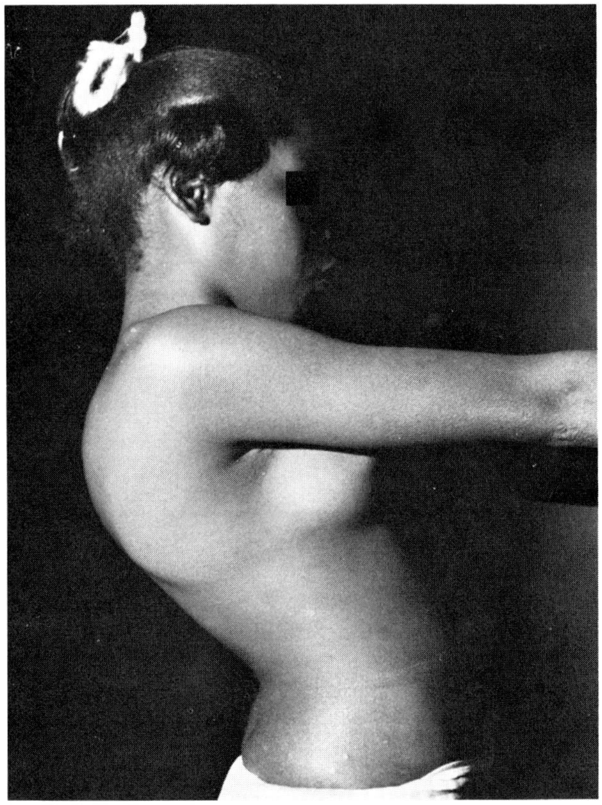

Fig. 8-31. Postural round back may cause shoulder pain in patients required to work with arms in the overhead position. The humerus impinges on the anterior structures about the glenoid because of the downward slope of the shoulder girdle. (Courtesy R. D. D'Ambrosia.)

Fibrositis of the shoulder girdle is poorly understood. Many cases diagnosed as fibrositis of the shoulder girdle are actually cases of cervical spondylosis. Some authorities believe that small herniations of fat, unmyelinated nerves, or small blood vessels through the superficial fascia may cause this entity. The problem is characterized by pain in the region of the trapezius muscles and trigger points which reproduce the patient's symptoms. Relief is obtained by injecting these trigger points with a local anesthetic and is considered diagnostic. Two characteristic locations of fibrositis of the shoulder girdle are the superior medial border of the scapula in the region of the rhomboids (suprascapular syndrome) and the inferior medial border of the scapula (lower trapezius syndrome) (Fig. 8-32).

The snapping scapula is an interesting entity caused by an outgrowth on the undersurface of the scapula which interferes with its movement across the thoracic cage. A definite bump or snap of the scapula, usually painful, is noted as the patient abducts his shoulder. The cause of this syndrome most often is an osteophyte or bony spur which occurs on the superior medial border of the scapula, and the diagnosis is confirmed by roentgenogram (Fig. 8-33).

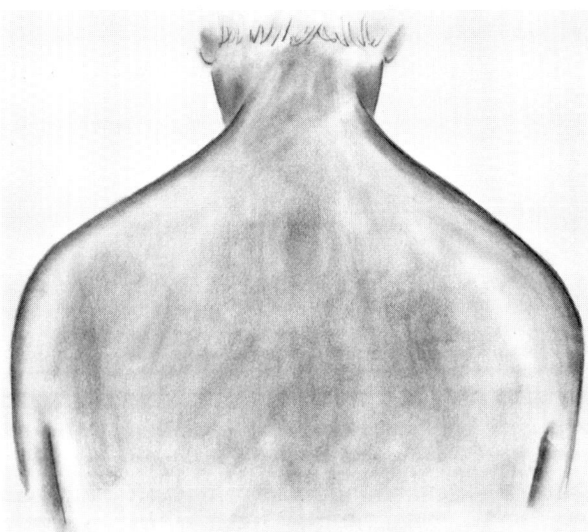

Fig. 8-30. Patients with long sloping shoulders may experience chronic pain in the trapezius muscle. This position places the muscle at a mechanical disadvantage, causing muscle fatigue.

Diseases of the abdominal or thoracic viscera can refer pain to the shoulder and neck region. Lesions of the apical portion of the lung, such as a Pancoast's tumor, will produce pain in the shoulder and base of the neck. Myocardial infarction can cause pain in the base of the neck or shoulder with radiation down the left arm and occasionally the right. Gall bladder disease, subphrenic abscess, lesions of the stomach, and hiatal hernia are just several abdominal problems which produce pain in

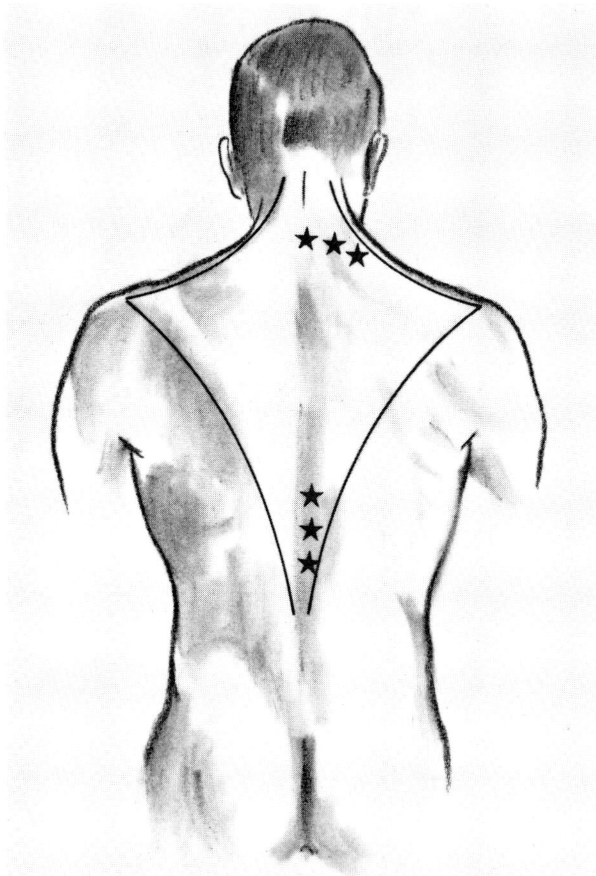

Fig. 8-32. Fibrositis. The location of common trigger points that reproduce the patient's complaints. The cephalad locations are called the suprascapular syndrome. The trigger points of the caudal border of the trapezius are found in the trapezius syndrome.

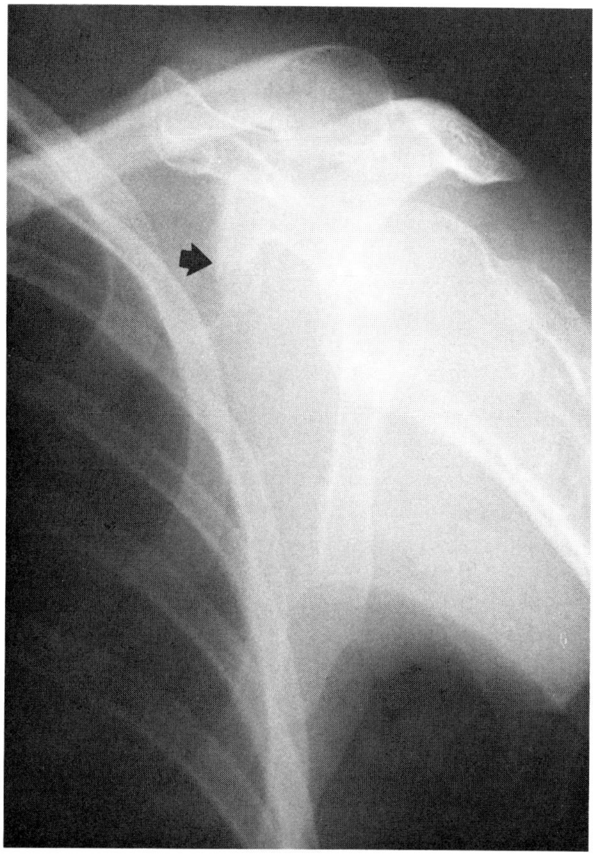

Fig. 8-33. Snapping scapula caused by a large osteochondroma (*arrow*) on the undersurface of the scapula.

the shoulder by diaphragmatic irritation. Usually with referred pain from the thoracic or abdominal viscera the examiner can find sufficient symptoms in the chest or abdomen which lead to the correct diagnosis.

Lesions Which Produce Pain Predominantly in the Shoulder

Subdeltoid bursitis results from degenerative changes in the rotator cuff which is the floor of the subdeltoid bursa (see Fig. 8-18). Degenerative changes in this area followed by calcium deposits can produce an acute inflammatory reaction in the subdeltoid bursa. The onset of pain is usually acute and severe, most often occurring in the fifth decade of life. Shoulder movement, particularly abduction, is painful and the patient can demonstrate an area of exquisite tenderness in the region of the subdeltoid bursa. Roentgenograms of the shoulder in the anteroposterior projection, with the humerus in internal and external rotation, may demonstrate a calcium deposit in the subdeltoid bursa and confirm the diagnosis (Fig. 8-34). Subdeltoid bursitis frequently goes into subacute and chronic phases. The patient's symptoms are much less severe in the subacute phase. Tenderness about the shoulder is more generalized with limitation of abduction and external rotation. In the chronic phase of this disease an adhesive capsulitis may occur in which the patient experiences pain in the shoulder only with certain motions. Rather marked limitation of motion of the shoulder usually in abduction and external rotation

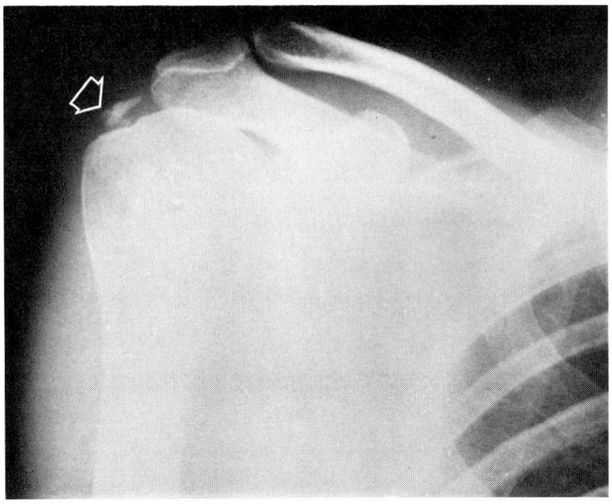

Fig. 8-34. Roentgenogram of the shoulder in a patient with acute bursitis. Calcium deposits can be seen in the region of the subdeltoid bursa (*arrow*). (Courtesy R. D. D'Ambrosia.)

can develop, and attempts to move the shoulder into these positions aggravate the patient's symptoms. The patient is usually comfortable at rest. The most common cause of chronic adhesive capsulitis is subdeltoid bursitis, but any condition in which there is limitation of shoulder motion for prolonged periods may result in capsular contraction and adhesions.

Bicipital tenosynovitis can be difficult to differentiate from subacute subdeltoid bursitis because the pain is in the same general area. The long head of the biceps tendon extends through the bicipital groove across the joint of the shoulder intrasynovially to attach to the superior rim of the glenoid. It is subjected to chronic degenerative changes similar to those of the rotator cuff because of its long intraarticular course. The patient exhibits pain in the bicipital groove on palpation, and the result of the Yergason's test (Fig. 8-35) is positive. The test is performed by having the patient supinate the forearm against resistance and, in so doing, pain is produced in the bicipital groove. The biceps muscle is a forearm supinator which contracts when supinating the forearm, thereby irritating the proximal origin of the muscle. Subluxations of the biceps tendon are also a cause of chronic tenosynovitis. The diagnosis is made by palpating the tendon in the bicipital groove with the arm abducted. The tendon can be felt as it subluxates from the groove on internal and external rotation of the arm in the abduction position. Roentgenograms depicting the bicipital groove (Fig. 8-36) may show spurring or degenerative changes in the groove.

Chronic irritation of the biceps tendon over a prolonged period may cause rupture of the tendon and distal retraction of the muscle mass with a diagnostic lump in the forearm (Fig. 8-37). Rupture occa-

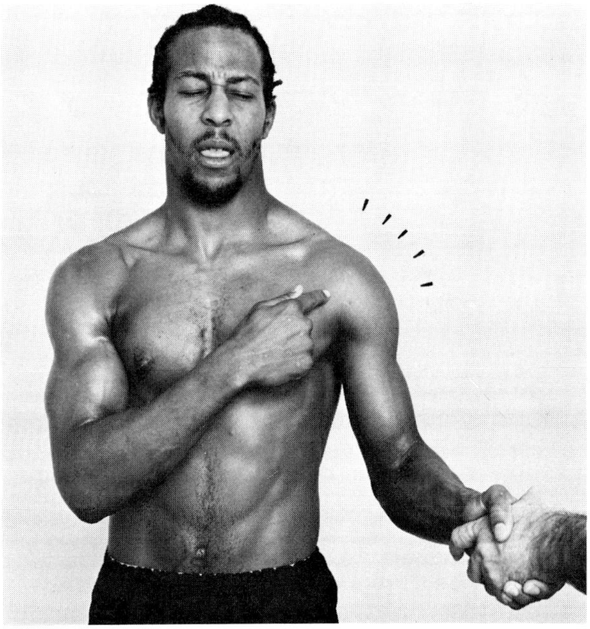

Fig. 8-35. Yergason's test for bicipital tenosynovitis. Supination of the forearm against resistance produces pain in the biceps tendon of the bicipital groove.

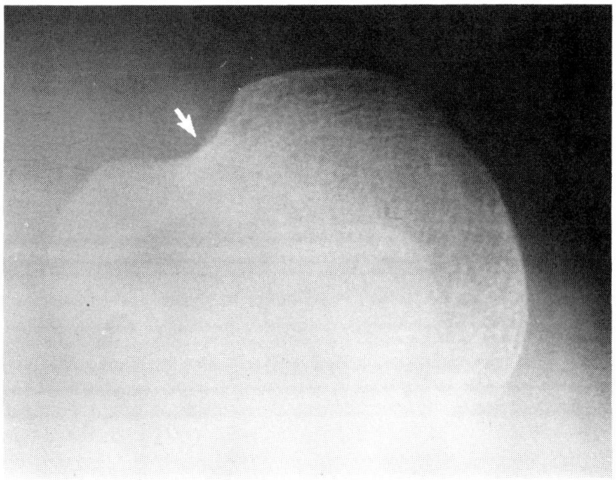

Fig. 8-36. Roentgenogram of the bicipital groove (*arrow*). Spurs or roughening of the groove may produce bicipital tenosynovitis.

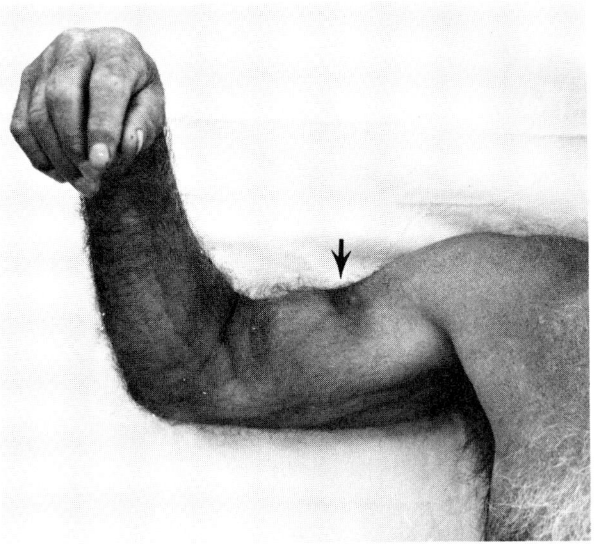

Fig. 8-37. Rupture of the long head of the biceps tendon. The characteristic bulge of the biceps muscle in the arm can be seen more distal from its former location (*arrow*). (Courtesy R. D. D'Ambrosia.)

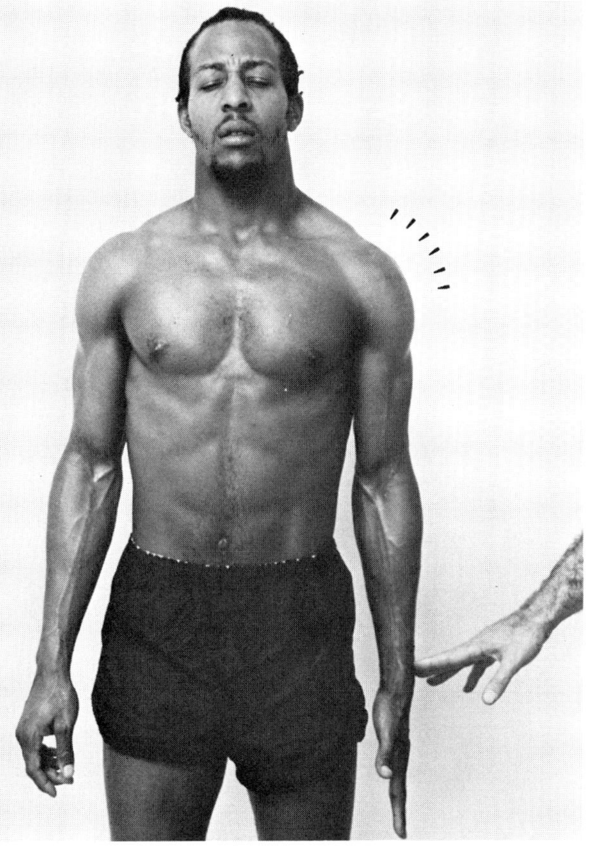

Fig. 8-38. Torn rotator cuff. Patient can not overcome the slightest resistance to elevation. Pain may be experienced in region of the rotator cuff.

sionally occurs distally where the tendon attaches to the bicipital tuberosity on the radius with proximal retraction of the muscle mass.

Tears of the rotator cuff can result from degenerative changes in the cuff which occur over many years, but the actual tear is usually the result of minor trauma in a middle-aged individual. The patient complains of pain in the deltoid area following the tear and is unable to abduct the shoulder even against slight resistance (Fig. 8-38). However, if the shoulder is brought to 90 degrees in the abducted position, it can usually be held there by the deltoid muscle if the pain is not severe. Physical evidence of atrophy of the supraspinatus and infraspinatus muscles is observed on the physical examination if the tear has been present for a long period of time. Arthrography of the shoulder is especially helpful in diagnosing complete ruptures of the rotator cuff. The radiopaque material introduced into the shoulder joint leaks through the tear in the rotator cuff to fill the subdeltoid bursa (Fig. 8-39).

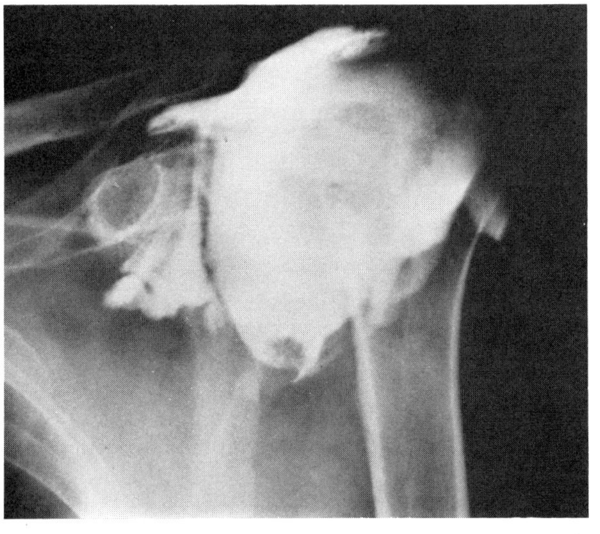

Fig. 8-39. Arthrogram of the shoulder in a patient with torn rotator cuff. The dye can be seen to leak into the subdeltoid bursa through the tear.

Arthritis of the glenohumeral, acromioclavicular, and sternoclavicular joints also causes localized pain about the shoulder. On physical examination, pain is usually localized to the joint and is accompanied by grating and some limitation of motion. Intraarticular injections of a local anesthetic produce temporary relief of the patient's symptoms, and roentgenograms of the joint usually confirm the arthritic process (Fig. 8-40).

Subluxations of the shoulder can cause shoulder pain and must be considered in the differential diagnosis, particularly in young athletes. The patient experiences momentary pain and discomfort in the shoulder in overhead motions in external rotation, such as swimming or throwing a ball. The diagnosis may be difficult if complete dislocation of the shoulder does not occur. The physical examination is usually within normal limits, although occasionally the patient may be able to reproduce a jerking sensation which can be felt by the examiner. Special roentgenograms of the inferior rim of the glenoid process (Fig. 8-41) may demonstrate small avulsion fractures in a large percentage of cases, and arthrograms sometimes show a large redundant capsule along the anteroinferior margin of the joint.

Tumors about the shoulder are either primary or metastatic and can occur in either soft tissue or bone. Soft tissue lesions are usually palpable on physical examination, and bony lesions, if large enough, may be palpable as well. Roentgenographic examination of the shoulder will usually identify bone lesions, and a biopsy will identify the type of tumor.

Lesions Producing Shoulder Pain with Radiation into the Arm

The cervical root syndrome may result from intraspinal tumors and tumors of the vertebrae which impinge upon the root; however, most cervical root syndromes are the result of degenerative disk disease or cervical spondylosis which cause root impingement. The cervical root is compressed as it exits from the spinal canal over the intervertebral disk beneath the facet joint and passes the joints of Luschka (see Chap. 6). The nerve root is surrounded by structures that can impinge upon it and these impingements are a common cause of shoulder and arm pain. The most common cervical roots involved are the fifth through eighth. Remember, in the cervical spine the roots exit superior to the vertebral body, except for the eighth cervical which exits between the seventh cervical and first thoracic vertebrae. With irritation of the fifth cervical nerve root (Table 8-1) pain is located in the neck, shoulder, medial

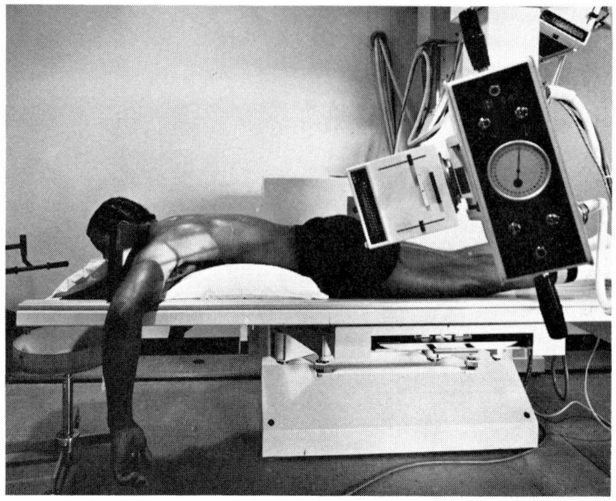

Fig. 8-41. Position of the patient to obtain a roentgenogram of the inferior glenoid rim in patients with suspected chronic recurring subluxations of the shoulder.

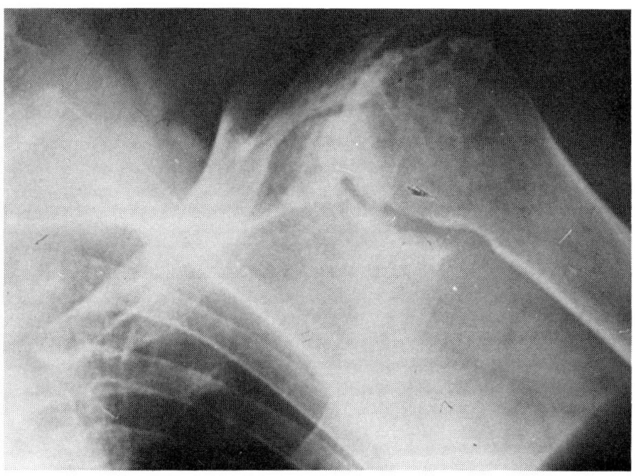

Fig. 8-40. Roentgenogram of a patient with degenerative joint disease of the glenohumeral joint.

Table 8-1. Physical Findings in Cervical Nerve Root Impingement Syndromes

Impinged Root	*Sensory Disturbances*	*Motor Weakness*	*Reflex Loss*
C5	Anterolateral forearm	Anterior deltoid	Biceps
C6	Thumb	Biceps Scapular muscles	Brachio radialis
C7	Index and long fingers	Triceps	Triceps
C8	Ring and little fingers	Intrinsic muscles of hand	—

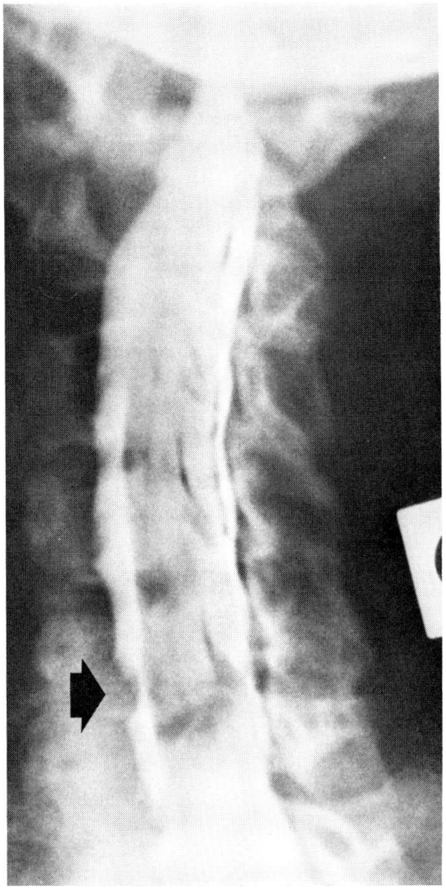

Fig. 8-42. Myelogram in a patient with a cervical disk protrusion. The indentation of the dye column can be seen (*arrow*).

border of the scapula, and lateral aspect of the arm. There may also be numbness over the lateral aspect of the arm, and, if motor weakness is present, it is found in the deltoid muscle. The finding of no biceps reflex is helpful in reaching a diagnosis. In the sixth cervical nerve root syndrome (Table 8-1), neck and shoulder pain are still present with pain along the medial border of the scapula, inner aspect of the arm, and dorsum of the forearm. Sensory changes may be present in the thumb and index finger, and there may be some weakness of the biceps muscle. The brachioradialis reflex may be absent. In the seventh cervical nerve root syndrome (Table 8-1), neck and arm pain are in approximately the same distribution as in the sixth cervical nerve root syndrome while the sensory changes will move to the index and long finger with weakness of the triceps muscle and absence of the triceps reflex. In the eighth cervical nerve root syndrome (Table 8-1), pain is in the medial aspect of the arm and forearm with numbness of the ring and little fingers, plus weakness of the intrinsic muscles of the hand. The triceps strength may be slightly diminished. The myelogram is most helpful in delineating cervical root syndrome by demonstrating an indentation of the dye column at the level of the protruded disk (Fig. 8-42). Electromyographic examination may also be helpful in identifying the level of the lesion.

The neurovascular compression syndromes of the shoulder are identified by the location of the compression. Some etiological causes are: cervical ribs, hypertrophy of the scalene muscles, and bony abnormalities of the clavicle or first thoracic rib. The patient complains of an aching sensation in the shoulder, arm, forearm, or hand when the extremity is placed in a particular position.

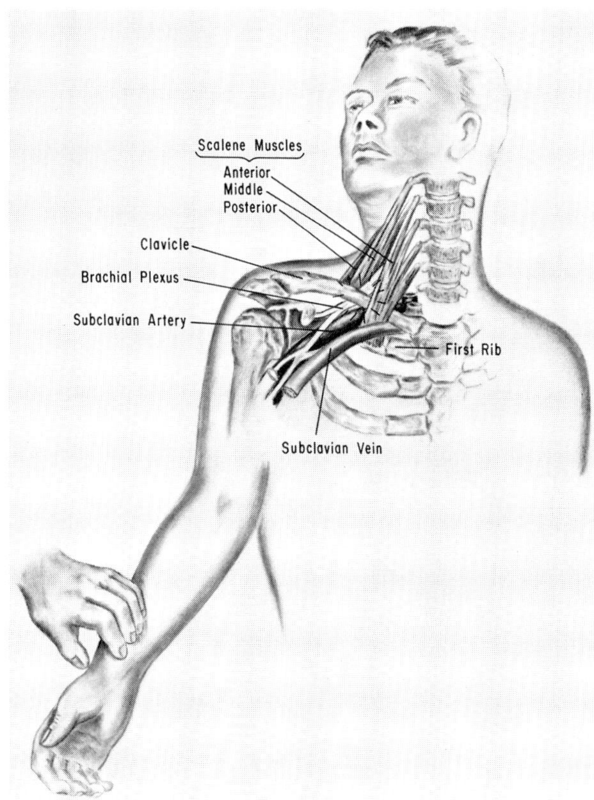

Fig. 8-43. Adson's test to reproduce compression of the neurovascular structures in the neck. The patient is asked to inhale deeply and turn his head to one side then the other. A diminution of the radial pulse and reproduction of the patient's symptoms indicates constriction of the neurovascular bundle in the scalene muscles.

Paresthesias and vascular disturbances result and on rare occasions gangrene of the extremity has been reported. The diagnosis is made when the patient's symptoms are reproduced and there is diminution of the pulse when the extremity is placed in the appropriate position. However, diminution of the pulse alone is not diagnostic as many normal persons will show a marked reduction of the pulse with certain positions of the arm and shoulder and yet have no symptoms. Compression of the neurovascular bundle by the scalene muscles may be reproduced by the Adson maneuver. In Adson's test (Fig. 8-43), the patient is asked to rotate his head toward the involved extremity while extending the neck and inhaling. Compression of the neurovascular bundle between the first rib and clavicle is performed by asking the patient to brace his shoulder as in the rigid military posture (Fig. 8-44). Compression of the neurovascular bundle by the coracoid process and pectoralis minor muscle is produced by hyperabduction of the arm high above the patient's head (Fig. 8-45). Roentgenograms of the lower cervical spine, clavicle, first rib, and shoulder should be obtained

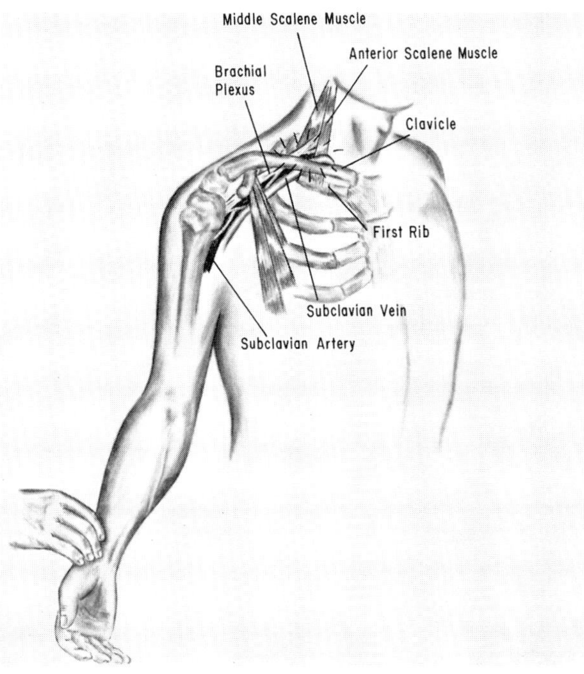

Fig. 8-44. Costoclavicular syndrome can be reproduced by asking the patient to adduct his scapula forcing the clavicle against the first rib. Symptoms should be reproduced with a diminished radial pulse to confirm the diagnosis.

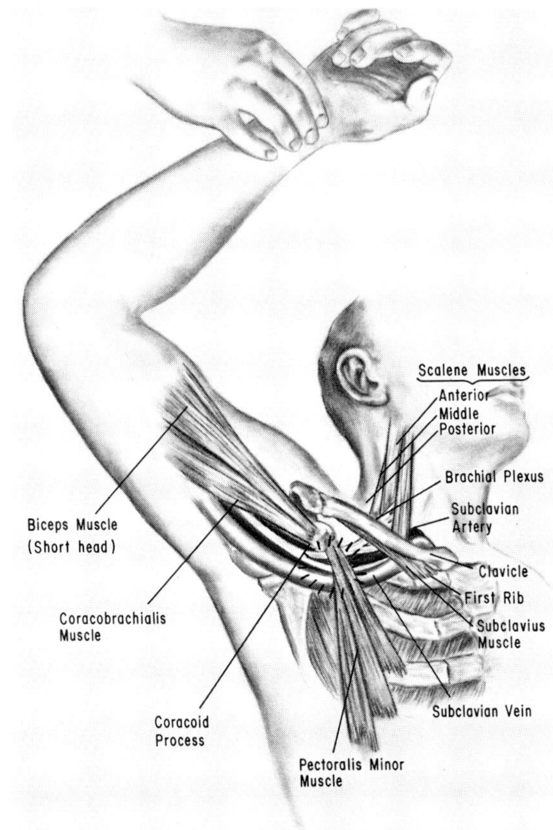

Fig. 8-45. Hyperabduction syndrome. The patient abducts his arm above his head. Where the neurovascular bundle is compressed under the coracoid process and pectoralis minor muscle, symptoms should be reproduced along with a diminished radial pulse.

and examined for abnormalities of these structures. A cervical rib is a more common cause of neurovascular compression syndrome (Fig. 8-46). Electrical studies or nerve conduction studies of the ulnar nerve by an experienced electromyographer may demonstrate delayed nerve conduction from the neck to the upper arm (Chap. 3), and angiography may demonstrate vascular compression.

The shoulder-hand syndrome is a poorly understood condition of the upper extremity and is believed to be caused by malfunction of the autonomic nervous system. The patient complains of severe and bizarre pains in the extremity associated with excessive sweating and coolness. There is glossiness of the skin with loss of normal skin texture and associated joint stiffness. This syndrome occurs

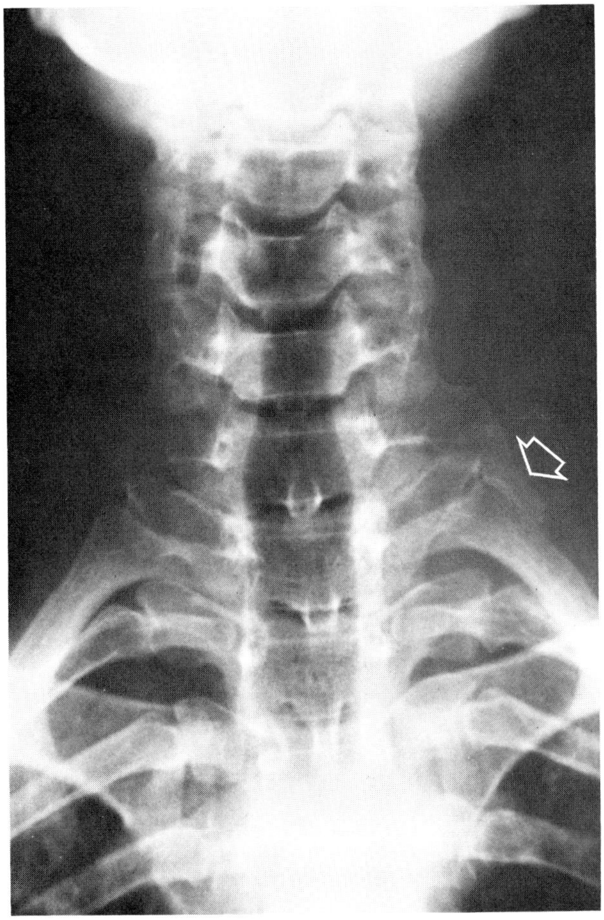

Fig. 8-46. Roentgenograms of the neck in a patient with a cervical rib (*arrow*). A cervical rib may produce a neurovascular disturbance in the upper extremity.

more commonly in people who are emotionally unstable and who have extremely low pain thresholds. The initiating factor may be trauma, often quite minor, or it may result from remote disease of the thoracic or abdominal viscera which causes referred pain to the shoulder and arm.

Many miscellaneous diseases can produce pain in the shoulder and arm, such as the nerve entrapment syndromes. The nerves most commonly involved are the dorsal scapular, suprascapular, and the long thoracic. Patients with entrapment of the dorsal scapular nerve present with pain along the medial border of the scapula radiating to the posterior aspect of the arm and forearm, sometimes as far as the thumb (Fig. 8-47). A trigger point may be demonstrated in the region of the brachial plexus

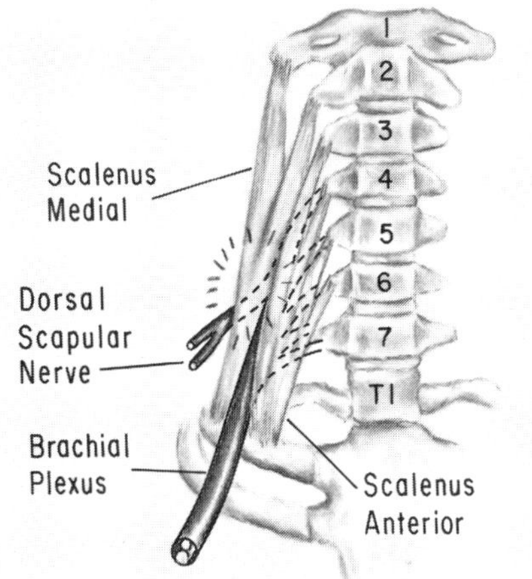

Fig. 8-47. Dorsal scapular nerve entrapment. The nerve is compressed as it passes through the scalenus medius. The patient experiences pain along the radial aspect of the arm and forearm with some slight winging of scapula. A trigger point may be found at the base of the neck over the brachial plexus.

which reproduces the symptoms. Suprascapular nerve entrapment symptoms are reproduced by adduction of the involved extremity across the chest (Fig. 8-48). The pain locates about the shoulder and scapula with some radiation into the arm. The diagnosis is made if symptoms are relieved by a suprascapular nerve block in the suprascapular notch. Injuries to the long thoracic nerve produce winging of the scapula and pain along the lateral border of the trunk (see Fig. 8-15). Various lesions have been reported responsible for injuries to the long thoracic nerves including viral infections, injections of antitoxin, and trauma. Other nerves of the brachial plexus may be similarly affected and produce different syndromes but are much less common.

Arterial and venous lesions of the upper extremity may also be a source of pain about the shoulder and arm. Assessment of the circulation by appropriate palpation of the pulses, examination of capillary filling, Doppler examination, venography, and arteriography assists in the diagnosis of these conditions.

Shoulder Problems in Children

Birth Trauma—Brachial Plexus Injuries. An infant can sustain a stretching injury to the brachial plexus at the time of delivery. The upper

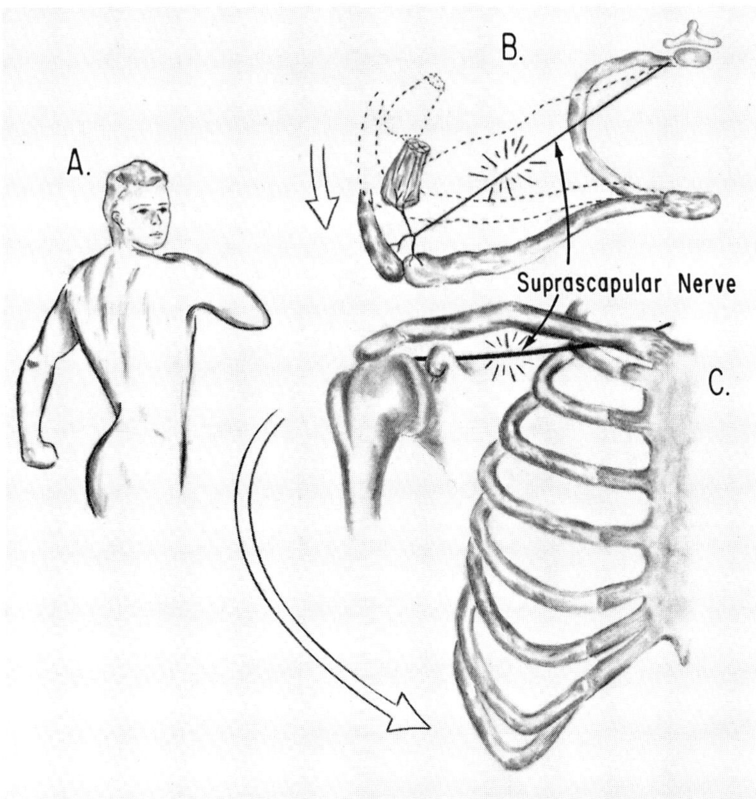

Fig. 8-48. Suprascapular nerve entrapment. The patient experiences pain on hyperadduction of the arms across the chest. Pain is poorly localized to the posterior aspect of the shoulder. Atrophy of the supraspinatus and infraspinatus may occur. A suprascapular nerve block should temporarily relieve symptoms.

roots are most often involved, and this is referred to as Erb's palsy (Fig. 8-49). The child has a lack of spontaneous movement in the extremity, specifically lack of abduction and external rotation. Movement in the hand, wrist, and forearm will appear normal. If the lesion does not resolve and no subsequent treatment is instituted an internal rotation adduction deformity of the shoulder plus a pronation deformity of the forearm due to muscle contraction secondary to the nerve loss will develop. When the entire plexus is involved, the child exhibits a paralysis of the entire extremity with no spontaneous movement. Injury to the lower roots of the brachial plexus occasionally occurs and is known as Klumpke's palsy. In this case the child shows a lack of spontaneous movement in the wrist, fingers, and forearm but has essentially normal shoulder motion.

Fractures of the proximal end of the humerus or clavicle also occur at birth and these injuries often imitate nerve root injuries causing a problem in differential diagnosis. However, fractures of the clavicle can usually be detected by palpation plus the presence of some swelling and ecchymosis over the bone. Fractures of the proximal end of the humerus are even more difficult to delineate as this area is cartilagenous and not visible on roentgenogram. The child exhibits a pseudoparalysis of the extremity because of pain closely resembling an Erb's palsy. It is imperative that roentgenograms be obtained several weeks after delivery; these will be diagnostic if healing bone and periosteal reaction are visible, indicating the presence of a fracture. Electrical studies of the muscle may also be helpful several weeks after birth for denervation potentials may be present.

Congenital deformities about the proximal humerus and scapula are uncommon but a large number exist. Congenital absence of muscle groups about the shoulder have been reported in all the muscles, but the most common is absence of the pectoralis major (Fig. 8-50). Depending on the muscle absent, the patient shows weakness or absence of the particular motion for which the muscle is responsible. There is lack of tissue or bulk in the area as well. This is difficult to recognize in a young child

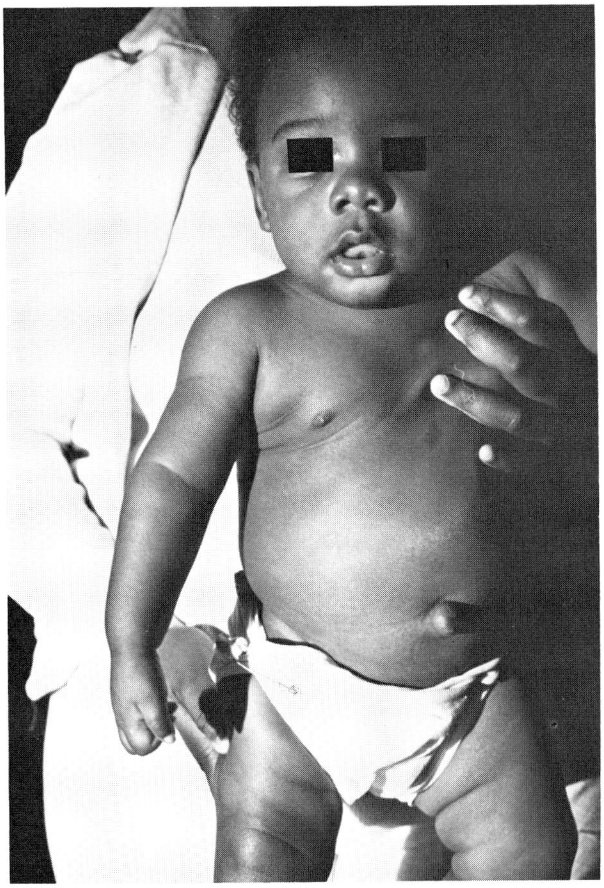

Fig. 8-49. Child with resolving Erb's palsy. The arm still lacks normal abduction and external rotation. (Courtesy R. D. D'Ambrosia.)

because of the large amount of adipose tissue present. Weakness of muscle groups found in the various muscle and nerve disorders may produce winging of the scapula suggesting an abnormality in the shoulder girdle. A more thorough evaluation of the child reveals weakness in all muscle groups and other stigmata of a more generalized disease, such as elevation of the muscle creatine phosphokinase (CPK), abnormal electromyogram and histological findings on muscle and nerve biopsy (see Chaps. 3 and 4).

Cleidocranial dysostosis (see Fig. 8-28) and *Sprengel's deformity* (see Fig. 8-27) are two of the more common congenital malformations of the upper extremity. In cleidocranial dysostosis, a defect is present in the formation of membranous bones with manifestations chiefly in the skull and clavicle with hypermobility of the shoulders, specifically scapular flexion. The skull also has a characteristic shape with numerous wormian bones. In Sprengel's deformity the scapula remains small because it fails to descend and is occasionally attached to the cervical spine by an omohyoid bone. The child has a small palpable scapula with an abnormal contour of the neck and limited abduction of the shoulder. Roentgenograms demonstrate the abnormal position and shape of the scapula and may reveal an attachment to the cervical spine by an omohyoid bone. This malformation is due to failure of normal descent of the shoulder girdle during embryonic development.

Abnormalities of the spine are occasionally mistaken for deformities of the shoulder, such as scoliosis with a prominent scapula over the rib hump, the Klippel-Feil syndrome with multiple anomalies of the cervical spine which produces a broad thick neck, and Turner's syndrome with webbing of the neck. These are just a few of the anomalies that may be mistaken for congenital deformities of the shoulder girdle (see Chap. 6).

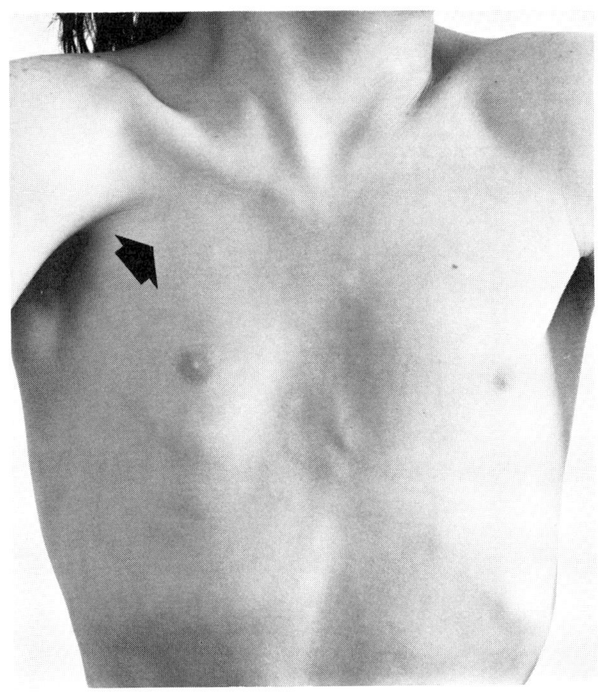

Fig. 8-50. Congenital absence of the right pectoralis major muscle. Note the flattening of the chest wall and absent right anterior axillary fold.

Infections in this area commonly are hematogenous osteomyelitis of the proximal part of the humerus or pyarthrosis of the shoulder joint (Fig. 8-51). The diagnosis may be difficult in infants as the classic manifestations of infection may be absent. The child may refuse to eat, be listless and hyperirritable. There may be no signs of acute localized pain or high fever. Careful observation reveals the lack of spontaneous motion in the affected extremity, and aspiration of the suspected area produces purulent fluid which on gram stain and culture reveals the offending organism. The more classic findings of heat, pain, fever, and limitation of motion are present in the older child. Roentgenograms reveal swelling in the joint space or destructive changes in the proximal part of the humerus indicative of osteomyelitis. As in infants, aspiration of the area is most helpful in diagnosis. Hematogenous osteomyelitis in children usually begins in the metaphyseal region of the bone, and, if intracapsular, early diagnosis and treatment are imperative to prevent rupture of the bone abscess into the joint capsule and a subsequent pyarthrosis. Half of the proximal metaphysis of the humerus is intracapsular and the potential of an osteomyelitis developing into a pyarthrosis much as in the hip (see Chap. 10) is present.

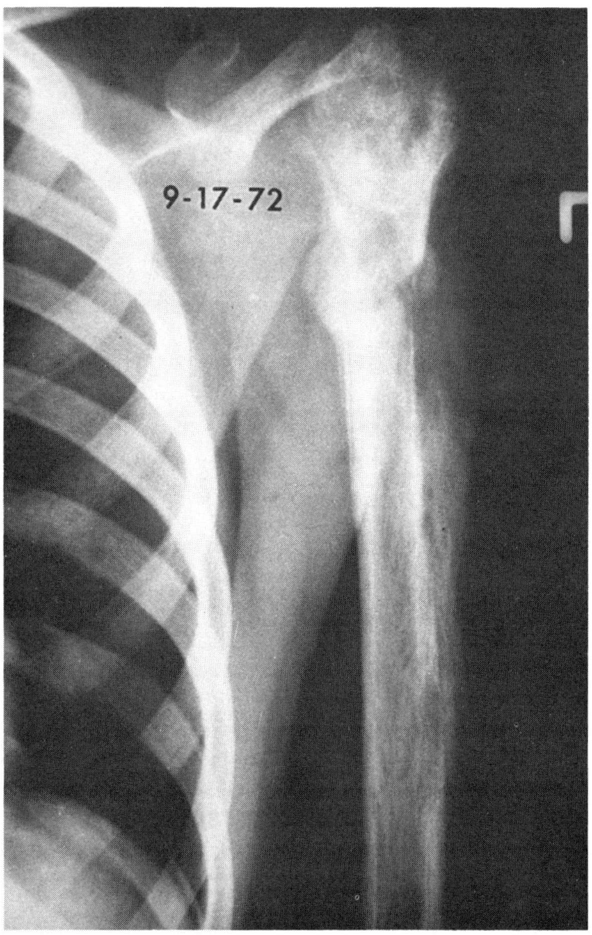

Fig. 8-51. Roentgenogram of a child's humerus several weeks after the onset of osteomyelitis. The periosteal reaction is obvious. Very early in the course of the disease the roentgenograms may show only slight soft tissue swelling. Bone changes require some time to develop.

Shoulder Trauma

Trauma to the shoulder and upper part of the arm produces a number of different types of injuries. Probably the simplest is muscular strain appearing in such muscles as the latissimus dorsi, biceps, triceps, and occasionally the anterior portions of the deltoid. More serious injuries, such as fractures and dislocations, also occur. The clavicle is the most frequently injured bone of the shoulder girdle, but fractures also occur in the proximal part of the humerus and scapula. The common dislocations are anterior dislocation of the glenohumeral joint and dislocations of the acromioclavicular joint. Sternoclavicular dislocations and posterior dislocations of the glenohumeral joint also occur but are rare.

Common Fractures

Fractures of the clavicle are more common in children but do occur in adults. They result from a fall on the shoulder or arm with a rotary component and forces are transmitted through the extremity to the trunk. A visible and palpable deformity is usually present because the clavicle is subcutaneous. There is also associated ecchymosis and pain. Diagnosis is confirmed by roentgenograms (Fig. 8-52). Fractures distal to the coracoid process present like an acromioclavicular separation with a prominence at the acromioclavicular joint and the proximal clavicle riding high above the acromion. This is an instance where a fracture can be easily confused with a dislocation.

Fractures of the proximal end of the humerus are also caused by a fall on the extremity or the outstretched hand. The force is transmitted

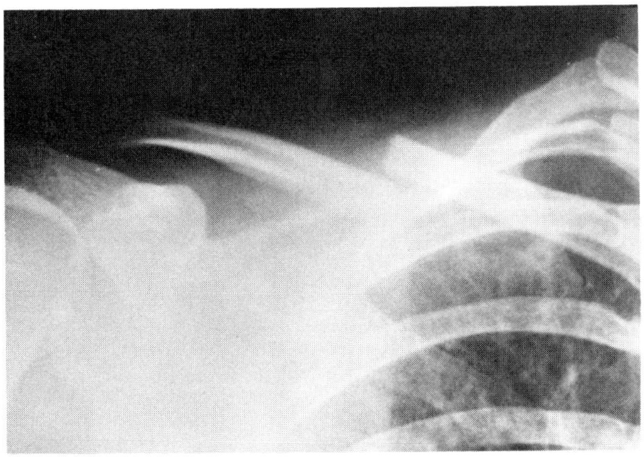

Fig. 8-52. Roentgenogram of the common type of fracture of the clavicle.

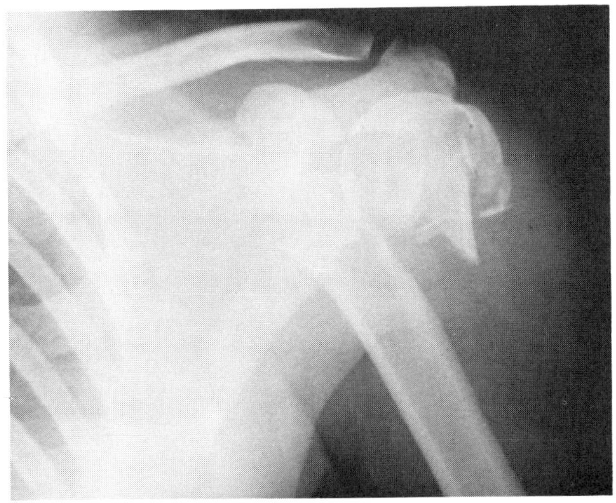

Fig. 8-53. Roentgenogram of a fracture of the proximal humerus.

along the axis of the upper extremity through the shoulder, and a rotary component is frequently involved. There are several classifications of fractures of the proximal end of the humerus, but they are more pertinent to the management of the problem rather than the diagnosis. The presenting symptoms are pain and discomfort with some swelling and occasional ecchymosis about the proximal part of the humerus. If the fracture is not impacted, false motion and crepitus may be elicited on clinical examination. Roentgenograms of the shoulder in both the anteroposterior and axillary plane should be obtained to confirm the diagnosis and distinguish the type of fracture (Fig. 8-53). On rare occasions an axillary view is not possible and a transthoracic lateral should be ordered as a substitute.

Fractures of the scapula fall into two groups: those that occur about the glenohumeral joint and coracoid process and those that occur elsewhere in the scapula. There is a presenting history of trauma, usually severe, and the patient has pain about the shoulder girdle with any motion of the upper extremity. Scapular fractures are frequently associated with more serious injuries to the chest wall, cervical spine, and brachial plexus, and one should always be alert for them. Fractures about the glenohumeral joint can result in moderate stiffening of the shoulder and limitation of motion but those in the body and elsewhere heal without any sequelae. The suspected diagnosis is confirmed by roentgenograms (Fig. 8-54).

Common Dislocations

Anterior Dislocations. The two common dislocations about the shoulder occur at the acromioclavicular and glenohumeral joints. Ninety-five percent of all glenohumeral dislocations are anterior and occur most commonly in young adult males (Fig. 8-55). They are the result of forced abduction external rotation injuries to the shoulder. The head of the humerus leaves the glenohumeral joint through a tear in the anterior inferior capsule (see

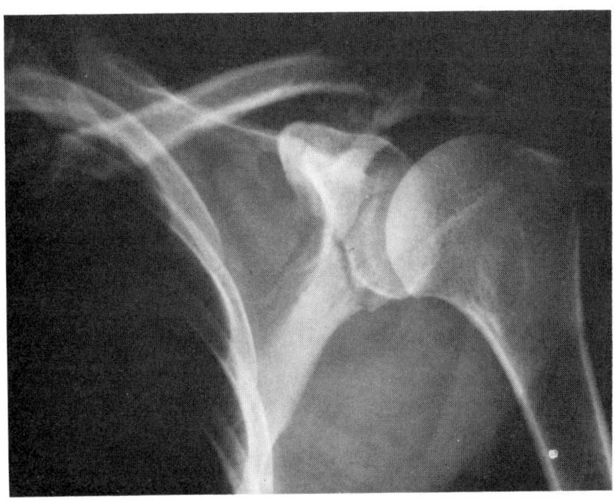

Fig. 8-54. Roentgenogram of a scapular fracture. Because of the involvement of the glenoid some residual shoulder stiffness can be expected.

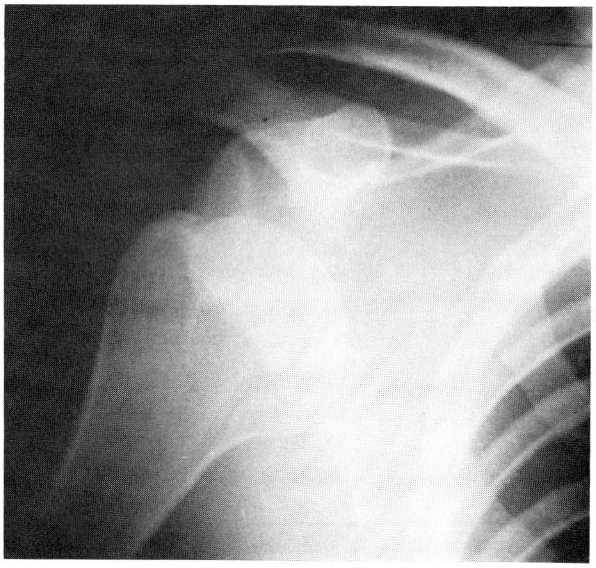

Fig. 8-55. Roentgenogram of an anterior dislocation of the shoulder. The head of the humerus lies anterior and below the coracoid process.

Fig. 8-25), a defect which usually does not heal. The patient is then subject to recurrent dislocations which occur whenever he abducts and externally rotates the extremity. In the acute lesion there is a history of trauma with pain and considerable discomfort over the glenohumeral joint when one attempts to move the upper extremity. Careful, early inspection reveals flattening and loss of the normal curvature of the shoulder, but swelling obliterates these findings later, and roentgenograms are necessary to confirm the diagnosis. When shoulder dislocation is suspected, an axillary view is paramount to distinguish the exact position of the head of the humerus in relation to the glenoid process (Fig. 8-56). Anterior dislocations of the shoulder can often be recognized on the anteroposterior roentgenogram, but posterior dislocations of the shoulder may frequently be in line with the glenoid process and be indistinguishable in this view. Therefore, the axillary lateral roentgenogram is necessary in all suspected shoulder dislocations to rule out the rare posterior dislocation.

Dislocations of the shoulder are occasionally accompanied by injury to the axillary nerve with resulting loss of function of the deltoid muscle. For this reason it is important to ascertain the function of the deltoid and particularly any sensory disturbance in the skin overlying the deltoid in shoulder dislocations. The area over the deltoid is innervated by the axillary nerve, and assessment of skin sensation will aid in predicting the subsequent function of the nerve. Dislocations of the shoulder rarely result in injury to other nerves and vessels of the upper extremity, although injuries of the posterior cord of the brachial plexus have been reported.

Dislocations of the acromioclavicular joint occur from a fall on the point of the shoulder. The coracoclavicular ligaments are the main stabiliz-

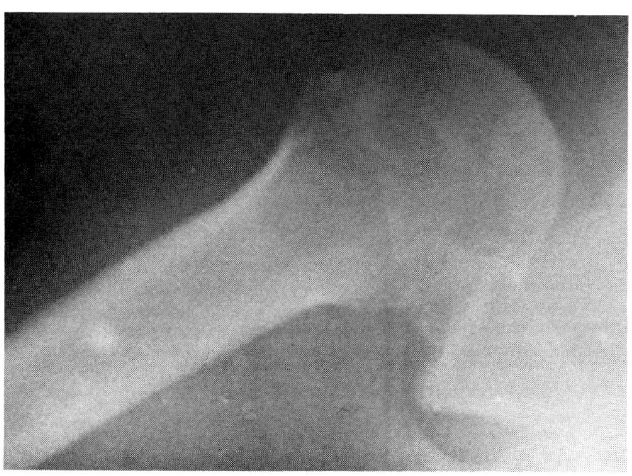

Fig. 8-56. Roentgenogram: axillary view of an anterior dislocation of the shoulder. The humeral head lies anterior to the glenoid. A large defect (compression fracture) is present in the posterior position of the humeral head (Hill-Sack lesion) caused by the rim of the glenoid.

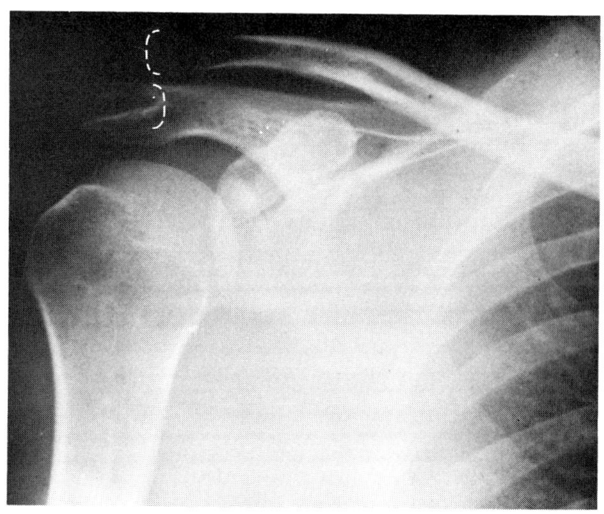

Fig. 8-57 Roentgenogram of a patient with a complete dislocation of the acromioclavicular joint.

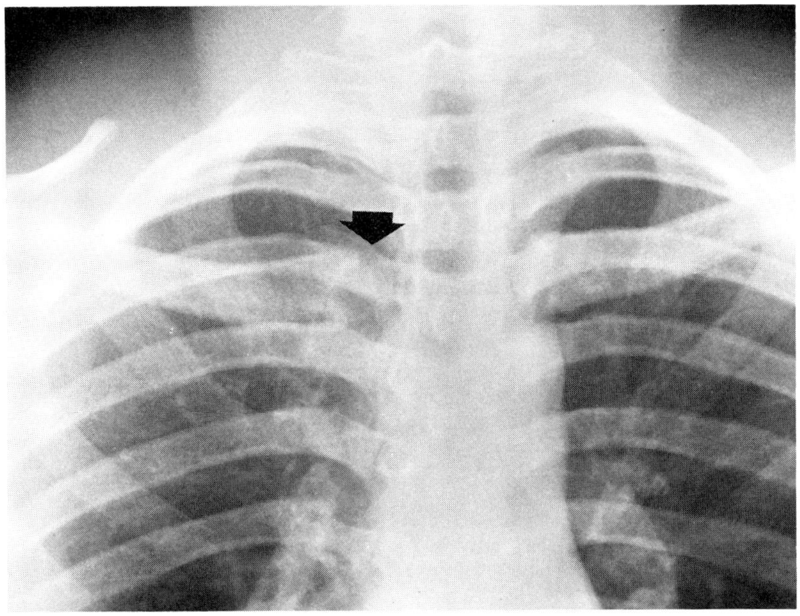

Fig. 8-58. Roentgenogram of a patient with a posterior dislocation of the right sternoclavicular joint (*arrow*).

ers of the acromioclavicular joint. Subluxation occurs when these ligaments are partially torn, and complete dislocations occur with total disruption. Patients with this injury present with pain and tenderness over the joint accompanied by ecchymosis. In complete disruption of the coracoclavicular ligaments, the distal end of the clavicle is visible and prominent. Diagnosis is confirmed by an anteroposterior roentgenogram of the acromioclavicular joint with a weight suspended from the patient's wrist (Fig. 8-57). The weight causes the upper extremity and shoulder girdle to separate from the clavicle accentuating the displacement of the acromion from the clavicle. A similar roentgenogram on the uninvolved side is obtained for comparison.

Sternoclavicular dislocations are rare and often difficult to diagnose. The patient complains of pain and tenderness in the region of the joint and there may be a prominence of the proximal end of the clavicle when compared with the opposite side. If routine roentgenograms of the sternoclavicular joint are not diagnostic, then serial laminograms are necessary to define minor displacements. Posterior dislocations of this joint can cause major damage to the subclavian vessels and may even obstruct the trachea causing respiratory embarrassment (Fig. 8-58).

SUGGESTED READINGS

1. Aid to the Investigation of Peripheral Nerve Injuries. ed. 2, rev. Medical Research, Memorandum #7. Her Majesty's Stationary Office, London.
2. Bateman, J. E.: The Shoulder and Neck. Philadelphia, W. B. Saunders, 1972.
3. Brain, A., and Wilkinson, M.: Cervical Spondylosis. Philadelphia W. B. Saunders, 1967.
4. Calliet, R.: Shoulder Pain. Philadelphia, F. A. Davis Company, 1966.
5. Compere, C. L., and Banks, S. W.: Pictorial Handbook of Fracture Treatment. ed. 5. Chicago, Year Book Medical Publishers, 1963.
6. Debakey, M. E., and Simeon, F. A.: Acute Battle Anterior Injuries in Surgery in World War II. Vascular Surgery, Medical Department, U.S. Army, Washington, U.S. Government Printing Office, 1965.
7. Kopell, H. P., and Thompson, W.: Peripheral Entrapment Neuropathies. Baltimore, Williams and Wilkins, 1973.
8. Lord, J. W., and Rosanti, L. M.: Neurovascular Compression Syndromes of the Upper Extremity. CIBA Clinical Symposium, Vol. 102, March-April, 1966.
9. Moseley, H. F.: Shoulder Lesions. ed. 3. Baltimore, Williams and Wilkins, 1969.
10. Rang, Mercer: Children's Fractures. Philadelphia, J. B. Lippincott Company, 1974.
11. Rockwood, C. A., Jr., and Green, D. P.: Fractures. vols. 1 and 2. Philadelphia, J. B. Lippincott Co., 1975.
12. Steindeler, A.: Lectures on the Interpretation of Pain in Orthopaedic Practice. Charles C Thomas, Ill., 1959.
13. Quiring, D. P.: Collateral Circulation. Philadelphia, Lea & Febiger, 1969.

9 The Upper Extremity: Elbow, Forearm, Wrist and Hand

Robert G. Chuinard, M.D.

The function of the hand is not only dependent on the bones, joints, and muscles of the hand but also on the integrity of the nervous system from the motor and sensory cortices in the brain out to the fingertips. When assessing function of the upper extremity, the examiner should keep in mind that peripheral manifestations of more proximal or central lesions must be considered as part of the differential diagnosis. These more proximal problems are discussed in the chapters on the cervical spine and the shoulder, so we will deal with the evaluation of the upper extremity from the elbow joint distally. Since the function of the upper extremity is to place the hand in a useful position, an appraisal of hand function requires a knowledge of the anatomy of the entire upper extremity.

ANATOMY

BONE AND JOINT

The three major bones of the upper extremity are the humerus, radius, and ulna. There are eight carpal bones in the wrist, and listed in order from the radial to ulnar side, in the proximal row there is the scaphoid (navicular), lunate, triquetrum, and the pisiform at the terminus of the flexor carpi ulnaris tendon. The bones of the distal row are the trapezium and trapezoid (the greater and lesser multangulars), capitate, and hamate. Distal to the carpus are the five metacarpals. The thumb has a proximal and distal phalanx; the index, middle, ring, and little fingers each have a proximal, middle, and distal phalanx (Fig. 9-1).

The elbow joint actually is comprised of three separate joints. The first (a hinge joint) is between the ulna and the humerus and this allows flexion and extension of the forearm through an arc of 0 degrees to approximately 160 degrees. The radiohumeral joint is primarily a gliding joint which allows flexion and extension of the forearm and also permits pronation and supination of the radius through an arc of approximately 180 degrees around the central limb of the ulna. Rotational motion of the radius around the ulna is also allowed by the third portion of the elbow joint, the proximal radioulnar joint.

The palpable bony landmarks about the elbow joint are the medial and lateral epicondyles of the humerus, the olecranon process of the ulna, and the radial head on the lateral aspect of the proximal forearm just distal to the lateral epicondyle (Fig. 9-2). The spheroidal-shaped capitulum on the lateral epicondyle fits into the cup-shaped radial head. The grooved trochlea on the medial epicondyle articulates with the trochlear notch of the proximal ulna. The lateral epicondyle is the most proximal point of origin of the extensor muscles of the forearm and hand, while the medial epicondyle is the most proximal point of origin for the flexor muscles of the forearm and hand. The elbow joint is completely invested in a capsular ligament which is stronger on its medial and lateral aspects than the anterior and posterior aspects. The lateral ligament takes its origin from the lateral epicondyle in close relation to the overlying common origin of the extensor muscles and passes distally to blend into the anular ligament of the radius as well as more distally on the lateral aspect of the olecranon process of the ulna. The medial ligament arises from the medial epicondyle with the common origin of the superficial flexor

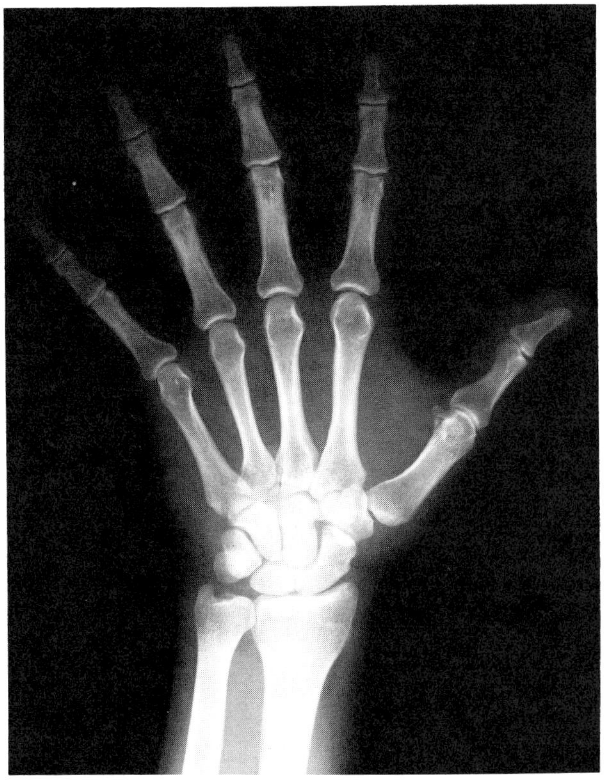

Fig. 9-1. Bones of the wrist and hand. The proximal carpal row from radial to ulnar side are the scaphoid, lunate, triquetrum, and pisiform. The distal carpal row from radial to ulnar side are the trapezium, trapezoid, capitate, and hamate. Distal to the carpus are the five metacarpals. The thumb has a proximal and distal phalanx; the index, middle, ring, and little fingers each have a proximal, middle, and distal phalanx.

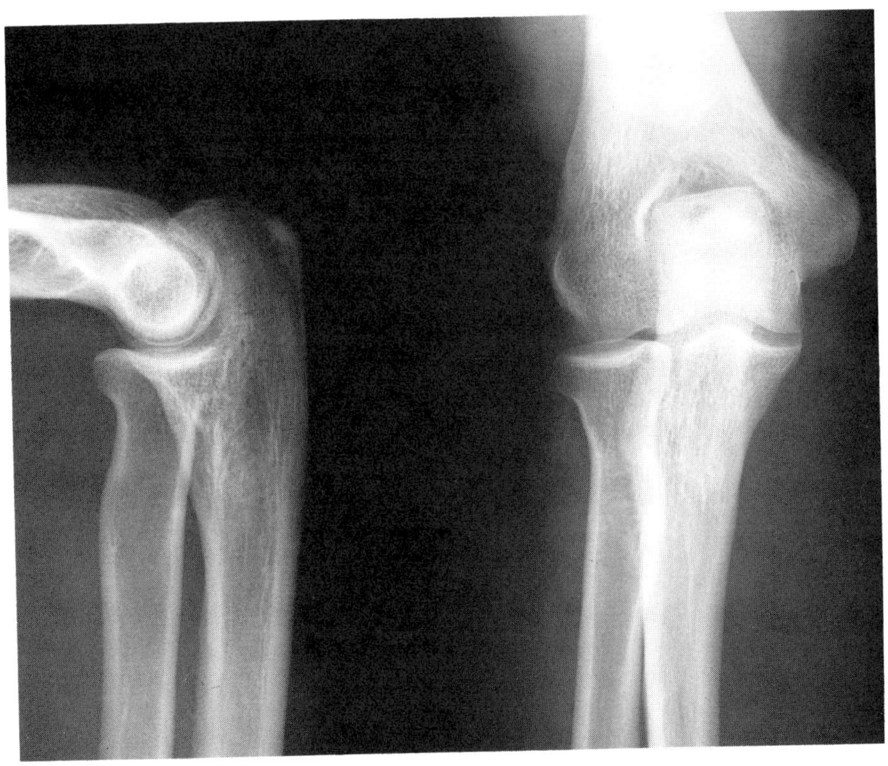

Fig. 9-2. Radiograph of elbow and forearm: (*left*) lateral view; (*right*) anteroposterior view. The palpable bony landmarks above the elbow joint are the medial and lateral epicondyles of the humerus, the olecranon process of the ulna, and the radial head on the lateral aspect of the proximal forearm just distal to the lateral epicondyle. The spheroidal-shaped capitulum on the lateral epicondyle fits into the cup-shaped radial head. The grooved trochlea on the medial epicondyle articulates with the trochlear notch of the proximal ulna.

muscles and passes distally to insert in the coronoid process and olecranon. A strong coronoid-olecranon ligament is also present which forms the base of the cubital tunnel through which the ulnar nerve penetrates from the arm into the forearm. The proximal radioulnar joint is a gliding type joint in which the head of the radius rotates in the radial notch of the medial aspect of the proximal ulnar. The anular ligament of the proximal radius is a well-defined, strong fibrous band which attaches to the anterior and posterior margins of the radial notch of the ulna and surrounds the head of the radius holding it firmly within the joint. Just distal to the proximal radioulnar joint is the tuberosity of the radius which serves as the point of insertion for the tendon of the biceps muscle. This tendon is easily palpable in the antecubital area in conjunction with the broad bicipital aponeurosis or lacertus fibrosus. The brachial artery can also be palpated approximately three finger breadths proximal to the medial epicondyle and medial to the biceps muscle and tendon.

In the anatomical position, the radial side of the forearm is lateral and the ulnar side is medial. With the ability of the forearm to pronate and supinate, this distinction sometimes becomes blurred when dealing with the actual examination of the patient. Therefore, for clarity, in the remainder of this chapter, the terms "medial" and "lateral" will only be used when no possibility of confusion exists. All relationships will be routinely defined as radial for lateral and ulnar for medial.

Proceeding distally in the forearm, the next joint encountered is the wrist which is a four-joint complex. The first part is the distal radioulnar joint which enables the forearm to pronate and supinate. The joint is formed by the distal end of the ulna and the ulnar notch on the distal radius. Weak transverse dorsal and volar capsular ligaments are present, but the chief uniting structure is the triangular-shaped articular disk called the triradiate cartilage.

The remaining wrist joint complex is comprised of three different levels (radiocarpal, intercarpal, and carpometacarpal) and should be considered as one unit. The major portion of wrist motion occurs at the radiocarpal joint and will be considered as the joint of reference. Normal flexion and extension movements at this joint are between 60 and 80 degrees, and when combined with approximately 35 degrees of ulnar deviation and 15 degrees of radial deviation, the hand is able to circumduct through a wide range of motion on the forearm.

The two most prominent bony landmarks about the wrist joint are the radial and ulnar styloid processes. Normally there is an 18 to 25 degree angle between the two styloids as measured from a direct transverse line, with the ulnar styloid lying more proximal. On the volar surface, just at the level of the distal wrist crease and proximal to the palm, is the easily palpable pisiform bone which is the terminus of the flexor carpi ulnaris tendon.

The carpometacarpal joints, with the exception of the first metacarpotrapezial joint, have little or no motion, especially between the second and third metacarpals and the trapezoid and capitate bones with which they articulate. Further discussion of the carpometacarpal relationships will be taken up later in the discussion of the arches of the hand.

The first metacarpotrapezial joint is a unique joint in the human body. It is located beneath the anatomical snuff box which is formed by the abductor pollicis longus, extensor pollicis brevis, and extensor pollicis longus tendons. The surfaces of the joint are each saddle-shaped, forming a reciprocal biconcave articulation. This particular configuration allows the thumb to move through a range of approximately 70 to 80 degrees of circumduction so that the tip of the thumb can be brought into a position of opposition to the tips of each of the fingers.

The metacarpophalangeal joints of the hand are easily palpable, and with the fingers in flexion, the heads of the second, third, fourth, and fifth metacarpals form the prominent knuckles. The proximal interphalangeal and distal interphalangeal joints are ginglymus (gliding-hinge) joints, just as are the metacarpophalangeal joints; however, radial and ulnar deviation (abduction and adduction) motions are not possible, as at the metacarpophalangeal joints. These joints are all invested by a circumferential capsular ligament and supported on the sides by strong radial and ulnar collateral ligaments.

There are two arches in the hand (Fig. 9-3). The longitudinal arch of the hand is the static arch around which all motion takes place. This arch is composed of the second and third metacarpal rays and their articulations with the trapezoid and capitate and with each other at their bases. The transverse arch of the hand is the mobile arch around which metacarpal motion occurs. On the radial side of the second and third metacarpals it is composed of the first metacarpal and its metacarpotrapezial joint which allow up to 80 degrees of circumduction. On the ulnar side it is composed of the heads of the fourth and fifth metacarpals; motion between the fourth and fifth metacarpal bases and the hamate allows an arc of approximately 30 degrees for the fifth metacarpal and approximately 15 degrees for the fourth metacarpal. Hence, the longitudinal arch is the support about which the mobile arch moves.

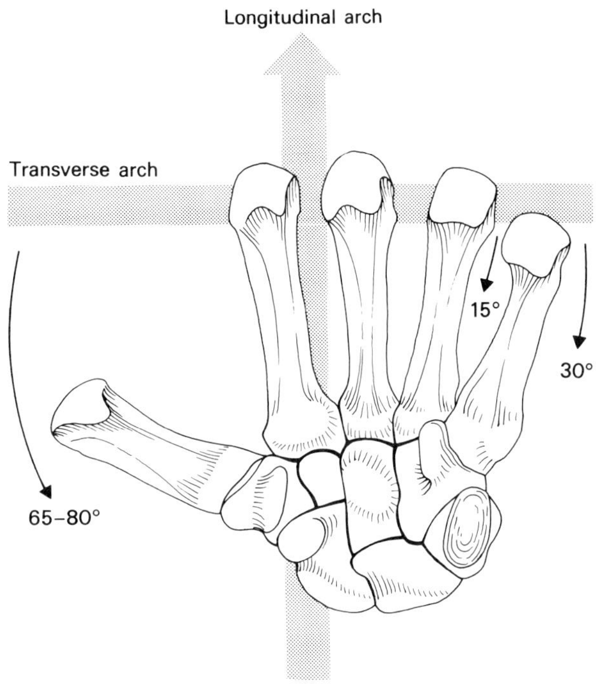

Fig. 9-3. Arches of the hand. The static longitudinal arch is composed of the second and third metacarpal rays and their articulations with the triquetrum and capitate. The transverse or adaptive arch of the hand is mobile; this motion occurs about the longitudinal arch.

MUSCLE AND TENDON

The principal muscles about the elbow joint are the biceps, triceps, and brachialis which have their origin in the upper arm and insert distally in the proximal forearm. The united bellies of the biceps insert through a strong tendon on the tubercle of the radius. From the anteromedial aspect of the tendon, a strong fibrous band spreads in an ulnar and distal direction over the hollow of the cubital fossa to attach in the fascia which covers the origins of the flexor and pronator muscles of the forearm. This is the bicipital aponeurosis or lacertus fibrosus. The more superficial fibers can be palpated in conjunction with the biceps tendon as it crosses in front of the brachial artery and median nerve.

The brachialis muscle at the level of the distal humerus is obscured by the body of the biceps. It inserts by a strong tendon onto the lower surface of the coronoid process and tuberosity of the ulna. The major portion of the insertion is covered by the pronator teres muscle.

The triceps muscle is the only muscle on the back of the arm. The three heads of origin insert through a common tendon, extending across the posterior aspect of the elbow joint, into the proximal surface of the olecranon process of the ulna. A second muscle aiding in extension of the elbow joint is the anconeus. This small triangular muscle has its origin on the distal part of the posterior aspect of the lateral epicondyle of the humerus and the posterior ligament of the elbow joint. It inserts by rather fleshy, nontendinous fibers onto the lateral side of the olecranon process.

The brachialis muscle is the most powerful flexor of the elbow joint but is assisted in this action by the biceps, brachioradialis, and pronator teres. The biceps also acts as a weak flexor of the shoulder and is a strong supinator of the proximal radioulnar joint. The triceps is the principal extensor of the elbow joint. The anconeus, while acting as an extensor, aids in seating the ulna into the trochlear groove of the humerus.

The muscles of the forearm will be discussed in two separate ways: first in terms of their anatomical relationships, both at the proximal level (Fig. 9-4) of their origin and again at the level of the wrist joint (Fig. 9-5); secondly, there will be a more or less schematic discussion with the neuromuscular relationships of the forearm and hand.

The flexor muscles of the forearm and hand are located on the anterior and anteromedial aspect of the forearm. At their origin (see Fig. 9-4) they are found in three more or less distinct layers: the superficial layer consists of those muscles which take their origin from a common tendon which attaches to the medial epicondyle of the humerus. From the radial to ulnar side they are: the pronator teres, flexor carpi radialis, palmaris longus and flexor carpi ulnaris. The

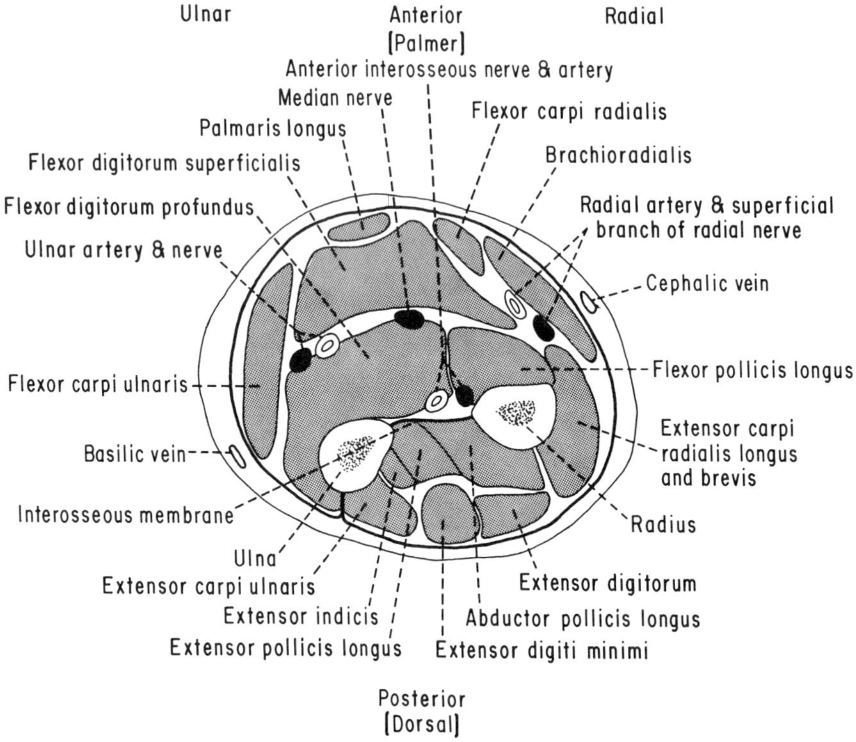

Fig. 9-4. Transverse section of right forearm at a level 2 cm. distal to the elbow joint viewed from proximal to distal.

intermediate muscle layer consists entirely of the flexor digitorum superficialis muscles. The deep layer consists of the flexor digitorum profundus, the flexor pollicis longus and pronator quadratus.

At the level of the wrist joint (see Fig. 9-5) the flexor muscle bellies have now given way to tendons. The most superficial tendon is the palmaris longus, and it can be palpated just proximal to its insertion into the palmar fascia. This tendon is unilaterally absent in 5 to 7 percent of the population and absent

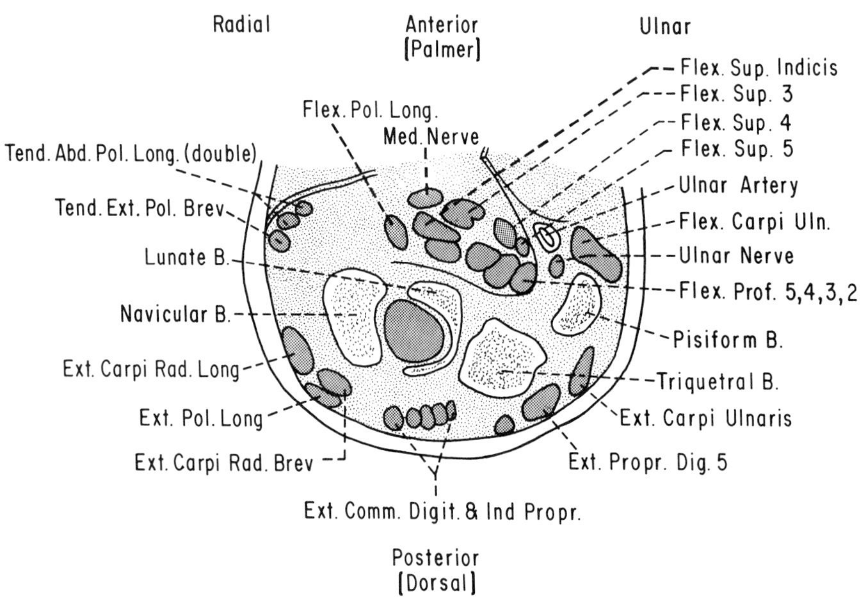

Fig. 9-5. Transverse section of right forearm at the level of carpal canal viewed from distal to proximal.

bilaterally in 11 percent of the population. When present, this tendon is of great importance in identifying the location of the median nerve; at the level of the wrist joint, the nerve lies directly beneath the palmaris longus tendon.

On the ulnar side of the wrist, the flexor carpi ulnaris tendon can be identified easily by palpation proximal to the pisiform. Distally, the tendon inserts through two tough fibrous bands; the first is the pisohamate ligament which forms the roof of the canal of Guyon, and the second is the pisometacarpal ligament which inserts into the base of the fifth metacarpal. On the radial aspect of the palmaris longus tendon, the flexor carpi radialis can be easily palpated as it traverses the wrist joint to insert onto the base of the second metacarpal. Just radial to the tendon of the flexor carpi radialis, the radial pulse can be palpated.

The remaining flexor tendons are those to the thumb and fingers. Along with the median nerve, they are contained within the carpal canal at the level of the wrist joint. The carpal canal is a bony arch formed by the tubercle of the scaphoid and crest of the trapezium on the radial side and the pisiform and the hook of the hamate on the ulnar side. The floor of the canal is formed by the bodies of the capitate and lunate bones, and the deep flexor retinaculum forms the anterior surface. The median nerve traverses the carpal canal in the most superficial radial position. Just beneath it on the radial side is the tendon of the flexor pollicis longus. On the floor of the carpal canal are the four profundus tendons to the index, middle, ring and little fingers. Lying superficial to the profundus tendons and ulnar to the median nerve are the four tendons of the superficialis group. They are arranged so that the superficial tendons to the middle and ring fingers lie on top of the superficial tendons to the index and little fingers.

The extensor muscles of the wrist and hand are found on the dorsum of the forearm. Proximally, at the level of the elbow joint (see Fig. 9-4) they are divided into a superficial and a deep layer. The superficial muscles extending from the radial to the ulnar side are the brachioradialis, extensor carpi radialis longus and brevis, extensor digitorum, extensor digiti minimi, and extensor carpi ulnaris. The five muscles of the deep layer are the supinator, extensor pollicis longus, extensor pollicis brevis, abductor pollicis longus, and extensor indicis.

At the level of the wrist (see Fig. 9-5) is a strong dorsal carpal ligament which varies from 2 to 3 cm. in width, and through various compartmentations in its deep layer, it contains the extensor tendons. Starting on the radial border of the wrist, the first tunnel contains the two tendons of the abductor pollicis longus and extensor pollicis brevis. Superficial to this is the tunnel for the extensor pollicis longus; as these three tendons triangulate from the level of the wrist joint, they form the anatomic snuff box. The next most ulnar compartment contains the two tendons of the extensor carpi radialis longus and brevis. The longus tendon can be palpated inserting into the base of the second metacarpal, and the brevis tendon can be palpated inserting into the base of the third metacarpal. The next most ulnar compartment contains the common extensor tendon with slips to the index, middle, ring, and little fingers, and beneath this the tendon of the extensor indicis proprius. The next compartment contains the tendon to the extensor digiti quinti, and the most ulnar and last compartment constains the tendon to the extensor carpi ulnaris. The compartments can be identified by remembering the following "number game": 2-1-2-2-1-1.

The muscles of the hand are primarily located on the volar surface, although the interossei, as their name implies, lie between the shafts of the metacarpals. The muscles in the hand can best be considered in three separate groups: the first group is comprised of the thenar muscles, the second group comprises the hypothenar muscles, and the third group comprise the interossei, lumbricals, and adductor of the thumb.

The abductor pollicis brevis is the most radial and superficial muscle of the thenar eminence. This muscle has a broad origin from the distal border of the volar carpal ligament and inserts through a small tendon which is adherent to the radial aspect of the joint capsule of the metacarpophalangeal joint of the thumb. The flexor pollicis brevis is located adjacent to the abductor brevis and on the ulnar aspect of the opponens pollicis. It has two heads of origin; the more superficial radial head takes its origin from the distal lateral border of the volar carpal ligament and the anterior surface of the tunnel of the flexor carpi radialis near the insertion of its tendon into the base of the second metacarpal. The deeper, more ulnar head, arises from the anterior surface of the trapezoid and appears continuous in its origin with the oblique portion of the adductor pollicis. The two heads unite and come to lie radial forming a trough for passage of the flexor pollicis longus tendon. The fibers of insertion extend the central length of the volar capsule of the metacarpophalangeal joint of the thumb where they also insert into the radial sesmoid of the flexor pollicis longus and the radial tubercle of the base of the proximal phalanx; a broad expansion is sent to the dorsal apparatus of the extensor mechanism of the thumb. The opponens pollicis muscle takes its origin immediately beneath the abductor pollicis brevis along the volar carpal ligament, ridge of the trapezium, and the capsule of the metacarpotrapezial joint. The tendon of insertion is broad; it runs in an oblique course in a radial and distal direction along the volar radial aspect of the first metacarpal.

The adductor pollicis muscle, although moving the thumb, is not of the thenar muscle group, and in terms of its nerve supply from the ulnar nerve, should be considered an intrinsic muscle. It has two heads of origin: a transverse head and oblique head. The transverse head originates from the crest of the third metacarpal in the area of the neck just proximal to the metacarpophalangeal joint. The oblique head arises from the intercarpal ligaments covering the capitate and trapezoid and the tunnel of the flexor carpi radialis as well as the volar fascia overlying the third metacarpal. The muscle traverses the deep part of the palm in an ulnar direction toward its insertion on the ulnar sesamoid of the flexor pollicis longus and the base of the proximal phalanx of the thumb.

The muscles of the hypothenar eminence consist of the abductor digiti quinti, the flexor digiti brevis, and opponens digiti quinti. The most important of these three muscles is the abductor digiti quinti which takes its origin primarily from the pisiform and the pisohamate ligament. The muscle inserts into the ulnar tubercle of the proximal phalanx of the little finger, with a secondary slip into the dorsal apparatus of the proximal joint of the little finger. The flexor digiti quinti brevis and the opponens digiti quinti both take their origin in the area of the hook of the hamate and insert into the ulnar aspect of the shaft of the metacarpal and the proximal phalanx.

The intrinsic muscles of the fingers are extremely important for normal function. They consist of the four dorsal interossei, the three volar interossei, and the four lumbricals. The distinction between palmar and dorsal interossei is based on the location of the origin on the metacarpal in relation to the longitudinal axis of the hand which passes through the third metacarpal and middle finger and the way it moves the finger away from or toward this central axis.

The dorsal interosseous muscles are bipenate muscles with each muscle belly originating from an adjacent metacarpal. The tendon inserts onto the side of the phalanx that is furthest from the longitudinal axis. In this way the dorsal interossei act as abductors of the fingers away from the midline. The key to understanding the function of the dorsal interossei is to remember that the middle finger can only abduct away from the longitudinal axis; that is, it abducts either in a radial direction or an ulnar direction. Radial abduction is performed by the second dorsal interosseous and ulnar abduction is performed by the third dorsal interosseous. Hence, the first dorsal interosseous muscle abducts the index finger in a radial direction, and the fourth dorsal interosseous muscle abducts the ring finger in an ulnar direction. The little finger is abducted by the abductor digiti quinti as noted above.

The volar interossei are unipenate muscles originating as a single muscle belly from the ulnar two thirds of the metacarpal shaft on the side of the metacarpal closest to the axis of the hand. Their insertion is on the same side of the proximal phalanx as that of their origin so that they act as adductors of the fingers. The first volar interosseous muscle adducts the index finger in an ulnar direction toward the midline. The second and third volar interosseous muscles adduct the ring and little fingers, respectively, toward the midline of the longitudial axis in a radial direction. Remember, the middle finger can only be abducted; therefore, no volar interosseous muscles are associated with its function.

The four lumbrical muscles take their origin from the radial side of the flexor digitorum profundus tendons to the index, middle, ring, and little fingers. The muscle fibers of the lumbricals run in conjunction with the flexor tendons toward the radial side of the fingers until the tendons enter the proximal pulleys at the level of the midpalmar crease. With the exception of the first lumbrical, the tendons cross the deep transverse intermetacarpal ligament with the digital nerves and vessels and insert as a portion of the wing tendon into the extensor apparatus on the dorsum of the finger. The first lumbrical has no intermetacarpal ligament in association with it; however, it does maintain its relationship with the neurovascular bundle. As the lumbricals pass from the palmar aspect of the hand they lie beneath the axis of rotation of the metacarpophalangeal joint. In this position, they function as active flexors of the metacarpophalangeal joint.

Nine flexor tendons pass through the carpal canal from the forearm into the hand, a common synovial sheath called the ulnar bursa surrounds the flexor digitorum profundus and superficialis tendons, and a separate synovial sheath called the radial bursa surrounds the flexor pollicis longus tendon. This latter synovial sheath continues out the length of the tendon into its point of insertion at the base of the distal phalanx of the thumb. Usually, the synovial sheath surrounding the flexor digitorum profundus and superficialis tendons has a continuation along the flexor tendons to the little finger out to its point of insertion. The synovial sheaths surrounding the flexors of the index, middle, and ring fingers usually are not connected to the wrist synovium but begin at the level of the proximal pulley and extend distally along the tendons to their point of insertion.

At the level of the midpalmar crease on the palm of the hand (which overlies the metacarpophalangeal joint) the flexor tendons enter a strong fibrous sheath which is divided into thick and thin areas. The thick areas comprise the pulleys. The proximal pulley is located near the base of the proximal phalanx; the middle pulley is located over the distal end of the proximal phalanx, and the distal pulley is located in the middle of the middle phalanx. At the level of the origin of the tendon sheath, the superficialis tendon lies in a volar position on top of the profundus tendon. At the level of the midportion of the proximal phalanx, the superficialis tendon splits and is penetrated by the profundus tendon. This split in the sublimis tendon is called the chiasm of Camper. The divided superficialis tendon then inserts along the volar aspect of the middle phalanx; the profundus tendon proceeds onto its insertion into the base of the distal phalanx.

The pulleys formed by the thickened portion of the flexor tendon sheath act as tethers holding the tendons against bone during active flexion. This maintains the mechanical advantage of the tendons, and prevents "bow-stringing" across the joint. The sheath is narrowest and most confining in the area from the metacarpophalangeal joint to the proximal interphalangeal joint. This is the area which Bunnell called "no man's land," indicating that no attempt at primary tendon repair should be made in this area.

The flexor digitorum profundus tendon has a specific function: flexing the distal joint of the finger. The profundus to the index finger has a separate muscle belly of origin; however, the profundus tendons to the middle, ring, and little fingers have a more or less common belly of origin. The flexor digitorum superficialis tendons, each originating from an individual muscle belly, have the specific function of flexing the proximal interphalangeal joint of the finger. The flexor pollicis longus tendon flexes the interphalangeal joint of the thumb.

The extensor mechanism of the fingers is somewhat more complex than that of the flexors. The extensor digitorum communis originates more or less as a common muscle belly and divides into four common extensor tendons to the index, middle, ring, and little fingers just distal to the dorsal retinaculum. Proximal to the metacarpophalangeal joints, short oblique slips, called the junctura tendinum, connect these common extensor tendons. Independent extension of the index and little fingers is provided by the extensor indicis proprius and extensor digiti quinti proprius tendons, respectively. At the level of the metacarpophalangeal joint, all extensor tendons become intimately involved with the "dorsal extensor apparatus." In conjunction with the tendons of the interossei and lumbricals, they form the extensor mechanism for the proximal and distal interphalangeal joints.

At the level of the metacarpophalangeal joint, the extensor digitorum communis tendon is held in the midline by the extensor hood. This hood is arcuate in appearance, with the fibers running more or less perpendicular to those of the extensor tendon. They attach directly into the substance of the extensor and help to keep it in a midline position. At the level of the metacarpophalangeal joint, small filamentous fibers from the extensor tendon insert into the capsule at the level of the base of the proximal phalanx. The fibers of the extensor hood fan out to form the dorsal aponeurotic membrane which essentially attaches the tendons of the interosseous and lumbrical muscles to the extensor mechanism over the proximal interphalangeal joint. Just proximal to the level of this joint, the extensor tendon provides slips to the lateral bands which are formed by a combination of these slips and the intrinsic muscle tendons. The central slip of the extensor tendon traverses across the proximal interphalangeal joint to insert into the dorsum of the proximal end of the middle phalanx. The lateral bands continue distally over the middle phalanx to insert across the distal interphalangeal joint into the base of the dorsum of the distal phalanx.

The extensor pollicis longus tendon traverses the wrist joint around Lister's tubercle and forms the dorsal border of the anatomical snuff box. At the level of the metacarpophalangeal joint of the thumb, it is held in position by the dorsal hood, similar to that of the metacarpophalangeal joints of the finger. It then proceeds across the interphalangeal joint of the thumb to insert at the base of the distal phalanx. The extensor pollicis brevis, along with the abductor pollicis longus, forms the volar margin of the anatomical snuff box at the level of the wrist joint. This tendon is the smaller of the two and is located dorsal to that of the abductor pollicis longus. It then runs along the radial aspect of the first metacarpal, crosses the metacarpophalangeal joint, and inserts into the dorsum of the base of the proximal phalanx of the thumb. The abductor pollicis longus forms the most inferior border of the anatomical snuff box. It inserts in the base of the first metacarpal, on the radial side, just distal to the metacarpotrapezial joint. An accessory tendon slip of the abductor pollicis longus inserts into the fascia overlying the abductor pollicis brevis.

VASCULAR

At the level of the elbow joint, the brachial artery divides into the radial and ulnar arteries which supply the vascularity to the forearm and hand. Just proximal to the elbow, the brachial artery can be palpated beneath the biceps tendon and lacertus fibrosus where it lies on the brachialis muscle. At this level, it is in close contact with the median nerve which lies just medial to it. After traversing the antecubital fossa, the brachial artery divides into the smaller radial artery and the larger ulnar artery.

Arising from the brachial artery at the level of the distal third of the humerus is the profunda brachii artery which turns posteriorly behind the humerus, dividing into anterior and posterior terminal branches just proximal to the supracondylar area. The anterior branch anastomoses with the radial recurrent artery, and the posterior branch anastomoses with the interosseous recurrent artery. These anastomoses form the recurrent arterial system on the radial side of the elbow joint.

Distal to the origin of the profunda brachii artery lies the origin of the ulnar collateral artery and the supratrochlear artery; these two arteries form the proximal side of the arterial anastomoses on the ulnar side of the elbow joint. Each of these arteries anastomoses with an ulnar recurrent artery which comes off immediately after the division of the brachial artery into the radial and ulnar arteries.

The radial artery traverses the forearm superficial to the radial portion of the flexor digitorum superficialis and flexor pollicis longus muscles; it lies beneath the brachioradialis muscle in the proximal half of the forearm and beneath the forearm skin and fascia in the distal half. As it traverses the forearm, it supplies the muscles on the radial side. At the level of the wrist, the artery divides into the deep branch and the superficial palmar branch which later anastomoses with the superficial ulnar artery to form the superficial palmar arch. The deep branch curves around the radial side to the dorsum of the wrist, beneath the tendons of the abductor pollicis longus, extensor pollicis brevis, and extensor pollicis longus and over the top of the scaphoid and trapezial bones. It penetrates the hand between the two heads of the first dorsal interosseous muscle and lies deep to the oblique head of the adductor pollicis. After giving off the princeps pollicis artery, which divides to form the digital arteries to the thumb, it anastomoses with the deep branch of the ulnar artery to form the deep palmar arch.

The ulnar artery begins in the cubital fossa and penetrates into the forearm beneath the ulnar head of the pronator teres. After giving off the ulnar recurrent arteries, the common interosseous artery is encountered. This branch divides to form the anterior and posterior interosseous arteries which lie on the volar and dorsal surfaces of the interosseous membrane, respectively. The main branch then comes to lie on top of the ulnar aspect of the flexor digitorum profundus muscle, beneath the flexor digitorum superficialis muscle, and just medial to the ulnar nerve.

The artery penetrates the hand, through Guyon's canal where it divides into the superficial and deep branches. As noted above, each branch anastomoses with the respective branch of the radial artery to form the superficial and deep palmar arches.

The superficial palmar arch, which lies just beneath the palmar fascia at the level of the base of the thumb, supplies the common digital arteries to the second, third, and fourth web spaces. These common digital arteries bifurcate at the level of the web space and supply the contiguous sides of adjacent fingers just as the digital nerves do. The ulnar side of the little finger is supplied by a separate digital artery which has its origin from the superficial branch of the ulnar artery.

The deep palmar arch, lying beneath the oblique head of the adductor pollicis at the level of the midpalmar crease, is the source of the previously noted princeps pollicis artery as well as the digital artery to the radial side of the index finger. The deep arch gives off three deep metacarpal arteries which are similar in configuration to the common digital arteries of the superficial arch. At the level of the metacarpophalangeal joints, there are usually anastomotic connections between the deep metacarpal arteries and the superficial common digital arteries.

RETINACULAR SYSTEM

As its name implies, the function of the retinacular system in the hand is to maintain the various anatomic parts of the hand in position for optimum function and to protect them from injury. This system of fascial layers serves as containers for the moving structures dividing the hand into functional or structural components.

Immediately beneath the skin over the thenar and hypothenar eminence lie the thick subcutaneous fat pads. These fat pads act as cushions, protecting the underlying neurovascular and muscular structures. They are compartmentalized by the fibrous strands which unite the skin to the underlying fascia of the muscles. These fibrous strands also attach the skin of the central palm to the thick palmar fascia. In the hypothenar fat pad are the fibers of the palmaris brevis muscle.

In the center of the palm, contiguous with the palmaris longus tendon insertion, is the thick midpalmar fascia. It is triangular in shape, extending from the deep transverse volar carpal ligament to the level of the metacarpophalangeal joints of the index, middle, ring, and little fingers. It consists of two layers. The longitudinal fibers, called the pretendinous bands, run parallel with and are superficial to the flexor tendons of the fingers. The longitudinal bands are connected by short vertical fibers from the overlying skin of the palm to the underlying tendon sheaths and bone. Lying between these longitudinal fibers are thin, strong transverse fibers which act as interconnectors between the pretendinous bands. These fibers blend into the transverse fibers of the superficial transverse ligament at the level of the metacarpophalangeal joints. Just distal to the transverse fibers are the natatory ligament fibers which band the interdigital folds between the fingers. The natatory ligament continues directly into the fingers investing the digital artery and nerve and combines with the skin ligaments of Clelland. These natatory ligament fibers connect the palmar fascia and the structurally similar digital fascia.

The fascial layers in the hand help to divide the palm of the hand into two important spaces: the thenar and midpalmar spaces. These potential spaces are deep within the hand and are located beneath the tendons and in front of the metacarpals. The thenar space occupies the radial side of the hand and is limited on the ulnar side by the fascial attachment of the flexor tendon sheath of the middle finger to the underlying third metacarpal. It lies essentially on top of, and is directed toward, the thumb, along the course of the adductor pollicis muscle. Distally, there is potential expansion into the inner-digital folds through the first and second lumbrical muscle canals. The midpalmar space lies ulnar to the septum attaching the middle finger flexor tendons to the third metacarpal and is limited on its ulnar border by the hypothenar fascia. This space also opens distally through the course of the third and fourth lumbrical muscles.

A third space, Parona's space, is located in the lower forearm and is directly juxtaposed to the distal radial and ulnar synovial bursas of the flexor tendons. It lies beneath the flexor digitorum profundus tendons and on top of the pronator quadratus fascia. Laterally it is limited by the flexor carpi radialis and medially by the flexor carpi ulnaris. The distal limit of the space is potentially open through the carpal canal into the hand. However, this communication is usually limited by the synovial bursas of the flexor tendons.

NEUROMUSCULAR RELATIONSHIPS

Paramount in examining the upper extremity is having a clear and correct understanding of the neuromuscular anatomy of the forearm and hand. A schematic type of diagram is helpful in remembering the relationships.

MEDIAN NERVE

The median nerve (Fig. 9-6) penetrates the forearm between the two heads of the pronator teres muscle to which it provides nerve supply. The nerve to the pronator teres branches off prior to penetration of the muscle and at the same time as the nerve to the flexor carpi radialis. The flexor carpi radialis and palmaris longus muscles along with the flexor digitorum superficialis muscle belly now lie anterior to the median nerve and are supplied by branches from the nerve. Shortly after exiting the pronator teres, the median nerve divides into the anterior interosseous

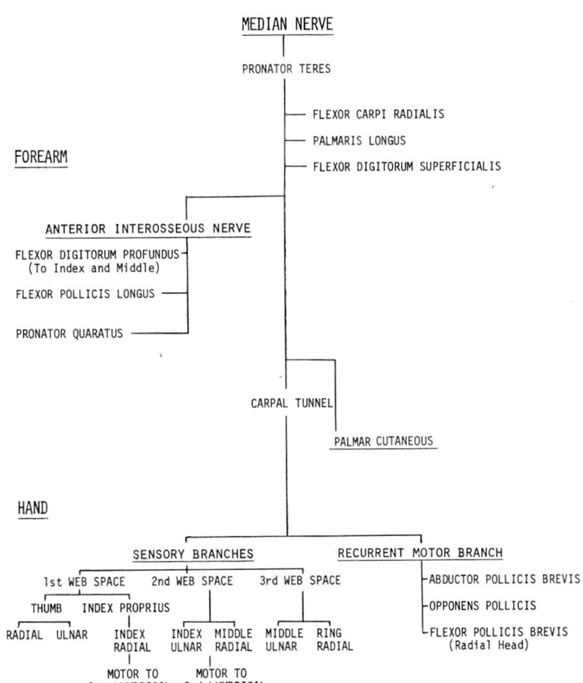

Fig. 9-6. Schematic representation of median nerve in the forearm and hand.

nerve and the continuation of the median nerve. The anterior interosseous nerve penetrates the body of the flexor digitorum profundus muscle belly to the index and middle fingers and supplies these two muscles. It continues on, lying anterior to the interosseous membrane in conjunction with the anterior interosseous artery, and supplies the flexor pollicis longus muscle and the pronator quadratus muscle. The anterior interosseous nerve terminates as small sensory twigs to the wrist joint.

The median nerve continues its course down the forearm lying superficial to the flexor digitorum profundus muscle bellies and beneath the flexor digitorum superficialis muscle belly. At the level of the wrist joint it comes to lie in a radial position relative to the tendons of the flexor digitorum superficialis and beneath the palmaris longus tendon. Immediately after coming out of the carpal canal, the median nerve gives off the recurrent motor branch from its radial dorsal margin. The recurrent motor branch provides the nerve supply to the abductor pollicis brevis, the opponens pollicis, and the radial head of the flexor pollicis brevis. Two small motor branches are also given off to supply the first and second lumbrical muscles.

The remaining function of the median nerve is purely sensory. Just distal to the carpal canal it gives off a common sensory nerve which splits to provide sensibility to the radial and ulnar aspect of the volar surface of the thumb. The next sensory branch is the indicis proprius which provides sensibility to the radial aspect of the index finger. Two more sensory branches, the common digital to the second web space and the common digital to the third web space, divide at approximately the level of the transverse metacarpal ligament. The common digital nerve to the second web space supplies the ulnar half of the index finger and the radial half of the middle finger. The common digital nerve to the third web space supplies the ulnar side of the middle and the radial side of the ring fingers. In this manner, sensibility to the volar surface of the thumb, index, middle, and radial half of the ring finger is provided.

ULNAR NERVE

The ulnar nerve (Fig. 9-7) penetrates the forearm in the cubital groove beneath the medial epicondyle of the humerus. As it enters the forearm it passes between the humeral and ulnar heads of the flexor carpi ulnaris muscle which it supplies. It then travels the length of the forearm beneath the muscle belly of the flexor carpi ulnaris and on top of the muscle belly of the flexor digitorum profundus in close concert with the ulnar artery. It provides the motor nerves to the profundus muscles of the ring and little fingers. At the level of the wrist, it passes in a slightly radial direction to the pisiform bone and enters the hand through the canal of Guyon formed by the pisohamate ligament. At or just distal to the level of Guyon's canal, the ulnar nerve trifurcates. A common sensory branch gives rise to the ulnar sensory nerve to the little finger and the common digital nerve to the fourth web space. This latter nerve divides at the level of the transverse metacarpal ligament and provides sensibility to the radial border of the little finger and the ulnar border of the ring finger. A second branch supplies the motor function for the hypothenar muscles including the palmaris brevis. The third branch, the deep motor branch, provides motor function for the majority of the intrinsic muscles of the hand. It supplies the motor function to the volar and dorsal interossei, the adductor of the thumb, the ulnar head of the short thumb flexor, and the third and fourth lumbricals to the ring and little fingers, respectively.

Approximately 1 to 2 cm. proximal or distal to the ulnar styloid, the dorsal sensory branch of the ulnar nerve divides from the main trunk and courses around to the dorsum of the ulnar side of the hand at the level of or just distal to the ulnar styloid. It supplies sensibility to the dorsum of the hand and the little and ring fingers in exactly the same distribution as on the volar surface.

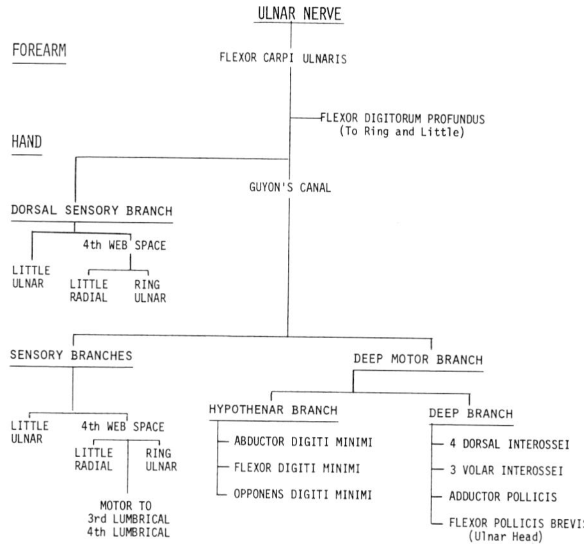

Fig. 9-7. Schematic representation of ulnar nerve in forearm and hand.

Radial Nerve

The radial nerve (Fig. 9-8) enters the forearm through the body of the supinator from a posteroradial position on the arm. As the nerve traverses the posterior aspect of the distal one third of the humerus through the spiral groove, it is subject to injury by fracture or trauma, and injury at this level usually produces a complete radial nerve palsy. Prior to penetrating the body of the supinator, the radial nerve gives off the nerve supply to the supinator, brachioradialis, and extensor carpi radialis longus. At a variable distance above or within the body of the supinator, the radial nerve divides into the posterior interosseous nerve and the dorsal radial sensory branch.

The dorsal sensory nerve continues distally on the dorsum of the forearm beneath the brachioradialis muscle belly and tendon. The nerve becomes superficial approximately 3 cm. proximal to the wrist joint, and at the level of the wrist joint it divides into multiple sensory branches which provide sensibility to the dorsum of the thumb, index, middle, and radial half of the ring fingers.

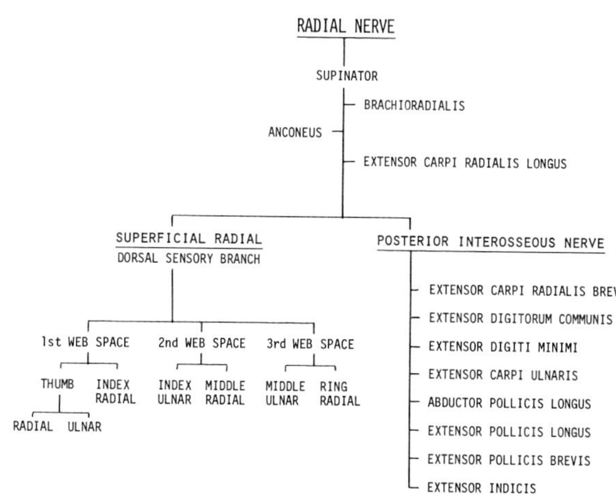

Fig. 9-8. Schematic representation of radial nerve in forearm and hand.

The posterior interosseous nerve continues down the forearm lying on the dorsal aspect of the interosseous membrane in conjunction with the posterior interosseous artery. This nerve supplies the motor function for the remainder of the extensor muscles of the forearm and hand. In order of supply from proximal to distal they are: the extensor carpi radialis brevis, extensor digitorum communis, extensor digiti quinti, extensor carpi ulnaris, extensor pollicis longus, extensor pollicis brevis, abductor pollicis longus, and extensor indicis.

REGIONAL EXAMINATION

The regional examination of the forearm and hand may be for a complaint in this area alone. However, problems more proximal to this region can be the underlying cause of signs and symptoms which are manifest in the hand. In any case, careful and detailed observations should be made, motions recorded, and comparisons made between the normal and abnormal extremities. If no differences exist, then a more central pathological condition should be expected. Qualifying adjectives, such as good, fair, and poor, should be eliminated whenever possible and precise measurements of motion and strength recorded on a flow sheet.

HISTORY

The first step in obtaining an accurate diagnosis is a careful and detailed history. Approximately 40 percent of all industrial injuries in this country today involve the hand, and a precise description of the mechanism of injury is a great aid in later evaluation of impairment of function and rating of the disability. If trauma is not involved, the date of onset of symptoms should be elicited. Once these facts have been established, close questioning as to the mechanism of the injury or the progression of symptoms should be done. Information as to swelling, bleeding, deformity, loss of function, and especially pain should be elicited. A detailed account of any previous treatment should be included in the history, and reports of previous operations should be obtained whenever possible. It is extremely important to elicit the history of any previous infection of the hand, especially postoperative infections. Included in the history are the occupation of the patient as well as his hobbies. The dominant hand should be recorded.

When questioning the patient, care should be taken to elicit a history of past trauma from which the patient has recovered. Late or tardy nerve palsies, tendon ruptures, and bony deformities may all be secondary to old trauma or trauma which the patient considered minor at the time. In this regard, old reoentgenograms can be a great help, especially for comparison to recent films.

Systemic diseases may be manifest in the hand by signs and symptoms which affect function. Such things as rheumatoid arthritis, diabetes, psoriasis, angina pectoris, and degenerative neuropathies may all affect the hand and forearm. It cannot be emphasized enough that careful questioning will help elicit an adequate history which will greatly aid in the diagnosis.

PHYSICAL EXAMINATION

Physical examination of the upper extremity actually begins in the cervical spine with the cervical nerve roots. It proceeds through an examination of the brachial plexus, shoulder joint region and continues with an examination of the upper arm. These areas are discussed in Chapters 6 and 8.

The examination should be conducted with the patient in a comfortable sitting position and the hands resting on a low examining table. The arms should be bare from at least the midarm distally.

Inspection

A visual examination is conducted of both upper extremities. Attention is first paid to the extremity about which the patient is complaining; this extremity is then compared with the opposite extremity. If the complaints are bilateral, symmetry or asymmetry between the involved areas is noted.

Deformity or Absence of Parts

Beginning at the elbow, the configuration of the carrying angle with the arm in full extension is noted. The normal carrying angle is a slight cubitus valgus which is greater in females than males. The normal is between 3 and 8 degrees; however, it can be as much as 15 or 20 degrees. Compare it with the opposite side and note any symmetry or asymmetry.

A reverse carrying angle or cubitus varus of anything more than 3 to 5 degrees is abnormal. Cubitus varus usually results from an incomplete or incorrect reduction of a lateral epicondylar or supracondylar fracture of the humerus which results in a malunion. It may also be due to dislocation of the radial head in a posterior position.

Deformity of the forearm is usually due to malunion of a fracture, although some congenital conditions, such as absence of the radius may cause some moderate to marked deformity. Wrist deformities are usually associated with old trauma, such as a malunited Colles' fracture or intraarticular disease processes such as rheumatoid arthritis or infectious arthritis. These deformities usually result in loss of motion.

Hand deformities are most often seen following severe trauma which results in amputation or in such disease processes as rheumatoid arthritis in which supportive structures about the joint are destroyed.

Congenital deformities and amputations about the upper extremity are usually associated with genetic defects or fetal insults. The former includes Down's syndrome, achondroplasia, and so forth, and the latter are associated with drug-induced deformities, as in the thalidomide cases, or by unknown causes as in the radial club hand or syndactyly.

Atrophy or Hypertrophy

In examining the upper extremity or the hand, atrophy must be differentiated from hypertrophy, although the latter is rare. When present, it is almost always on a congenital basis. Atrophy, however, is almost always associated with some form of underlying neurological or neuromuscular condition. Examples of neurological disease include median and ulnar nerve compression syndromes. Rheumatoid arthritis, almost universally, affects the small muscles of the hand, causing moderate to marked atrophy. Again, comparison with the opposite extremity is most important.

Appearance of the Skin

The appearance of the skin is often a key to an underlying pathological disease. In neuroanesthetic areas the skin is thin, hairless, and pale, and there is an absence of sweating. Edema and swelling often indicate the presence of an underlying infection, as well as being a sequela to trauma. Skin markings and skin creases, if abnormal or of unusual configuration, can indicate underlying systemic or genetic problems. The position of calluses and the texture of the palmar skin indicate the type of work performed by the patient. Position and consistency of scars are often an indication of contractures and impairment of function.

Palpation

Palpation begins in the region of the elbow over the bony prominences and the radial head. Any pain or tenderness should be noted. Palpation of the ulnar nerve is easily accomplished in the cubital groove and any paresthesias elicited should be noted. The brachial artery is palpated on the ulnar side of the biceps tendon, just anterior to the cubital fossa. It should be remembered that the median nerve is in close conjunction with the artery at this point. It is often helpful to palpate the forearm while having the patient squeeze the dynamometer during the grip strength test to determine if he is attempting to exert maximum force. Palpation is extremely useful in attempting to differentiate bony from soft tissue pain. Very often lateral pressure which does not put active compression on the underlying bony architecture will aid in differentiating soft tissue from bony pain. If a patient complains of pain when using the upper extremity against resistance, tendons in the area of the pain must always be palpated to rule out the possibility of a tendonitis as the cause. Palpation is used in association with inspection in determining anesthetic areas on the forearm and hand. Palpation often determines the boundary between sweating and dry skin, and can be used as a gross test of light touch and deep pressure in delineating areas of nerve damage. If stiff joints are carried through a passive range of motion, one can often determine whether or not the block is a firm bony block or a springy soft tissue block.

Function

Functional testing of the upper extremity includes tests for range of motion, grip strength, sensory function, and vascular function which are done at the time of the initial evaluation. Other tests of function are of a more specialized nature and are applied when indicated by the history and physical examination. These include electromyographic and nerve conduction studies, nerve blocks with a local anesthetic, and roentgenographic evaluation by arteriography for suspected vascular problems.

Range of Motion

Range of motion should be active in all cases, with an additional notation of passive motion where this is greater than the recorded active motion. It is measured with a goniometer and recorded to the precise degree. Such terms as good, better, decreased, and severe are never used in place of objective, precise motions obtained with the goniometer. Full extension is 0 degrees (not 180); lack of full extension is recorded as a minus number (i.e., a 30 degree flexion contracture of the elbow would be recorded as −30). Flexion is recorded as the number of degrees from 0 that comprises the arc of motion of the joint.

Elbow. Flexion and extension at the elbow joint are measured with the arms of the goniometer parallel to the humerus and radius and the center point over the lateral epicondyle. Normal extension is 0 degree although some loose jointed people may be able to hyperextend the elbow joint; in this case, it is recorded as a plus number, i.e., +10. Normal flexion varies but is somewhere between 150 and 165 degrees (Fig. 9-9).

Pronation and supination are measurements of both the elbow and wrist joint motion and are actually measured at the level of the wrist joint. The elbow is flexed to 90 degrees and held firmly fixed at the side of the patient. The measurement is obtained at the level of the carpus to eliminate measuring the slight extra mobility of the hand and fingers. Both pronation and supination are measured in degrees obtained from the neutral position in which the hand is held in a plane perpendicular to the transverse plane of the elbow joint. From this point, there is normally 90 degrees of pronation and supination (Fig. 9-10).

Wrist. With the patient's elbow resting firmly on the table, actively flex and extend (dorsiflex) the wrist (Fig. 9-11A). The goniometer is placed along the midline of the forearm and the midline of the third metacarpal, with the point of rotation centered over the wrist joint. Normal flexion and extension are measured from 70 degrees or greater. When measuring flexion and extension at the wrist, the fingers should be relaxed, as any tethering of the flexor or extensor tendons to the fingers can act as a check rein on motion.

Radial and ulnar deviation are checked with the patient's forearm and hand on the flat surface of the examining table (Fig. 9-11B). The goniometer is placed in the midline of the forearm and on the hand over the third metacarpal with the point of rotation over the wrist joint. Normally ulnar deviation is 35 to 40 degrees. Radial deviation is normally one half that of ulnar deviation, and care should be taken to maintain the palm firmly on the table as

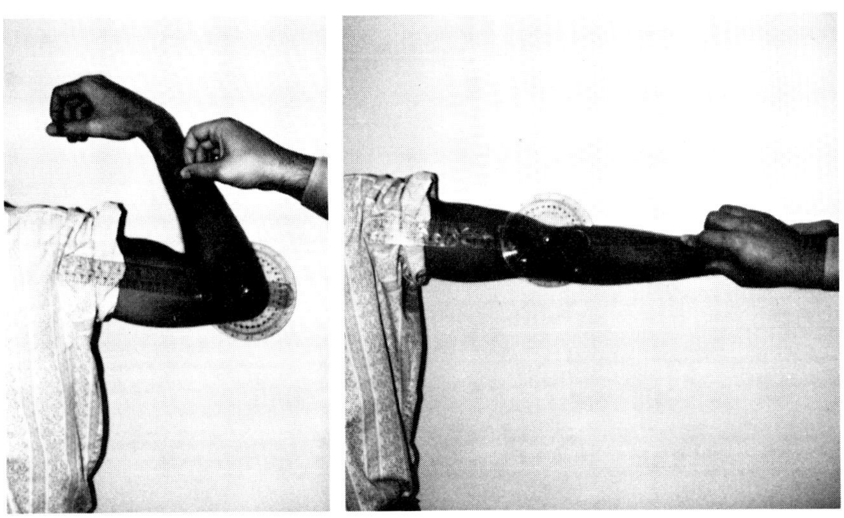

Fig. 9-9. Measurement of flexion and extension of the elbow joint.

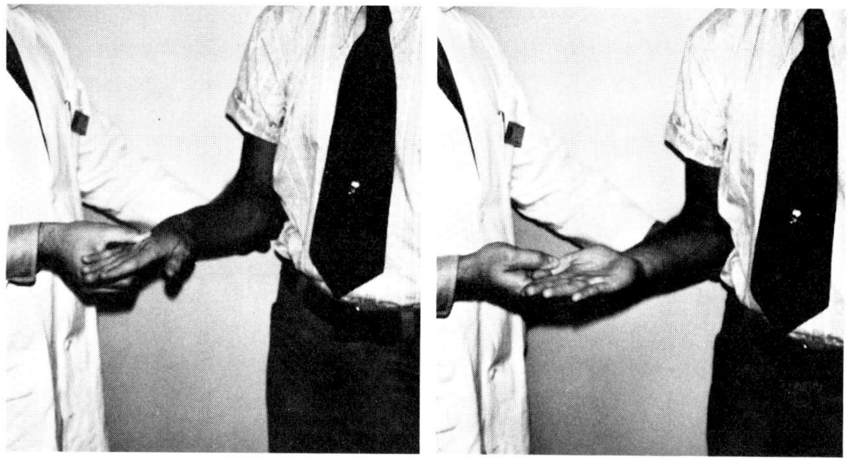

Fig. 9-10. Measurement of pronation and supination at the level of the wrist joint.

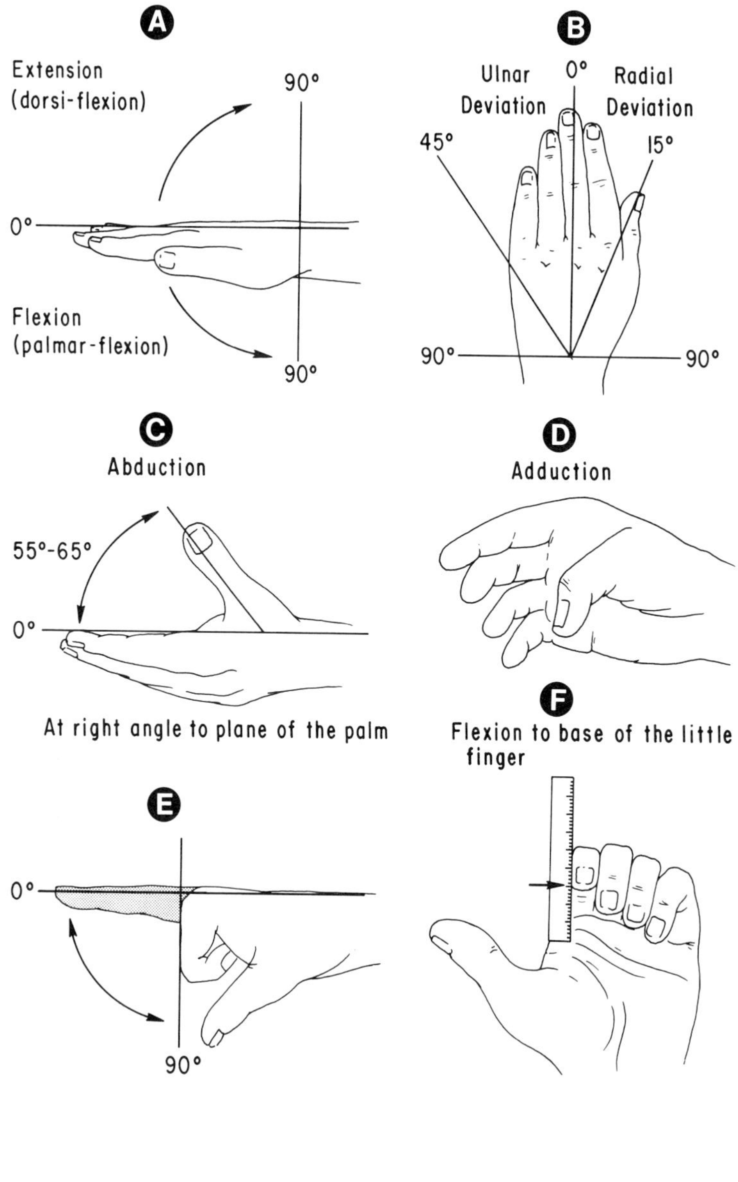

Fig. 9-11. (*A*) Measurement of flexion and extension of the wrist joint. (*B*) Measurement of radial and ulnar deviation of the wrist joint. (*C*) Measurement of abduction of the thumb. (*D*) Measurement of adduction of the thumb. (*E*) Measurement of flexion and extension of the finger joints. (*F*) Measurement of fingertip flexion to the level of the midpalmar crease.

radial deviation increases with supination and flexion at the wrist joint.

Thumb. Extension and flexion of the proximal and distal joints of the thumb are measured plus abduction and adduction. These additional two measurements give an indication of the patient's ability to oppose the thumb to the fingertips. Abduction is the angle between the first and second metacarpals with the thumb perpendicular to the plane of the palm. This is normally 50 to 65 degrees (Fig. 9-11C). Adduction is not measured in degrees. The patient is asked to touch the tip of the thumb to the base of the little finger (Fig. 9-11D). If he can do so, this is normal and is recorded as 0. However, if he is unable to adduct the thumb completely, the distance between the pulp of the thumb and the base of the little finger is recorded in centimeters, and this is recorded as a lack of flexion-adduction.

Range of motion of the proximal and distal joints of the thumb is measured and recorded. Normal extension of each joint is listed as 0 although the distal joint of the thumb quite normally is able to hyperextend up to 30 degrees beyond neutral. Lack of full extension is recorded as a minus number. When recording flexion, it is important to stabilize the joint being recorded by firmly holding the segment proximal to that joint in a neutral position. This should also be done when measuring flexion of the finger joints. All flexion measurements are carried out with the goniometer on the dorsum of the thumb or finger.

Flexion of the proximal joint of the thumb is variable. If severly limited, hyperflexion may be present at the distal joint. The reverse can also be true with hyperflexion at the proximal joint and limited flexion at the distal joint. Regardless, both sides should be essentially equal and the resultant summation of flexion should allow the patient to adduct-flex the thumb enabling him to touch the base of the little finger.

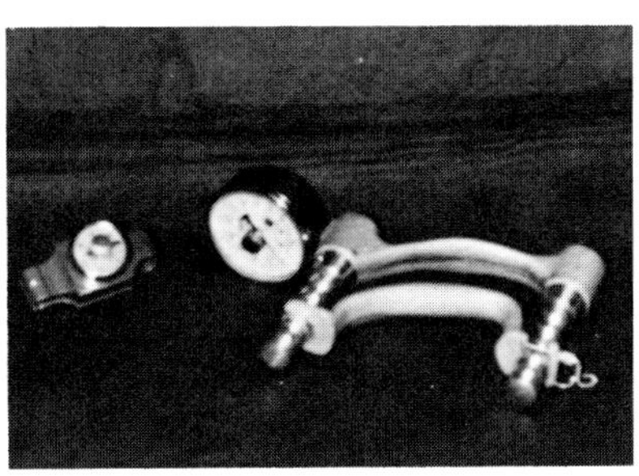

Fig. 9-12. Instruments for measuring pinch strength (*left*) and grip strength (*right*).

Fingers. Extension of the proximal, middle, and distal joints of the fingers (Fig. 9-11E) is measured and recorded with normal full extension being 0 degrees. Patients with hypermobile joints will be able to hyperextend the metacarpophalangeal joints. However, hyperextension does not need to be measured if it is essentially equal in all fingers of both hands. Lack of full extension is recorded as a minus number.

Flexion of each joint is measured by stabilizing the segment proximal to that joint in a neutral position. Normal flexion of the metacarpophalangeal joints ranges between 85 and 100 degrees. Normal flexion of the proximal interphalangeal joints ranges from 90 to 110 degrees. Normal flexion of the distal interphalangeal joints ranges up to 65 degrees. The important aspect of flexion is that the summation of flexion in all joints should allow the fingertip to touch the mid-palmar crease (Fig. 9-11F). Failure to do so should be measured between the pulp of the fingertip and the midpalmar crease and recorded in centimeters.

If abnormal motion of any joint is observed in the upper extremity, it must always be compared with motion in the opposite joint. This is true, even if the opposite joint does not have a normal range of motion. A simplified method of notation is to record the motions as a fraction, with the involved side as the numerator and the comparison side as the denominator.

Grip Strength

Grip strength is a more or less gross measurement of overall hand function. It is obtained subjectively by asking the patient to squeeze the examiner's index and middle finger, and the examiner subjectively compares one side to the other. A more objective measurement can be obtained by using a dynamometer and a pinch meter (Fig. 9-12). The dynamometer is adjusted to fit the patient's hand comfortably, and he is asked to squeeze the handles forcefully and then relax on three separate measurements. These measurements are recorded and compared with similar measurements obtained on the uninvolved side. The examiner should help stabilize the dynamometer with one hand and with the other hand palpate the muscle contraction of the flexors and extensors on the proximal forearm. This aids in determining whether or not the patient is applying the full force of which he is capable. Pinch is tested on the pinch meter. It should be noted whether the patient is able to pinch pulp-to-pulp or whether he uses thumb-pulp-to-side of index, the so-called "key pinch" position. These measurements should be obtained in three separate trials on each hand and recorded as grip strength.

Contractures

Contractures are secondary to cicatrix of the skin, joint stiffness, and/or loss of excursion of a tendon. The hand should be carefully examined to determine the underlying cause of the contracture. Most are flexion contractures, but occasionally an extension contracture is encountered.

The most obvious cause of a contracture is cicatrix of the skin. The location and size of the scar are identified and recorded by measurement and accurate sketches. The quality of the scar is examined both visually and by palpation, and notations should be made as to whether it is hypertrophic, firm and indurate, or soft and pliable. Scars which cross flexion creases at or approaching the perpendicular will tend to hypertrophy and contract due to the tension placed on them during active extension (Fig. 9-13). Revision of these scars by z-plasty or skin graft is usually required to prevent further contracture of the underlying joint.

Joint stiffness is another cause of contracture. Most often it is caused by prolonged immobilization of the small joints of the hand, and active physical therapy is usually all that is required to regain normal function. Immobilization of the joints of the hand, except in special circumstances, should be accomplished in the "functional position." This position has the wrist in approximately 20 degrees of dorsiflexion, the metacarpophalangeal joint in approximately 35 to 45 degrees of flexion, the proximal interphalangeal joints in approximately 30 degrees of flexion, the distal phalangeal joints in approximately 15 degrees of flexion, and the thumb placed in a comfortable position of abduction-opposition.

Other causes of joint stiffness include direct trauma to the joint and inappropriate vasomotor responses secondary to upper extremity injury. If the joint stiffness is long standing, surgical intervention may be required to reestablish motion.

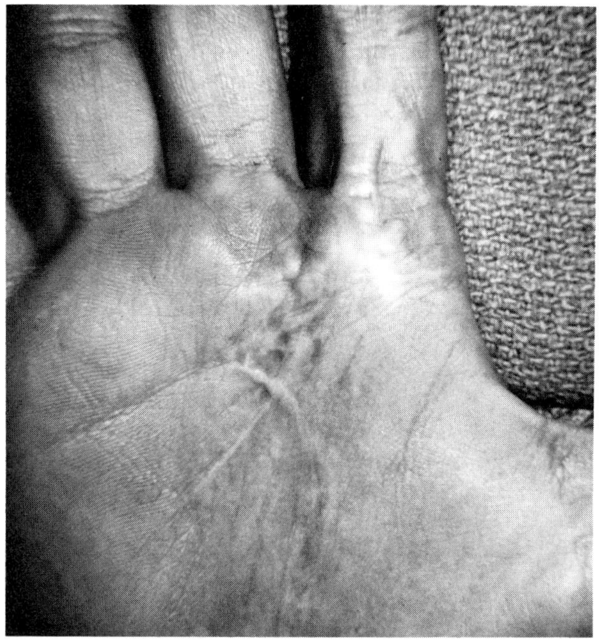

Fig. 9-13. Joint contracture due to cicatrix. Note the broad, shiny, hypertrophic scar on the ulnar aspect of the proximal joint of the index finger; longitudinal lines of tension can be noted in the skin distal to the thickened cicatrix.

Tendon injury, especially in the areas of the flexor pulleys, can cause scar tissue formation about the tendons which prevents their normal gliding. This type of injury usually produces a flexion contracture, with the tendon acting as a check rein preventing either active or passive extension beyond the point of contracture. Further flexion from the point of contracture is often severely limited, due to the scar formation. Correction of this type of contracture almost always must be obtained surgically by tendolysis. Adhesions of the extensor tendon are the most common cause of an extension contracture in which the tethered extensor tendon acts as a check rein to flexion.

Tendons

The tendons of the hand and wrist are usually palpable beneath the skin, especially if motion is obtained against some resistance. When palpating the tendons, areas of pain and tenderness should be noted and recorded. Careful palpation of the flexor tendons in the palm at the level of the metacarpophalangeal joints and of the thumb at the same level often elicits the presence of a nodule which may be causing the pain. The patient should be tested for independent profundus or superficialis function. Superficialis function is tested by holding the distal joints of the fingers in full extension and asking the patient to flex the finger to be tested. This immobilizes the profundus tendons, and flexion of the middle joint is obtained through superficialis function. Profundus function is checked by blocking flexion of the proximal interphalangeal joints and allowing flexion only at the distal joints. Each finger should be checked independently of the others.

Neurological

Neurological function is divided into tests for sensibility and motor function. Sensibility is used to indicate the objective findings indicative of decreased sensory function. Sensation is the subjective appreciation by the patient of a stimulus applied to an area in the distribution of the nerve being evaluated.

The test for light touch is easily performed using a cotton swab. Deep pressure is tested by squeezing the area being examined between the examiner's fingers. Areas of diminished or hypersensibility should be carefully plotted and recorded on a diagram of the hand. Two point discrimination over the fingertips can be tested with a caliper or if this instrument is not available, a simple bent paper clip will suffice. Normal two-point discrimination ranges between 3 and 5 mm. and is abnormal if greater than 6 mm. Tests for disruption in motor nerve function can be indicative of muscle function abnormality, and care must be taken to differentiate between the two.

The neurological examination of the upper extremity should cover the three nerves supplying the forearm and hand. Motor and sensory function for the median, ulnar, and radial nerves should be evaluated separately and recorded.

There are several ways to differentiate a high median nerve palsy due to damage or division at or proximal to the level of the elbow joint from a lesion involving the anterior interosseous nerve. With involvement of the anterior interosseous nerve only, median nerve sensibility in the hand is normal, while it is diminished or absent with high nerve involvement. The anterior interosseous nerve supplies the flexor pollicis longus and flexor digitorum profundus muscles to the index and middle fingers. Loss of this nerve makes thumb-index pinch weak, and the distal joints of the thumb and index finger are characteristically in hyperextension when forceful pinch is attempted. In interosseous nerve palsy, thenar motor function is normal while it is absent in high median nerve involvement.

Low median nerve damage distal to the distal one third of the forearm results in absent thenar function and diminished or absent sensibility in the median nerve distribution to the hand. The flexor pollicis longus, flexor digitorum superficialis, and flexor digitorum profundus function will all be intact. A variable amount of thumb abduction may remain present in low median nerve palsy; this is due to action of the ulnar head of the short flexor which is supplied by the ulnar nerve. Normal abduction-opposition is absent.

High ulnar nerve palsy gives complete absence of sensibility in the ulnar nerve distribution, and depending on the level, presents with varying amounts of weakness of the flexor carpi ulnaris. Flexor digitorum profundus function to the ring and little fingers is absent, but superficialis function is present as these muscles are supplied by the median nerve. Intrinsic motor loss results in atrophy of the hypothenar eminence, interossei, and adductor of the thumb. The hand assumes the classic claw deformity in the resting position, with hyperextension of the metacarpophalangeal joints of the ring and little fingers and flexion of the proximal interphalangeal and distal interphalangeal joints. The index and middle fingers do not assume the claw position as the lumbrical muscles to these two fingers continue to flex the metacarpophalangeal joints, thereby opposing the long extensor. Without the balance of opposing intrinsic muscles, the long extensor exerts all its force at the metacarpophalangeal joint, pulling it into hyperextension, and the unopposed superficialis and profundus tendons at the middle and distal joint pull them into flexion. The classic sign of ulnar palsy, Froment's sign, is elicited by placing a piece of paper between the thumb and index finger at the level of the metacarpophalangeal joint. The patient is asked to squeeze the paper while the examiner attempts to pull it out. Because of the inability to strongly adduct the thumb or abduct the index finger, the paper can be easily removed. Froment's pinch, often confused with Froment's sign, demonstrates the patient's inability to obtain thumb-index pulp-to-pulp pinch. This pinch is also very weak as the patient is unable to stabilize the index finger due to absence of the first dorsal interosseous, and he is unable to apply opposing pressure from the thumb as he has lost the adductor. The patient will also usually hyperflex the interphalangeal joint of the thumb and the middle and distal joints of the index finger, as all of his power of pinch is through the extrinsic flexor pollicis longus and flexor digitorum superficialis and profundus.

A low ulnar palsy usually preserves the sensibility on the dorsum of the hand as the dorsal sensory branch often splits from the main trunk of the ulnar nerve proximal to the level of the lesion at the wrist or at the canal of Guyon. The remaining motor and sensory losses are the same as a high palsy except for absence of involvement of the flexor carpi ulnaris and profundus tendons to the ring and little fingers.

High radial nerve palsy usually occurs secondary to radial nerve injury above the elbow joint. The triceps function is preserved, but the remaining motor function is lost below the level of the lesion. Although the brachioradialis does not function, elbow flexion is unaffected as the brachialis and biceps continue to work. The patient will be unable to extend the wrist or fingers completely, and there is absence of sensibility over the dorsoradial aspect of the hand. Low radial nerve palsy is referred to as the posterior interosseous nerve syndrome. However, the interruption of the nerve can occur proximal to the level of division into the radial sensory branch and the posterior interosseous nerve. In this instance, the brachioradialis muscle is functioning, and the patient is able to extend his wrist, as the extensor carpi radialis longus and possibly the extensor carpi radialis brevis muscle will be functioning because their nerve supply comes off above the level of the supinator.

Special Tests

Intrinsic-Plus Test. The intrinsic-plus test is useful and specific when examining the hand of a patient with rheumatoid arthritis. In this test, the intrinsic muscles are put in a position of maximum passive stretch (not motion) by hyperextending the metacarpophalangeal joint of the finger being tested. Passively, the middle and distal joints will achieve a position of slight flexion. The examiner then further attempts to passively flex the proximal interphalangeal joint of the finger being tested. If there is no intrinsic muscle contracture or tightness, the proximal interphalangeal joint can be completely passively flexed to at least 90 degrees with minimal resistance. If, on the other hand, there is intrinsic tightness or contracture, further passive flexion of the proximal interphalangeal joint will be either severely restricted or impossible. This test is usually positive even in the early stages of rheumatoid disease prior to any destruction or deformity of the hand.

Finklestein Test. This test is useful in examining a patient with complaints of pain on the radial aspect of the wrist joint. The test is used to differentiate involvement of the abductor pollicis longus and extensor pollicis brevis tendons from other tendons in the area, such as the extensor pollicis longus and radial wrist extensors and flexors. In this test, the examiner holds the patient's hand and wrist in a neutral position with his thumb stabilizing the patient's first metacarpal. The patient then attempts to abduct the first metacarpal and extend the proximal joint of the thumb. If the patient experiences pain, this is recorded as a positive Finklestein test and is indicative of De Quervain's disease (see below).

Allen Test. This test is an extremely important part of the routine examination of the upper extremity and should be performed on every patient. The anatomy of the vascular arches of the hand has been discussed above. In some instances there is a singular vascular arch or a failure of connection between the ulnar and radial arches in the palm. If this latter condition is present, division or a ligation of the radial or ulnar arteries could have disastrous results. This test is performed to determine the patency of the vascular communication in the hand.

The examiner first palpates and occludes with whatever pressure is necessary, the radial artery. If the ulnar artery is not palpable, it can be occluded by applying pressure on the radial side of the flexor carpi ulnaris tendon at the level of the wrist joint, just proximal to the pisiform. After manual occlusion of both arteries, the patient is then asked to open and close his fingers rapidly from three to five times. This will cause the palmar skin to blanch. Pressure is then released from either the radial or ulnar artery, and the rapidity with which the hand regains color is noted. The test is then repeated with occulusion of both arteries, and this time the opposite artery is released from pressure. Again, the rapidity of vascular refill is noted, and any failure of fill is also noted.

A positive Allen's test indicates that there is a diminished or absent communication between the superficial ulnar arch and the deep radial arch. When this condition exists, it usually is exhibited by persistent blanching of the thumb or radial side of the hand. In this case, all circulation to the thumb is from the radial artery with no cross communication between the ulnar arch and the princeps pollicis artery. Division of the radial artery could, therefore, result in gangrene and loss of either all or a portion of the thumb.

A negative Allen test indicates that the normal cross communication between the radial and ulnar arches is present.

LABORATORY

Electromyographic and Nerve Conduction Studies

These should be obtained on all patients in whom nerve lesions or muscle disease are suspected or have been diagnosed. They are obtained at the time of initial examination and repeated again at appropriate intervals to follow the progression of healing or degeneration. They should be performed by a physician trained to interpret the information. An in-depth appreciation of these examinations is covered in Chapter 3.

ROENTGENOGRAPHY

Even if the patient has no complaints indicative of bony involvement, roentgenograms of the hand and wrist should always be obtained at the initial examination, if only as a base-line. Often soft tissue calcification, abnormal shadows, bony erosions, or other unsuspected findings indicate more severe disease or offer a clue to the underlying cause of the patient's complaints.

Examination of the elbow by roentgenography is not mandatory, but should be done if there are any limitations of motion of the elbow joint or of pronation and supination. Anteroposterior and lateral roentgenograms are usually sufficient but occasionally positional roentgenograms are indicated to demonstrate bony abnormalities of the medial or lateral epicondyle or the radial head.

Roentgenograms of the wrist and hand should always include anteroposterior, lateral, and oblique views. When dealing with finger injuries, especially, both right and left oblique views may be indicated.

Other special roentgenographic views of the hand may be ordered when indicated. The carpal tunnel view is warranted if the patient has complaints which indicate compression of the median nerve at the wrist level. This projection silhouettes the scaphoid tubercle, greater multangular, pisiform, and hook of the hamate and may demonstrate some bony abnormalities not seen on routine roentgenograms. In patients with rheumatoid disease or any disease causing bony destruction of the metacarpal heads, a Brewerton's projection is helpful which outlines the heads and necks of the metacarpal. If there are complaints of ulnar nerve palsy, with signs and symptoms indicative of nerve entrapment at the elbow joint, a posterior cubital tunnel view will outline the bony parameters of the ulnar groove.

DIFFERENTIAL DIAGNOSIS

CONGENITAL DEFORMITIES

Congenital deformities present an enormous challenge to the physician not only in diagnosis but in family and genetic counseling as well. Some easily identifiable congenital defects are associated with other much less readily apparent deformities which can be life-threatening to an infant. A careful physical evaluation is imperative so they are not overlooked. Compassionate family counseling aids the parent and other siblings to adjust to the situation, and in the cases of hereditary disorders, genetic counseling is invaluable. Congenital deformities of the upper extremity and hand are not rare and occur in approximately 5.5 to 6 per 1,000 live births. Most deformities are minor and in no way impair the functional use of the hand and arm.

A simplified classification for upper extremity deformities has been adopted by the International Federation of Hand Societies. The defects are grouped into six divisions, and each indicates a specific embryological failure. The six divisions are: (1) Failure of differentiation of parts, including such things as radioulnar synostosis, failure of segmentation of the carpal bones, failure of differentiation of muscles or ligaments, and deviation due to asymmetrical development. (2) Arrest of development of parts. Developmental arrest can occur in a transverse direction, resulting in congenital amputation or intermediate segmental arrest as seen in phocomelia, and longitudinal arrests including congenital absence of the radius, ulna, or fingers. (3) Focal defects. These can involve the skin, fascia, muscles, or neurovascular structures. (4) Duplications. Examples include polydactyly and bifid thumbs. (5) Overgrowth. Gigantism of the entire upper extremity, as well as megalodactyly involving only one finger. (6) Generalized skeletal defects. These include the generalized osteochondral dystrophies such as achondroplasia, mucopolysaccharidoses, and congenital syphilis.

Positive factors of congenital deformities are grouped into two broad categories. The first is the hereditary or endogenous type implying some defect in the germ plasm. The second category is the acquired or exogenous type indicating some insult to the developing fetus at a particular time of embryonic life. The mode of transmission of most congenital defects affecting the extremities is by simple mendelian inheritance with varying degrees of penetrance which makes inheritance patterns difficult to assess: A careful family history and examination of other family members is invaluable in these instances. Acquired or exogenous anomalies are usually associated with some abnormal intrauterine condition. Defects secondary to some teratogenic insult of the fetus are more common than the defects from heredity. Etiological agents include drugs, chemicals, hormones, physical agents, viruses, nutritional deficiencies, and many others. They may be directly toxic to the fetus or may interfere with metabolic processes by acting as antimetabolites or interfering with the endocrine balance.

Whatever the teratogenic agent, it is known that exposure during certain periods of fetal life will lead to subsequent specific deformities. Exposure during the third and fourth week will lead to absence of the entire limb. If the insult occurs during the fifth and

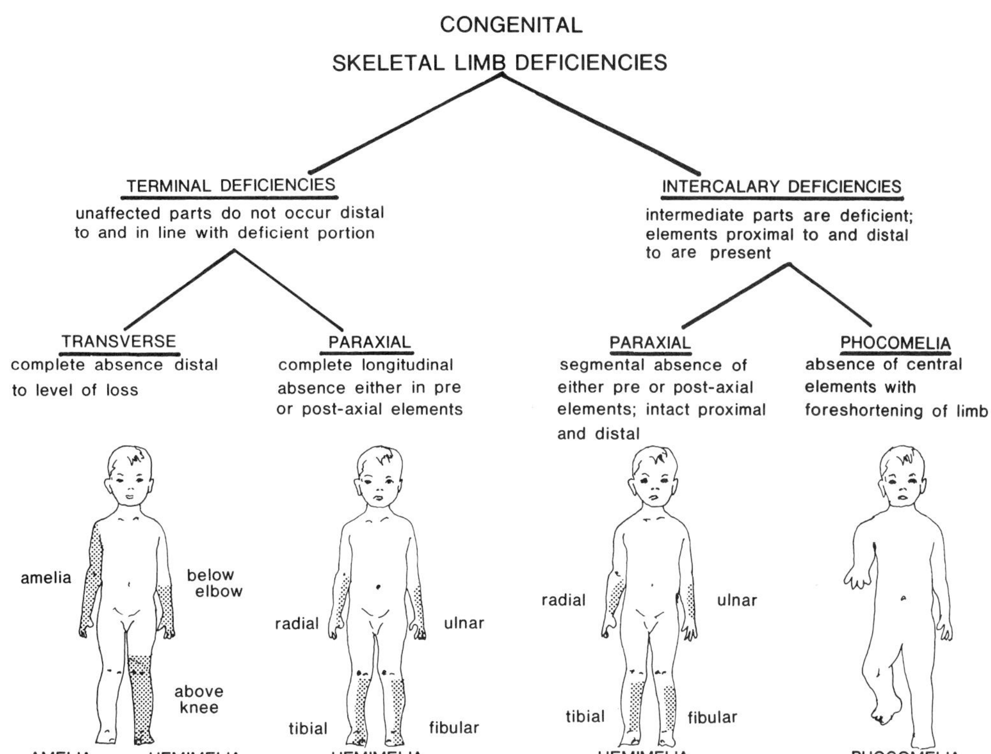

Fig. 9-14. Classification of longitudinal and transverse defects in limb bud development. (Adapted from O'Rahilly: Am. J. Anat. 89, Sept. 1951.)

sixth week, absence of a portion of the forearm or some or all of the hand results. A seventh week insult will disrupt finger formation, and an insult occurring in the eighth week produces digital stunting.

A system of classification of longitudinal and transverse defects in the limb buds has been developed by Franz and O'Rahilly. This system is useful in explaining, on an anatomic basis, most of the acquired congenital deficiencies (Fig. 9-14).

Radial Club Hand

A defect in the radial aspect of the upper extremity limb bud can result in a hemimelia, which is usually terminal, but may be intercalary in that a hypoplastic or normal thumb may be present (Fig. 9-15). This condition is usually unilateral by a ratio of ten to one, with no sex preference, and is much more common than absence of the ulna. If hereditary, it is often bilateral and associated with other systemic problems, such as anemia and splenomegaly (Fanconi's syndrome).

On physical examination, the entire upper extremity is usually foreshortened. The elbow joint is usually abnormal, and the ulna and humerus may be ankylosed. The ulna is short and bowed. The hand is usually a four-fingered hand but may include a hypoplastic thumb. The hand sits on the radial side of the end of the ulna in marked radial deviation, often at right angles to the ulna at the level of the wrist.

Laboratory studies are usually normal; however, if Fanconi's syndrome is present, a microchromic anemia is noted. However, this does not usually manifest itself until the end of the first decade of life. The earlier the anemia occurs, the more grave is the prognosis for survival of the child.

Roentgenographically there may be complete absence of the radius or some portion thereof may be present; if present, it is usually a portion of the proximal radius. Not only is the radius absent, but the carpal scaphoid and trapezium are also absent along with the first and sometimes the second metacarpal rays. In this latter condition, the thumb and index finger are also absent. Occasionally the thumb is present and is usually hypoplastic.

The Floating Thumb

This condition is a more distal manifestation of an insult to the radial limb bud. It occurs later in fetal life and is really a focal defect in bony development. The thumb is hypoplastic and can be considered vestigial. It usually contains a proximal and distal phalanx, a fingernail, and normal neurovascular structures, but it lacks a flexor and extensor tendon. Roentgenographically there is absence of all or part of the first metacarpal, and there may be absence of the trapezium and the scaphoid. This condition occurs spontaneously or in association with the more severe radial agenesis. Regardless, the patient has no active control of thumb function.

Radioulnar Synostosis

This condition is not uncommon and occasionally is hereditary; 70 percent of the time it is bilateral.

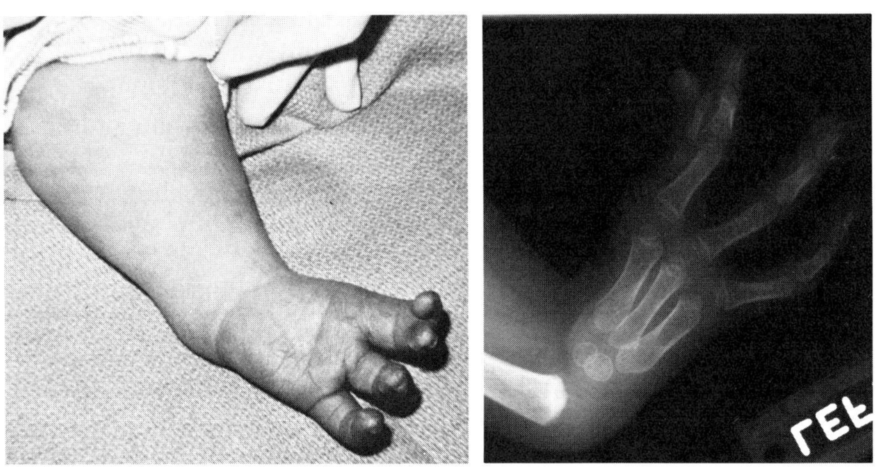

Fig. 9-15. Preoperative photo and radiograph of radial club hand. There is complete absence of the radius and first and second metacarpals. The index finger is hypoplastic and syndactylized to the radial border of the middle finger. The carpus articulates with the radial side of the distal ulna.

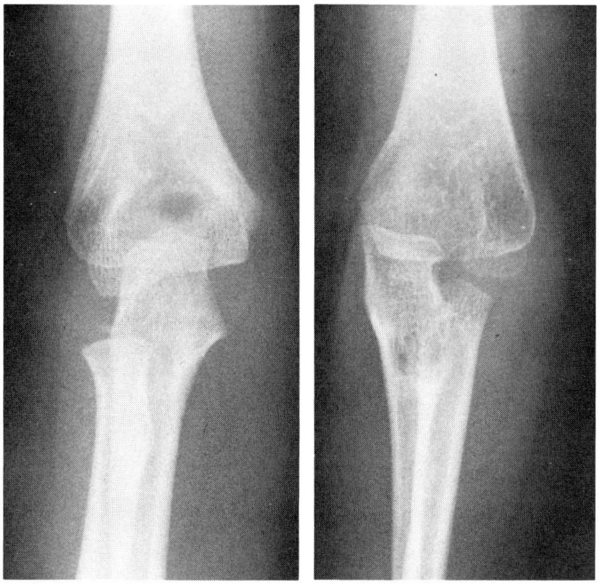

Fig. 9-16. Radioulnar synostosis. The radiograph on the right demonstrates coalescence of the proximal radius with the proximal ulna in the area of the coracoid process. A radiograph of a normal elbow is included on the left for comparison.

The synostosis usually occurs at the proximal end in the area of the proximal radioulnar joint (Fig. 9-16). However, it has been reported to occur at both ends. Often the radial head is dislocated in a posterior direction, and as growth occurs, a cubitus valgus deformity results. Fortunately the fusion almost always occurs with the wrist in the neutral position so that adequate pronation and supination of the hand can be obtained by abduction or adduction of the shoulder joint. Most activities of daily living are accomplished with the hands in pronation.

Roentgen examination demonstrates the presence of the synostosis between the radius and ulna at the level of the proximal joint. The synostosis can be broad or narrow, and in the very young child may be simply a cartilagenous bar which ossifies as the child matures. Occasionally this fusion will extend across the elbow joint and involve the humeroulnar joint as well.

Finger Deformities

Finger deformities may be due to skin abnormalities, joint abnormalities, bony defects, or all three conditions existing at the same time. For purpose of the discussion, they will be considered individually.

Polydactyly is the most common congenital malformation of the hand. It is frequently hereditary and is often accompanied by other hand deformities. The most common example of polydactyly is the bifid thumb (Fig. 9-17). The bifid thumb can occur at any level, although it is usually at the level of the distal joint. The extra thumb may be symmetrical and equal in length to the other thumb, or it may be a rudimentary protrusion containing a nail but no tendon at the base of either the proximal or distal phalanx on the radial side.

Syndactyly is the second most common hand deformity (Fig. 9-18). It is actually a focal deficiency due to failure of segmentation during the seventh to eighth week of fetal life. It is often hereditary and is twice as frequent in males. Syndactyly may involve only one web space or it may involve all the web

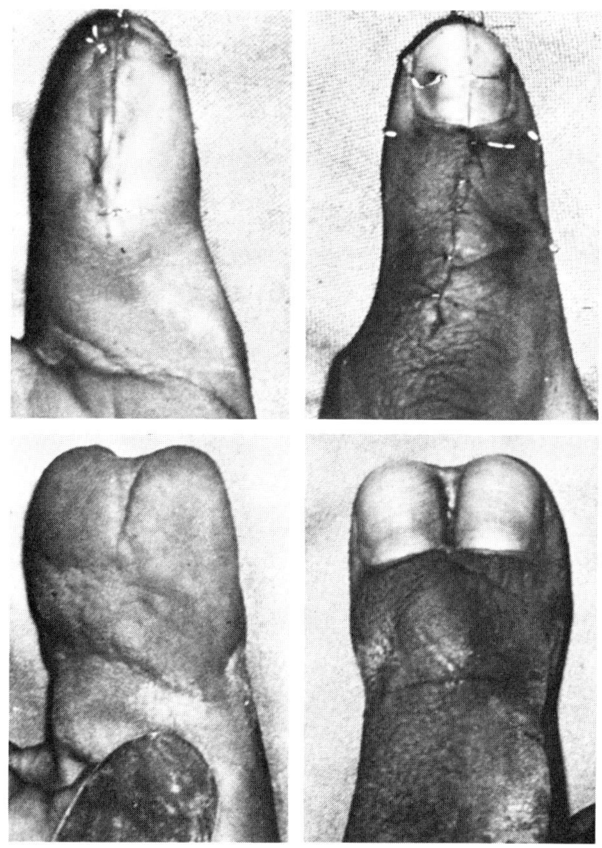

Fig. 9-17. Polydactyly. The lower two photographs show a bifid thumb. The upper two photographs show the thumb following surgical correction.

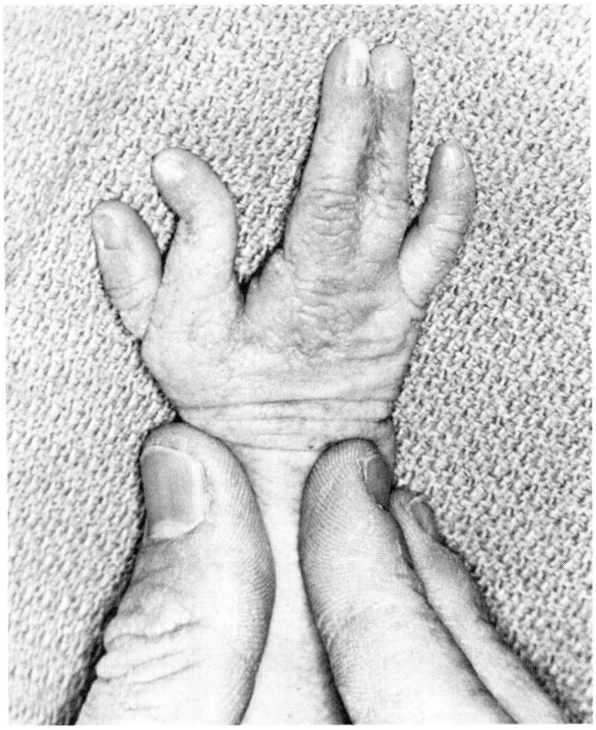

Fig. 9-18. Syndactyly and clinarthrosis. There is complete syndactylization of the middle and ring fingers. The hand also exhibits other congenital anomalies. There is a deep cleft between the index and middle fingers. There is clinarthrosis of the middle joint of the index finger, and there is a floating thumb.

spaces; however, it rarely involves the first web space. The skin web normally extends, on the volar surface of the hand, to the level of the middle one third of the proximal phalanx but may extend to the level of the proximal interphalangeal joint of a single web space or may involve the entire web space. If the entire web space is involved, it is possible that the underlying neurovascular bundle does not bifurcate in a normal manner at the level of transverse metacarpal ligament, and this possibility must be remembered during surgical correction. This condition most commonly involves the third web space between the middle and ring fingers and is usually symmetrical. It is frequently associated with other hand anomalies of a minor or major nature, and in Poland's syndrome is associated with absence of the pectoralis major muscle.

Clinarthrosis is deviation or malalignment of joints (Fig. 9-18). It may be secondary to defects in bony development in which a rudimentary or wedge-shaped delta phalanx intrudes between more normal appearing phalanges. It also occurs in conditions that disrupt or delay soft tissue or epiphyseal development at the joint level. The physical findings are confined to the joint area. The finger may be either ulnarly or radially deviated at the joint level, and the underlying cause is apparent on roentgenogram.

Constrictions and Amputations

The cause of these defects (Fig. 9-19) is still subject to controversy. One theory of etiology is that the fetal mesenchyme during a very specific stage of development undergoes necrosis which then organizes into scar causing an anular constriction band. If the insult is not too severe, growth distal to the band may occur. Another theory holds that the constriction bands are secondary to amniotic disruption in which the fetal part is protruded through the amnion which prevents normal growth at the level of the constriction ring but, if not too deep, allows

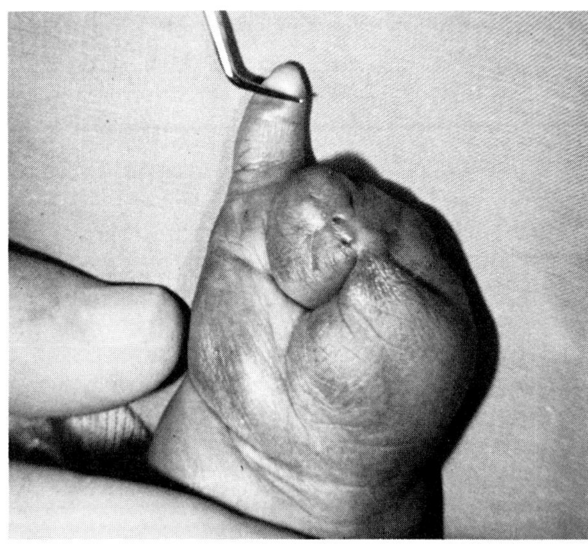

Fig. 9-19. Constrictions and amputations. Right hand of a three-month-old baby. The probe is on the normal little finger. Congenital amputations of the ring, middle, and index fingers at the level of the proximal interphalangeal joints and amputation of the thumb at the level of the interphalangeal joint is noted. There is a thin, secondary web of skin joining the tip of the residual thumb to the tip of the index stump. Note the two skin dimples which are constriction ring residuals.

development distally. If the constriction band is too deep, strangulation of neurovascular structures leads to subsequent gangrene and intrauterine amputation.

The rings may be shallow, involving only the skin and subcutaneous tissue, or they may involve the fascia down to the level of the bone. In the latter case, either arterial supply or venous drainage is disrupted, and the part either becomes necrotic or grossly edematous secondary to venostasis. They may be single or multiple, and may involve any part of the upper or lower extremity. Regardless of theory, the causative factor was present before or during the eighth week of fetal development.

Megalodactyly

This is an uncommon congenital anomaly which may affect the entire limb and involve both the soft tissue and sketetal elements or the bony elements alone. However, it is more commonly associated with tortuous nerves, as in neurofibromatosis, excess fat and lymphatic tissue, and occasionally hemangiomas.

The index and middle fingers are more commonly involved, but occasionally the thumb may be involved as well. If only a finger is involved, the metacarpal ray to that finger is rarely involved. The condition is rarely associated with other congenital anomalies, seldom bilateral, and only on occasion hereditary. Etiologically, the only known causes are in association with neurofibromatosis or hemangioma.

Arthrogryposis

This is a strange and uncommon congenital anomaly of unknown etiology. It presents as a syndrome of varying severity in which multiple joints of the extremity are either fixed in severe flexion or extension contractures. It is associated with absent or markedly hypoplastic musculature which is often replaced with increased amounts of subcutaneous fat and, in one pathological report, with a decrease or absence of anterior horn cells in the spinal cord. In the hand and upper extremity, there are usually three distinct categories of involvement.

The first category contains the least severely involved patients. They usually have a pronation deformity of the forearm, a flexion contracture of the wrist with a thumb-clutched hand. Symphalangism is often associated with this form of the disease. Joints proximal to the hand have more or less normal configuration and function. Roentgenograms of the involved hand often show absence of the small joints with phalangeal or metacarpophalangeal joint synostosis. The intrinsic musculature in the hand is hypoplastic or completely atrophic, with the extrinsic musculature usually present in varying degrees.

The second category of the disease is more severe. The joints of the entire extremity are involved, with the more proximal extensors, such as the triceps, usually stronger than the opposing flexors. Varying amounts of muscle tissue are present, and some limited functional use of the extremities is possible.

In the third form of the disease, all extremity muscle tissue is completely absent or replaced by fatty tissue. Quite often these patients have completely flaccid extremities with marked extension contractures.

Congenital Trigger Thumb

This condition is common, has no sex difference, and no known etiology. The underlying pathology is due to a large nodule on the flexor pollicis longus tendon of the thumb which is hung up on the proximal flexor pulley at the level of the metacarpophalangeal joint. This nodule prevents any active or passive extension of the interphalangeal joint and, to some extent, motion at the metacarpophalangeal joint. Since the thumb is held in the thumb-clutched position in the palm (Fig. 9-20), it must be differentiated from a flexion-adduction contracture of the thumb. This rare condition is probably associated with a sex-linked recessive gene, much more common in males and frequently bilateral. It is usually due to congenital absence of or weakness of the extensor pollicis brevis and occasionally an associated absent extensor pollicis longus. No other congenital anomalies are associated with this deformity.

BONE AND JOINT PAIN OR SWELLING

Infectious Arthritis

Infectious arthritis is often confused with noninfectious arthritis. Such diseases as rheumatoid arthritis, gouty arthritis, and the arthritis of rheumatic

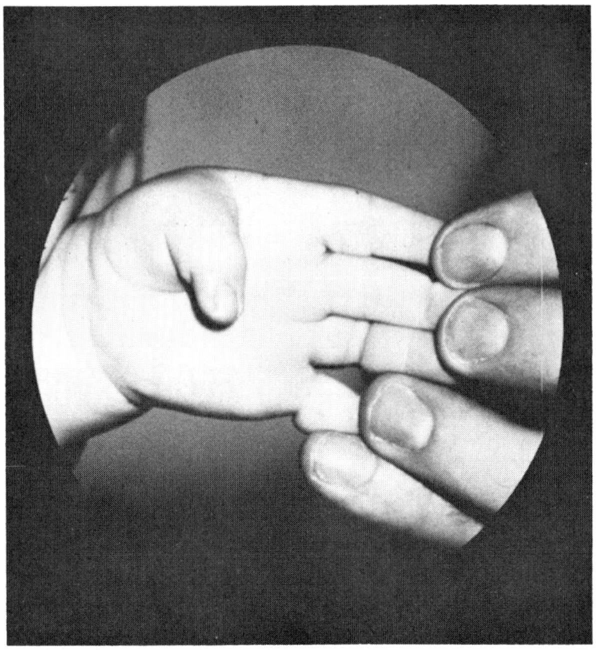

Fig. 9-20. Congenital trigger thumb. The thumb is held in an acutely flexed position at the metacarpophalangeal joint. The metacarpal and phalanges are normal in configuration and development.

fever (especially in the adult) often present with a single red hot swollen joint. Only by careful history and physical examination and correct evaluation of the laboratory studies can the diagnosis be correctly ascertained.

Pyogenic Arthritis (Prototype—Staphylococcus Aureus)

Acute septic arthritis in the upper extremity is most common in the wrist joint. However, the elbow joint and the metacarpophalangeal joints of the hand are frequently involved. When evaluating a patient for infection in the wrist joint or hand, associated tendon sheath infections must be considered present until proven otherwise. Even if the overlying tendons are not involved, a reactive synovitis about the tendon sheath will often produce signs and symptoms making it difficult to rule out the presence of infection.

Pyogenic arthritis involving the elbow, wrist, and less frequently the small joints of the hand, can be due to blood-borne inoculation, direct inoculation from a penetrating wound, or direct contiguous spread from an adjacent osteomyelitis which ruptures into the joint. The blood-borne route is by far the most common method of inoculation.

The presenting symptom is invariably pain which is present at rest and is exacerbated with any attempted motion. If in the elbow joint, it is held in 90 degrees of flexion, and if in the wrist, in 30 degrees of flexion; the fingers assume the position of function. The skin over the involved area is erythematous and warm and edema is obvious. At the elbow the easiest place to examine the joint is the level of the radial head where the joint capsule bulges and is tender to palpation. At the wrist level the pain and tenderness are most marked on the dorsum of the hand and motion of the extensor tendons is painful. If the small joints of the hand, bulging occurs on the dorsal lateral surface, on either side of the extensor mechanism, which is the weakest point in the joint capsule. Palpation of the underlying flexor tendons may elicit a painful response, indicating either a tendon sheath infection or a sympathetic synovial response. Tendon sheath involvement is best determined by moving the tip of the finger while stabilizing the infected joint. This maneuver allows the tendons to glide within the flexor tendon sheath, and they will do so without pain if there is no tendon sheath infection.

Inoculation by penetrating wounds is obvious for large objects like a kitchen knife, screwdriver, nail, or any other household or occupational object. However, such innocuous things as a rose thorn, palm thorn, sliver of wood, sewing needle, or a staple can act as the hypodermic vehicle introducing the bacteria. Although a patient may deny any gross injury, close questioning as to exposure to any of the possible smaller inoculating vehicles should be undertaken.

Dog bites are not uncommon, but are rarely causes of intraarticular infection, if the wound is treated correctly. Dog bites should be left open to heal by secondary intension; usually no supplemental antibiotic therapy is necessary. The two worst bites are those of the domestic cat and the human. Cat bites should be thoroughly evaluated, and never closed, and occasionally, open drainage is required. Direct inoculation of a joint via a human bite can be extremely serious, and subsequent infection can completely destroy the bone, joint, and the tendons around it. There are approximately 20 known species of bacteria present in the human mouth, and all, under proper conditions, are capable of causing severe infection. Since human bite inoculations most often occur during a fist fight, the joint should be examined with the finger in flexion. In this way any underlying tendon and joint laceration will be at the same level as the skin laceration, but it may be missed if examined only in extension. If eight hours old, human bite inoculation should be treated surgically.

As in other joint infections, the routine laboratory examination will reveal an elevated white blood cell count, with a moderate to marked left shift of 80 to 100 percent polymorphonuclear leukocytes. The sedimentation rate will be elevated to about 45 or 50 mm. an hour. Aspiration of the joint will obtain a thick mucoid pus which on gram stain is filled with polymorphonuclear leukocytes and in most cases a moderate to large number of bacteria. Culture and sensitivity study should be performed immediately, and the results should be available within 24 to 36 hours.

Roentgenographic examination early in the disease will usually be nonspecific. Early capsular distention may be noted as a soft tissue shadow with associated distraction or subluxation of the joint, compared with the normal or uninvolved side. Later in long-standing infection, evidence of osteomyelitis, cartilage necrosis, and bony necrosis may be present.

Nonpyogenic Infectious Arthritis (Prototype—Tuberculosis)

Although tuberculosis is considered the prototypic granulomatous infection, the differential should include coccidioidomycosis, blastomycosis, and actinomycosis. Depending on the region of the United States in which the patient has lived, coccidioidomycosis may be more common than tuberculosis.

The historic presentation of this disease is almost always one of insidious onset and chronic progression. The elbow joint is less frequently involved with tuberculosis, but is more commonly involved with coccidioidomycosis. Although the small joints of the hand can be involved with tuberculosis, the wrist joint is the most commonly affected joint in the upper extremity, and our discussion will be confined primarily to the wrist. The route of inoculation is always by hematogenous deposition of the organisms into the synovium of the joint. A previous history of tuberculous infection may or may not be present. However, there is invariably evidence of old pulmonary disease on roentgenographic examination.

The initial manifestation is swelling which is boggy in consistency, and never elicits an overlying hyperemic skin response (Fig. 9-21). Initially, wrist motion is limited, with gradual progression of restriction, and is almost never painful. Tendon function is not restricted, and any loss of range of motion is due to the bulk of the synovium rather than tendon rupture which rarely occurs. Swelling is progressive, and enlargement of the wrist joint further decreases motion. Pain is a late symptom and is associated with underlying bony destruction seen on roentgenogram. By this stage, the patient complains of some weakness and loss of grip strength. Other nonspecific findings of systemic illness, such as night sweats, weight loss, and easy fatigability, may be present.

The peripheral hematological picture is of a nonspecific infection. The patient may have a microcytic-normochromic anemia with or without a leukocytosis, which if present, shows a moderate shift

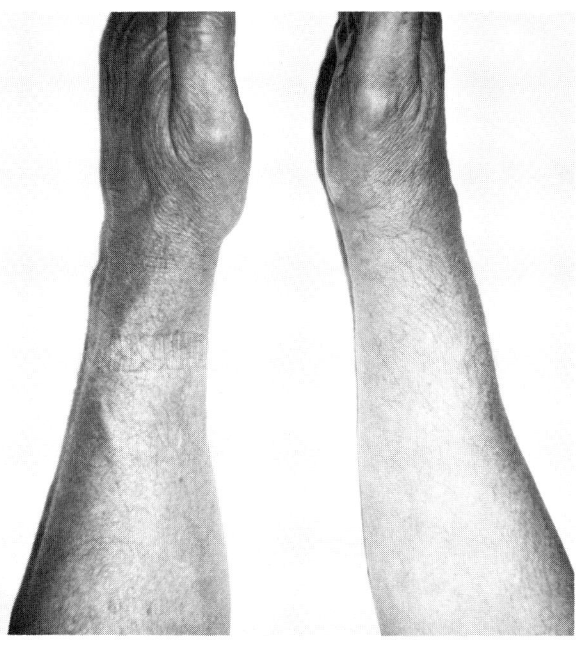

Fig. 9-21. Tuberculous infection of the wrist joint. The right wrist is enlarged and loss of normal soft tissue landmarks such as the extensor pollicis longus tendon and extensor tendons is apparent when compared to the normal left wrist.

to the right in the lymphocytic series. The erythrocyte sedimentation rate is elevated, and the tuberculin skin test is usually positive.

Joint aspiration is usually not helpful, as the mass of diseased synovium prevents the needle from penetrating the joint space cavity itself. Even if an aspirant is obtained, a smear may or may not demonstrate the presence of acid-fast bacilli. Cultures are more apt to be positive. Microscopic examination of the synovium reveals classic granulomatous tubercles consisting of areas of central caseation necrosis surrounded by epithelioid and Langhans' giant cells. The synovium will also be infiltrated with lymphocytes and numerous plasma cells.

Roentgenographically, the earliest signs are nonspecific and consist of soft tissue swelling and possibly some osteoporosis of the small bones of the wrist. Irregular joint space narrowings may be present throughout the entire distal radius and carpal bones. Eventual ankylosis of the wrist joint is a late manifestation.

Tuberculous Tenosynovitis. It should be remembered that tuberculous infection of the wrist is a synovial infection; hence, any synovial tissue can be infected. The extensor and flexor tendons are surrounded by synovial tissue on the dorsum and volar surface of the hand, wrist joint, and in the area of the tendon sheaths in the finger. A tuberculous tenosynovitis in these areas without joint involvement is possible. The disease presents much the same way as it does with joint involvement. The principal complaint is a painless swelling with decreasing motion. Tendon rupture is late and is secondary to pressure necrosis rather than infection. Diagnosis is made by excisional biopsy, and the pathological findings are consistent with those noted in the wrist. Roentgenographically, soft tissue swelling is the only persistent nonspecific finding.

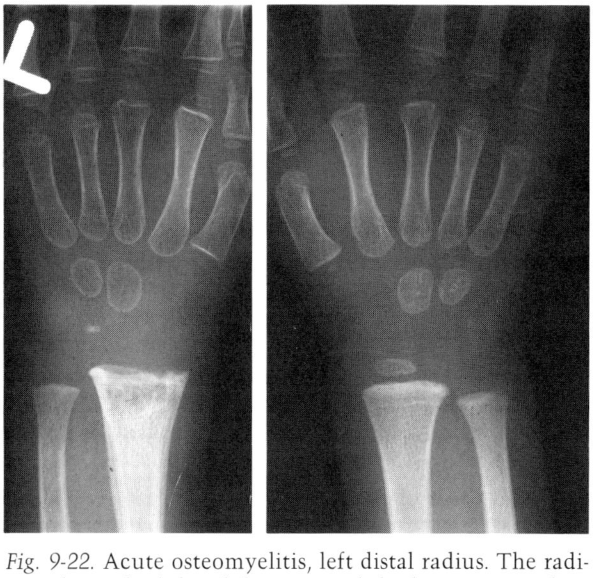

Fig. 9-22. Acute osteomyelitis, left distal radius. The radiograph on the left exhibits cortical thickening secondary to periosteal elevation about the distal radius. There is cavitation of the distal radius and loss of the distal radial epiphysis when compared to the right.

Acute and Chronic Osteomyelitis

Acute osteomyelitic infection can be difficult to differentiate from acute pyogenic arthritis. They usually result from blood-borne bacteria in the metaphyseal area. The classic location of osteomyelitis in the forearm and hand is the distal radius (Fig. 9-22). The small carpal bones, metacarpals, and occasionally the distal humerus about the elbow joint are involved. A more common manifestation of osteomyelitis in the upper extremity is dactylitis. This is more of an infection of the periosteum rather than the underlying bone. It is more commonly seen in children than adults, and is usually associated with tuberculosis or syphilis.

Chronic osteomyelitis of the forearm and hand is usually secondary to a granulomatous infection. Tuberculous osteomyelitis almost invariably is accompanied with tuberculous arthritis. This infection is commonly found in the epiphysis, as opposed to the metaphyses in acute pyogenic osteomyelitis.

Noninfectious Arthritis

The noninfectious arthritides cover a broad spectrum of systemic, metabolic, and idiopathic diseases which have manifestations in the upper extremities as well as in other regions. Grouping of these diseases is possible because they have many overlapping characteristics.

Rheumatoid arthritis is the prototype disease for the systemic arthritides, but psoriasis, lupus, and gout have some unique characteristics. Primary osteoarthritis is an idiopathic disease with probably some genetic predetermination and must be differentiated from degenerative arthritis secondary to posttrau-

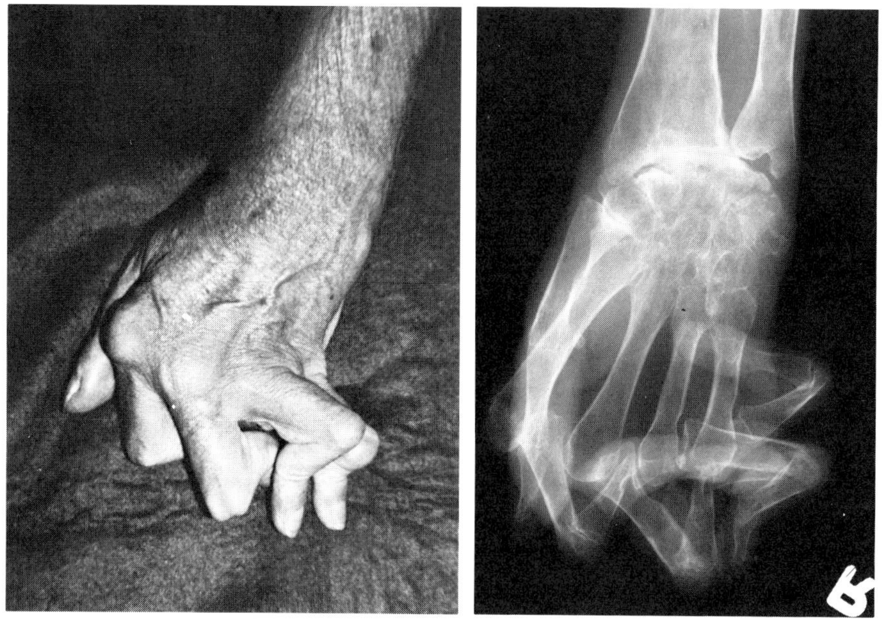

Fig. 9-23. Rheumatoid arthritis. Photograph and radiograph of a 43-year-old woman with an 11-year history of rheumatoid arthritis. The metacarpophalangeal joint of the thumb had been fused eight years prior to these roentgenograms. There is complete dislocation of all metacarpophalangeal joints, the index and middle fingers are in a volar position, and the ring and little fingers are in a dorsal position. All fingers demonstrate severe boutonniere deformities with destruction of the proximal interphalangeal joints apparent on roentgenogram. The fingers are in ulnar drift and the wrist is in a radial position. There is coalescence and collapse of all the carpal bones.

matic joint changes. The avascular necroses, while idiopathic in etiology, are fairly specific in their location and manifestations in the upper extremity.

Rheumatoid Arthritis

This is a systemic disease whose early manifestations include fatigue, morning stiffness, anemia, possibly some loss of appetite and weight, and, above all, painful joint swellings. The small joints of the hands and feet are usually the first to be involved with this disease.

Rheumatoid arthritis of the upper extremity usually begins in the metacarpophalangeal joints of the hand (Fig. 9-23). It often involves all the metacarpophalangeal joints of one hand, and may present in both hands simultaneously. Rarely, it presents as an isolated swelling of one of the proximal interphalangeal joints, where it subsides over a few weeks to several months, to be followed later with the more classic presentation in the metacarpophalangeal joints. This disease almost never involves the distal interphalangeal joints, which is significant in differentiating it from primary osteoarthritis. Initially, the metacarpophalangeal joints are swollen, boggy to palpation, and filled with obvious fluid. The overlying skin is mildly erythematous and warmer to touch than the surrounding skin. There is stiffness and pain with motion or rest. Both the metacarpophalangeal and interphalangeal joints of the thumb may be involved, but the first metacarpotrapezial joint is rarely involved early in the disease.

Early involvement of the wrist joint is accompanied by pain and swelling, usually on the dorsum of the hand, much as infectious arthritis. Early involvement of the synovium of the extensor tendons is also a concomitant finding. Flexor tendon involvement is a later manifestation and is much less apparent than extensor involvement. Involvement of the distal radioulnar joint is an early manifestation accompanied by pain and a clicking or catching sensation with pronation and supination of the forearm.

The elbow joint is rarely the primary locus, but it becomes involved as the disease progresses. Signs and symptoms of synovial inflammation, characterized by swelling in the area of the radial head on the lateral side of the elbow joint, are present as in infectious arthritis. With synovial proliferation, gradual destruction of the medial and lateral collateral ligaments of the elbow joint and the annular ligament about the radial head leads to progressive atrophy and destruction of the elbow joint. Motion of the elbow joint becomes progressively more painful, which ultimately results in a marked decrease in range of motion or ankylosis.

Synovial proliferation about the extensor and flexor tendons at the wrist ultimately leads to tendon rupture secondary to direct synovial invasion and lysis of the tendon itself. Tendon rupture usually begins on the ulnar side of the hand, and the extensor digitorum communis tendons are the first to be involved. The extensor indicis proprius is usually the last extensor tendon to rupture, and rupture of the extensor pollicis longus is variable since it is contained in a separate extensor tunnel. The flexor tendons may be involved at the level of the wrist joint or the fingers within the flexor tendon sheaths. Because of their deep location, it is often difficult to diagnose flexor tendon involvement prior to rupture. The flexor pollicis longus tendon is the most common flexor tendon to rupture. Very often the proliferating synovium causes pressure on the median nerve in the carpal canal, and the patient presents with a carpal tunnel syndrome.

Early in the disease, a consistent finding is a positive intrinsic-plus test. The ulnar intrinsics are tighter than the radial intrinsics which contributes to the ulnar deviation seen in the fingers of a rheumatoid hand. This intrinsic tightness contributes to the development of boutonniere and swan neck deformities, commonly seen in the rheumatoid hand. The boutonniere deformity (see Fig. 9-23) is seen in patients with long standing rheumatoid arthritis who have sustained destruction or laxity of the extensor mechanism at the proximal interphalangeal joint. Swelling of the joint produces stretching of the central slip and lateral band mechanism, attenuation of the collateral ligament supporting structures, and occasionally complete disruption of the central tendon. Stretching of the support fibers of the extensor mechanism over the middle joint allows the lateral bands to assume a more volar position beneath the axis of rotation of the proximal interphalangeal joint. Now, tension on the tendons by the intrinsic muscles causes flexion of the proximal interphalangeal joint and a concurrent hyperextension of the distal joint as the full power of the intrinsic muscles is transferred distally. The patient is unable to extend the middle joint actively, although passive extension is possible in the early stages. Hyperextension of the distal joint is apparent and is fixed if the deformity is of long standing. The patient still can flex the middle joint fully from the point of the flexion contracture. Although classically seen in rheumatoid arthritis, a boutonniere deformity can be secondary to traumatic disruption of the central slip of the extensor mechanism at the proximal interphalangeal joint.

The swan neck deformity is essentially the antithesis of the boutonniere deformity and is commonly seen in rheumatoid arthritis. In this instance, the volar plate mechanism which acts as a check rein to hyperextension, becomes attenuated secondary to joint swelling. The pull of the tight intrinsic mechanism at the level of the proximal interphalangeal joint exaggerates the propensity to hyperextension. The dissipation of the intrinsic pull at this level allows the profundus tendon to overpull the weak extensor force at the distal joint, and the distal joint assumes a position of flexion. The swan neck deformity also can be secondary to trauma but is much rarer than a traumatic boutonniere deformity. It is usually secondary to an avulsion of the volar plate mechanism at its insertion on the base of the middle phalanx. This allows the middle phalanx to assume a dorsally dislocated position, and the intrinsic pull is then concentrated on the dorsal aspect of the proximal interphalangeal joint.

With continued progression of the rheumatoid disease, the involved joint capsules and restraining ligaments become attenuated and atrophic. At the level of the metacarpophalangeal joint, the extensor tendons dislocate in an ulnar direction into the valleys between the metacarpal heads. This, plus the tight ulnar intrinsics and underlying bony erosion, contributes to the ulnar drift of the fingers.

Rheumatoid nodules often accompany this disease and are a middle or late manifestation of the systemic problem. These nodules are a subcutaneous collection of rheumatoid lymphocytes and on biopsy show nonspecific changes of central fibrinous necrosis surrounded by masses of lymphocytes. They invariably occur on the extensor surfaces about the olecranon process and proximal bony prominence of the ulna, and the extensor aspects of the metacarpophalangeal and proximal interphalangeal joints. They are firm, occasionally tender if active, and are easily differentiated from boggy synovium by palpation.

In particularly severe cases of rheumatoid arthritis, rheumatoid vasculitis is present. In these cases, the small vessels of the hand are affected, which can lead to the serious sequelas of cell death, tissue necrosis, and gangrene.

Varying degrees of osteolysis of the carpal bones are evident on roentgenograms (see Fig. 9-23). The wrist assumes a position of radial deviation of 15 to 20 degrees. Complete collapse of the proximal carpal row can be seen accompanied by subluxation or complete dislocation of the wrist joint in a volar direction relative to the distal radius. Metacarpal head erosion is present with or without complete metacarpal head destruction. The capsular attenuation and bony destruction allow subluxation or complete dislocation of the metacarpophalangeal joints.

Juvenile rheumatoid arthritis usually presents as a pauciarticular arthritis involving the larger joints of the body. If the disease becomes persistent, the hands become involved. Characteristically, the proximal interphalangeal joints of the hand are involved before the metacarpophalangeal or wrist joints. The joints may be warm with superficial erythema but are rarely swollen. The principal complaints are pain, marked stiffness, and limited motion. The arthritis is a dry, constrictive type tending to involve the joints in a proximal migration with each succeeding flare of the disease. There is little or no involvement of the extensor and flexor tendon synovial sheaths. The joint changes are usually those seen with cartilage necrosis and bony erosion. Ankylosis and contracture are common sequelae. Progression into the adult type of rheumatoid arthritis is not common and, if seen, the juvenile form has usually occurred close to or at the time of puberty.

Psoriatic and Lupus Arthritis

Occasionally, these two systemic autoimmune diseases present as arthritis involving the small joints of the hand. With the exception of systemic lupus erythematosus, in which the hip joints are commonly involved, the large joints of the body are rarely affected. The hallmark of differentiation between rheumatoid arthritis and these two arthritides is that these are "dry" and there is no proliferating boggy synovium. They also begin in the distal interphalangeal joints. They are invariably accompanied by fingernail changes, especially in psoriatic arthritis and although the overlying skin may be warm and erythematous, there is no apparent swelling. This also differentiates these arthritides from primary osteoarthritis which also begins in the distal interphalangeal joints. Psoriatic arthritis usually proceeds from the distal interphalangeal joints to the proximal interphalangeal joints to the metacarpophalangeal joints in a direct proximal progression. Joint destruction is severe, and complete destruction of the phalanges is not uncommon (Fig. 9-24).

On the roentgenographic examination of psoriatic arthritis, the hallmark manifestation is the so-called "opera glass" deformity in which the distal joint surface becomes egg cupped in shape and the proximal

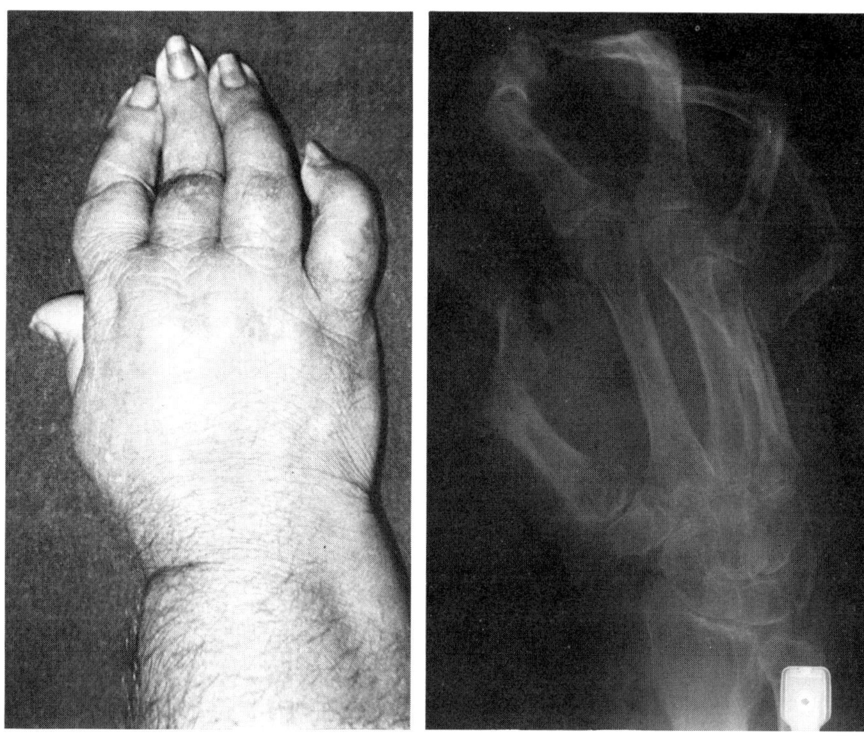

Fig. 9-24. Psoriatic arthritis. The photograph shows the hand of a 52-year-old woman with a 35-year history of psoriasis. The radiograph demonstrates the accompanying joint destruction. There is involvement of all the small joints of the fingers and thumb and involvement of the intercarpal and carporadial joints.

joint surface becomes rounded and fits like a ball into a socket. Lupus arthritis has little bone destruction but commonly a great amount of cartilage necrosis and joint space narrowing. In lupus arthritis, the more proximal the joint, the milder the involvement.

Gouty Arthritis

Gout is a systemic disease of purine metabolism in which uric acid, the terminal product of the nucleotide pathway, is deposited into tissues about the joint or in the synovium of the joint itself. The uric acid accumulation is either a result of overproduction or underexcretion. The disease is much more common in males than females and occurs with increasing incidence after the third decade of life. The pathogenesis of the disease is thought to be a deposition of uric acid from the supersaturated serum into the soft tissues where they form tophi or into the synovium of the joint. Release of the crystals into the joint causes a chemotactic reaction in which the polymorphonuclear neutrophils digest the uric acid crystals, undergo lysis, thus releasing lysosomes into the joint. This precipitates an attack of acute gout. Although the joints of the lower extremity are more commonly involved (the proximal joint of the great toe is the pathognomonic joint) the small joints of the hand, and especially the interphalangeal joints are often afflicted.

The diagnosis is made in the laboratory where uric acid crystals in the joint fluid are easily identified under polarized light and are pathognomonic of the disease. The other positive laboratory finding is an elevated blood uric acid, which may not be present. The tophus, histologically, is a multicentric deposit of urate crystals surrounded by a typical foreign body granuloma with epithelioid cells and foreign body giant cells.

Roentgenographic examination of the hand during an attack of acute gouty arthritis reveals soft tissue swelling and distention of the involved joint. In chronic disease, uric acid crystals are deposited in the superficial portions of the articular cartilage, synovial and capsular tissues, periarticular tissues,

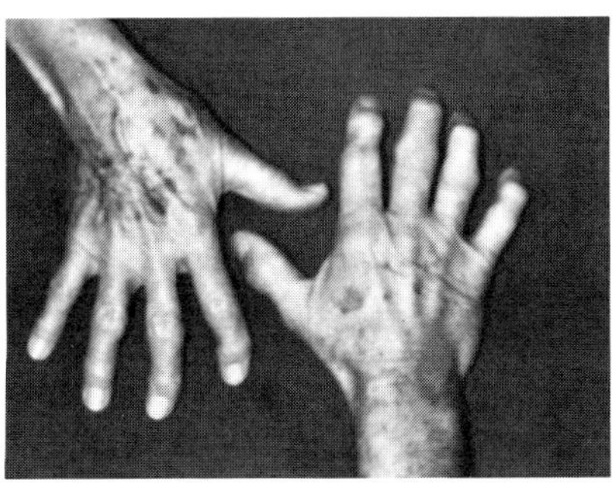

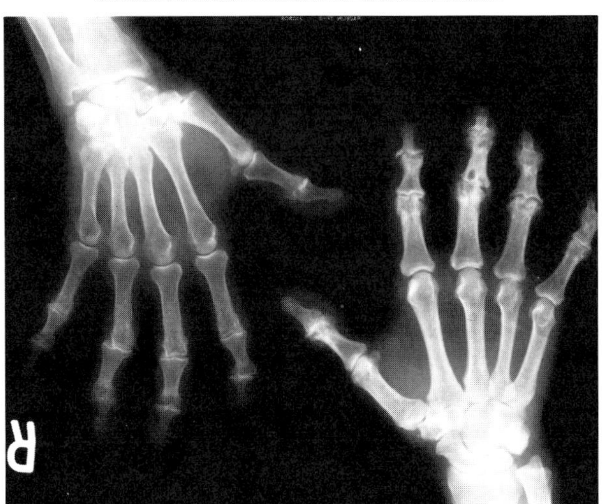

Fig. 9-25. Osteoarthritis. The photograph and accompanying radiograph are of the hands of a 70-year-old woman (*top and bottom, left*) and 72-year-old man (*top and bottom, right*). Note the deformity of the proximal and distal interphalangeal joints with complete sparing of the metacarpophalangeal joints. Heberden's nodes are particularly apparent on the distal joints of both index fingers and a Bouchard's node is apparent on the proximal interphalangeal joint of the middle finger of the man's hand. The radiographs demonstrate moderate to marked destruction and ankylosis of the proximal and distal interphalangeal joints of both hands. The radiolucent area in the proximal portion of the middle plananx of the middle finger of the man's hand is consistent with gouty joint destruction. The radiolucent area represents an interosseous tophaceous deposit. There is mild first metacarpotrapezial joint arthritis evidenced on the radiograph of the woman's hand.

and in the subchondral marrow spaces of bone. Involved cartilage undergoes nonspecific degenerative changes, and punched out lucent lesions occur in the bone, usually in epiphyseal areas (Fig. 9-25). These represent tophaceous deposits which have replaced the normal bony calcium salts. Late in the disease there is eventual collapse and coalescence of contiguous joints. In the skin, typical tophi formation occurs in the pinna of the ear over the olecranon bursa and in the area of the Achilles tendon.

Primary Hypertrophic Osteoarthritis

Although this disease is most often seen by the physician when the patient presents with complaints of pain in the weight-bearing joints, it is common to elicit a history of pain in the small joints of the hand, usually the distal interphalangeal joints, which began sometime toward the end of the fourth decade of life. A family history is usually positive in a high percentage of these patients and they recall that their parents or grandparents suffered from "crippling arthritis" of the hands.

The first manifestation of this disease is usually a painful, nodular-type swelling on the dorsum of the distal interphalangeal joint of the fingers but rarely the thumb. The joints are stiff and painful to move, and the nodule itself is often quite tender to palpation. The pain and tenderness gradually subside but the node persists. They may also develop insidiously over a number of months or years and be completely unassociated with any pain whatsoever. These are called Heberden's nodes. Gradual destruction of the supporting ligamentous structures of the distal joints leads to instability and deformation of these joints and, eventually, bony ankylosis may occur (see Fig. 9-25). In severe cases, proximal interphalangeal joints of the fingers may become involved. Similar nodular formations at the proximal interphalangeal joint are called Bouchard's nodes. The soft tissue swelling at the middle joints is more fusiform, more painful, and severely limits flexion.

The only proximal joint of the hand which may be involved in primary osteoarthritis is the first metacarpotrapezial joint. The patients present with a complaint of pain when attempting to use the hand as in opening a door, turning a key, opening a jar, and especially when opening the door latch of an automobile. The initial finding is usually a tensely swollen joint which is painful to palpation and painful when pressure is applied on the first metacarpal in the so-called "grind test." Heberden's nodes never form at this joint. Due to pull of the abductor pollicis longus tendon and laxity of the joint capsule, the first metacarpal may sublux or even completely dislocate at the level of the metacarpotrapezial joint. Subluxation is in a radial and proximal direction, and the head of the metacarpal assumes an adducted position. Due to the loss of range of motion at the metacarpotrapezial joint, the patient is unable to abduct the first metacarpal and develops a hyperextension deformity at the metacarpophalangeal joints. Following this, the distal joint goes into flexion in order to balance the tendon forces. This produces the so-called "z-collapse" thumb (Fig. 9-26).

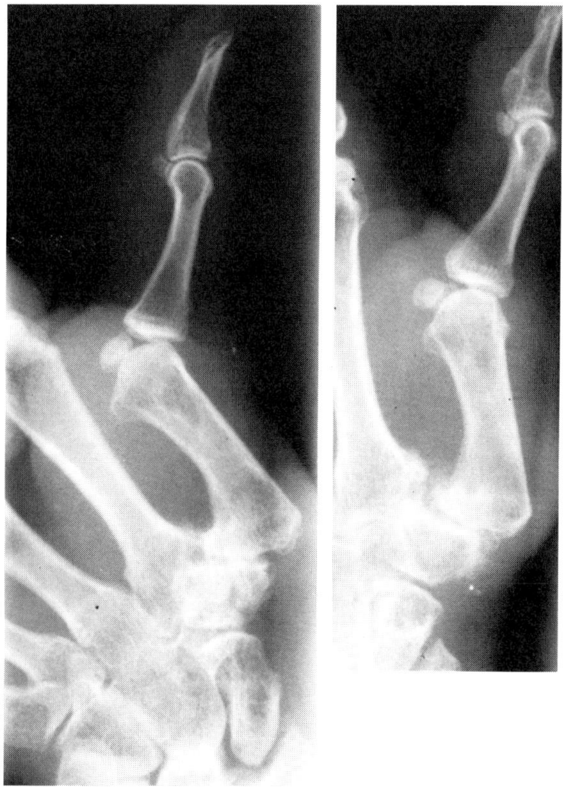

Fig. 9-26. An anteroposterior and oblique roentgenogram of the first metacarpotrapezial joint of a 67-year-old female with primary osteoarthritis of the basal joint of the thumb. There is sclerosis and collapse of the joint with proximal subluxation of the first metacarpal. This condition has created a classic "Z" collapse deformity of the thumb with hyperextension of the metacarpophalangeal joint and flexion of the interphalangeal joint. Moderate osteophyte formation and moderate osteosclerosis and boney collapse of the trapezium are apparent. The trapezioscaphoid joint, however, is free of arthritis.

Roentgenograms of the distal finger joints, obtained early, will often demonstrate the presence of an amorphous radiodensity, indicative of acute calcium deposition; this forms a Heberden's node. Roentgenographic changes at the proximal interphalangeal joint (Bouchard's nodes) are similar to those seen at the distal joints, and bony ankylosis may eventually occur (see Fig. 9-25). Although an acute Heberden's node may resemble an acute gouty tophus at the level of the distal joint, the roentgenographic findings make differentiation easy. The joint location and the quality of the swelling make it easy to differentiate this form of arthritis from rheumatoid arthritis. Roentgenograms of the metacarpotrapezial joint early in the disease may show simple joint distention, but as the disease progresses and symptoms persist, a gradual wearing away of the radial tubercle of the trapezium occurs (see Fig. 9-26). This is accompanied by osteophyte formation both dorsally and laterally.

Degenerative (Posttraumatic) Arthritis

A brief discussion of this entity is warranted as it must be differentiated from primary osteoarthritis.

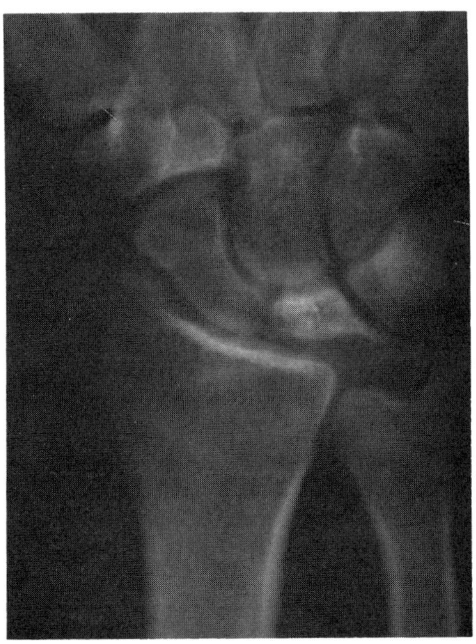

Fig. 9-27. Kienbock's disease. This radiograph demonstrates the classic findings in Kienbock's disease with sclerosis and collapse of the carpal lunate secondary to avascular necrosis.

Historically, some prior injury to the joint can be recalled, such as subluxation or complete dislocation or possibly only a mild sprain, often without treatment. The principal complaint of the patient at the time he seeks medical attention is stiffness and loss of motion with or without pain. Roentgenograms obtained at this time will often demonstrate evidence of old healed chipped fractures which are indicative of tendon or ligamentous rupture.

Avascular Necrosis

This is not a specific disease entity. Multiple joints are involved and usually there is a history of trauma. The most common areas are the elbow, lunate, and scaphoid.

Osteochondritis dissecans of the elbow usually presents with complaints of mild pain on the lateral aspect. Roentgenograms usually indicate an apparent area of fragmentation in the capitellum. Occasionally there is evidence of an osteochondral fracture at the trochlea. The most severe form of this disorder occurs when the entire medial epiphysis is involved and is known as "little league elbow."

Kienbock's disease is avascular necrosis of the carpal lunate bone (Fig. 9-27). The patient presents with pain in the wrist which is exaggerated with flexion and extension of the wrist and forced grasp. Pain is elicited with palpation in the area of the carpal lunate and is the principal cause of functional loss in the disease. There are no roentgenographic findings early because the first signs of avascularity are subtle and easily missed even by an experienced examiner. Early signs include slight increase in radiodensity and occasionally osteophyte formation of less than 1 mm. in diameter in the area of the scapholunate joint. With progression, further sclerosis of the lunate becomes obvious, accompanied by small areas of radiolucency indicating hypermic attempts at bony repair. The lunate eventually collapses, and the patient experiences progressive limitation of wrist motion.

Preiser's disease is avascular necrosis of the carpal scaphoid (Fig. 9-28) and is rare. The presenting symptom is usually pain in the area of the anatomical snuff box and over the flexor carpi radialis tendon following some trauma to the wrist joint. The clinical and radiographic presentation of the disease follows much the same course as that seen in Kienbock's disease.

Old scaphoid fracture with nonunion and avascular necrosis of the proximal segment is the most common avascular entity seen in the upper extremity. A definite history of old trauma is present, and quite often the patient has been treated for varying periods of time by cast immobilization. It results from a lack of blood supply to the proximal pole of the fractured scaphoid. Anatomically, the nutrient artery enters through the radioscaphoid ligament and the distal joint capsule into the distal pole of the scaphoid. A fracture through the waist or proximal one third of the scaphoid severs the blood supply to the proximal pole. Avascular necrosis does not always result, but it is a common sequela. The presenting symptom is pain with motion and forced grip and may persist at rest. Like Preiser's disease, there is tenderness in the anatomical snuff box and motion of the wrist is restricted due to pain. Grip strength is diminished. Roentgenograms first demonstrate nonunion of the scaphoid, followed by increasing radiodensity of the proximal pole. Collapse of the proximal fragment results with obvious degenerative changes in the proximal scaphoradial joint (Fig. 9-29).

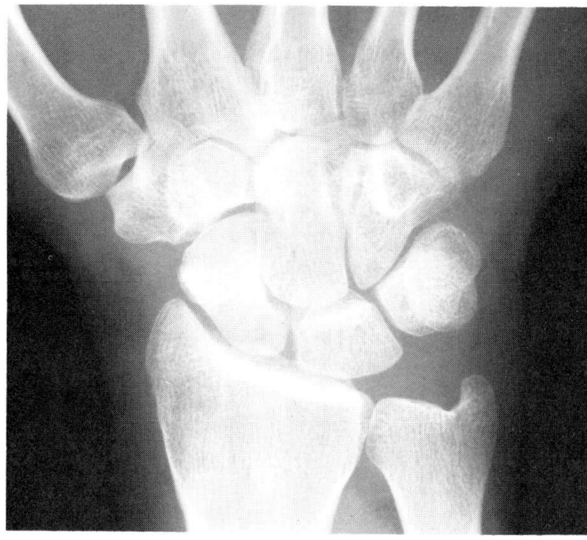

Fig. 9-28. Preiser's disease. Careful inspection of this radiograph demonstrates disruption of the normal trabecular pattern in the proximal pole of the scaphoid. There is some narrowing of the normal scapholunate joint.

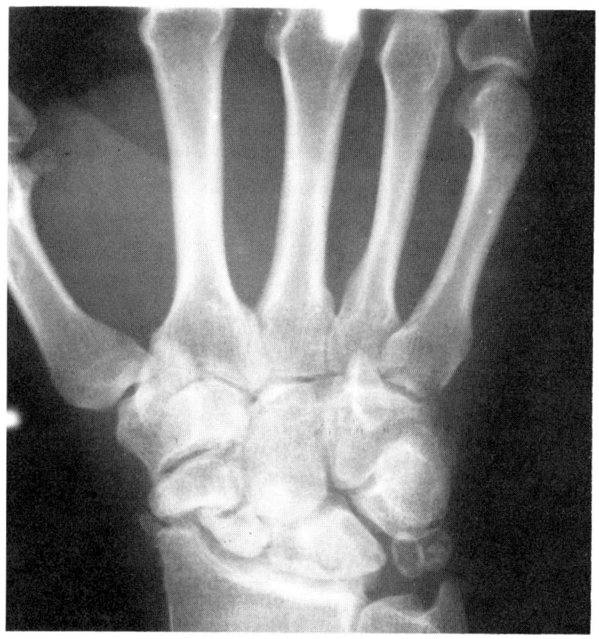

Fig. 9-29. This radiograph demonstrates severe carporadial degenerative arthritis secondary to an old fracture of the scaphoid. The proximal pole of the scaphoid is avascular, sclerotic, and has collapsed, allowing it to impinge on the radial styloid; note the small osteophyte on the radial side of the styloid. There is also early avascular necrotic changes present in the carpal lunate.

SOFT TISSUE PAIN OR SWELLING

INFECTION (PYOGENIC AND GRANULOMATOUS)

Infections of the soft tissues can be pyogenic or granulomatous. It is important to rule out contiguous bone or joint involvement as soft tissue manifestations are often secondary to underlying bone or joint infection. However, the skin, subcutaneous tissue, tendon sheaths, and tissue spaces can be infected independently. The areas most commonly involved are the olecranon bursa, the fingernail, the pulp space of the finger or thumb, the tendon sheath, and the hand spaces.

Olecranon bursitis is an inflammation of the potential space lying over the bony prominence of the olecranon process. Patients with gout or rheumatoid arthritis often have an acute inflammation of this bursa without infection. If it becomes infected, it is usually by direct inoculation. Clinically, there is moderate to marked swelling over the extensor surface of the elbow joint. The skin is erythematous and warm, and there is pain to palpation. If pyogenic, there is a febrile course and laboratory examination reveals an elevated white count with a shift to the left, and the erythrocyte sedimentation rate is elevated.

Perionychium infection involves the soft tissues directly overlying and adjacent to the side of the fingernail. This is the most common hand infection and is usually secondary to a hangnail. The causative organism is usually Staphylococcus aureus. If the infection extends over the soft tissues overlying the dorsum of the nail, it is called an eponychium, and results from direct contiguous spread. The tissues on the side and base of the nail are swollen, erythematous, purplish in color, and exquisitely tender to palpation. Acutely, there is a cellulitis of the overlying skin, but chronically there is little cellulitis, and the area is only slightly tender to palpation. Chronic perionychiums are usually indicative of a subungual abscess, osteomyelitis of the distal phalanx, or a retained foreign body.

Subungual tuberculosis and carcinoma of the nail bed, although rare, need to be included in the differential diagnosis. Both conditions will show bony destruction on roentgenographic examination not seen in the usual perionychium. A nonsuppurative perionychium is usually caused by a mycotic infection, and the eponychial area is also involved. The fingernail bed ultimately is destroyed resulting in a condition called onychomycosis.

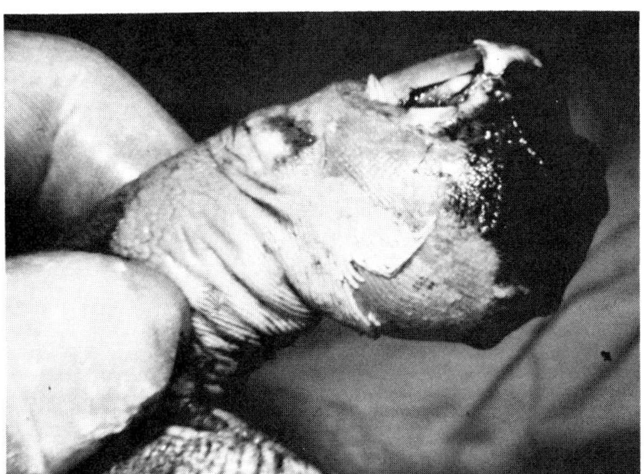

Fig. 9-30. The severe coagulation necrosis of the tip of the thumb apparent in this photograph is secondary to inadequate primary treatment of a felon. The infection was secondary to Staphylococcus aureus. Perionychial and eponychial involvement is also apparent in this photograph. Treatment was by amputation.

A felon is a specific infection of the pulp space of a finger or thumb tip (Fig. 9-30). Anatomically, the space is filled with fatty tissue which contains numerous fascial trabeculations that anchor the overlying skin to the bone. It, therefore, acts as a closed, confined space and subsequent swelling and edema, secondary to the infection, cause a great amount of pain. It usually results from a puncture wound to the fingertip, but may develop secondary to deep perionychial infection which becomes sealed off from the dorsum. The patient presents with his hand held above the level of his heart, because if he lets it hang down, there is a constant throbbing pain. The volar aspect of the fingertip is swollen and exquisitely tender to palpation. A roentgenogram will demonstrate soft tissue swelling and indicates if osteomyelitis or bone necrosis is present.

Tendon Sheath. Acute suppurative tenosynovitis of the flexor tendon sheaths in the fingers and thumb is almost always secondary to a work-related injury or rupture of a felon, as the profundus tendon inserts into bone at the base of the proximal phalanx. The offending organism is usually Staphylococcus aureus, most often introduced directly into the tendon sheath by a penetrating wound. Pain on motion, but not at rest, is the presenting complaint. The finger will be swollen in its entire length with moderate to marked pain to palpation over the course of the flexor tendon from the fingertip into the palm (Fig. 9-31). The finger is held in a position of mild flexion, and passive extension elicits severe pain; this latter finding is pathognomonic of a tendon sheath infection. It can be differentiated from a joint infection by direct palpation of the joint. With a tendon sheath infection the metacarpophalangeal joint can be flexed with only mild discomfort because flexion is secondary to intrinsic muscle function, and is not accomplished by the long flexors.

Hand space infections involve either of the two major fascial compartments of the hand: the thenar or midpalmar spaces. The division between the two lies in the longitudinal plane of the third metacarpal in conjunction with the origin of the adductor pollicis muscle. A fascial septum separates the two compartments which is attached to the entire length of the third metacarpal. Although a thin structure, it is adequate enough to keep the infection confined to one space or the other. These infections usually result from a direct puncture wound with

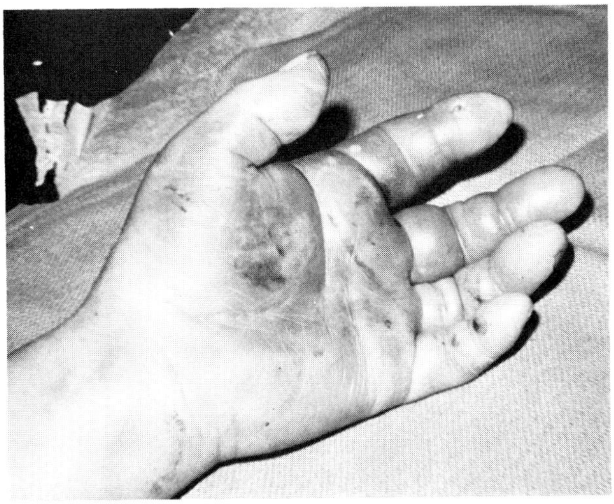

Fig. 9-31. This preoperative photograph shows the presentation of a thenar and midpalmar space infection which involves the flexor tendon sheaths to the index and middle fingers. Note the tense shiney quality of the skin and the position of mild flexion of the fingers.

bacterial inoculation but can follow an acute suppurative tenosynovitis, septic abrasion, or extension of a collar button abscess.

Pain with motion and palpation along with varying degrees of swelling are the usual presenting symptoms. Swelling on the palmar surface (see Fig. 9-31) is tense and confined to the fascial compartment. Dorsal swelling varies from moderate to marked and is secondary, or reactive, in nature because the major venous and lymphatic drainage is toward the dorsum of the hand. If a thenar space infection is present, the index finger is almost always held in flexion, and passive or active motion of the thumb is painful. If a midpalmar space infection is present there is obliteration of the normal cup-shape of the palm, with prominent bulging over the base of the middle and ring fingers. The long and ring fingers will be held in the flexed position. The thumb and little fingers are usually spared from involvement with hand space infections because the flexor tendon synovium of the digit is contiguous with that of the carpal space. The third space on the volar aspect of the hand is the hypothenar space which encloses the hypothenar muscle. It is rarely involved but, if present, the abscess presents on the dorsal ulnar border of the hand. Although not in the hand, the quadrilateral space in the distal forearm, Parona's space, can become secondarily infected through rupture from a thumb or a little finger synovial sheath infection. This potential space lies beneath the fascia of the profundus muscles separating it from the pronator quadratus muscle. It results from an extension of infection from the radial bursa of the flexor pollicis longus or the ulnar bursa of the profundus tendons and produces a firm indurated swelling in the forearm. The wrist is held in the flexed position, and pain in the area is elicited with passive or active extension of the wrist joint.

The patient exhibits signs of systemic illness, with fever to 104 F, an elevated leukocyte count, and shift to the left on differential. The sedimentation rate is elevated. Aspiration of the infected space is often nonproductive, but material for bacterial study can be obtained at the time of open drainage. Approximately 80 percent of hand space infections are secondary to Staphylococcus aureus, 10 percent to streptococci, and the remainder to gram-negative organisms.

A collar-button abscess is the most common type of infection involving the palm. It presents in the area of the metacarpal head beneath a hard callus. (Fig. 9-32). Penetration of the callus is the usual

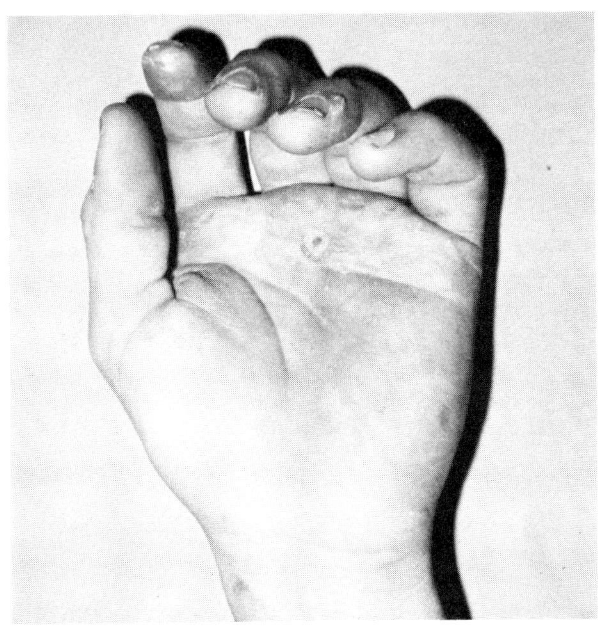

Fig. 9-32. A small furuncle is present at the base of the third web space between the heads of the third and fourth metacarpals. This is the usual place of presentation of a collar-button abscess. Note the moderate swelling of the entire hand.

method of inoculation of bacteria into the subepithelial area. The infection then spreads in a dorsal direction through a hole in the palmar fascia hence the name "collar-button." It may further spread to the underlying palmar spaces or to the dorsal area of the web space through the natatory ligament. The presenting complaint is pain and swelling in the palm over the metacarpal head. The skin, especially on the dorsum, is erythematous and motion is limited at the metacarpophalangeal joint. If long standing, there may be signs of tendon sheaths involvement and palmar space involvement.

A web space infection usually arises in the same way as the collar button abscess from an infected callus over the metacarpal head in the palm. However, following penetration of the natatory ligaments, the infection involves the lumbrical space and canal as it exits volar to the transverse metacarpal ligament and dorsal to the natatory ligament. There is pain, tenderness, and swelling in the web space between the involved fingers which are held in an abducted position. There may be reactive lymphedema in the dorsum of the hand, and rarely, in neglected cases, there is extension into the palmar spaces through the lumbrical canal.

Inflammation

Inflammatory affectations in the upper extremity, not involving the joints, are usually limited to the tendons, and are idiopathic in etiology. There is usually no history of predisposing trauma and no evidence of systemic illness. Nonspecific tenosynovitis is an inflammation of the synovial bursas about the flexor and extensor tendons in the upper extremity in which all possible etiological factors have been ruled out. It usually has a spontaneous, rapid onset, and uneventful recovery. Clinically, active motion of the tendon is painful; however, with passive motion of the contiguous joints, movement of the tendon is not painful. This sign aids in the differential diagnosis between acute suppurative tenosynovitis and nonspecific inflammation. The overlying skin may be warm and erythematous with moderate swelling. The laboratory and roentgenographic examinations are normal.

Two syndromes invloving a nonspecific synovitis are De Quervain's and trigger finger.

De Quervain's syndrome is involvement of the abductor pollicis longus and extensor pollicis brevis in the common tendon sheath on the radial side of the wrist just proximal to the radial styloid. Swelling and inflammation of the surrounding synovium, contained within the tight tendon sheath, produces pain on abduction of the thumb. Pain is also produced with any synergistic action of the abductor pollicis longus and extensor pollicis brevis tendons, as in stabilization of the base of the thumb when unscrewing a jar lid, opening a car door, or turning a key. The Finklestein test is positive and diagnostic. Simple ulnar deviation of the wrist joint, with the thumb held in the adducted position, is usually sufficient to apply enough passive tension to the abductor pollicis longus tendon to elicit moderate to marked pain.

Trigger or snapping finger is usually associated with a secondary, nonspecific reactive synovitis. The synovitis, as well as the triggering phenomenon, is caused by a nodule on the flexor tendon at the level of the proximal end of the tendon sheath in the palm of the hand. The nodule is secondary to small tears in the substance of the flexor tendon which then ball-up and round-off. The resultant nodule slips through the tendon sheath with difficulty, and when the finger is flexed, hangs up on the edge of the sheath. This interrupts the smooth flow of finger motion and the increased tension necessary to force the nodule beyond the point of obstruction causes the finger to snap or trigger into extension. This triggering phenomenon is painful. Occasionally the finger will stick in the flexed position and have to be extended manually with the other hand. There is usually pain to palpation in the palm and along the area of the flexor tendons over the proximal 2 or 3 cm. of the tendon sheath in the finger. As the patient wiggles the finger, the nodule can be felt passing beneath the examining fingertip. Tendon nodularity and triggering are often seen in patients with diabetes and rheumatoid arthritis long before the disease has been diagnosed clinically. Patients who present with isolated complaints of a trigger finger should be evaluated for diabetes mellitus and rheumatoid arthritis.

Tennis elbow or radial epicondylitis is a symptom complex which presents with pain about the elbow, especially with extension of the wrist or fingers against resistance. It is usually due to a tear in the conjoined tendon of the extensor muscles, and is often associated with a bone chip or spur on the lateral epicondyle of the humerus. Direct compression of the dorsal interosseous nerve at or distal to the level of the supinator can also give the same symptoms.

On palpation, there is pain in the area of the lateral epicondyle and continuing down the dorsal aspect of the forearm over the muscle bellies of the wrist extensors and the extensor digitorum communis. The patient should be tested by having him extend his wrist against resistance with the fingers flexed to eliminate action of the extensor digitorum communis, and then have him extend the middle finger against resistance with the wrist held in a neutral position. This will differentiate between tears in the origin of the extensor carpi radialis longus and the extensor digitorum communis.

Etiological factors include direct trauma to the elbow joint in the area of the lateral epicondyle, or more commonly a muscle strain secondary to athletic activities. If direct trauma is determined as the underlying etiology, tangential roentgenograms of the lateral epicondyle should be obtained. They may demonstrate the presence of small osteophytes within the substance of the conjoined tendon, as well as cortical irregularity of the epicondyle.

Occasionally, medial epicondylitis is encountered. This usually has the same etiology as tennis elbow and involves either the medial epicondyle or the common tendon flexor origin.

Nerve Compression Syndromes

Nerve compression syndromes in the upper extremity are discussed in Chapter 5. This section will relate the physical findings of nerve compression in the forearm relative to its effect on hand function.

Median Nerve

The pronator syndrome is entrapment of the median nerve as it traverses the elbow joint in the area of the pronator muscle. It is usually caused by an aberrant course of the nerve beneath both heads of the pronator teres rather than between them. There is weakness of all forearm and thenar muscles supplied by the median nerve. Paresthesias in the median nerve distribution to the hand are present. It is differentiated from compression of the median nerve at the wrist, a carpal tunnel syndrome, by its involvement of the forearm flexor muscles. Nerve conduction studies demonstrate slowed conduction velocities in the area of the proximal forearm with no involvement of the nerve across the wrist joint.

Anterior Interosseous Nerve Syndrome. After supplying the pronator teres, flexor carpi radialis, palmeris longus, and flexor digitorum sublimis muscles, the median nerve divides into the main trunk which continues into the hand, and the anterior interosseous branch, which supplies the flexor pollicis longus, the flexor digitorum profundus to the index and middle fingers, and the pronator quadratus. Compression of the anterior interosseous branch of the median nerve in the forearm, usually secondary to anomalous muscle and tendon origins, produces the anterior interosseous nerve syndrome. The characteristic physical finding is paresis or paralysis of the muscles which it supplies. On physical examination, there is weakness of grip and a characteristic pinch in which the index finger is extended at the distal interphalangeal joint with hyperflexion of the proximal interphalangeal joint; the metacarpophalangeal joint of the thumb has increased flexion and the interphalangeal joint is hyperextended. Thenar muscle function and sensory function in the median nerve distribution are normal.

In the anterior interosseous nerve syndrome, the pronator quadratus is nonfunctioning and pronation is accomplished entirely by the pronator teres, and selective pronation tests are positive in varying degrees. They are based on the fact that the pronator teres muscle is strongest with the elbow joint in extension, and weaker with the elbow flexed to 145 degrees. The patient is asked to pronate against resistance and if the pronator quadratus is nonfunctioning, the patient will have more pronation power with the arm extended, where the pronator teres is at its maximum advantage, than with the elbow flexed, when the pronator quadratus contributes its force to pronation.

The carpal tunnel syndrome is the most common nerve compression syndrome in the upper extremity and is produced by compression of the median nerve. Any condition which causes synovial hypertrophy (such as rheumatoid arthritis), systemic diseases (such as hypothyroidism, gout, and diabetes), tumors (such as ganglia or lipomas), pregnancy, and direct trauma can cause narrowing of the carpal canal and impingement of the nerve.

The presenting complaint is usually pain, numbness, or tingling in the median nerve distribution which awakens the patient at night. It is produced by the patient sleeping with the wrist in a flexed position, and the face resting on the dorsum of the hand. The carpal canal is narrowed and pressure is placed on the median nerve. This is the basis of the Phalen's test which is performed by holding the patient's wrist in an acutely flexed position. If symptoms of numbness, tingling, or pain occur within 60 seconds, the test is considered positive.

Persistent pressure on the nerve over a long period of time will produce a neuropraxia. Tinel's sign is now positive, and if the carpal canal is tapped, the patient will complain of tingling or electric shock sensations radiating into the fingers and thumb in the median nerve distribution. Tinel's sign is nonspecific, but it does indicate that the nerve is irritable and has sustained some damage. If the compression is allowed to persist, the numbness becomes quite dense, the tingling disappears, and thenar atrophy ensues. The abductor pollicis brevis becomes atrophic, and the radial border of the thenar eminence assumes a dish-shaped concavity.

Electromyographic studies indicate denervation of the thenar muscles, and nerve conduction studies demonstrate slowed conduction velocities across the wrist joint. No laboratory studies are specifically associated with this syndrome unless the underlying cause is of a systemic nature, and tests relative to these diseases may well be positive.

A neuroma in continuity in the digital nerve of the thumb on the ulnar side is known as bowler's thumb. When a bowling ball is gripped by the ulnar border of the thumb at the level of the metacarpophalangeal joint, the underlying nerve is subject to direct trauma. This can cause a neuropraxia, or an axonotmesis. The normal reparative processes produce a neuroma in continuity which on stimulation produces pain or discomforting electric shocks in the nerve distribution. The neuroma is usually palpable just distal to the metacarpophalangeal joint of the thumb.

Ulnar Nerve

Cubital Tunnel Syndrome. Pressure on the ulnar nerve as it exits the arm and passes beneath the medial epicondyle in the cubital tunnel produces the cubital tunnel syndrome. At this location the nerve is essentially subcutaneous and easily subject to external pressure or damage. Pain and hyperesthesias extend down the ulnar border of the forearm and the ulnar aspect of the hand, along with transient weakness in the intrinsic muscles of the hand. It may be caused by direct trauma, or be of insidious onset as seen in patients who are subject to prolonged bed rest who constantly prop themselves into sitting position with their elbows.

Positive physical findings include a Tinel's sign in the area of the ulnar groove, diminution in grip strength, and a positive Froment's sign. If long standing, intrinsic muscle wasting is obvious in the interosseous spaces on the dorsum of the hand, and there is a dish-shaped depression in the area of the atrophied first dorsal interosseous muscle. Pinch, grip strength, and finger adduction and abduction are weak.

Electromyographic studies show the denervation potentials in the muscles innervated by the ulnar nerve, and conduction velocities are slowed across the elbow joint. Charcot-Marie-Tooth disease affects the ulnar nerve first in the upper extremities and is differentiated from a cubital tunnel syndrome by the fact that it is symmetrical, and nerve conduction studies are abnormal across both the elbow and wrist joint. It must also be differentiated from compression of the ulnar nerve at the wrist by the fact that the flexor carpi ulnaris and the flexor digitorum profundus muscles to the ring and little fingers are also weak.

Guyon's canal compression is produced by pressure on the ulnar nerve as it enters the hand through the canal of Guyon. The canal is formed by the pisiform and hamate bones and surfaced by the pisohamate ligament. The nerve is accompanied by the ulnar artery as it traverses the canal, and thrombosis or aneurysm of the artery will produce this syndrome, in addition to fracture of the hook of the hamate. The presenting complaint is pain or numbness in the ulnar distribution of the volar surface of the ring and little fingers. It is differentiated from a high ulnar nerve palsy by the fact that there is no weakness of the flexor carpi ulnaris and flexor digitorum profundus and dorsal ulnar sensibility is intact. Electromyographic studies of the small muscles of the hand show the same findings as seen in the high ulnar palsy; however, nerve conduction velocities are diminished, and nerve conduction times are increased at the level of the wrist and normal at the elbow.

Radial Nerve

Complete radial palsy is secondary to disruption of the radial nerve in the area of the spiral groove in the distal one third of the humerus. All muscles in the forearm supplied by the radial nerve are nonfunctioning, and there is absence of sensibility on the dorsum of the hand in the radial nerve distribution. Although the brachioradialis and supinator muscles are involved, elbow flexion and supination are not appreciably weakened because the biceps muscle provides both functions. Supination is weaker with the elbow in extension, as this is the position of greatest mechanical advantage of the supinator.

The attitude of the forearm, hand and wrist is that of pronation with no ability to extend the wrist, metacarpophalangeal joints of the fingers, or distal joint of the thumb. The thumb also cannot be abducted in the plane of the palm. Grip strength is weakened because of the inability to stabilize the wrist in a neutral or extended position where the flexor tendons have a greater mechanical advantage. Extension of the fingers at the proximal and distal interphalangeal joints is possible because the interossei and lumbrical muscles are still functioning.

The posterior interosseous nerve syndrome is differentiated from complete radial nerve palsy by the presence of a functioning brachioradialis, extensor carpi radialis longus, and supinator. The nerve supply to these three muscles comes off the radial nerve prior to penetration into the supinator. The patient is able to extend the wrist, but not the metacarpophalangeal joints of the fingers, the distal joint of the thumb, or abduct the thumb in the plane of the palm. Sensibility on the dorsum of the hand may be intact as the dorsal sensory branch of the radial nerve may not be involved. Posterior interosseous nerve compression is usually secondary to hypertrophy of constricting fascial bands or various anatomical anomalies.

SOFT TISSUE INJURIES

TENDON RUPTURE

Acute tendon rupture in the upper extremity is usually secondary to trauma but bony incongruity due to old trauma may lead to tendon rupture by chronic attrition.

Profundus Tendon

The most common tendon to rupture in the hand is the profundus tendon to the ring finger. It occurs when an incomplete grip is obtained on a rapidly moving object, which suddenly tears from the patient's grasp. A classic example is an unsuccessful jersey tackle in football. It results from a sudden hyperextension of the involved finger at the time maximum grip force is being applied. The tendon is torn from its insertion on the proximal volar aspect of the distal phalanx, and retracts toward the palm. There is hemorrhage into the finger and tendon sheath with superficial ecchymotic discoloration, and pain on flexion of the involved finger. The tendon can be palpated within the tendon sheath, and the patient classically is unable to flex the distal phalanx.

Mallet Finger

Mallet finger is produced by a direct blow to the distal phalanx of the involved finger, when the joint is in slight to moderate flexion. The acute force of

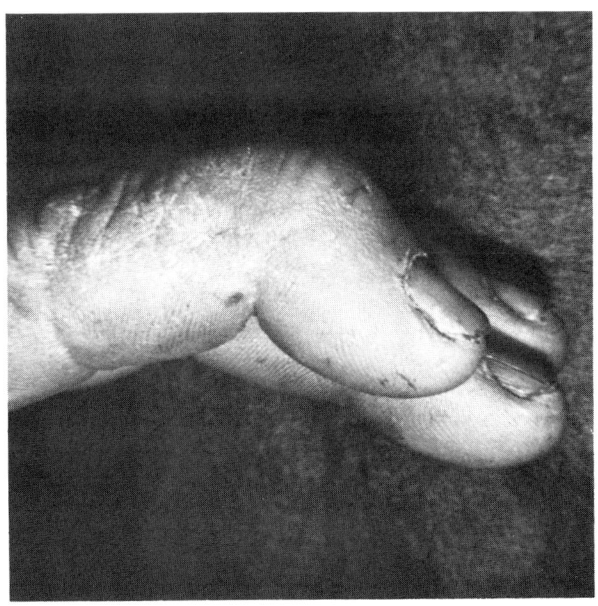

Fig. 9-33. The acute flexion deformity of the distal joint of the index finger indicates disruption of the extensor tendon mechanism from the dorsum of the distal phalanx. The hyperflexed position is due to the unbalanced pull of the flexor digitorum profundus tendon.

the blow hyperflexes the distal joint and the extensor tendon is avulsed from its insertion in the dorsum of the distal phalanx. The patient is unable to extend the distal phalanx, and it is held at an attitude of 35 to 45 degrees of flexion by the pull of the unopposed profundus tendon (Fig. 9-33). There is pain and swelling over the distal joint, and the area is tender to palpation.

All mallet finger injuries should have roentgenograms, even though no underlying fracture is suspected because the force of the traumatic blow may be sufficient to avulse a portion of the dorsal cortex and joint surface of the proximal end of the distal phalanx.

Extensor Pollicis Longus

Rupture of the extensor pollicis longus tendon can occur as it crosses the wrist joint because its fibrous sheath is attached to Lister's tubercle on the dorsum of the radius. A fracture in this area can result in disruption of the normally smooth gliding surface of the tendon, and the rough bony fragments can cause wear attrition and eventual rupture of the tendon. When it occurs there is an immediate flexion deformity of the distal joint of the thumb. The patient is unable to extend the distal joint of the thumb when the proximal joint is in extension. However, there is weak extension power of the distal joint when the proximal joint is held in flexion, as the extensor pollicis brevis can provide some power through the dorsal extensor mechanism of the intrinsic muscles.

Sprains

Finger Joints

Joint sprains are generally defined as partial or complete disruption of the ligamentous supporting structures of a joint. Sprains of the elbow and wrist joint are relatively uncommon, but sprains of the finger joints are very common. They usually result from being struck on the finger by a ball (baseball, softball, basketball, volleyball, etc.) or falling with the finger in an extended position. It can involve either the radial or ulnar collateral ligament and results in pain and tenderness on the involved side with swelling of the entire joint. The finger is examined in the extended position and at 45 degrees of flexion. Laxity of the involved ligament will be apparent when compared with the uninvolved side, when lateral stress is applied by the examiner.

Gamekeeper's Thumb

Gamekeeper's thumb is an eponym applied to a specific sprain or disruption of the ulnar collateral ligament of the metacarpophalangeal joint of the thumb. It was first described as an occupational hazard of people who break rabbit's necks. In our society, it is secondary to a fall during an athletic event in which the thumb is jammed onto a hard surface, or if the thumb is acutely abducted at the metacarpophalangeal joint.

The ulnar collateral ligament avulses from its distal insertion on the base of the proximal phalanx. There may be a small articular fracture as well (see Fig. 9-39B). There is pain, tenderness, and moderate swelling in the area, but ecchymosis is rarely present. On examination, the metacarpophalangeal joint is held in full extension and the thumb can be abducted often up to 90 degrees. Comparison with the opposite side is paramount because some people are more loose jointed than others.

Roentgenograms should always be obtained as a portion of the ulnar cortex of the proximal end of the phalanx, including a portion of the joint surface, can be avulsed with the ligament.

Dislocations

Dislocations result from trauma, and an accurate history of the mechanism of injury is important in arriving at the correct diagnosis. It is usually inappropriate to examine the area of pain, and unnecessary if the deformity is apparent on inspection. However, it is imperative to perform a gentle examination of the joints proximal and distal to the area of injury to rule out less obvious accompanying injuries. It is also necessary to ascertain the neurovascular status proximal and distal to the area of trauma. A missed brachial artery occlusion can result in a Volkmann's ischemic contracture, or a missed nerve compression can result in permanent loss of muscle function. It is imperative that roentgenograms be obtained of all dislocated joints, not only to make a correct diagnosis, but also to rule out accompanying minor or major fractures.

Elbow

The elbow joint is almost always dislocated posteriorly, with the olecranon process ultimately lying behind the distal humeral condyle. The radial head dislocates from the capitellum in a posterior lateral position. The biceps tendon is rarely ruptured and acts as a restraining force to further proximal migration of the radius and ulna. The forearm is shortened with a prominent bulge in the antecubital fossa. The arm is in moderate extension, and the olecranon process is palpable in a more proximal position. The median and ulnar nerves are in jeopardy and the brachial artery is subject to trauma. Although rarely torn it may go into reflex spasm or become occluded from pressure over the humeral condyle. Prolonged disruption of circulation to the forearm results in the condition known as Volkmann's ischemic contracture. Roentgenograms should be obtained to rule out associated fractures of the coronold process of the ulna and radial head. Humeral fractures rarely accompany elbow dislocation.

Wrist

The two most common wrist dislocations involve the lunate bone. Both are produced by a fall or blow on the outstretched hand, in which the major force of trauma is on the base of the palm. In a simple lunate dislocation (Fig. 9-34), the lunate rotates volarward on the radiolunar ligament through the anterior wrist joint capsule. The rest of the carpus remains intact in a normal position. Roentgenograms are dificult to interpret, but on the lateral view the lunate lies volar to the rest of the carpus with the superior pole pointing in a volar direction. Median nerve compression is a complication.

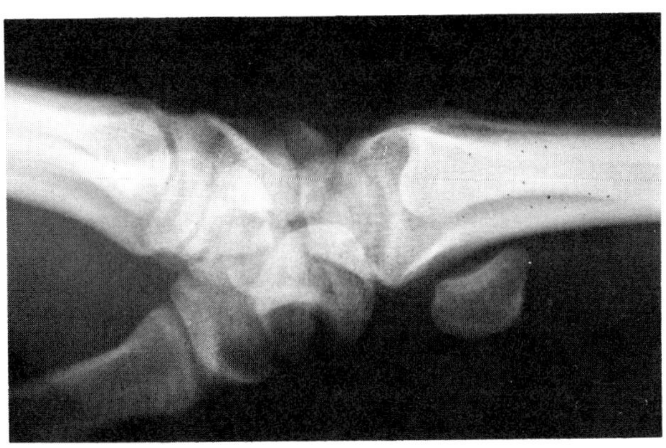

Fig. 9-34. This lateral roentgenogram demonstrates a lunate dislocation. The lunate has rotated to point in a volar direction just distal to the end of the radius. The dorsal pole of the lunate can be seen pointing towards the base of the thumb. The boney fragment beneath the distal end of the radius is the proximal pole of the scaphoid. This patient had a trans-scaphoid-lunate fracture-dislocation.

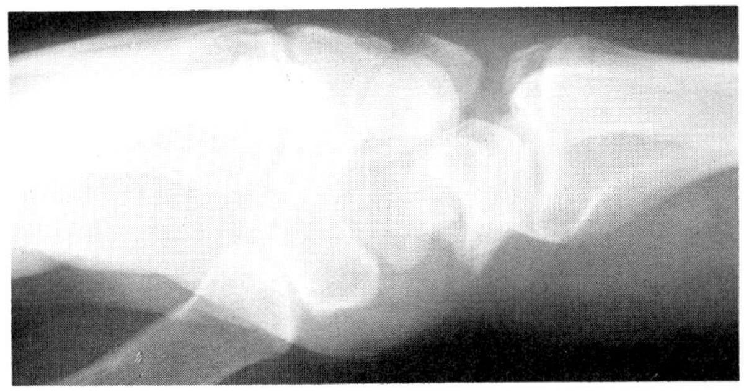

Fig. 9-35. This lateral roentgenogram demonstrates the lunate in its normal position of articulation with the distal radius with the palmar pole pointing in its normal direction, although slightly flexed. The remainder of the carpus, including the base of the capitate, can be seen riding dorsally on top of the slightly rotated lunate. The entire carpus is foreshortened.

In a perilunate dislocation (Fig. 9-35), the lunate remains in its normal relationship with the distal radius, and the remainder of the carpus dislocates dorsally around it. The lateral roentgenogram is most beneficial. It shows the lunate in essentially a normal configuration and position, but the remainder of the carpus is in a dorsal position relative to the lunate. If this dislocation is accompanied by a fracture of the scaphoid through its waist it is termed a trans-scaphoid perilunate fracture-dislocation. The scaphoid fracture is apparent on the anteroposterior roentgenogram.

Finger Joints

Metacarpophalangeal Joint. Dislocation of the metacarpophalangeal joint is almost always dorsal. It results from a fall in which the fingers are hyperextended at the metacarpophalangeal level. The metacarpal head penetrates the volar joint capsule and avulses the volar plate from its metacarpal attachment. The proximal phalanx assumes a dorsal position, and the volar plate becomes a hinge between the base of the proximal phalanx and the dorsal aspect of the metacarpal head (Fig. 9-36). This, plus the collar button effect of the ruptured volar

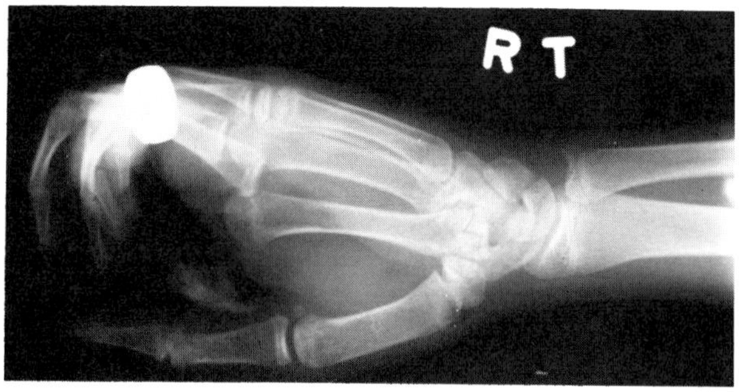

Fig. 9-36. The dorsal dislocation of the proximal phalanx of the index finger onto the dorsum of the head of the second metacarpal is readily apparent. The normal articular configuration of the metacarpophalangeal joint of the middle, ring, and little fingers is also apparent.

capsule, acts as a restraint to closed reduction. The index and middle fingers are most commonly involved.

On examination the metacarpal head is prominent in the palm in a subcutaneous position. The finger is in a cocked position on the dorsum of the metacarpal head and is painful to motion. There is little or no volar swelling, but there may be some dorsal swelling.

Volar dislocations of the metacarpophalangeal joint are almost always secondary to chronic destructive joint disease, such as rheumatoid arthritis.

Proximal Interphalangeal Joint. Dislocations of the proximal interphalangeal joint are classified as either volar or dorsal.

In a volar dislocation the middle phalanx lies volar to the proximal phalanx, as a result of disruption of the extensor mechanism at the proximal interphalangeal joint level. The central slip is avulsed from its insertion on the dorsal base of the middle phalanx, and the lateral bands are pulled volarly.

Dorsal dislocation of the proximal interphalangeal joint is far more common than a volar dislocation. It is often associated with radial or ulnar collateral ligament sprain or avulsion. The volar plate is usually torn from its insertion under the head of the proximal phalanx, and may flip up into the joint. Occasionally it is avulsed from its origin on the volar base of the middle phalanx with a chip of bone which is readily apparent on roentgenogram.

Distal Interphalangeal Joint. Distal interphalangeal joint dislocations are rare. The most common injury to this joint is an avulsion of the extensor tendon which results in a mallet finger. If associated with an avulsion of one of the collateral ligaments, the distal joint subluxes in a volar direction.

FRACTURES

ELBOW

All three bones which comprise the elbow joint can be involved with fractures. Roentgenographic examination provides the definitive diagnosis. it is imperative that a careful neurological and vascular status examination of the arm and hand be performed, as fractures about the elbow joint, especially the distal humerus, can lacerate or occlude the brachial artery. This results in a condition of forearm ischemia and muscle death known as Volkmann's ischemic contracture.

Volkmann's Ischemic Contracture

The *sine qua non* of this condition is absence of the radial pulse. It may be absent at the time of initial examination or after reduction and stabilization of the fracture. If absent, manipulation of the forearm into a different position may allow recovery of the pulse. Pain, increasing out of proportion to that expected from the fracture, is the next presenting symptom. The pain is described as deep within the forearm, constant, and aching in nature. It is exacerbated by passive extension of the fingers and is accompanied by increasing numbness in the median nerve distribution. With progression, the wrist and fingers are drawn into a flexion posture, and the forearm becomes tense and swollen secondary to muscle edema. Cell death begins at six hours after the onset of ischemia and continues until the pressure in the forearm is relieved and circulation restored. In severe cases, both the deep and superficial layers of the flexor muscles are involved along with both the median and ulnar nerves. Fibrous scar tissue which contracts replaces dead muscle producing strangulation of the median and ulnar nerves. The wrist is drawn into flexion, the thumb into abduction and extension, and the fingers assume the claw deformity due to lack of intrinsic muscle function of the hand.

WRIST

Colles' Fracture

Colles' fracture is named for Abraham Colles, Professor of Surgery at Dublin University, who first described this fracture in 1814. It involves a fracture of the distal 1.5 inches of the radius with dorsal angulation of the distal fragment, and fracture of the ulnar styloid (Fig. 9-37). It is produced by a fall on the outstretched hand usually in older people. There is moderate to marked swelling with dorsal angulation of the distal fragment resulting in a deformity similar to that of an upside-down dinner fork. Colles' fracture can be complicated by acute and chronic median nerve compression, rupture of the extensor pollicis longus tendon, and foreshortening of the radius. The last condition results in decreased motion of the wrist, prominence of the distal ulna, and radial deviation of the hand.

Smith's Fracture

Smith's fracture of the distal radius was first described in 1847 and is commonly called the reverse Colles' fracture. It is sustained by a fall on the flexed wrist. The distal fragment assumes a volar position with the ulnar styloid fractured.

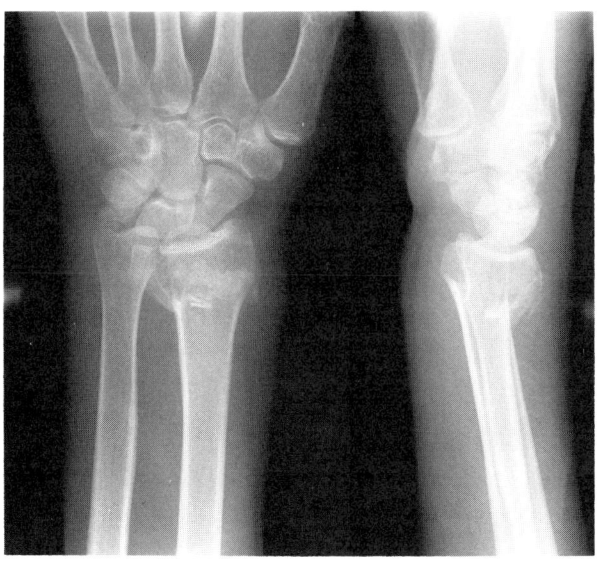

Fig. 9-37. These roentgenograms demonstrate an anteroposterior and lateral view of a Colles' fracture. On the anteroposterior view the fracture through the ulnar styloid is apparent. On the lateral view the dorsal angulation and silver fork deformity of the carpus and distal radius is apparent.

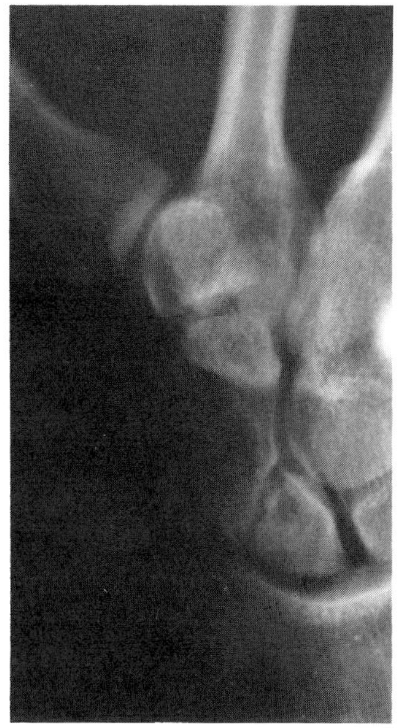

Fig. 9-38. There is a transverse fracture at the level of the proximal one-third of the carpal scaphoid.

Carpal Scaphoid

Fracture of the carpal scaphoid usually occurs in younger people who sustained the same trauma that produces a Colles' fracture in older people. Presenting symptoms include mild swelling, pain on wrist flexion or radial deviation and tenderness to palpation over the anatomical snuff box and volar aspect of the radial side of the wrist. Patients usually present with a one or two-week history of the above symptoms, and roentgenographic examination demonstrates the presence of the scaphoid fracture (Fig. 9-38). Sometimes roentgenographic examination at the time of the injury will not demonstrate the fracture. Subsequent examination, 10 to 14 days later, reveals early reabsorption at the fracture line providing the diagnosis. Fracture of the carpal scaphoid can accompany a perilunate dislocation.

HAND

Metacarpal and phalangeal fractures can be grouped together under three types: spiral, transverse, and articular.

Spiral Fractures

Spiral fractures of the metacarpals or phalanges are usually the result of a twisting injury to the finger or hand. The fracture is long and oblique with disruption of both cortices (Fig. 9-39A). It is basically unstable with shortening of the bone by proximal migration of the distal fragment. Because of the spiral nature, it twists around the fracture line, leading to a rotary deformity of the digit, distal to the fracture site. Evidence for malrotation should be determined by flexing the involved fingers individually toward the base of the palm. Normally, each finger rotates to a point at the base of the thumb on the radial side of the thenar crease. Involved fingers should be gently flexed to determine the presence or absence of malrotation and compared with the normal finger on the opposite hand.

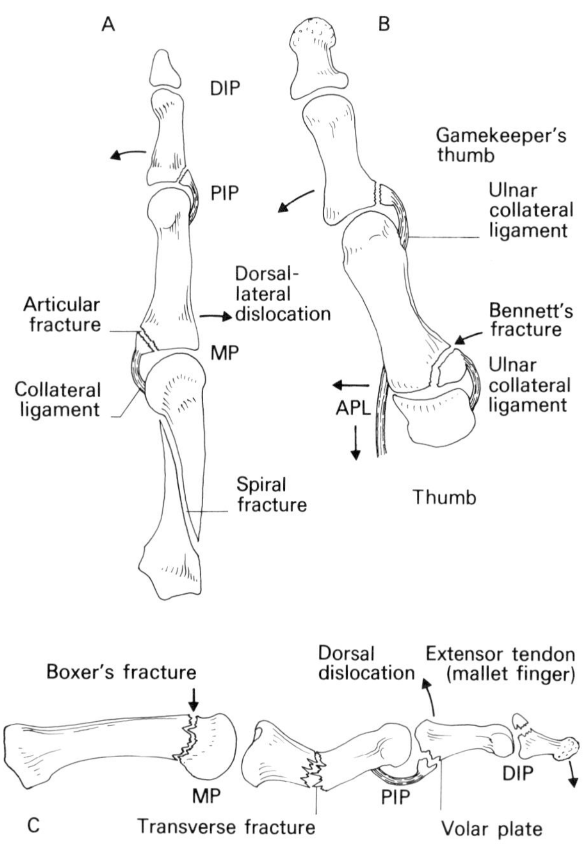

Fig. 9-39. Schematic diagram of hand fractures and dislocations. See text for explanations.

Transverse Fractures

Boxer's Fracture. Transverse fractures are usually stable. Boxer's fracture is the most common transverse fracture (see Fig. 9-39C). It usually involves the fifth metacarpal, just proximal to the head. There is volar angulation of the distal fragment, and if severe, the metacarpal head can be palpated in the palm. The metacarpophalangeal joint is usually mobile enough that the volar position of the distal fragment will not impede extension of the metacarpophalangeal joint.

Transverse fractures at the base of the proximal phalanx, especially with any volar angulation at the fracture site, can lead to fibrosis and restriction of the flexor tendon (see Fig. 9-39C). The thick proximal flexor pulley is located on the volar aspect of the proximal metacarpal, and any fracture in this area, especially with volar angulation, narrows the pulley. With healing, callus formation can further impinge the flexor tendons within the pulley limiting function of the finger in both flexion and extension.

Articular Fractures

Articular fractures of the small joints of the hand, if not recognized, can lead to very serious sequelae in terms of joint laxity, instability, and loss of function. Most articular fractures involve the supporting structures of the joints or tendon insertions at the joint level. Roentgenographic examination of the involved digit must always include anteroposterior, lateral, and at least one oblique view.

Lateral articular fractures are seen on anteroposterior roentgenogram and involve the articular surface of the phalanx on the distal side of the joint (see Fig. 9-39A). They are produced by lateral force injuries in which the collateral ligament of the joint remains intact but is avulsed along with a portion of the bone into which it inserts. These fractures can be properly positioned by flexing the finger to the functional position.

Dorsal articular fractures occur at the proximal interphalangeal and distal interphalangeal joints. They represent an avulsion of the insertions of the extensor tendon along with a fragment of bone into Which the tendon inserts (see Fig. 9-39C). At the proximal interphalangeal joint level it is the central slip of the extensor, and at the distal interphalangeal joint level it is the confluence of the lateral bands. A boutonniere deformity results at the proximal interphalangeal joint, and a classic mallet finger deformity results at the distal interphalangeal joint.

Volar articular fractures are seen on lateral roentgenogram. They usually occur from the distal phalangeal side of the joint and represent a disruption of the volar plate mechanism (see Fig. 9-39C). They usually occur secondary to a dorsal dislocation of the involved joint and may be accompanied by disruption of the collateral ligament mechanism on one side of the joint as well.

Bennett's fracture represents a specific articular fracture involving the metacarpotrapezial joint at the base of the thumb. It is an oblique fracture through the base of the thumb involving the articular surface of the proximal end of the first metacarpal (see Fig. 9-39B). The mechanism of injury is a fall on the outstretched hand which places the thumb in a position of excessive abduction. The ulnar collateral ligament of the metacarpotrapezial joint, which inserts on the ulnar aspect of the base of the first metacarpal, is essentially stronger than the bone.

The small proximal fragment is maintained in position by the ulnar collateral ligament, and the distal fragment is drawn into a proximal position by the abductor pollicis longus and extensor pollicis brevis tendons and an adducted position by the abductor pollicis muscle.

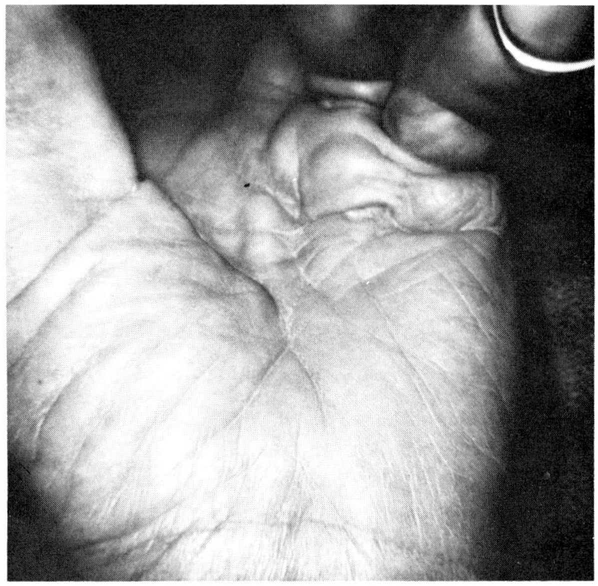

Fig. 9-40. This close-up photograph of the palm of a 67-year-old man demonstrates marked involvement with Dupuytren's disease. A thick fibrous band can be seen extending from the midpalm up across the base of the thumb to the left of the picture. The little and ring fingers are being extended to their maximum by the loops of a clamp. Note the dense thickening of the subcutaneous tissue at the base of the ring and little fingers. Also note the pitting of the skin where the fascia has grown into it.

TUMORS AND TUMOR-LIKE CONDITIONS

Dupuytren's Contracture

Dupuytren's contracture is named for the French surgeon Baron Guillaume Dupuytren. It is not a true tumor, but consists of a thickening of the palmar fascia (Fig. 9-40). It occurs primarily in caucasian males of northern European extraction with an onset between 40 and 60 years of age. It is bilateral in almost half of the patients, although rarely is there symmetrical involvement. The etiology remains unknown although there is a definite hereditary factor appearing as a simple mendelian dominant with varying penetrance. There is a statistically significant association of Dupuytren's contracture with epileptics and diabetics. Attempts at correlating the disease with manual labor have failed.

The disease usually begins at the base of the ring or little finger as a small lump or nodule in the pretendinous fascias about the level of the midpalmar crease. The nodule becomes incorporated in the thickened pretendinous band which contracts. Secondary nodules may appear in the digital fascia of the involved finger. The ring and little fingers are most commonly involved, with the middle, thumb, and index finger involved in descending order. The resulting contracture can involve the proximal and middle joint of the finger but rarely the distal joint.

Microscopic examination of the hand reveals greatly thickened strands of fascial connective tissue, with essentially normal cellular elements. The nodule has marked cellularity and hyperplasia of fibroblasts with little connective tissue between the cells and moderate pleomorphism. In some cases it resembles a low grade fibrosarcoma, but no instances of malignant degeneration have been recorded.

Ganglion

The most common tumor of the hand is a ganglion which probably results from repetitive minor trauma to the wrist joint. It usually occurs on the dorsum of the wrist joint (Fig. 9-41), but the volar radial aspect of the wrist and the metcarpophalangeal joint of the fingers are also sites of presentation. The borders of the tumor are easily outlined by transillumination with a flashlight in a darkened room. This tumor consists of several layers of flattened fibrous cells which usually form one large and several small loculations containing a jellylike substance which is clear and acellular. On the dorsum of the wrist, the most common area of origin is the dorsal scapholunate ligament. On the volar surface it is the volar scapholunate ligament. At the metacarpophalangeal level, a rent in the proximal pulley apparently allows extrusion of the synovial lining of the flexor tendons which then becomes sealed off and forms a small tumor. The patient complains of pain in the area of the tumor, especially with forced grip, and extremes of wrist motion are painful. A dorsal ganglion is readily apparent with maximum volar flexion and is prominent on the back of the wrist, usually on the radial side. The tumor is palpated as a firm, rubbery lump, located distal to the extensor retinaculum usually between the tendon of the long extensor of the thumb and the long extensor of the wrist.

Volar wrist ganglions can be brought into prominence by extending the wrist. They are usually located on the radial side between the flexor carpi radialis tendon and the radial artery. The radial pulse can be palpated in the ganglion by transmission, and occasionally the ganglion will completely surround the artery itself. Volar wrist ganglions can present into the carpal canal causing median nerve compression and signs and symptoms of a carpal tunnel syndrome.

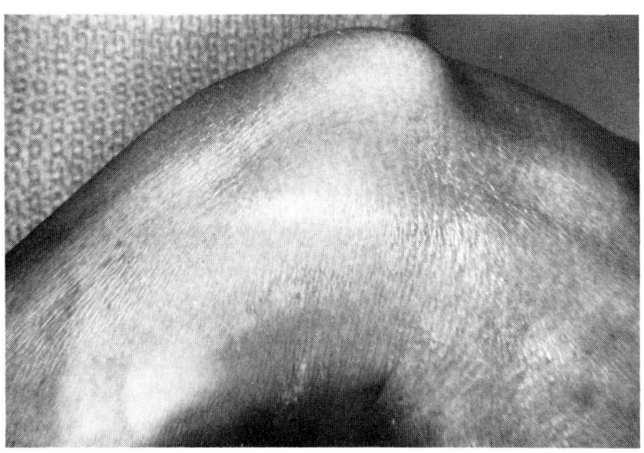

Fig. 9-41. This photograph shows a dorsal wrist ganglion made more prominent by flexing the wrist joint.

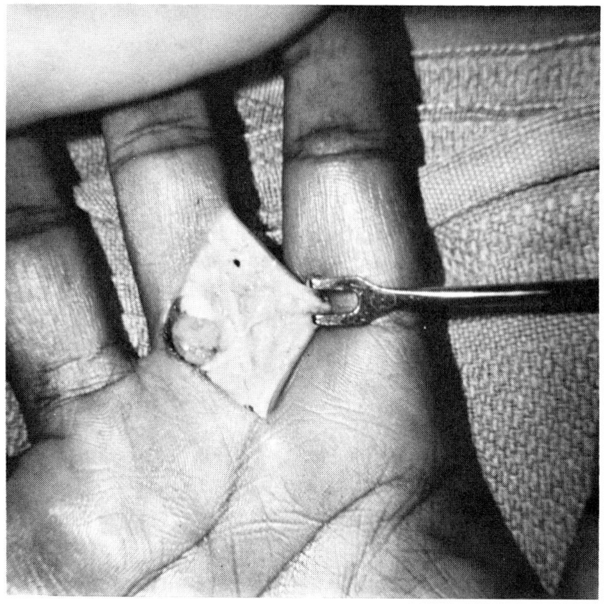

Fig. 9-42. This operative photograph shows a small ganglion presenting at the level of the metacarpophalangeal joint from the flexor tendon sheath. The ganglion is located at the apex of the incision; the neurovascular bundle can be seen traversing the surgical field just to the right of the ganglion.

Ganglions of the flexor tendon sheath at the metacarpophalangeal joint level are easily palpable on the radial or ulnar side of the joint. They are usually painful and cause symptoms of nerve irritation in the digital nerve on the involved side of the finger (Fig. 9-42). The differential diagnosis of these tumors includes xanthomas, fibromas, and epithelial inclusion cysts. Xanthomas move with motion of the tendon but ganglions do not. Fibromas and inclusion cysts are usually adherent to the overlying skin but ganglions are not.

Xanthoma (Giant Cell Tumor of Tendon Sheath)

Next to ganglions, giant cell tumors of tendon sheath are the most common tumor seen in the hand. They appear to originate from the tendon sheath, but there is some evidence that they may originate from the proximal interphalangeal or distal interphalangeal joints. Although of unknown etiology, they are thought to be secondary to trauma. They occur after the fortieth year of life with an equal sex incidence. The index or middle finger is usually involved, on the volar surface, in the right hand.

This benign tumor is rubbery-firm to palpation, does not transilluminate, and is eccentrically located on the volar aspect of the finger (Fig. 9-43). If palpable in the palm they usually have a connection with, or an extension to, a tumor in the finger. The tumor is painless but can mechanically interfere with function. If long standing, roentgenographic examination might demonstrate some bony erosion due to pressure from the contiguous tumor. Grossly it is a well encapsulated grayish-white to yellow-brown and histologically there is a predominance of fibroblasts with carotene and xanthophyll pigments in lipoid tissue accounting for the yellowish to brown color.

Epidermoid Cysts

Epidermoid cysts are the result of trauma and can occur anywhere on the forearm and hand but usually on the volar aspect. The theory is that at the

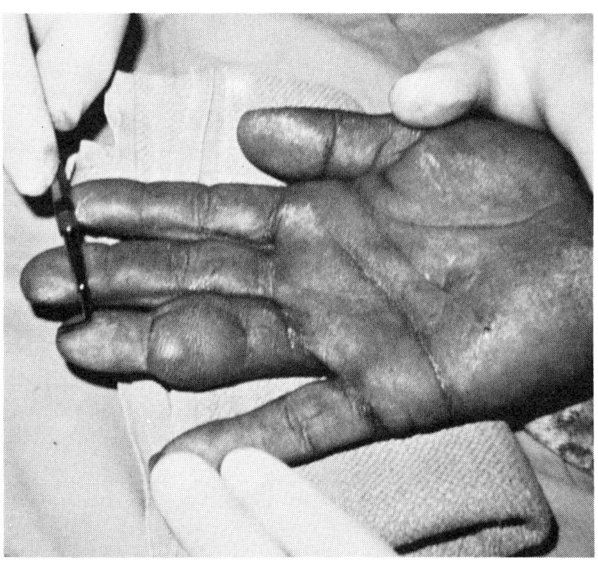

Fig. 9-43. This preoperative photograph shows the presence of a large xanthoma overlying the flexor tendons at the level of the middle phalanx of the ring finger.

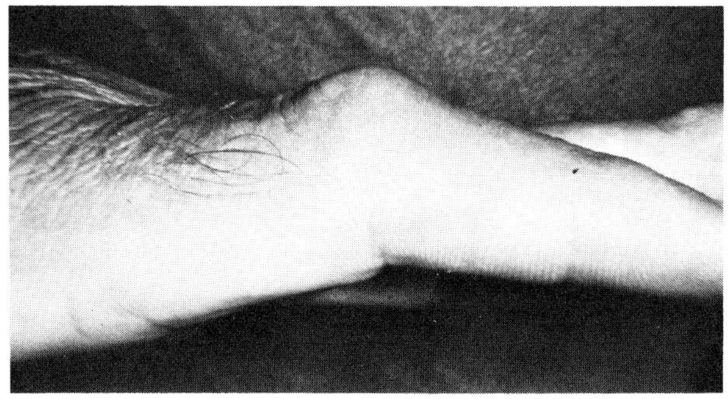

Fig. 9-44. This photograph shows the prominent knuckle pad on the dorsum of the little finger. The underlying epidermoid inclusion cyst was secondary to retained pieces of a small wood splinter.

time of trauma, small amounts of epidermis are implanted subcutaneously and proceed to enlarge and grow. The tumor is firm and rubbery and appears adherent to the overlying skin (Fig. 9-44). They do not transilluminate, are nonpainful, and are only symptomatic when located in a position interfering with function.

Grossly they are round or ovoid and variable in size with thick walls filled with a pearly white, somewhat caseous material. Histologically, the cyst has an extremely thick fibrous tissue wall lined with squamous epithelium with a keratin layer present in places. They are sometimes difficult to differentiate from a ganglion and xanthoma.

Chondroma

Although uncommon, chondromas are the most common bony tumors of the hand. They are congenital and probably secondary to cartilage rests which develop during fetal life at the time of joint differentiation. Single or multiple, they are usually confined to the phalanges, but if multiple there will be metacarpal involvement as well. They do not become malignant. The patient rarely presents with symptoms, unless a fracture through the tumor has been sustained. Often they are discovered as an incidental finding on a roentgenogram.

The lesion is highly characteristic by roentgenographic appearance and location. A benign bone cyst is about the only other condition considered in the differential diagnosis. They have a "ground-glass" appearance of amorphous radiodensity. Although

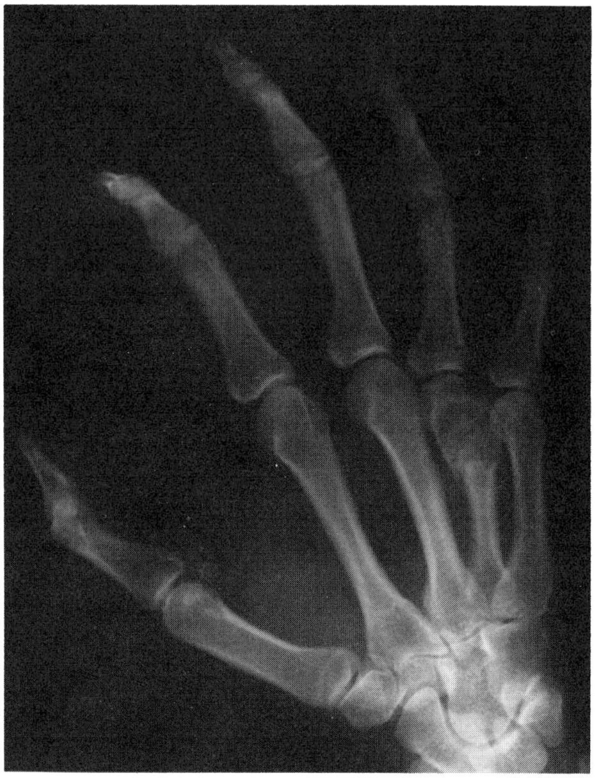

Fig. 9-45. This roentgenogram demonstrates an enchondroma just proximal to the head of the fourth metacarpal. Careful inspection will demonstrate the presence of a fracture through the enchondroma, as evidenced by some mild displacement and shortening and disruption of the cortical margins.

the bone may be slightly expanded, the tumor is usually well contained by a thin cortical shell (Fig. 9-45).

Epithelioma

Epithelioma is a malignant tumor of the skin and is the most common malignant tumor originating in the hand. It is associated with chronic or persistent irritation to the skin. Irritative agents include roentgen rays, sunlight, chemical or thermal burns, chronic infections, and even mechanical irritation of a repetitive and prolonged nature. The tumor can occur anywhere on the hand, but most often the dorsum is involved.

Grossly, the tumor is usually a heaped up, fungating ulcer with an area of drainage from an underlying chronic infection (Fig. 9-46). However, it may take the form of a small crack or fissure in an area of hyperkeratosis. Microscopically, these tumors are of the squamous or basal cell type and are of varying malignancy. The cancer spreads locally by invasion and metastasizes fairly late. Underlying fixation and destruction of deep tissues usually precedes metastasis. The great majority of the lesions occur on the back of the hand where they are readily visible and are accompanied by some pain. Ulcerations, when present, may become secondarily infected.

The differential diagnosis includes senile hyperkeratosis with keratoacanthoma formation. However, these lesions themselves are precancerous.

Carcinoma of the Nailbed

More rare than epithelioma of the hand, they are secondary to old trauma in and about the nail which has healed poorly. It is often secondary to chronic peronychial infection especially if there is underlying osteomyelitis of the distal phalanx. It is a low

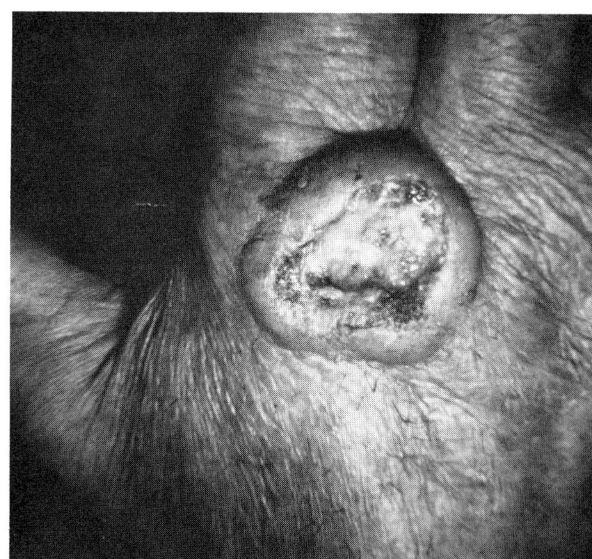

Fig. 9-46. This large heaped-up ulcerated lesion on the dorsum of the hand is a picture of a squamous cell carcinoma of approximately 2½ years' duration. Note the small areas of necrosis in the central crater and the large indurated heaped-up margins.

Table 9-1. Other Tumors Encountered in the Hand

1. Vascular a. Capillary hemangioma b. Cavernous hemangioma c. Glomus tumor of nailbed 2. Neurological a. Neurofibromatosis b. Neuroma c. Neurolemmoma 3. Bone a. Osteocartilagenous exostosis b. Osteoid osteoma c. Giant cell tumor d. Osteosarcoma e. Ewing's tumor	4. Soft tissue a. Sebaceous cyst b. Mucous cyst of fingernail c. Fibroma d. Lipoma e. Fibrosarcoma f. Malignant melanoma g. Synovioma

grade malignancy usually only locally invasive. In this regard, the differential diagnosis is primarily osteomyelitis of the distal phalanx.

Metastatic Tumor

The most common malignant tumor in the hand is of metastatic origin from a malignancy elsewhere in the body. The metastases are usually found in the phalanges, primarily the terminal phalanx. The most common source is bronchogenic carcinoma, usually of the oat-cell type, but breast tumor metastases are also common. Diagnostically, the metastasis will mimic an infection and even look like osteomyelitis on roentgenogram. Other tumors encountered in the hand are summarized in Table 9-1.

SUGGESTED READINGS

1. Boyes, J. H.: Bunnell's Surgery of the Hand. ed. 5. Philadelphia, J. B. Lippincott, 1970.
2. Brash, J. C. (ed.): Cunningham's Textbook of Anatomy, ed. 9. London, Oxford University Press, 1951.
3. Flynn, J. E. (ed.): Hand Surgery, ed. 2. Baltimore, Williams & Wilkins, 1975.
4. Kaplan, E. B.: Functional and Surgical Anatomy of the Hand, ed. 2. Philadelphia, J. B. Lippincott, 1965.
5. Spinner, M.: Injuries to the Major Branches of Peripheral Nerves of the Forearm. Philadelphia, W. B. Saunders, 1972.

10 The Hip

Robert D. D'Ambrosia, M.D.

The hip is a most challenging region to examine. It is a ball and socket joint which allows a wide range of motion that is surpassed only by the shoulder. It provides marked stability because of the close fit of the head of the femur in the acetabulum with its deepened lip, the glenoid labrum. Further stability is provided by the tough capsular ligaments plus the fact that the strongest muscles in the body go across this joint. It is the most deeply situated joint in the body and therein lies some of the real problems of examination and diagnosis of disorders of this joint.

ANATOMY

BONY LANDMARKS, MUSCLES, BURSAE

The hip joins the pelvis with the lower extremity. Grossly, the skin over the thigh medially and anteriorly (Fig. 10-1) is thin, fine, and loosely attached whereas the skin of the gluteal region (Fig. 10-2) is tough, coarse, thick, and poorly vascularized making it a common site for carbuncles. Anteriorly, the hip is flat (see Fig. 10-1); laterally, it is slightly rounded (Fig. 10-3); and posteriorly, it is quite rounded (see Fig. 10-2). The inner boundary of the hip is the innominate bone, which is formed by the junction of the ilium, ischium, and pubis. At their junction is a hollow cavity called the acetabulum. It provides the socket for the ball (head) of the femur. The crest of the ilium is palpable throughout its entire length. The anterior limit of the crest is the anterior superior iliac spine. It gives attachment to the inguinal ligament and the sartorius muscle (see Fig. 10-1). The posterior limit of the crest is the posterior superior iliac spine (see Fig. 10-2). It can be felt in the depths of the dimple of the skin lying at the level of the second sacral spine and opposite the mid-portion of the sacroiliac articulation. The prominence lateral to the hip joint is the greater trochanter (see Fig. 10-3), which is felt just below the fascia lata. The fascia lata is part of the iliotibial band that extends from the crest of the ilium to the head of the fibula and lateral condyle of the tibia (see Fig. 10-3). The iliotibial band can be felt when the thigh is adducted or abducted against resistance. The tensor fasciae latae muscle (see Fig. 10-3) originates from the anterior portion of the crest of the ilium and inserts into the fascia lata distal to the greater trochanter. It is felt when the thigh is abducted against resistance in slight flexion.

In the buttock, the rounded posterior appearance of the hip joint is predominantly gluteus maximus (see Fig. 10-2). It originates from the posterior portion of the ilium and lateral part of the sacrum to insert into the fascia lata and gluteal tuberosity of the femur just distal to the greater trochanter (see Fig. 10-3). The gluteus maximus can be felt when the thigh is extended or externally rotated against resistance. The gluteus medius lies just between the gluteus maximus and tensor fasciae latae muscle (Fig. 10-4), and can be felt when the hip is abducted against resistance. It originates from the wing of the ilium and inserts into the greater trochanter. Just below it is the gluteus minimus, which has a similar function. Below the gluteus maximus are the small external rotator muscles (piriformis, gemellus inferior, gemellus superior, obturator internus, and quadratus femoris), which can be considered as one muscle. They pass from the greater sciatic notch of the innominate bone to the back of the greater tro-

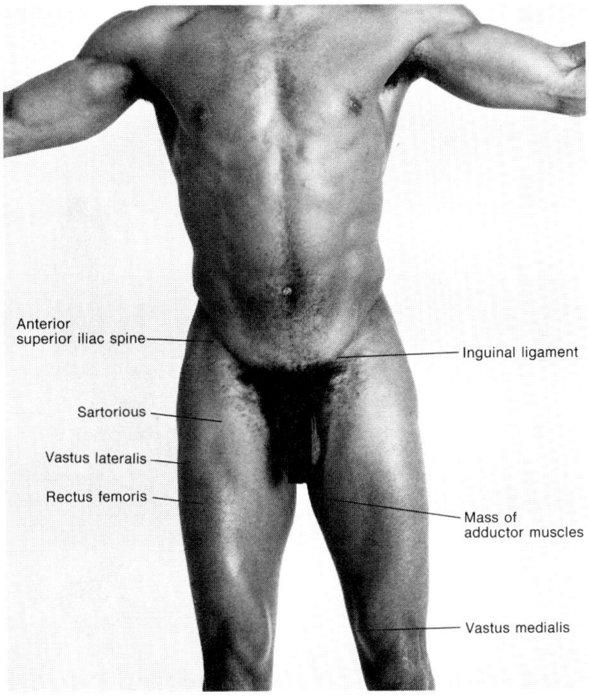

Fig. 10-1. Anterior aspect of hip is covered by thin skin which is loosely attached. Important landmarks on the anterior aspect of the hip are: anterior superior iliac spine, inguinal ligament, sartorius muscle, rectus femoris muscle, and adductor muscle mass.

chanter. They lie too deep for one to feel their power externally. The sciatic nerve leaves the sciatic notch between the piriformis and superior gemellus, posterior to the neck of the femur and midway between the ischial tuberosity and greater trochanter below the gluteus maximus; it then enters the thigh beneath the long head of the biceps femoris. It is important to know its location so that injection or incision into the posterior aspect of the hip joint will not damage it. Over the greater trochanter and immediately underneath the fascia lata lies the trochanter bursa. This area is often inflamed, and it is important to differentiate lesions here as a source of hip pain. Bursitis in this area can cause pain with any motion of the hip joint.

The sartorius muscle arises from the anterior superior iliac spine and extends to the medial aspect of the tibia (see Fig. 10-1). It is visible on the front of the hip joint when the thigh is flexed, abducted, and laterally rotated. Lateral to and just below the sartorius muscle is the bulky rectus femoris, which can be felt by setting the quadriceps muscle as in straight leg-raising (see Fig. 10-1). Medial to the sartorius muscle lies the adductor group of muscles of the thigh (gracilis, pectineus, adductor longus, adductor brevis, adductor magnus, and obturator externus) (Fig. 10-5). They arise from the external surfaces of the pubic ramus and the ramus of the ischium. They are supplied by the obturator nerve and are readily visible upon resisted adduction of the hip.

ARTICULAR CAPSULE AND LIGAMENTS

Stripped of its external musculature, the hip is visualized as a mass of capsular tissue holding the ball (head of femur) in the rounded socket (acetabulum) (Fig. 10-6). The head of the femur forms two

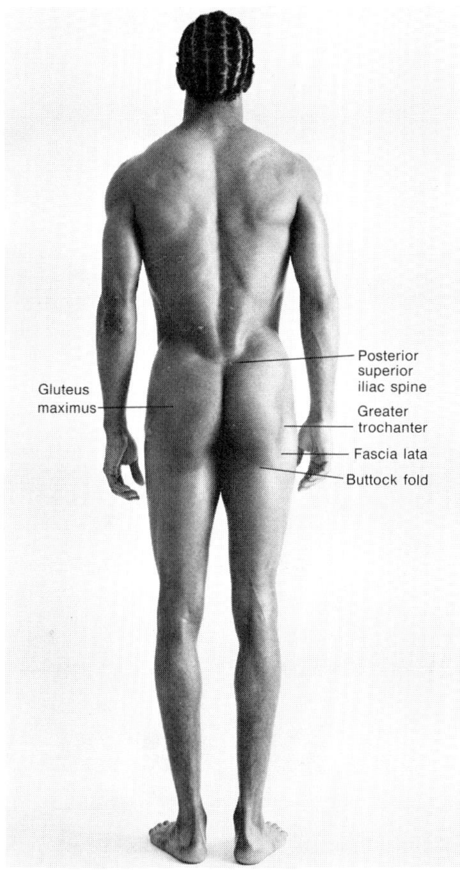

Fig. 10-2. Posterior aspect of the hip is covered by the gluteus maximus muscle. Important landmarks on the posterior aspect of the hip are: posterior superior iliac spine and buttock fold.

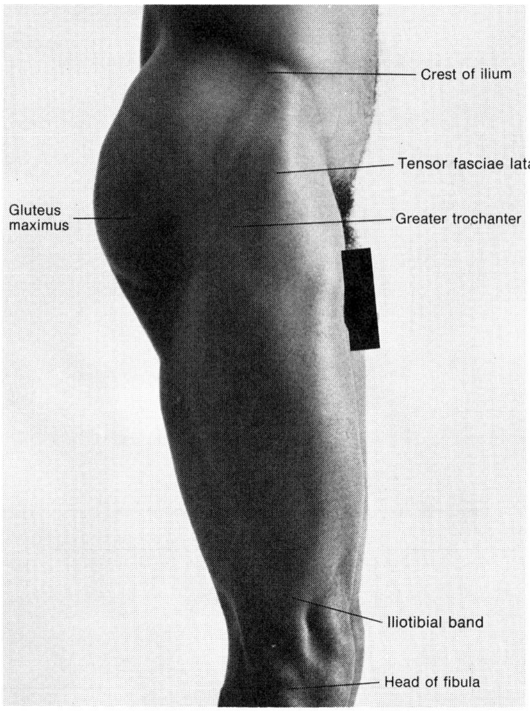

Fig. 10-3. Lateral aspect of the hip which is slightly rounded. The lateral prominence is the greater trochanter.

thirds of a sphere which is covered by articular cartilage. The cartilage is thickest superiorly in the line of weight-bearing and thins to an irregular termination at the junction with the neck of the femur. It is loosely attached to the acetabulum by the ligamentum teres which passes from the lower portion of the acetabulum to the center of the head. It has no function in the normal use of the hip but does act as a checkrein limiting the extremes of rotation and adduction.

The articular surface of the acetabulum is horseshoe in shape and arches around the acetabular fossa. Its cartilage is thickest superiorly and thins out at the border of the fossa. The fossa lodges a fat mass called the haversian gland, which is covered by synovium, and the transverse ligament of the acetabulum closes the fossa below. The acetabulum is deepened superiorly by the fibrocartilage glenoid labrum, which is attached to the bony rim and the transverse ligament. The free edge of this lip cups around the head of the femur, thus holding the ball firmly in the socket. The acetabulum is strongest superiorly and posteriorly where the greatest strain is on weight-bearing. Anteriorly and inferiorly, where there is little strain, it is shallow and thin.

The hip joint is surrounded by a cylinder of ligaments that forms a heavy strong capsule which encloses the hip joint and prevents the head from moving laterally out of the acetabulum (Figs. 10-7, 10-8). The capsule is attached to the bony rim of the acetabulum and extends distally to insert on the femur in the area of the intertrochanteric line. The capsule is shorter posteriorly and limits internal rotation. The capsule is also reinforced by several

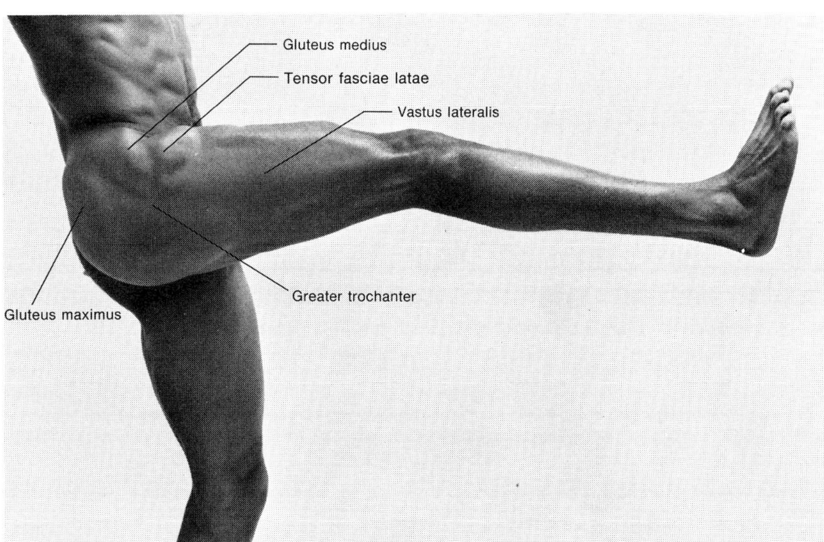

Fig. 10-4. Lateral aspect of the hip. The gluteus medius muscle is prominent lying between the gluteus maximus and tensor fasciae latae muscles.

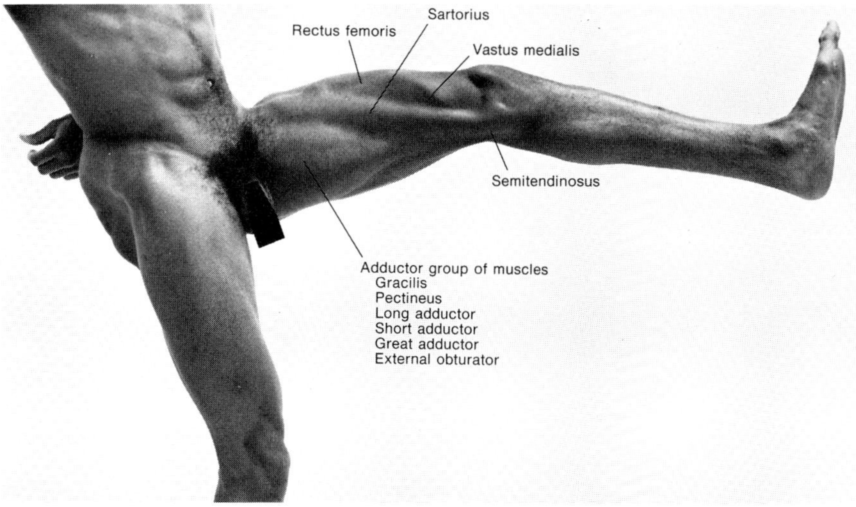

Fig. 10-5. Medial aspect of the hip. The adductor mass of muscles lies medial to the sartorius muscle.

strong bands. The orbicular ligament runs in a circular manner in contrast to the ischiofemoral and capsular fibers, which are longitudinal and most prominent posteriorly (see Fig. 10-8). This all aids in holding the head of the femur in the acetabulum. The fibers of the capsule, therefore, wind downward and forward anteriorly in a spiral course which is continued onto the posterior aspect of the capsule. As the thigh becomes fully extended, the capsule shortens and twists the head of the femur, which is guided like a screw into the socket. In full extension, the head is most congruent with the acetabulum and provides the hip its greatest stability. Adding strength to the articular capsule are three accessory bands: iliofemoral, pubofemoral, and ischiofemoral ligaments. The *iliofemoral* ligament lies on the anterior surface of the capsule forming an inverted Y (λ). The stem is attached to the anterior inferior iliac spine and the diverging ends of the Y are attached to the entire length of the intertrochanteric line. It is tightest in full extension. The *pubofemoral* ligament reinforces the capsule on its medial inferior surface. It also is tightest in extension and limits abduction. The *ischiofemoral* ligament reinforces the posterior aspect of the capsule.

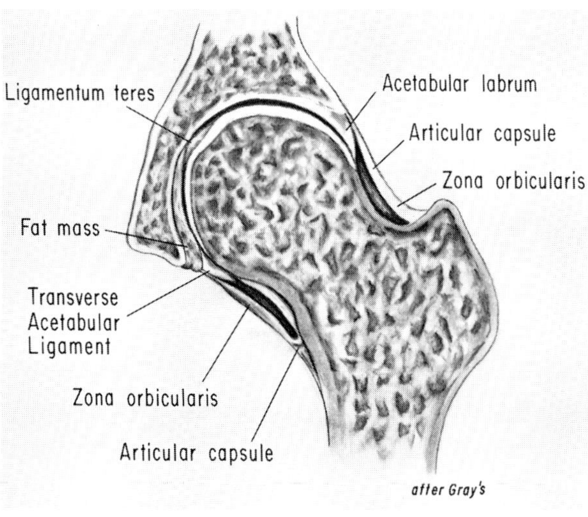

Fig. 10-6. Sagittal section through hip joint.

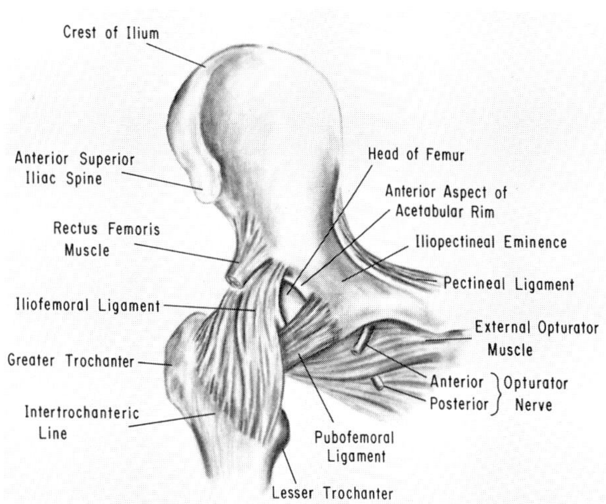

Fig. 10-7. Ligaments of the hip joint—anterior.

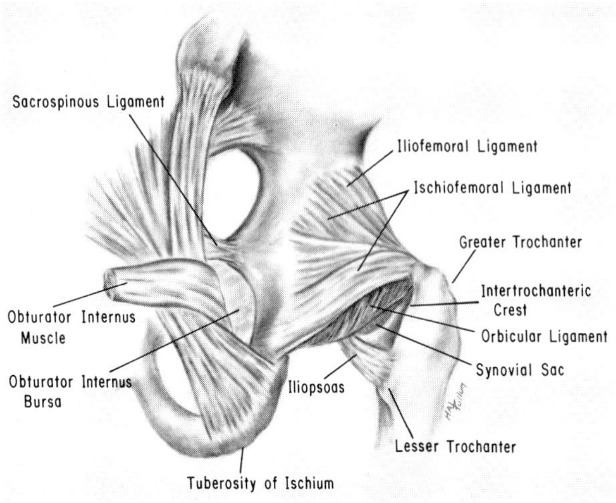

Fig. 10-8. Ligaments of the hip joint—posterior.

VASCULAR ANATOMY OF THE FEMORAL HEAD

There are three primary sources of blood supply to the adult femoral head which have been carefully worked out by Trueta (Fig. 10-9). The most important and main vascular supply is from the *retinacular* vessels, which reach the femoral head from a posterior lateral direction with the superior branch (lateral epiphyseal artery) being the most important. It arises from the medial femoral circumflex artery.

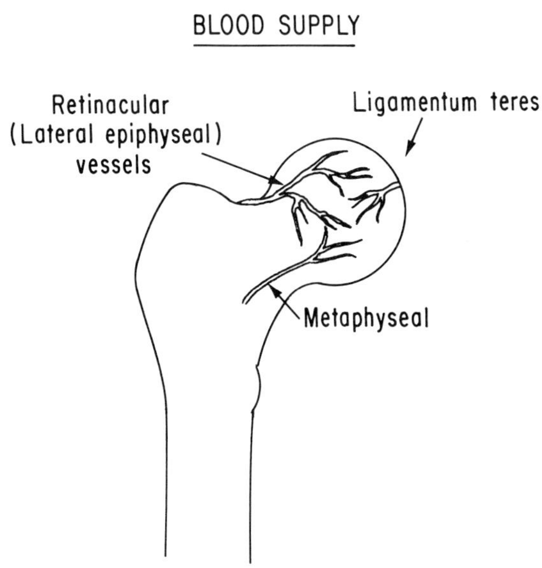

Fig. 10-9. Vascular anatomy of the femoral head.

There is an anterior retinacular artery arising from the lateral femoral circumflex artery, but it is inconsistent. The other two sources of blood supply are the *ligamentum teres* and *metaphyseal* vessels. They are supplemental sources and are usually unimportant, but in some instances can be vital.

The ligamentum teres usually arises from the obturator artery and, occasionally, the medial femoral circumflex. The metaphyseal vessels are terminations of the nutrient artery of the femur, which ascends in the medullary cavity before crossing the metaphysis.

In childhood the vascular supply is variable and several childhood diseases of the hip have been related to this variability. In the infantile period from four months to four years the predominant supply is from the metaphyseal vessels with the lateral epiphyseal vessels being secondary. There are no vessels from the ligamentum teres at this point.

In the intermediate period from four to seven years the epiphyseal plate becomes established, thus effectively blocking the metaphyseal vessels. The ligamentum teres vessels are still absent and, therefore, the only source of blood is from the lateral epiphyseal vessels. If they should become obstructed by trauma or inflammation we have Legg-Calvé-Perthes disease.

In preadolescence (nine to ten years) the arteries from the ligamentum teres finally become consistent but the growth plate continues to block the metaphyseal vessels. Legg-Calvé-Perthes disease also becomes less common with the arrival of this supplemental source of blood.

In adolescence (11 to 15 years) the epiphyseal plate begins to break down with metaphyseal vessels beginning to cross over the former barrier. This period of great vascular activity on the metaphyseal side of the growth plate may account for the occurrence of slipped capital femoral epiphysis. Once epiphyseal fusion takes place the three sources of blood supply characteristic of the adult are present.

NECK—SHAFT ANGLE

The hip with its attached capsule, ligaments, and muscles will move as a ball and socket joint within the range of a half sphere. At birth, the hip is in flexion, lacking full extension by 20 degrees. The neck of the femur is also twisted so that anteversion of 25 degrees is present, which is the same position noted in four-legged animals. During the first two years of life, the position of extension is assumed, and anteversion is reduced to 5 to 15 degrees. Often, the anteversion persists in later life and is manifested in intoeing. It is also abnormally increased in persons with congenital dislocation of the hip (see Fig. 10-11).

REGIONAL EXAMINATION OF THE HIP

HISTORY

The first step in assessing hip disease is to take an accurate and complete history. Problems about the hip will usually be manifest as pain, loss of joint motion, muscle weakness which causes a peculiar gait, and joint disturbances which produce deformity; all these problems characteristically occur at certain ages.

The presence or absence of pain should be noted. Although most hip problems involve pain, a few are characterized by the absence of pain, for example, congenital dislocation of the hip, coxa vara, and Charcot's joint. The hip joint is supplied by three nerves: obturator, femoral, and sciatic. Therefore, pain in the hip joint can be felt medially, anteriorly, or posteriorly or it may be referred along the course of any of these nerves. Because of this, pain in the region of the hip joint is usually misleading. Hip pain is usually felt in the groin or in the front or inner part of the thigh, but pain in the knee can be the predominant feature. There are a number of entities that will mimic hip pain. Pain in the spine or pelvis will often be referred to the hip, and there will be no connection with the hip joint whatsoever. The hip pain referred from the lower lumbar vertebrae and sacrum will usually be felt in the gluteal region with radiation often down the back or outer side of the thigh. In contrast, lesions in the upper lumbar vertebrae will often refer pain into the anterior aspect of the thigh. True hip pain is made worse by walking, whereas hip pain referred from the spine will usually be aggravated by such activities as stooping and lifting and will often be relieved by walking. Hernias and various problems in the lower part of the abdomen will often refer pain into the groin and proximal part of the thigh. Thrombophlebitis, blood clots, or problems of insufficient blood supply will often be associated with pain in the buttock and anterior aspect of the thigh.

Almost all disorders of the hip will eventually result in some loss of joint motion. The very young patient cannot tell you this, and the older patient will usually relate it as an inability to tie shoes or put on trousers.

Muscles in certain areas of the hip can become weak and present a characteristic gait. Particular joint disturbances, such as osteoarthritis, will produce characteristic deformities of the hip brought about by flexion and external rotation contractures. Usually these conditions will be related to the physician in unusual manners.

Age is very important in assessing hip disease, especially in children. During certain age periods, one characteristically sees specific problems that will not be seen at other times (Table 10-1).

PHYSICAL EXAMINATION

For the hip joint to be examined adequately, the patient should remove all clothing except for undergarments and a sheet or towel is placed between his legs. It is important to proceed with the examination in a systematic and routine manner so that important parts of the examination are not overlooked. You will also find that a routine, orderly manner will make the maximum use of your time, thus enhancing your efficiency. A problem-oriented physical examination, as in the musculoskeletal consultation, is highly recommended.

Table 10-1. Hip Disorders in Relation to Age

Disease	*Age at Diagnosis*
CDH	Infancy
Coxa vara	Infancy or later
Infection	Infancy and childhood but can occur later
Legg-Calvé-Perthes	3–12
Toxic synovitis	2–9
Slipped capital femoral epiphysis	10–15
Osteoid osteoma	5–30
Trauma	All ages
Malignancy	All ages
Rheumatoid arthritis	All ages
Aseptic necrosis	All ages
Degenerative arthritis	Above 40
Neuropathic joint	Above 40

GROSS INSPECTION

With the patient standing, observe and inspect the posture, both in the front and back, for the presence of any fixed deformity. Note the level of the iliac crests, anterior iliac spines, posterior iliac spines, position of the knee, and if both feet are flat and on the floor. Any deformity of the hip joint will affect the patient's posture.

Pelvic Extremity Relationships

Causes of Iliac Crest Elevation. If there is a unilateral elevation of the iliac crests, one must take into account and look for possible causes such as:

Lumbar Scoliosis. If the patient has a fixed structural lumbar scoliosis, the unilateral elevation of one crest will be seen (Fig. 10-10). It is, therefore, important to observe the patient's back for this deformity.

Adduction Contracture. If there is an adduction contracture, the affected limb will be physiologically shortened, because when the patient stands he would have to cross his adducted foot over the normal side. The patient will raise the pelvis on the side of the fixed adduction deformity to compensate for this deformity, causing apparent shortening of that extremity. The pelvic tilt causes an apparent shortening of the leg.

Abduction Contracture. This is less common than an adduction contracture but when it does occur it causes that limb to be physiologically lengthened. The patient compensates by raising the pelvis on the opposite side causing that extremity to look shorter.

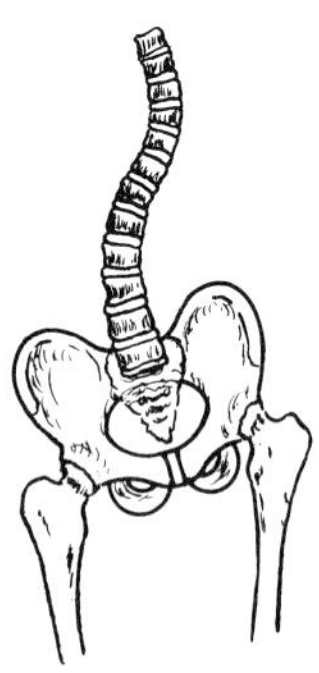

Fig. 10-10. A fixed structural lumbar scoliosis can produce unilateral elevation of one crest. It is just one of several causes for iliac crest elevation. No hip pathology is present and the problem is in the back.

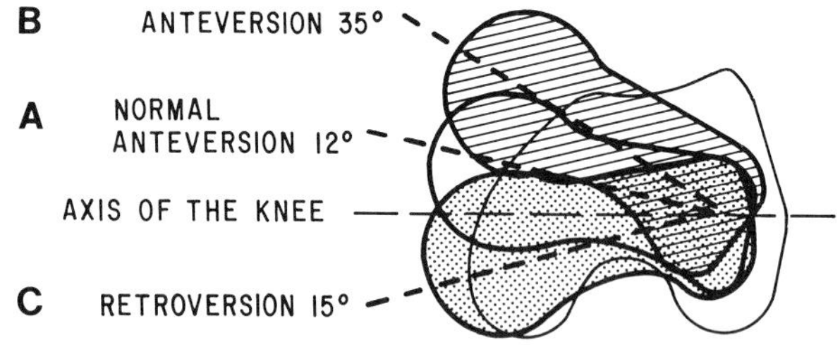

Fig. 10-11. Version at the neck of the femur is evaluated by looking down on the hip and knee joint with the femoral head superimposed on the knee joint. The angle made between the axis of the knee and axis of the neck of the femur is described as version of the neck of the femur. If this angle is in the anterior plane, it is known as anteversion and in normal subjects this averages out to 12 degrees (*A*). Pronounced anteversion is seen in congenital dislocated hip and most in-toeing problems (*B*). If the angle is in the posterior plane it is known as retroversion (*C*). Retroversion is occasionally seen in the person who out-toes (duck walker).

The patient can also compensate for the deformity by bending the knee on the involved side or standing on the toes (equinus position) of the opposite side.

Leg Length Inequality. There may be actual leg length differences, but with a mobile spine and hip joint as much as 1 inch of shortening can be masked even without bending the opposite knee or standing in the equinus position. This can be accomplished by tilting the pelvis and assuming an abducted position at the hip joint on the involved side or adducted position in the opposite extremity (see Fig. 10-12).

Version at Neck of Femur. There may be version problems at the neck of the femur which will manifest either as an out-toeing (laterally rotated) due to retroversion or an in-toeing (internally rotated) due to anteversion (Fig. 10-11).

Version problems are best detected by observing the position of the patellas during a walking exercise. A patella that points straight ahead usually denotes neither hip nor thigh abnormality, and the problem is below the knee. If the neck of the femur is in anteversion, the head of the femur will be uncovered anteriorly. For this patient to bear weight adequately the leg will be rotated medially to cover the head of the femur completely. In this individual the patella will point medially when walking. If the neck of the femur is in retroversion, the head of the femur will be inadequately covered posteriorly. For this patient to bear weight adequately, the leg must be rotated laterally to better cover the head of the femur. The patella will point laterally when walking.

Gait

As the patient walks to the examining table observe the gait. Gait analysis will often disclose obvious problems of the hip area. There are several gaits characteristic of hip disease.

Antalgic (Painful) Hip Gait. The patient will move slowly and gingerly with a short stance phase.

Ankylosed (Stiff) Hip Gait. Stride is restricted and a circumducted gait is characteristic.

Extensor Thrust Gait. This occurs secondary to loss of gluteus maximus muscle power and is apparent in patients who cannot halt their stride because of the defective extensor musculature; therefore, the upper torso attempts to slow down the stride.

Trendelenburg Gait. This is secondary to weakness of abductor muscles and causes an instability of the hip joint so that when the patient is walking on the affected hip, he throws his body over the affected hip to bring his center of gravity over the hip.

Careful Inspection and Palpation

A solid, sturdy table which does not fold is the best type for a hip examination. With the patient supine, the first step is to be sure the pelvis is lying square with the limbs. This is done by observing the anterior iliac spines and their relationship with the limbs. Attempts to set the pelvis square may be impossible because of a fixed pelvis tilt secondary to fixed adduction or abduction contractures. If there is fixed pelvic deformity, this must be kept in mind during the subsequent course of the examination. Carefully observe and palpate the bony and soft tissue contours. The hip joint is such that obvious swelling in the hip joint secondary to an irritation will be totally masked by the soft tissues. Patients with synovial irritation and swelling, however, will unwind their hip to provide maximum room for the increased fluid, thus bringing their extremity into a flexed, abducted, externally rotated position. Look for previous surgical scars, traumatic scars, or sinus tracts from previous infection in the area of the hip. Inspect the skin about the hip anteriorly and posteriorly for color and texture. Compare it with the opposite hip. Carefully palpate the bony and muscular contours as described earlier. Note any abnormalities of bone or soft tissue. While palpating about the hip note any areas of tenderness and be very specific as to location for it is the first step in delineating the source of the problem. If there is marked tenderness in the area of the greater trochanter, focus in on that area to explain the nature of the pain. Be aware of skin temperature differences by constant comparison with the opposite side.

Leg Length Measurements

True and Apparent Leg Lengths

Measure limb lengths and differentiate the true or real lengths from the apparent lengths which may give a false appearance because of a fixed pelvic tilt (Fig. 10-12). To measure the true length accurately, one should measure from the center of the hip joint to the medial malleolus. Since there is no surface landmark for the hip joint, the anterior superior iliac spine is used; this is obvious lateral to the hip joint. For the measurement to be accurate, the angle between limb and pelvis must be the same on both sides. Both limbs must be placed in a symmetrically

DIFFERENTIATION OF TRUE FROM APPARENT LIMB LENGTH

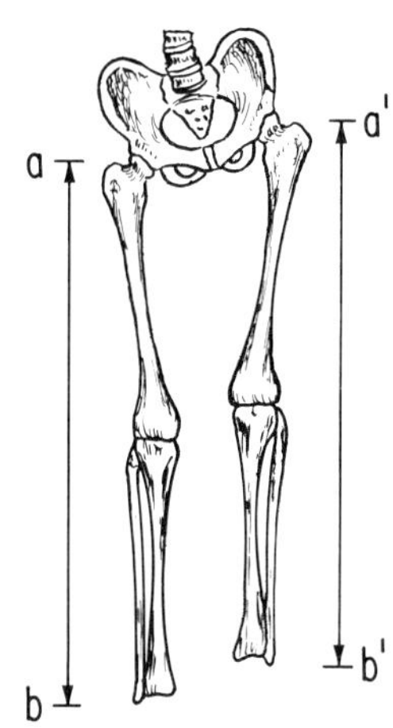

Fig. 10-12. Differentiation of true from apparent limb length. The true length of the right limb (a-b) and left limb (a′-b′) are equal. The apparent limb length is different because the pelvis is not square. If the pelvis was made square the apparent and true limb lengths would be equal.

comparable position in relation to the pelvis. For example, if there is a fixed adduction contracture on one side, the opposite limb should go into the same adducted position when it is measured because if the limb is adducted, the medial malleolus is carried farther away from the anterosuperior iliac spine, and if abducted, it is brought closer to the anterosuperior iliac spine. Next, compare the true length with the apparent limb length. This is done by measureing from a point in the midline above the hip joint to the medial malleolus. The most common point used is the xiphisternum.

Tests for Extremity Shortening Above Trochanter Level

If there is evidence of shortening of the limb, it should be determined if it is in the hip joint area. If the shortening has occurred between the anterosuperior iliac spine and the trochanteric level, the shortening can be ascribed to an abnormality at or near the hip joint. There are several tests which can be used to determine if there is shortening above the trochanteric level. The more common ones used are presented in the order of their use.

Nélaton's Line. An imaginary line is drawn from the anterosuperior iliac spine to the ischial tuberosity (Fig. 10-13). Normally, the greater trochanter lies just distal to this line. If the greater trochanter is at the level of the line, subluxation or coxa vara is suggested, but this can be normal in some individuals. If the greater trochanter is above Nélaton's line, the femur has definitely displaced upward, and this could be due to congenital dislocation of the hip, coxa vara, or epiphyseal arrest of the proximal femur from several causes.

Bryant's Triangle. This is constructed by dropping a perpendicular from the anterosuperior iliac spine, projecting a second perpendicular up from the tip of the greater trochanter. The triangle is then constructed from the intersection of the perpendiculars, the anterosuperior iliac spine, and greater trochanter. The distance measured is the distance from the intersection of the perpendicular to the greater trochanter (Fig. 10-14). This measurement is then compared with the opposite side. If both sides are abnormal, this measurement, of course, is useless.

Schoemaker's Line. Imaginary lines are drawn from the tip of the greater trochanters through the anterosuperior iliac spines and projected upward (Fig. 10-15). The two lines should meet in the midline above the umbilicus. If one femur is displaced upward, the two lines intersect away from the mid-

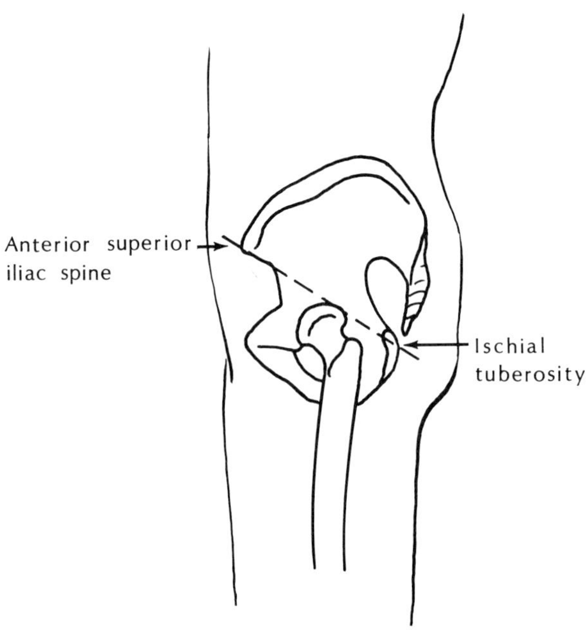

Fig. 10-13. Nélaton's line.

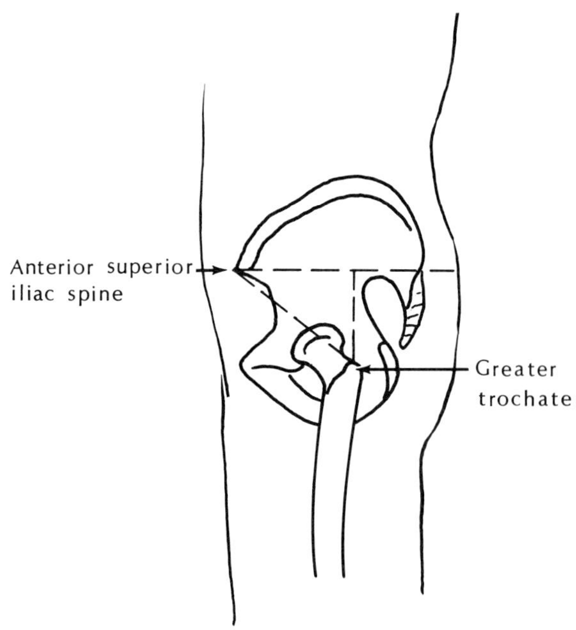

Fig. 10-14. Bryant's triangle.

line on the normal side. If both femurs are displaced upward, the two lines will intersect close to the midline but below the umbilicus.

Fixed Deformities

With the patient on a firm table, avoiding soft beds or collapsible tables, accurately record any fixed deformities which you may have noticed in the earlier part of your examination. Contractures of the capsule or muscle commonly occur about the hip joint, thus preventing the hip from coming to a neutral position.

Adduction-Abduction

Fixed adduction or abduction of the hip is determined by drawing an imaginary line between the two anterior iliac spines and seeing the relationship of each limb with the pelvis. If a perpendicular is formed, there is no fixed contracture. If the angle formed is less than 90 degrees, there is an adduction contracture, and if it is more than 90 degrees, there is a fixed abduction contracture.

Fixed Flexion

If there is a fixed flexion contracture at the hip, the patient compensates for it by arching the spine and pelvis into an exaggerated lordosis. Lordosis is often hereditary, however, and does not, by itself, denote a fixed hip flexion contracture. Therefore, before checking for flexion at the hip joint, routinely place your hand between the lumbar vertebrae and table to check for lordosis. If there is no lordosis, there can be no fixed flexion deformity. If, however, lordosis is present, the fixed flexion contracture is determined by means of the Thomas test. The normal hip is flexed maximally so that the pelvis and spine rotate until the arching of the pelvis and spine is obliterated. If there is a fixed flexion deformity, the affected limb will be lifted from the table, and the angle the thigh makes with the table is the degree of flexion contracture present.

Fixed Rotation

Fixed rotation contractures are best determined by carefully observing the position of the patella. With the hip in a neutral position, the patella will normally point straight upward. If there is a fixed rotation deformity, the limb will be unable to rotate into the neutral position with the patella pointing straight up. The angle by which the patella falls short of neutral is the degree of fixed rotational contracture. Lateral rotation contractures are most commonly observed because of their development with osteoarthritis.

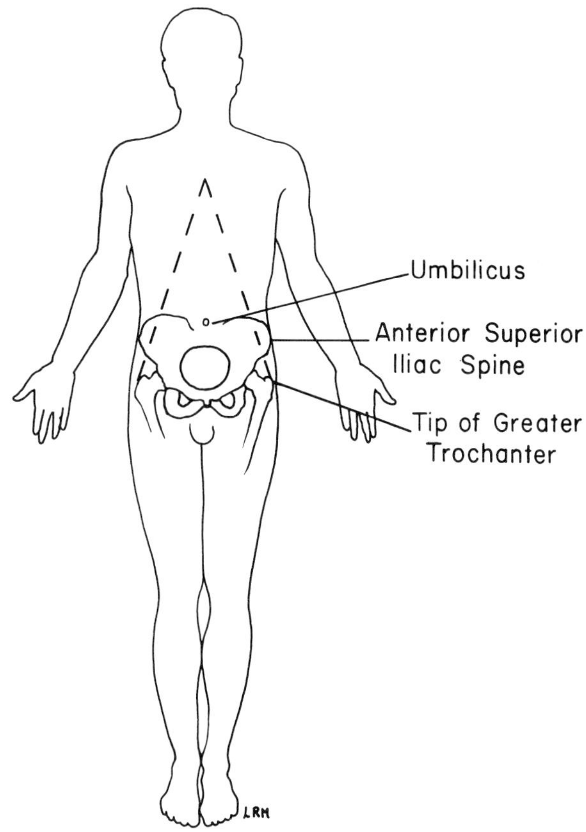

Fig. 10-15. Schoemaker's lines.

Range of Motion

Motion of the hip should be accurately recorded. Be careful that small restrictions of hip motion are not being masked by motion of the pelvis. Therefore, during your examination for motion at the hip joint, it is essential that one hand be kept on the pelvis to be sure compensatory motion is not being performed at the pelvis.

Flexion

Flexion is first tested for after the presence or absence of a flexion contracture has been deter-

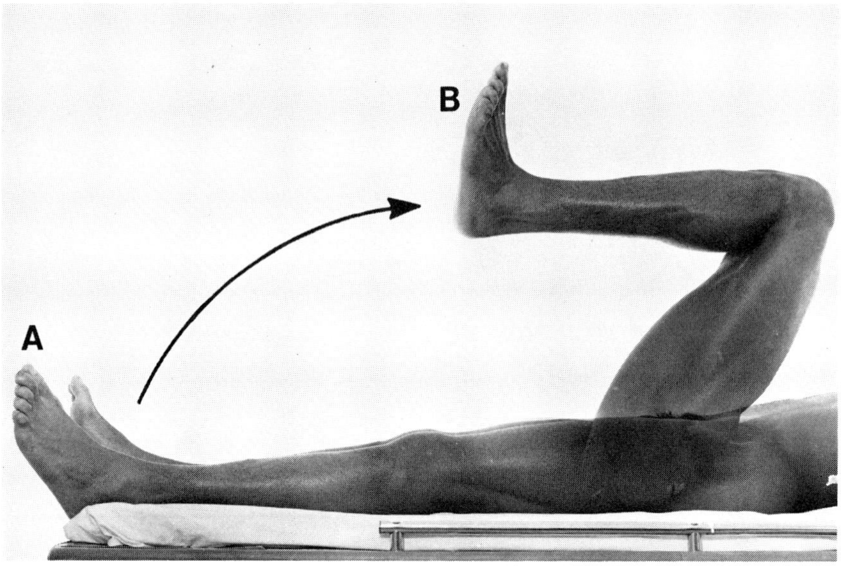

Fig. 10-16. Flexion at the hip is measured with the patient supine on a flat surface (*A*). The hip is then flexed maximally (*B*) with the examiner keeping one hand on the iliac crest noting when the pelvis begins to rotate.

mined. Normal flexion will be 120 to 135 degrees (Fig. 10-16). Flexion is increased 10 to 15 degrees in children.

Abduction

Abduction is then measured in both extension (Fig. 10-17) and flexion (Fig. 10-18). The limb being examined is held with one hand while the opposite hand is on the pelvis so that false measurements are not imparted due to pelvic tilt. Abduction in extension in the adult is approximately 35 to 40 degrees, and abduction in flexion is 70 to 75 degrees. Abduction is increased 10 to 20 degrees in children. Coxa vara will often be associated with more limited abduction in extension than in flexion because the greater trochanter abuts against the pelvis in extension.

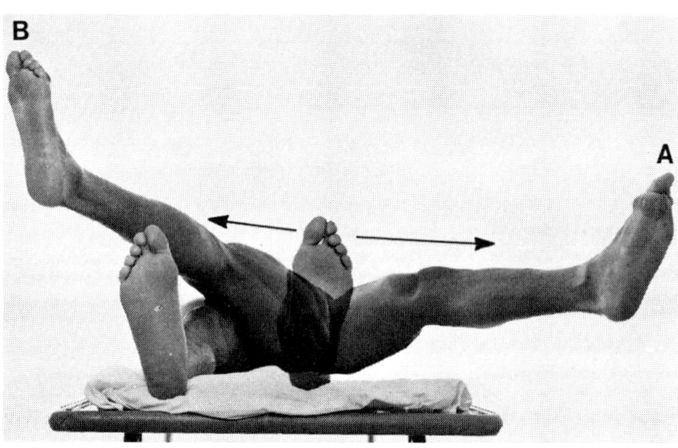

Fig. 10-17. Abduction (*A*) and adduction (*B*) of the hip joint measured in extension. The patient is supine on a flat surface with the feet at right angles to the pelvis. Outward motion of the extremity is abduction (*A*) and inward motion of the extremity is adduction (*B*).

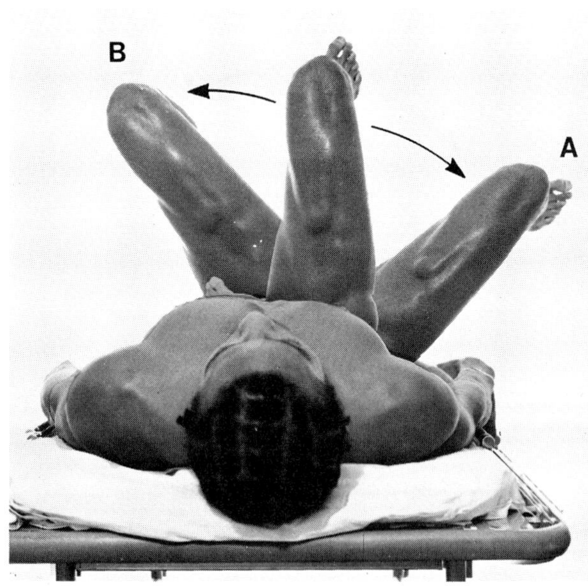

Fig. 10-18. Abduction (*A*) and adduction (*B*) of the hip joint measured in 90 degrees of flexion. Outward motion of the extremity is abduction (*A*) and inward motion of the extremity is adduction (*B*).

Adduction

Adduction is measured by crossing the leg to be measured over the opposite leg and simultaneously keeping one hand on the pelvis to avoid pelvic tilt (see Figs. 10-17 and 10-18). Adduction is normally 25 to 30 degrees.

Rotation

Internal and external rotation can be measured both in extension (Fig. 10-19) and flexion (Fig. 10-20). However, be sure to use an imaginary line drawn through the knee and not in relation to the foot or abnormally increased measurements will result. Both internal and external rotation are approximately 45 degrees in the young adult. There is greater internal rotation in the child than in the older adult.

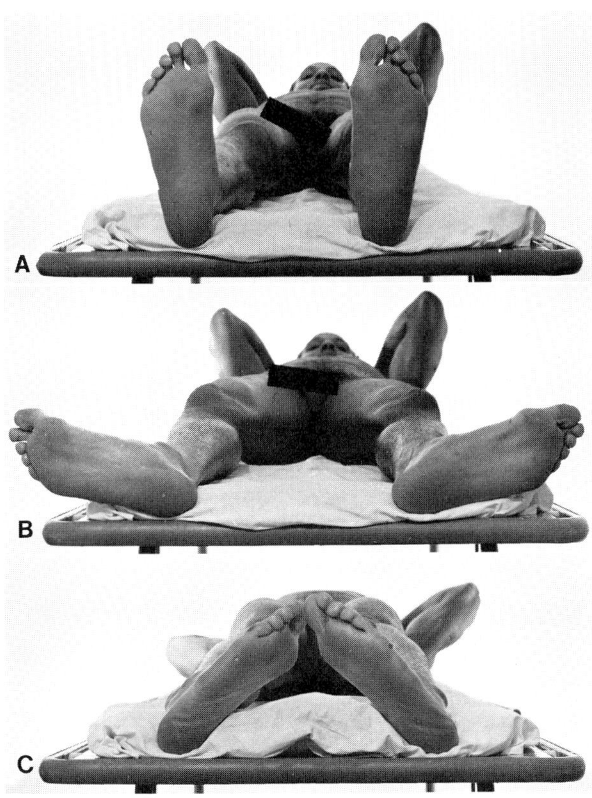

Fig. 10-19. Rotation of the hip joint in extension. The patient is supine on a flat surface (*A*) and external rotation is measured by rotating the leg outward (*B*) and internal rotation is measured by rotating the leg inward (*C*).

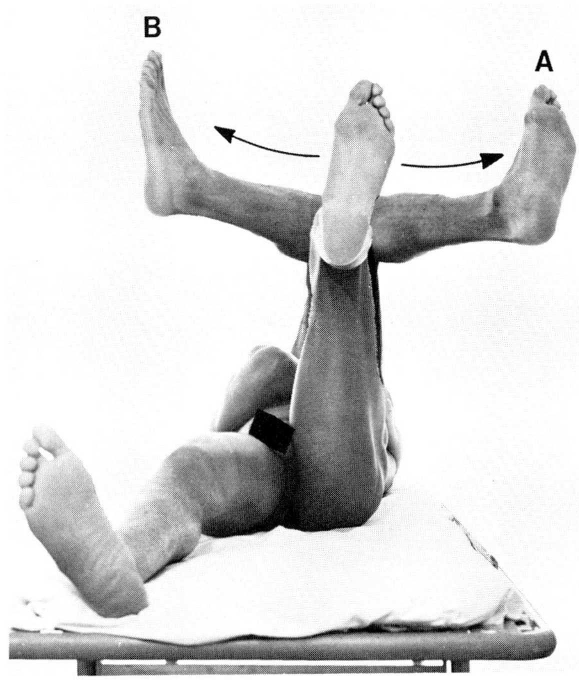

Fig. 10-20. Rotation of the hip joint in flexion. The patient is supine with the hip in 90 degrees of flexion. Internal rotation is measured by rotating the leg inward (*A*) and external rotation is measured by rotating the leg outward (*B*).

Extension

Extension is measured by having the patient lie prone and then lifting the limb with one hand on the pelvis (Fig. 10-21). Normal extension is 20 to 30 degrees in the hip joint, and if motions greater than this are obtained, it is usually due to movement in the spine and pelvis.

Postural Stability

The gluteus medius and minimus are hip abductors that stabilize the pelvis on the femur, and their action during walking is to tilt the pelvis upward on the opposite side when that leg is raised from the ground. If there is any abnormality, the pelvis on the opposite side will droop when the opposite leg is raised from the ground. The Trendelenburg test is performed by having the patient stand with his back toward you (Fig. 10-22A, B, C). Pick two identical points on the posterior iliac spine and mark them with your fingers or a pen. Have the patient first

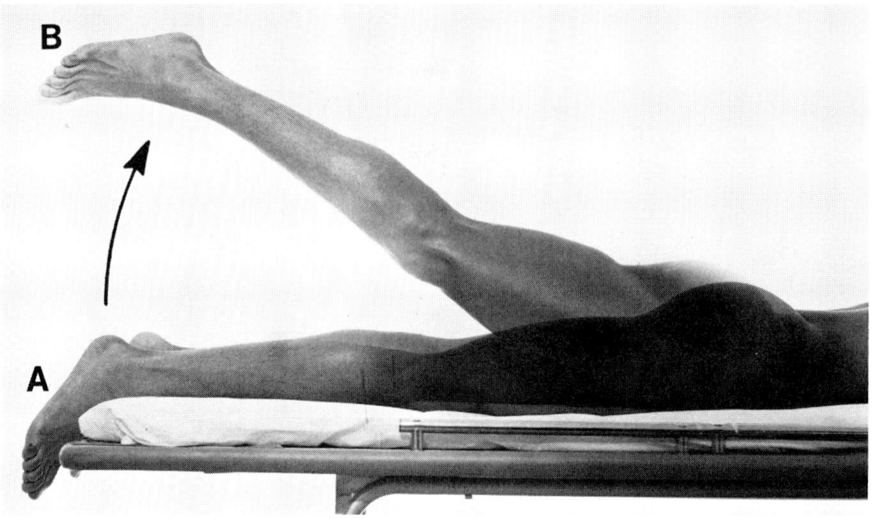

Fig. 10-21. Extension of the hip joint is measured with the patient prone on a flat surface (*A*). The leg is extended with the knee straight (*B*).

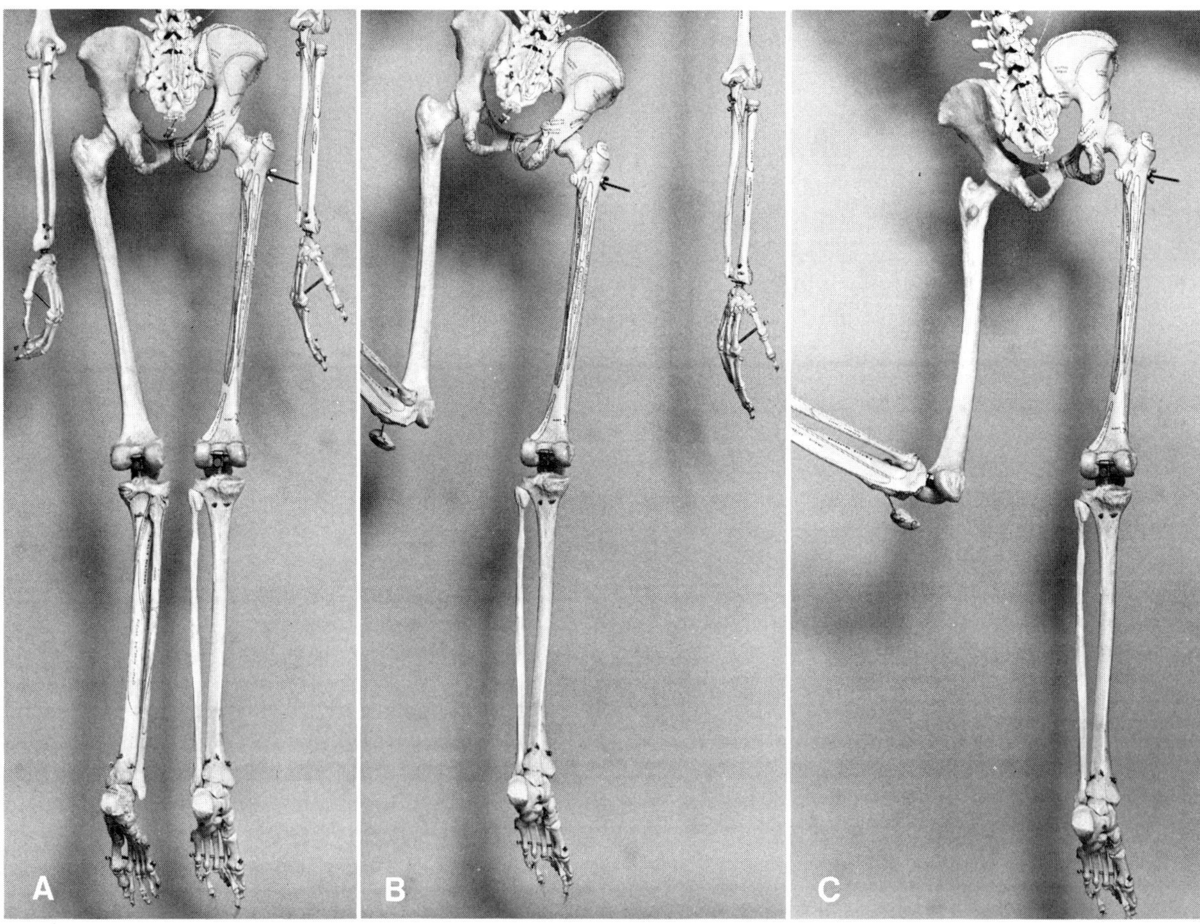

Fig. 10-22. Trendelenburg test designed to test hip stability and particularly the gluteus medius mechanism. The erect position (*A*). If one foot is raised from the ground normally the pelvis tilts upwards on that side (*B*) indicating normal function of the hip abductors on the standing limb and a negative test. If the abductors are deficient on the standing limb when the opposite foot is raised from the ground the pelvis drops (*C*).

stand on the normal limb and raise the abnormal one from the ground; then have him stand on the abnormal limb and raise the normal one from the ground. The limb on which the patient is standing is the one being tested. Therefore, if the pelvis falls on the side of the foot which is off the ground, the finding is positive. The result will be positive in any muscle disease state which affects the abductor muscles; the most common in the past has been poliomyelitis. The result will also be positive in any disease state which mechanically shortens the abductor muscles. This would include congenital dislocation of the hip, coxa vara, Legg-Calvé-Perthes disease, or an abnormality in the proximal femoral epiphysis. It can also be positive if a bony abnormality is present in the proximal part of the femur, such as a neck fracture or slipped capital epiphysis when there is loss of stability of the bone on which the abductor muscles work.

Special Tests

Erichsen's Sign

The iliac bones are grasped between the examiner's two hands and pressed together. If pain results, sacroiliac disease rather than hip disease should be suspected (Fig. 10-23).

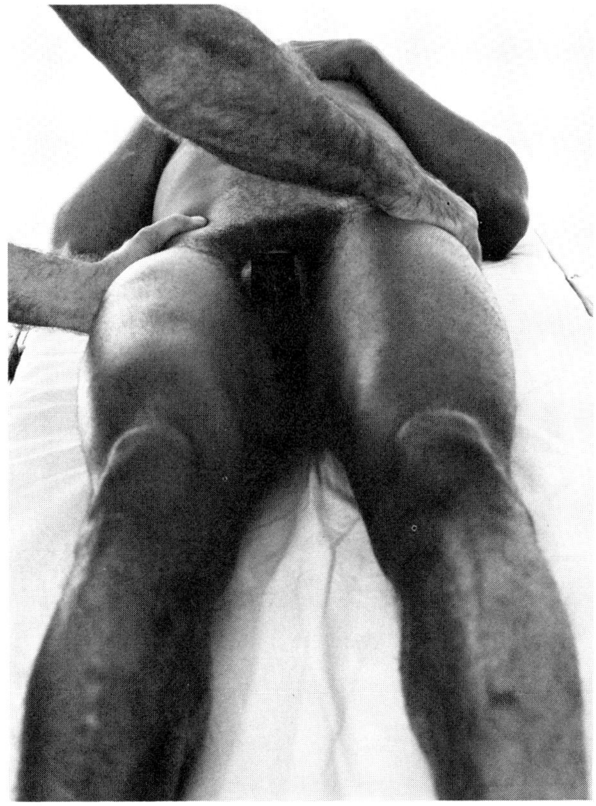

Fig. 10-23. Erichsen's sign designed to test for the presence of sacroiliac disease.

Ludloff's Sign

Swelling and ecchymosis at the base of Scarpa's triangle, accompanied by inability to raise the thigh while in the sitting position, indicates traumatic separation at the epiphysis of the lesser trochanter.

Ober's Test

This test is performed while the patient is lying on his side. The bottom leg is flexed to eliminate lordosis, and the top leg, which is being tested, is abducted, extended, and flexed to 90 degrees. The top leg is then allowed to drop to the table and, if it doesn't, the test indicates contracture of the iliotibial band (Fig. 10-24).

Patrick's Test

With the patient lying flat on the table, the hip and knee are flexed with the external malleolus resting on the opposite knee just above the patella. In this position, the knee is depressed, and if pain is produced, arthritis of the hip is indicated (Fig. 10-25).

Other Areas

A hip examination is not complete without inspection of the spine, sacroiliac joints, lower part of the abdomen, pelvis, rectum, and peripheral pulses. In addition, a neurological examination should be performed. There are many extrinsic causes of hip disease other than the hip joint, and lack of inspection in these areas will often lead to misdiagnosis.

Roentgenography

Routine roentgenography includes an anteroposterior view of the pelvis, including both hips, and lateral of the involved hip. If indicated, roentgenograms of the spine, sacroiliac joints, and femur should be obtained.

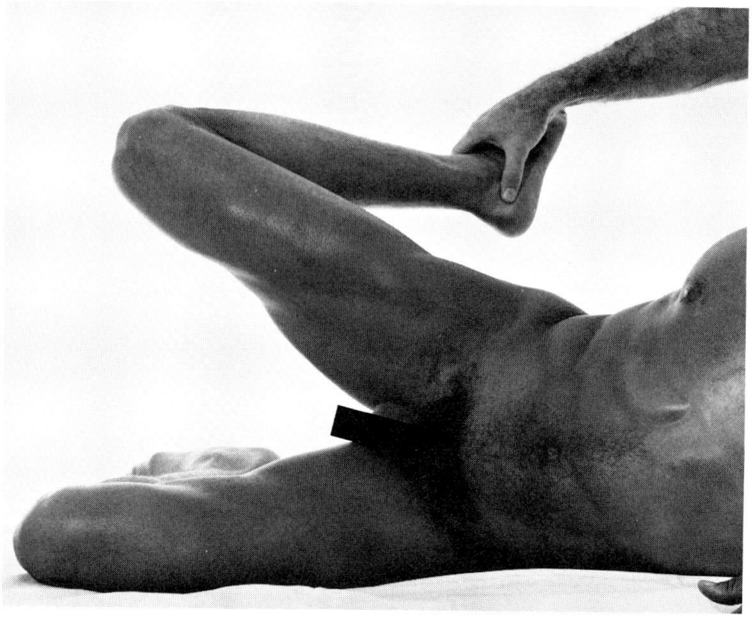

Fig. 10-24. Ober's test is designed to evaluate for the presence of contracture of the iliotibial band.

DIFFERENTIAL DIAGNOSIS

CHILDREN

PAINFUL HIP WITH TEMPERATURE ELEVATION

Pyogenic Arthritis (Prototype—Staphylococcus Aureus)

Septic arthritis of the hip joint can occur at any age, but it is most frequently seen in childhood and especially infancy. The earlier the disease presents in infancy, the fewer are the signs and symptoms, and the only early symptom may just be irritability of an infant with a temperature elevation. The older the child, however, the more clearcut are the symptoms.

Pyogenic arthritis of the hip can be blood-borne, by direct extension from osteomyelitis of the femur, or by direct introduction. The usual route of entry in infants and children is hematogenous. It usually occurs as a complication of some generalized septicemia elsewhere in the body with the hematogenous spread of microorganisms from a distant focus. The primary focus is usually the ear (from otitis media), but it may be the lungs, skin, gastrointestinal tract, or umbilical vein. There may be a primary synovial

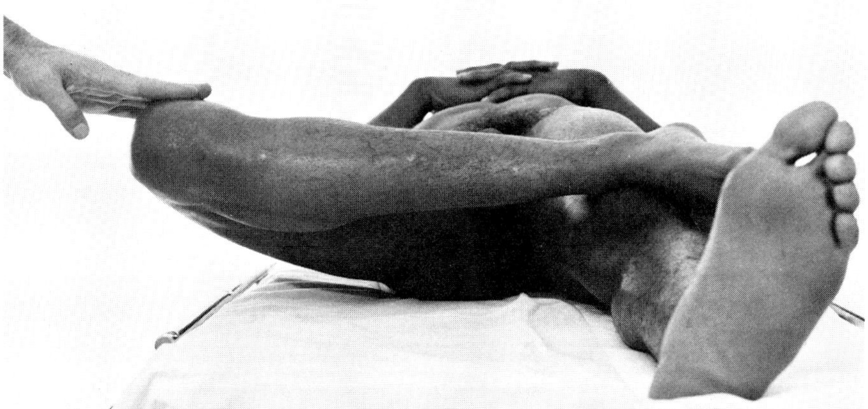

Fig. 10-25. Patrick's test is designed to evaluate the presence of arthritis of the hip.

infection, but more commonly, it lodges in a metaphyseal area.

The entry can be by direct extension of the organisms from osteomyelitis of the metaphysis of the proximal part of the femur when rupture of the cortical bone and periosteum occurs and pus breaks directly into the joint. The hip joint is unique in that the metaphysis of the neck of the femur is contained within the hip joint capsule.

Direct implementation by femoral vein puncture is occasionally reported in the literature but is an unusual occurrence.

On physical examination, the initial finding may be just irritability, but as the infection progresses, the child becomes toxic and severely ill. The infection presents rather acutely as a rule. In the very young infant, there is often only a slight elevation in temperature, usually less than 100 degrees F, but in the older child, the usual presentation is extreme pyrexia. The pulse rate and respiratory rate increase, and there is a fall in blood pressure.

Hip motion will be limited, and motion causes pain. The hip is usually held in some flexion, abduction, and external rotation. This position increases the intracapsular volume, which decreases the intracapsular pressure within the hip joint. Swelling of the groin, upper part of the thigh, or trochanteric area may be present. This swelling obscures bony prominences and makes palpation of the anterior aspect of the head of the femur virtually impossible. Palpation will reveal tenderness anteriorly and posteriorly over the hip joint. Later in the disease, frank dislocation secondary to the pus will occur with restricted abduction, deeper transverse crease, or an extra thigh crease.

Laboratory findings will reveal an elevation of the leukocyte count of 10,000 to 40,000, except in cases of overwhelming sepsis or partially treated infection. The count will reveal a preponderance of polymorphs. The erythrocyte sedimentation rate will be raised. Joint aspiration on gram stain will reveal many polymorphs and bacteria, and on the following day the particular organism may be determined by culture. Positive blood culture will confirm the diagnosis.

During the first week, roentgenograms will reveal signs in the soft tissues only, without bony change (Fig. 10-26). There will be distension of the capsular shadows and a widening of the joint space. Occasionally, swelling occurs along the inner wall of the pelvis which is secondary to effusion in the obturator internus. Within seven to fourteen days, the first signs of bony changes will be noted in the form of either periosteal new bone formation or rarefaction in the metaphysis, which eventually results in destruction of bone. In the younger child, the head of the femur may be completely resorbed, dislocated, or appear very dense, showing signs of avascular necrosis. In the older child and adult, dislocation or resorption is not usually seen; instead, joint space narrowing is the characteristic finding. Late sequelae on roentgenograms include degenerative joint disease, growth disturbances, and fibrous or even bony ankylosis (Fig. 10-27).

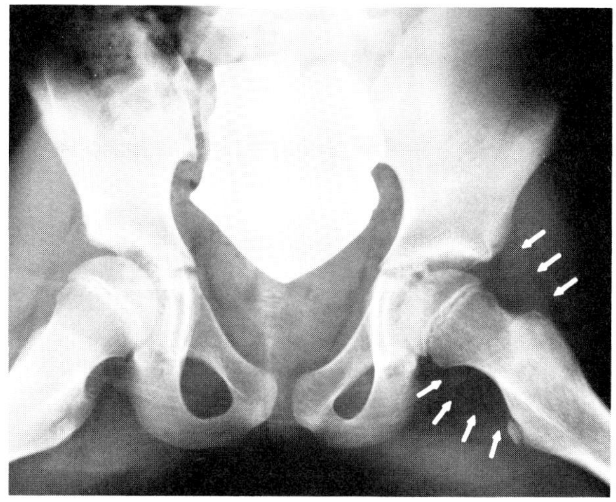

Fig. 10-26. Anteroposterior roentgenogram depicting capsular distention caused by an accumulation of fluid within the hip joint. This roentgenogram taken during the first week of a patient with symptoms of painful hip with temperature elevation could actually be the first radiographic sign seen with all six diseases in this section.

Nonpyogenic Arthritis (Prototype—Tuberculosis)

In children, tuberculosis of the hip joint occurs with about the same frequency as tuberculosis of the small bones of the hands and feet, but is more serious because of the pressure system within the hip joint. The signs and symptoms may present acutely, but as a rule they appear insidiously and are more chronic than the pyogenic type of infection. As many as 5 percent of all patients with tuberculosis have bone lesions.

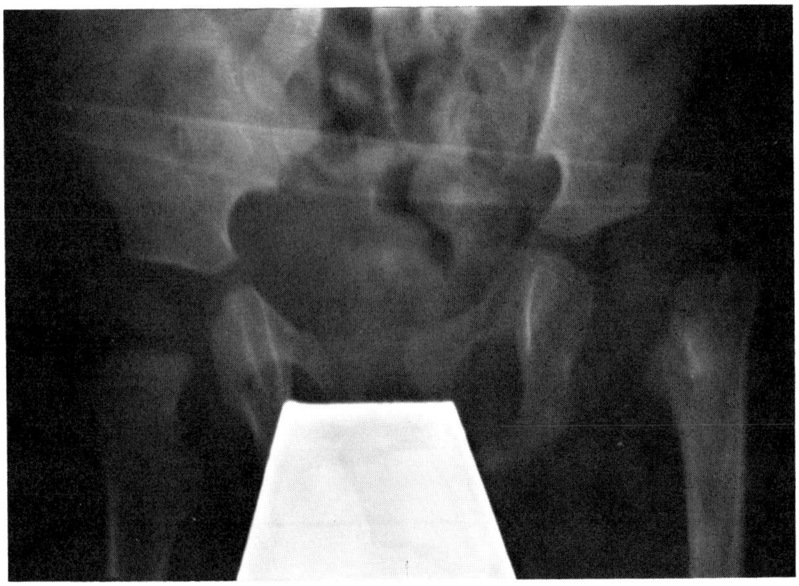

Fig. 10-27. Growth disturbance of the proximal femur resulting from infection. Fibrous ankylosis was also present.

In most cases, the organisms are deposited hematogenously in the synovium, but they can also deposit in the epiphysis or metaphysis of the hip joint area, usually in the superior part of the acetabulum or inferior part of the neck. These deposits are secondary to a focus elsewhere in the body and are disseminated in the blood stream. The organisms can shower from a healed lesion which is not necessarily active. Tuberculosis of the genitourinary or gastrointestinal tract may also travel to the hip via the lymphatics.

The initial symptoms will present insidiously with the patient appearing chronically ill and with a limp of prolonged duration. The patient will have intermittent elevations with or without night sweats. Groin pain which increases with hip motion will be present with some protective muscle spasm. There may be other nonspecific symptoms, such as weight loss, general fatigability, and anorexia.

Hip motion will be slightly limited in the course of the disease, but this will increase later on. The hip will be held in slight flexion and abduction, and the results of the Thomas test will be positive. Swelling does not usually present until very late. Because of its chronic nature, there will usually be muscle wasting at the time of presentment. Night pain sometimes occurs. During the day, muscle spasm can mask hip pain, but with disappearance of the muscle spasm during sleep, there will be a sudden awakening with night pain. Late findings will reveal limb shortening due to loss of bone or premature epiphyseal closure. There may even be a draining abscess through the skin.

Laboratory findings will reveal anemia with or without leukocytosis. If leukocytosis is present, it will not be shifted to the left as in pyogenic infection. The lymphocyte is the most common cell seen. The sedimentation rate will be raised and can be used to indicate the stage of the disease.

Acid-fast stain of aspirated joint fluid may show tubercle bacillus. If not, the bacillus may be cultured during the next few weeks. Synovial biopsy will be diagnostic, revealing masses of lymphocytes and plasma cells, mixed with fibrous and vascular tissue, infiltrating the epithelioid granulomatous tissue. Tubercles may be present in areas of caseation necrosis and will be surrounded by epithelioid and giant cells. The results of a tuberculin test will probably be positive.

Roentgenographically, the earliest changes will be soft tissue swelling with capsular distention. Diffuse osteoporosis of both sides of the joint will gradually appear. Joint space narrowing will occur even though no proteolytic enzymes are present to digest cartilage, as in the pyogenic infection. The cartilage loss is gradual, probably on a nutritional basis.

Active destruction of bone will be present which is very irregular and usually on both sides of the joint.

Subchondral bone destruction will occur and is often accompanied by complete separation of cartilage, which becomes free bodies in the joint. Fibrous ankylosis is often a late sequela.

Osteomyelitis of the Proximal Femur

This condition occcurs hematogenously like pyogenic hip infection. The physical findings are similar to pyogenic hip infection, except usually not as marked. There will be capsular distention as a result of sympathetic swelling to the irritated metaphyseal focus (Fig. 10-28).

The laboratory findings are the same as in pyogenic hip infection, except there is no joint space narrowing.

Bone scan will reveal a localized area of active destruction, characterized as a hot spot, even before bony changes occur on roentgenograms. Roentgenography will reveal soft tissue swelling and/or periosteal elevation over the area of active bone destruction in the metaphysis.

Transient Synovitis (Observation Hip, Toxic Synovitis)

This is the most common cause of acute pain in the hips of children. It is a benign, self-limiting disease which occurs in three to ten year olds and is usually seen in boys (80%). Its symptoms range from mild to severe with the severe cases closely mimicking a septic hip. Symptoms usually last seven to ten days and rarely over two weeks.

The etiology remains unknown although many factors have been proposed, including infection, allergic reaction, and trauma, but none has been proved. Its short, self-limiting course suggests synovial pinching or entrapment with subsequent synovial irritation and effusion secondary to the irritation.

On physical examination, the pain is usually in the hip but may be referred to the knee, and the patient will have an antalgic gait and limp. There will be limitation of motion with the hip abducted, flexed, and externally rotated, which is the position giving maximum hip joint capacity. There will usually be a low grade fever (101° F) with an occasional rise to 103 degrees F, with tenderness of the hip joint to both anterior and posterior palpation.

A complete blood count will usually show no leukocytosis except for mild elevations to the 12,000 range. If a joint aspiration is performed, the results will be negative. Normality of laboratory studies is consistent with this diagnosis.

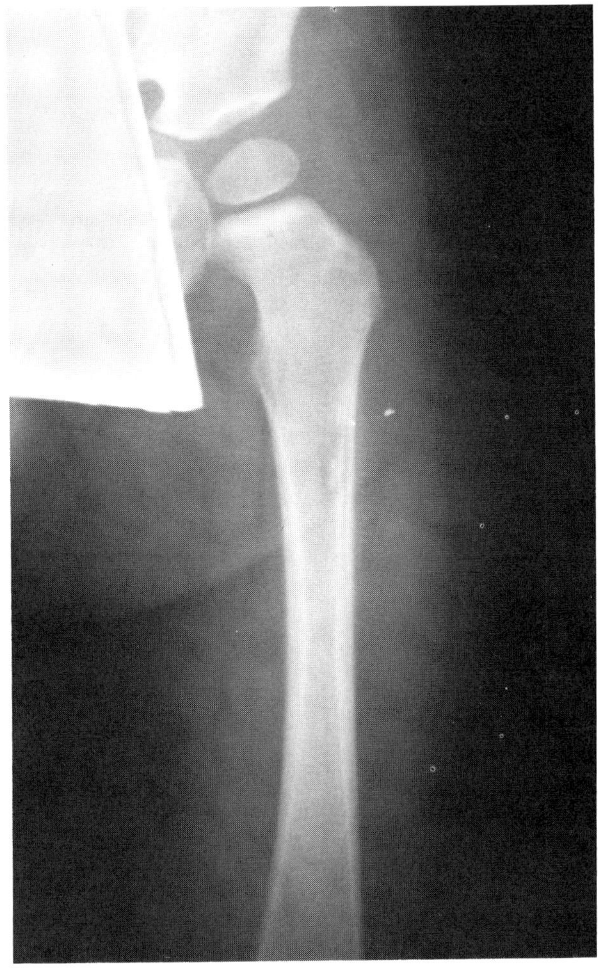

Fig. 10-28. Osteomyelitis of the proximal femur. The patient presented with a limp and painful motion at the hip not detected on the original anteroposterior roentgenogram of the hip joint which was cut off proximal to the lesion.

On roentgenograms, swelling of capsular shadows about the hip is seen laterally on the superior aspect and medially on the inferior aspect. This is accompanied by a widening of medial inferior hip joint space (Waldenstrom's sign).

Pauciarticular Arthritis

This is the term given to rheumatoid arthritis which presents in a single joint, and it often leads to confusion in diagnosis because of its similarities to other entities in this section. The most common joint to be affected is the knee, but the hips, ankles, and elbows are often involved. Its onset is usually insidious, but it has been known to present rather acutely. It is most predominant in girls (2:1) under four years of age.

The cause remains unknown although various theories have been proposed, including infection (virus and bacteria have been implicated), but an autoimmune response to body collagen or an immune response to certain bacteria enjoys the greatest favor at present. On physical examination, pauciarticular arthritis does not present in the same manner as the severe metabolic disease, Still's disease, with systemic involvement of liver, spleen, anemia and malnutrition. Therefore, diagnosis is usually difficult. There will be swelling associated with warmth in the groin or over the greater trochanter. Motion is limited and painful. Early in the disease, flexion contracture is present with the limb in some abduction. Later in the course of the disease, there is an adduction contracture with flexion contracture and marked restriction of rotation. Temperature elevation may be low grade or moderate.

Twenty-five percent of patients develop iridocyclitis at various times during their disease, and it is characteristically chronic and may result in permanent ocular damage. The sedimentation rate is moderately elevated and latex fixation is usually negative. Febrile agglutinins, ASO titer, and blood cultures are usually negative. C-reactive protein may be positive.

Synovial fluid is slightly cloudy with increased cell count, predominantly polymorphonuclear, and there is a poor mucin precipitation test with acetic acid. A compliment fixation test may be diagnostic.

Early roentgenography reveals an effusion manifested by capsular swelling and widening of the medial joint line. As the disease progresses, osteoporosis will be evident on both sides of the joint due to resorption secondary to hyperemia. Later, there is joint space narrowing with the appearance of subchondral cysts often not in the line of weight-bearing. Fibrous ankylosis may be present late in the disease.

Rheumatic Fever

Joint involvement is the most common manifestation of rheumatic fever. Initially, one joint is involved and others gradually become affected. Each joint may be active for two to seven days, and as other joints become involved, earlier ones quiet down. There may be monoarticular involvement for the first day or two without other symptoms, and this can present serious problems in differential diagnosis. The usual presentation, however, is for many joints to be affected in quick succession for short periods of time. The hip is involved only 15 percent of the time compared with 75 percent for knees and 50 percent for ankles.

Fifty percent of rheumatic fever attacks are preceded by streptococcal pharyngitis. The latent period between pharyngitis and rheumatic fever usually varies from 6 to 35 days.

On physical examination arthralgia, joint pain without any objective signs of inflammation, is present. Joint pain with objective signs of inflammation, such as swelling, erythema, heat, and limited motion, is indicative of arthritis. There is marked tenderness to palpation of the joint characterized by extreme pain and limited motion which is always out of proportion to the swelling, erythema, or heat evoked by the disease. These patients will have a fever over 100 degrees F which responds to aspirin. The diagnosis can be easy if there are other presenting symptoms, such as carditis, chorea, erythema margination, and subcutaneous nodules.

Laboratory findings consist of an ASO titer above 25 in adults and more than 333 in children. Elevation of acute phase reactants, erythrocyte sedimentation rate (ESR), and C-reactive protein (CRP) may be present, but neither is specific for rheumatic fever, particularly the CRP. Other findings are elevated white blood cell count, prolonged PR interval on electrocardiogram, and positive throat culture for group A streptococcus. Serum concentrations of gamma globulins, alpha-2 globulins, mucoproteins, and polysaccharides are increased, and albumin is decreased. Gamma-1-A globulin is disproportionately high.

Aspiration of synovial fluid can cause a great deal of confusion because of the high cell count with turbidity. The absence of bacteria and positive culture are extremely helpful in differentiating rheumatic fever from an acutely infected joint.

Painful Hip with Gait Disturbance (Limp)

Legg-Calvé-Perthes Disease

Known also as osteochondritis deformans juvenilis or coxa plana, this disease is largely limited by age and sex. The disease was described separately in the United States, Germany, and France by Legg (1910), Perthes (1910), and Calvé (1910). It is seen almost exclusively in children three to twelve years of age, but has been reported in children as young as two, and in others as old as 18, with boys being affected over girls by a ratio of 4:1. It is usually unilateral (85 percent). A familial history was reported in 20 percent of the patients seen by Goff.

The most widely accepted cause is interruption of the blood supply to the head of the femur which is thought to be produced by excessive fluid pressure of a synovial effusion in the hip joint. Trueta has shown that the head of the femur is at risk between ages three and ten because of the three blood supplies to the femoral head, only the lateral epiphyseal vessels are functional during this period. Tucker also has shown by injection studies that the blood supply varies to different segments of the head of the femur, with the blood supply to the posterior segment being more generous than that to the anterior segment. This correlates with the fact that the posterior portion of the head of the femur is often spared from this disease.

Caffey has demonstrated subchondral fractures early in the disease and postulates the fracture as being the initiating factor in a sequence of events that results in Legg-Calvé-Perthes disease.

Abnormal blood clotting processes caused by substances creating a state of hypercoagulability are thought to result in formation of platelet aggregations and fibrin thrombi which could block the limited vascular supply to the head of the femur.

Ferguson and Howorth have suggested a relationship between previous transient synovitis or other inflammatory processes because of the presence of thickened blood vessels and capsule in surgically observed cases.

On physical examination, pain can range from mild to severe and will be felt in the groin, thigh, and very often in the knee. This is associated with a limp or slight abnormality of gait. The gait is antalgic in which the patient tries to protect the hips by rapidly shifting body weight off the foot on the involved side.

With a flexion contracture (positive Thomas test) motion at the hip is limited, particularly abduction, internal rotation, extension, and flexion. There is muscle spasm of adductor and psoas muscle, muscle wasting of thigh and buttock, and the anterior and/or posterior aspects of the hip joint may be tender.

The sedimentation rate might be elevated, but the results of other laboratory investigations are normal.

There are usually four separate stages of radiological appearances which will be tabulated, but it is important to realize that these all overlap and are not discrete stages (Fig. 10-29).

In the first stage there is capsular swelling about

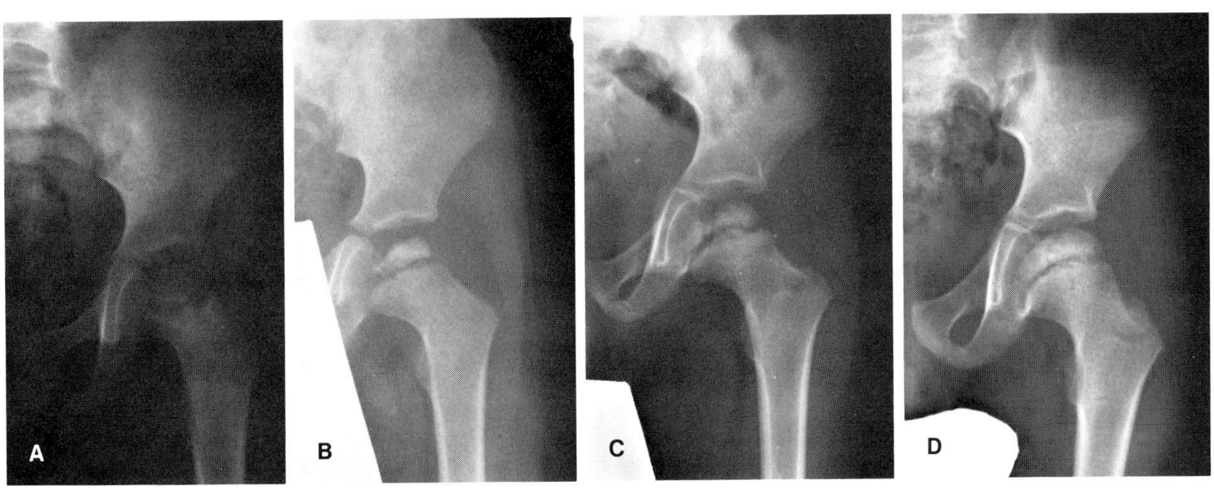

Fig. 10-29. The four stages of Legg-Calvé-Perthes disease. The first changes are capsular swelling, increased joint space, and demineralization at the metaphyseal-epiphyseal junction (*A*). This is followed by increase in density of the head (*B*) which flows into stage 3 where radiolucent areas are present (*C*). Ultimately the patient has an enlarged deformed femoral head, with widening of the neck of the femur (*D*).

the hip, joint space widening, and a porosis demineralization of the femoral metaphysis immediately adjacent to the epiphyseal line (Fig. 10-29A).

The second stage is characterized by an increase in the density of the head of the femur in its entirety or some portion of it (Fig. 10-29B).

The third stage will be marked by radiolucent areas in the epiphysis which are areas of dead bone removal, fragmentation of epiphysis with cyst-like spaces, and possible widening of the epiphysis and the neck of the femur (Fig. 10-29C).

The final or fourth stage is characterized by enlargement of the head of the femur (coxa magna), deformity of the head, widening of the neck of the femur, and an acetabulum that might be deformed (Fig. 10-29D).

Slipped Capital Femoral Epiphysis

This disease primarily occurs in adolescents nine to seventeen years of age, and 60 to 80 percent of the patients will be boys. It is seen in the earlier age ranges in females because of their advanced skeletal maturity and at the latter age range in boys. Clinically and roentgenographically there will be bilateral involvement in 40 percent of the patients.

Various theories of how this disease occurs have been proposed. Hormones have been implicated, with Harris demonstrating that growth hormone decreases and sex hormone increases the resistance of the epiphyseal line to shearing force, i.e., a tall thin child has increased growth hormone and a Froehlich child has decreased sex hormone.

Ponseti and McClintock theorize it is a result of cohesion loss of cartilage matrix from a biochemical alteration of ground substance arising from an abnormality of protein metabolism. It has been pointed out by Ghormley that the epiphyseal plate changes from a horizontal to an oblique position at adolescence. This mechanical alteration of the epiphyseal line makes it subject to more shearing stresses than any other epiphysis.

These patients will have typical physical findings. The patient may have a Froehlich-type body with female fat distribution and sexual underdevelopment. He can be tall and thin with long extremities and will have a history of rapid adolescent growth. There is mild discomfort but no severe pain in the groin, thigh or knee and there will be tenderness to palpation over the hip joint. This is associated with a mild limp of antalgic nature or awkward gait with the affected foot turned outward from external rotation at the hip. In severe slip, there may be a waddling Trendelenburg-type gait. If the thigh is flexed, the leg rides into external rotation and usually cannot be brought to neutral. Motion is limited, particularly internal rotation and abduction, with or without a flexion contracture. Extension of the hip may be increased consistent with the amount of slip. Careful examination of the limb above the greater trochanter will reveal shortening of 0.5 inch or more.

There will be roentgenographic evidence of widening of the epiphyseal line, usually the earliest change, with prominent capsular shadows and irregular demineralization of an area adjacent to the epiphyseal line, but the actual displacement of the head relative to the neck of the femur is most apparent on lateral projection (Fig. 10-30B). When obvious on the anteroposterior view, the epiphysis appears sickle-shaped with the lower border of the head projecting below the lower border of the neck (Fig. 10-30A).

The head of the femur maintains its relationship with the acetabulum throughout the process, and the neck of the femur is seen in various stages of displacement. Late in the disease, the epiphysis may appear dense with loss of cartilage space; this is termed cartilage necrosis and can occur in untreated patients but is more common in those who have undergone a surgical procedure.

Sickle-Cell and Hemoglobin Diseases

Infarcts or avascular necrosis of the hip are most commonly reported in SS (sickle-cell anemia) and in SC (sickle cell hemoglobin C disease), but it has been reported in at least five variations of the hemoglobin diseases. Although generally thought of as a disease of Negroes of African heritage, it or its variants have been reported in the Mediterranean, Middle East, and some eastern countries, such as India, Ceylon, Burma, and Indonesia. The cause of this disease is a direct result of interruption of the vascular supply to the head of the femur. Systemic factors cause the red blood cells to sickle with subsequent blockage of blood vessels.

Clinical features reveal pain in the hip, tenderness to palpation over the hip joint, limp characterized as an antalgic gait, and limitation of motion similar to Legg-Calvé-Perthes disease. It usually presents in chil-

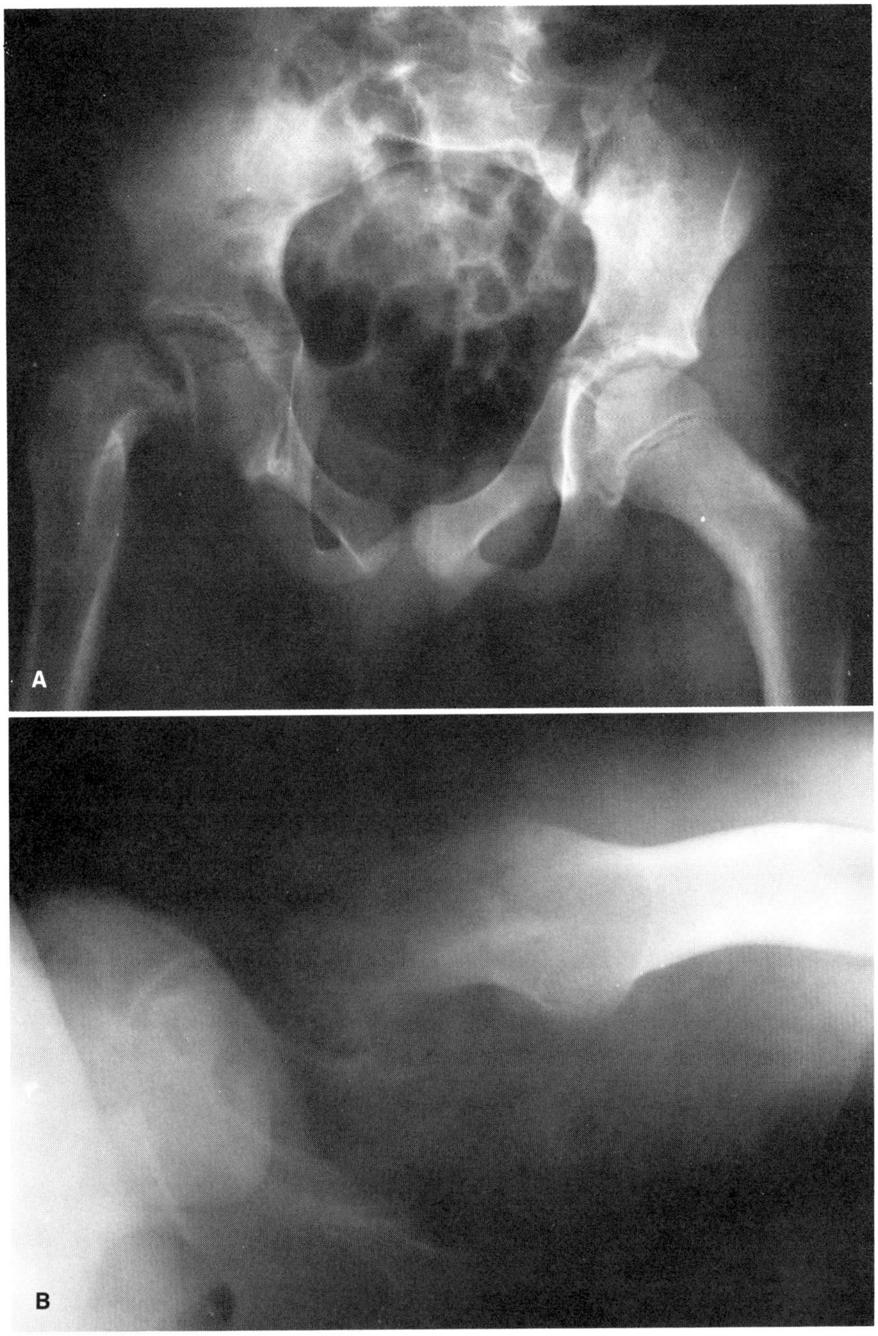

Fig. 10-30. Anteroposterior (*A*) and lateral (*B*) roentgenogram of a patient with slipped capital femoral epiphysis. Note the sickle-shaped epiphysis on the anteroposterior view (*A*).

dren more than three months of age, after the fetal hemoglobin has been replaced by the abnormal hemoglobin.

There also may be other systemic problems associated with a history of abdominal pain or sickle cell crisis. On closer inspection, anemia or pallor will be present with enlargement of the spleen.

Laboratory findings will reveal normocytic or microcytic anemia and the red blood cells sickle with the reducing agent sodium bisulfite, and hemoglobin electrophoresis will determine the specific disease. Increased bilirubin and increased urobilinogen will be present in urine and feces. Blood smear reveals reticulocytosis, polychromatophilia, normoblasts, leukocytosis with "shift to the left" in myeloid series, and increased platelets.

The avascular necrosis of the head of the femur is very characteristic on roentgenogram, closely resembling Legg-Calvé-Perthes disease except for the absence of changes in the metaphysis, which clearly distinguishes it from Perthes disease (Fig. 10-31).

Hemophilia

Hemophilia includes a broad group of diseases, each one characterized by some specific defect in the clotting mechanism. The majority are sex-linked recessive disorders which occur in males but are passed on by females. The two most common forms are Factor VIII (hemophilia A) and Factor IX (Christmas disease). The manifestations of the disease are not seen in the neonatal period and usually do not appear until after six months of age. Hemophilic disorders cause four hip-related problems, and these are examined separately.

Hemarthrosis. The physical findings consist of pain in the groin and thigh. This is associated with a fullness in the hip joint both anterior in the groin and over the greater trochanter, and there is limited motion with the hip assuming the flexed, abducted, externally rotated position which allows the most room for the blood in the capsule of the joint.

A battery of tests can be performed, including bleeding time, tourniquet test, whole blood clotting time, one stage prothrombin time, prothrombin consumption test, platelet count, blood grouping, and specific assays of Factors VIII and IX when indicated.

Roentgenography reveals swelling of capsular shadows around the hip joint with an associated increase in the joint space.

Hemorrhage into Iliacus. Pain will begin in the groin and gradually spread to the lumbar region and thigh, and will be associated with a swelling mass in the iliac fossa. Hip motion will be limited with the hip held in flexion, abduction, and external rotation, but there will be severe pain if the hip is extended, helping to distinguish it from hemorrhage into the hip joint. There may be palsy of the femoral nerve with attendant sensory and motor deficit.

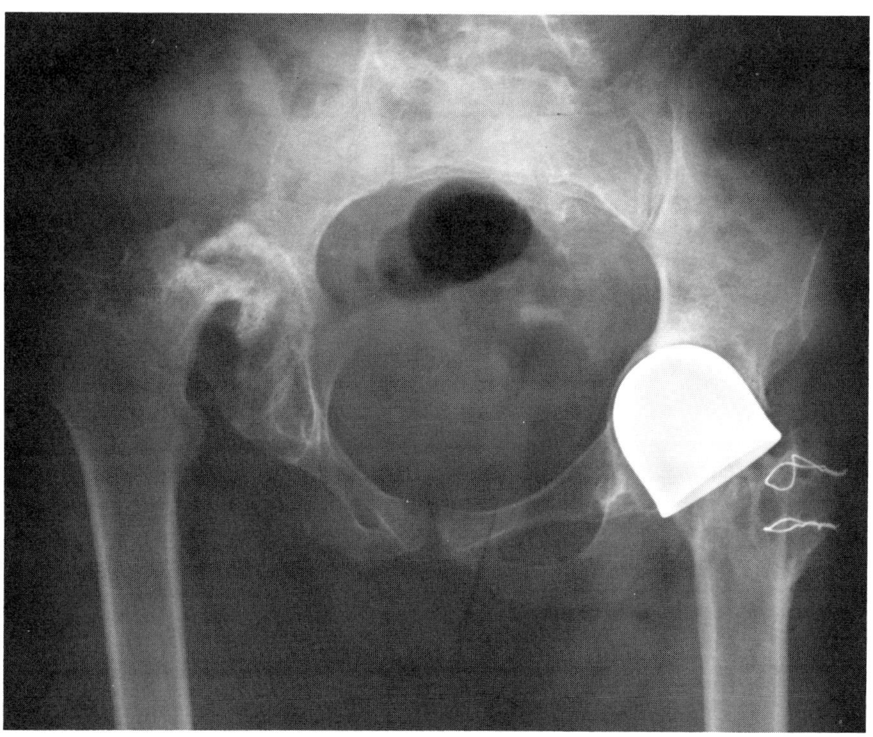

Fig. 10-31. Anteroposterior roentgenogram of a patient with sickle cell disease and the late sequelae of avascular necrosis; there is complete destruction of the right femoral head with subsequent shortening. A cup arthroplatsy was performed previously on the left.

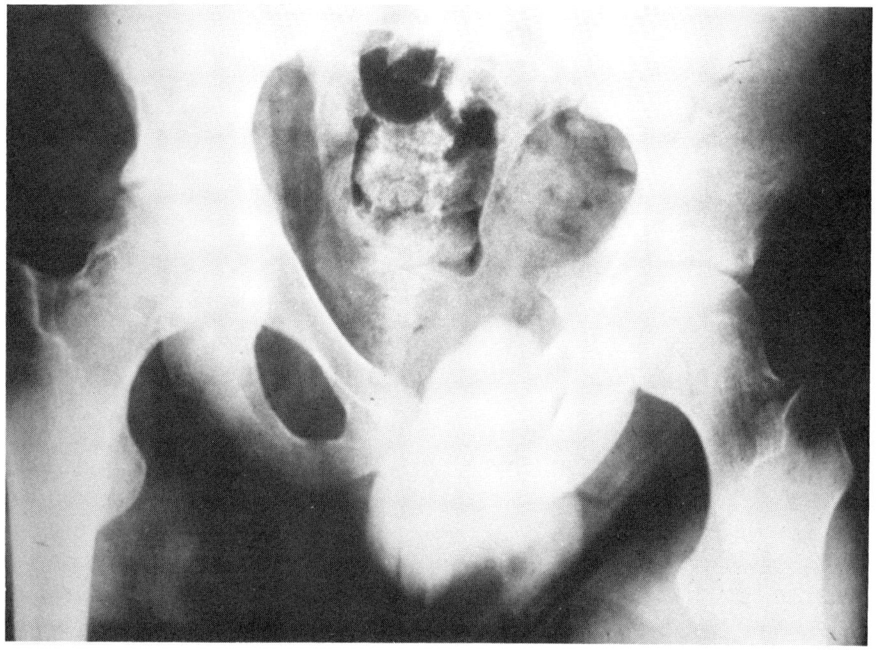

Fig. 10-32. Anteroposterior roentgenogram of a patient with hemophilia. The right hip demonstrates the end result of multiple bleeds with avascular necrosis and cyst formation. (Courtesy of Kurt M. Niemann.)

Neither increase in the joint space nor swelling of capsular shadows at the hip will be evident on roentgenograms. There will, however, be blurring of the hip joint from hemorrhage into the iliacus muscle.

Avascular Necrosis. There is pain in the groin, thigh, or knee which is associated with a limp and antalgic gait. Hip motion is decreased primarily in flexion, internal rotation, and abduction.

Roentgenographic findings are similar to those in patients with Legg-Calvé-Perthes disease except for absence of changes in the metaphysis (Fig. 10-32).

Pseudotumor. The physical findings are similar to those of avascular necrosis with groin pain, limp, and painful motion; however, there will be roentgenographic evidence of an enlarging bone cyst due to subperiosteal hemorrhage.

Painless Deformity of Hip or Gait Abnormality

Congenital Dislocation of the Hip

Congenital dislocation of the hip may be noted at birth by the pediatrician, or it may not be discovered until much later, when ambulation occurs. It is six times more frequent in females and is bilateral in one third of the patients. There is a hereditary predisposition, with 5 percent of siblings and 40 percent of monozygotic twins affected with the disease. Certain geographical areas are endemic for the disease, such as Holland, Southern France, and Northern Italy, while in other areas of Asia and Africa it is extremely rare. Dislocation is reported ten times higher in breech deliveries.

Various etiological factors have been implicated in congenital dislocation of the hip. The one factor common to all dislocations or dislocated hips is laxity of the joint capsule. It has been suggested that hormones derived from the maternal circulation cause this laxity. The presence of contracture or actual shortness of the iliopsoas is thought to play a major role. The acetabular dysplasia present causes the acetabulum to no longer act as a buttress, and when it slopes too much and does not contain the head, it predisposes to dislocation. At birth, if the limbus is underdeveloped and because most of the covering for the head of the femur is limbus, the head will be less contoured.

Anteversion (both acetabular and femoral) has been described, and if there is an excessive amount of anteversion, the head of the femur has decreased coverage. There is a predisposition to dislocation when the in-utero flexed position is suddenly changed to extension after birth. An enlarged ligamentum teres and haversian fat pad could be primary or secondary following dislocation and there will be subsequent filling of the vacuum. One, however, must recognize the role of heredity, for there is no doubt that genes predispose to the disease although its exact role has not been worked out.

On physical examination in the newborn, there are two tests which are helpful in the diagnosis of congenital dislocation of the hip. The Ortolani test in the newborn is demonstrated by placing the baby on the examining table with his knees together and both hips flexed at 90 degrees, held firmly by the examiner. As both hips are slowly abducted, before the 90 degree angle is obtained, the dislocated hip will relocate with a palpable and sometimes audible click. This should not be confused with the movement of the fascia lata over the greater trochanter. There are two parts to the Barlow test, the first part being only a slight modification of Ortolani's test. The baby's hips are flexed to 90 degrees and the knees are fully flexed. The examiner's middle finger of each hand is placed on the greater trochanter while his thumb applies counterpressure on the thigh at the level of the lesser trochanter. As the child's thighs are abducted to mid-position, the examiner's middle finger tries to relocate the hip by forcing pressure on the greater trochanter. The second part of the test is to try to dislocate the hip with thumb pressure on the lesser trochanter.

There is limited abduction with an adduction contracture. This is usually not seen at birth but develops soon thereafter and is probably a second development to the dislocation. One must keep in mind, however, the 20 percent of all normal children have limited abduction. Internal rotation may be increased because of increased anteversion. The skin folds of the thigh do not approximate and are asymmetrical, but this is also present in one third of normal babies. The buttock fold is also higher on the side that is dislocated. If the thigh is completely dislocated, you will be unable to palpate the head of the femur in the groin, and a hollow area will be felt, but it may be palpated in the buttocks. The greater trochanter will be above Nélaton's line. If both the hip and knees are flexed to 90 degrees, one knee will lie below the other knee; however, this sign, called the Galeazzi sign, is only good for unilateral dislocation.

The femur telescopes when it is moved to and fro in line with its long axis. In bilateral dislocations, a wide perineum will be noted. The extremity will be shorter on measurement. If the child can stand, the Trendelenburg test will be positive. If the patient is walking, a Trendelenburg waddling gait will be evi-

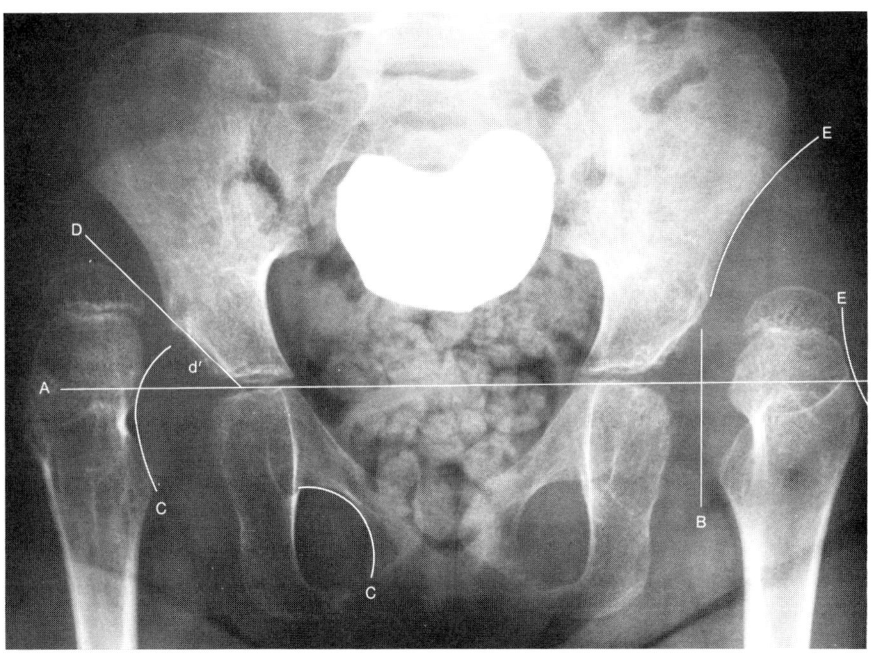

Fig. 10-33. Anteroposterior roentgenogram of a 6-year-old patient with bilateral dislocated hips. Hilgenreiner's line (*A*) is drawn through the two triradiate cartilages. A line (*B*) dropped perpendicular from the anteroinferior iliac spine will divide the hip joint into four quadrants. Interruption of Shenton's (*C*) and Simon's line (*E*) are suggestive of subluxation or dislocation. A line drawn from the tip of the ilium to the superior outer edge of the acetabulum (*D*) forms an angle with Hilgenreiner's line (*A*) known as the acetabular index (*d′*).

dent. Gait abnormality is frequently the first sign of dislocation manifested to unknowing parents. The normal lumbar lordosis is accentuated if there is fixed flexion at the hip.

Numerous identifying features have been used to recognize this entity on roentgenogram (Fig. 10-33). A line, known as Hilgenreiner's (Fig. 10-33A) is drawn between the two triradiate cartilages. A second line is dropped perpendicular from the anteroinferior iliac spine (Fig. 10-33B). Normally, the epiphyseal and the medial portion of the metaphysis are in the lower inner quadrant. In frank dislocation, the epiphysis will be in the upper outer quadrant. This sign is obviously more valuable after ossification of the epiphysis. Shenton described a line (Fig. 10-33C) which is drawn on the inner surface of the neck of the femur and is continued along the superior border of the obturator foramen; this should form a uniform, uninterrupted, curved line. If a line is drawn from the tip of the ilium to the superior outer edge of the acetabulum, it will make an angle with Hilgenreiner's line; this is known as the acetabular index (Fig. 10-33D). This index is normal up to 25 degrees. It was originally thought that anything over 25 degrees was indicative of congenital dislocation of the hip, especially indices in the range of 40 degrees. Caffey, however, has shown that normal children can have angles in this range. The test, therefore, should be interpreted in proper perspective with the other roentgenographic signs. Simons described a line drawn from the outer lateral surface of the neck of the femur which if extended upward to the outer surface of the acetabulum and lateral margin of the ilium should be uniform and uninterrupted. Interruption of this line is suggestive of dislocation (Fig. 10-33E).

On an anteroposterior roentgenogram of the pelvis with the patella straight up, the hips will be in some external rotation, suggesting anteversion. This can be differentiated from valgus in that the distance from the head of the femur to the greater trochanter will not be increased. In valgus this distance will be increased. A true lateral roentgenogram, however, clearly denotes the degree of anteversion of the neck of the femur.

Coxa Vara

The angle between the shaft and the neck of the femur in the adult is usually between 120 to 140 degrees and is slightly greater in children (135 to 145 degrees). When the shaft of the neck decreases below this range it is referred to as coxa vara, usually known as infantile, developmental, idiopathic, or congenital as opposed to the acquired type, which is usually secondary to some underlying growth disorder, such as rickets, achondrodysplasia, dysplasia, epiphyseal multiplex, or epiphyseal arrest from infection or trauma. Congenital or developmental coxa vara is rare and occurs only once in every 25,000 live births. Unilateral involvement is at least twice as common as bilateral. It is probably familial, and there appears to be no relationship to geography, sex, or race.

We do not know what causes coxa vara and there have been many plausible theories cited; therefore, the idiopathic terminology is often linked synonymously with the disease. Those who believe the disease to be congenital have theorized it as the result of lack of uterine space, which causes bending of the neck of the femur, an abnormality in endochondral ossification, or embryonic circulation to the neck of the femur, but none of these theories is based on laboratory information. The fact that there is a triangular piece of bone at the neck which may come from an ossification center has given basis that it is the result of some developmental error.

Clinically, when the child first begins to walk, between the ages of one and three, a gait abnormality is noted. With unilateral involvement, the gait is a gluteus medius lurching type, and with bilateral involvement, it is more of a waddling type. The gait is not at all unlike that seen in congenital dislocation of the hip. The Trendelenburg test is positive because the distance from the greater trochanter to the iliac spine is shortened. With unilateral involvement there will be a slight leg length discrepancy. The greater trochanter will lie above Nélaton's line.

Motion is most limited in abduction, usually more so with the hip at full extension than at 90 degrees' flexion. There is an attendant adduction contracture. There may be some mild limitation of flexion, adduction, extension, and internal and external rotation, but this is very little compared with the limited abduction. There is widening of the perineum in bilateral involvement.

Most of the aforementioned symptoms are present in congenital dislocation of the hip, but to the uninitiated observer, they can be a source of real confusion. The fact, however, that the head of the femur can be palpated in its normal position, along with the absence of hip instability and no evidence of telescoping, can serve to differentiate this disease from congenital dislocation of the hip.

There are no distinguishing laboratory findings in congenital or developmental coxa vara. In the acquired forms of the disease, such as in rickets, one can be helped by the laboratory.

There is a decrease in the neck shaft angle below 135 degrees on roentgenogram, and most often a right angle is formed (Fig. 10-34). A widened epiphyseal line assumes a more vertical position and is referred to as the inverted Y fragment. The Y fragment is formed by the isolation of a triangular segment of bone occurring at a fissure defect at the inferior neck just below the epiphyseal line. Later in the disease, the epiphyseal line can become thin and fragmented, often with premature closure. The neck shortens, the shaft narrows, the greater trochanter enlarges, and the head and acetabulum become progressively deformed. If left untreated, the entire proximal end of the femur becomes grossly deformed.

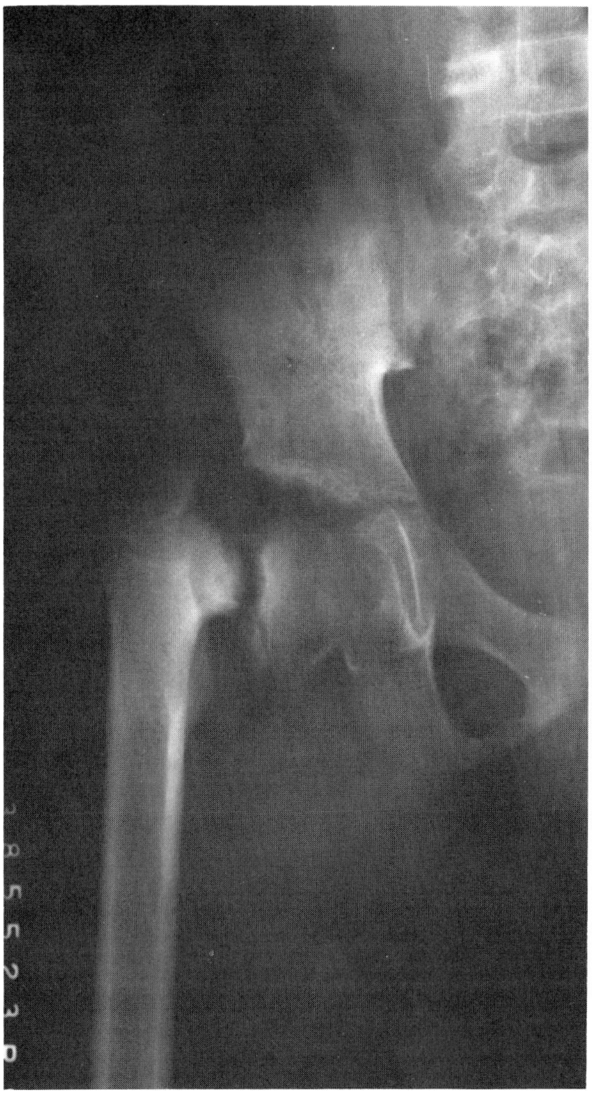

Fig. 10-34. Coxa vara in a 12-year-old male with a history of progressive limp and shortening of the extremity for three years. The neck shaft angle has decreased below the 135 degree norm to below 90 degrees. The epiphyseal line has widened with the formation of an inverted Y fragment.

Proximal Femoral Focal Deficiency

According to the classification of Aiken, there are four types of proximal femoral focal deficiency of increasing severity (Fig. 10-35). We will allude only to Type A in this discussion because of its possible confusion with coxa vara in the very young. However, as the child grows older and the leg length discrepancy becomes obvious, the confusion should no longer exist. In fact, several investigators believe that congenital coxa vara may be just the first stage of defects in the proximal part of the femur.

This defect probably develops very early in the embryonic period at the time of formation of the hip joint cleft. Duraiswami was able to produce defects of the proximal portion of the femur by injecting insulin into the yolk sac of a six-day-old chick embryo.

On physical examination, the leg length discrepancy is usually greater than 1 inch, whereas with coxa vara it is less than 1 inch, and if sufficient shortening exists, there will be a short leg gait. The greater trochanter lies above Nélaton's line, and the results of the Trendelenburg test will be positive. The hip will have flexion, abduction, and external rotation contracture. With increasing severity, the thigh may be shortened and appear to have increased muscle bulk.

Roentgenographic findings will include coxa vara, fragmentation and flattening of the femoral epiphysis, delayed ossification of the head of the femur, and

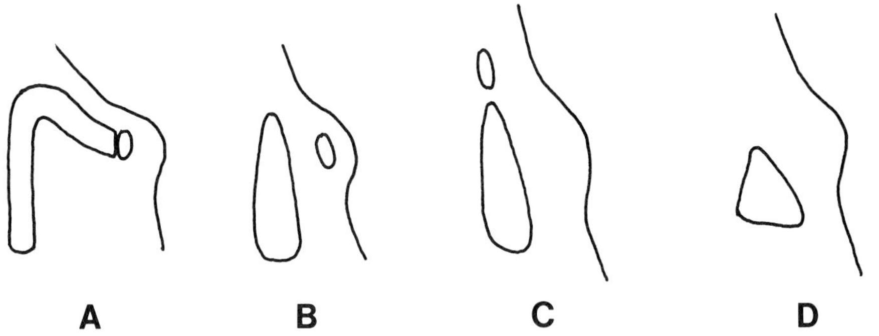

Fig. 10-35. Classification of proximal femoral joint deficiency. (Modified from Aitken, G. T. [ed.]: Proximal Femoral Focal Deficiency, A Congenital Anomaly. Symposium, Washington, D.C., June 13, 1968. National Academy Sciences, 1969.)

a narrowing and sclerosis of the upper part of the shaft of the femur.

Paralytic Hip of Cerebral Palsy

The severe cases of paralytic hip abnormality pose no difficulty in diagnosis when the many facets of the disease with its other stigmas are present. The milder cases, however, can be of some confusion to the physician. Our discussion will limit itself to the patient with mild cerebral palsy and hip abnormality. For further information on the polio and myelomeningocele deformities, the reader is referred to Sharrard's text of *Paediatric Orthopaedics and Fractures.*

Cerebral palsy is caused by interference of the motor system control through a central nervous system lesion. The incoordination of the extremity can be classed according to the type of involvement, for example, flaccidity, rigidity, tremor, athetosis, ataxia, or spasticity. We will limit our discussion to the spastic type which affects the hip and, specifically, the milder type which may give some problem in diagnosis.

The underlying defect is upper motor neuron damage in the brain or spinal cord and can occur before or after birth. If it occurs at birth, the patient will usually have a history of prematurity and associated birth trauma with anoxia or hemorrhage. Complications of delivery with forceps pressure or unnecessary traction on the neck may be elicited. Infections, such as encephalitis or convulsions and dehydration in the first six months can also cause this problem.

The physical findings are first noted by the mother who becomes aware of some difficulty in applying diapers because of the spasticity in the adductors. Some cases can be detected early but other milder cases may not be recognized until ages four or five. At the hip there are variations of flexion, adduction, and internal rotation deformities. Abduction is limited and is associated with an adduction contracture. The flexion contracture of the hip is associated with increased lumbar lordosis. The hip contractures often cause pelvic obliquity and secondary scoliosis. A scissoring type gait is obvious in the severe spastic, but the milder forms with minimal adductor tightness can be difficult to recognize if you are not cognizant of this disease.

A careful neurological examination may reveal other abnormal reflexes and signs which will confirm the physician's suspicions. An accurate history is important because if convulsions, speech abnormalities, balance problems, and symptoms of mental deficiency are present, the problem of diagnosis is easy, and these signs are important when assessing mild cases with a gait problem attributed to the hip.

There may be some abnormal electroencephalographic findings.

On roentgenogram there is a valgus deformity of the neck of the femur—possibly with some anteversion (Fig. 10-36). The hip joint may be subluxated with the earliest sign being a break in Shenton's line.

Less Common Causes

There are several other entities which will not be specifically elucidated but could pose some problem in diagnosing a painless limp if a careful history is not taken or one is not aware of the other stigmas of a specific disease. Limited abduction of the hip will be apparent with chondrodystrophies, such as Morquio's or Hurler's disease. The diagnosis, however, becomes obvious with the classic facies and other characteristics of these diseases.

Unrecognized trauma at birth to the proximal

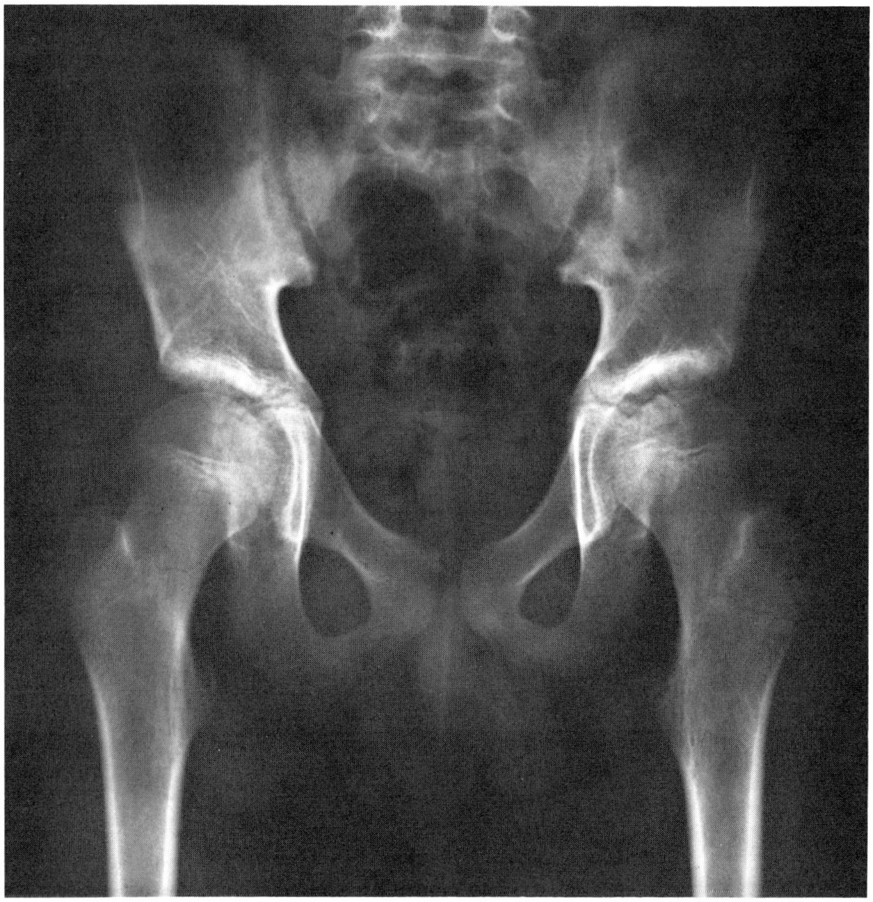

Fig. 10-36. Bilateral valgus hip in cerebral palsy with some anteversion.

growth centers of the hip, with limb length discrepancy, may only become obvious when the child begins to walk. Septic arthritis of the hip joint which may have arrested itself with subsequent epiphyseal arrest or disintegration of the proximal end of the femur may have occurred.

Congenital scoliosis with the development of pelvic obliquity and subsequent adduction deformity of the hip can be easily diagnosed by looking at the back.

ADULT

Acute Pain in the Lateral Soft Tissues

Trochanteric Bursitis

There are numerous bursae about the hip joint which are connective tissue sacs lined with a synovial-like membrane. These overlie a bony prominence or separate a tendon from a muscle. They are thought to serve as a gliding mechanism which reduces friction and pressure between two adjacent surfaces. All of these bursae are subject to various inflammatory processes and the cause varies from infection to systemic diseases but most often is nonspecific. The bursa overlying the greater trochanter is the most commonly involved. Iliopsoas and ischiogluteal bursitis will be discussed later in this chapter.

The cause is usually a nonspecific, sterile inflammation but can be a pyogenic infection such as staphylococcus, nonpyogenic infection such as tuberculosis, or a systemic disease such as gout or rheumatoid arthritis.

On physical examination, pain is present at or usually just posterior to the greater trochanter in an area between the gluteus maximus tendon and lateral surface of the greater trochanter. Tenderness can be elicited by direct palpation over this area. On internal and external rotation of the hip there is guarding, and the pain is localized at the greater trochanter. Hip motion is usually normal without a flexion contracture. However, if inflammation is marked in the area of the gluteus maximus tendons, the hip may have an external rotation contracture to reduce the tension on the gluteus maximus tendons.

If infection is suspected and pus is present in aspirated fluid, it should be cultured and tested for both pyogenic and nonpyogenic organisms, as this is a common site for tuberculosis. Systemic disease, such as gout and rheumatoid arthritis, is frequently present in this area, so uric acid and latex fixation tests should be performed routinely.

Roentgenograms are usually normal except for soft tissue swelling or an area of calcification in the area of the trochanteric bursa (Fig. 10-37). The area of the bony greater trochanter should be observed for areas of active destruction from osteomyelitis or tumor, as bursal pain may be the initial presenting complaint.

Snapping Hip

This is the term given to the audible or palpable click felt on the lateral surface of the thigh in the area of the greater trochanter. Usually it does not produce pain unless sufficient irritation is present, and its symptoms present as a trochanteric bursitis. It is caused by a tight fascia lata slipping over the bony prominence of the greater trochanter. When the hand is held over the greater trochanter, the band can be felt slipping forward and backward over the greater trochanter.

Roentgenograms are usually normal, but osteochondritis dissecans of the greater trochanter and osteochondromas have been reported.

Meralgia Paresthetica

Meralgia paresthetica is the name given to an inflammation of the lateral cutaneous nerve of the femur. The nerve is a direct branch of the lumbar plexus and is formed by the posterior branches of the second and third lumbar nerves. It appears at the lateral border of the psoas muscle then crosses the iliacus muscle just deep to its fascia in a direction toward the anterior iliac spine. It then passes under the lateral side of the inguinal ligament just medial to the anterior superior spine; it becomes subcutaneous and divides into an anterior and posterior branch. The anterior branch is usually the larger of the two and supplies the skin on the lateral aspect of the thigh to the knee. The smaller posterior branch supplies the skin of the lateral buttock distal to the greater trochanter. Meralgia paresthetica is caused by direct blunt trauma, that is, a plaster body jacket too closely molded to the anterior spine of the pelvis, corsets, belts, or a surgical scar from an anterior approach to the hip.

On physical examination there are dysesthesias affecting either or both branches of the nerve along its course described as burning or "pins and needles" sensations or hypesthesia. If a neuroma is present a positive Tinel's sign may be elicited by direct palpation.

Laboratory and roentgenography do not aid in the differential diagnosis.

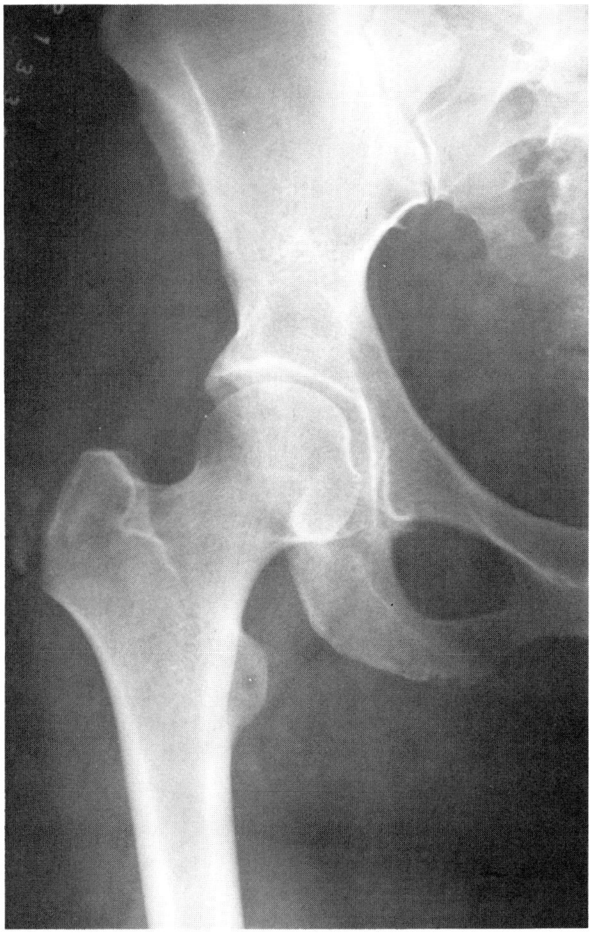

Fig. 10-37. Calcification in greater trochanteric bursa.

Sprain of the Iliotibial Band

This syndrome was described by Cyriax and occurs only in dancers and athletes, causing symptoms similar to trochanteric bursitis. He lists four characteristics of this syndrome: pain on the involved side with flexion toward the painless side which increases if the patient crosses his legs before he bends sideways; pain on full passive adduction of the hip; no pain on any other passive motion; and no pain on resisted abduction of the hip.

Gluteal Muscle Bruise

This is caused by direct trauma to the gluteus maximus muscle, and a history of such can be elicited. Occasionally, a hematoma can be palpated in the muscle mass.

Claudication Pain Secondary to Obstruction of Internal Iliac Artery

Vascular obstruction of the internal iliac artery from hematoma or atherosclerotic plaque will often present initially as pain in the gluteal muscles. This pain may be lateral or posterior.

The disease is usually seen in men between the ages of 50 and 70, when there is some degree of atherosclerosis of the aorta. The lumen narrows, becomes stenotic, and when blood flow decreases below 90 percent claudication pain symptoms occur. Symptoms occur after the patient walks two to three blocks.

Claudication symptoms secondary to ischemia of the gluteal muscles are often the most predominant feature on physical examination. These symptoms are also confused with lumbar spine lesions. Usually, there will be symptoms of claudication equally in both lower extremities with involvement of leg and thigh muscles. There will be absence or diminution of the femoral pulses combined with absence of popliteal and pedal pulses. Palpation of the abdomen will reveal pulsation of the abdominal aorta. A systolic bruit is audible over the aorta or iliac arteries. Signs of chronic ischemia in legs or feet will be manifested by the absence of hair and brittle nails, or the presence of rubor. Sustained gluteal contraction produces pain in the gluteal muscle while passive motion of extension and abduction does not cause pain. Impotence of varying severity is often a complaint.

Electrocardiography is helpful in assessing the presence of concomitant coronary artery disease. Aortography can definitely establish the diagnosis as well as the extent of occlusive disease present.

A flat plate or roentgenogram of the abdomen will often reveal calcification in the wall of the aorta.

Herniated Disk

A herniated lumbar disk lesion can transmit pain to the lateral side of the hip and may be confused with trochanteric bursitis. However, it is more apt to be referred to the posterior aspect of the buttocks. Disk lesions are discussed in Chapter 7.

Avulsion of the Greater Trochanter

This may be seen following a history of direct trauma. It is more apt to be seen in the young athlete with an open epiphysis due to severe, forceful muscle contracture of the abductors. There will be pain and tenderness at the greater trochanter, and on resisted abduction the pain will point directly to the avulsion.

Acute Pain in the Posterior Buttocks

Ischiogluteal Bursitis

The ischiogluteal bursa lies between the tuberosity of the ischium and the gluteus maximus. A sterile inflammation of this bursa often develops in persons whose occupation requires prolonged sitting. The name originally given to this bursitis was "weaver's bottom." The pain will appear as soon as the ischium touches the chair and be relieved the minute the patient arises. The cause is similar to that of trochanteric bursitis, and the physical findings are pain and tenderness over or just above the ischial tuberosity. Roentgenograms are normal except when osteomyelitis is present, in which case active destruction of bone would be seen.

Proximal Hamstring Sprain or Rupture

This can occur to one or all three of the hamstring muscle group (semitendinous, semimembranous, or biceps femoris). They all have in common their origin from the ischial tuberosity and their nerve supply from the tibial division of the sciatic. A history of sudden contracture of the hamstring muscle group followed by acute pain at their origin will usually be elicited. The physical findings are pain and tenderness usually in the tendinous origin of the hamstrings with or without a palpable hematoma.

Resisted flexion of the knee will produce pain in the area of the affected hamstring musculature. Laboratory and roentgenographic findings are normal.

Herniated Lumbar Disk

Pressure from disk protrusion of the nerve root at the level of the fourth or fifth lumbar vertebra is a common cause of referred pain to the buttock area. The problem of diagnosing a disk lesion is discussed in more detail in Chapter 7.

Acute Pain in the Medial Soft Tissues

Iliopsoas Bursitis

The iliopsoas is probably the largest of the bursae lying between the iliopsoas muscle and tendon anteriorly and the pelvis and capsule of the hip joint posteriorly. It communicates with the hip joint and lies next to the femoral nerve, often irritating it.

It is usually caused by a nonspecific, sterile inflammation but can become inflamed from a pyogenic infection such as staphylococcus, nonpyogenic infection such as tuberculosis, or a systemic disease.

Physical findings will include pain, tenderness, and swelling in the area of Scarpa's triangle. There may be signs of femoral nerve compression with pain referable to the knee, similar to hip disease. The pain is worse when the thigh is flexed or extended, both of which stretch the iliopsoas muscle. The most painful movement, however, is adduction in flexion in which the bursa is actually squeezed. When examining this area, a high index of suspicion must be present for both an obturator hernia or a psoas abscess, which both present with swelling in Scarpa's triangle. Because of the possible communication with the joint, such proliferative synovial diseases as rheumatoid arthritis and pigmented vilonodular synovitis must be considered. Acute hemorrhage into the iliopsoas bursa can occur, and diagnosis is made by needle aspiration. The typical history will include a sudden jarring of the thigh followed by immediate pain and swelling and an inability to flex the hip joint.

If infection is thought to be present, aspiration and culture are necessary for an accurate diagnosis.

On roentgenogram there may be obliteration of the iliopsoas muscle which is present on the anteroposterior view of the pelvis.

Adductor Longus Rupture or Sprain

Adductor longus rupture or sprain occurs following a history of sudden, forced adduction at the hip. The rupture is usually partial. Formerly it was thought to be a hazard only in horsemen. The novice first learning to ride a horse will often complain of pain in the adductor area. Pain on resisted adduction will localize at the site of the injury.

Iliopsoas Rupture or Lesser Trochanter Avulsion

Iliopsoas rupture can occur following a history of severe, violent flexion at the hip. In the younger patient with an open epiphysis, an avulsion of the lesser trochanter may occur. Pain on resisted flexion at the hip will localize at the point of rupture or avulsion. Hematoma formation will cause swelling in the soft tissue just above the lesser trochanter.

Intraabdominal Lesion

Multiple disease entities in the lower part of the abdomen often have hip pain as their presenting symptom; therefore, careful examination of the lower part of the abdomen is essential in a hip evaluation. The usual presentation is to the groin or medial thigh area. For example, appendicitis sometimes irritates the iliopsoas muscle to such an extent that the leg goes into spasm with the hip held in a flexed, externally rotated position. Pelvic inflammatory disease or a peritoneal abscess may irritate the iliopsoas or the obturator internus muscle. If the obturator internus is irritated and goes into spasm, the patient will have marked pain and discomfort when the leg is rotated internally. It should be emphasized that pain in the hip does not rule out intraabdominal lesions.

Acute Pain in Anterior Soft Tissues

Rectus Femoris Rupture

Of all the muscles in the area of the hip, the rectus femoris is the most prone to rupture. This condition usually occurs in young athletes. Following a violent muscular contraction of the quadriceps, the patient feels something giving way in the anterior aspect of the hip. The pain, although not severe at the time, will be intolerable in the morning.

With the patient lying prone, there will be pain

and tenderness anteriorly in the groin on resisted extension. This is diagnostic. A hematoma may or may not be present. Knee flexion will be limited with the patient in the prone position, but if the patient lies supine, there is a normal range of knee flexion. This is explained by the fact that the tension in the quadriceps distally from knee flexion is released by the relaxation proximally from hip flexion. Protrusion of the third lumbar disk can mimic this when knee flexion is also altered whether or not the hip is flexed. In a disk lesion, however, one often does not see pain with quadriceps weakness.

Laboratory findings are not helpful, but a lateral roentgenogram may reveal a hematoma in the soft tissues anterior to the hip.

Sartorius Rupture

It is doubtful if rupture of the sartorius tendon alone ever occurs. Erroneously, the term "cricket-leg" was ascribed to sartorius rupture, but, in fact, quadriceps rupture has since been shown to be the real culprit. An avulsion of the sartorius with a piece of the anterosuperior iliac spine often occurs. It invariably is in an adolescent male who is running and suddenly feels a painful snap laterally in the upper part of the groin. The most painful hip motion following this injury is resisted flexion and external rotation. The tenderness is localized to the area of the anterosuperior iliac spine.

Intraabdominal lesions and meralgia paresthetica are also often referred anteriorly to the hip joint and were discussed earlier.

Acute and Chronic Pain in the Hip

Osteoarthritis

Osteoarthritis can occur in many joints, but it is more commonly seen in the weight-bearing joints such as the hips or knees. The first changes probably occur in the articular cartilage with clear documentation of a decrease in the ratio of chondroitin sulfate to keratosulfate. Ultimately, it involves the subchondral bone capsule and contiguous structures. The disease appears to be familial and unquestionably increases with advancing years. There are also constitutional factors, such as obesity, which do not initiate the process, but certainly aggravate existing degeneration.

The predominant symptom is progressive pain, described as a constant gnawing made worse with movement and relieved by rest. There is usually stiffness after rest which disappears on movement. There is tenderness to palpation which the patient describes as deep in the groin and also lateral and posterior. Active and passive motion of the joint are restricted, with the most marked restrictions being flexion, internal rotation, and abduction. Flexion, external rotation, and adduction contractures usually develop. Crepitation will be elicited, often both audible and palpable. There is an antalgic gait which may have a Trendelenburg component late in the disease. If muscle atrophy is present, swelling may be palpable in the groin or over the greater trochanter The effusion present in the joints may overflow into the bursae which communicate with the hip joint. Osteoarthritis of the hip is associated with Heberden's nodes, which occur at the distal interphalangeal joint of the fingers, so one should always observe the hands.

There are no laboratory tests diagnostic for osteoarthritis. Specific tests, such as uric acid for gout and latex fixation for rheumatoid arthritis, may aid in the differential diagnosis.

On roentgenogram, there is narrowing of the joint space which in reality is the cartilage present on both sides of the joint. The subchondral bone becomes sclerotic on both sides of the joint beginning in the superior lateral weight-bearing portion and gradually expanding. Pseudocysts develop in the sclerosing bone, and osteophytes will form on the joint margins (Fig. 10-38). As the disease progresses, the neck of the femur becomes grossly distorted into a coxa magna situation, and distortion of the acetabulum occurs concurrently.

Rheumatoid Arthritis

Rheumatoid arthritis is a systemic disease involving mesenchymal tissue throughout the body and is not a disease of articular cartilage like osteoarthritis, which is more often confined to one joint. Rheumatoid arthritis can begin in the hip joint and subsequently involve other joints, but this is unusual for its presentation. Many etiological factors have been incriminated, but the bulk of the evidence points to an autoimmune disease. On clinical presentation, the disease is polyarticular, particularly involving the small joints of the hands and feet; it does not usually present in the hip only. Pain and stiffness are the main complaints, particularly when arising in the morning. There is tenderness to palpation in all areas of the hip joint—anterior, posterior, and lateral. All motions of the hip joint become restricted because of pain, and contractures develop, particularly flexion and adduction. The gait is antalgic with involvement of multiple joints, and because there is an inability to come off one limb due to pain in the other, the patient walks with a shuffling gait, attempting not to place too much weight on either limb. Low grade fever is usually present with nonspecific symptoms, such as weight loss, anemia, tiredness, and depression. Because it is a systemic disease there are multiple associated problems in other areas of the body, including the skin, arteries, nerves, lungs, pleura, and heart. The tendons and bursae adjacent to the hip, which are mesenchymal are inflamed, as is the synovium.

There is a normochromic or hypochromic normocytic anemia. White blood cell counts are usually normal but can be slightly to moderately elevated. The erythrocyte sedimentation rate is elevated in direct relationship to the activity of the disease. The presence of rheumatoid factor in the serum is usually seen in 70 percent of these patients. Serum complement levels are normal or mildly increased but markedly decreased in the joint fluid. There is poor mucin precipitation of the joint fluid when dropped into acetic acid (see Fig. 1-7).

Roentgenograms will show early soft tissue swelling and effusion with distention of the capsular tissues about the hip. The decreased cartilage space is concentric and is decreased medially as well as in the superior weight-bearing portion of the hip. Osteoporosis is present on both sides of the joint. As the disease progresses, marginal erosions appear along the joints. Subchondral cyst formation appears and protrusio acetabuli can be noted (Fig. 10-39). Total disintegration of the joint similar to a neuropathic joint is seen late in the disease and may be associated with the administration of steroids and pain medication.

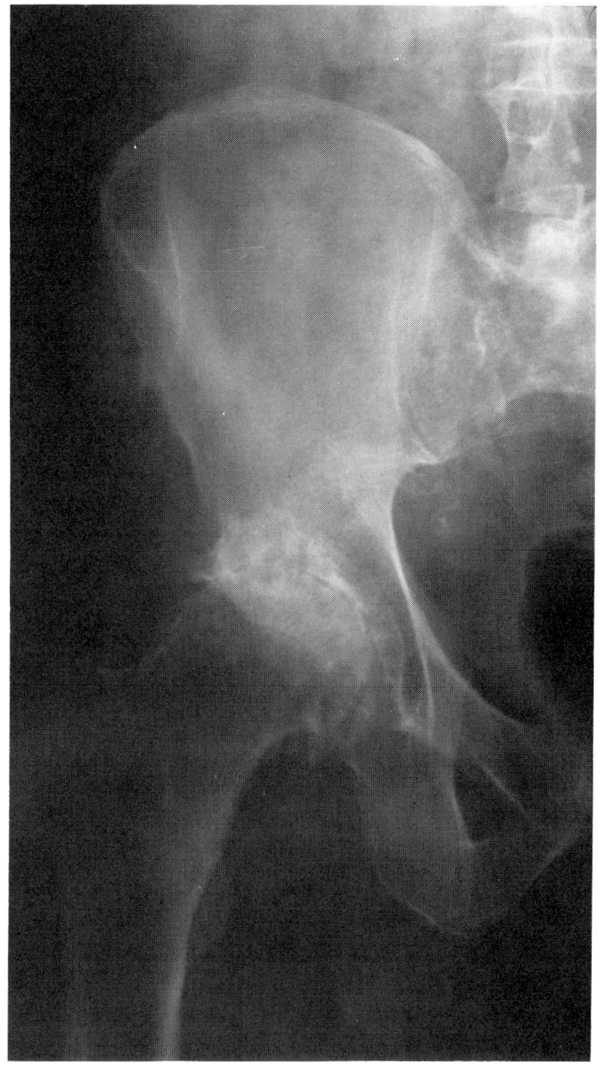

Fig. 10-38. Osteoarthritis of hip. Note the sclerosing bone with pseudocysts in the superior lateral weight bearing portion of the bone. The cartilage space is narrowed and osteophytes are present on the joint margins.

Avascular Necrosis

The term avascular necrosis is not a disease state but instead is the term ascribed to the head of the femur which has lost its blood supply and has become sclerotic as seen on roentgenograms. There have been multiple factors associated with this affliction of the head of the femur: fracture of the neck of the femur, dislocation of the hip, steroid administration, renal transplantation, alcoholism, sickle cell and other hemoglobin diseases, caisson disease, Gaucher's disease, radiation, arteriosclerosis, gout, and prolonged administration of pain medications. In all these conditions the basic lesson implicated is mechanical interruption of the blood supply to the head of the femur.

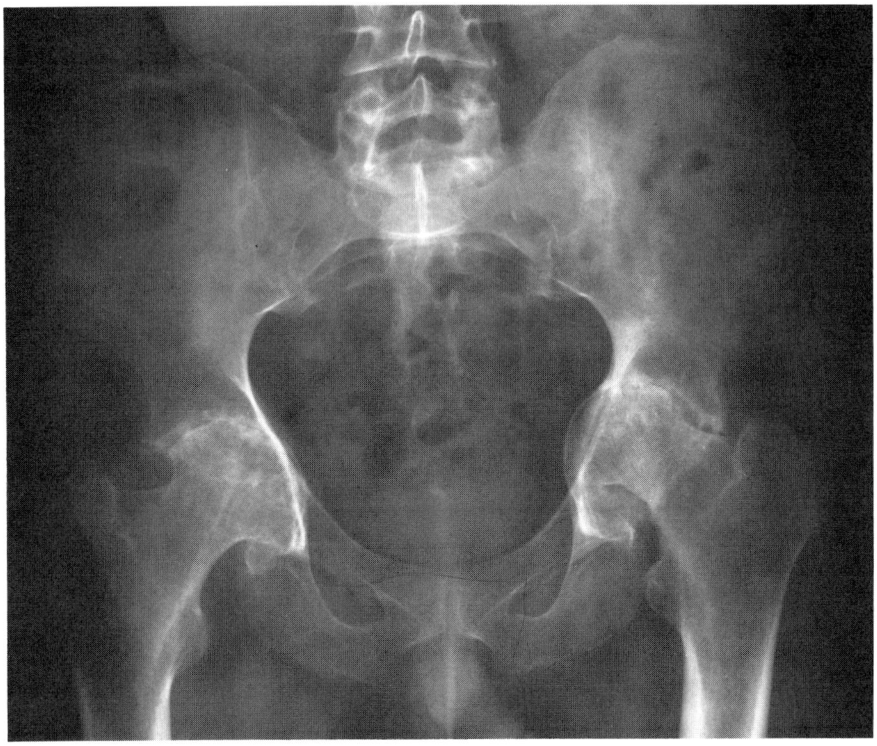

Fig. 10-39. Rheumatoid arthritis with protrusion. The cartilage space is concentric and is decreased medially as well as in the superior weight bearing portion of the bone. Osteoporosis and subchondral cyst formation is present on both sides of the joint.

Clinically, there is an insidious onset of chronic pain which occurs more often in males in their fourth decade of life. About 50 percent of these patients have an onset of similar pain in the opposite hip within several years. Motion of the hip joint remains normal until secondary degenerative arthritis develops, and in most patients an antalgic gait with short stance phase will be noted on the side of the involved extremity.

The first change noted on roentgenograms is increased density (sclerosis) of a portion or the entire head of the femur, but this will not be seen until several months after the vascular insult (Fig. 10-40). Osteoporosis of the acetabulum and adjacent neck of the femur probably develops secondary to disuse. Segmental collapse and flattening of the vascular area of the neck of the femur appear, along with areas of radiolucency within the sclerotic bone related to resorption and repair of the devascularized area. Pseudocyst formation will develop, and late in the disease all the changes of degenerative arthritis are present including osteophytes, joint narrowing, and marked sclerosis.

Ankylosing Spondylitis

This disease is covered in Chapter 7, but is mentioned here because although primarily an arthritis of the spine, one fifth of the patients will notice the first symptoms in the peripheral joints and approximately one third of these will ultimately have hip disease. Late in the disease, marked flexion contractures are present in the hips, and bony ankylosis of the hip often results.

Paget's Disease

This disease manifests itself with increasing frequency after age 40, and its etiology remains an enigma to investigators. Phosphorus appears to play a role in its manifestation because geographic areas where dietary phosphorus is low have a decreased incidence of Paget's disease.

This disease should always be considered in the differential of hip pain in the older adult. Twenty percent of patients with Paget's disease present with insidious progressive pain in the hip or thigh area not unlike the symptoms of osteoarthritis. It characteristically is aggravated by exercise and is more severe when sleeping. The patient will often complain of muscle cramps in and around the hip. The bone mass is increased but it is not normal bone and, therefore, structurally much weaker. Because the bone is weaker and more prone to stress, a coxa vara at the hip with a concurrent bending in the femur produces characteristic bowing of the lower extremity. This effect on the femur plus a curving spine, and pelvic involvement in the advanced stages, combine to give these patients a characteristic waddle and uneven gait. If suspicious of this disease, one must always ask the patient who wears a hat if he has had an increase in his hat size. This disease characteristically attacks the skull and adds bone mass to the calvarium. Spontaneous stress fractures in the proximal femur are not uncommon, and fractures occurring with minimal trauma in this area require careful consideration of Paget's disease as the underlying primary disease. Symptoms referable to cranial nerves and spinal cord encroachment because of decrease in the lumen or foramen from expanding bone mass are not uncommon.

The characteristic laboratory finding is marked elevation of alkaline phosphatase, especially in active generalized disease. Because of the marked osteoplastic activity, alkaline phosphatase elevation is not unexpected. There is a destructive osteolytic phase to the disease, but even then a normal serum calcium and phosphorus is found as in all stages. If an elevated serum calcium is found, it is secondary to disuse atrophy, as seen in the immobilized patient. The findings on microscopic sections of bone are pathognomonic. The characteristic mosaic pattern, vascularity with large numbers of osteoclasts in the adult bone, is seen. The other disease which must be considered when large numbers of osteoclasts are present in adult bone is parathyroid adenoma.

Roentgenographically, the osteoclastic and osteoblastic activity of the disease is reflected in the bony

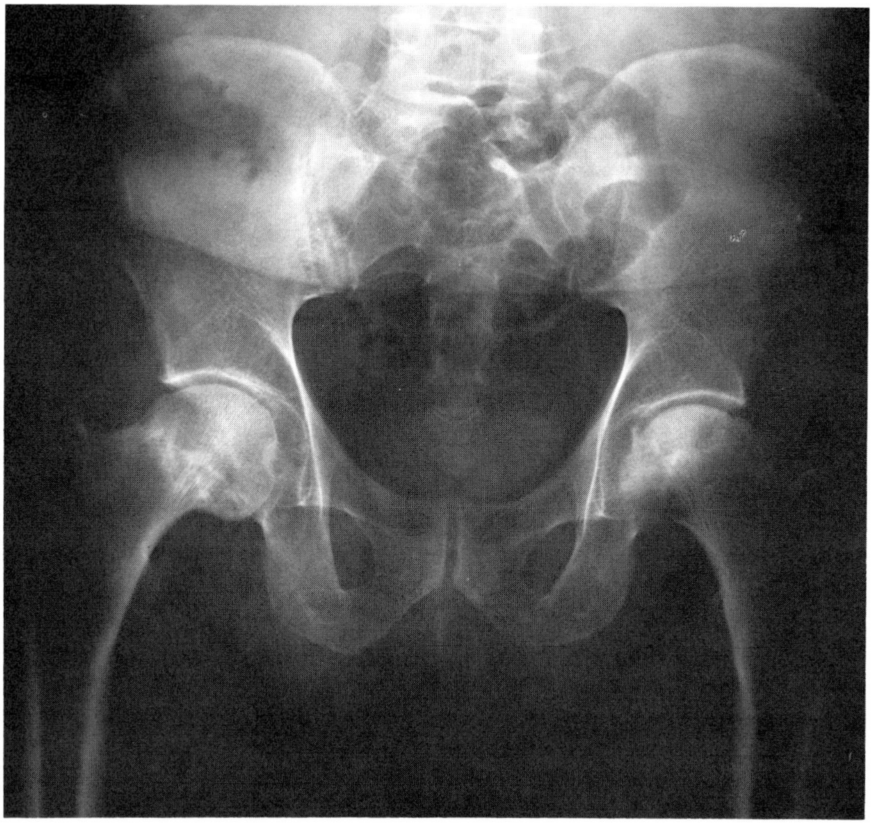

Fig. 10-40. Avascular necrosis in a kidney transplant patient. Note the increased density (sclerosis) of the superior portion of the femoral head, particularly on the left.

picture of radiolucency and opacity. The femur is thicker, opaque, and bowed (Fig. 10-41), and, not uncommonly, pseudofractures are seen.

Pigmented Villonodular Synovitis

This disease will manifest either as a benign tumor or inflammatory granuloma. The etiology is obscure, but because of the large hemosiderin deposits in the synovia, hemorrhage was thought to be a factor. There is no higher incidence in the patient with hemophilia so its pathogenesis remains an enigma.

When the hip joint is involved the symptoms are intermittent pain and swelling of a prolonged duration. Aspiration of the joint reveals a dark brown fluid, and biopsy reveals the characteristic hemosiderin deposits in the lining. The proliferating synovia can penetrate and actually replace cancellous bone in both the acetabulum and femoral head. Roentgenographically, then, this disease should always be suspected in patients with obvious disease in the hip joint, plus irregular areas of radiolucency in the subchondral bones of both the acetabulum and head and neck of the femur.

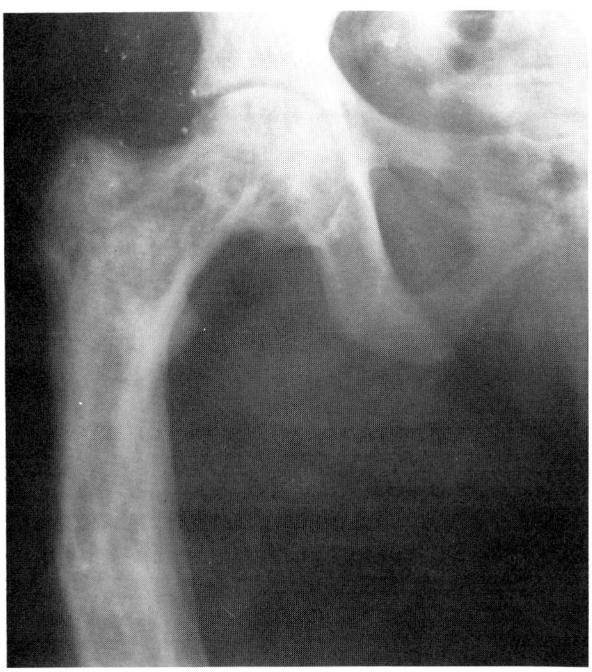

Fig. 10-41. Paget's disease with bowing of the femur. The bony picture of radiolucency and opacity reflects both the osteoclastic and osteoblastic activity of the disease. Pseudofractures are seen in the thicker bowed femur.

Tumor

Benign and malignant tumors can present with chronic type pain in the hip and are usually diagnosed by roentgenography. While malignant tumors will have active bone destruction and an associated tumor mass (see Chap. 2), the benign tumors are well circumscribed with a sclerotic rim of bone (see Chap. 2).

Gout

Gout is a disease more frequently seen in males over age 20 and is not usually seen in women until menopause. The hip is not usually involved, but it does occur. Initially, it may present as an acute attack clearing completely in one to two weeks, but it will present again later and often progress to a chronic pain. Avascular necrosis of the head of the femur can be associated with gout.

Uric acid elevation is indicative of gout, but the diagnosis depends on clinical findings plus identifying the urate crystals with a polarizing microscope. Roentgenograms are helpful if subchondral bone erosions or radiopaque-tophaceous deposits are present.

Fracture-Dislocations of the Hip

Fractures

All of the fracture-dislocations of the hip have in common a history of severe trauma. The type of trauma and the mechanism of injury are extremely important in differentiating the disease. Physical examination and simple observation of the attitude of the limp will aid in differentiating the type of fracture-dislocation even before roentgenography. Laboratory data are usually of no help unless there are extremely low hemoglobin and hematocrit counts, then the possibility of pelvic fracture must be paramount because enormous quantities of blood can be lost in the retroperitoneal area from pelvic fractures. The reader is referred to Rockwood and Green's *Fractures* for more detailed information on these problems.

Head of the Femur. Fractures of the head of the femur (Fig. 10-42) usually occur in association with a dislocation of the head of the femur, but have been known to occur without a dislocation. There is nothing unique about their presentation that aids in

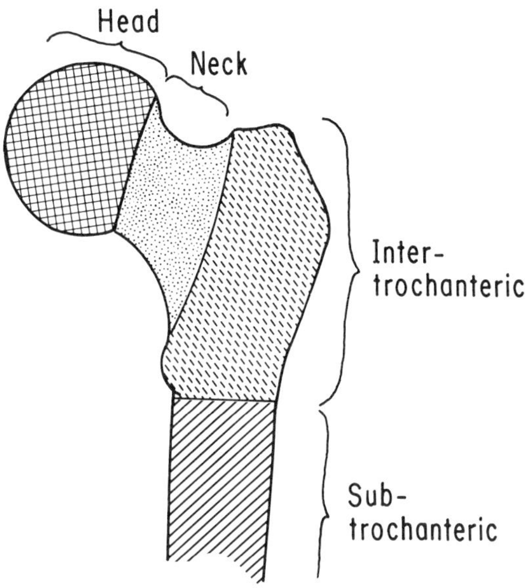

Fig. 10-42. Fractures of the hip can occur in the head, neck, intertrochanteric, and subtrochanteric areas as indicated on the diagram.

their differentiation, and one must rely on good roentgenography to depict the fracture. One should look for fractures of the superior aspect of the head of the femur with anterior dislocations and fractures of the inferior aspect with posterior dislocations.

Neck of the Femur. Fractures of the neck of the femur (see Fig. 10-42) may be displaced or undisplaced. The undisplaced fractures are due to stress (usually young athletic individuals), impaction (minor trauma with associated osteoporosis), or postirradiation of the pelvis for cervical cancer. The patients present with mild to moderate pain in the groin, no rotational deformity, or length discrepancy of the extremity, and often they are able to walk but have an antalgic gait. Routine anteroposterior roentgenograms of the hip will often be normal, so if your index of suspicion is high, oblique roentgenograms and tomograms are indicated.

Displaced fractures of the neck of the femur, on the other hand, have a usual mode of presentation. They occur in osteoporotic individuals, usually older women, and are associated with a minor fall and, only rarely, severe trauma. These patients have severe pain throughout the hip, and the leg is held in some external rotation and mild abduction, and there is some shortening. Roentgenograms are diagnostic and readily apparent with the displacement and disruption of Shenton's line (Fig. 10-43).

Intertrochanteric Fractures. These fractures (see Fig. 10-42) occur in slightly older persons than do the neck fractures, average age being 70 years. They are more common in females, and the incidence has been reported to be as high as eight times. They usually occur in a major fall or an associated automobile injury, with both direct and indirect forces acting on the hip. The indirect forces are the iliopsoas with its attachment on the lesser trochanter and the abductors with their attachment on the greater trochanter, and this explains why there are often separate fragments with this injury. There will be marked external rotation of the extremity, especially in the comminuted fracture, with the foot

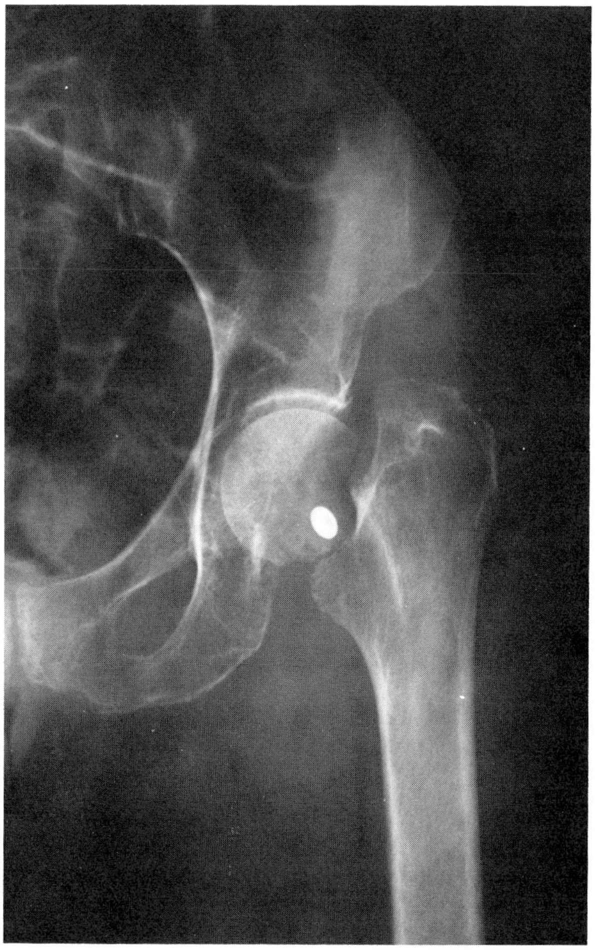

Fig. 10-43. Fracture of neck of femur.

often resting on its lateral surface. This occurs because of the attachment of the iliopsoas, which because of the fracture can now rotate the shaft of the femur externally. The leg shortening varies with the degree of comminution. Obvious swelling of the hip is present in distinction to that of a fracture of the neck of the femur, and, if seen late, ecchymosis can be noted, especially laterally. Roentgenograms are diagnostic (Fig. 10-44).

Subtrochanteric Fractures. Patients with subtrochanteric fractures (see Fig. 10-42) are usually younger than those with neck or intertrochanteric fractures. More force is required to produce this fracture than the intertrochanteric. The physical findings are the same, and the differentiation can only be made by roentgenography.

Dislocations

Posterior Dislocation of the Hip. Posterior dislocation is the most common dislocation at the hip and usually occurs in association with automobile-related accidents, but are occasionally seen in athletic injuries. The patients are usually passengers in the front seat, and the injury occurs when the knee hits the dashboard. The knee and hip are flexed and the hip is either neutral or in adduction. If the hip is in slight abduction or hip flexion is less than 90 degrees, there may be an associated posterior acetabular fracture. Classically, the patient presents with a shortened extremity, with the hip internally rotated and adducted. Usually the involved side will rest on the uninvolved thigh (Fig. 10-45). With dashboard injuries, one must look carefully for injuries of the shaft of the femur and knee, as these frequently occur.

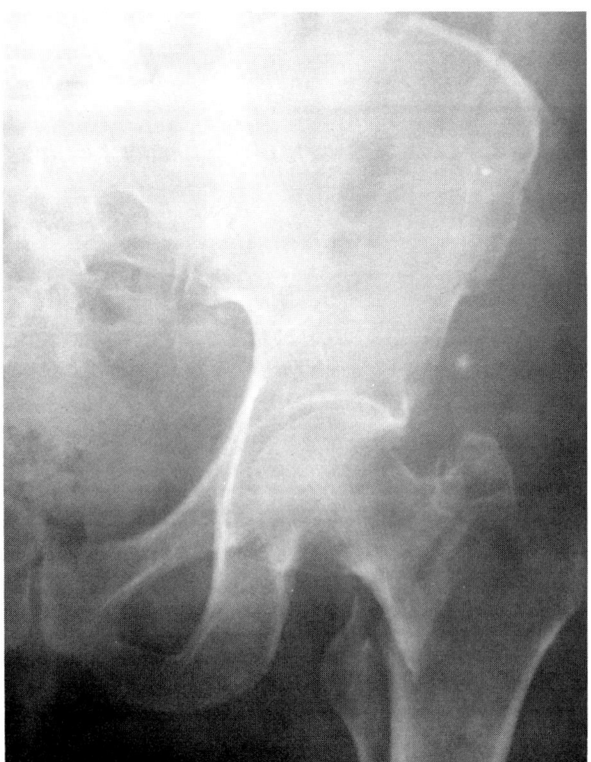

Fig. 10-44. Intertrochanteric femur fracture.

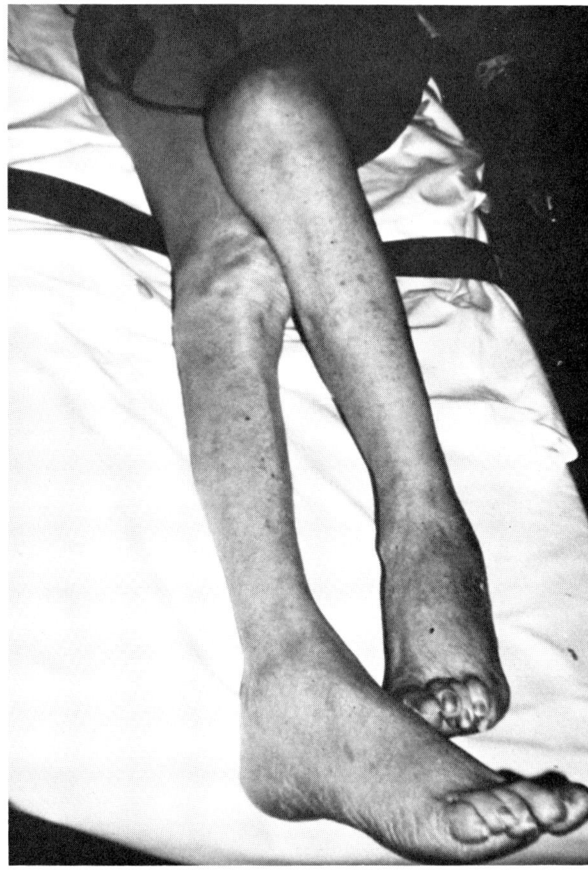

Fig. 10-45. Posterior dislocation of hip. The extremity is shortened with the hip flexed, internally rotated, and adducted. The involved extremity is resting on the uninvolved thigh.

Roentgenography invariably confirms the physical examination (Fig. 10-46).

Anterior Dislocation of the Hip. Like posterior dislocations, anterior dislocations are usually automobile-related, but in this instance the major

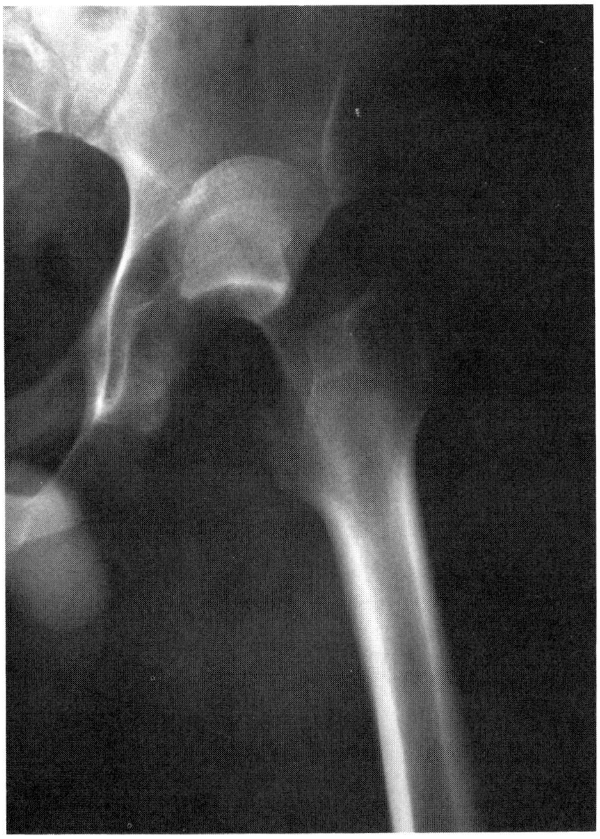

Fig. 10-46. Posterior dislocation of hip—x-ray.

factor in producing an anterior dislocation is forced abduction. They have also been reported to occur in falls from heights or a blow to the back when the patient is in a squatting position. Abduction is always necessary, following which the neck or trochanter impinges on the acetabular rim levering the head out through a tear in the anterior capsule. The attitude of the hip determines if an obturator or pubic dislocation occurs. If the hip is flexed, obturator dislocation occurs and if extended a pubic dislocation results.

On physical examination, there is seldom detection of any shortening with either the obturator or pubic type. In both instances, abduction and external rotation are present (Fig. 10-47). In a pubic dislocation, however, the hip is extended instead of flexed. The head of the femur can be palpated near the anterosuperior iliac spine in a pubic type dislocation and in the groin in an obturator dislocation.

Roentgenography will confirm the physical findings.

Central Fracture-Dislocations of the Hip. Central fracture-dislocations of the hip are more common than anterior dislocations but not as frequent as posterior dislocations. They are usually automobile-related, and severe force is necessary for them to occur. It results either from direct force acting on the greater trochanter or force acting along the long axis of the femur when abduction of the hip is present.

The physical findings are inconsistent and not specific. All hip motion is usually restricted with marked muscle spasm. If the fracture is displaced to any degree, limb shortening will be present. It is important to realize its association with other severe injuries to the head, chest, and abdomen and, therefore, it is easy to see how it may be easily overlooked. An anteroposterior view of the pelvis should be obtained in all patients with serious trauma to avoid misdiagnosis (Fig. 10-48). When unexplained severe

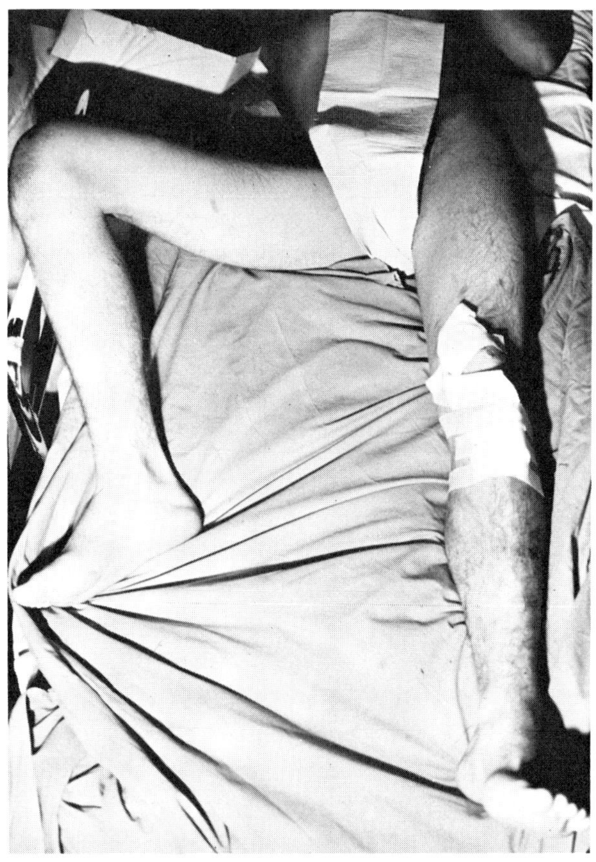

Fig. 10-47. Anterior dislocation of hip. Note the flexed, abducted, and externally rotated position of the extremity.

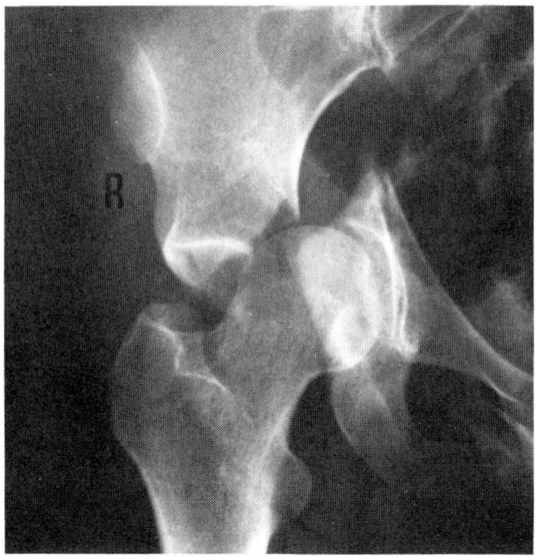

Fig. 10-48. Central fracture-dislocation of hip.

blood loss is involved in any patient without an open injury, one should always consider an acetabular fracture which may be causing loss of large quantities of blood into the pelvis.

SUGGESTED READINGS

1. Adams, J. A.: Transient synovitis of the hip joint in children. J. Bone Joint Surg. *45-B:*471, 1963.
2. Aitken, G. T.: Surgical amputation in children. Chap. 26. *In* Instructional Course Lectures. Vol. 18, J2. pp. 271–277. The American Academy of Orthopaedic Surgeons, 1962–1969.
3. Aitken, G. T. (ed.): Proximal Femoral Focal Deficiency, A Congenital Anomaly. Symposium, Washington, D.C., June 13, 1968. National Academy Sciences, 1969.
4. Almond, G. A.: Familial infantile coxa vara. J. Bone Joint Surg. *38-B:*539, 1956.
5. American Orthopaedic Association: Manual of Orthopaedic Surgery, 1966.
6. Baitch, A.: Recent observations of acute suppurative arthritis. Clin. Orthop. *22:*157, 1962.
7. Barlow, T. G.: Early diagnosis and treatment of congenital dislocation of the hip. J. Bone Joint Surg. *44-B:*292, 1962.
8. Blair, W.: Psoas myositis or fibrositis in the differential diagnosis of lower abdominal disease. Am. J. Surg. *22:*505, 1956.
9. Borella, L., Goobar, J. E., Summitt, R. L., and Clark, G. M.: Septic arthritis in childhood. J. Pediatr. *62:*742, 1963.
10. Bosworth, D. M.: Bone and joint tuberculosis in childhood. Recent advances in diagnosis and treatment. Pediatr. Clin. N. Am. *2:*1129, 1955.
11. Brinkhous, K. M., and Scarborough, D. E.: Some mechanisms of thrombus formation and hemorrhage following trauma. J. Trauma *9:*684, 1969.
12. Burrows, H. J.: Slipped upper femoral epiphysis. Characteristics of a hundred cases. J. Bone Joint Surg. *39-B:*641, 1957.
13. Caffey, J.: The early roentgenographic changes in essential coxa plana: Their significance in pathogenesis. Am. J. Roentgenol. Radium Ther. Nucl. Med. *103:*620, 1968.
14. Calvé, J.: Sur une forme particuliere de pseudo-coxalgie greffee sur des deformations caracteristique de l'extremite superieure du femur. Rev. Chir. *30:*54, 1910.
15. Catto, M.: The histological appearances of late segmental collapse of the femoral head after transcervical fracture. J. Bone Joint Surg. *47-B:*777, 1965.
16. Chung, S. M. K., and Ralston, E. L.: Necrosis of the femoral head associated with sickle-cell anemia and its genetic variants. A review of the literature and study of 13 cases. J. Bone Joint Surg. *51-A:*33, 1969.
17. Cleveland, M., Bosworth, D. M., Thompson, F. R., Wilson, H. J., and Ishizuka, T.: A ten year analysis of intertrochanteric fractures of the femur. J. Bone Joint Surg. *41-A:*1939, 1959.
18. Cozen, L.: Trochanteric bursitis. Am. J. Orthop. *7:*70, 1965.
19. Cruess, R. L., Bennerhassett, J., MacDonald, F. R., Maclean, L. D., and Dossetor, J.: Aseptic necrosis following renal transplantation. J. Bone Joint Surg. *50-A:*1577, 1968.
20. Cyriax, J.: Textbook of Orthopaedic Medicine. ed. 5 p. 649. Baltimore, Williams & Wilkins Co., 1969.
21. Davidson, P. T., and Horowitz, I.: Skeletal tuberculosis, a review with patient presentations and discussions. Am. J. Med. *48:*77, 1970.
22. Donaldson, W. F.: Transient synovitis of the hip joint. Pediatr. Clin. N. Am. *2:*1073, 1955.
23. Drey, L.: A roentgenographic study of transitory synovitis of the hip joint. Radiology *60:*588, 1953.
24. Duncan, H. G.: Congenital coxa vara occurring in identical twins. Am. J. Surg. *37:*112, 1937.
25. Duraiswami, P. K.: Experimental causation of congenital skeletal defects and its significance in orthopedic surgery. J. Bone Joint Surg. *34-B:*646, 1952.
26. Duthie, R. B., and Ferguson, A. B., Jr.: Mercer's Orthopaedic Surgery. ed. 7. Baltimore, Williams & Wilkins Co., 1973.
27. Edwards, E. G.: Transient synovitis of the hip joint in children. Report of 13 cases. JAMA *148:*30, 1952.
28. Epstein, H. C.: Traumatic dislocations of the hip. Clin. Orthop. *92:*116, 1973.
29. Eyre-Brook, A. L.: Septic arthritis of the hip and osteomyelitis of the upper end of the femur in infants. J. Bone Joint Surg. *42-B:*11, 1960.
30. Eyring, M. J. (ed.): Report of the Seminar on the Role of the Orthopaedist in the Management of Juvenile Rheumatoid Arthritis. Apr. 27–29, 1972. Glen Cove, N.Y., Harrison House, 1972.
31. Fairbank, H. A. T.: Infantile or cervical coxa vara. *In* Milford, Humphrey (ed.): The Robert Jones Birthday Volume. A Collection of Surgical Essays. London, Oxford University Press, 1928.
32. Ferguson, A. B., Jr.: Orthopaedic Surgery in Infancy and Childhood. ed. 4. Baltimore, Williams & Wilkins Co., 1974.
33. Ferguson, A. B., and Howorth, M. B.: Coxa plana and related conditions at the hip. J. Bone Joint Surg. *16:*781, 1934.
34. Gardner, E., Gray, D. J., and O'Rahilly, R.: Anatomy: A Regional Study of Human Structure. ed. 4. Philadelphia, E. B. Saunders Co., 1975.
35. Ghormley, R. K., and Fairchild, R. D.: The diagnosis and treatment of slipped epiphysis. JAMA *114:*229, 1940.
36. Gill, G. G.: The cause of discrepancy in length of the limbs following tuberculosis of the hip in children. Arrest of growth from premature central closure of the epiphyseal cartilages about the knee. J. Bone Joint Surg. *26:*272, 1944.
37. Goff, C. W., Shutkin, N. E., and Hersey, M. R.: Legg-Calvé-Perthes Syndrome and Related Osteochondroses of Youth. Springfield, Ill., Charles C Thomas, 1954.
38. Golding, J. S. R., MacIver, J. E., and Went, L. N.: The bone changes in sickle cell anaemia and its genetic variants. J. Bone Joint Surg. *41-B:*711, 1959.

39. Goodfellow, J., Fearn, C. B., and Matthews, J. M.: Iliacus haematoma. A common complication of haemophilia. J. Bone Joint Surg. *49-B:*748, 1967.
40. Grant, J. C. Boileau: An Atlas of Anatomy. ed. 4. Baltimore, Williams & Wilkins Co., 1956.
41. Greenberg, M. S., Kass, E. H., and Castle, W. B.: Studies on the destruction of red blood cells XII. Factors influencing the role of hemoglobin in the pathologic physiology of sickle cell anemia and related disorders. J. Clin. Invest. *36:*833, 1957.
42. Hardinge, K.: The etiology of transient synovitis of the hip in childhood. J. Bone Joint Surg. *52-B:*100, 1970.
43. Harris, W. R.: The endocrine basis for slipping of the upper femoral epiphysis. An experimental study. J. Bone Joint Surg. *32-B:*5, 1950.
44. Hass, J.: Congenital Dislocation of the Hip. Springfield, Ill., Charles C Thomas, 1951.
45. Heimann, W. G., and Freiberger, R. H.: Avascular necrosis of the femoral and humeral heads after high-dosage corticosteroid therapy. N. Engl. J. Med. *263:*672, 1960.
46. Hilgenreiner, H.: Early diagnosis and early treatment of congenital dislocation of the hip. (Zur Friihdiagnose and Friihbehandlung der Angelborenen Hiiftgelenkverrenkung). Med. Klin. *21:*1385, 1925.
47. Hollander, J. L., and McCarty, D. J. (eds.): Arthritis and Allied Conditions. Philadelphia, Lea & Febiger, 1974.
48. Hong, R., and West, C. D.: Gamma-1 globulin levels in rheumatic fever. Arthritis Rheum. *7:*128, 1964.
49. Hoyt, W. A., Jr., and Greenberg, B. J.: Congenital coxa vara. Chap. 7. *In* Tronzo, Raymond G.: Surgery of the Hip Joint. Philadelphia, Lea & Febiger, 1973.
50. Hucherson, B. C., and Freeman, G. E.: Iliopectineal bursitis. A cause of hip pain frequently unrecognized. Am. J. Orthop. *4:*220, 1962.
51. Jacobs, B. W.: Synovitis of the hip in children and its significance. Pediatrics *47:*558, 1971.
52. Johanning, K.: Coxa vara infantum, clinical appearance and aetiological problems. Acta Orthop. Scand. *21:*273, 1951.
53. Jones, J. P., Jr., and Engleman, E. P.: Osseous avascular necrosis associated with systemic abnormalities. Arthritis Rheum. 9:728, 1966.
54. Jones, T. D.: The diagnosis of rheumatic fever. JAMA *126:*481, 1944.
55. Jonsater, S.: Coxa plana. A histo-pathological and angiografic study. Acta Orthop. Scand. Suppl. 12, 1953.
56. Judet, R., Judet, J., and Letournel, E.: Fractures of the acetabulum: Classification and surgical approaches to open reduction. Preliminary report. J. Bone Joint Surg. *46-A:*1615, 1964.
57. Klein, A., Joplin, R., Reidy, J., and Honelin, J.: Slipped Capital Femoral Epiphysis. Springfield, Ill., Charles C Thomas, 1953.
58. Larson, C. B.: Fracture-dislocations of the hip. Clin. Orthop. *92:*147, 1973.
59. Legg, A. T.: An obscure affection of the hip joint. Boston Med. Surg. J. *162:*202, 1910.
60. Lotke, P. A.: Soft tissue lesions affecting the hip joint. Chap. 14. *In* Tronzo, R. G. (ed.): Surgery of the Hip Joint. Philadelphia, Lea & Febiger, 1973.
61. Magnusson, R.: Coxa vara infantum. Acta Orthop. Scand. *23:*284, 1954.
62. Mankin, H. J., Dorfman, H., Lippielo, L., and Zarins, A.: Biochemical and metabolic abnormalities in articular cartilage from osteo-arthritic human hips. II. Correlation of morphology with biochemical and metabolic data. J. Bone Joint Surg. *53-A:*523, 1971.
63. McCarroll, H. R., and Schwartzmann, J. R.: Spastic paralysis and allied disorders. J. Bone Joint Surg. *25:*745, 1943.
64. McKibbin, B.: Anatomical factors in the stability of the hip joint in the newborn. J. Bone Joint Surg. *52-B:*148, 1970.
65. Mercer, W.: The management of the tuberculous hip joint. J. Bone Joint Surg. *36-A:*1123, 1954.
66. Mills, T. J., Owen, R., and Strach, E. H.: Early diagnosis of bone and joint tuberculosis in children. Lancet *271:*57, 1956.
67. Monty, C. P.: Prognosis of "observation hip" in children. Arch. Dis. Child. *37:*539, 1962.
68. Nicholson, J. T.: Pyogenic arthritis with pathologic dislocation of the hip in infants. JAMA *141:*826, 1949.
69. Ortolani, M.: Un segno poco noto e sua inportanza per la diagnosi precoce di prelussazione congenita dell' anca. Pediatria *45:*129, 1937.
70. Palmen, K.: Preluxation of the hip joint. Diagnosis and treatment in the newborn and the diagnosis of congenital dislocation of the hip joint in Sweden during the years 1948–1960. Acta Paediatr. Scand. (Suppl.) 50:129, 1961.
71. Perthes, G.: Ueber Arthritis Deformans Juvenilis. Dtsch. Z. Chir. *107:*111, 1910.
72. Phelps, W. M.: Characteristic psychological variations in cerebral palsy. Nerv. Child. *7:*10, 1948.
73. Ponseti, I. V., and McClintock, R.: The pathology of slipping of the upper femoral epiphysis. J. Bone Joint Surg. *38-A:*71, 1956.
74. Potter, C. M. C.: Osteomyelitis in the new-born. J. Bone Joint Surg. *36-B:*578, 1954.
75. Pylkkanen, P. V.: Coxa vara infantum. Acta Orthop. Scand. (suppl.) 48: 1–120, 1960.
76. Rockwood, C. A., Jr., and Green, D. P. (eds.): Fractures. Philadelphia, J. B. Lippincott Co., 1975.
77. Rowe, C. R., and Lowell, J. D.: Prognosis of fractures of the acetabulum. J. Bone Joint Surg. *43-A:*30, 1961.
78. Sharrard, W. J. W.: Paediatric Orthopaedics and Fractures. Oxford, Blackwell Scientific Publications, 1971.
79. Simon, G.: Principles of Bone X-Ray Diagnosis. ed. 2. London, Butterworths, 1965.
80. Slowick, F. A.: Purulent infections of the hip joint. An analysis of sixty cases. N. Engl. J. Med. *212:*672, 1935.
81. Stetson, J. W., DePonte, R. J., and Southwick, W. O.: Acute septic arthritis of the hip in children. Clin. Orthop. *56:*105, 1968.
82. Steward, M. J., and Milford, L. W.: Fracture-dislocation of the hip. An end-result study. J. Bone Joint Surg. *36-A:*315, 1954.
83. Stollerman, G. H., Markowitz, M., Toranta, A., Wonnamaker, L. W., and Whittemore, R.: Committee report. Jones criteria (revised) for guidance in the diagnosis of rheumatic fever. Circulation *32:*664, 1965.
84. Tipton, W. W., D'Ambrosia, R.D., and Ryle, G. P.: Nonoperative management of central fracture-dislocations of the hip. J. Bone Joint Surg. *57-A:*888, 1975.
85. Tronzo, R. G.: Trochanteric bursitis confused with referred pain from herniated lumbar disc lesions. Philadelphia, Philadelphia Orthopaedic Society, 1969.
86. Tronzo, R. G.: Surgery of the Hip Joint. Philadelphia, Lea & Febiger, 1973.
87. Trueta, J.: The normal vascular anatomy of the human femoral head during growth. J. Bone Joint Surg. *39-B:*358, 1957.
88. Tucker, F. R.: Arterial supply to the femoral head and its clinical importance. J. Bone Joint Surg. *31-B:*82, 1949.
89. Walker, G. F.: Failure of early recognition of skeletal tuberculosis. Br. Med. J. *1:*682, 1968.
90. Winston, M. E.: Haemophilic arthropathy of the hip. J. Bone Joint Surg. *34-B:*412, 1952.
91. Woodburne, R. T.: Essentials of Human Anatomy. New York, Oxford University Press, 1957.

11 The Knee

Stanley L. James, M.D.

The knee is the largest and one of the most complex joints in the human body. Although its location makes it readily available for examination, diagnosis is often difficult because of its complex nature. As in other areas, proper evaluation of the knee is dependent upon three factors: a thorough understanding of functional anatomy, a systematic and orderly examination, and an understanding of the various pathological entities affecting the knee. A complete understanding of these three factors is necessary to obtain a logical differential diagnosis. The sequence of examination discussed is not absolute and is only a reference for adapting personal needs and desires. Everyone develops his own technique with experience and the earlier a pattern is developed, the easier becomes the examination and the less the likelihood of overlooking important findings.

ANATOMY

The knee was originally thought of as a simple hinge joint but, in fact, is more complex because aside from flexion and extension, it also has significant rotary components to its motion. It is three joints in one, with a joint between the patella and femoral condyles and between each femoral condyle and tibial plateau. The osseous structures are secured in their proper relationship by the surrounding capsule, ligaments, and musculotendinous units. Pathological conditions may affect any or all three articulations as well as the surrounding soft tissue structures.

The Osseous Structures

The femoral condyles are two rounded eminences eccentrically curved with the anterior portion being part of an oval and the posterior portion a section of a sphere. They are more curved posteriorly than anteriorly and anteriorly are somewhat flattened, with the lateral being slightly more so than the medial condyle. Anteriorly between the two femoral condyles is the patellofemoral groove or sulcus through which the patella glides with flexion and extension of the knee. Inferiorly and posteriorly, the condyles are separated by the intercondylar notch, which houses the cruciate ligaments.

The proximal end of the tibia is flattened to form two surfaces, or condyles, which articulate with the femoral condyles. In the midline they are separated by the intercondylar eminence with a medial and lateral intercondylar tubercle. Anterior and posterior to the intercondylar eminence are the intercondylar areas where the cruciate ligaments and menisci are attached. The articular surface of the medial plateau is flat while the lateral plateau is more rounded or convex.

The patella is a somewhat triangular-shaped sesamoid bone which is wider proximally than distally. The articular surface is divided by a longitudinal ridge, creating a medial and lateral facet.

The Extensor Mechanism

The extensor mechanism consists of the quadriceps muscles, the quadriceps tendon, the patella, the medial and lateral retinacula, the patellar tendon, and the tibial tubercle (Fig. 11-1). The quadriceps muscles and, more specifically, the distal portion of the vastus medialis, referred to as the vastus medialis obliquus, plays a dynamic role in stabilizing the patella and holding it in its midline position. Statically, the joint contour and congruity between the patella and femoral condyles as well as the integrity of the medial and lateral retinacula, the patellar femoral ligaments, the patellotibial bands, and the patellar tendon combine to help stabilize the patella. The tendons of the quadriceps fuse together immediately above the patella to form the quadriceps tendon. Medial and lateral to the patella lie the medial and lateral retinacula. The medial retinaculum overlies the joint capsule and is an aponeurotic expansion of the vastus medialis. The lateral retinaculum is composed of the aponeurotic expansion of the vastus lateralis, iliotibial tract, and some contribution from the biceps tendon. The quadriceps tendon inserts into the proximal pole and the patellar tendon into the distal pole of the patella. The patella is divided into a medial and larger lateral facet which are separated by a thick, median ridge of articular cartilage. In full extension and in early flexion, the more distal portion of the patellar facets articulate with the femoral condyles, while the more proximal portion rests on the supracondylar fat pad. As the knee progresses into flexion, the contact area on the patella moves more proximally so that with complete flexion only the more proximal portions of the articular facets are in contact with the femoral condyles. The function of the patella is to increase the mechanical advantage of the quadriceps mechanism. This is most apparent in the mid-ranges of motion and is less at the extremes of extension or flexion. Although all elements of the quadriceps aid in extension of the knee, the primary function of the vastus medialis obliquus is to dynamically guide the patella medially and to resist forces which have a tendency to displace the patella laterally. It is not the primary extensor for the last 15 degrees of extension, as has often been reported in the literature. Fibers of the vastus medialis obliquus are oriented more obliquely toward the midline than the more proximal fibers of the vastus medialis and blend into the medial retinaculum which inserts along the medial margin of the patella and medial margin of the patellar tendon. The capsule thickens medially and laterally forming a ligamentous band called the patellofemoral ligament. It extends from the midportion of the patella to the femoral condyles medially and laterally, acting as a static stabilizing band to prevent either medial or lateral displacement of the patella. The femoral sulcus is formed in the midline by the two condyles of the femur which come together, with the lateral condyle being slightly higher. The patella fits congruently into this sulcus and is maintained in the sulcus by the previously described dynamic and static stabilizing elements. The patella has a tendency to subluxate or displace laterally when the knee is flexed at 40 to 50 degrees, the tibia is externally rotated, and the quadriceps is under

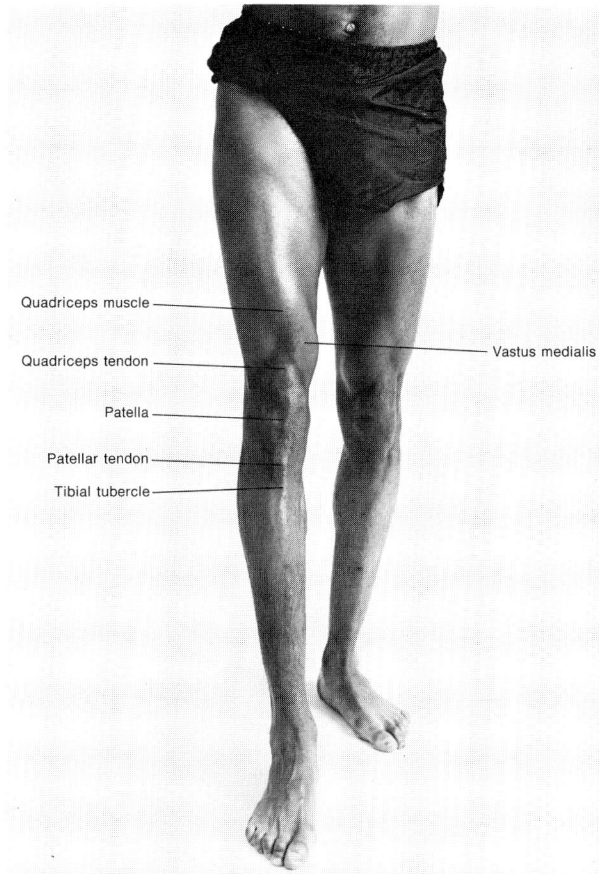

Fig. 11-1. Extensor mechanism (anterior view). Subject is "setting" the quadriceps or extensor mechanism. The extensor mechanism consists of the quadriceps muscles, quadriceps tendon, patella, medial retinacula, lateral retinaculum, patellar tendon, and tibial tubercle.

forceful contraction. All elements must then be in perfect balance to stabilize the patella and prevent lateral subluxation or dislocation.

THE SUPPORTING STRUCTURES

The Medial Complex

Superficially the medial aspect of the knee is limited by the quadriceps tendon, patella, and patella tendon anteriorly, and posteriorly by the pes anserinus and medial head of the gastrocnemius (Fig. 11-2). The capsule forms a sleeve completely covering all sides of the knee with a defect anteriorly filled in by the extensor mechanism. It is convenient to divide the medial aspect of the knee into three segments. The anterior segment, which extends from the medial border of the patellar tendon and the patella to the tibial collateral ligament anteriorly, consists of the medial retinaculum as well as the underlying joint capsule. The middle segment consists of the superficial tibial collateral ligament and the underlying capsule known as the deep capsular ligament. The posterior segment extends from the tibial collateral ligament and blends with the posterior capsule to form a sling about the medial femoral condyle which becomes taut in full extension but relaxed with flexion.

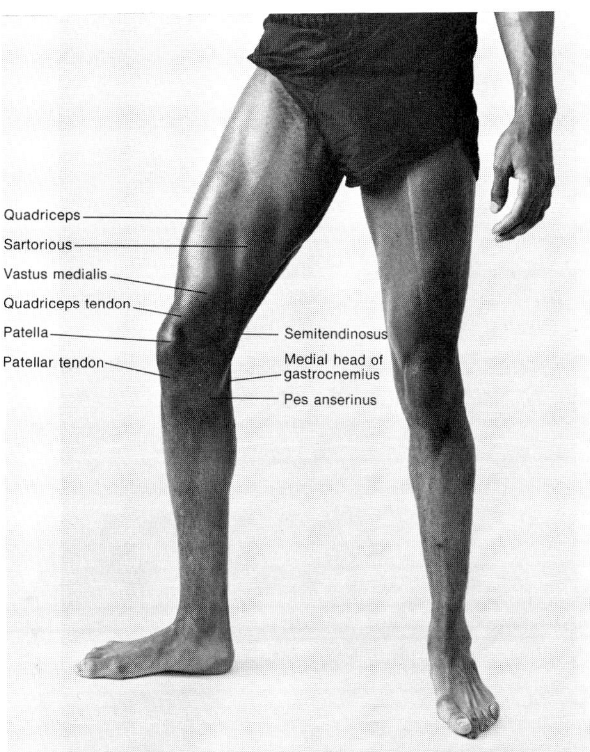

Fig. 11-2. Medial aspect of knee. Anterior limits are the quadriceps tendon, patella, and patella tendon. Posterior limits are the pes anserinus (sartorius, gracilis, and semitendinosus), and medial head of gastrocnemius.

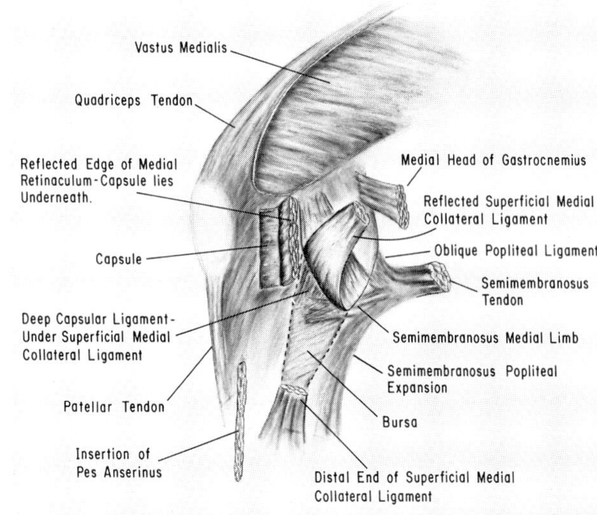

Fig. 11-3. The medial complex.

The superficial tibial collateral ligament originates from the medial aspect of the femoral condyle and inserts 8 to 10 cm. below the knee joint onto the anterior medial aspect of the tibia (Fig. 11-3). The anterior border is sharply delineated and often is palpable, but posteriorly it blends with the capsule. It is not adherent to the underlying deep capsular ligament but is separated from it by a bursa. Acute tears may occur in the deep capsular ligament and/or the superficial tibial collateral ligament, and in different areas from proximal to distal. The superficial and deep tibial collateral ligaments both stabilize the knee against excessive external rotation of the tibia. If both the superficial and deep portions are torn, then valgus and rotary instability will occur in the knee, but in this situation the anterior cruciate is usually also ruptured. It is possible to have the deep capsular ligament torn while the superficial is intact, with the tibia having excessive external rotation indicative of anterior, external, rotary instability but no valgus instability because of the intact superficial ligament.

The semimembranosus tendon (Fig. 11-3) has several ramifications and is the primary dynamic stabilizing element for the posterior medial aspect of the knee. The first limb extends laterally and obliquely across the posterior capsule to form a thickened ligamentous structure called the oblique popliteal ligament. The second limb attaches to the posterior capsule and the posterior portion of the medial meniscus. This segment dynamically aids in displacing the medial meniscus posteriorly. The third slip passes medially along the proximal portion of the tibia and disappears under the superficial portion of the tibial collateral ligament. It is a definite tendinous-appearing structure, and in many anatomy texts is identified as the semimembranosus tendon without mention of the other ramifications. A fourth segment attaches directly into the posterior medial tibial tuberosity about 1 to 2 cm. below the joint line. A fifth branch passes distally and blends into the popliteal fascia.

The three medial hamstring muscles, sartorius, gracilis, and semitendinosus, have a conjoined tendon which inserts onto the medial proximal aspect of the tibia just anterior to the insertion of the tibial collateral ligament and form the pes anserinus (see Fig. 11-3). A bursa is located between the distal portion of the superficial tibial collateral ligament and the overlying pes anserinus. The pes anserinus is primarily a flexor of the knee, an internal rotator of the tibia, and dynamically resists valgus and external rotational forces applied to the knee.

The Posterior Complex

Superior to the joint crease the posterior aspect of the knee is delimited by the semitendinosus medially and the biceps tendon laterally. Inferiorly the medial and lateral heads of the gastrocnemius are prominent (Fig. 11-4). With these muscles removed the posterior aspect of the knee consists mostly of capsule. The oblique popliteal ligament (Fig. 11-5), one of the ramifications of the semimembranosus, passes obliquely from medial to lateral and from distal to proximal across the posterior aspect of the capsule. Therefore, as tension is applied to the semimembranosus tendon when the knee flexes, it is also applied to the oblique popliteal ligament and the posterior capsule. The posterior capsule arches over the popliteus muscle laterally and forms an arcuate ligament which inserts onto the fibular styloid. The

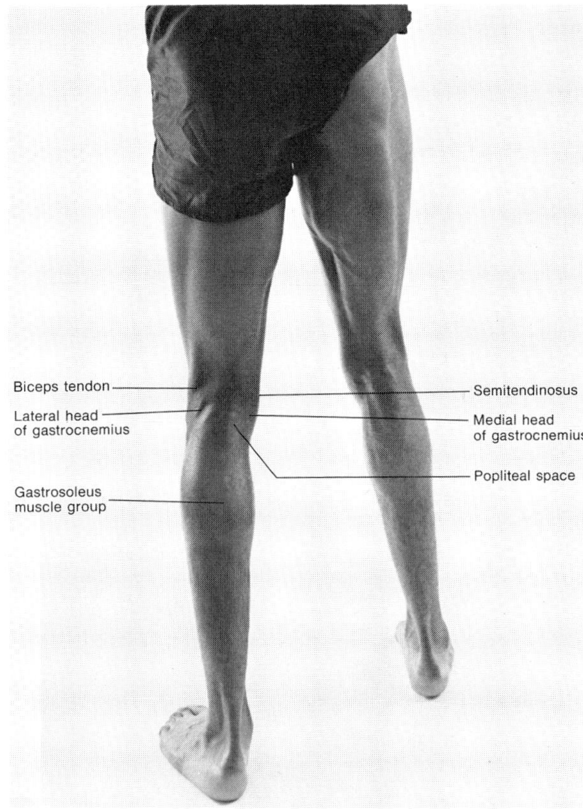

Fig. 11-4. Posterior aspect of knee. Superiorly the medial limit is the semitendinosis, and laterally it is the biceps tendon, inferiorly, the medial and lateral head of the gastrocnemius. The bulge in the middle directly posterior is the popliteal space.

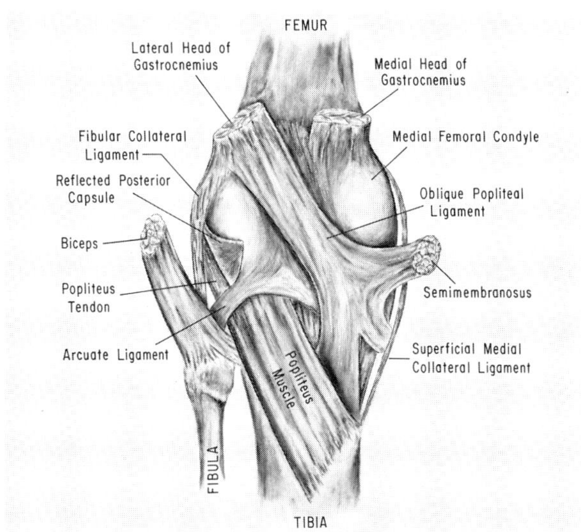

Fig. 11-5. The posterior complex.

arcuate ligament plays a significant role in stabilizing the "posterior lateral corner" of the knee. The popliteus muscle lies on the posterior aspect of the tibia and is oriented obliquely running proximally and laterally. The medial two thirds of the popliteus inserts into the arcuate ligament and the posterior portion of the lateral meniscus, while the lateral one third sends a tendinous structure deep to the fibular collateral ligament to insert onto the lateral femoral condyle. The popliteus is an internal rotator of the tibia in relation to the femur, actively displacing the lateral meniscus posteriorly during flexion, and it also prevents forward displacement of the femur on the tibia during flexion of the knee. As long as the posterior capsule remains intact all ligamentous structures can be disrupted, yet when the knee is forced into full extension there is no medial or lateral instability. This anatomical fact is important clinically because when stressing the knee for ligament continuity, the knee must be flexed slightly in order to relax the posterior capsule to assess the integrity of the collateral ligaments adequately. The two heads of the gastrocnemius which insert above the medial and lateral femoral condyles respectively make up the remaining posterior supporting structure.

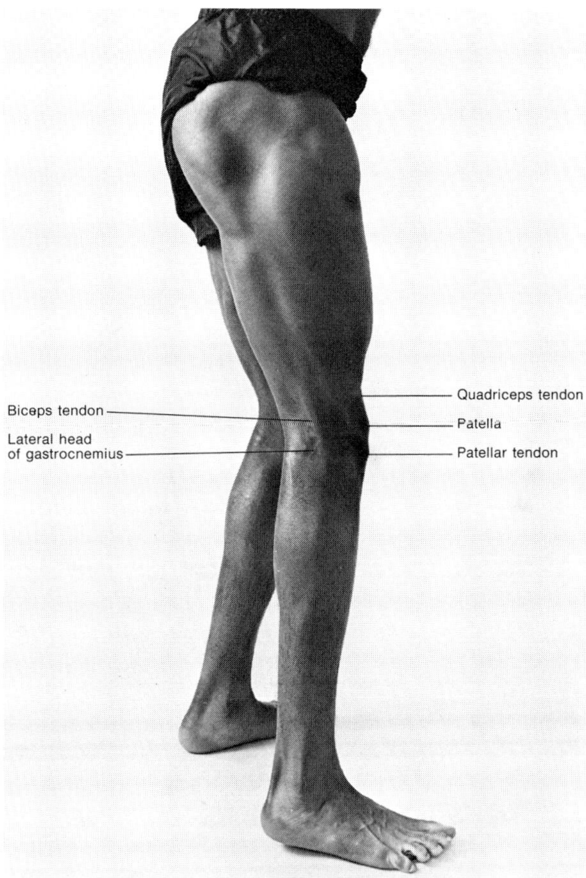

Fig. 11-6. Lateral aspect of knee. Posterior limits are the biceps tendon and lateral head of gastrocnemius. Anterior limits are the quadriceps tendon, patella and patellar tendon.

The Lateral Complex

The lateral aspect of the knee is bound by the biceps tendon and lateral head of gastrocnemius posteriorly and the quadriceps tendon, patella, and patellar tendon anteriorly (Fig. 11-6). There are four significant structures which contribute to knee stability laterally. They are the fibular collateral ligament, biceps tendon, the popliteus tendon, and the very important iliotibial tract (Fig. 11-7). The fibular collateral ligament is a rather small, tendinous-like structure extending from the lateral femoral condyle distally to insert onto the head of the fibula. It is probably the least important stabilizing structure. Clinically the fibular collateral ligament is easily located by having the patient cross his leg over the opposite knee and allowing the hip to fall into external rotation. This maneuver places a varus stress on the knee in flexion and tenses the fibular collateral ligament, making it palpable subcutaneously. The heavy tendon of the biceps also inserts onto the head of the fibula and has important extensions onto the lateral aspect of the tibia, both behind and in front of the fibular collateral ligament and head of the fibula. Dynamically the biceps and popliteus tendons help stabilize the lateral side of the knee.

The iliotibial tract, however, is the most important structure from the standpoint of static stability. It has a firm attachment to the intermuscular septum just proximal to the lateral femoral condyle and inserts distally onto the anterior lateral aspect of the proximal tibia. It is free to glide back and forth with flexion and extension. The mid-lateral capsule is easily palpated between the posterior or trailing edge of the iliotibial tract and the fibular collateral ligament. The lateral head of the gastrocnemius inserts just superior to the lateral femoral condyle and blends with the posterior capsule in this area.

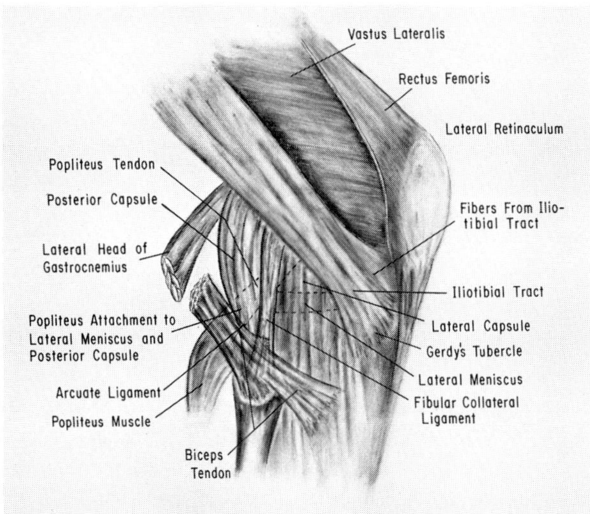

Fig. 11-7. The lateral complex.

The Cruciates

The cruciate ligaments, which are intraarticular but extrasynovial, are approximately 4 cm. in length and are found within the knee joint (Fig. 11-8). The anterior cruciate ligament arises from the tibia, courses posteriorly, superiorly, and laterally to insert onto the lateral femoral condyle posteriorly near its articular margin. Immediately behind the anterior cruciate ligament is the heavier posterior cruciate ligament, which passes anteriorly and obliquely to insert onto the lateral aspect of the medial femoral condyle anteriorly near the articular margin. It is larger and functionally more significant than the anterior cruciate ligament. The cruciate ligaments wrap around each other with internal rotation of the tibia in relation to the femur forcing the femoral condyles firmly against the tibial plateaus, enhancing stability of the knee. Their specific function is difficult to describe thoroughly because it cannot be isolated from that of the other ligamentous structures about the knee. The anterior cruciate ligament certainly stabilizes the tibia from anterior displacement in relation to the femoral condyles. In the past, disruption of the anterior cruciate ligament was thought to be the primary element in creating an anterior drawer sign, which is subluxation anteriorly of the tibia in relation to the femoral condyles when a force is applied behind the calf with the knee flexed. The anterior cruciate ligament plays a role in this type of instability, but it appears that there must also be additional injury to the collateral structures to create a positive anterior drawer sign.

Basically, the posterior cruciate ligament prevents posterior displacement or subluxation of the tibial plateaus in relation to the femoral condyles. It is located close to the vertical axis of rotation of the knee and is one of the key elements in stabilizing the knee about its vertical axis. The collateral ligaments, however, are located farther from the vertical axis of rotation and, thus, are better able to resist rotational forces.

The Menisci

The menisci are two semilunar shaped pieces of fibrocartilage which are wedge-shaped in cross-section, with the base along the periphery attached to the adjacent tissues by the coronary ligament (see Fig. 11-8). The lateral inferior geniculate artery runs within the substance of the lateral coronary ligament and is easily cut during the course of lateral meniscectomy. The medial meniscus is more firmly attached about the periphery and is closely adherent to the capsular structures via the coronary ligament. Consequently, it is less mobile than the lateral meniscus and more subject to injury. The lateral meniscus, on the other hand, is not as firmly attached on the periphery and is more mobile. It is under the dynamic control of the popliteal muscle which retracts it posteriorly with knee flexion. The medial meniscus is larger than the lateral and more C-shaped while the lateral is more oval. Both menisci

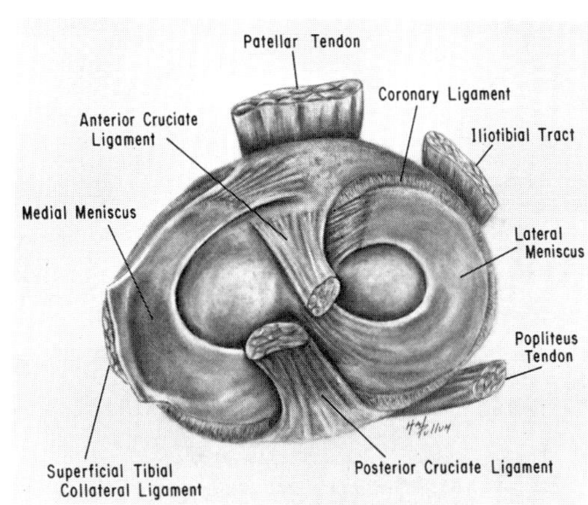

Fig. 11-8. The cruciates and menisci.

have tibial attachments at their anterior and posterior horns. The posterior portion of the lateral meniscus sometimes has two additional attachments to the lateral aspect of the medial femoral condyle. One is via the ligament of Wrisberg, which lies on the posterior aspect of the posterior cruciate ligament somewhat paralleling its course, and less frequently the ligament of Humphry, which lies anterior to the posterior cruciate. Perhaps these small ligaments act as restraints while guiding the motion of the lateral meniscus.

REGIONAL EXAMINATION

History

A thorough history is probably the most significant portion of the knee examination. It should be taken in an orderly sequence and in a consistent manner so that important questions and areas of inquiry are not overlooked. The age and sex of the patient suggest conditions more prevalent in certain age groups or in one sex. The chief complaints fall into the categories of pain, swelling, limitation of motion, deformity, instability, catching, or locking. It is important to determine the duration of the problem in order to differentiate a disease process from an injury. If an injury is involved, question the patient to determine the mechanism of injury. This often leads the examiner to suspect certain pathological conditions which result from forces applied at the time of injury. A previous severe injury to the knee is important in evaluating the status of ligament stability because it may indicate previous damage to the ligaments. It is also helpful to know what type of treatment was administered for the injury and by whom. The knee symptoms are classified as acute, chronic, or intermittent. Ascertain the location, type, and severity of pain and whether it occurs with activity, after activity, or has no relationship to activity. People with chondromalacia of the patella frequently complain of an aching sensation about the patella when sitting for long periods of time or when going up and down stairs or hills. An arthritic knee is often symptomatic during periods of activity and is relieved by rest. Patients with a horizontal cleavage lesion of the medial meniscus complain of swelling and pain posteromedially over the joint line at night, and subsequent examination reveals tenderness in this region. If swelling is a major complaint, the patient should be questioned to determine the frequency and degree of swelling and specifically if it is related to an injury. Immediate swelling (within an hour) after injury denotes a bloody effusion within the joint. Traumatic hemarthrosis occurs with rupture of the synovial membrane, intraarticular fracture, rupture of the anterior cruciate ligament, or a peripheral meniscal tear. Hemarthrosis may also occur with a hemorrhagic diathesis, such as hemophilia, either after trauma or spontaneously. Swelling which occurs several hours later, or rather insidiously, may simply be an accumulation of synovial fluid secondary to a synovitis from trauma or disease. A warm swollen knee accompanied by a history of fever and chills suggests a septic joint but must be differentiated from acute synovitis with gout, pseudogout, or rheumatoid arthritis.

Patients with an arthritic condition will often state that they have difficulty arising from a chair, particularly one which is very low. Arising from a sitting position places excessive stress upon the joint, creating discomfort. Any limitation of motion in extension or flexion should be determined. Question the patient concerning his or her standing tolerance and its relationship to pain, fatigue, and type of standing surface.

The patient's walking tolerance provides important information. There may be no problem walking on a smooth surface but considerable difficulty may be encountered on a rough, uneven surface or even prolonged walking on a smooth surface in the presence of degenerative changes. Find out how far the patient can walk before a rest is required. Going up or down stairs or hills places additional stress on the knees, particularly impact loading going down, and may be troublesome. Some patients may be unable to negotiate stairs at all, and others may have to lead with their uninvolved extremity rather than going foot over foot.

The complaint of weakness is a rather nondescript complaint but is often secondary to quadriceps insufficiency from disuse atrophy following an injury or disease. "Giving away" is a frequent complaint with many knee conditions. It may or may not be accompanied by pain and is often associated with some activity or circumstance placing the knee in a vulnerable posture. It can be caused by intermittent impingement of a torn meniscus or loose body, patellar subluxation, ligament instability (particularly the rotary type), or simply quadriceps insufficiency. Instability is difficult to differentiate from giving way or buckling and for practical purposes need not be, but this term refers more specifically to ligament instability. Some patients are explicit in the description of their knee feeling loose, insecure, or wobbly with certain motions, particularly twisting or pivoting, implicating ligament instability.

The assessment of the ability to run certainly would not be applicable to a 75-year-old woman with rheumatoid arthritis but may be a significant factor in the history of a young athlete with a chronic knee problem. Whether or not the patient can run at top speed and has the ability to stop, start, cut, pivot, and twist could prove to be significant. An individual with chronic ligament laxity of the knee may have noticed that running straight is no problem, but a sudden change in direction with cutting, pivoting, or twisting creates a feeling of instability. This suggests a rotary instability of the knee. Mild to moderate pure medial or lateral instability is often tolerable, but even mild amounts of rotational instability (abnormal tibial rotation) can be troublesome.

One of the most common complaints misinterpreted by the patient and the physician is "locking." This term is associated with a bucket handle tear of the meniscus which becomes interposed between joint surfaces, preventing complete extension of the knee. "Locking" should apply only to the inability to extend the knee completely, particularly the last 5 to 10 degrees. If the patient states the knee locks in full flexion or at some angle greater than perhaps the last 30 to 40 degrees of extension, be cautious about placing any significance to this complaint, specifically as it relates to a torn meniscus. With a locking episode, the patient may find that by manipulating the knee or having someone tug on the leg, the knee may suddenly straighten accompanied by a snap or pop which is described as "something slipped back into place." Locking from impingement of a loose body is usually transient and unexpected. Occasionally, the stump of a torn anterior cruciate ligament can simulate a locking phenomenon as it becomes impinged anteriorly between the joint surfaces upon extension. There are many conditions which prevent full extension and are confused with locking, such as joint effusions, patellofemoral arthritis, degenerative arthritis, lesions of the infrapatellar fat pad, and hamstring spasm with acute knee injuries.

Catching, snapping, popping, and grinding are frequent complaints but are rather nonspecific. For a woman or young child complaining of snapping or popping, a congenital discoid lateral meniscus should be suspected. It is more subject to injury than a normally shaped meniscus. Snapping may be difficult for the patient to localize, and the examiner should be aware of extraarticular causes such as a hamstring tendon snapping over a bony prominence. Catching, snapping, or popping are symptoms present with the occasional symptomatic suprapatellar plica as it snaps over the proximal prominence of the medial femoral condyle or becomes impinged between the condyle and the medial patellar facet. Grinding indicates wear with attendant roughening and irregularity of the articular surfaces which may cause a recurrent catching sensation, particularly in the patellofemoral joint with chondromalacia or degenerative arthritis.

It is also important to ask patients if they have noted anything loose moving about in the knee. Some patients with a loose body from osteochondritis dissecans or an osteochondral fracture may feel or be able to palpate a movable mass subcutaneously about the knee and may or may not associate this with catching or locking episodes.

A complete patellar dislocation may be graphically described by the patient, making the diagnosis obvious. Others, however, are unaware of what happened, particularly if the patella reduces spontaneously. Then they may have nonspecific complaints of pain, giving way, something slipping out, and swelling. Some people will describe the patella as being displaced to the inside or medial aspect of the knee. In view of the fact that patellar dislocations in humans almost invariably go laterally, this complaint should be viewed with some suspicion. Patellar subluxations, on the other hand, are frequently difficult to diagnose by history alone. The complaints are diffuse and vary from giving way to catching, popping, or recurrent painful episodes with or without swelling. This is a condition that must be kept in mind by the examiner. Often it can be verified during the course of the physical examination.

Physical Examination

Before proceeding with the physical examination be sure the patient is appropriately undressed with the entire lower extremity visible. Any attempts to examine a knee with the pant leg rolled up are entirely inadequate. The height, weight, body build, and general physical condition are first recorded.

Alignment

The standing alignment of the lower extremities is examined with the patient facing the examiner, then turning sideways, and finally facing away. Abnormalities in alignment may be developmental or acquired from injury or disease. The common deformities are genu varum, genu valgum, genu recurvatum, and a flexion contracture. Genu varum refers to a bowleg deformity often seen with degenerative arthritis involving the medial compartment. Genu valgum is a knock-knee deformity, and genu recurvatum refers to hyperextension of the knee. A flexion contracture is present if the patient is unable to extend the knee completely. Genu recurvatum, or "back-knee" deformity, may be congenital, secondary to quadriceps contracture, acquired from posterior capsule or cruciate rupture, or in some instances iatrogenic following tibial tubercle transplant for a dislocating patella prior to closure of the proximal tibial epiphyseal plate (Fig. 11-9). This may cause premature closure of the epiphyseal plate, creating forward tilt of the tibial plateaus as growth continues posteriorly. Patients often demonstrate a bilateral genu recurvatum deformity which is congenital in nature, and it is frequently associated with patella alta (high riding patella), an unstable patella, and ligamentous laxity of the knee.

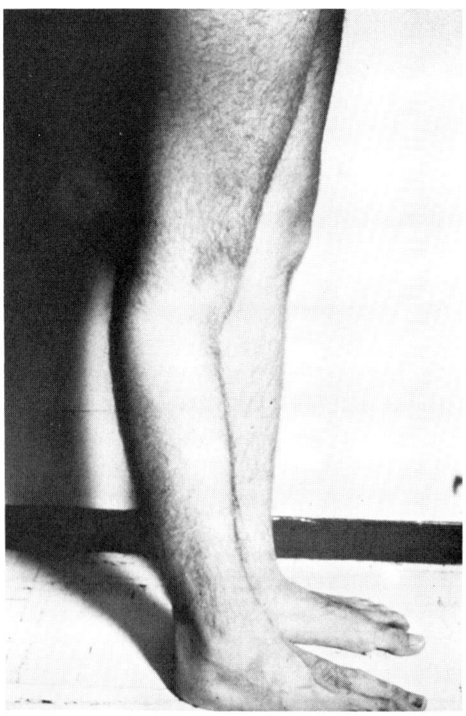

Fig. 11-9. Genu recurvatum. An acquired deformity of the right knee secondary to early closure of the anterior portion of the proximal tibial epiphyseal plate causing forward inclination of the tibial plateaus.

A flexion deformity is easily detected from the side. The knee is held in a semiflexed position, and the patient's heel will probably not make contact with the supporting surface because of his inability to extend the knee completely. Functionally, this deformity creates a shorter lower extremity. The most frequent cause for a fixed flexion contracture is either primary or secondary degenerative arthritis.

Tibial torsional or rotational deformities are usually seen in children. Most will spontaneously correct by maturity. Tibial torsion is estimated by having the patient sit with the legs dangling free. The relative position of the ankle axis (a line between the malleoli) is determined by placing the thumb on the medial malleolus and the index finger on the lateral malleolus and comparing this to the transverse axis of the knee. Most babies have about 2 degrees external tibial torsion which gradually increases until the adult normal of about 22 degrees is reached. Another method is to notice the alignment of the tibial tubercle in relation to the second metatarsal. Normally, they should be in line with the foot held in the neutral position.

Functional Tests

Functional tests are an essential part of the examination but must be adapted to the capabilities of the patient. Some patients with a painful knee may not be able to perform any functional tests and require use of a wheelchair or crutches. Others with less severe but chronic problems may actually be able to demonstrate their ability to run. Patients should be observed during walking to determine a limp and the degree of knee motion present. Additional functional tests may include the stationary jog, the lean-

Fig. 11-10. The leaning hop test (*A*) which can be valuable in assessing ligamentous instability. The duck waddle test (*B*) is helpful in determining functional flexion and patients with torn menisci find it difficult to perform.

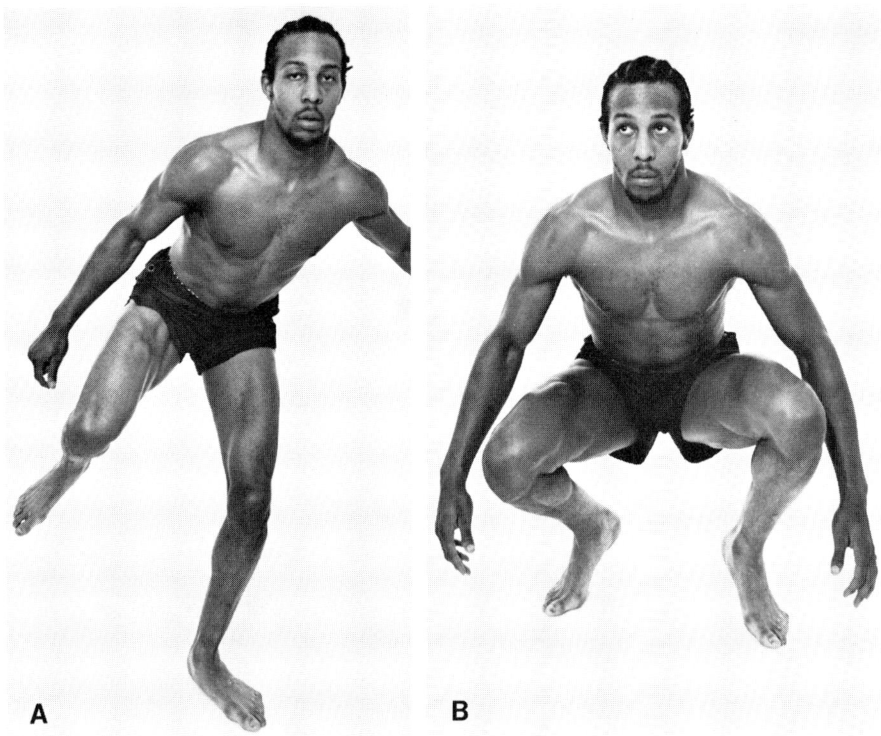

ing hop test, squatting, kneeling, and duck waddling. The leaning hop test is performed with the patient standing on the involved lower extremity, abducting the other extremity, and then hopping (Fig. 11-10A). This places significant valgus stress upon the knee and in instances of ligamentous laxity may cause the feeling of giving way or instability. The squat and duck waddle tests are also helpful in determining the degree of functional flexion. This position places considerable stress upon the extensor mechanism as well as the capsular and ligamentous structures and will often cause posterior discomfort and perhaps a click with a posterior horn tear of a meniscus (Fig. 11-10B).

Measurements

Measurements about the knee should be a routine procedure. Mid-calf, mid-patellar, 4 cm. proximal to the patella, and mid-thigh measurements (Fig. 11-11) should be taken. The mid-thigh position is selected by measuring approximately 20 cm. above the medial joint line; the measurement is taken with the muscles tensed. Measurement 4 cm. proximal to the patella, again with the quadriceps tense, gives an index of vastus medialis obliquus bulk. Length is measured from the anterosuperior spine of the ilium to the tip of the medial malleolus. A discrepancy in extremity length may be observed in a patient with a knee flexion contracture which creates an apparent leg

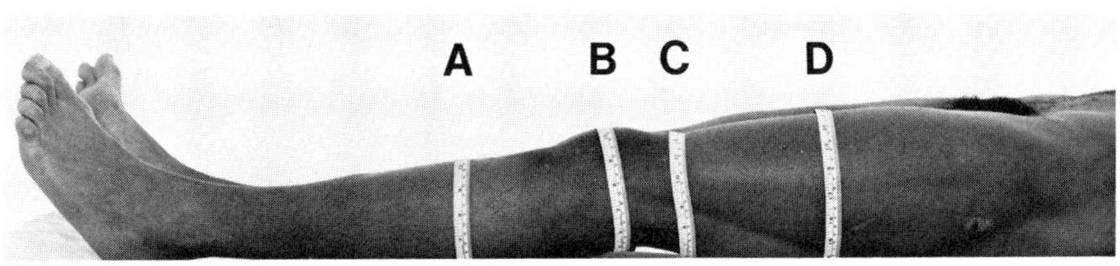

Fig. 11-11. Measurements about the knee: mid-calf (*A*), mid-patellar (*B*), 4 cm, proximal to the patella (*C*), and mid-thigh (*D*).

length discrepancy rather than an actual discrepancy because of pelvic tilt.

Motion

Knee motion should be examined both actively and passively and recorded (Fig. 11-12). Discomfort at the extremes of motion should be noted as well as pain and crepitation during motion. The knee should be passively stressed into maximum extension and maximum flexion by the examiner. A knee assumes a slightly flexed position after an acute injury. This position places the supporting structures under the least stress and is a position of relative comfort. Pain on forced extension is often present with joint effusions, meniscal lesions with locking, a peripheral meniscal tear with a hematoma, popliteal space hematomas, arthritis, and ligamentous and capsular injuries. Pain with forced flexion is also caused by similar conditions but in addition quadriceps contracture, patellofemoral arthritis, and posterior meniscal tears are implicated. If genu recurvatum has been previously detected, frequently an extensor lag is also present and is expressed in degrees. Extensor lag is the amount of passive extension beyond active extension of the knee. It is tested by asking the patient to actively extend the knee completely, and then the examiner passively attempts to extend the knee a bit further, revealing the amount of lag present. Some lag is usually present with a significant genu recurvatum and may be related to patellar instability. It is commonly present to some degree following a patellectomy. Finally, test knee motion with a varus (adduction) and valgus (abduction) stress placed upon the knee. Valgus stress testing with motion is best accomplished by having the patient in the supine position with the leg secured to the examiner's side (Fig. 11-13). The examiner's hand then exerts pressure over the lateral aspect of the knee, creating a valgus stress on the knee as it is moved through a range of motion. This maneuver compresses the joint laterally and places the medial supporting structures under tension. Lateral pain and

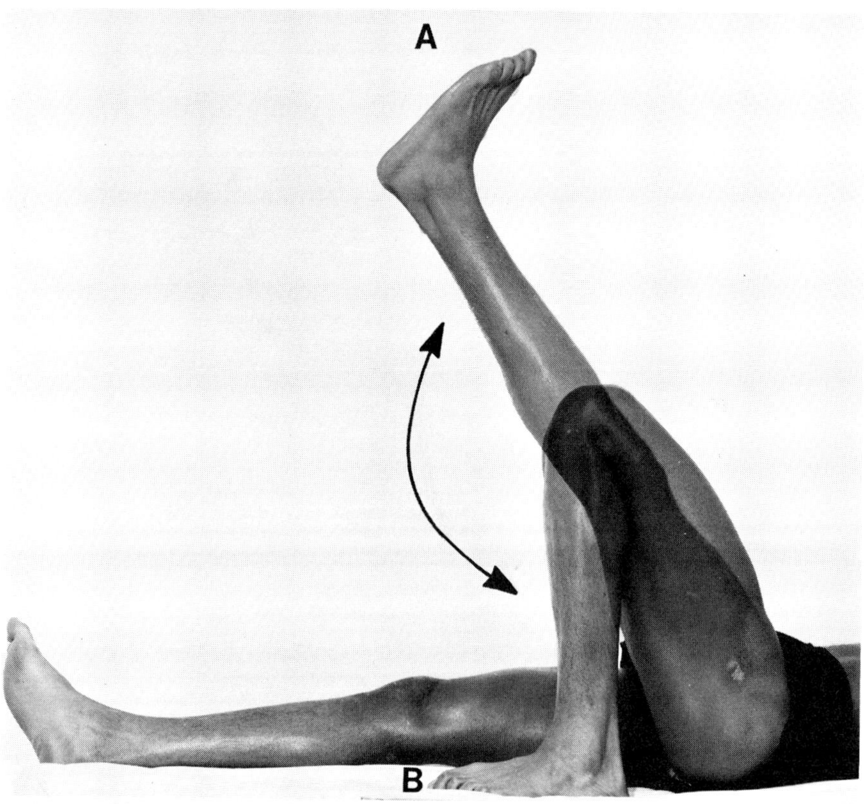

Fig. 11-12. Knee motion is measured from the neutral or zero starting position (*A*) to maximum flexion (*B*). Hyperextension is degrees beyond the neutral opposite to that of flexion.

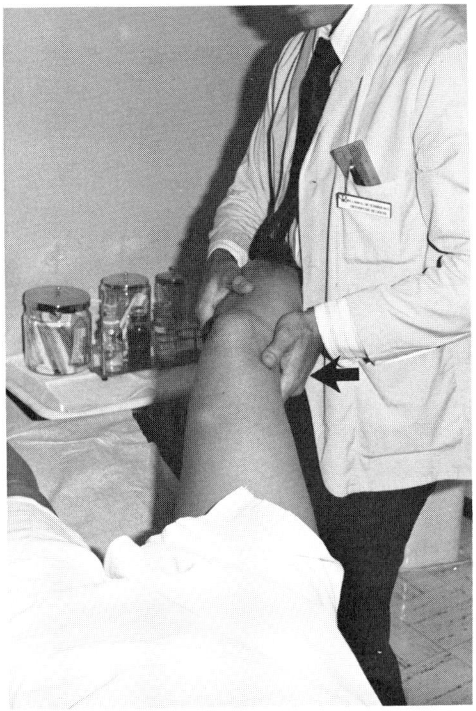

Fig. 11-13. Motion with valgus stress. The patient lies supine with the leg supported by the examiner's one hand while the other hand applies a valgus stress to the knee as it is moved back and forth through a range of motion. This places a compression force on the lateral compartment and tension on the medial ligaments either of which may produce pain.

crepitation may be elicited with degenerative changes of the lateral joint surface or meniscal lesions. Patients may also complain of medial pain if the taut capsule is rubbed over marginal femoral osteophytes.

Varus stress with motion testing is accomplished with the patient in the same position but with the extremity externally rotated at the hip and, again, the leg secured to the examiner's side (Fig. 11-14). Pressure may then be exerted over the medial aspect of the knee, creating a varus stress compressing the medial joint and stretching the lateral capsule and ligaments with similar findings, as discussed above. These tests are particularly helpful with degenerative meniscal lesions.

Swelling

The knee should be observed for swelling and a determination made between intraarticular and extraarticular swelling. Extraarticular swelling may be easily distinguished from intraarticular swelling by palpating the knee. A mushy, spongy consistency anterior to the patella indicates extraarticular swelling in the prepatellar bursa or soft tissues, and the patella cannot be ballotted or pushed up and down against the femoral condyles as though it were floating. With intraarticular swelling, the patella is easily palpable subcutaneously, the retinaculum is usually tense, the suprapatellar pouch distended, the knee held in slight flexion, and the patella can be ballotted (patellar tap test). Rapid swelling following a knee injury indicates bleeding within the joint while chronic swelling is secondary to accumulation of synovial fluid from a synovitis. If there is some doubt as to the type of fluid, joint aspiration is indicated. Bloody fluid with definite fat globules floating in it implicates an intraarticular fracture. A septic knee yields purulent-appearing, cloudy fluid, and the diagnosis is confirmed with appropriate laboratory

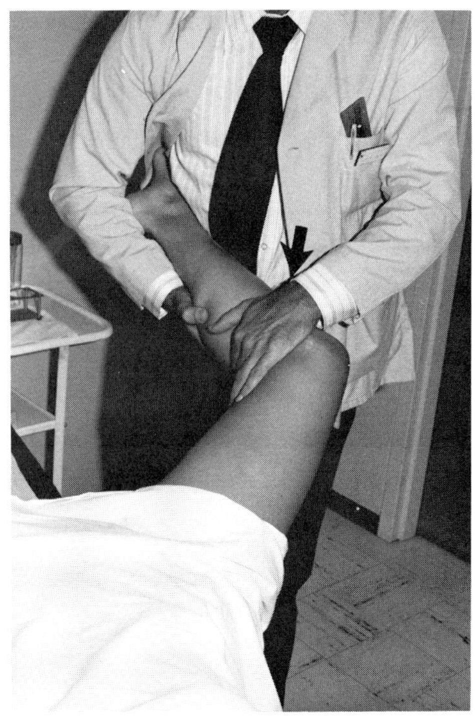

Fig. 11-14. Motion with varus stress. The leg is supported by the examiner and the extremity is allowed to fall into external rotation at the hip. One hand applies pressure over the medial joint as the knee is moved through a range of motion this time compressing the medial joint and placing the lateral ligaments under tension.

analysis (stain, cell count, and culture). Chronic synovitis presents with swelling but a mushy consistency, and generally, the results of the patellar tap test will be negative with little effusion.

Extensor Mechanism

Examination of the extensor mechanism starts with evaluation of the quadriceps muscles. Measurements of thigh circumference generally give some index of quadriceps development, but sometimes actual measurement does not fully indicate the quality of the quadriceps. The measurements may be equal, but upon inspection it is obvious that a quadriceps muscle mass is not as soundly developed as its counterpart, and palpation reveals that the tone is likewise diminished. The vastus medialis obliquus is obvious when the quadriceps are tense and the knee extended. Its development and position in relation to the patella should be inspected. The retinaculum may heal in an elongated fashion after a severe injury to the medial retinaculum and ligamentous structures of the knee, allowing the vastus medialis to migrate proximally (Fig. 11-15). This reduces its effectiveness as a dynamic stabilizer.

With the patient standing, facing the examiner, and the quadriceps tensed, the alignment of the quadriceps, patella, patellar tendon, and tibia may be assessed. The patellae should be facing straight ahead with the feet parallel, but with malalignment of the extensor mechanism the patellae may be inclined medially or laterally. With external tibial torsion and the feet placed parallel, the patellae point toward each other. Lateral placement of the tibial tubercle causes the patellar tendon to incline laterally, thus creating a "bayonet" or "zig-zag" aligment of the extensor mechanism. These people frequently have femoral neck anteversion, mild genu varum, chondromalacia of the patella, and pronated feet.

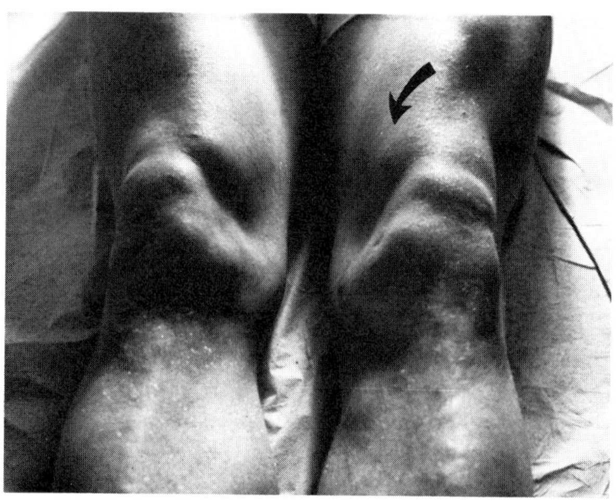

Fig. 11-15. The vastus medialis obliquus on the left is atrophied and has migrated slightly proximal following a severe medial ligament injury. The patella was clinically unstable.

The patella is next observed with the patient in a sitting position with the legs dangling over the edge of the examining table. The position of the patellae in relation to the tibial tubercles is noted. Normally the tibial tubercle is lined up with the midline of the patella but in some instances the patella is displaced lateral to the tibial tubercle, thus creating a condition known as "grasshopper eye patellae." This type patella is frequently associated with lateral subluxation and chondromalacia of the patella.

Some assessment of the height of the patella above the joint line should be made clinically. Unfortunately, there are no precise guidelines, either clinically or roentgenographically, to determine if a patella is too high or too low. The extremes are easy to detect, but small degrees from normal are difficult. A patella alta, or high riding patella, is often associated with genu recurvatum, a prominent fat pad, and a rather small patella. In addition, the patella is often unstable to lateral displacement. A significantly lowered patella, or patella baja, is also easy to detect clinically. It sometimes is seen after a tibial tubercle transplant in which the tibial tubercle has been moved too far distally. When present, excessive pressure is exerted on the articular surface of the patella with attendant chondromalacia.

Patellar mobility is tested with the knee in extension and at 30 degrees of flexion. Most patellae will demonstrate a moderate amount of lateral mobility in full extension but generally speaking no more than about one half the width of the patella. If the patella displaces more then half its width, increased lateral patellar instability is present. With the knee flexed to 30 degrees and with the patient in the supine position, again attempt to displace the patella laterally (Fig. 11-16). The patella normally is secure in the sulcus at this degree of flexion with little or no displacement present. If there is a grossly unstable patella, it may be possible to dislocate it; however, the patient often becomes apprehensive when this

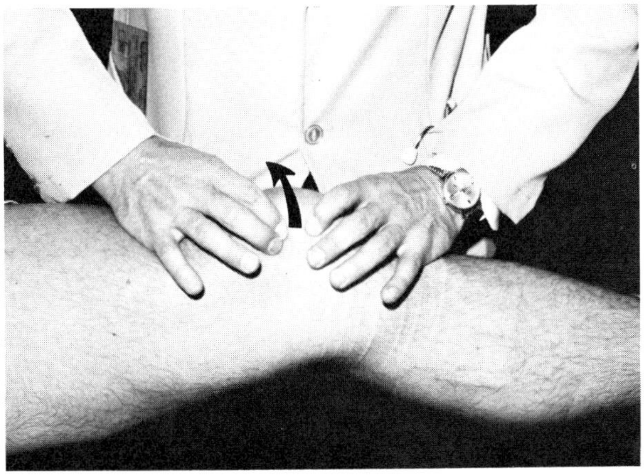

Fig. 11-16. Patellar stability test. The knee is flexed 30 to 40 degrees and medial pressure applied to the patella. An unstable patella will displace laterally, often making the patient very apprehensive.

maneuver is performed. The patient may state that this is the sensation felt in the past with episodes of giving way.

The patella should be thoroughly palpated about its periphery for tenderness. The facets are examined by displacing the patella medially and laterally with the knee extended and palpating the border of the medial and lateral facets (Perkin's test). With chondromalacia this maneuver will reveal varying degrees of tenderness. The patella should also be compressed against the femoral condyle by the examiner's hand, while the patient is tensing the quadriceps. Frequently, this will elicit discomfort in the presence of chondromalacia. During this maneuver, the examiner should also be aware of any crepitation that might be present. The patella is palpated as the knee is actively moved through a range of motion, preferably while the patient does a series of half-squats or knee extension against resistance. Frequently, minimal or no crepitation is present as the knee is flexed and extended passively, but with the patient performing half-squats, crepitation may be apparent. The mere presence of crepitation does not always indicate associated pain. Often, there can be either marked pain with minimal crepitation or minimal pain with marked crepitation. Palpation over the femoral condyle just medial to the proximal pole of the patella may reveal tenderness and a snapping sensation indicative of a thickened suprapatella plica.

Examination of the patella following an acute dislocation will usually reveal tenderness along the medial border of the patella and also along the lateral femoral condyle articular margin where an osteochondral fracture may occur during reduction of the patella. At times, pain will not be localized along the medial border of the patella following acute dislocation but more posteriorly over the femoral condyle at the attachment of the patellofemoral ligament where the tear has occurred. The diagnosis of patellar dislocation is easily made with the patella completely displaced laterally over the lateral femoral condyle; however, it often reduces spontaneously and the diagnosis is not so readily apparent (Fig. 11-17A, B). Medial dislocation of the patella is extremely rare in humans but can occur following a tibial tubercle

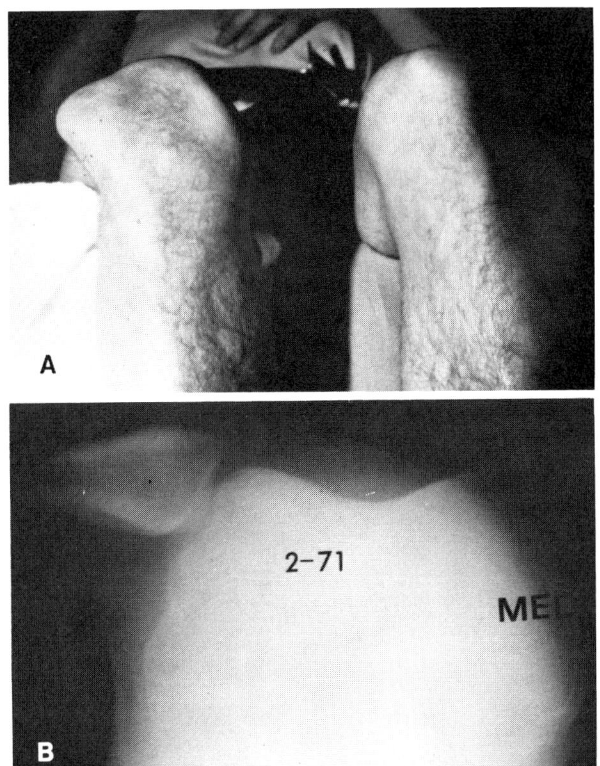

Fig. 11-17. (*A*) The right patella has been acutely dislocated and lies on the lateral aspect of the lateral femoral condyle. (*B*) A tangential roentgenogram shows the medial facet impinged on the lateral femoral condyle. During reduction, shear stress may create an osteochondral fracture of the medial patellar facet or from the lateral margin of the lateral femoral condyle.

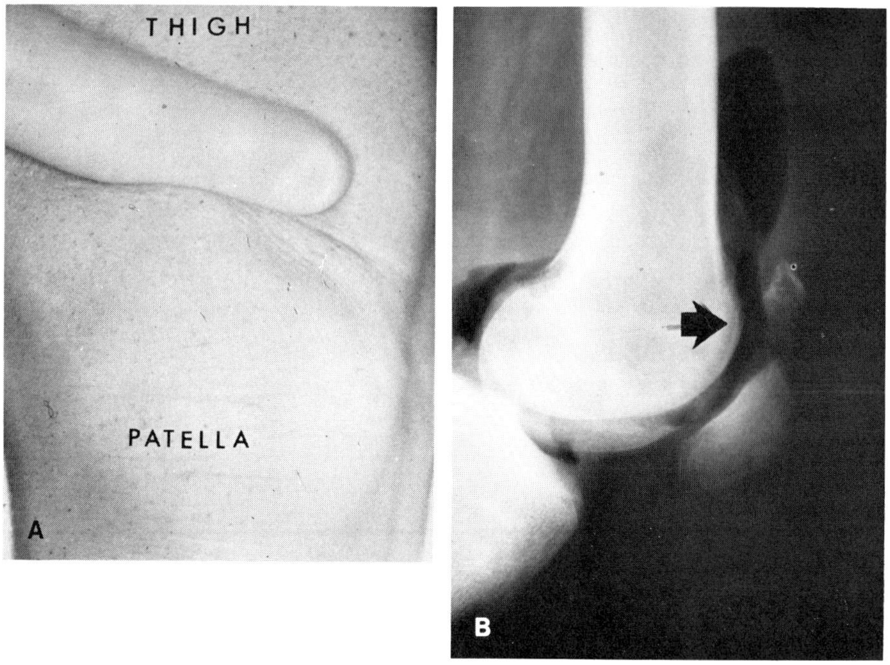

Fig. 11-18. (*A*) The examiner's finger has been placed into a defect in the quadriceps tendon. The patella lies immediately below. (*B*) This patient had an old untreated rupture of the quadriceps tendon and has ectopic ossification at the site of injury just proximal to the patella (*arrow*). The roentgenogram was taken after injecting air into the joint (air arthrogram) to delineate the synovial confines. The air shows as dark areas beneath the patella and in the suprapatellar pouch. This reveals that the ectopic bone is extraarticular and not a loose body.

transfer in which the tibial tubercle is displaced too far medially or after too vigorous reefing of the medial retinaculum. An osteochondral fracture from the lateral femoral condyle or medial facet of the patella can complicate a dislocation of the patella. This occurs during spontaneous reduction of the patella when a sheer stress is placed on the medial facet as it snaps over the lateral femoral condyle where there is impingement. Recurrent catching and locking are common symptoms when loose bodies become impinged between the joint surfaces.

Palpation assesses the integrity of the patellar and quadriceps tendons. Elderly patients commonly rupture the quadriceps tendon secondary to a forceful contraction from a misstep. Palpation of this area will reveal a defect, indicating a loss of continuity of the quadriceps tendon (Fig. 11-18A, B). Patellar tendon ruptures are infrequent but do occur in athletes with vigorous quadriceps contraction. A defect in the tendon is easily palpable, the patient is unable to extend the knee actively, and the patella rides high (Figs. 11-19). This is usually preceded by chronic tendinitis of the patellar tendon or "jumper's knee," characterized by pain and tenderness at the distal pole of the patella which is aggravated by activity.

The tibial tubercle should be examined for tender-

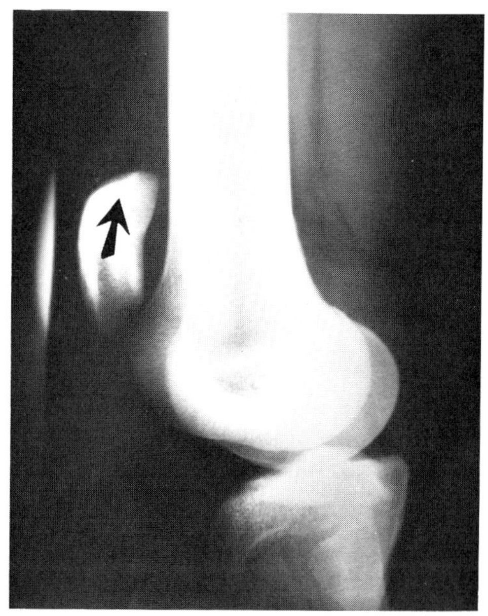

Fig. 11-19. A lateral roentgenogram of a knee with acute rupture of the patellar tendon. The patella is located much more proximal than normal. This patient had chronic patellar tendinitis for a number of years preceding the rupture. Clinically, a palpable defect was present over the patellar tendon area, and at operation the patellar tendon and the medial and lateral retinacula were disrupted at the level of the distal pole.

ness, swelling, and prominence. Children are often afflicted with a condition called Osgood-Schlatter's disease (traction epiphysitis) characterized by pain and swelling over the tibial tubercle region. It is most likely secondary to minute avulsions of the patellar tendon insertion into the tibial tubercle. Roentgenography usually reveals ectopic bone formation over the tibial tubercle (Fig. 11-20).

Prominence of the anterior fat pad has already been mentioned in relation to genu recurvatum and patella alta. Fat pad lesions are a clinical entity but not very common. This appears to be caused by an enlarged fat pad, perhaps secondary to trauma, or a normal-sized pad with less space available due to a degenerative process in the joint. Both situations result in pinching the overlying synovium as it is pushed into the joint with extension. There may be tenderness to palpation and pain anteriorly with extension.

A clinical measurement associated with extensor mechanism alignment is the quadriceps (Q) angle. The Q-angle is the angle between the long axis of the femoral shaft and a line from the middle of the patella to the tibial tubercle. In women this angle generally measures approximately 15 degrees and in men 10 degrees. The Q-angle may be measured by placing a goniometer directly over the center of the patella with one arm aimed at the anterosuperior spine of the ilium and the other in line with the center of the patellar tendon (Fig. 11-21). The Q-angle may be dynamically increased with external tibial rotation, and in some individuals with an excessive amount of external rotation, it may become quite marked. When the tibia is externally rotated, the tibial tubercle is displaced laterally, thus increasing the Q-angle, and with a vigorous quadriceps contraction, the increased resultant force tends to displace the patella laterally. If the patient should have a rather shallow sulcus and insufficient medial stabilizing elements, a patellar subluxation or dislocation may occur. Patellar dislocation usually occurs when an individual is vigorously extending the flexed knee with the leg externally rotated.

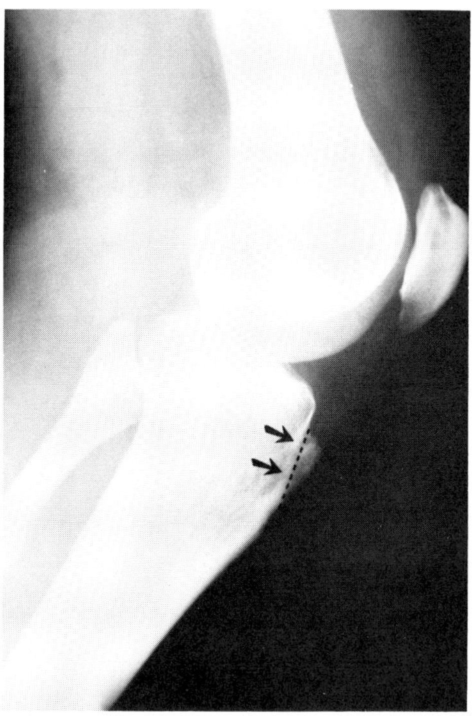

Fig. 11-20. Bony prominence of the tibial tubercle (*arrows*) secondary to "traction tendinitis" (Osgood-Schlatter's disease). Often small ectopic fragments are noted adjacent to the tibial tubercle rather than just an enlargement of the tubercle as depicted here.

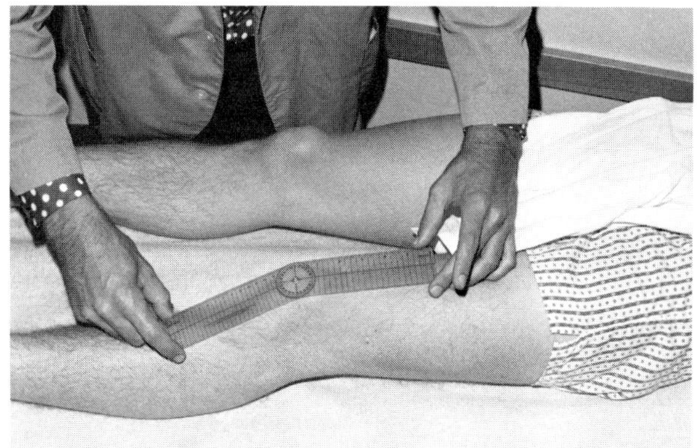

Fig. 11-21. The Q-angle (quadriceps angle) is measured by placing a goniometer over the middle of the patella with one arm pointing to the anterosuperior spine of the ilium and the other over the center of the tibial tubercle. The normal value for women is approximately 15 degrees and for men 10 degrees.

Joint Palpation

The knee should be thoroughly palpated for areas of tenderness along the medial capsule, the course of the tibial collateral ligament, the lateral capsule, and lateral ligaments. In addition, the joint line should be thoroughly palpated both medially and laterally with points of tenderness and osteophytes noted. A cyst of the meniscus frequently presents as a mass along the lateral joint immediately anterior to the lateral collateral ligament or medially immediately anterior or posterior to the tibial collateral ligament. Acute ligament tears can frequently be localized by point tenderness, and tears of the medial or lateral meniscus are often identified by tenderness directly over the joint line at the site of the lesion. A midlateral meniscal tear will occasionally present as a bulge or pseudocyst at the lateral joint line with the patient holding the knee at 45 degrees flexion.

Ligament Instability

Ligamentous instability of the knee is a complex subject which cannot be thoroughly covered in a short discussion. Ligament instability may be defined as abnormal rotational and/or translational motion of the tibial plateaus in relation to the femoral condyles, occurring about one or more axes or in one or more planes of motion, resulting in a *functional deficit.* The key to evaluating ligament instability is the term functional deficit. Although two patients may have identical degrees of ligamentous instability, the functional deficit in each is not necessarily the same because of the demands which they place upon the knee. A moderate amount of instability in an individual desiring to take part in a vigorous physical activity may create a serious handicap while a more sedentary individual may find it no serious problem whatsoever.

Stability of the knee is provided by static and dynamic elements which work together as an integrated mechanism. Static support is a function of the ligaments, capsule, menisci, and bony contour of the joint and dynamic support is a function of the surrounding muscles. Attempting to assign a specific function to each ligament has led to a great deal of confusion in evaluating ligamentous instability. The examiner must bear in mind that the static stabilizers are an integral part of a mechanism which must provide support to an inherently unstable joint subject to a great variety of forces. Rarely does an injury affect a single element in this complex system but rather directly or indirectly influences one or more of the other structures as well. The knee joint is not merely a hinge joint allowing flexion and extension but also has the element of rotation and even some valgus and varus motion.

Knee stability, even with normal ligaments, is at best a rather tenuous situation without the dynamic support of the various muscles of the thigh and calf which protect the static elements. The static structures define the limits of motion while the musculotendinous units control motion through voluntary and kinesthetic mechanisms, thus creating appropriate motion and simultaneously serving as an energy-absorbing mechanism for extrinsic and intrinsic forces which might otherwise injure the static structures.

Testing for ligamentous instability must be carried out methodically and carefully. Examination of an acute ligament injury is best performed as soon as possible after the injury. If delayed, hamstring muscle spasm may give the impression of a stable knee while masking a severe ligament injury. Frequently, patients with acute ligament injury may walk even with severe ligament damage by simply splinting the knee with their muscles, thus deluding the unwary examiner into assuming there is no serious problem. When adequate muscle relaxation is impossible, the knee must be examined under some form of anesthetic. Occasionally, satisfactory anesthesia is accomplished with instillation of a local anesthetic agent intra-articularly or directly into the area of maximum tenderness. Another possible trap for the uninitiated is lack of swelling with a severe ligament injury. This is not uncommon, because the fluid can escape into the surrounding soft tissues.

When examining the knee for ligamentous instability, the patient should be placed at ease and the uninvolved knee examined first. The patient should be lying comfortably on his back in a totally relaxed position.

Varus and Valgus Instability. The patient should be lying comfortably supine, totally relaxed, and on an examining table at a convenient height for the examiner. Examine the normal knee first to place the patient at ease and give him some idea of what to expect from the examination.

The patient's proximal leg is grasped with both hands by the examiner while the ankle is secured between the examiner's arm and side (Fig. 11-22). This provides good stable control of the extremity. The knee is first tested in full extension. Many of the old textbooks emphasized testing the knee in full extension only, but if the posterior capsule and posterior cruciate ligament are intact, no ligamentous

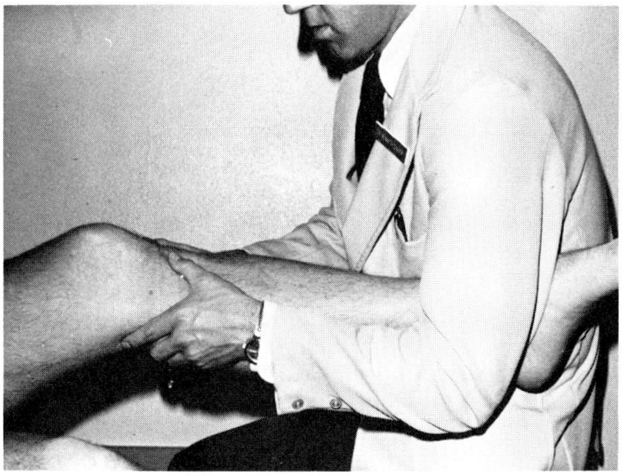

Fig. 11-22. Varus-valgus stress test. The leg is secured to the examiner's side and the proximal part of the leg grasped with both hands. Initially, the test is performed with the knee in extension to determine the integrity of the posterior capsule and then at 30 degrees of flexion to stress the collateral structures. A valgus stress (abduct the leg) and then a varus stress (adduct the leg) are applied, and the amount of instability, if any, is noted. Medial stability is tested with valgus stress and lateral stability with varus stress.

instability will be demonstrated even if the collateral ligaments are totally ruptured. If on the other hand, the knee does demonstrate varus or valgus instability in full extension, this means that not only are the collateral ligaments injured but that a portion or all of the posterior capsule and posterior cruciate ligament has been injured as well. A valgus and then varus stress is applied to the knee by applying pressure to first one side and then the other of the proximal leg so that the leg is abducted and adducted in relation to the knee and any instability is noted. Once this maneuver has been completed with the knee in full extension, the knee is flexed to 30 degrees to relax the posterior capsule and the test is repeated again noting if there is any medial or lateral instability. Often a certain amount of tibial rotation accompanies varus or valgus instability. With medial instability, the valgus test seems to increase if the tibia is externally rotated and decreases when the tibia is internally rotated. The reason for this is that with internal tibial rotation, the posterior cruciate increases the stability of the knee by becoming tighter and reducing the amount of valgus instability. This effect is diminished with external tibial rotation by allowing the posterior cruciate ligament to become more lax and thus giving the appearance that the valgus instability increases. There is often a slight amount of varus laxity present normally and this should be determined by examination of the normal knee. It should also be kept in mind that some people's knees are naturally more lax than others and this should not be mistaken for pathological instability.

Rotary Instability Testing (Anterior Drawer Test). Rotational instability of the knee refers to abnormal rotation of the tibia in relation to the femoral condyles. Normally the vertical axis of rotation is located just medial to the tibial spines but with ligament injury it may shift position, allowing abnormal internal or external rotation of the tibial plateaus in relation to the femoral condyles depending upon the ligament combination involved.

Rotary instability testing is performed by placing the patient in a supine position with the hip flexed 45 degrees, the knee flexed to 90 degrees, and the foot resting on the examining table (Fig. 11-23). The

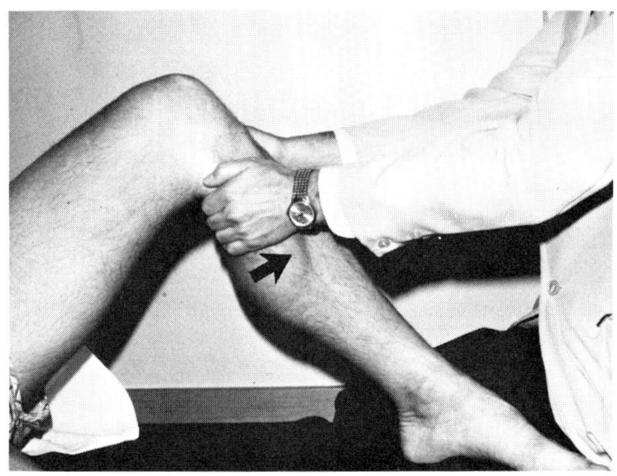

Fig. 11-23. Rotary instability test. The patient lies supine with the knee flexed 90 degrees, and the examiner sits across the forefoot. The test is performed by pulling forward on the proximal part of the calf first with the leg and foot internally rotated 30 degrees, then externally rotated 15 degrees, and finally in neutral position. The tibial plateaus are observed for any abnormal anterior displacement. With injury to the medial capsule, superficial tibial collateral ligament and often the anterior cruciate ligament, the medial tibial plateau will sublux anteriorly and rotate externally when the test is done with the leg and foot externally rotated 15 degrees. This indicates anteromedial rotary instability, which is the most common type.

examiner secures the patient's foot by sitting across the forefoot and then grasps the proximal calf with both hands. A push and pull force is applied to the proximal leg and the tibia is noted for abnormal motion in relation to the femoral condyles. Initially the foot and leg are positioned in 30 degrees of internal rotation and an anterior force applied to the proximal part of the leg with the hamstrings relaxed. Any hamstring tightness or spasm will invalidate the test. The tibia is then observed for possible anterior shift in relation to the femoral condyles. With an intact posterior cruciate ligament and lateral collateral ligaments, the femoral condyles are held securely to the tibial plateaus and no abnormal motion will be detected. Should the lateral plateau shift anteriorly and rotate internally, the test indicates pathological anterior and internal rotation of the tibia implicating an injury to the posterior cruciate and the lateral ligamentous structures.

The foot and leg are repositioned into 15 degrees of external rotation and the test repeated. This stresses the medial ligaments and the anterior cruciate ligament. If these structures have been injured, the medial tibial plateau will shift anteriorly and rotate laterally in relation to the medial femoral condyle. The amount of instability increases with serial rupture of the deep capsular ligament, the

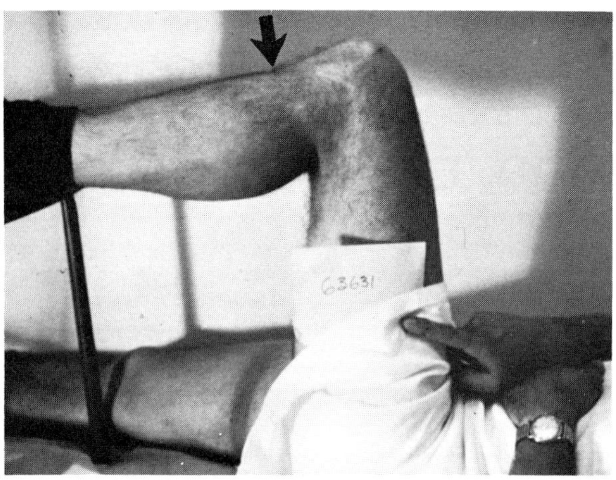

Fig. 11-24. Ninety-degree position for testing the posterior cruciate. The patient lies supine with the foot supported and the knee and hip flexed 90 degrees. The mere weight of the leg causes a posterior sag of the tibia with an incompetent posterior cruciate ligament. In addition, however, this patient had severe instability of the collateral ligaments.

superficial portion of the tibial collateral ligament, and finally the anterior cruciate ligament. If these structures are mildy injured, the test may not be positive because the posterior horn of the medial meniscus can block forward and outward rotation of the medial tibial plateau. The test may subsequently become positive following a meniscectomy or attrition of the posterior horn. The test is finally repeated with the leg in neutral rotation and the foot positioned straight ahead. This is what has been classically referred to as the "anterior drawer sign" for anterior cruciate instability. The test is repeated by pulling forward on the proximal leg, and the tibia noted for abnormal anterior shift in relation to the femoral condyles. This test does indicate some degree of anterior cruciate ligament incompetency but a significant anterior shift also implicates injury of the collateral structures on one side or the other as well. If the tibia subluxes directly anteriorly with both plateaus coming forward an equal amount (one plane anterior instability) it is quite likely that in addition to an injury of the anterior cruciate ligament that both the medial and lateral capsular structures have been injured.

Isolated tears of the anterior cruciate ligament have been reported in the literature but are still seriously questioned by many authorities on knee ligament injuries. The proposed mechanism is one of internal tibial rotation with the knee close to full extension or a hyperextension injury. There are instances reported in which the anterior drawer sign has been clinically negative preoperatively only to find the anterior cruciate ligament absent or severely injured at the time of surgery. For practical purposes one may consider that a significantly positive anterior drawer sign indicates some degree of injury to the anterior cruciate ligament, but keep in mind that there may be associated collateral ligament injuries as well.

The Posterior Drawer Sign. The posterior drawer sign is a physical sign in which the tibia sags posteriorly in relation to the femoral condyles, indicating incompetency of the posterior cruciate ligament and some degree of collateral ligament injury as well (one plane posterior instability). The test is performed by positioning the patient as one would for the anterior drawer test with the tibia in neutral rotation (Fig. 11-25). A posterior force is applied to the proximal part of the tibia and any posterior sag of the tibia is noted. It is particularly important that the starting position of the tibia in relation to the femoral condyles is noted for proper interpretation of the test. The problem arises in that with incompetency of the posterior cruciate ligament, the tibia may sag posteriorly by simply positioning the patient for the test. The uninitiated examiner may then apply an anterior force to the proximal tibia which subluxes forward into its *normal* relationship with the femoral condyles, but the examiner may not realize that the tibia was actually posterior at the start of the test and incorrectly interprets this as being a positive anterior drawer sign. When the tibia does displace posteriorly with a positive test, the femoral condyles will be felt to bulge anteriorly in front of the tibial plateaus, and the contour of the knee as seen from the side reveals a concave profile.

Another method of testing for a posterior drawer sign is to have the patient lying supine with the foot supported at the heel and the hip and the knee flexed to 90 degrees. The knee is observed from the side for a posterior sag of the proximal tibia in relation to the femoral condyles (Fig. 11-24).

The External Rotation-Recurvatum Test. The patient is postioned supine and the lower extremity is grasped with one hand under the heel and the other supporting the calf. The knee is allowed to pass from about 10 degrees of flexion into full extension. A positive test is indicated when the knee assumes a position of slight recurvatum, the tibia externally rotates, and there is increased tibia vara. This indicates injury to the arcuate complex (arcuate ligament, popliteus, and fibular collateral ligament), lateral one half of the posterior capsule, and some degree of injury to the posterior cruciate ligament.

Types of Instability. A thorough discussion of the various types of instability is beyond the scope of this chapter. Medial instabilities generally consist of some degree of valgus instability accompanied by abnormal tibial rotation. Medial rotational instability can be *anteromedial rotary instability* in which there is anterior, external rotational instability of the medial tibial plateau or *posteromedial rotary instability* with abnormal posterior displacement of the medial tibial plateau. The most common type of medial instability is valgus and anteromedial rotary instability. This is a result of injury to the deep capsular ligament, superficial tibial collateral ligament, and the anterior cruciate ligament. It is diagnosed with a positive valgus stress test at 30 degrees of flexion and a positive rotary instability test performed with the leg in 15 degrees of external rotation. The medial tibial plateau subluxes anteriorly in relation to the medial femoral condyle while the lateral tibial plateau remains relatively stable.

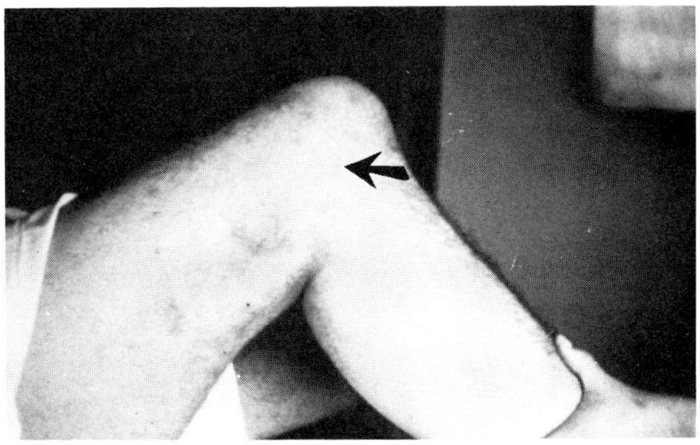

Fig. 11-25. The posterior drawer test performed with the patient supine and the extremity positioned similar to the rotary instability test. The tibia is pushed posteriorly. The femoral condyles become prominent anteriorly as the tibia subluxes posteriorly, indicative of posterior cruciate injury and usually some injury to the collateral ligaments as well.

Lateral instabilities of the knee may consist of both varus instability and rotational instability. The rotational instabilities are *anterolateral rotary instability* with the lateral tibial plateau displacing anteriorly and *posterolateral rotary instability* in which the lateral tibial plateau displaces posteriorly. The most frequently encountered lateral instability is anterolateral rotary instability. You can perform the rotary instability test with the leg in neutral position noting that the lateral tibial plateau displaces anteriorly farther than does the medial tibial plateau thus indicating abnormal internal tibial rotation.

McIntosh has described a lateral rotary instability which he calls the "lateral pivot shift." This should not, however, be confused as something other than anterolateral rotary instability. Clinically it is characterized by a giving way as the patient decelerates suddenly and pivots on the involved extremity.

The McIntosh test for anterolateral rotary instability is performed with the patient lying supine and the lower extremity supported at the heel by the examiner's one hand. The other hand is placed laterally over the proximal tibia just distal to the knee. The more proximal hand applies a valgus stress and internally rotates the tibia as the knee is gradually moved from a position of full extension into flexion. At about 30 to 40 degrees of flexion a sudden jump is noted as the lateral tibial plateau which has subluxed anteriorly in relation to the femoral condyle suddenly reduces. The McIntosh type of test for anterolateral rotary instability is dependent upon an *intact iliotibial tract,* and the mechanism of this will be discussed later.

My preferred technique for demonstrating anterolateral rotary instability is performed in the following fashion and described for examination of the patient's right knee. With the examiner's right arm and hand the distal leg is secured to the examiner's side while (Fig. 11-26) the left hand is placed over the lateral, proximal aspect of the leg just distal to the knee. With the knee in full extension, a valgus stress is applied and the leg internally rotated as the knee is gradually flexed. Within the first 5 to 10 degrees of flexion, the lateral tibial plateau can be felt to sublux

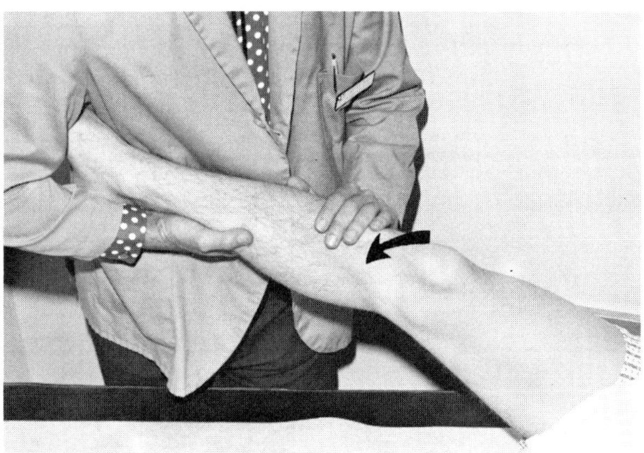

Fig. 11-26. Anterolateral rotary instability test (pivot shift). The leg is grasped with one hand and the other is placed over the lateral, proximal aspect of the leg. With the knee in extension, a valgus stress is applied and the leg internally rotated as the knee is flexed. As the knee flexes, the lateral tibial plateau can be felt to sublux anteriorly in relation to the lateral condyle; there is slight resistance to flexion, lateral crepitation is sometimes felt, and the iliotibial tract becomes very tight. At about 30 to 40 degress of flexion, the iliotibial tract becomes tight, passes behind the transverse axis of rotation (the instant center of rotation appears to be fixed as the tibial plateau hinges on the femoral condyle), and the tibial plateau is suddenly reduced, frequently with a "clunking" sensation.

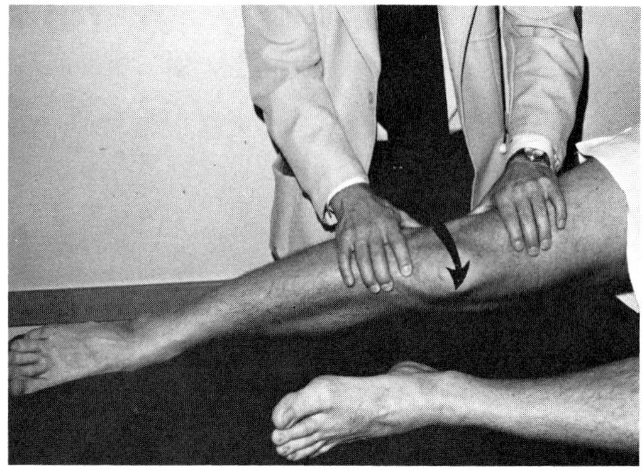

Fig. 11-27. Anterolateral rotary instability test modified by Slocum. The patient lies in the lateral position with the involved knee uppermost and the other extremity flexed 90 degrees at the hip and knee. The pelvis is rotated slightly posterior with the weight of the extremity supported by the inner aspect of the foot and heel. The weight of the extremity creates a valgus stress at the knee, and the relative position of the pelvis and foot cause slight internal rotation of the leg. The examiner grasps the distal thigh with one hand and the proximal part of the leg with the other hand while pressing behind the head of the fibula and femoral condyle with the thumbs. The knee is pushed into flexion and again as the iliotibial tract passes behind the transverse axis of rotation, the lateral tibial plateau is reduced with a palpable "clunk." In some instances the test is quite subtle with a gentle slipping or giving way sensation. If the test is applied with some finesse, a point can be found where the tibial plateau can be slipped back and forth in relation to the femoral condyle.

anteriorly in relation to the lateral condyle and to translocate slightly medially. With continued flexion a slight resistance is often encountered and frequently lateral crepitation is felt over the joint line. The iliotibial tract becomes very taut at this point. At about 30 to 40 degrees of flexion it glides posterior to the transverse axis of rotation and the tibial plateau is suddenly reduced with a jumping sensation. With practice, very subtle anterolateral rotary instabilities can be detected with this technique.

Slocum has further modified the test for anterolateral rotary instability as described by McIntosh (Fig. 11-27). The patient lies in the lateral position with the involved knee upper-most and the other extremity flexed 90 degrees at the hip and knee. The pelvis and torso are rotated slightly posterior (about 30 degrees) with the weight of the extremity supported by the inner aspect of the foot and heel. The weight of the extremity creates a valgus stress at the knee and the relative position of the pelvis and foot cause slight internal rotation of the leg. The examiner grasps the distal thigh with one hand and the proximal part of the leg with the other while pressing behind the head of the fibula and the femoral condyle with the thumbs. The knee is then gently pushed from extension into flexion and again as the iliotibial tract passes behind the transverse axis of rotation at about 30 to 40, degrees of flexion, the lateral tibial plateau, which has subluxed forward, is reduced with a palpable jumping sensation.

Hughston has further modified the McIntosh test for anterolateral rotary instability and refers to it as the "jerk sign." In this instance the extremity is grasped at the foot with one hand while the other hand rests over the proximal, lateral aspect of the leg just distal to the knee with the knee flexed at 90 degrees. Again a valgus stress is applied to the knee and the tibia internally rotated. The knee is gradually extended. Initially the lateral tibial plateau is in a reduced position to the femoral condyle but as the knee extends and passes through about 30 to 40 degrees of flexion, the lateral tibial plateau suddenly subluxes forward in relation to the femoral condyle and does so with a jerking sensation; thus the name "jerk sign." As the knee continues on into extension, the lateral plateau gradually resumes a reduced position which is complete at termination of full extension.

All forms of the McIntosh tests demonstrate the same type of instability, namely anterolateral rotary instability. In spite of the fact that each has a different approach, the basic mechanism behind each test is very similar. When the knee is in full extension, the lateral tibial plateau is in a reduced position. Within the first 5 to 10 degrees of flexion and with valgus stress being applied to the knee as well as internal tibial rotation, the lateral tibial plateau begins to gradually sublux anteriorly and the lateral femoral condyle rocks posteriorly over the convex surface of the tibial plateau. The maximum position of subluxation is reached at about 30 to 40 degrees of knee flexion. The iliotibial tract becomes very tight with knee flexion and glides posteriorly. At 30 to 40 degrees of flexion it passes behind the transverse instant center rotation of the knee and suddenly pulls the lateral tibial plateau posteriorly reducing it in relation to the femoral condyle creating a sudden jumping sensation which is easily detectable. This particular sign is dependent upon an intact iliotibial tract to demonstrate anterolateral rotary instability in this particular fashion. If the test is performed by starting with the knee flexed at 90 degrees as described by Hughston, these events take place in reverse order. Initially the lateral tibial plateau is in a reduced position but at 30 to 40 degrees of flexion as the iliotibial tract passes anterior to the instant center of rotation, the tibia suddenly subluxes anteriorly in relation to the lateral femoral condyle and then as knee extension is continued the lateral plateau gradually reduces itself with reduction complete upon accomplishment of full extension. Anterolateral rotary instability is created by incompetency of the anterior cruciate ligament, perhaps the midlateral capsule, some degree of laxity of the arcuate ligament and occasionally laxity of the iliotibial tract. Again it must be stressed that if the iliotibial tract has been stretched or injured then the McIntosh type of test for anterolateral rotary instability will not be positive with the classical jumping sensation. In most anterolateral rotary instabilities, the iliotibial tract is intact and the instability can be more graphically demonstrated with some form of the McIntosh test.

Posterolateral rotary instability is a posterior shift of the lateral tibial plateau in relation to the lateral femoral condyle with abnormal external tibial rotation. This type of instability is created by laxity of the arcuate complex, the lateral one half of the posterior capsule, and usually some incompetency of the posterior cruciate ligament. It is diagnosed with a positive external rotation-recurvatum test and a positive posterior drawer test noting excessive posterior sag of the lateral tibial plateau accompanied by external tibial rotation. The medial tibial plateau remains relatively stable and does not sag posteriorly.

Frequent combination rotational instabilities are (1) anteromedial and anterolateral rotary instability and (2) anterolateral and posterolateral rotary instability.

It is essential to accurately identify the type or types of instability which are present. Although differentiating the various types of instability may seem most difficult, an additional problem to the examiner is that of learning to quantitate the findings so they are meaningful. Ligament injuries are graded on a basis of I to III with I being a mild sprain with minimal or no instability and little or no functional deficit; a grade II with moderate instability and a rather moderate functional deficit; and grade III which is gross instability and significant functional deficit. As a general rule, a grade I or III type of instability is not difficult to diagnose and the course of therapy is quite clearcut. Grade I may generally be treated conservatively and the grade III will probably require surgical repair or reconstruction. The grade II, however, presents an enigma to the examiner in attempting to decide whether to proceed conservatively or surgically, particularly in the young vigorous individual desirous of being able to perform strenuous activities. I use the following criteria as a helpful rule of thumb in evaluating acute ligament injuries. Experience has shown me that even successfully repaired ligaments usually have some residual laxity (a mild grade II) and if an acutely injured knee demonstrates a degree of laxity similar to this, a conservative course is followed. Only after classifying the type of instability, grading it, and then determining the functional deficit can a physician decide upon a course of action and determine the proper treatment. Experience in evaluating chronic ligament instability and correlating the findings with functional deficit provides an invaluable background to evaluate acute ligament injuries. The examiner acquires a basis for comparison and the capability of determining what the prognosis is likely to be. There is no short cut in learning to evaluate ligament instabilities.

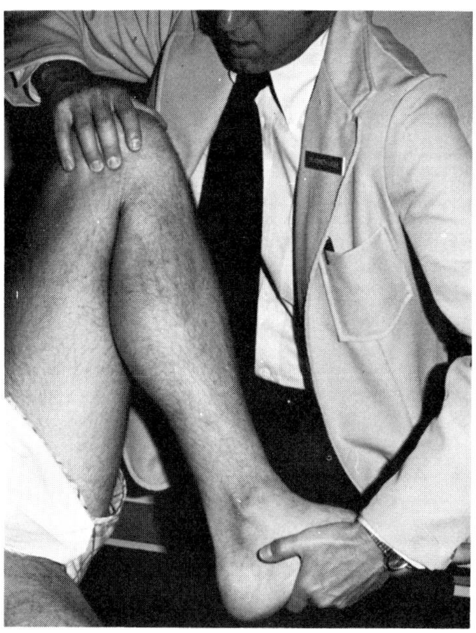

Fig. 11-28. McMurray test. The patient lies supine while the examiner grasps the foot with one hand and palpates the joint line with the other. The knee is acutely flexed, the tibia rotated back and forth, and then held alternately in internal and external rotation as the knee is extended. A click or crepitation may be felt over the joint line with a posterior meniscal lesion as the knee is extended.

Ligament instabilities are classified as acute or chronic. The acute cases are considered to be within two weeks of injury and the chronic in excess of three months. The time period of two weeks has been arbitrarily selected based upon the maximum time following injury when surgical repair is technically feasible. Beyond about two weeks, the healing process has progressed to a point where it becomes very difficult to repair the ligament because of abundant granulations and friability of the tissues. After 2 weeks, it is perhaps best to delay any plans for surgical intervention until the healing process has resolved and then if necessary, a reconstructive procedure may be planned in an effort to restore the functional deficit. Reconstructive procedures as a rule are not as successful as acute repairs, which emphasizes the importance of proper diagnosis during the acute phase in determining what the prognosis is likely to be.

Meniscal Tears

One of the most common problems of the knee is a meniscal lesion in which one or more of the menisci is torn. Various tests have been designed to detect a torn meniscus. Unfortunately, none of these is totally reliable. Three of the more common tests utilized are the McMurray test, the Apley grinding test, and the Helfet sign.

The McMurray test is performed with the patient in the supine position and the knee acutely flexed (Fig. 11-28). The examiner grasps the foot with one hand, flexes the knee, and then extends the knee holding the tibia either internally or externally rotated. If there is a tear of the posterior horn of the medial meniscus or the lateral meniscus, a clicking or crepitant sensation will often be elicited over the appropriate side, but there are false-positive clicks which this test will elicit and care must be taken in interpreting the sign.

Theoretically if a click occurs with the tibia externally rotated, it is indicative of a tear posteriorly in the medial meniscus, and if a click occurs with internal tibial rotation, the tear supposedly involves the posterior aspect of the lateral meniscus. In performing this test, it is often helpful to rotate the tibia back and forth rapidly with the knee in full flexion before beginning extension in either internal or external rotation. This will sometimes cause impingement of the meniscus and elicit the sign more readily.

The Apley grinding test is performed with the patient in the prone position, the knee flexed to 90 degrees, and the leg pointing toward the ceiling (Fig. 11-29). The examiner then applies a direct pressure downward on the foot and rotates the tibia first inward and then outward. This may elicit a grinding sensation on the involved side, reproducing the symptoms for the patient and indicating a torn meniscus. This test is then repeated by applying a distraction to the leg, and if pain is elicited it is theoretically indicative of ligamentous injury rather than a meniscal injury.

The Helfet sign is based upon the fact that as the normal knee goes into full extension, the tibia rotates externally in relation to the femoral condyles; this motion is described as a "screw home" mechanism. With a torn meniscus blocking the joint, the screw home mechanism is blocked so that when the knee is placed into extension, the tibial tubercle remains slightly medial in relation to the patella, and the final limit of external rotation is prevented. Normally the tibial tubercle will line up with the lateral half of the patella in complete extension. The medial femoral condyle in complete extension is also flush with the medial tibial plateau, but if the screw home mechanism is blocked, the femoral condyle may protrude slightly over the anterior margin of the medial tibial plateau. This test, like the others, may be helpful, but none of these tests is absolutely diagnostic for a torn meniscus.

Popliteal Space

The popliteal space is the last part of the knee to be examined. The most frequent condition encountered in this area is a Baker's cyst, or more properly a popliteal cyst, which usually arises from the semimembranosus tendon bursa, although other bursae may be involved (Fig. 11-30). They may communicate with the joint and are frequently associated with a posterior lesion of the medial meniscus. Often they fluctuate in size, depending upon the patient's activities, and, although benign, can at times become a nuisance with discomfort. Occasionally an aneurysm will be encountered but can be differentiated from a popliteal cyst by auscultation and listening for a bruit.

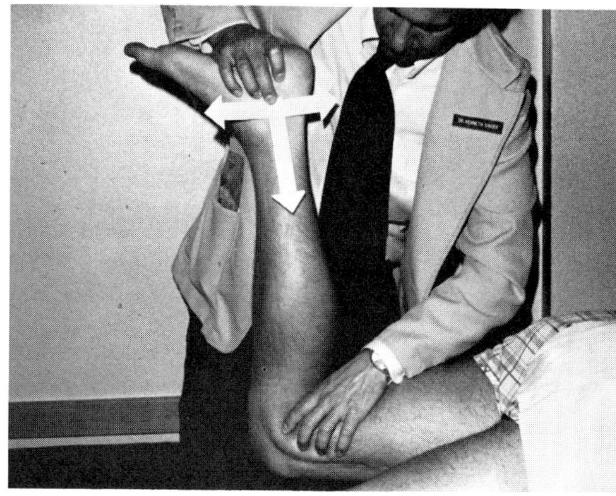

Fig. 11-29. Apley grinding test. The patient lies prone with the knee flexed 90 degrees. The examiner pushes down on the foot and rotates the tibia back and forth while palpating the joint line with the other hand feeling for crepitation.

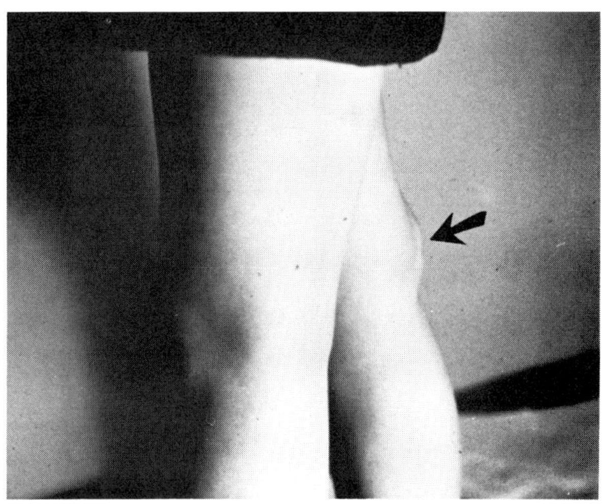

Fig. 11-30. Popliteal cyst. The cystic enlargement in the right popliteal space (*arrow*) communicated with the semimembranosus bursa.

A condition involving the posterior lateral aspect of the knee is popliteal tendon tenosynovitis. This is common in distance runners and joggers. It is characterized by recurring pain over the posterior lateral aspect of the knee, generally brought on by activity. Clinically, there is tenderness directly over the popliteal tendon but rarely is swelling observed. The popliteal tendon is best palpated with the patient lying supine, the knee flexed 90 degrees, and the involved extremity crossed over the opposite extremity at the knee (Fig. 11-31). This is the same position as previously described for examining the fibular collateral ligament. The tendon lying just posterior to the ligament may actually be rolled under the examiner's finger, eliciting tenderness.

Roentgenographic Examination

Roentgenograms are an integral part of the knee examination. A standardized technique is essential for producing consistent results and facilitating their interpretation. For a routine series the following views are recommended:

Anteroposterior Standing. Weight-bearing gives a better indication of alignment across the joint and also the status of the joint space. The feet should always be placed parallel and adjacent to each other (Fig. 11-32).

Lateral. The lateral femoral condyle has a more flattened curve and a characteristic notch. The posterior contour of the lateral tibial plateau is more squared off than the medial (Fig. 11-33A, B).

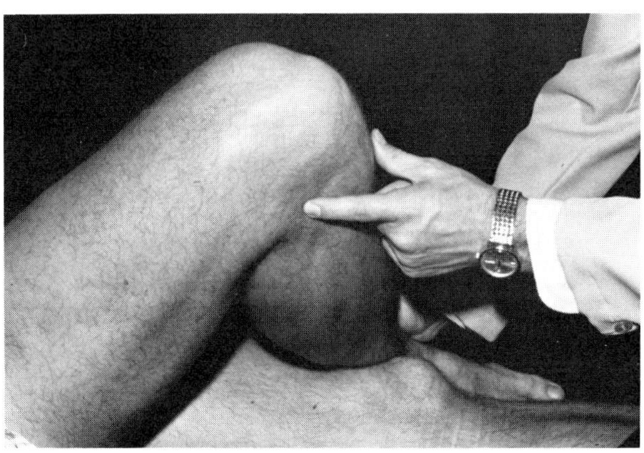

Fig. 11-31. Crossed leg position for examining the fibular collateral ligament which is stretched tight. The popliteal tendon lies immediately posterior to the ligament. The mid-lateral joint line is also readily palpable anterior to the ligament and posterior to the iliotibial tract.

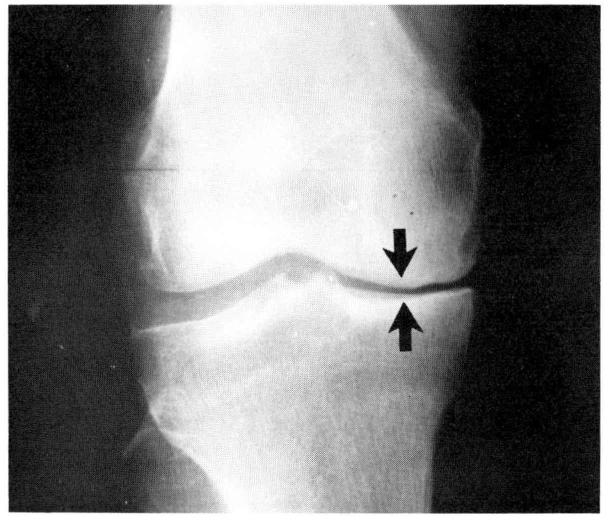

Fig. 11-32. Standing anteroposterior roentgenogram of the knee. Loss of medial joint space is quite apparent with weight-bearing (*arrows*) whereas a nonweight-bearing view showed no loss of medial joint space.

Posteroanterior Intercondylar. Displays the intercondylar notch not seen on the AP view (Fig. 11-34A). This view is important in defining areas of osteochondritis dissecans (Fig. 11-34B).

Tangential Patellar View. Numerous techniques are available, but one should be chosen which displays the patella in the femoral sulcus at about 30 to 40 degrees of knee flexion. This positions the patella in the sulcus where it is most likely to sublux or dislocate (Fig. 11-35A, B).

The configuration of the femoral sulcus normally provides additional stability to the patellofemoral articulations. The most important feature is the height of the medial and lateral condyles in relation to the bottom of the sulcus and also the steepness of the sides of the sulcus. Normally, the lateral condyle projects higher than the medial condyle, helping to prevent lateral patellar subluxation or dislocation, but the relative height cannot be determined accurately with the routine patellar views. A significant clinical measurement roentgenographically is the *sulcus angle*. It is determined by drawing a line from the bottom of the sulcus to the apex of the medial and lateral femoral condyles and measuring the angle between the two lines (see Fig. 11-35A). A normal

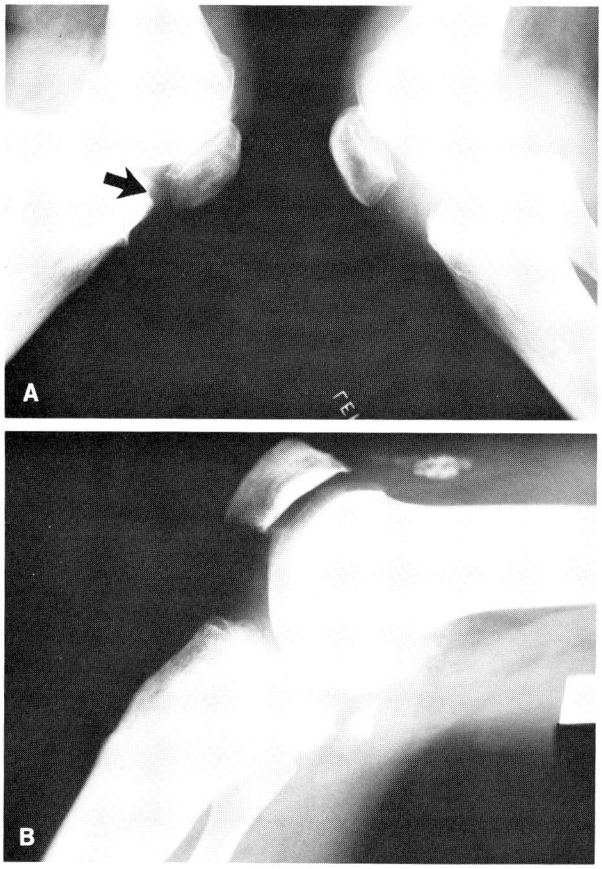

Fig. 11-33. (*A*) Lateral roentgenogram of the knees showing a patella baja (low riding patella) on the left (*arrow*) and normal position on the right. (*B*) Lateral view revealing a loose body in the suprapatellar pouch and posterior compartment.

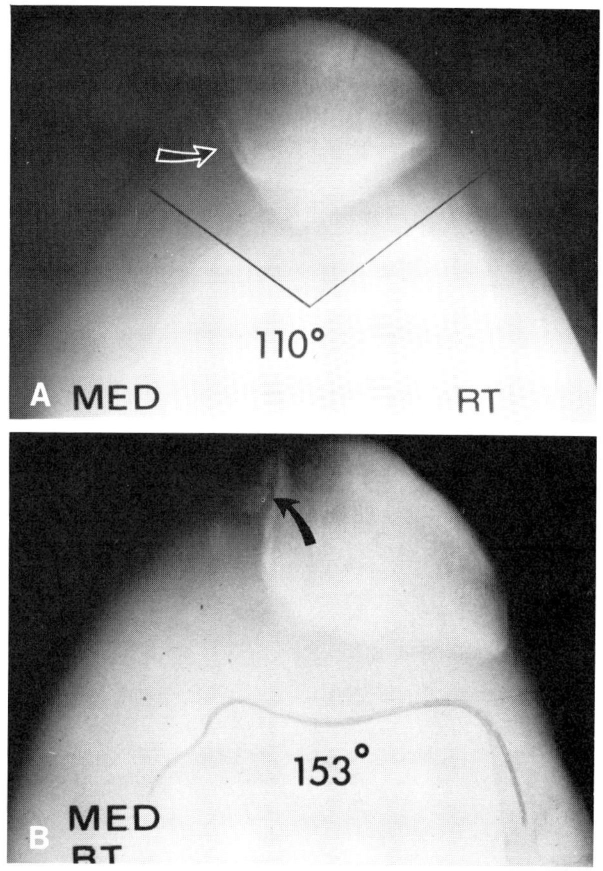

Fig. 11-35. (*A, B*) Tangential patellar view. This view shows the patella in relation to the femoral sulcus. (*A*) A sulcus angle of 110 degrees well within normal limits for the technique used (Hughston view) with a symmetrically placed patella. The arrow, however, indicates a medial avulsion fracture suggestive of an old subluxation or dislocation. (*B*) Tangential view with a very shallow sulcus, the patella is tilted slightly lateral and a medial avulsion fracture is seen. The patella was clinically unstable.

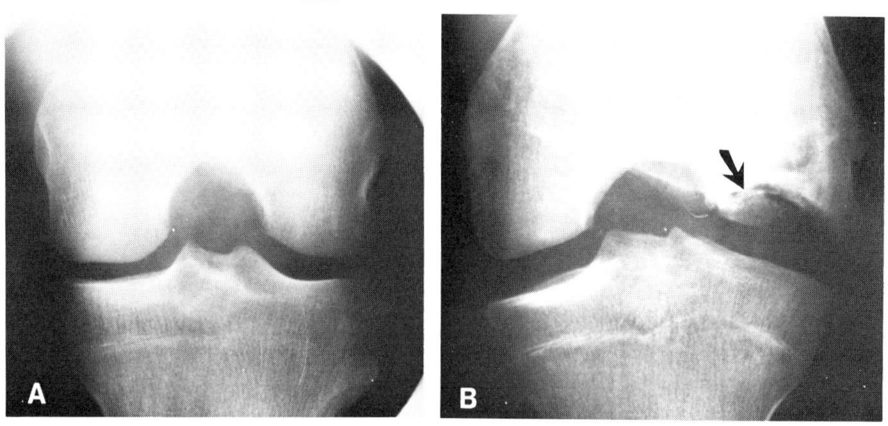

Fig. 11-34. (*A, B*) Posteroanterior notch or tunnel view. (*A*) Normal notch view showing the notch and more posterior aspects of the femoral condyles not seen on the anteroposterior view. (*B*) Steroid osteochondritis dissecans of the lateral femoral condyle (*arrow*).

sulcus angle must be determined for whatever technique is used on the tangential patellar view. A large angle (shallow sulcus) suggests less stabilizing effect while the opposite is true with a smaller angle which indicates a sulcus with steeper sides.

Some indication of patellofemoral joint congruency can also be obtained from the tangential view. Patellar tilt or asymmetrical placement of the patella in the sulcus (see Fig. 11-35B) often correlates with chondromalacia. A position of subluxation over the lateral femoral condyle supports the clinical impression of recurrent subluxation or dislocation. An avulsion fracture is frequently seen along the medial border of the patella with these conditions.

Additional views of the knee are often helpful for certain conditions. A valgus stress view to demonstrate medial ligament laxity (Fig. 11-36) is useful particularly in the preadult patient to differentiate between a medial ligament tear and fracture subluxation of the distal femoral epiphysis which clinically presents as medial ligament instability. A varus

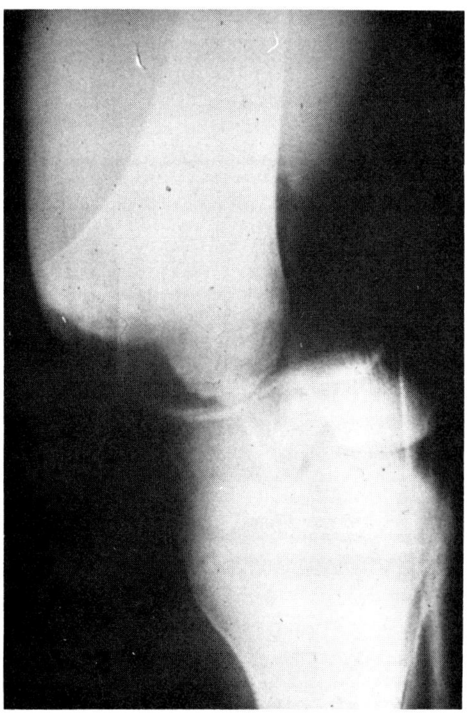

Fig. 11-36. Fracture-dislocation of the distal femoral epiphysis. A valgus stress view on roentgenogram clearly differentiates this injury from a medial ligament injury in the teenage patient.

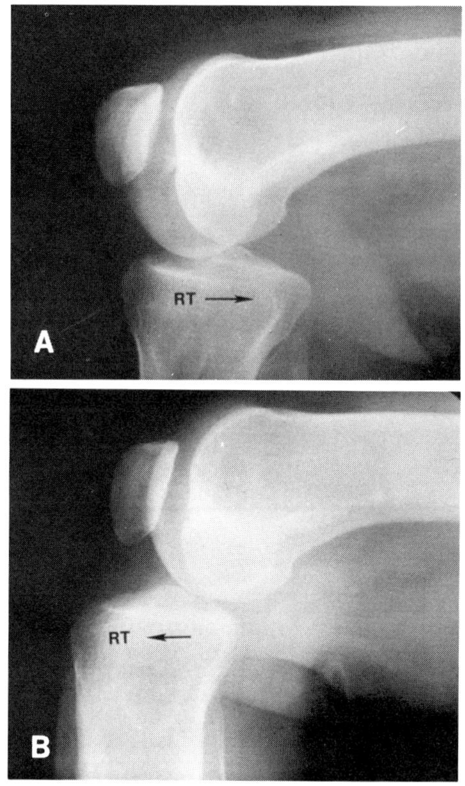

Fig. 11-37. (*A, B*) Sagittal stress roentgenogram of the knee. (*A*) The tibia has a normal relationship to the femoral condyles when a posterior drawer test is done. (*B*) With anterior stress, the tibia subluxes forward. This patient had a chronic valgus and anteromedial rotary instability.

stress view may be taken to display lateral ligament instability.

As a corollary to the rotary instability test and posterior drawer sign, a lateral view of the knee with anterior and then posterior stress applied to the proximal tibia may be done to reveal the amount of sagittal displacement of the tibial plateaus in relation to the femoral condyles (Fig. 11-37A, B). This gives an objective measurement of anteroposterior instability.

Nonstandard views are often necessary to display certain areas of the knee not revealed on the routine views. An astute roentgen technician informed of the problem can usually devise a technique to display the involved area satisfactorily.

Arthrography

Knee arthrography has become an extremely valuable diagnostic tool. It is not infallible but is accurate if performed by a capable radiologist with scrupulous attention to technique and experience in interpretation. Arthrograms are particularly useful in detecting meniscal lesions (Fig. 11-38) They are also helpful in evaluating the anterior cruciate ligament, the collateral ligaments, and the capsule with acute injuries. Arthrograms often display a popliteal bursa which communicates with the joint, nonopaque loose bodies, and synovial tumors. The most difficult area to interpret is the posterior horn of the lateral meniscus because of the many recesses and bursa which create overlapping of the contrast material. The orthopaedist should review each arthrogram ordered and not depend solely on the radiologist's interpretation.

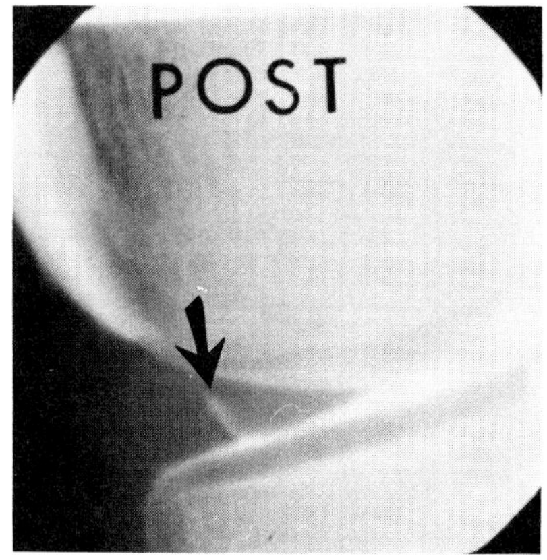

Fig. 11-38. Arthrogram showing a vertical tear (*arrow*) in the medial meniscus. The contrast medium outlines the wedge-shaped meniscus and flows into the defect.

Arthroscopy

Arthroscopy is a diagnostic aid which compliments arthrography. If performed by an orthopaedist familiar with the technique, considerable information can be gained without the necessity of arthrotomy. The status of the menisci (including the posterior horn of the lateral meniscus), synovium, anterior cruciate ligament, and articular cartilage of the patella and femoral condyles can be appraised. Again, it must be emphasized that as in arthrography, the value of the procedure is directly dependent upon the technique and experience of the operator.

DIFFERENTIAL DIAGNOSIS OF DISORDERS OF THE KNEE

INTERNAL DERANGEMENTS OF THE KNEE

Meniscal Lesions

The term internal derangement refers to conditions causing a malfuction on a mechanical basis. One of the most common problems under this category is a meniscal lesion in which one or more of the menisci is torn. The function of the two menisci is not completely understood, but the following functions have been attributed to them: weight-bearing, control of motion, increase of joint contact area, and shock absorption. Except for the congenitally deformed discoid lateral meniscus, meniscal lesions are unusual in children under 15 years of age. Most lesions involve the medial meniscus since it is more firmly attached about its periphery and consequently less mobile than the lateral meniscus making it more subject to injury. The lateral meniscus, on the other hand, is quite mobile, not as firmly attached about its periphery, and is under the dynamic control of the popliteus muscle which can retract it posteriorly when the knee is flexed, protecting it from injury. The mechanism of injury to the meniscus is thought primarily to be a combination of compression and rotation.

With this mechanism the meniscus is frequently split down the middle creating the *bucket-handle lesion* so often found in young active people (Fig. 11-39). The inner portion of the bucket-handle is frequently displaced into the middle of the joint blocking complete extension and creating a locking phenomenon.

A more common type of injury to the menisci, particularly in the middle aged and elderly, is a tear involving the posterior portion of the medial meniscus called a *horizontal cleavage lesion.* This is

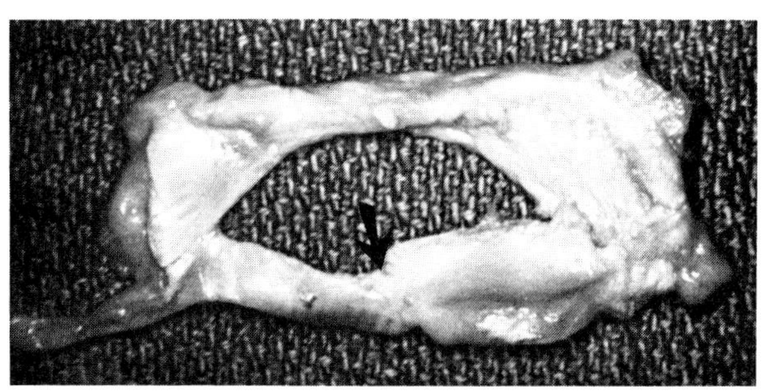

Fig. 11-39. A bucket handle tear of the medial meniscus. The bucket handle portion (*arrow*) had dislocated into the notch creating a locking phenomenon.

caused by repeated shear stresses which create a transverse lesion within the meniscus as it becomes impinged between the tibial plateau and the medial femoral condyle.

The congenital discoid lateral meniscus is a condition in which the meniscus assumes a discoid or semi-oval shape rather than the normal semilunar shape. It rarely occurs medially but can be bilateral and is more frequently found in children and adult women. Its abnormal shape and mechanics make it more susceptible to injury.

Symptoms of a torn meniscus are locking, giving way, swelling, pain, tenderness, and frequently a click or clunk within the joint. The characteristic complaint of a discoid lateral meniscus is a click or snapping in the knee which is similar to that found with other internal derangements. The diagnosis in this case is often made by a high index of suspicion because of the patient's age or sex and lateral location of the snapping. The locking phenomena is the most pathognomonic feature of a torn meniscus but unfortunately is not always present. True locking is the inability of the patient to extend the knee completely because the torn portion of the meniscus blocks the joint and prevents full extension. This occurs only with a typical bucket-handle tear which we have previously discussed. Giving way is a common complaint and occurs with transient impingement of the torn meniscus between the articular surfaces. With the initial injury, effusion is common, but in the horizontal cleavage lesion, an effusion may not be present, and in old lesions of the menisci, effusions are frequently not present even with recurrent locking episodes. Quadriceps atrophy accompanies the chronically torn meniscus. Tenderness over the lesion is an important diagnostic sign and a positive McMurray's test, Apley grinding test, or Helfet sign will add credibility to the diagnosis. Arthrography and arthroscopy are particularly useful when the clinical findings are less obvious.

Recurrent Subluxation and Dislocation of the Patella

A repeated partial or complete lateral dislocation of the patella is secondary to dynamic and/or static patellar instability. This condition may affect any age group but is more frequent in the second and third decades with a higher incidence occurring in females than males. More recent evidence implicates this condition in males more frequently than has been thought in the past. It is unusual that one etiological factor can be singled out.

The symptoms associated with patellar subluxation or dislocation are not unique. Pain, giving way, swelling, "something slipping out," catching, and grinding are the more common complaints. Many times, however, the complaints are vague and can implicate almost any form of internal derangement.

There are a number of factors which combine to produce patellar instability. Direct trauma to the patella creating a frank lateral dislocation is an occurrence in contact sports. Even with this, however, there may be anatomical variations predisposing to a patellar dislocation. Other factors to consider are extensor mechanism malalignment; a shallow femoral sulcus; vastus medialis obliquus weakness or atrophy; an excessive Q-angle; patella alta; femoral and/or tibial torsional problems; incompetence of the medial retinaculum or medial patellofemoral ligament; patellofemoral joint incongruity; and dynamic overload when the knee is flexed 30 to 40 degrees and the leg externally rotated in the presence of a vigorously contracting quadriceps muscle.

A complete lateral dislocation is apparent to both the patient and the examiner (see Fig. 11-17A), but the patella often spontaneously reduces itself and the patient is not aware of what happened. The examiner must have a high index of suspicion particularly since recurrent subluxation has rather subtle findings. Increased lateral patellar mobility with medial pressure on the patella applied with the knee flexed 30 to 40 degrees is a significant sign. The patient may become apprehensive when this test is performed. Hemarthrosis usually accompanies an initial episode of dislocation but does not necessarily occur with subsequent episodes. The initial episode of dislocation tears the medial retinaculum, either along the medial patellar border or more posteriorly at the insertion of the patellofemoral ligament into the medial femoral condyle. These areas are tender to palpation but once healed in an elongated fashion, subsequent dislocations or subluxations may occur without significant damage to the retinaculum.

In this situation, there is no hemarthrosis and little localized tenderness. Chondromalacia of the patella with retropatellar crepitation and pain on compression is a usual finding with subluxation or recurrent dislocation of the patella. Patellar instability is also associated with patella alta characterized by a rather small patella, genu recurvatum, some extensor lag, and a prominent fat pad. The role of dynamic stability afforded by the vastus medialis obliquus has already been discussed. Atrophy of this muscle is associated with diminished stabilization of the patella allowing its lateral displacement. Some people, such as professional dancers, have increased external tibial rotation which dynamically increases the Q-angle, thus potentially enhancing the tendency for lateral displacement of the patella. A Q-angle of over 25 degrees measured with the knee in extension may be considered abnormal. Genu valgum has long been implicated in patellar instability but more likely assumes a secondary role in subluxation or dislocation. In infancy the cause is usually fibrosis of the iliotibial tract which pulls the patella laterally. Familial joint laxity is another contributing factor with a history of other family members having recurrent dislocation or subluxation.

The routine four views of the knee should be taken with special attention given to the tangential view. The patella may be tilted laterally, subluxed, or actually dislocated. An avulsion fracture from the medial border of the patella is frequently noted and if present is a most significant clue to the examiner. A defect in the subchondral bone of the medial patellar facet or along the lateral margin of the lateral femoral condyle indicates the site of a tangential osteochondral fracture. The roentgenograms should be thoroughly scrutinized for the fragment. A shallow sulcus angle raises the index of suspicion for patellar instability, particularly if the patella is tilted laterally or subluxed.

Chondromalacia of the Patella

Chondromalacia of the patella is a softening of the articular cartilage of the patella accompanied by some degree of fibrillation, fissuring, and, in severe situations, erosion to the extent that the entire articular surface of the patella may be destroyed. The patellar mechanics are extremely sensitive and slight abnormalities of knee function can produce secondary chondromalacia of the patella. Therefore, it is often associated secondarily with many forms of internal derangement. In its pure or primary form the symptoms are suggestive of other forms of internal derangement. The etiological factors are numerous and include direct trauma, patellofemoral joint incongruity, recurrent subluxation and dislocation, meniscal lesions, transverse plane rotational abnormalities secondary to femoral or tibial torsion, extensor mechanism malalignment, postsurgery or postimmobilization syndromes, and a prominent medial femoral condylar ridge (Outerbridge's ridge).

The characteristic symptom of chondromalacia is pain with sitting, climbing stairs or hills, and prolonged walking or running. Distance runners frequently complain of retropatellar pain. Patients will often complain of a catching sensation simulating other types of internal derangement. They also have grating, recurrent swelling, and pain upon squatting which places considerable force on the patellofemoral joint. Stiffness in the knee after a rest, particularly while sitting, is a characteristic complaint. However, the symptoms are often vague and difficult to evaluate.

The clinical findings are peripatellar, retropatellar, or facet tenderness accompanied by retropatellar crepitation upon compression of the patella. Associated findings may be lateral placement of the patella secondary to patellar instability, patella baja, malalignment of the extensor mechanism, and a chronic knee effusion in some instances of severe chondromalacia.

Patellar Tendon Tendinitis

Another condition related to the patella, which must be differentiated from chondromalacia of the patella, is patellar tendinitis or "jumper's knee." The etiology of this condition is repeated stress applied to the insertion of the quadriceps tendon proximally or the patellar tendon insertion at the distal pole of the patella. Pathologically, microruptures of the tendon at the insertion site and/or local tendon degeneration occur.

Symptomatically, there is pain about the patella with aching after exercise, particularly with vigorous repetitive activity requiring jumping, running, and climbing. The condition is often progressive and may become disabling as far as vigorous activity is concerned. Occasionally, there is swelling over the involved site and with chronicity can result in patellar tendon or quadriceps tendon rupture.

The classic physical finding is tenderness directly over the proximal or more commonly the distal patellar pole. Roentgenographic examination may reveal some periosteal reaction at the involved site, an elongated distal pole, and irregularity of the subchondral bone. Most often, however, nothing abnormal is found.

Loose Bodies

Loose bodies or "joint mice" are most commonly osteocartilaginous fragments of traumatic origin from tangential osteochondral fractures but can also originate from a pathological process, such as osteochondritis dissecans (see Fig. 11-33B). Other types of loose bodies may consist of chondral fragments (pieces of articular cartilage), remnants of menisci, foreign bodies, fibrous tissue, and intraarticular tumors. Some loose bodies may obtain a synovial attachment while more commonly they remain loose in the joint. A tangential osteochondral fragment with its normal bone is more likely to become attached to the synovium than is a fragment from osteochondritis dissecans with its necrotic bone fragment. Fragments of articular cartilage can enlarge as they are nourished by the synovial fluid. Small loose bodies are more likely to cause symptoms than larger ones, since the former may be more easily impinged between articular surfaces.

The most likely site of origin for a loose body in a teenage male is (1) osteochondritis dissecans at the classic site, (2) a marginal fracture from the lateral margin of the lateral femoral condyle secondary to direct trauma and/or patellar dislocation and (3) a medial tangential osteochondral fracture of the patella from dislocation. This order is reversed in the female patient.

Osteochondritis dissecans is an ischemic condition involving the subchondral bone, probably either the result of or in association with repeated trauma to the area. The involved area of ischemic bone demarcates and may eventually separate along with the overlying articular cartilage leaving behind a defect with the fragment becoming a loose body within the joint. The knee is the most commonly involved joint and the incidence is higher in men than in women. The most common sites are (1) the lateral border of the medial femoral condyle (the classic site); (2) the inferior, central area of the lateral femoral condyle; and (3) the inferior, central region of the medial femoral condyle. It is postulated that osteochondritis dissecans occurs at the classic site by repeated trauma to the area from contact with a prominent medial tibial spine. The central lesions in the femoral condyles are usually associated with a meniscal lesion which traumatizes the area. Often there is a family history of osteochondritis dissecans, and it is not unusual for both knees to be involved.

Classically the problem occurs in a teenage male with complaints of pain and giving way in the knee. There may be effusions and transient episodes of locking as opposed to a more persistent locking seen with a torn meniscus. Before the fragment separates there is nothing diagnostic in the complaints, but after the fragment separates, episodes of transient locking are frequent, and the patient may be aware of "something loose" in the knee.

At physical examination, tenderness over the lesion may be present even before it separates. The classic site is palpated by acutely flexing the knee and applying pressure along the lateral margin of the medial femoral condyle. Some patients assume a gait with the tibia externally rotated; this prevents contact between the classic site and the medial tibial spine. In these situations, internal rotation of the tibia with the knee flexed about 30 degrees may create pain by bringing the tibial spine into contact with the involved area.

The diagnosis of osteochondritis dissecans is a radiological diagnosis before the fragment separates. There will be a defect in the subchondral bone with a fragment of sclerotic bone separated by an area of rarefaction. The radiological differential diagnosis should include anomalies of ossification, osteochondral fracture, steroid osteochondritis, and spontaneous osteonecrosis.

Anomalies of ossification are areas of irregular ossification of the femoral condyles; they are often found in children and generally disappear by age 10 in boys and age 5 in girls. Persistence beyond these ages should be viewed with suspicion as possible osteochondritis dissecans.

Osteochondral fractures are the result of a traumatic fracture involving a living piece of subchondral bone and the overlying articular cartilage. These lesions involve and cross the margin of the lateral femoral condyle while osteochondritis dissecans does not break the lateral margin. Osteochondritis dissecans of the patella is located more centrally and does not involve the articular margin as does an osteochondral fracture.

Roentgenographically, steroid osteochondritis dissecans resembles osteochondritis dissecans. Patients taking steroids may develop this condition after oral administration or following repeated injections of steroid into the knee. The history of steroid administration is extremely helpful in this diagnosis.

Osteonecrosis or osteochondritis dissecans of the elderly usually involves the femoral condyles. It is probably associated with a torn meniscus which produces repeated microtraumas to the area resulting in the development of an ischemic bone fragment.

Roentgenographically, the notch or tunnel view is particularly helpful, especially when the lesion is located at the classic site. In some instances multiple views or tomograms may be necessary to delineate the lesion clearly.

Suprapatellar Plica

A condition creating internal derangement of the knee, but not as common as those just discussed, is a snapping suprapatellar plica. The suprapatellar plica is a fold of synovial tissue separating the suprapatellar bursa from the suprapatellar pouch. It can create a complete diaphragm or allow a communication between the suprapatellar pouch and bursa, and, in this latter situation, the synovial fold is referred to as a suprapatellar plica. The plica starts laterally originating from the undersurface of the quadriceps tendon and then courses medially across the joint to curve distally medial to the patella and inserts into the synovium covering the fat pad. It can become taut, as it is pulled over the superior margin of the medial femoral condyle with flexing the knee. With chronic irritation from impingement between the femoral condyle and patella, the plica becomes thickened and fibrotic. The patients complain of pain and swelling frequently accompanied by catching, snapping, or clicking which resembles many other types of internal derangement.

On physical examination the plica can be felt snapping across the medial and sometimes lateral femoral condyle proximal to the superior pole of the patella as the knee is flexed. A thickened cord-like structure can sometimes be palpated. Often the snapping sensation is ill-defined and may even occur with performance of the McMurray test, thus giving rise to suspicion of a torn meniscus. Chondromalacia of the patella usually accompanies this condition, and it must be differentiated from a loose body or subluxation of the patella.

Infrapatellar Fat Pad Lesions

Another condition not frequently encountered but nevertheless one that must be taken into consideration concerns lesions of the infrapatellar fat pad. The fat pad is interarticular but extrasynovial. It has a strand of tissue connecting it to the intercondylar area of the femur called the ligamentum mucosum which, in turn, has two extensions medially and laterally called the alar ligaments. Smillie emphasized the importance of the infrapatellar fat pad as a source of anterior joint pain. Any condition creating compression of the fat pad anteriorly, either endogenous to the fat pad itself creating enlargement or exogenous encroaching upon the fat pad space, may result in irritation of the overlying synovial membrane. Etiological factors to consider are direct trauma to the fat pad with subsequent swelling secondary to hemorrhage; edema of the fat pad, as might be found in premenstrual women with water retention syndrome; a space-occupying lesion of the fat pad; compromise of the anterior compartment by a displaced bucket-handle tear of the medial meniscus; or osteoarthritic changes anteriorly in the joint with spur formation reducing the space. There also appears to be some relationship to genu recurvatum which diminishes the anterior compartment space and may result in small fronds or villi of the synovial membrane becoming impinged with extension of the knee.

The clinical feature of an anterior fat pad lesion is one of anterior knee pain usually of long duration. This must be differentiated from chondromalacia of the patella, patellar tendon tendinitis, Osgood-Schlatter's disease, and lesions involving the anterior one half of the menisci. Pain is the most outstanding clinical complaint and is usually related to activity and relieved by rest, as is chondromalacia. Women may note some relief by wearing high heeled shoes which keeps the knee in slight flexion, thus relieving any impingement caused by full extension.

Swelling may be present in some instances, and there may be repeated effusions of the joint with activity. The patient may have also noted that there is generalized tenderness anteriorly about the patellar tendon. Generally speaking, however, the tenderness in this condition is well localized to the patellar tendon itself or the fat pad on either side but not directly over the joint line, as one would find with meniscal lesions. It can usually be differentiated from chondromalacia of the patella which has facet tenderness medially or laterally along with crepitation retropatellarly. In "jumper's knee" the tenderness is discreet over the distal pole of the patella, and in Osgood-Schlatter's disease prominence and tenderness of the tibial tubercle are evident. Recurrent impingement of a synovial tag or frond can produce symptoms of giving way, such as with recurrent subluxation of the patella, meniscal lesions, or transient impingement of a loose body.

THE SWOLLEN KNEE

The swollen knee deals with conditions which create an inflammatory response of the synovial membrane. The basic inflammatory process in each condition is similar and if left to proceed unhindered, eventuates in secondary degenerative changes of the joint. The differential diagnosis of these conditions may seem difficult at the onset but with sufficient information, the diagnosis usually becomes quite apparent.

Traumatic Effusion or Hemarthrosis

Undoubtedly trauma is the most common cause of effusion within the knee joint. It may be caused by such intrinsic factors as internal derangements which damage the synovial membrane, creating bleeding within the joint, or from extrinsic factors, such as a direct blow to the knee or a twisting injury. In most instances of trauma, the history itself is sufficient to make a diagnosis of a traumatic effusion or hemarthrosis. This may not be apparent, however, in the infant or young child who is unable to communicate. It also is not apparent in the adult in whom the effusion is secondary to repeated microtrauma. The microtrauma may be secondary to some activity related to the individual's occupation, such as one requiring repeated use of the knee to perform a certain maneuver, or repeated minor blows to the knee, which to the patient may not seem to be of any significance.

Traumatic Synovitis

The so-called "idiopathic" effusion usually has its beginning as a traumatic synovitis creating a synovial effusion leading to rest and immobility with resultant quadriceps wasting. The loss of muscle protection makes the knees more susceptible to the minor trauma of every day usage with reinjury creating repeated synovial effusions and setting up a vicious cycle which promotes a chronic synovitis. Clinically, the patient presents with a painful swollen knee held in a semiflexed position, the position of maximum comfort. The suprapatellar pouch may be distended and quite tense. The patella is ballotable, and the knee may be somewhat warm but yet does not give the appearance of a septic joint. Motion is generally resisted because attempts at flexion or extension create more tension within the joint causing pain.

Differentiation of traumatic hemarthrosis from traumatic synovitis can be a diagnostic problem. Generally swelling from a traumatic hemarthrosis begins within a few minutes after the injury while a traumatic synovial effusion begins several hours after the injury and progresses more slowly. The aspiration of blood from the joint confirms a traumatic hemarthrosis, and fat globules floating in the blood indicate an interarticular fracture as well. A traumatic synovial effusion, on the other hand, may have essentially normal appearing synovial fluid, although in some instances it may be slightly tinged with blood. The joint is somewhat warmer than usual to the touch but yet does not have the warmth nor redness of the skin found with an acute septic arthritis.

Rheumatoid Arthritis

Adult rheumatoid arthritis is a generalized, systemic disease with joint involvement characterized by a nonsuppurative inflammation of the synovial membrane. The knee is the most frequently involved large joint. Generally, multiple joints are involved and characteristically in a symmetrical fashion. Females are more frequently affected than males, and the onset in adults is generally between 30 and 45 years of age; however, rheumatoid arthritis can be found in any age group. The onset may be spontaneous or insidious. An acute onset is often accompanied by polyarticular involvement with fever, malaise, fatigue, and multiple swollen, painful joints. Clinically, at the onset, the knee is warm, swollen, and painful with a mild to moderate effusion and is held in a semiflexed position. Although warm to touch, the overlying skin is not erythematous. Quadriceps atrophy and weakness appear early. Palpation of the joint reveals a boggy sensation secondary to synovitis, and a fine crepitance is felt with motion.

Joint involvement may range from transient synovitis with mild discomfort and disability to complete joint destruction in the more extreme cases. Chronic synovitis eventually promotes secondary changes with joint deformity and instability ensuing. The mechanics of the joint are disrupted causing abnormal forces which enhance further secondary degenerative changes. Typically, the knee assumes a valgus deformity with external tibial rotation (Fig. 11-40). Crepitation is quite apparent with joint motion; this is caused by the bone-on-bone contact following the loss of articular cartilage. The patella can assume a subluxed position overhanging the lateral femoral condyle with marked retropatellar crepitation on motion. Instability and deformity may become so severe that the patient is incapable of weight-bearing on the joint.

There is no specific laboratory test diagnostic of rheumatoid arthritis. The rheumatoid factor detected by latex fixation or sensitized sheep cell agglutination test is positive in some 70 to 80 percent of established adult cases, but the test is not specific. It may be positive with infectious hepatitis, subacute bacterial endocarditis, chronic pulmonary tuberculosis, and some leukemias, to mention only a few. The erythrocyte sedimentation rate is generally elevated, but this test is nonspecific. The C-reactive protein sometimes is positive, and the patients generally have a secondary hypochromic, normocytic anemia.

Examination of the synovial fluid generally reveals it to be somewhat cloudy forming a very poor mucin clot, and there is a lowered glucose level (see Table 1-2). The rheumatoid factor may be present. Total complement is depressed, but this is also true with systemic lupus erythematosus. The leukocyte count is usually elevated, but the differential count reveals fewer polymorphonuclear leukocytes than septic arthritis.

The early roentgenographic findings are simply those of soft tissue swelling, capsular distention, and periarticular osteoporosis. Once established, subchondral erosions at the capsular junction are seen. Later typical changes of secondary degenerative arthritis are noted with joint space narrowing and marginal osteophyte formation.

Juvenile Rheumatoid Arthritis. The juvenile form of rheumatoid arthritis is more common in

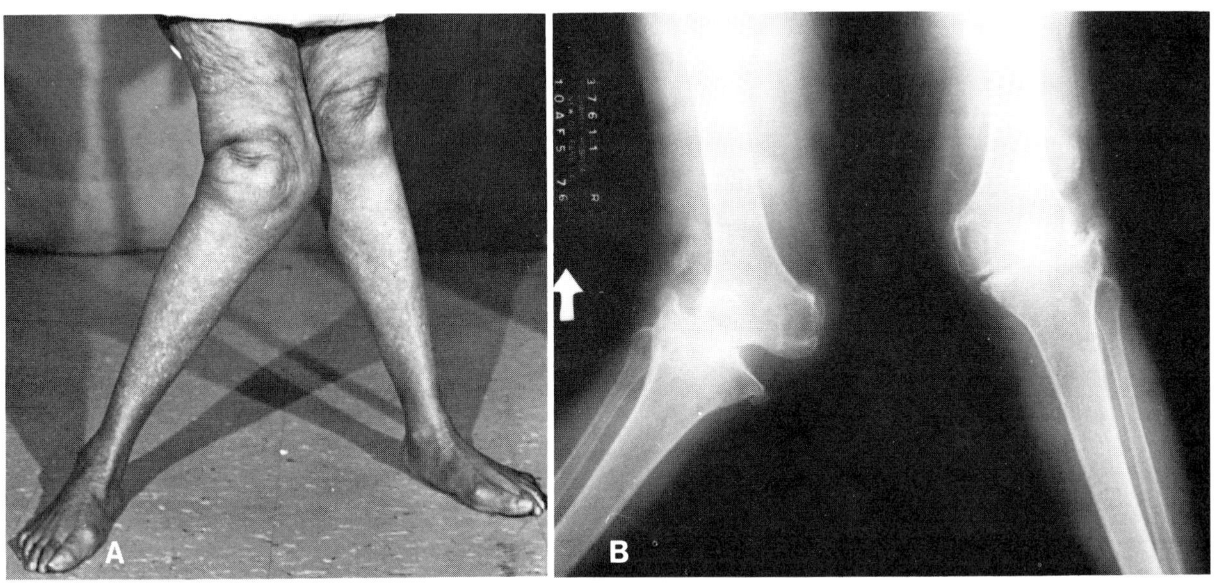

Fig. 11-40. (*A*) Valgus deformity of the knee in a patient with rheumatoid arthritis. (*B*) Weight bearing anteroposterior roentgenogram of same patient. (Courtesy R. D. D'Ambrosia.)

girls than boys. The incidence is greatest between ages 2 and 4, with over 50 percent of the patients having their onset before the fourth year. It is characterized by involvement of a few large joints. The onset is usually insidious with swelling, stiffness, and pain. Overgrowth of a limb may result from the chronic synovitis. In general, the clinical course with this type of involvement is rather benign, and in most patients the duration of the process is less than two years, but it can become chronic in some cases.

It can occur very acutely with severe systemic manifestations and is known as Felty's syndrome. It generally runs a stormy course with acute exacerbations lasting for weeks to months with variable periods of partial remissions. In some patients, the disease may progress relentlessly to total disability.

Laboratory findings are generally similar to that in the adult except that the rheumatoid factor is present in less than 20 percent of the children. It is important to remember that there are no specific diagnostic laboratory findings.

Monoarticular Arthritis. The monoarticular (pauciarticular) form of the disease is difficult to differentiate from a traumatic arthritis in the early stages. Its presentation as an acute inflammatory process makes it difficult to differentiate from acute suppurative arthritis, gout, or pseudogout. There may be fever and signs and symptoms of systemic illness which further complicate the differential diagnosis. In rheumatoid arthritis, however, the febrile course is not as elevated, and the knee is not as warm nor quite as tender.

In the early stages, the differentiation between a traumatic synovitis and rheumatoid arthritis is probably not so important since the general treatment is much the same, but this is not the case with an acute suppurative arthritis which demands immediate institution of appropriate antibiotic therapy and frequently incision and drainage. Joint aspiration with stains and cultures will usually differentiate suppurative arthritis from rheumatoid arthritis. It is important to remember that 25 percent of patients with monoarticular arthritis develop iridocyclitis during the course of their disease which is chronic and may progress to permanent ocular damage.

Acute Suppurative Arthritis

Acute suppurative arthritis is an inflammatory process secondary to a bacterial invasion. It can occur in any age group but is most common at age one or two, with males predominating over females. The hip joint is the most commonly involved, but it frequently occurs in the knee. Staphylococcus aureus is the usual organism with the bacteria gaining entrance hematogenously from a distant focus of infection, by direct extension from a nearby infection, such as osteomyelitis of the distal femur or proximal tibia, or by direct introduction into the knee joint from an injury. In the infant, umbilical sepsis with a subsequent septicemia may hematogenously seed the knee joint. Otitis media, furunculosis, and pneumonia commonly precede a septic joint.

Clinically, the onset is usually acute with a febrile course accompanied by pain and swelling. The involved joint becomes tense, warm, and the overlying skin erythematous. If the patient is still able to walk, he does so with an antalgic gait. As with other inflammatory processes, the joint is held in a moderate degree of flexion, a position of relative comfort, and the joint is diffusely tender. The patient resists active or passive motion. The diagnosis is usually confirmed with joint aspiration. The synovial fluid is usually turbid and purulent appearing (see Table 1-2). The total white count is markedly elevated to 60,000 or more and has a high polymorphonuclear leukocyte count. The joint fluid glucose and the mucin clot are decreased. A specimen should be submitted for culture and sensitivities and also a gram stain done immediately which may help select the appropriate antibiotic.

Initially, roentgenographic findings are nonspecific, showing a distended joint capsule with fluid. Later bone atrophy appears and if the articular cartilage has been involved, joint space narrowing will be evident.

Osteomyelitis of Distal Femur or Proximal Tibia

In children, osteomyelitis commonly involves the metaphyseal area of the distal femur and proximal tibia and is easily confused with a septic joint. The systemic course is similar, and frequently there is joint effusion with osteomyelitis due to the proximity of the joint. The joint is not as tender with osteomyelitis as with septic arthritis nor is it quite as painful to move. The maximum area of tenderness in osteomyelitis is over the distal femoral metaphysis or proximal tibial metaphysis rather than over the joint, and the entire limb is rather swollen as opposed to just the joint with septic arthritis. Aspiration of a swollen joint accompanying an osteomyelitis will generally reveal clear synovial fluid without a significantly elevated leukocyte count. When differentiating osteomyelitis from a septic joint, the joint should be aspirated *before* attempting to aspirate the metaphyseal areas so that there is no contamination of the joint.

Rheumatic Fever

Rheumatic fever may be easily confused with septic arthritis in the early stages; however, the joint involvement is usually fleeting and subsequent characteristic cardiac changes will help differentiate it from a suppurative joint. The reader is referred to Chapter 10.

Gonococcal Arthritis

A septic knee joint can be caused by a variety of other organisms aside from Staphylococcus aureus, and one which should be considered, although it has not been a frequent offender in the recent past, is that of gonococcal arthritis. Gonorrhea is increasing in our country so the incidence of gonococcal arthritis will probably rise in the future. This usually takes the form of a polyarthritis but may be limited to one joint. The onset is usually around ten days following a urethritis. The joint becomes swollen, painful, and warm. A history of gonorrhea aids in making the diagnosis, but definitive diagnosis is dependent upon joint aspiration and culture of gonococcus although it is often difficult to culture gonococcus from the fluid.

Gout

Gout and pseudogout characteristically present as an acutely painful, swollen, warm knee joint in the adult. Gout typically has its onset in the middle aged or elderly adult male. About 50 percent of the patients have a family history of gout and male members of the family have serum uric acid levels slightly above normal for their age. The presence of hyperuricemia alone does not mean that gout is clinically manifest in the subject. The onset of an attack of gout is characteristically associated with overeating, particularly foods rich in nuclear proteins. It also occurs following injestion of alcoholic beverages. Typically the onset is with intense pain often accompanied by a mild fever much like a septic arthritis. The involved joint is exquisitely tender and becomes rapidly swollen. The skin appears rather purplish red and shiny. Although the great toe has classically been implicated as the site of initial involvement, other joints, such as the knee, may be the initial site. A dramatic response to colchicine aids in the diagnosis.

Joint aspirate reveals a cloudy synovial fluid with poor mucin clot and slight leukocytosis (see Table 1-2). The diagnosis is confirmed if urate crystals are found in the fluid by examining the aspirate under a polarized light microscope which reveals strongly negative birefringent monosodium urate crystals of gout. Serum uric acid levels are often elevated.

Early radiological examination is not diagnostic, but with the development of chronic gouty arthritis, marked destructive changes in the joint may occur. Although there are no characteristic roentgenographic findings which occur in the knee joint, small punched out areas, about 5 mm. in diameter, may appear in the subchondral bone.

Chondrocalcinosis

Pseudogout or chondrocalcinosis is a crystal synovitis clinically similar to gout but caused by the precipitation of calcium pyrophosphate in the joint as opposed to sodium urate crystals and also pressure from joint distention. Roentgenographic examination may prove to be definitive in the diagnosis since the calcium pyrophosphate crystals are radiopaque, and calcification of the menisci, articular cartilage, or synovial membrane may be present (Fig. 11-41). The diagnosis can generally be made readily upon examination of joint aspirate with the polarized light microscope, revealing weakly positive birefringent calcium pyrophosphate crystals of pseudogout.

Hemophilia

Hemophilia is a hereditary coagulation defect due to lack of coagulation Factors VIII, IX, or XI. Recurrent hemarthrosis in the knee joint is common in this condition and, at times, is precipitated by relatively minor trauma or occurs spontaneously. The joint becomes grossly distended with blood, and the bleeding continues until the hydrostatic pressure of the blood within the joint acts as a tamponade and prevents further bleeding. These joints become grossly swollen and painful. Repeated bleeding into a

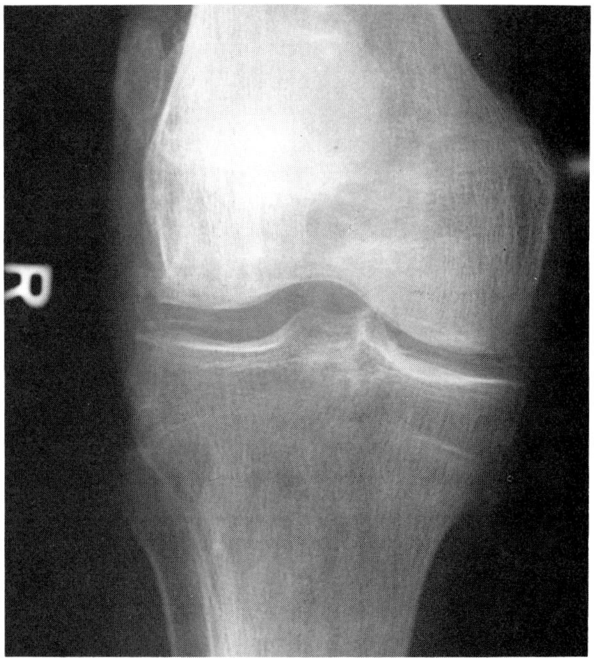

Fig. 11-41. Calcification of meniscus in chondrocalcinosis. (Courtesy R. D. D'Ambrosia.)

joint may result in a bony overgrowth due to increased circulation about the epiphyseal plate and epiphysis.

Roentgenographically, there is soft tissue swelling about the joint secondary to capsular distention. With repeated bleeding, chronic synovitis ensues with bony osteoporosis, subchondral cysts, and narrowing of the joint space. The eventual consequence is fibrous ankylosis of the joint for the poorly managed or intractable cases. See also Chapter 10.

MALALIGNMENT

Alignment problems are either torsional with rotational deformities or angular. In the child abnormal forces or pressures applied to the bone result in disturbances in growth particularly if the epiphyseal plate is affected. In the adult malalignment is characteristic of secondary degenerative arthritis involving a single compartment of the knee from a disease process, such as rheumatoid arthritis, or trauma creating a defect in the joint surfaces with subsequent angular deformity. Torsional deformities as well as angular deformities anywhere in the lower extremity can affect knee function.

Etiological factors creating torsional forces with subsequent deformities in the child are persistent fetal alignment, heredity, and certain habitual positions in sitting or sleeping. In the adult external tibial rotation is often seen in rheumatoid arthritis and can be caused iatrogenically by transferring a tibial tubercle too far medially when this procedure is done to correct recurrent dislocation or subluxation of the patella.

Rotational Deformities

Femoral torsion or femoral neck anteversion can create an alignment problem of the entire extremity. Children with anteversion of the neck of the femur have a toed-in gait and are usually brought to the orthopaedist because they walk "pidgeon-toed." The knees and the patellae are rotated inward, and the child's gait may be clumsy. There is significantly more internal hip rotation than external. When these children stand, they appear to be somewhat bowlegged with the patellae turned toward each other or facing inward. If the patellae are positioned straight ahead, the apparent bowing in the leg disappears, but the feet are externally rotated. This is not an unusual clinical picture associated with chondromalacia of the patella. These children develop a valgus deformity of the heel, pronation of the foot, and lateral torsion of the tibia which are secondary changes in an attempt to accommodate to the hip anteversion.

Tibial Torsion. Torsional deformity of the tibia can likewise affect knee function. The tibia may be internally or externally rotated. It is estimated by having the patient sit with the legs dangling over the edge of the examining table and noting the relative relationship of the medial and lateral malleolus in relation to the transcondylar plane of the tibial plateau. Most babies have slight external tibial torsion which gradually increases at about 1.3 degrees per year until adulthood when the normal tibial torsion is about 20 to 25 degrees external torsion. Internal tibial torsion in the adult is less than 5 percent.

Internal tibial torsion in the child is generally characterized by a toed-in position when walking or standing. The deformity becomes more noticeable when the child first begins to walk. On examination the medial malleolus is located posterior to the lateral malleolus, and the involvement is generally bilateral.

Angular Deformities

Developmental. Angular deformities of the lower extremities must be carefully considered in light of the evolutionary changes which take place as the child grows. The newborn has a moderate degree of genu varum which slowly diminishes in the first two years and then the legs become quite straight. At about two and one-half years a significant majority will progress to physiological genu valgum (Fig. 11-42) and by the age of seven, 95 percent of the genu valgum deformities will disappear. Roentgenographic evidence consistent with developmental genu varum, which generally corrects itself, is typified by a medial tilting of the transverse plane of the knee and the ankle joint; thickened medial cortices of the tibia and femur; medial angulation of the tibia; normal appearance of the epiphyseal line and the epiphysis; and the involvement is generally symmetrical. If deformity at the tibia is asymmetrical, other causes should be sought. Persistent severe genu valgum with an intermalleolar distance greater than 9 or 10 cm. persisting into adolescence may well demand corrective measures.

Epiphyseal Plate Injury. Angular deformity can occur in children secondary to injury of the epiphyseal plate of the distal part of the femur or proximal end of the tibia. A discrepancy of growth occurring on either side of the epiphyseal plate causes angulation with continued growth. Fractures involving the epiphyseal plate are generally quite evident, and the child should be followed for several months to determine whether or not any growth disturbance ensues. Compression injury of the epiphyseal plate is not apparent on roentgenograms but should be suspected by the nature of the injury. If suspected, the patient should be followed for several months to determine if any growth disturbance occurs.

Tibia Vara. A nondevelopmental type of genu varum involving a disturbance at the medial side of the proximal tibial epiphyseal plate is tibia vara (Blount's disease) or osteochondrosis deformans tibiae. The etiology of this process is unknown. There is progressive medial angulation of the tibia secondary to the disturbance in growth and ossification of the medial portion of the proximal tibial epiphysis. Two variations have been described, an infantile and an adolescent type, with the infantile being the more severe form creating greater deformity and more likely requiring operative intervention. At the onset, the infantile type may be difficult to differentiate from developmental genu varum. Involvement is more likely to be bilateral, however, and is characterized by progressive bowing without the spontaneous correction normally observed. Associated findings are obesity, internal tibial torsion, and pronation of the feet.

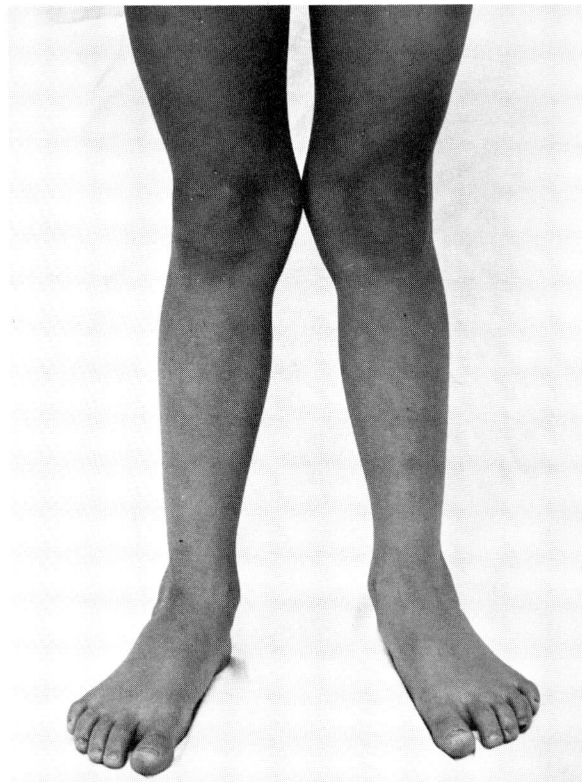

Fig. 11-42. Physiological genu valgum. This deformity will usually correct by age seven. (Courtesy R. D. D'Ambrosia.)

The adolescent type has its onset between 8 and 13 years of age, and a vast majority demonstrate unilateral involvement rather than bilateral. The deformity is generally not as marked as the infantile type, and the associated findings of obesity, internal tibial torsion, and foot pronation are not found. Adolescent tibia vara may well be due to arrest of the epiphyseal plate medially while the infantile type is considered a dysplasia of growth. The adolescent variety may also demonstrate a significant shortening in leg length, whereas this is very slight in the infantile type. Pain and tenderness over the medial metaphyseal area of the proximal tibia are present in the adolescent type and absent in the infantile type.

Characteristic roentgenographic features are present during progressive stages of the infantile variety. The changes take place in the medial epiphyseal and metaphyseal areas (Fig. 11-43). There is acute medial tibial angulation in the metaphyseal area along with development of a medial beak. Irregular areas of ossification appear in the epiphyseal plate, and the epiphysis becomes wedged medially. The beak then fragments and eventually a step-off occurs medially in the metaphyseal area which is filled in by cartilage with some narrowing of the epiphyseal plate, producing a very distinct downward slope of the metaphysis medially. This gives the appearance that the medial epiphyseal cartilage has been bent downward into the depressed area. There is still a propensity for spontaneous correction during the early stages up to age 10. With progression, however, the step-off in the medial metaphysis becomes more apparent, and the medial epiphysis becomes more wedge-shaped. The medial half of the epiphysis displays delayed ossification and becomes angulated distally creating a distinct medial slope to the joint. During the later stages, the epiphyseal plate seems to separate the downward angulated portion of the epiphysis from the more normally formed lateral portion. This gives the appearance of two epiphyses. The entire medial articular surface of the joint slopes distally. By age 13, the two portions of the deformed epiphysis unite and the changes are irrevocable.

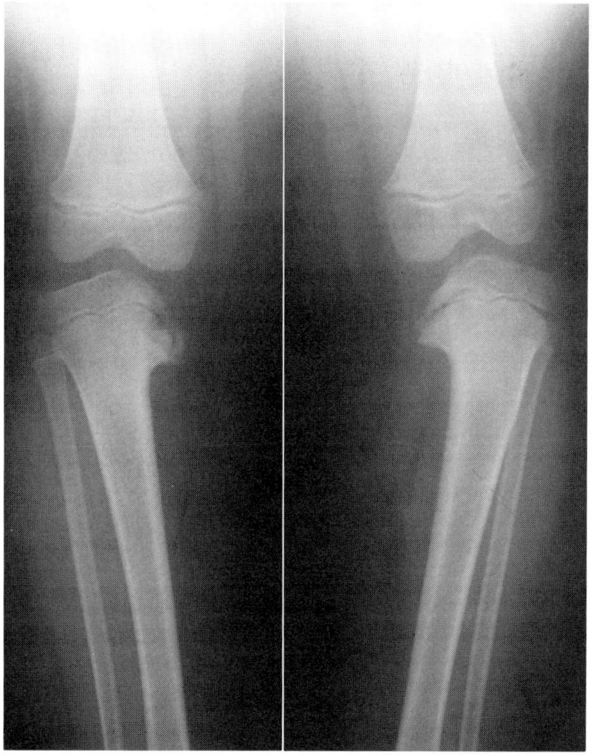

Fig. 11-43. Bilateral Blount's disease caused by a disturbance at the medial epiphyseal plate. Acute medial tibial angulation occurs in the metaphysis with development of a characteristic medial beak. (Courtesy R. D. D'Ambrosia.)

Rickets. Genu valgum or genu varum deformities of the knees in children may occur with a simple vitamin D deficiency, rickets. This disease is no longer common but can occassionally occur in destitute areas where starvation and poor diet are common or in parts of our society where fadish diets deficient in vitamin D may be in vogue. Vitamin D is essential for normal calcium and phosphorus metabolism, and without it there is deficient calcification at the zone of provisional calcification. This results in increased thickness of the epiphyseal plate and failure of ossification of osteoid tissue.

Rickets can be caused by a dietary deficiency or defective absorption of vitamin D, such as in celiac disease. It may also be secondary to renal tubular insufficiency with inadequate resorption of phosphorus resulting in hypophosphatemic vitamin D refractory rickets which has several variations biochemically.

The abnormally formed tissue of rickets in the growing skeleton bends under the stress of weight-bearing creating the typical deformities of genu varum or genu valgum. Greenstick fractures of the femur and tibia can occur. Besides the long bone deformities there is progressive enlargement of the ankle, knees, and wrists; pidgeon-breast deformity; delayed developmental landmarks; muscular weakness; rib deformities; and craniotabes.

Roentgenogically, the epiphyseal plate becomes thickened and hazy while the metaphysis adjacent to the epiphyseal plate displays a brush-like appearance. The epiphyses become widened, and the diaphyses of the long bones become rarified with wide spaces between the bony trabeculae (Fig. 11-44).

The various types of rickets can be differentiated biochemically. In the vitamin D deficient form of rickets, the serum calcium may be low or normal but phosphorus is low and alkaline phosphatase is high. Vitamin D resistance rickets secondary to inadequate resorption of phosphorus reveals a normal calcium, low phosphorus, high alkaline phosphatase, thus making the biochemical findings very similar to vitamin D deficient rickets. The primary point in differential diagnosis is that it does not respond to normal doses of vitamin D but requires unusually high dosages. The other forms of rickets secondary to renal tubular insufficiency can be differentiated by the detection of abnormal animo acids in the urine.

Degenerative Arthritis. Although the vast majority of angular or torsional deformities during the growth period are spontaneously corrected, some persist into adulthood which with time may lead to secondary osteoarthrosis of the knee because of abnormal forces due to the altered mechanics.

Degenerative arthritis or osteoarthritis is probably the most common cause of angular deformities in the adult, and the knee is the most commonly involved joint. Primary osteoarthrosis is defined as that which has no known etiology while secondary osteoarthrosis can be traced to abnormal mechanics of the joint. The abnormal knee mechanics produce secondary changes in the articular cartilage, subchondral bone, and supportive structures of the knee. There is some evidence that even osteoarthritis probably is a physiological response to repetitive, longitudinal impulse loading of the joint. Degenerative arthritis may involve either the medial or lateral compartment of the knee or the patellofemoral joint or be panarticular, involving all three areas.

An angular deformity of only 10 degrees increases the weight-bearing per unit area in the knee by a factor of three. A varus deformity of the knee results in increased medial compartment forces which can subsequently lead to a horizontal cleavage lesion of the medial meniscus. This produces degenerative changes in the articular cartilage enhancing the varus deformity of the knee, thus leading to further degenerative changes involving the subchondral bone. These changes eventually affect the ligamentous structures of the knee further enhancing the problem. The clinical features of primary and secondary osteoarthritis are the same. The primary complaint is usually pain which may be muscular, capsular, or perhaps venous in origin. The muscles of the thigh, particularly the quadriceps become painful as a fixed flexion contracture of the knee develops

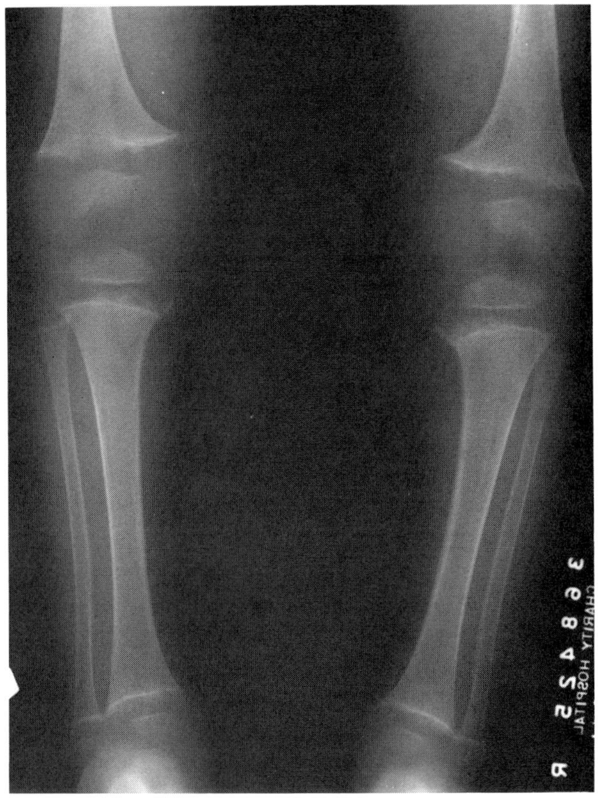

Fig. 11-44. Anteroposterior roentgenogram of a four-year-old male who presented with marked bowing of the legs. The epiphyseal plate is thickened and hazy while the metaphysis has a brush-like appearance characteristic of rickets. (Courtesy R. D. D'Ambrosia.)

requiring more muscular effort for knee stability. The capsular pain is from irritation of the capsule and synovium from rubbing on osteophytes and rough irregular surfaces. Increased venous pressure in the medullary canal of the proximal tibia is also thought to be a cause of pain. It is postulated that the pain relief following proximal tibial osteotomy is due to disruption of the vascular channels which reduces the venous pressure in the area.

Stiffness is also a common complaint secondary to several factors, including muscle weakness, synovitis, increased frictional forces within the joint, and perhaps swelling. As the deformity increases there is loss of joint flexion with subsequent development of a fixed flexion contracture secondary to bony blockage from deformity of the articular surfaces. The loss of articular cartilage reducing the joint space and actual bony deformity increases the ligamentous laxity.

This is not due to stretching of the ligamentous structures but from a relative lengthening of the ligaments following articular cartilage (joint space) loss. The tibial plateau often assumes a cup-shape deformity as the femoral condyle sinks into it.

An insecure knee results in giving way episodes which may be secondary to muscle fatigue, transient severe pain secondary to minor trauma which may be the result of a misstep, loose bodies, or momentary impingement of degenerated menisci. The pain is aggravated with activity or weight-bearing, but occasionally there is even pain at rest, particularly if the knee is held in one position for a prolonged period of time. When the patient rises, his knee is stiff and painful; this is relieved after motion but again becomes painful once the weight-bearing tolerance of the joint is exceeded by prolonged walking or standing.

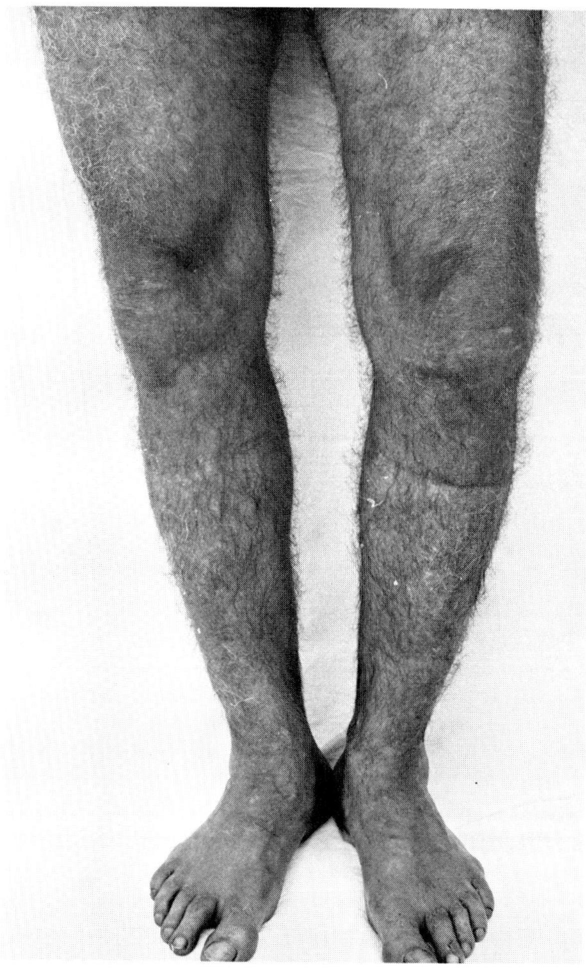

Fig. 11-45. Degenerative arthritis of the left knee. The medial compartment is more involved in this man with less of the medial joint space and resultant genu varum. Genu varum is more common than genu valgum in osteoarthritis. (Courtesy R. D. D'Ambrosia.)

The most frequent alteration in alignment of the osteoarthritic knee is a varus deformity (Fig. 11-45). This is often associated with internal tibial torsion of the tibia. People with interal tibial torsion attempt to walk with their feet straight ahead by externally rotating the tibia. This results in increased forces in the medial compartment of the knee which create a degenerative lesion of the medial meniscus and subsequent degenerative changes of the medial compartment, but later panarticular. Torsional malalignment also produces patellofemoral arthritis and subsequent abnormal mechanics of the extensor mechanism.

Any condition resulting in a loss of rotation at the hip, such as a hip fusion, will eliminate the screw home mechanism of the knee and result in vastus medialis obliquus atrophy, lateral tibial rotation, increased ligamentous laxity of the knee, and eventual genu valgum deformity. The abnormal mechanics of this combination eventually produces degenerative changes in the knee.

A flexed knee gait often results from a leg length discrepancy in the opposite shorter extremity not compensated for with a built up shoe. The patient, therefore, walks with the uninvolved extremity flexed at the knee and this results in increased patellofemoral joint forces leading to excessive wear and degenerative changes in the joint.

Examination of the extensor mechanism in an osteoarthritic knee reveals quadriceps atrophy, parapatellar tenderness, retropatellar pain with compression, and retropatellar crepitation. If genu valgum is present lateral subluxation of the patella is not unusual.

In unicompartmental degenerative arthritis, joint compression and motion with the appropriate varus or valgus stress to the knee elicits pain. In addition, crepitation is palpable over the involved side. Marginal osteophytes along the femoral condyles are also palpable and are sites of capsular tenderness due to local irritation.

The roentgenographic examination is helpful in assessing the degree of degenerative changes in the knee. It should be remembered, however, that changes in the articular cartilage are quite extensive before bony changes are first seen on roentgenogram. Standing or weight-bearing views of the knee are essential. A non-weight-bearing anteroposterior view of the knee may demonstrate good joint space while a standing or weight-bearing view of the same knee will reveal diminished cartilage (joint) space. In addition to the routine four views of the knee, varus and valgus stress roentgenograms are valuable in the unicompartmental type of arthritis to assess adequately the joint space of the opposite compartment. As an example, weight-bearing views of the knee with genu varum will show diminished medial joint space while the lateral compartment may appear to have good joint space. With valgus stress of the knee, however, the lateral compartment is loaded and may also show diminished joint space secondary to articular cartilage wear. This information is particularly helpful when considering a tibial osteotomy. The typical roentgenographic changes with established degenerative arthritis of the knee are subchondral sclerosis, loss of joint space, marginal spurring, bony deformity, and perhaps loose bodies.

Differential Diagnosis of Common Fracture-Dislocations about the Knee

Fractures of the knee include the supracondylar area of the distal femur to the proximal metaphysis of the tibia. They are classified as supracondylar and condylar femoral fractures and fractures of the tibial plateaus, tibial eminence, tibial tubercle, tibial metaphysis, and patellar fractures. Due to the extreme violence often associated with fractures in this region, more than one of these areas may be involved, and many are intraarticular in nature. The propensity for subsequent traumatic arthritis with intraarticular fractures, particularly involving a weight-bearing joint, such as the knee, makes the proper diagnosis and selection of a subsequent course of treatment particularly important.

There is generally a history of severe violence to the knee, with many fractures being caused by vehicular accidents or a fall from a height. The forces involved may be angular with a varus or valgus stress, torsional, compressive, or a combination of the three. Patients complain of pain, swelling, and the inability to bear weight. Patients with severe ligament injury may actually be able to bear weight, but this is seldom true with a knee fracture.

The clinical findings are quite similar regardless of the area fractured, and, thus, the final nature of the injury awaits roentgenographic examination. Swelling, crepitation, tenderness, deformity, and false motion are typical findings. The knee is splinted by the surrounding muscles to resist motion. Hemarthrosis may be present with intraarticular fractures, but if the capsule is ruptured, the extent of the hemarthrosis may be quite minimal. Neurovascular injuries are not frequent but must be considered in order to prevent their disastrous consequences if undiagnosed. Sensation and peripheral pulses are evaluated immediately. Instability may be present and must be differentiated from ligamentous injuries, although both may be present. Specifically, a fracture dislocation of the distal femoral epiphysis in a child must be differentiated from collateral ligament injury with instability. Do not be deceived into assuming that a fracture is not present when the history does not include direct violence to the knee. Indirect forces with the knee being forced into flexion against a vigorously contracting quadriceps can create a fracture, particularly involving the patella or tibial tubercle.

Although one may have a high index of suspicion of a fracture from physical examination, the final determination depends upon adequate roentgenographic examination. Routine anteroposterior and lateral roentgenograms should be acquired as soon as possible, but frequently additional roentgenograms, in nonstandard projections, are necessary to elucidate fully the nature of the fracture.

Supracondylar fractures of the distal femur may be undisplaced, impacted (Fig. 11-46), displaced, or comminuted and, in many instances, are also associated with T or Y fractures of the femoral condyles. Fractures in this area are influenced initially by the forces applied at the time of the injury and secondarily by forces applied from the muscles about the knee. The powerful quadriceps and hamstring muscles have a tendency to create shortening, often driving the femoral shaft down between fractured femoral condyles or displacing it into the suprapatellar pouch. The attachment of the medial and lateral gastrocnemius muscle heads superior to the femoral condyles produces a characteristic deformity, with the distal fragment rotated posteriorly in relation to

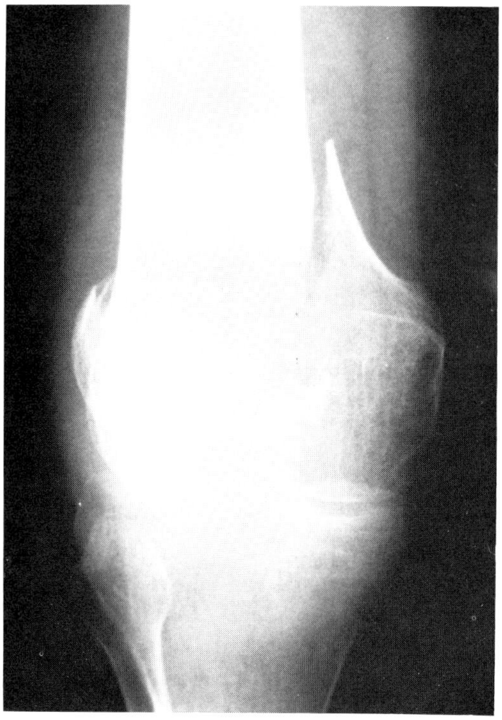

Fig. 11-46. An impacted supracondylar femoral fracture with the shaft driven into the cancellous bone of the femoral condyles. The alignment remained satisfactory.

the proximal fragment. The adductor muscles of the thigh, with their insertions predominately on the proximal fragment, often create a valgus deformity, and there is a tendency for the proximal fragment to rotate externally.

Condylar fractures (Fig. 11-47) of the femur may be in the sagittal or coronal plane and involve one or both condyles. These fractures are intraarticular and, therefore, have a potentially serious consequence as far as future knee function is concerned.

Tibial eminence fractures (Fig. 11-48) most frequently occur in patients before skeletal maturity has been achieved. This fracture is actually an avulsion fracture of the anterior cruciate ligament from its insertion onto the tibia just anterior to the tibial eminences. It is the result of a direct blow to the tibia, forcing it anteriorly or from hyperextension of the knee. The displacement may be very minimal to quite marked with the anterior portion of the avulsion fragment being tilted into an almost vertical position. The fragment displaces proximally and posteriorly in line with the course of the anterior cruciate ligament.

Tibial tubercle fractures (Fig. 11-49) may occur in

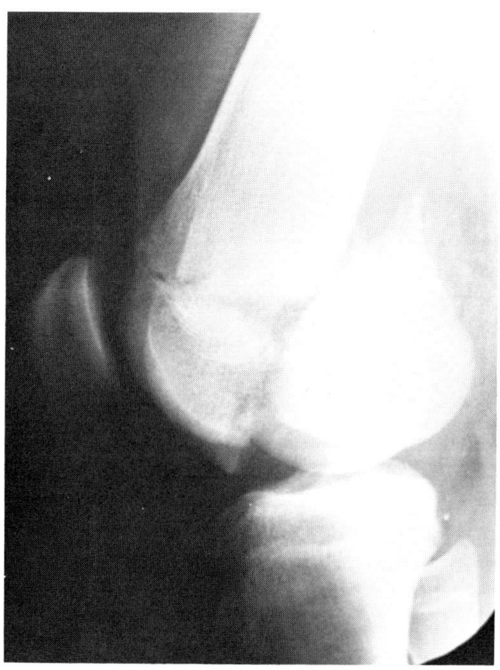

Fig. 11-47. Bilateral condylar fractures of the femur in a teenage girl injured in an auto accident.

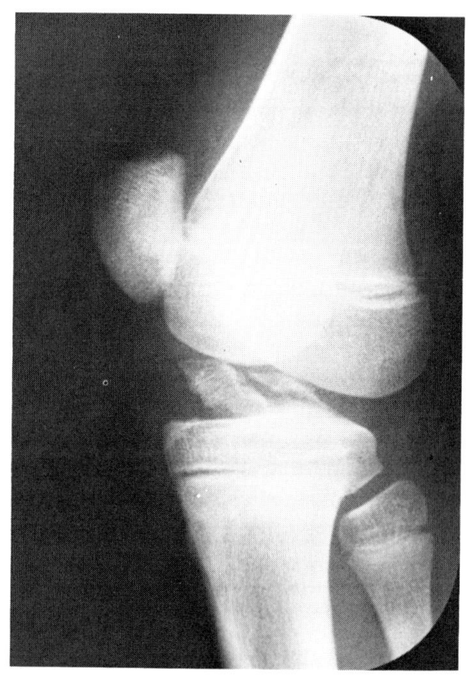

Fig. 11-48. Avulsion fracture of the tibial eminence in a 12-year-old girl injured in a motorbike accident.

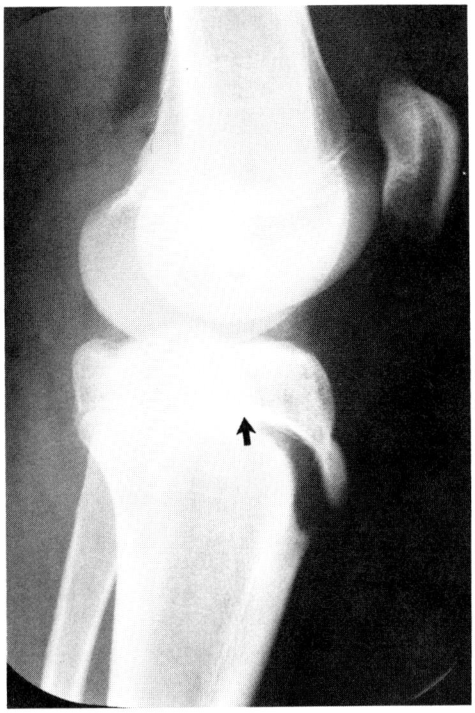

Fig. 11-49. Avulsion fracture of the tibial tubercle.

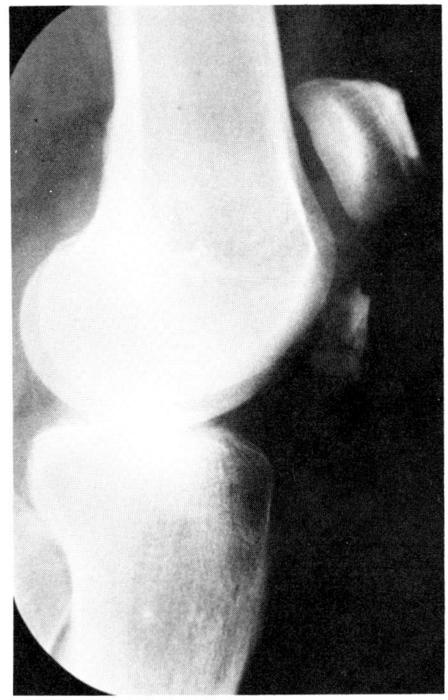

Fig. 11-50. Fracture involving the distal third of the patella in a 55-year-old woman who fell on her knee.

adults but, again, are more likely in the preadolescent or adolescent group and represent an avulsion type fracture, involving the insertion of the patellar ligament onto the tibial tubercle. This type of injury occurs with an extremely vigorous contraction of the quadriceps muscles, as might occur with a misstep or in athletic endeavors, avulsing the tibial tubercle which seems to be the weakest link of the extensor mechanism in this particular age group. Displacement may be very minimal, involving only the tibial tubercle itself, or quite marked with the fracture line extending proximally into the joint.

Patellar fractures (Fig. 11-50) usually are the result of direct violence but may also be caused by indirect forces due to quadriceps contraction. These fractures involve a variety of configurations, with some being very simple transverse fractures with minimal displacement and others having complete displacement, in which case the medial and lateral retinacula are disrupted. With a severe blow, the patella is often badly comminuted, making salvage in some instances impossible. Clinically this condition is typified by acute swelling in the knee secondary to hemarthrosis, and often a defect can be palpated over the patella accompanied by crepitation and tenderness. Knee aspiration will most likely reveal fat globules floating on the blood, indicative of an intra-articular fracture.

Tibial plateau fractures (Fig. 11-51) come in a number of configurations which may be classified as compression, undisplaced, split fracture, split compression fracture, total condylar depression, and a comminuted fracture. The anteroposterior view of a tibial plateau fracture should be taken at an angle of 115 degrees to a line drawn along the anterior crest of the tibia, thus reducing distortion of the tibial plateau to a minimum and giving a more accurate picture of fracture-fragment relationships (Fig. 11-52 A, B). Due to the high incidence of collateral ligament injuries associated with tibial plateau fractures, varus and valgus stress views under general anesthesia should be performed to establish the integrity of the collateral ligamentous structures. Widening of the medial or lateral joint space with varus or valgus stress implicates a rupture of the collateral ligament. If there is some question as to whether or not the widening is significant, comparable views of the uninjured knee may be taken for comparison.

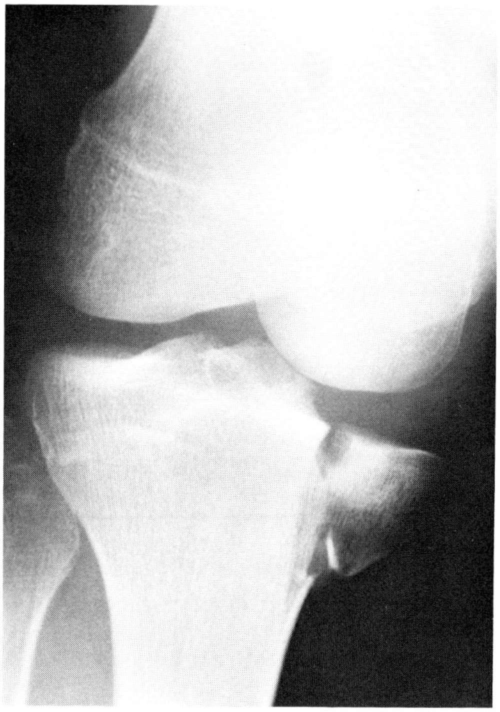

Fig. 11-51. Medial tibial plateau fracture in a 19-year-old gymnast who landed from a vault off balance and on an extended knee.

Meniscal injuries are also associated with tibial plateau fractures. The meniscus may be torn peripherally within its substance or, in some instances, impinged between fracture fragments. If an open reduction of the fracture is not required, the meniscal injury may not be suspected until a later date when the patient begins having typical symptoms.

A femorotibial dislocation is the ultimate in a severe knee sprain. This is the result of violent forces disrupting the ligaments and completely displacing the tibia in relation to the femoral condyles. The titia may move anteriorly, posteriorly, or to either side (Fig. 11-53).

Perhaps the most difficult dislocation to actually diagnose, either clinically or roentgenographically, is a posterolateral dislocation. In this type of dislocation the tibia rotates externally as well as displacing posteriorly in relation to the femoral condyles. The medial femoral condyle may rupture through the medial capsule and become impinged by infolding of the capsular ligament, thus trapping the condyle and making reduction very difficult by closed techniques. The displacement of the tibia in relation to the femoral condyles is not quite as marked as with

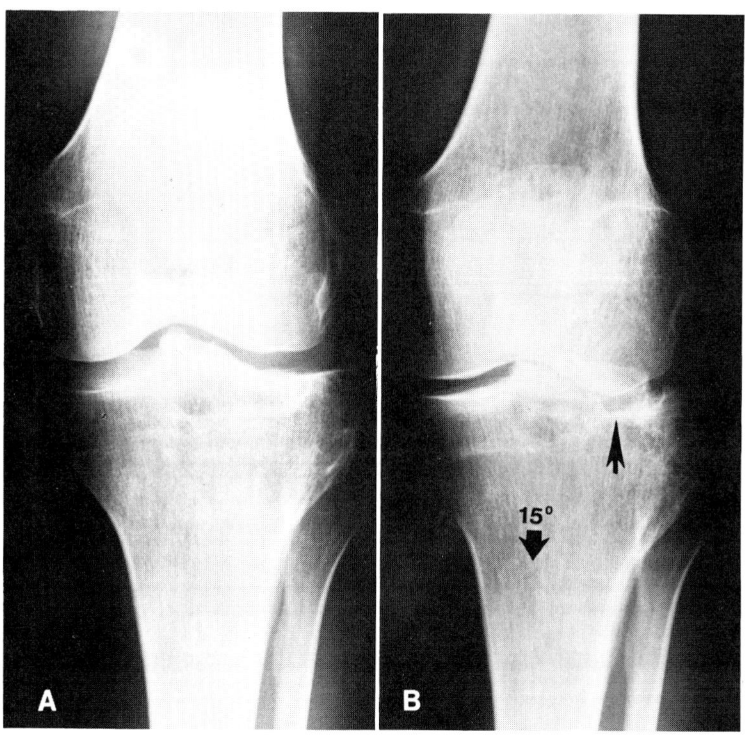

Fig. 11-52. (*A*) Routine AP view of a tibial plateau fracture showing minimal displacement. (*B*) The same fracture but with the x-ray tube angled 115 degrees to the tibial crest. A depression in the central portion of the lateral tibial plateau is revealed.

the other varieties of dislocations, making the diagnosis of a knee dislocation less obvious upon examination. Even with roentgenogram examination the diagnosis is somewhat difficult due to the appearance of the tibia in relation to the femoral condyles. The medial femoral condyle appears to be displaced disproportionately more medially in relation to the tibia than the lateral tibial plateau, laterally in relation to the lateral femoral condyle. This should be the tip off to this particular dislocation. It should also be borne in mind that a peroneal nerve injury has its greatest incidence with this type of dislocation.

A grossly unstable knee with both cruciates torn even though reduced when initially examined, was probably dislocated at the time of injury and spontaneously reduced. Careful early examination will give insight into the pathological condition present and help plan the course of treatment. The importance of assessing the peripheral vascular supply cannot be overstressed. The popliteal artery is frequently injured and even an intact peripheral pulse can be misleading in the early stages. The artery may be damaged and result in a mural thrombus with obliteration of the vascular supply some hours after injury, a potential disaster if unrecognized. Anterior dislocations have the highest incidence of popliteal artery injuries because the popliteal artery is fixed above and below the knee, and marked anterior displacement of the tibia can create a severe stretch injury to the artery.

If the knee is still dislocated when initially examined, the diagnosis is apparent. Peripheral pulses, warmth, and sensation should be immediately investigated. Beware of arterial injury even when encountering a warm foot. Sensory disturbance and paralysis should be looked for, but it may be difficult to differentiate a pure nerve injury from ischemic changes. Once initial roentgenograms and examination have been completed, reduction should be carried out carefully and efficiently. In the event of vascular compromise, reduction should be accomplished as soon as possible. If there should be some question concerning vascular integrity, an arteriogram should be done and preparation made for open exploration, if indicated. Examination of ligamentous instability should be carried out cautiously to avoid redislocation and adding further insult.

When suspecting a knee dislocation one should not assume that there are no associated fractures, and roentgenograms are always mandatory. The presence of abnormal motion on clinical examination must not be interpreted as being indicative of ligamentous instability until roentgenographic examination has eliminated the presence of an associated fracture.

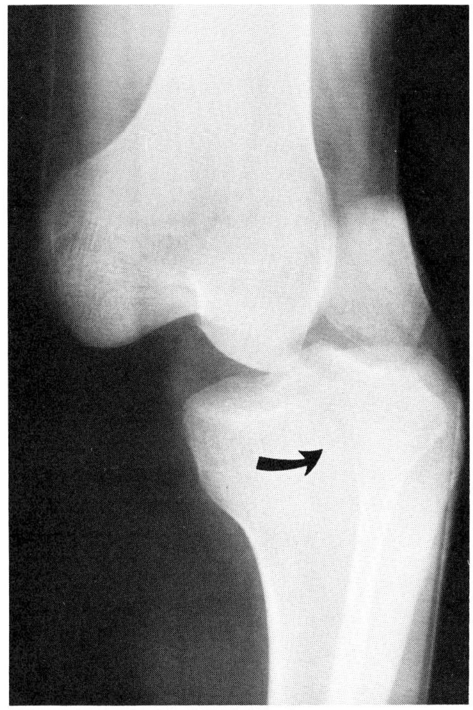

Fig. 11-53. A lateral femorotibial dislocation. In this instance, there were no neurovascular complications. The fibular collateral ligament, arcuate ligament, popliteus tendon, and posterior lateral capsule remained intact while the medial ligaments, posterior medial capsule, cruciates, medial retinaculum, and epicondylar attachment of the iliotibial tract were torn.

SUGGESTED READINGS

1. Andrews, J. R.: The Suprapatellar Plica and Internal Derangement. Given at Am. Acad. Ortho. Surg. Post-grad. Course "The Injured Knee in Sports." Eugene, Oregon, July 1973.
2. Bently, G.: Chondromalacia patella. J. Bone Joint Surg. 52-*A*:221, 1970.
3. Blazina, M. E., Kerlan, R. K., Jobe, F. W., Carter, V. S., and Carlson, G. J.: Jumper's Knee. Orthop. Clin. N. Am. *4*:665, 1973.
4. Brantigan, O. C., and Voshell, A. F.: The mechanics of the ligaments and menisci of the knee joint. J. Bone Joint Surg. 23:44, 1941.
5. Brattstrom, H.: Shape of the intercondylar groove normally

and in recurrent dislocation of the patella. Acta Orthop. Scand. (Suppl.) 68:1, 1964.
6. Furman, W., Marshall, J. L., and Girgis, F. G.: The anterior cruciate ligament. A functional analysis based on postmortem studies. J. Bone Joint Surg. *58-A*:179, 1976.
7. Galway, R. D., Beaupre, A., and McIntosh, D. L.: Pivot shift: A clinical sign of symptomatic anterior cruciate insufficiency. J. Bone Joint, Surg. *54-B*:763, 1972.
8. Hand, W. L., Hand, C. R., and Dunn, A. W.: Avulsion fractures of the tibial tubercle. J. Bone Joint Surg. *53-A*:1579, 1971.
9. Helfet, A. J.: Disorders of the Knee. Philadelphia, J. B. Lippincott Co., 1974.
10. Hohl, M.: Tibial condylar fractures. J. Bone Joint Surg. *49-A*:1455, 1967.
11. Hohl, M., and Larson, R. L.: Fractures and dislocations of the knee. *In* Rockwood, C. A., Jr., and Green, D. P. (eds.): Fractures. vol. II. Philadelphia, J. B. Lippincott Co., 1975.
12. Hollinshead, W. H.: The back and limbs. *In* Anatomy for Surgeons. vol. III. ed. 2. pp. 763–787.
13. Hughston, J. C.: Subluxation of the patella. J. Bone Joint Surg. *50-A*:1003, 1968.
14. Hughston, J. C., and Eilers, A. F.: The role of the posterior oblique ligament in repairs of acute medial (collateral) ligament tears of the knee. J. Bone Joint Surg. *55-A*:923, 1973.
15. Hughston, J. C., Andrews, J. R., Cross, M. J., and Moschi, A.: Classification of knee ligament instabilities, Parts I and II. J. Bone Joint Surg. *58-A*:159, 1976.
16. Jaffe, H. L.: Metabolic, Degenerative, and Inflammatory Diseases of Bones and Joints. Philadelphia, Lea & Febiger, 1972.
17. James, S. L., and Larson, R. L.: Surgical Anatomy of the Knee. Instructional Course Lecture, Am. Acad. Orthop. Surg.
18. Kennedy, J. C.: Complete dislocation of the knee joint. J. Bone Joint Surg. *45-A*:889, 1963.
19. Kennedy, J. C., and Fowler, P. J.: Medial and anterior instability of the knee. An anatomical and clinical study using stress machines. J. Bone Joint Surg. *53-A*:1257, 1971.
20. Kennedy, J. C., Weinberg, H. D., and Wilson, A. S.: The anatomy and function of the anterior cruciate ligament. As determined by clinical and morphological studies. J. Bone Joint Surg. *56-A*:223, 1974.
21. Lee, P., Rooney, P. J., Sturrock, R. D., Kennedy, A. C., and Dick, W. C.: The etiology and pathogenesis of osteoarthrosis: A review. Semin. Arthritis Rheum. 3:189, 1974.
22. Lieb, F. J., and Perry, J.: Quadriceps function. An electromyographic study under isometric conditions. J. Bone Joint Surg. *53-A*:749, 1971.
23. Marshall, J. L., Girgis, F., and Zelco, R. R.: The biceps femoris tendon and its functional significance. J. Bone Joint Surg. *54-A*:1444, 1972.
24. Merchant, A. C., Mercer, R. L., Jacobsen, R. H., and Cool, C. R.: Roentgenographic analysis of patellofemoral congruence. J. Bone Joint Surg. *56-A*:1391, 1974.
25. Moore, T. M., and Harvey, J. T.: Roentgenographic measurement of tibial plateau depression due to fracture. J. Bone Joint Surg. *56-A*:155, 1964.
26. Nicholas, J. A.: The five-one reconstruction for anteromedial instability of the knee. Indications, technique, and the results in fifty-two patients. J. Bone Joint Surg. *55-A*:899, 1973.
27. Nicholas, J. A., Freiberger, R. H., and Killoran, P. J.: Double contrast arthrography of the knee. Its value in the management of two hundred and twenty-five knee derangements. J. Bone Joint Surg. *52-A*:203, 1970.
28. O'Donoghue, D. H.: Surgical treatment of fresh injuries to the major ligaments of the knee. J. Bone Joint Surg. *32-A*:721, 1950.
29. O'Donoghue, D. H.: Treatment of injuries to Athletes. ed. 2. Philadelphia, W. B. Saunders Co., 1970.
30. Outerbridge, R. E.: The etiology of chondromalacia of the patella. J. Bone Joint Surg. *43-B*:752, 1961.
31. Palmer, I.: On the injuries to the ligaments of the knee joint. A clinical study. Acta Chir. Scand. (Suppl.) *53*:8, 1938.
32. Slocum, D. B., Larson, R. L., and James, S. L.: Late reconstruction of ligamentous injuries of the medial compartment of the knee. Clin. Orthop. *100*:23, 1974.
33. Slocum, D. B.: Personal communication.
34. Slocum, D. B., and Larson, R. L.: Rotary Instability of the knee. Its pathogenesis and a clinical test to determine its presence. J. Bone Joint Surg. *50-A*:211, 1968.
35. Smillie, I. S.: Injuries of the Knee Joint. ed. 4. Baltimore, Williams & Wilkins, 1970.
36. Smillie, I. S.: Diseases of the Knee Joint. London, Churchill Livingstone, 1974.
37. Stewart, M. J., Sisk, T. D., and Wallace, S. L., Jr.: Fractures of the distal third of the femur. J. Bone Joint Surg. *48-A*:784, 1966.
38. Tachdjian, M. O.: Pediatric Orthopaedics. Philadelphia, W. B. Saunders Co., 1972.
39. Wang, C. J., and Walker, P. S.: Rotary laxity of the human knee joint. J. Bone Joint Surg. *56-A*:161, 1974.
40. Wang, J. B., Rubin, R. M., and Marshall, J. L.: A mechanism of isolated anterior cruciate ligament rupture. J. Bone Joint Surg. *57-A*:411, 1975.
41. Warren, L. F., Marshall, J. L., and Girgis, F.: The prime static stabilizer of the medial side of the knee. J. Bone Joint Surg. *56-A*:665, 1974.
42. Wiberg, G.: Roentgenographic and anatomic studies on the femoropatellar joint. Acta Orthop. Scand. 12:319, 1941.

12 The Foot and Ankle

Hiromu Shoji, M.D.

ANATOMY

The soft tissue structures and bones of the foot are similar in many aspects to those of the pronated hand, but there are some very obvious differences. The third finger ray of the hand is the functional central axis, whereas in the foot, the second ray is the central axis because of its weight-bearing function. The bones of the ankle and foot consist of the tarsus, metatarsals, and phalanges.

Bones

The tarsus is composed of seven bones: talus, calcaneus, cuboid, navicular, and three cuneiforms. The talus is the most posterior and rests on the calcaneus. Superiorly, it also articulates with the tibia and fibula. The talus and calcaneus represent the hindfoot; the remainder of the foot is known as the forefoot. The most proximal row of the forefoot is composed of the three cuneiforms and cuboid bone. The navicular bone connects with this proximal row of the forefoot bones (Fig. 12-1).

The talus has no tendon insertions and can be divided into three parts: body, neck, and head. The trochlea, the superior aspect of the body, articulates with the tibia and fibula. The medial surface articulates with the medial malleolus of the tibia, the superior surface with the distal end of the tibia, and the lateral surface with the lateral malleolus. The trochlea is wider in front than in back, thus making the ankle joint more stable to rotational stress when it is dorsiflexed. The posterior process is the narrow part of the body projecting behind the trochlea. A groove is formed at the end of the posterior process and within the groove runs the flexor hallucis longus. The medial side of the posterior process is called the medial tubercle and the lateral side, the lateral tubercle. The head and neck of the talus direct forward and medially about 15 degrees in the adult, so that the extension of its axis approximately follows the shaft of the first metatarsal (Fig. 12-2). The neck of the talus rests on the sustentaculum tali and the head on a strong ligament known as the spring ligament, which runs between the tuberosity of the navicular and sustentaculum tali (Figs. 12-1 and 12-3). A depression is formed in the lateral aspect of the neck; this is the roof of the sinus tarsi. The floor of the sinus tarsi is formed by the calcaneus. It narrows medially and extends as the tarsal canal toward the back of the sustentaculum tali. This structure is important because the major nutrient vessels to the body of the talus run through this sinus and canal. The articulation of the talus with the calcaneus is known as the subtalar joint, and there are three facets. The posterior facet is posterior to the tarsal canal; the middle facet is anterior; and an anterior facet is continuous with the convex articular surface of the head, and, in fact, forms the talocalcaneonavicular joint (Fig. 12-4).

The calcaneus is the largest tarsal bone and transmits much of the weight of the body from the talus to the ground. The front half of the upper aspect of the calcaneus is prolonged medially and is called the sustentaculum tali. It is palpable just below the medial malleolus. The groove for the flexor hallucis longus is below and behind the sustentaculum tali. This portion forms the middle facet of the subtalar joint. The smaller facet is anterior and the larger posterior. The posterior facet is located in the middle

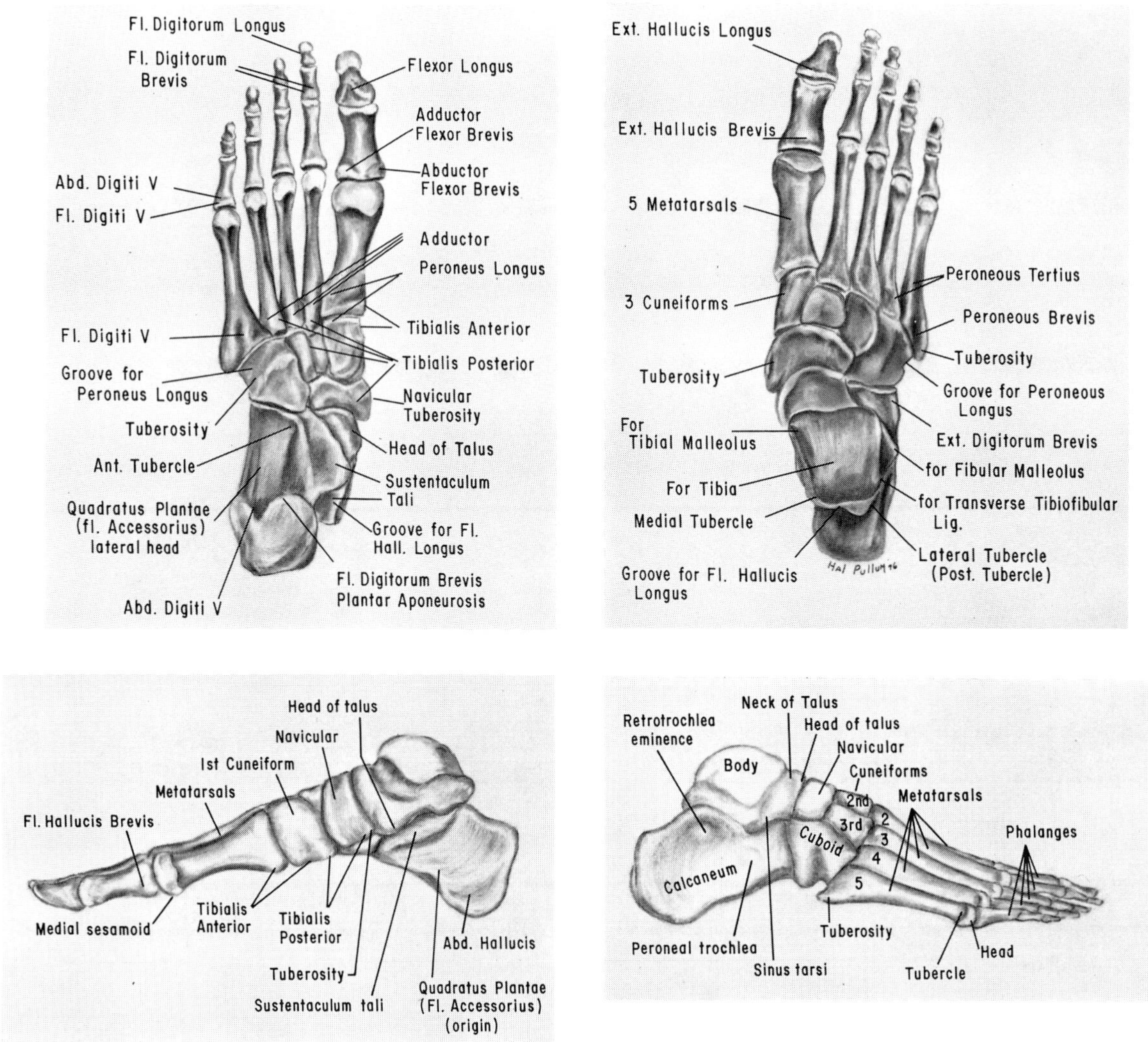

Fig. 12-1. Bones and tendon insertions of the foot.

of the calcaneus just posterior to the sinus tarsi. The fibulocalcaneal ligament attaches to the retrotrochlear eminence on the lateral side. The peroneus longus and brevis tendons pass anterior to this eminence, between which a small projection called the peroneal trochlea may be present. This trochlea is attached to the tendonous sheath of the peroneal muscles (see Fig. 12-1). The posterior aspect of the calcaneus projects downward and is known as the tuber calcanei, which supports the weight on the heel. An apophysis appears in the posterior aspect of the tuber calcanei at about age 10 and fuses at about age 13. The Achilles tendon attaches to the edge of the calcaneus but not to the apophysis. The calcaneocu-

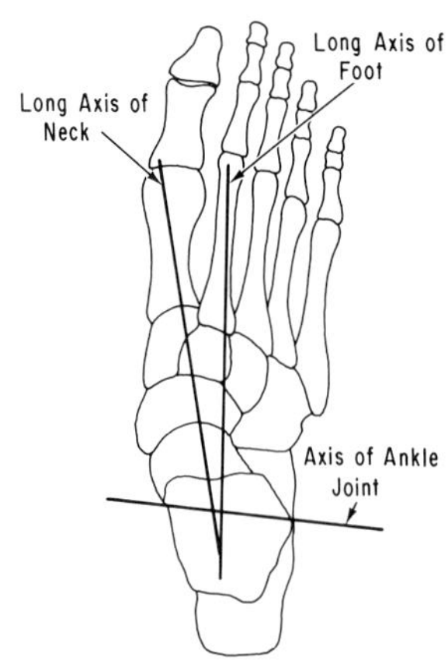

Fig. 12-2. Axes of the foot.

boid joint is formed on the anterolateral surface. The direction of the body of the calcaneus is slightly lateral, and the angle formed by the neck of the talus and calcaneal body is between 20 and 40 degrees.

The cuboid bone is palpable on the lateral aspect of the foot. In the normal foot, the outer margin of the cuboid is almost level with the calcaneus. The posterior portion of the cuboid bone articulates with the calcaneus and the anterior, with the fourth and fifth metatarsals. The medial surface articulates with the third cuneiform and occasionally also with the navicular bone. The peroneus longus courses in a groove on the lower surface of the cuboid.

The navicular bone articulates with the three cuneiforms anteriorly and with the talus posteriorly. The medial surface of the navicular has a palpable prominence directed downward, known as the tuberosity of the navicular bone.

The three cuneiforms articulate with the first, second, and third metatarsals. The transverse arch of the foot is formed by the navicular, cuneiforms, cuboid, and metatarsals. The longitudinal arch of the foot is formed by these bones plus the calcaneus and talus. There is very little motion present in the intertarsal and metatarsotarsal joints. Nonetheless, these joints are important because they maintain a strong arch for weight-bearing and yet on sudden impact or excessive static stress, can provide the elasticity to make the whole system more durable. The arches of the foot which transmit the weight to the calcaneus and metatarsal heads on standing (1:1 ratio) and are further reinforced by the plantar aponeurosis and strong intertarsal ligaments (Fig. 12-3). The phalanges articulate with the corresponding metatarsals.

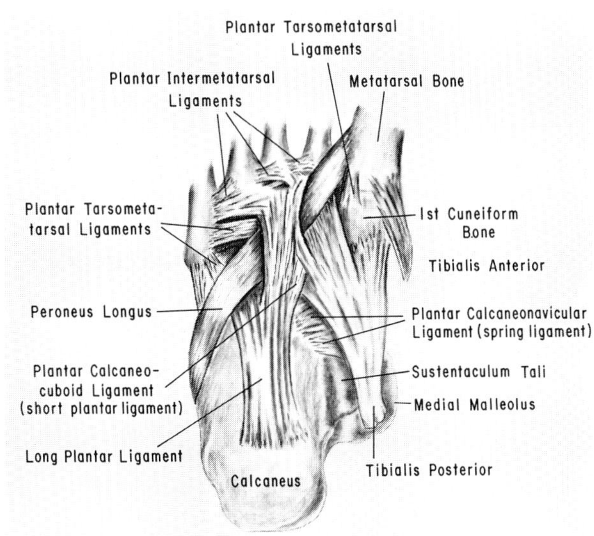

Fig. 12-3. Ligament and tendon insertions of the sole.

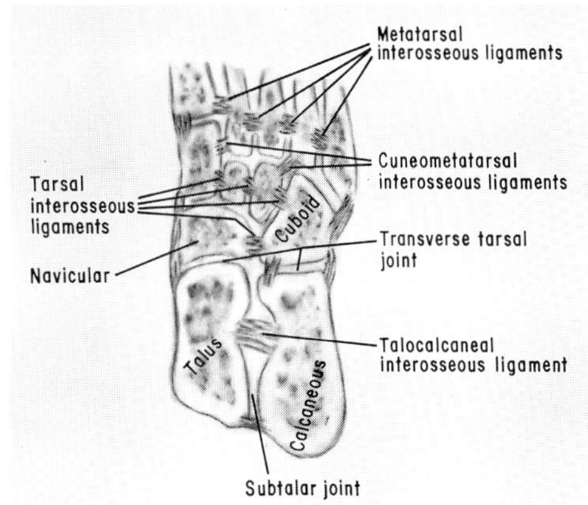

Fig. 12-4. Schematic drawing of interosseous ligaments.

Digital Sesamoids and Accessory Tarsals

Digital sesamoids of the foot are common; sesamoids are always present at the first metatarsophalangeal joint, and at the first interphalangeal joint 5 percent of the time (Fig. 12-5). The less common locations are the second metatarsophalangeal, second proximal interphalangeal, and the fifth metatarsophalangeal joints. The sesamoids at the first metatarsophalangeal joint are the most important because of the role they play in weight-bearing. In the erect posture, the weight of the body is distributed evenly between the calcaneus and the metatarsal heads. One third of the weight on the metatarsal heads is carried on the first metatarsal head; the remaining two thirds is evenly distributed on the other metatarsal heads. There are two grooves on the plantar aspect of the first metatarsal head by ligaments. The most medial slip of the plantar aponeurosis divides in two, and each joins to the sesamoid plantar ligament complex, thus extending its effect to the base of the proximal phalanx.

Because of their location, the first metatarsophalangeal sesamoids have a significant role in weight-bearing, especially during push-off in stance phase. The soft tissue over the ball of the first metatarsal head and the sesamoids reduces direct stress over the first metatarsal head.

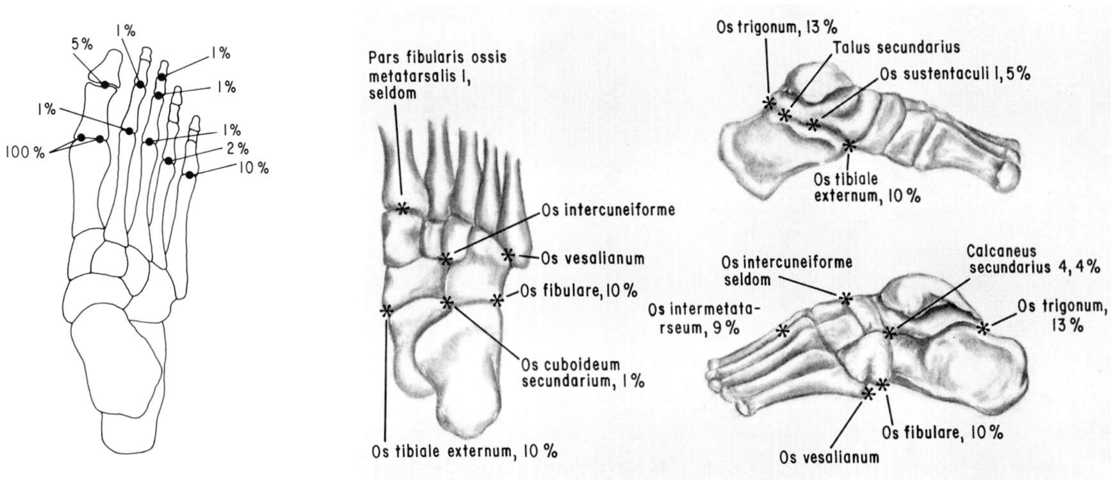

Fig. 12-5. Accessory tarsals and digital sesamoids. The frequency of the presence of digital sesamoids is expressed on the basis of roentgenograms.

There are many accessory tarsals, but the most common are the os trigonum, os intermetatarseum at the metatarsal base, the os tibiale externum, and the peroneal sesamoid. The os vesalianum, which is a separate tuberosity of the fifth metatarsal, is occasionally present but is not common. Knowledge of the sesamoids and their locations is important in differentiating such conditions as avulsion fractures (see Fig. 12-5).

Joints

Ankle Joint

The ankle is a type of hinge joint. It is formed by the tibia superiorly and medially, by the fibula laterally, and by the trochlea of the talus inferiorly. The lateral malleolus is located slightly below and posterior to the medial malleolus. The mediolateral axis of the ankle joint is not parallel to the knee joint because of tibial torsion, which is manifested by the more posterior location of the lateral malleolus compared with the medial malleolus. A lateral torsion of approximately 20 degrees is present, and it may vary from 0 to 40 degrees in a normal tibia without significant impairment of function or appearance. This torsion develops between birth and seven years of age. Most people consequently have approximately 10 degrees of toe-out, and the axis of the ankle joint is about 120 degrees in relation to the line of progression, compared with 90 degrees at the knee joint. The malleoli have a gripping effect upon the talus. The trochlea of the talus, which articulates with the tibia, has a broader arch anterior and is narrower in the posterior area. Because of this anatomy, although the joint imitates a hinge, it pronates slightly on dorsiflexion and supinates on plantar flexion. The gripping effect of the malleoli on a narrower area in plantar flexion is less, and the ankle joint is, therefore, less stable in this position and more stable in dorsiflexion because of a firmer grip on the broader trochlea. These factors also enable the joint to resist anterior subluxation of the tibia. The malleoli are bound strongly anteriorly and posteriorly by the strong inferior tibiofibular ligament (Fig. 12-7).

The center of gravity of the body falls just in front of the ankle joint, and this tends to make the tibia dislocate forward. This is accentuated by standing on the toes. This tendency is blocked, however, because of the anatomical structure just mentioned.

The ankle joint capsule is reinforced medially and laterally for stability by strong ligaments (Figs. 12-6 and 12-7). The deltoid ligament, which is medial, originates from the medial malleolus and attaches to the talus, navicular, and calcaneus. The anterior portion reaches to the neck of the talus and navicular. The posterior portion, the deepest part of the deltoid ligament, attaches to the medial side of the talus. The midportion attaches to the sustentaculum tali of the calcaneus. For practical purposes, the three parts of the deltoid ligament are not separable. The lateral ligament, however, has three distinct separable ligaments. The anterior talofibular ligament originates at the anterior lateral malleolus and inserts into the neck of the talus. The posterior talofibular ligament arises from the posterior lateral malleolus and inserts on the posterior tubercle of the talus. The fibulocalcaneal ligament arises from the midportion of the lateral malleolus and inserts into the calcaneal eminence. Nerve innervation of the ankle joint is through branches of the sural, deep peroneal, and saphenous nerves. The maximum range of ankle motion is variable, but the motion required for normal walking is between 10 degrees of dorsiflexion and 20 degrees of plantar flexion. The kinematic pattern of motion is a gliding type, and rolling motion is rare.

Intertarsal Joints

The intertarsal joints have very little range of motion because their main function for the foot is to provide stability except for eversion and inversion. This is the most important motion taking place in the intertarsal joints and occurs as the talus moves as a unit with the rest of the leg. The most important intertarsal joints are the subtalar, talocalcaneonavicular, and the calcaneocuboid joints, which are the joints fused in a triple arthrodesis. The last two are known as the midtarsal joints (see Fig. 12-4).

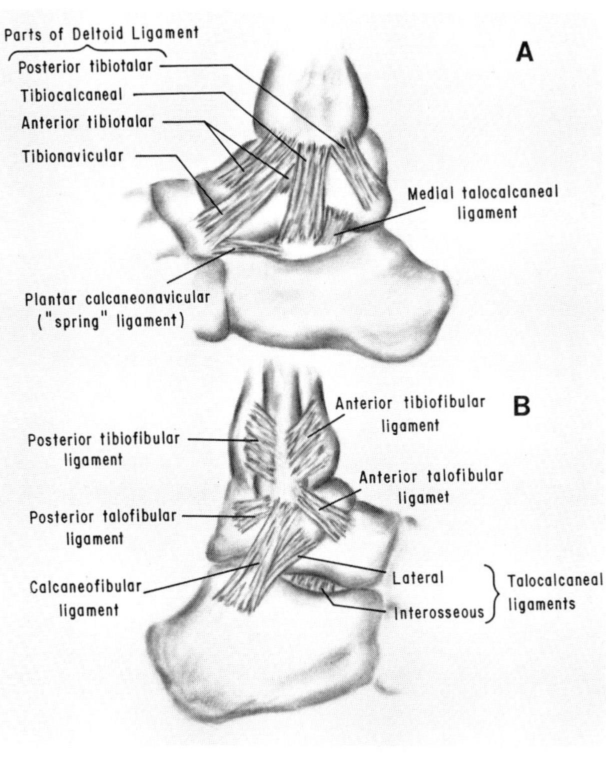

Fig. 12-6. Ligaments at the medial (*A*) and lateral (*B*) aspects of the ankle.

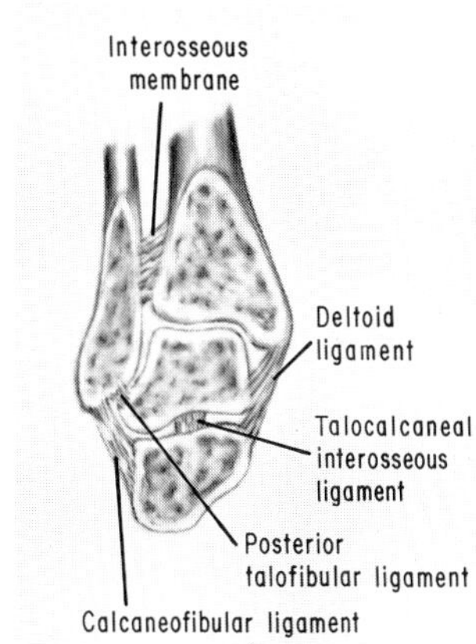

Fig. 12-7. Ligaments of the hindfoot in the coronal plane.

The Subtalar Joint. This joint is formed by the inferior surface of the talus and the superior surface of the calcaneus and has three articular facets: anterior, middle, and posterior. Anatomically, the anterior facet is separated from the latter two by the strong talocalcaneal ligament. Actually the anterior facet belongs in the joint cavity of the talocalcaneonavicular joint.

Talocalcaneonavicular Joint. This joint resembles a ball and socket joint because the head of the talus fits into a shallow socket in the navicular in front and the calcaneus lateral and below. However, unlike the ball and socket joints of the hip and shoulder joints, mobility is very limited. A strong plantar calcaneonavicular ligament, known as the spring ligament, connects the sustentaculum tali of the calcaneus with the navicular and functions in withstanding stresses placed upon the medial longitudinal arch.

Calcaneocuboid Joint. This joint has the configuration of a saddle joint, but motion is very limited. The strong bifurcate ligament reinforces the superior capsule. It arises from the upper part of the calcaneus in the floor of the sinus tarsi and inserts into the cuboid and navicular bones. The inferior capsule is reinforced by the long and short plantar ligaments which arise from the plantar surface of the calcaneus to insert into the cuboid. These ligaments stabilize the hindfoot against weight-bearing. These intertarsal ligamentous structures are further reinforced by the plantar aponeurosis and the tendon insertions of the tibialis posterior and peroneus longus, which fan out.

Cuneocuboid, Intercuneiform, and Cuneonavicular Joints. Although individually these joints are relatively unimportant structures in terms of motion, together with the other tarsal bones and joints they help maintain flexibility while providing stability for the middle and posterior portion of the foot.

The motions of inversion and eversion (Fig. 12-8), although taking place primarily in the subtalar joint, are augmented by other intertarsal joints. Each of these joints has an anatomical axis in a different direction with reinforcing capsule and ligamentous structures so that the pure motions of flexion-extension, abduction-adduction, and supination-pronation cannot occur by themselves. The inversion and eversion motions which take place at the intertarsal joints are just a combination of pure motions. Inversion is a combination of supination and adduction with the ankle in plantar flexion. Eversion is a combination of pronation and abduction augmented with the ankle in dorsiflexion. There has been some confusion in the past because various authors have used pronation to mean eversion and supination to describe inversion.

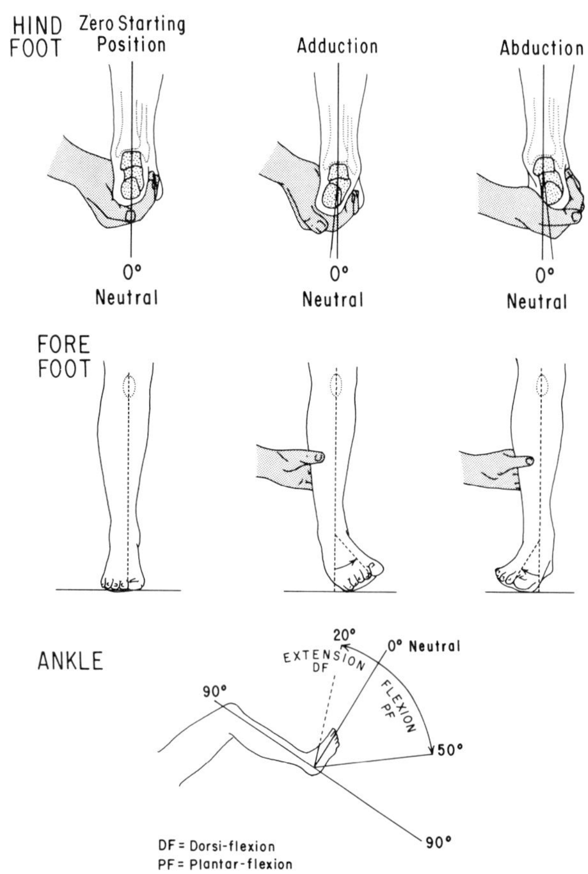

Fig. 12-8. Motions of the foot and ankle.

Tarsometatarsal Joints

The tarsometatarsal joints are formed between the bases of the metatarsals and the front ends of the three cuneiforms and the cuboid and consist of three joint cavities: the first is formed by the first metatarsal and first cuneiform, the second by the second and third metatarsals and the second and third cuneiforms, and the third by the fourth and fifth metatarsals and cuboid. The three joint cavities are separated by interosseous ligaments (see Fig. 12-4). The motion at each joint is minimal, but together they provide some flexibility of the foot by allowing a twisting to occur at the forefoot which increases any motion begun at the intertarsal joints.

Metatarsophalangeal and Interphalangeal Joints

These joints resemble those of the hand, and the basic anatomical structures are the same (see Chap. 9). The metatarsophalangeal joints have more lateral mobility than the interphalangeal joints, which act more like a hinge. The mobility at the metatarsophalangeal joints occurs because of the semisphericity of the head of the metatarsal facing the base of the neck. The collateral ligaments limit this lateral mobility and extend from the base of the proximal phalanx to the neck of the metatarsal head and the thickened plantar capsule called the plantar ligament. The plantar ligament is equivalent to the volar plate of the hand. The plantar ligaments are connected by the deep transverse metatarsal ligament, which helps prevent the metatarsal heads from spreading apart on weight-bearing. The digital nerves pass over this ligament between the metatarsal heads. Like the hand, the dorsum of the metatarsophalangeal joint is reinforced by the hood of the extensor mechanism; however, the fibers from the extensor hood in the foot are directed in such a manner that clawing of the metatarsophalangeal joint develops more easily than in the hand.

The interphalangeal joints also have collateral ligaments and plantar ligaments. The flexor and extensor mechanisms of the toes are similar to the hand, but the delicate motion that results from this complex anatomical arrangement in the hand is not present in the foot.

The motion at the metatarsophalangeal joint of the foot, like the hand, includes flexion, extension, abduction, and adduction, but unlike the hand, extension is greater than flexion and abduction-adduction is minimal. The joint assumes a slightly dorsiflexed position when resting which is the result of the weight-bearing and locomotor functions of the foot. This natural position of the metatarsophalangeal joint in slight dorsiflexion and the less well developed intrinsic muscles compared to the hand makes for a strong propensity for the development of claw and hammer toes in the foot.

Muscles, Tendons, and Nerves

The motions at the ankle joint are plantar flexion and dorsiflexion (see Fig. 12-8). The muscles in the posterior compartment, innervated by the tibial nerve (L5-S2), are primarily responsible for plantar flexion motion. The major muscles for plantar flexion are the gastrocnemius and soleus and they are supplemented by the tibialis posterior, peroneus longus, flexor digitorum longus, and flexor hallucis longus. The power of the gastrosoleus is weakened when the knee is in flexion since the gastrocnemius is a two-joint muscle. However, with the knee in flexion, passive range of dorsiflexion increases slightly. The muscles in the anterior compartment, innervated by the deep peroneal nerve (L4-S1), are primarily responsible for dorsiflexion motion. Dorsiflexion is performed by the tibialis anterior and the extensor digitorum longus. When these two muscles act together, their individual actions of inversion and eversion are neutralized. The extensor hallucis longus and peroneus tertius also aid in dorsiflexion.

The prime motions at the intertarsal joints are inversion and eversion and occur primarily at the subtalar joint (see Fig. 12-8). Inversion is achieved principally by the tibialis posterior and tibialis anterior but supplemented by the long toe flexors and gastrosoleus. Eversion is achieved primarily by the peroneus brevis and peroneus longus, innervated by the superficial peroneal nerve L5-S1, and is supplemented by the extensor digitorum longus and peroneus tertius.

The main motions at the metatarsophalangeal and interphalangeal joints are flexion and extension. Flexion of the metatarsophalangeal joint is achieved primarily by the lumbricals, interossei, and flexor hallucis brevis with augmentation by the flexor hallucis longus, and flexor digitorum longus and brevis. Extension of these joints is achieved by the extensor digitorum longus, extensor hallucis longus with supplementation by the extensor digitorum brevis and extensor hallucis brevis.

The interphalangeal joints are essentially hinge joints which allow flexion and extension but more flexion than extension. Flexion is achieved by the flexor digitorum longus at the distal interphalangeal joint and is supplemented by the flexor digitorum brevis at the proximal interphalangeal joint. In the hand, extension of the interphalangeal joints is performed by a complex extensor mechanism (see Chap. 9). However, in the foot this complex anatomical structure is still present, but the fine movements derived from this mechanism are virtually lost.

There are many intrinsic muscles about the foot, but only two are on the dorsal aspect: the extensor digitorum brevis and extensor hallucis brevis. Both are innervated by the deep peroneal nerve. The musculotendinous structure of the sole is divided into four layers. The first layer is composed of abductor hallucis, flexor digitorum brevis, and abductor digiti minimi. The second layer is composed of flexor hallucis longus, flexor digitorum longus, lumbricals, and quadratus plantae. The neurovascular bundle from the tibial nerve and vessels branches out between the first and second layers at the level of the tarsus. The third layer consists of adductor hallucis, flexor hallucis brevis, and flexor digiti minimi. The fourth layer is composed of the interossei and fanned out tendons of the peroneus longus. The medial plantar nerve which is one of the two major branches of the tibial nerve below the ankle and equivalent to the motor branch of the median nerve in the hand,

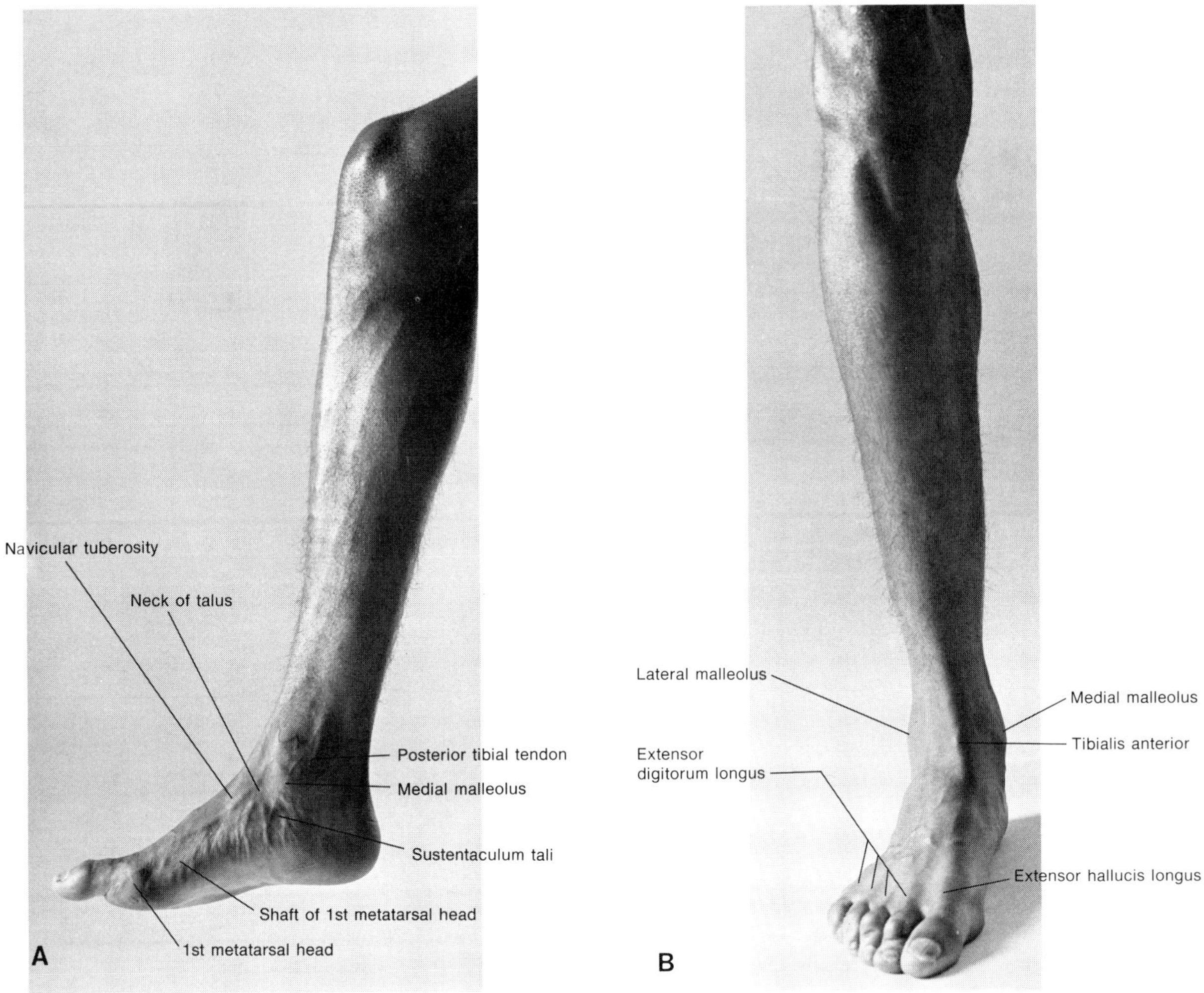

Fig. 12-9. Surface anatomy of the foot and ankle region. (*A*) Medial aspect. (*B*) Anterior aspect.

innervates the abductor hallucis, flexor hallucis brevis, first lumbrical, and the flexor digitorum brevis. The remaining muscles in the sole, except for such extrinsic muscles as the long flexors and peroneus longus, are innervated by the lateral plantar nerve. The tibial nerve at the level of the medial malleolus lies between the flexor digitorum longus and flexor hallucis in a very narrow canal. The digital nerves proper pass over the deep transverse metatarsal ligaments between the metatarsal heads. The anatomical relationship of these nerves to the surrounding structures is important and bears clinical significance, because they may be impinged, causing specific symptoms.

Surface Anatomy

It is important to bear in mind the location of the bones, joints, and muscles of the foot and ankle surface anatomy as they relate to the proper physical examination and diagnosis. On the medial side (Fig. 12-9), the palpable bony landmarks are the medial malleolus, sustentaculum tali, navicular tuberosity, neck of the talus, base, shaft and head of the first metatarsal, tendon of the tibialis posterior, and, on occasion, the flexor digitorum longus, which is just posterior to the posterior tibial tendon. The posterior tibial artery is palpable just posterior to the flexor digitorum longus. On the anterior aspect, the tibialis anterior and essentially all the long extensors of the

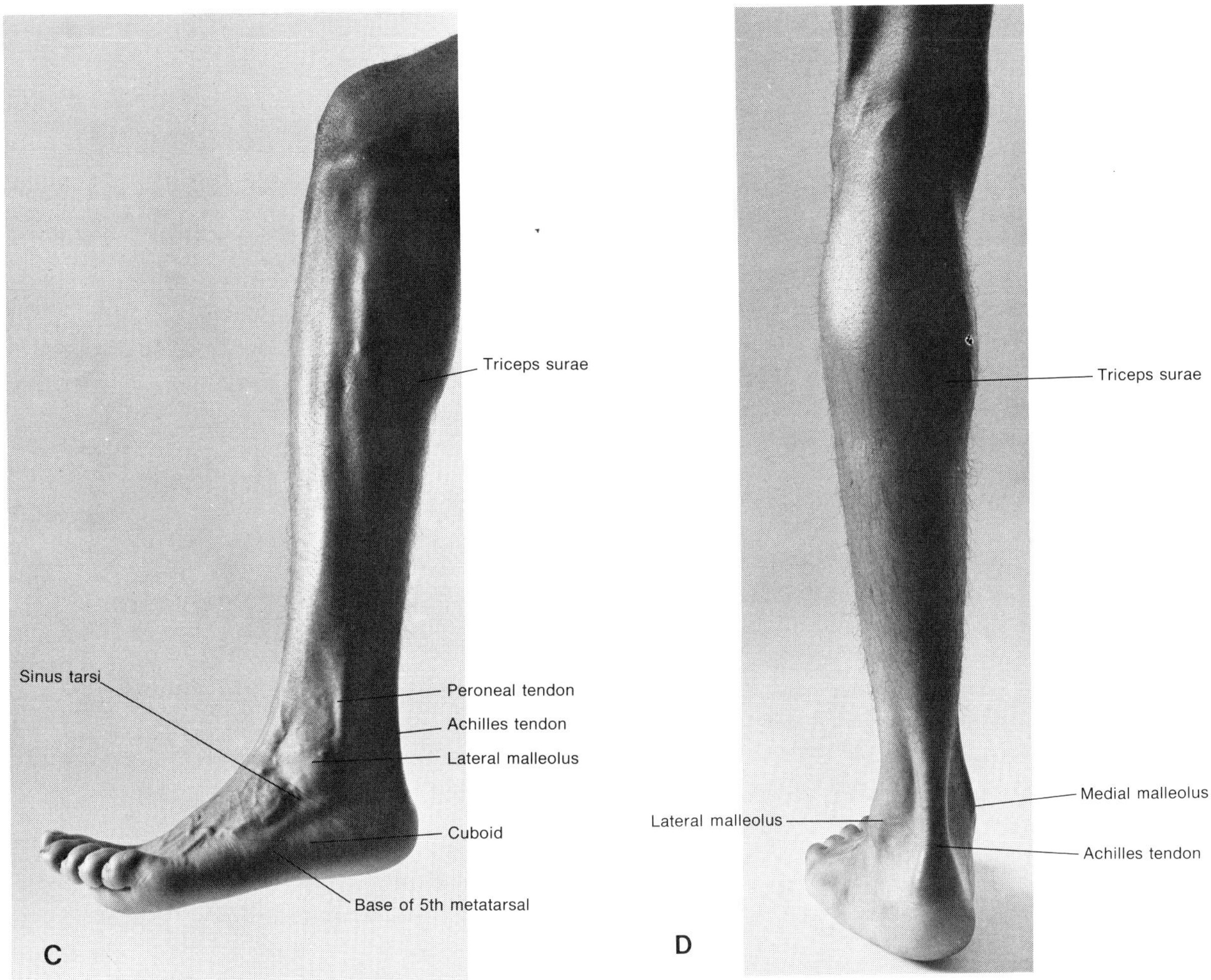

Fig. 12-9 (Continued). (*C*) Lateral aspect. (*D*) Posterior aspect.

ankle and toes are palpable (Fig. 12-9B). The dorsal pedal artery, with occasional variations, is usually palpable between the extensor hallucis and extensor digitorum longus just distal to the ankle joint. The deltoid ligament is palpable immediately below the medial malleolus.

On the lateral side (Fig. 12-9C), the lateral malleolus, base, shaft, and head of fifth metatarsals, and the trochlear process of the calcaneus are palpable. The cuboid bone, located between the prominent fifth metatarsal base and calcaneus, is palpable but not prominent. If prominent, a pathological condition such as clubfoot or forefoot adductus is probably present. The sinus tarsi, an important landmark, is a depression just anterior to the lateral malleolus. The peroneal tendons are palpable posterior and inferior to the lateral malleolus. The lateral ligaments of the ankle are not palpable except for the fibulocalcaneal portion which is palpable below the lateral malleolus. Posteriorly the Achilles tendon and triceps surae are easily palpable (Fig. 12-9D).

The locations, size, and geographic interrelationship of these described landmarks are important because unusual observations frequently are clues to the suspected diagnosis.

Development of the Normal Foot

The preceding sections of this chapter have dealt with the anatomy of the adult foot. Because many of the foot disorders occur in childhood, it is important to have some knowledge of the development of normal feet and the systemic neuromuscular system, disturbances of which can cause foot deformities. However, the development of the neuromuscular system is beyond the scope of this text, and the reader is referred to standard textbooks on pediatric neurology.

At birth, the foot at rest is either in neutral, right angle, or slight dorsiflexion and eversion. When the examiner picks up an infant's foot, the reaction is withdrawal of the foot, accompanied by increased dorsiflexion of the ankle and fanning out of the toes. The position of the calcaneus is neutral or slight valgus. The longitudinal arch of the foot does not noticeably develop during the first 12 months. The bones visible at birth on roentgenogram are: the talus, calcaneus, cuboid, and all the metatarsals and phalanges, except for the distal two phalanges of the fifth digit (Fig. 12-10). The third cuneiform appears at the age of two and one-half months in a female and at three months in a male. The navicular bone appears at three years in a female and at three years, eight months in a male. The calcaneal apophysis appears at six years in a female and at eight years in a male. The sesamoids in the first metatarsal head appear at 10 years in the female and at 13 years in the male.

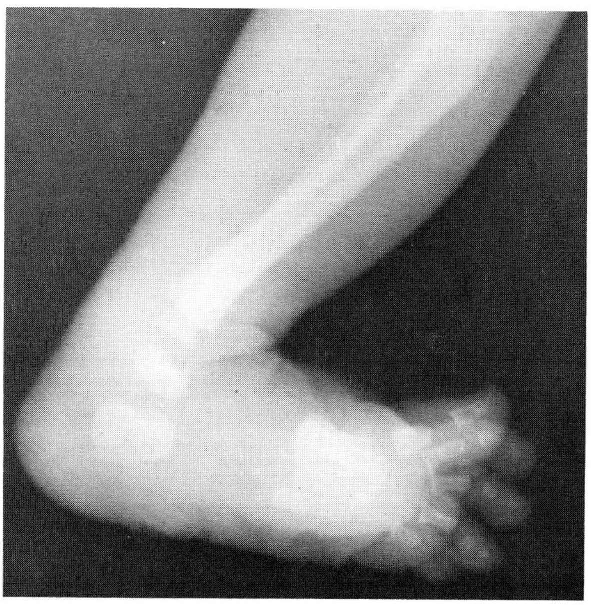

Fig. 12-10. Roentgenograms of a newborn foot.

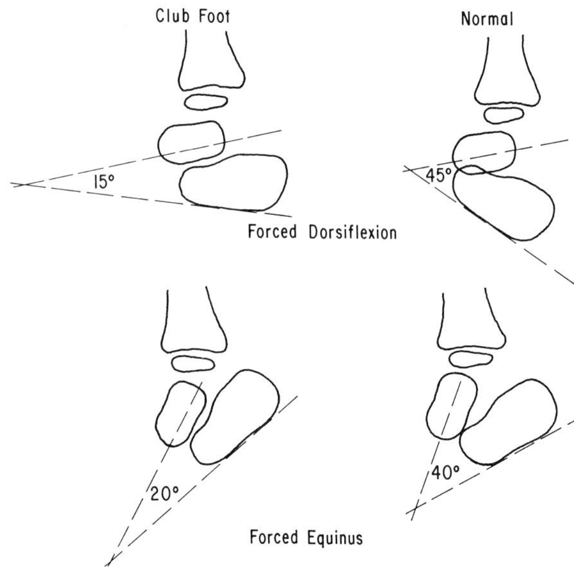

Fig. 12-11. Lateral talocalcaneal angles at dorsiflexion and plantar flexion in the normal and clubfoot. (Modified from Heywood, A. W. B.: The mechanics of the hindfoot in clubfoot as demonstrated radiographically. J. Bone Joint Surg., *46B*:105, 1964)

The anteroposterior roentgenogram of a normal infant's foot in 30 degrees plantar flexion describes the long axis of the talus pointing toward the first metatarsal and the long axis of the calcaneus toward the fifth metatarsal which normally forms a talocalcaneal angle of 20 to 40 degrees. A talocalcaneal angle of 35 to 50 degrees, formed by the long axis of talus and a tangent to the bottom of calcaneus, will be evident on the lateral roentgenogram. This angle increases but not beyond 50 degrees when a roentgenogram is taken with the ankle dorsiflexed, whereas the reverse is seen in a case of congenital clubfoot (Fig. 12-11).

REGIONAL EXAMINATION

History

Eighty-five million people in the United States are afflicted with abnormalities of the foot. From 80 to 90 percent of these abnormalities are in the forefoot of adults which result from ill-fitted shoes. However, in the child many foot problems are primary or congenital and not acquired. For this reason, foot problems of the child and adult are discussed separately.

The parent, not the child, provides the history,

and such essential items as events in early pregnancy, for example, rubella, histoplasmosis, and so forth, accidents during the pregnancy, events at delivery, and prematurity must be covered. A thorough family history must be taken because congenital foot deformities, bow legs, and other heritable disorders which manifest as foot problems may be noted in the family history and can help in treatment and genetic counseling. Childhood foot problems are not usually painful but instead present with deformity or abnormality of motion. If pain is present, an infant cannot complain in words; instead the parents express it as: "does not want to move," "cries with passive motion," "does not sleep," or "restlessness."

It is important to be familiar with the child's pattern of normal physical development, as found in standard pediatric or pediatric-orthopedic texts. The timing of walking, pattern of walking, shape and posture of the lower extremities, as well as sleeping and sitting patterns of the patient all must be reviewed and contrasted with the developmental pattern of the neuromuscular system in normal children.

When interviewing a patient for what appears to be a foot problem, do not ignore the other joints of the lower extremity, particularly the hip and knee. A painful ankle or foot is sometimes secondary to such systemic diseases as juvenile rheumatoid arthritis or septic arthritis. Foot intoeing in the child is frequently due to an abnormality in anteversion at the hip (see Chap. 10).

In contrast to that in the child, the presenting symptom in the adult patient is foot pain. The pain may be related to recent or past injury but more frequently it is related to a static problem secondary to the anatomical nature of the foot or ill-fitted shoes. Congenital deformities or those deformities acquired at an early age, which were either untreated or ill-treated and formerly painless, may now be a source of pain. The characteristics of the pain, such as being constant or intermittent, relationship with weight-bearing and activity, and the degree of limitation of activities of daily living, are important. A personal past and family history are also important in the adult. A history of neuromuscular problems, such as poliomyelitis, cerebral palsy, Charcot-Marie-Tooth disease, and Friedreich's ataxia, can provide important clues to the present disturbance. Occupation, type of shoes worn by the patient, past treatment of specific foot problems, and hygienic care of the foot must be investigated. Circumstances regarding smoking, pregnancy, and disorders in the pelvic region may be significant, as they may be related to Buerger's disease or venous varicosities which can cause secondary foot problems. A past or family history of gout, rheumatoid arthritis, tuberculosis, sarcoidosis, and venereal diseases is important since these conditions have a sociofamilial influence and often affect the foot and ankle. Sociogeographic history is also significant where endemic diseases, such as coccidioidomycosis or echinococcosis, flourish.

Physical Examination

The physical examination of the foot requires modification in each individual case, depending on such factors as the age of the patient or presence of an injury. The history and review of systems is a reflection of how narrow or how broad the differential diagnosis is at the onset. Paying attention to the minute details of each question or particular aspect of the physical examination will also reflect the frame of reference for the differential diagnosis.

Inspection

Adequate inspection requires visualization of the entire lower extremity in the resting, standing, and walking positions. The positional interrelationships of the hip, knee, and ankle joints and the intervening bones should be carefully observed. With the knowledge that no hip or knee abnormality is present one can focus on the foot if, indeed, the problem is in the foot or ankle.

The positional relationship of both malleoli to the front-pointing patella and the direction of the foot in relation to the ankle joint should be evaluated. Internal torsion of the tibia, if present, is easily discernible from this evaluation alone. Normally, the heels and metatarsal heads have equal contact with the ground. The weight distribution of a normal foot between the calcaneus and metatarsal heads is a 1:1 ratio in the erect position. If the heel loses contact with the ground, there is increased weight-bearing at the metatarsal heads, and stronger than usual tension is exerted on the plantar ligamentous structures. This condition is present in a fixed flexion contracture of the ankle. There are numerous conditions in which the heel loses contact with the ground on standing, including pain in any joint of the lower extremity. It may also be a result of flexion contracture of the hip or knee or leg length discrepancy. Subsequent examination of the passive range of motion of the ankle will ultimately differentiate these entities.

Neuromuscular diseases, such as arthrogryposis or cerebral palsy, are often associated with knee and hip flexion contractures and may present in this manner. When one stands, the weight-bearing line of the body falls slightly behind the hip joint rotation center but slightly forward of the rotational centers of the knee and ankle. Therefore, the ligamentous structures must reinforce these joints in such a way as to prevent collapse of the lower extremity. No matter what the etiology, if a patient cannot put his heel on the ground because of a flexion deformity, he must deviate from the normal erect posture by altering the position of the knee, hip, and spine.

Carefully observe the heel at rest and whether it is in a neutral, valgus, or varus position. The heel is normally neutral or in slight valgus. The varus position is always indicative of a pathological condition. Heel varus most often is secondary to a neuromuscular disorder, clubfoot, or some systemic congenital deformity. Heel varus may also be the result of past injury or improper healing sequela to the hindfoot from such causes as injury or infection. Early in infancy, prior to the development of a heel pad, it is difficult to recognize heel varus. Excessive heel valgus is also pathological. To evaluate heel valgus adequately, the heel position must be observed in weight-bearing and non-weight-bearing positions. Systemic connective tissue disorders with generalized joint laxity result in excessive hindfoot valgus,

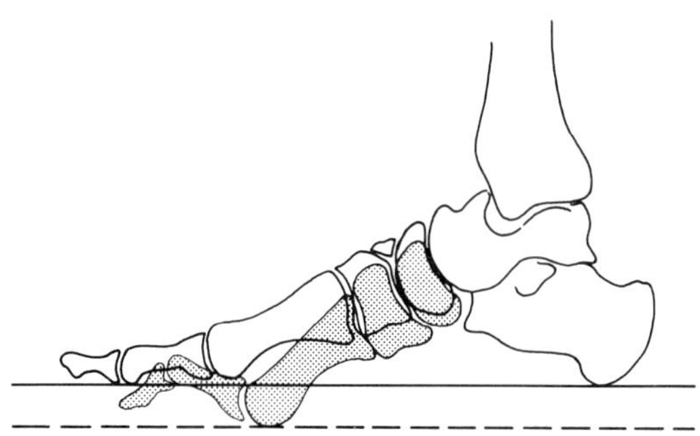

Fig. 12-12. Comparison of normal foot with pes cavus foot (cross-hatched area). (Modified from Tachdjian M. O.: Pediatric Orthopaedics. Philadelphia, W. B. Saunders, 1972)

but the planovalgus pronated foot (flatfoot) is the most common cause of excessive heel valgus. It is also seen in congenital vertical talus, tarsal coalition, or even neuromuscular disorders.

Examine the longitudinal and transverse arches of the foot. The best way to demonstrate sole-to-ground patterns is the foot print method or, even better, observation of the sole of the foot through a transparent glass from the bottom. Many disorders with heel valgus have an associated dropped arch. A knowledge of surface and internal anatomy aids in evaluating which joints forming the arch are most responsible for this deformity. An excessively high arch is known as pes cavus and is abnormal; it implies forefoot equinus (Fig. 12-12). When a person stands, his ankle joint compensates by dorsiflexing to maintain heel-metatarsal head weight-bearing which results in a high arch. A thorough neurological examination must be performed if pes cavus is noted in the young child or preadolescent because it results from muscle imbalance, and one should be suspicious of neuromuscular disorders, such as Charcot-Marie-Tooth disease, poliomyelitis, Friedreich's ataxia, cerebral palsy, Roussy-Levy syndrome, and meningomyelocele. Muscle atrophy should be evaluated not only in the lower but also in the upper extremities. Presence of thenar atrophy may be suggestive of Charcot-Marie-Tooth disease. Patients with pes cavus develop metatarsophalangeal joint hyperextension in the swing phase of gait clawing, and it can remain even when standing. It is important to remember that complex congenital deformities like clubfoot or metatarsus adductus are often associated with pes cavus. Talipes calcaneus, or dropped calcaneus, is frequently seen following poliomyelitis and imitates a pes cavus, and both may even occur simultaneously (Fig. 12-13). It is differentiated by careful examination of the relationship of the calcaneus to the other tarsal and metatarsal bones.

Observe the relationship of the forefoot to the hindfoot. Normally, the longitudinal axis of the neck of the talus extends into the first metatarsal, and the extension of the lateral border of the body of the calcaneus roughly follows the medial border of the fifth metatarsal shaft.

The elements of the forefoot may be adducted or abducted with or without tight soft tissue contractures. Forefoot adduction may be due to a congenital clubfoot or metatarsus varus. Congenital metatarsus

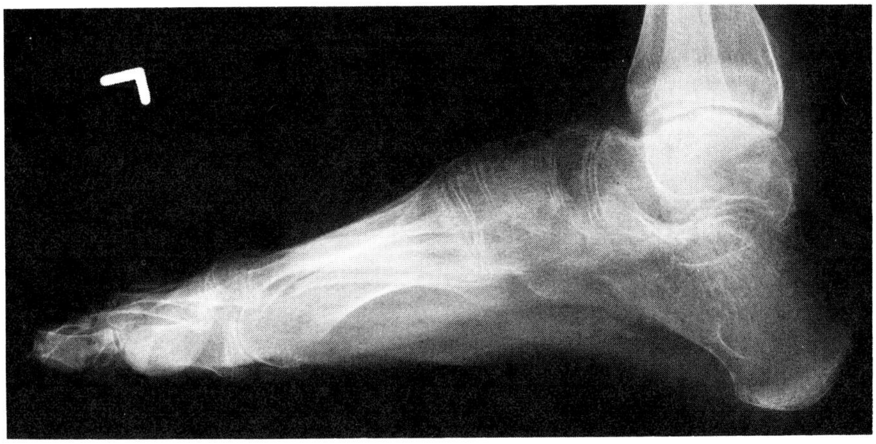

Fig. 12-13. Talipes calcaneus. Note the increased talocalcaneal angle.

varus sometimes is difficult to differentiate from a mild clubfoot with prominent metatarsus varus with lesser expression of the other deformities. Roentgenograms may be needed to show that in a typical clubfoot there is medial displacement of the navicular which is not the case in pure metatarsus varus. The base of the fifth metatarsal and cuboid bone is excessively prominent in forefoot adduction.

If metatarsus adductus only involves the first ray, with the other metatarsals in normal position, it is known as metatarsus primus varus. Hallux valgus may develop later with the first phalanx pointing toward the other phalanges. Metatarsus abductus is usually not a single deformity and is associated with hind foot deformities as in congenital vertical talus or severe pes planus.

In the coronal plane, observe the level of the metatarsophalangeal joints. The first metatarsophalangeal joint is located slightly more proximal than the second to maintain the normal weight-bearing distribution pattern of the metatarsal heads. The metatarsophalangeal joints support 50 percent of the total body weight in normal standing. If the first metatarsus is too short, it will cause too much pressure on the second and third metatarsal heads and can result in painful metatarsalgia, although a short first metatarsal is not always the major cause of metatarsalgia. A short fourth and fifth metatarsal may be an isolated finding and is suggestive of pseudohypoparathyroidism or mucopolysaccharidosis. Numerous deformities involving the metatarsophalangeal and interphalangeal joints, both congenital and acquired, are discussed in the differential diagnosis section.

Observe the joints for swelling, and also note the condition of the skin and nails. Skin inspection may reveal the results of improperly fitted shoes, and bony prominences should be correlated with skin problems and vice versa. The skin may be hypertrophied or more severe complications, such as infection and fistula formation, may be present. Patients with combined systemic disease, such as diabetes or arteriosclerosis, often have secondary changes in the skin.

Observe for abnormalities of gait. These may be due to foot, hip, or knee disorders. When an antalgic gait is secondary to a foot problem, the patient avoids ground contact with the painful area and, thus, shortens the stance phase which is normally 60 percent of the gait cycle. An abnormal stance phase pattern is not always secondary to an antalgic gait. It may result from a neuromuscular disorder which is basically pain-free or from a fixed equinus position of the foot. The best functional opportunity to assess dorsiflexion ability is during swing phase. A patient with a drop foot at the ankle or fixed equinus deformity will either circumduct or raise the foot higher than normal to raise it off the floor. Observe the toe-in or toe-out walking which may be a manifestation of abnormalities in the hip, knee, tibia or foot.

Palpation

Careful palpation of the foot will reveal tender areas, abnormal bony prominences and masses, as well as abnormal relationships of the bones and joint. An abnormal bony prominence often becomes tender when shoes are worn. When a normal bony prominence like the fifth metatarsal base becomes tender, an avulsion fracture by the peroneus brevis should be suspected. However, there is usually a history of injury.

The area of pain is not always the area of primary problem, for in some diseases, such as circulatory or causalgic disorders, there may be no tenderness in the area of pain. Each joint should be carefully palpated with particular attention to those that are symptomatic. Tenderness is present in joints affected with arthritis or osteochondritis dissecans, with or without fluid accumulation or synovial thickening. The recognition of joint fluid accumulation or synovial thickening is obvious in the anterior aspect of the ankle joint, but this is not the case in other joints of the foot. Tenderness present in the nonprominent areas without apparent history of trauma may be from metabolic bone diseases, bone tumors, or stress fractures which commonly occur in the tarsals. Tenderness in the calcaneal area may be indicative of retrocalcaneal bursitis, calcaneal spur, or fibrositis at the origin of the plantar fascia and requires further delineation. Tenderness at the Achilles tendon may be from tendonitis, avulsion fracture, exostosis, or Achilles tendon rupture; therefore, the location of the tenderness becomes very important.

The first metatarsophalangeal joint is frequently painful and tender. Bursitis, hallux valgus, ganglionic cyst, displaced sesamoid, gout, and hallux rigidus are just a few diseases which are common at this location.

Tenderness at the metatarsal heads on weightbearing is called metatarsalgia. Metatarsalgia is usually from excessive stress on the metatarsal heads, but may be a manifestation of Freiberg's disease or rheumatoid arthritis.

While palpating, try to differentiate whether the tenderness is from bone, tendon, tendon sheath, articular structures, ligaments, or nerve entrapment. This differentiation is important in dealing with adult foot problems. If an abnormal mass is noted, differentiate whether the mass is originating from the bone or soft tissue through palpation. Examine the mass for the presence or absence of local heat, fluctuation, tenderness, and moveability.

Range of Motion

The joints to be examined for range of motion are ankle, intertarsal, tarsometatarsal, metatarsophalangeal, and interphalangeal joints. As described in the section on anatomy, the range of motion of individual components of the intertarsal and tarsometatarsal joints is minimal, but as a whole, this joint complex allows some motion, particularly inversion-eversion and abduction-adduction.

Ranges of motion for the ankle, as well as for the intertarsal and metatarsotarsal joints are shown in Figure 12-8. The range of motion of metatarsophalangeal and interphalangeal joints may not be as important as their counterparts in the hand. However, it should not be neglected. Limited passive range of motion of the first metatarsophalangeal joint is an important sign of hallux rigidus or gout. If it is noted in the second metatarsophalangeal joint, it may indicate Freiberg's disease.

Range of motion of the ankle joint should be examined both with the knee in full extension and at 90 degrees flexion. If passive dorsiflexion of the ankle is significantly less with the knee in full extension than with the knee at 90 degrees flexion, tightening of the gastrocnemius component of triceps surae is indicated. If passive dorsiflexion is limited even with the knee fixed at 90 degrees, then all components of the triceps surae are tight, including both soleus and gastrocnemius muscles. Because of the effect of the triceps surae on the calcaneus when examining for inversion-eversion of the hindfoot or abduction-adduction of the forefoot, the knee should be at 90 degrees flexion in order to minimize their effect. Severe limitation of passive inversion in hindfoot valgus is indicative of a tarsal coalition.

Range of motion should be checked in both the active and passive ranges. Limited active range of motion can be from a painful joint, joint contracture, weak muscle power, or coordination disturbance due to neurological disorders. If the joint is painful or a contracture is present, passive range of motion is also limited. When active range of motion is decreased because of weak muscle power or coordination disturbance there is no limited passive range of motion unless joint contracture has developed secondarily.

Ligamentous Stability

Lateral and medial as well as anterior and posterior stability of the ankle joint are tested by exerting stress in each direction with the foot held firmly in the palm of the hand. Normally, the talus should not significantly move in any direction in relation to the tibia. Significant instability may indicate ligamentous injury, Charcot joint, connective tissue disorders, such as Ehlers-Danlos syndrome, ball and socket joint, or be the residual of malunion of old fractures around the ankle joint. The stability examination should always be performed on both ankles, as the comparison is invaluable in determining the degree of instability in patients with unilateral problems. In questionable cases, it is usually necessary to obtain stress roentgenograms of both ankles for comparison.

Muscle Testing

Muscle power around the foot and ankle should always be tested bilaterally. The muscles to be tested are the tibialis anterior, extensor digitorum longus, extensor hallucis longus, tibialis posterior, flexor hallucis longus, flexor digitorum longus, peroneus longus, peroneus brevis, and triceps surae. All muscle testing at the ankle has to be done with the knee in flexion to minimize the effect of the triceps surae. The tibialis anterior is tested by exerting a counterforce to the dorsiflexion and inversion movement of the foot and ankle performed by this muscle. The muscle power of the long toe extensors is tested by exerting the counterforce to the toes while the patient extends the metatarsophalangeal joints. The tibialis posterior is evaluated by exerting a counterforce to the foot while the patient inverts and plantar flexes the foot. The peroneus longus is tested by exerting a counterforce to a foot which is held in plantar flexion while the patient actively everts it. The peroneus brevis is evaluated in the same way except the foot is held in neutral flexion. The long toe flexors are tested by exerting a counterforce to the tip of the toes while the patient flexes the interphalangeal joints.

The soleus and gastrocnemius should be evaluated separately. The soleus is evaluated by applying a dorsiflexion force to the foot while the patient plantar flexes the foot with the knee in flexion. The same maneuver is then performed with the knee in extension to evaluate the muscle power of the gastrocnemius. The muscle testing is most important in dealing with neuromuscular disorders which can cause various deformities of the foot.

Neurological Examinations

Muscle testing is just one part of the neurological examination which also includes evaluation of sensorium and tendon reflexes. Achilles tendon reflex and ankle clonus should always be checked. Pathological reflexes, such as Babinski's, Oppenheim's, Chaddock's, Gordon's, Rossolimo's, and Schaeffer's signs, should also be tested. The sensory deficit is evaluated in relation to the dermogram of the foot and ankle (Fig. 12-14).

When evaluating a patient with metatarsalgia, one should always examine the sensorium of the digital nerve. Symptoms which appear to be from a metatarsalgia may be from a Morton's neuroma in which there is a sensory deficit of the involved digital nerve. Tenderness can be more severe in the plantar surface of the web space rather than the metatarsal heads. Morton's neuroma is most common between the third and fourth toes. When evaluating for pain on the medial side of the ankle, one should always be aware of the possibility of a tarsal tunnel syndrome. Therefore a Tinel's test and palpation over the posterior tibial nerve at the posterior aspect of the medial malleolus should be performed. There are many causes for this entrapment syndrome, but old fractures of the ankle and diabetes mellitus are the most common. Sensory disturbances which do not fit a dermographic distribution pattern are commonly seen in peripheral neuritis or in circulatory disturbances.

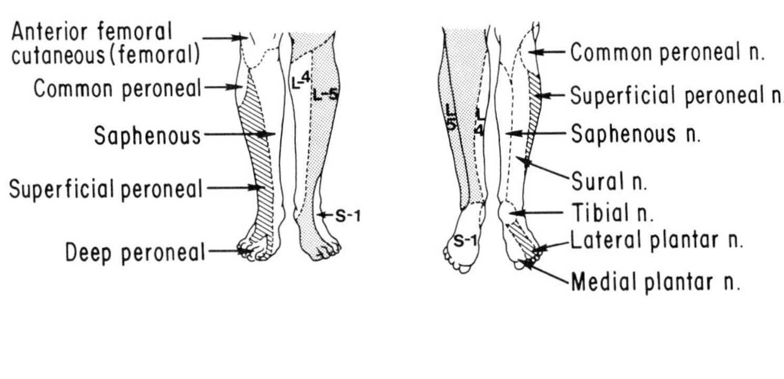

Fig. 12-14. Dermogram of foot and ankle.

Vascular Examination

The vascular status should be evaluated in terms of the arterial, venous, and lymphatic circulation. One should palpate the dorsalis pedis in the dorsum of the foot and the tibialis posterior at the posterior aspect of the medial malleolus and note their intensity. Capillary filling of the toes should also be checked. The color of the skin, temperature, and trophic changes of the toes should be noted.

Swelling or edema of the foot and ankle should be confirmed through palpation and measurement. Recent injury or acute arthritis may be an obvious cause. However, the ankle and foot are the most common sites for edema or swelling due to gravity. The swelling may be secondary to a disturbance of the venous or lymphatic return system, such as varicose veins, venous thrombosis, pregnancy, or lymphangitis. It may also be secondary to such systemic diseases as renal disorders, cardiac problems, hypothyroidism, or diabetes mellitus. Edema caused by these systemic disorders is characterized by their bilateralism in contrast to a unilateral problem secondary to local problems.

Special Tests and Signs

Homans' Sign. This test was designed to detect deep venous thrombosis in the lower part of the leg. It is positive if sudden increase of pain in the calf and/or popliteal space is noted on passive dorsiflexion of the ankle.

Thompson's Test. This test was designed to detect rupture of the Achilles tendon. The patient is placed in the prone position or kneels with his feet extending over the edge of the bed and the middle third of the calf muscle is squeezed. If the Achilles tendon, particularly the soleus portion, is ruptured, the squeeze does not cause a normal plantar flexion response.

Examination of the Shoes

Never neglect the examination of the shoes; this is a unique aspect in the examination of the foot and ankle. It is particularly important when dealing with disorders of the toes and metatarsophalangeal joints in the adult. Frequently a pair of shoes with an ill-fitted toe box or an excessively high heel can cause severe problems. A bony prominence from a primary deformity of the foot may cause secondary soft tissue problems due to tight-fitting shoes. When inspecting a shoe, observe the pattern of wear of the sole and heel. Note any abnormal deformation of the dorsum of the shoes and attempt to correlate it with the foot problem.

Roentgenographic Examination

Roentgenograms of the ankle joint should include anteroposterior, lateral, and oblique views. For the foot, anteroposterior and lateral views are routine. When a congenital deformity of the foot is present in children and preadolescents, modified additional views are usually necessary. These will be described in the differential diagnosis section with the particular diseases.

DIFFERENTIAL DIAGNOSIS OF FOOT AND ANKLE

The problems of children and adults are considered separately in view of the difference of the incidence and fundamental nature of the diseases occurring in the two groups. Congenital deformities of the foot in children seldom present with pain as a complaint. However, the same congenital deformity with superimposed secondary problems will present with pain when seen in adult life. The secondary problems may be the result of neglected disease or maltreatment. The classification described in Table 12-1 is based on generality, and the reader should not be misled into believing that these classified diseases always apply to a particular age group or the bone disease always causes the same deformity. It is also important to realize that diseases noted as painless disorders may also cause pain and that various types of hindfoot and forefoot deformities are frequently present concomitantly. In adults, the problems of the foot and ankle are almost always associated with pain, except for some of the primary dermatological disorders. When considering the differential diagnosis of adult foot and ankle disorders, it is most important to anatomically localize the source of pain and make a classification based on anatomical structure.

Table 12-1. Differential Diagnosis of Foot Deformities in Children

A. Hind Foot
  1. *Heel Varus* (heel inverted)
     a. Talipes equinovarus
     b. Talipes varus
     c. Arthrogryposis
     d. Poliomyelitis
     e. Friedreich's ataxia
     f. Meningomyelocele
     g. Post-injury sequelae to brain, spinal cord, peripheral nerve
     h. Cerebral palsy
     i. Congenital contracture of triceps surae
     j. Charcot joint
     k. Charcot-Marie-Tooth disease
     l. Diastematomyelia
     m. Myotonic dystrophy
     n. Osteogenesis imperfecta
     o. Congenital indifference to pain (results of trauma)
     p. Rickets
     q. Trisomy 13–15, 18
     r. Neurofibromatosis
  2. *Heel Valgus* (heel everted)
     a. Pes planus (pronated foot, so-called flatfoot)
     b. Vertical talus
     c. Arthrogryposis
     d. Talipes calcaneovalgus
     e. Talipes equinovalgus
     f. Tarsal coalition
     g. Meningomyelocele
     h. Poliomyelitis
     i. Cerebral palsy
     j. Post-injury sequelae to brain, spinal cord, peripheral nerve
     k. Charcot joint
     l. Diastematomyelia
     m. Ehlers-Danlos syndrome
     n. Osteogenesis imperfecta
     o. Congenital indifference to pain (results of trauma)
     p. Maltreated metatarsus varus
     q. Trisomy 13–15, 18
     r. Neurofibromatosis
  3. *Equinus Foot*
     a. Talipes equinovarus
     b. Talipes equinovalgus
     c. Vertical talus
     d. Arthrogryposis
     e. Cerebral palsy
     f. Friedreich's ataxia
     g. Poliomyelitis
     h. Post-injury sequelae to brain, spinal cord, peripheral nerve
     i. Meningomyelocele
     j. Congenital contracture of triceps surae
     k. Diastematomyelia
     l. Myotonic dystrophy
     m. Osteogenesis imperfecta
     n. Congenital indifference to pain (results of trauma)
     o. Trisomy 13–15, 18
     p. Neurofibromatosis
  4. *Calcaneus Deformity*
     a. Poliomyelitis
     b. Talipes calcaneovalgus
     c. Post-injury sequelae to the posterior tibial nerve
     d. Meningomyelocele
     e. Neurofibromatosis

B. Midtarsus and Metatarsus
  1. *Adduction deformity*
     a. Congenital clubfoot
     b. Congenital metatarsus varus
     c. Metatarsus primus varus
     d. Metatarsus primus atavicus when associated with clubfoot or metatarsus varus
  2. *Dropped Arch* (pes planus)
     a. Pronated foot (pes planus)
     b. Vertical talus
     c. Connective tissue disorders causing laxity such as Ehlers-Danlos syndrome
     d. Maltreated heel equinus deformity
     e. Secondary to heel valgus deformity of various etiology
  3. *High Arch* (pes cavus)
     a. Neuromuscular diseases
        1. Charcot-Marie-Tooth disease
        2. Dejerine-Sottas interstitial hypertrophic neuritis
        3. Meningomyelocele
        4. Neurofibromatosis
        5. Diastematomyelia
        6. Post-traumatic sequelae to brain, spinal cord, peripheral nerve
        7. Poliomyelitis
        8. Spinal cord tumor
        9. Friedreich's ataxia
        10. Roussy-Lévy syndrome
        11. Cerebral palsy
     b. Congenital club foot
     c. Congenital metatarsal adductus
     d. Idiopathic pes cavus
  4. *Abduction Deformity*
     a. Secondary to dropped arch of various causes; typically vertical talus, talipes calcaneovalgus

C. Toe
  1. Claw toes (pes cavus)
  2. Congenital curly toe
  3. Hammer toe
  4. Congenital overriding of toes
  5. Polydactylism
  6. Syndactylism
  7. Macrodactyly
  8. Mallet toe
  9. Microdactylism
  10. Valgus deformity of hallus at interphalangeal joint
  11. Hallux valgus
  12. Hallux varus

D. Ankle
  1. Charcot joint
  2. Congenital indifference to pain
  3. Congenital epiphyseal dysplasia such as dysplasia epiphysealis hemimelica
  4. Some bone and soft tissue tumors (osteochondroma, lipoma, etc.)

Painless Deformity of Ankle and Foot in Children

Congenital Clubfoot (Talipes Equinovarus, Talipes Varus)

It is composed of an equinus (plantar flexed) and varus (inverted) hindfoot and an adducted forefoot. The medial side of the forefoot has a cavus deformity (high foot arch). The deformity may or may not involve all these elements. The word "talipes" is derived from the Latin "talus" (ankle) and "pes" (foot). The primary deformity of a clubfoot is in the hindfoot, and, thus, the Latin description of the hindfoot deformity is traditionally used when referring to this disease. Talipes equinovarus is more common than talipes varus.

The etiology is unknown but it appears that it is a combination of genetic and in utero environments. Boys are affected twice as often as are girls. The primary skeletal deformity is probably in the anterior part of the talus, which is deviated in a medial and plantar direction. The general contour of the calcaneus is normal, but the talocalcaneal relationship is secondarily distorted resulting in varus and equinus of the calcaneus. The navicular and cuboid are displaced inward, causing metatarsus adductus. No abnormality of the tibiotalar relationship has been shown. Soft tissue changes are thought to be a secondary adaptation to the primary bony abnormalities, but the soft tissue structures in the medial and posterior aspect of the foot and ankle are shortened and do not develop normally. Contractures can occur in the posterior, medial, subtalar, and plantar soft tissue and are sometimes severe. In posterior contractures, the posterior capsule of the ankle and subtalar joint, the posterior talofibular ligament, and the triceps surae are shortened. The Achilles tendon inserts more medially, increasing the varus tendency. Medially, the deltoid, tibionavicular, and calcaneonavicular ligaments, plus the talonavicular joint capsule are shortened. The tibialis posterior, flexor digitorum longus and flexor hallucis muscles, and the neurovascular bundle are also tightened. In the subtalar area, the talocalcaneal interosseous ligament and bifurcated ligament (extending from the calcaneus to the lateral border of navicular and to the medial border of the cuboid) are shortened. The plantar fascia, abductor hallucis, and short toe flexors are shortened plantarward.

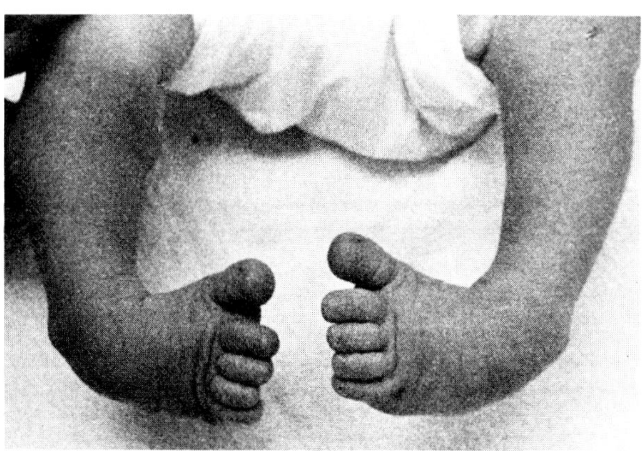

Fig. 12-15. Photograph of clubfoot. (Courtesy of Dr. Richard Kendrick)

The deformity is present at birth with varying degrees of severity. Those patients with poorly developed musculature and a small heel revealing a hindfoot in severe equinovarus and a forefoot in marked adductus have the worst prognosis. In the severe cases, the deformities are rigid, and it is extremely difficult to bring the heel to the neutral position. The flexible type of clubfoot with less severe deformity and contracture may be correctable to the neutral position on manipulation. The musculature development in such cases is good, without evidence of calf atrophy.

There are obvious characteristics readily observed because of the anatomical deformities. The hindfoot points downward with the heel drawn up under the talus in an inverted position. There are deepened skin creases on the posterior aspect of the ankle. The forefoot is adducted and inverted (Fig. 12-15). The head of the talus is very prominent laterally on the dorsum of the foot. The cuboid bone and fifth metatarsal base are prominent on the lateral border of the foot and point to the ground. The lateral malleolus is more prominent than the medial malleolus. The navicular bone is medially displaced and palpated on the innerside of the head of the talus. The tightened soft tissue structures are easily palpated on passive dorsiflexion and eversion of the foot.

When evaluating a patient with clubfoot deformity, all other joints, particularly the hip, must be carefully examined for subluxation or dislocation because of the association of clubfoot deformity with arthrogryposis. The spine should be carefully inspected during the neurological examination to rule out such primary neurological disorders as cerebral palsy, Charcot-Marie-Tooth disease, intraspinal tumor, or disorders at the spine, such as meningomyelocele and diastematomyelia, which are often associated with a clubfoot deformity.

The roentgenograms are used to determine the degree of deformity and serve as a guide for follow-up assessment during and after treatment, rather than for the purpose of diagnosis which is obvious on clinical examination (Figs. 12-11 and 12-16). Anteroposterior and lateral roentgenograms should be obtained. The lateral view is taken in plantar flexion and maximum dorsiflexion. In the older patient, standing weight-bearing films should always be taken. In the anteroposterior roentgenogram, the talocalcaneal angle is diminished below the normal of 20 to 40 degrees. In the lateral roentgenogram the talocalcaneal angle is decreased below the normal of 35 to 50 degrees. On maximum dorsiflexion this angle is diminished even further (increases in normal foot) (see Fig. 12-11).

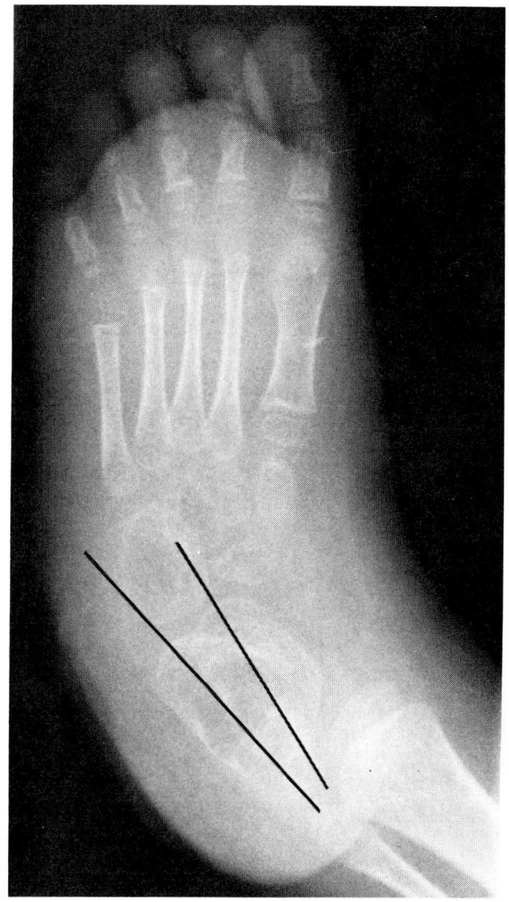

Fig. 12-16. Anteroposterior roentgenogram of a clubfoot. The talocalcaneal angle is significantly decreased.

Arthrogryposis

Arthrogryposis is a syndrome characterized by multiple contractures of various joints. The etiology has yet to be delineated but in utero, developmental, or environmental theories appear to be generally accepted. Sporadic reports of a hereditary incidence of the disease have been discussed, but the role of heredity has not been established. There is general agreement that the disease can be classified into three types: 1) neuropathic form, in which the anterior horn cells are decreased, the size of the spinal cord is decreased, and denervation with muscle atrophy is present; 2) myogenic form, in which the muscle biopsy reveals a fibrofatty change with no demonstrable change in the nervous system; and 3) mixed types with a combination of 1 and 2.

The clinical picture is present at birth. Both the extremities and trunk can be affected, but this is not always the case. Certain clinical features are very characteristic of the disease. They include atrophied muscles, multiple joint contractures with decreased active and passive range of motion, and tight and shiny skin which forms a flexed contracture webbing around the joint. There is no sensory deficit, but deep tendon reflexes are reduced or absent; mentality is generally normal. Typical deformities include dislocated hips and knees and talipes equinovalgus or a typical talipes equinovarus in the foot. The shoulder is usually in internal rotation, with forearm pronation, wrist flexion, and adduction of the thumb into the palm.

Vertical Talus (Congenital Convex Pes Valgus)

Vertical talus is essentially a primary dislocation of the talonavicular joint following which the navicular abnormally articulates with the dorsum of the talus, thus locking the talus in a plantar-flexed vertical position. The subsequent result is a rocker-bottom foot deformity which is present at birth giving the sole a convex appearance. Vertical talus may occur as an isolated primary deformity or in association with arthrogryposis, trisomy 13-5, trisomy-18, or meningomyelocele. Vertical talus may also be associated with dislocation of the hip, neurofibromatosis, and pollex varus.

Vertical talus is a rare disease, more common in males. The vertical position of the talus produces overstretching of the spring ligament, the dorsal talonavicular ligament, and shortening of the anterior part of the deltoid ligament. The anterior part of the calcaneus is pushed laterally, and the sustentaculum tali no longer supports the talus. The head of the talus is markedly prominent on the medial plantar aspect of the foot. The forefoot is abducted and dorsiflexed at the intertarsal joints, but the forefoot interrelationship is not disturbed. Along with the rocker-bottom deformity, the anterior tibial, extensor hallucis longus, extensor digitorum longus, peroneus brevis, and triceps surae muscles are all contracted. The posterior tibial and peroneal tendons are usually displaced anteriorly and function as dorsiflexors rather than plantar flexors as they do normally. The hindfoot is in equinovalgus with a contracted triceps surae and an everted and plantar flexed calcaneus. As a result of the above deformities, the ankle joint has limited plantar flexion and the subtalar joint, limited inversion.

The distorted talonavicular relationship produces a deep skin crease on the dorsolateral aspect of the foot near the ankle joint. When the patient stands, the head of the talus touches the ground but the heel may not. Lateral roentgenograms taken in maximum plantar flexion reveal a vertically positioned talus in relation to the calcaneus, confirming the diagnosis (Fig. 12-17). The talocalcaneal angle in the anteroposterior roentgenogram will be increased. The differential diagnosis includes any disorder which causes equinovalgus of the foot, dropped arch, and abduction of the forefoot. The disorders commonly mimicking vertical talus on clinical examination are talipes calcaneovalgus, tarsal coalition, and maltreated clubfoot. Talipes calcaneovalgus has an os calcis and talus which are dorsiflexed and flexible, and the ankle joint is easily plantar flexed. Tarsal coalition has a very rigid subtalar joint with heel valgus but good ankle motion. The rocker-bottom deformity seen with maltreated clubfoot is the result of a forefoot forcibly dorsiflexed without correction of hindfoot equinus. A thorough clinical examination is usually sufficient to differentiate the disorders, but roentgenographic examination will confirm the diagnosis.

Pes Planus (Pronated Foot)

Pes planus (pronated foot) is the normal appearance of feet seen in many cultures of the world and is commonly referred to as flatfeet in our culture. Some authors prefer to use pronated foot as the terminology for the disorder and pes planus as the descriptive term for the deformity. Pes planus assumes heel valgus and dropped arch on weight-bearing but on nonweight-bearing the deformity often disappears or becomes very mild. The child with pes planus often learns to walk with a toe-in gait, so that the weight-bearing line falls in the center, rather than on the medial side of the foot normally seen in patients. This pattern of walking protects the ligamentous weakness of the arch support. No joint contractures are present and active range of motion is not limited in either the ankle or foot. Other possible causes of toe-in walking must be differentiated particularly that due to hip anteversion or tibial torsion. Connective tissue disorders causing ligamentous laxity must also be ruled out. The rigid

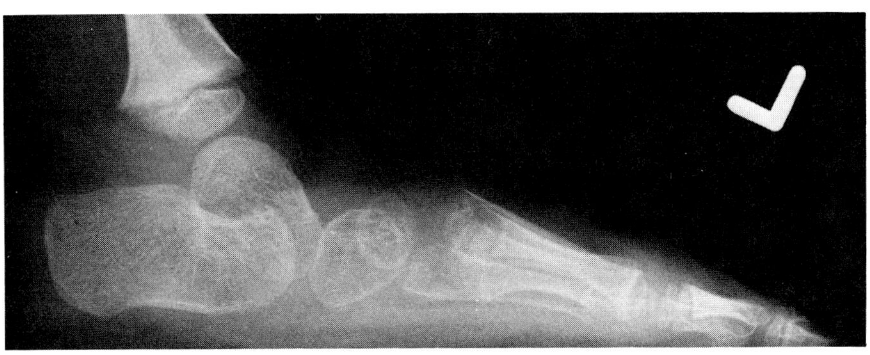

Fig. 12-17. Lateral roentgenogram of a vertical talus.

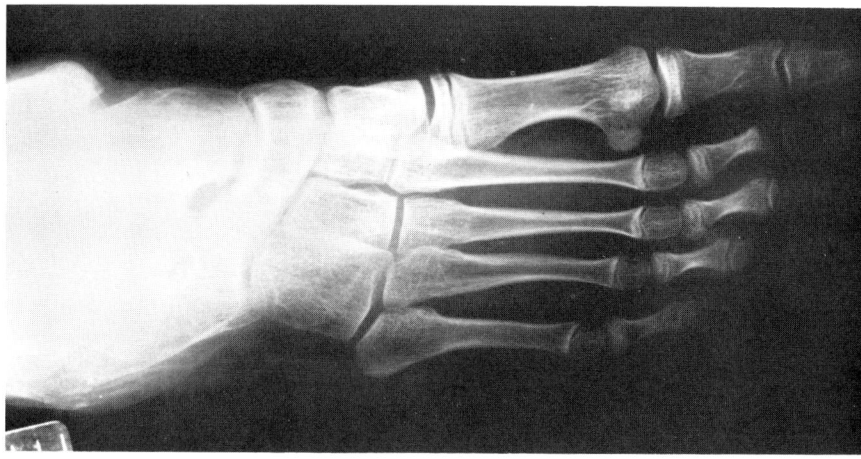

Fig. 12-18. Oblique roentgenogram of a foot showing a calcanconavicular coalition. (Courtesy of Dr. Jerremy Kaye)

flatfoot of tarsal coalition is sometimes confused with the more common flexible flatfoot of pes planus if flexibility is not assessed.

Tarsal Coalition

Tarsal coalition is caused by varying degrees of union (osseous, cartilaginous, fibrous, or a combination) which occur between two or more tarsal bones, producing a rigid planovalgus foot. The intertarsal fusions may be talocalcaneal (anterior, middle, or posterior facet), calcaneonavicular, talonavicular, calcaneocuboid, cubonavicular, or multiple and massive in type. It is thought to result from a failure of differentiation and segmentation of the primary mesenchyme which produces abnormal joint formation between the tarsal bones. Some evidence of heredity has been suggested. The talocalcaneal coalition is most common followed by calcaneonavicular and multiple coalition. The vast majority of rigid flatfeet are talocalcaneal and calcaneonavicular coalitions. The disease is usually not suspected before the patient begins walking and presents as parents become concerned over restricted motion at the involved tarsus. Most frequently the patient will present himself with pain in adolescence or early adult life, with restricted motion in the subtalar and midtarsal joints. The planovalgus deformity and rigidity are more severe in the talocalcaneal than in the calcaneonavicular coalition. Peroneal muscle spasticity is frequently noted at some time during the course of the disease. The patient with talonavicular coalition usually presents with a complaint of a prominence on the medial side of the foot, rather than pain. The arch of the foot is maintained.

If a tarsal coalition is suspected, special views must be obtained in addition to the routine anteroposterior and lateral roentgenograms. Calcaneonavicular coalition is best demonstrated on a 45 degree oblique view taken with the foot on the film with the roentgenogram beam projected from lateral to medial, at the middle of the foot (Fig. 12-18). For talocalcaneal coalition, particularly for middle and posterior facet evaluation, a 45 degree angle axial view of the calcaneus should be obtained (Fig. 12-19). One should remember that in the child, a good part of the bone is cartilaginous and even in the adult, when ossification is complete, the bars causing coalition may not necessarily be ossified. The roentgenograms are not a substitute for but must be used in conjunction with the clinical examination.

Talipes Calcaneovalgus

This disorder is noted at birth and has an incidence of 1 in 1,000 births, about the same as clubfoot. The cause of this disorder may be in utero environmental with a slightly greater predilection in females. The entire foot is dorsiflexed and everted but flexible and can be corrected easily on physical examination. It must be differentiated from vertical talus, in which the hindfoot is fixed in an equinus position, the talus vertically locked and a forefoot which is everted and abducted. Both conditions have a rocker-bottom deformity but of different severity. Careful roentgenographic studies, as outlined under

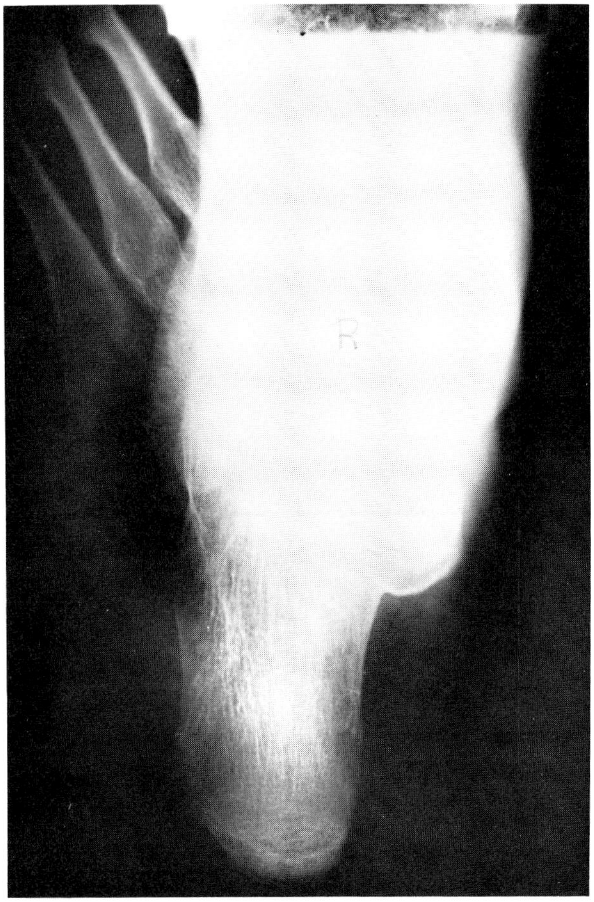

Fig. 12-19. An axial view roentgenogram of a calcaneus showing a talocalcaneal coalition. (Courtesy of Dr. Jerremy Kaye)

vertical talus, should be performed. Neurogenic disorders must be ruled out, and it is important to demonstrate functioning gastrosoleus, posterior tibial, and toe flexor muscle groups.

Congenital Metatarsus Varus

Congenital metatarsus varus presents at birth and is thought to be secondary to both genetic and environmental influences. The incidence is about 1 in 1,000 births with a slight predominance in females. All five metatarsals are adducted and inverted at the tarsometatarsal joints. The hindfoot is in neutral or a slight valgus position. Unlike the forefoot adduction of congenital clubfoot, the navicular is usually not displaced medially from the neck of the talus. The great toe is usually widely separated from the second toe. The medial border of the foot is concave and the lateral, convex. The arch of the foot tends to be high. Remember that normal infants have an active plantar grasp reflex revealing a tendency to forefoot adduction, but there is no fixed forefoot adduction. Anteroposterior roentgenograms reveal a normal or slightly increased talocalcaneal angle. Since the ossification center of the navicular bone does not appear until three years of age, one cannot visualize the naviculotalar relationship on roentgenograms until the age of three years (Fig. 12-20). After age three the navicular can be seen and is noted to be in normal relationship to the talus. A lateral roentgenogram reveals a talus and calcaneus which are not in plantar flexion.

Metatarsus Primus Varus

This condition is hereditary, manifesting at birth, with a marked predisposition to females. In contradistinction to metatarsus adductus, only the first metatarsal is deviated medially, with other metatarsals maintaining normal alignment. The deformity is trivial and is often neglected at early childhood. It often presents in later childhood with an associated hallux valgus causing difficulty with shoe wear.

Pes Cavus

By definition, pes cavus is a fixed equinus deformity of the forefoot in relation to the hindfoot regardless of the presence of hindfoot deformity (see Fig.

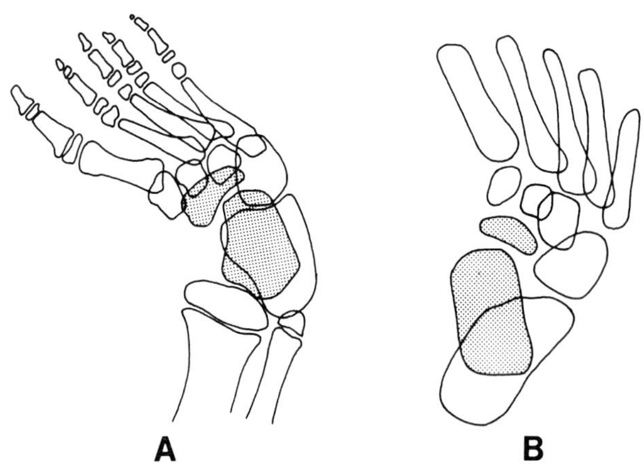

Fig. 12-20. Schematic representation of the talonavicular relationship in a clubfoot (*A*) and congenital metatarsus adductus (*B*). In a clubfoot the navicular bone is also adducted with the forefoot.

12-12). Congenital deformities, such as clubfoot, may have a pes cavus deformity, but it is the neuromuscular disease entities which must be ruled out when seeing patients with pes cavus. Muscle imbalance in and around the foot is considered responsible for the deformity. It is not usually due to increased strength of some muscle group but rather a matter of relativeness or a compensatory over-reaction. The muscle imbalance theories include imbalance between a strong peroneus longus and a weak anterior tibial muscle, intrinsic muscle paralysis, and a weak triceps surae which causes overaction of the other plantar flexors.

Pes cavus may or may not be associated with other types of deformity. The common types of pes cavus are simple pes cavus, pes cavovarus (medial column of the forefoot is dropped and lateral column is normal), calcaneocavus, and pes equinocavus. Calcaneocavus is seen in patients with meningomyelocele or poliomyelitis who have a flaccid paralysis of the gastrosoleus muscle. Pes equinocavus is common in clubfoot. The first cuneiform is most prominent in the cavus foot and, less frequently, the navicular bone forms the apex. Secondarily the toes exhibit a claw toe deformity (metatarsophalangeal hyperextension) which becomes exaggerated during the swing phase of gait. Pain in the dorsum of the interphalangeal joints of the toes or metatarsalgia with keratotic skin over these areas may be the chief complaint in later childhood or in adults. The plantar soft tissue structures are contracted and are best demonstrated on dorsiflexion of the forefoot. Every patient with pes cavus should have roentgenograms of the entire spine plus an anteroposterior and lateral weight-bearing and nonweight-bearing roentgenogram of the foot.

Metatarsus Primus Atavicus (Congenital Short First Metatarsal)

A shortened first metatarsal can occur as an isolated deformity or in association with metatarsus varus or clubfoot. It was first noted by Morton and, thus, is sometimes called Morton's toe. As an isolated deformity, it usually goes unnoticed until adolescence or adult life. If it is an element of associated deformities, the other deformities prompt attention rather than the metatarsus primus atavicus. Shortening of the first metatarsal in adults may cause more weight-bearing than usual on the second or third toe which may produce metatarsalgia. However, it is not the most frequent cause of metatarsalgia.

Congenital Contracture of Triceps Surae

This disorder is noted soon after the patient begins to walk. In normal children, a heel-to-toe walking pattern is established within six months after he or she has started to walk. Persistent toe walking in the child is usually secondary to contracture of the gastrosoleus with associated limited dorsiflexion of the ankle joint. An abnormally low insertion of the hypertrophied soleus can be palpated. Although the results of neurological examinations are usually negative, one should always rule out such disorders as cerebral palsy.

Congenital Indifference to Pain

Congenital indifference to pain is a rare disorder. The patients have no response to painful stimuli with an otherwise intact central and peripheral nervous systems. Without pain sensation, patients are unaware of being hurt and may continue their usual activities despite the injury. The end result of the repeated unnoticed trauma is various deformities of the bones and joints of the foot and ankle. The repeated trauma to the joints results in effusion hemarthrosis, synovial thickening, and joint laxity. The advanced situation reveals the same pathological and radiological manifestations as Charcot's joint.

In a child, unrecognized epiphyseal separation may heal in a malformed fashion, and the ankle joint is one of the more common locations. If a Charcot joint-type deformity is noted in a child, one should always consider this rather rare disease in the differential diagnosis. Skeletal survey roentgenograms are sometimes necessary to discover silent fractures if the diagnosis is seriously suspected. Once the patients have grown and realize the seriousness of the condition, they are more careful of injury.

Congenital Ball and Socket Ankle Joint

In this rare congenital disorder, the talus is dome-shaped in the sagittal and coronal planes, forming a ball-like articulating surface with the tibia. Lateral and medial instability of the ankle joint is inherent, and the patients are prone to ligamentous injury. It is sometimes associated with congenital hypoplasia or absence of the fibula and failure of segmentation of the vertebrae. An anteroposterior roentgenogram of the ankle joint confirms the diagnosis.

Painful Disorders Involving Epiphysis or Subchondral Bone in Children

Juvenile Osteochondroses

This is a group of conditions, commonly seen at puberty, in which the primary or secondary ossification center undergoes spontaneous aseptic necrosis. Following the avascular insult, a secondary reconstructive process takes place around the dead bone. It occurs in the epiphysis and apophysis of the long bones or ossification centers of the flat bones. The common locations in the foot are the second metatarsal head, calcaneal apophysis, and navicular bone. Many people, however, consider juvenile osteochondroses in the navicular bone (Kohler's disease) or calcaneal apophysis (Sever's disease) merely as irregular ossification patterns in normal development. There is pain and tenderness over these bones, and soft tissue swelling over these areas is often present. When it occurs in the metatarsal head, it is known as Freiberg's disease, and the usual complaints are increased pain in the affected metatarsal head on walking or athletic activity. The pain eases with rest, but movement of the affected metatarsophalangeal joint increases the pain. Roentgenograms demonstrate the irregular fragmentation of the epiphysis of the metatarsal bone, thus confirming the diagnosis (Fig. 12-21).

Osteochondritis Dissecans

Osteochondritis dissecans in the foot and ankle is most common in the dome of the talus and the first metatarsal head respectively. It commonly occurs in adolescents with or without a history of injury. Sometimes a fragment of the osteochondral segment separates from the underlying bone substance and becomes detached to form a loose body. Whether the osteochondral fragment becomes necrotic before or after the separation is not known. The patient will complain of increasing pain in the involved area on walking or during an athletic activity and obtain relief at rest. There is tenderness over the involved area often with a joint effusion, and range of motion is limited because of the pain. Persistent pain in the

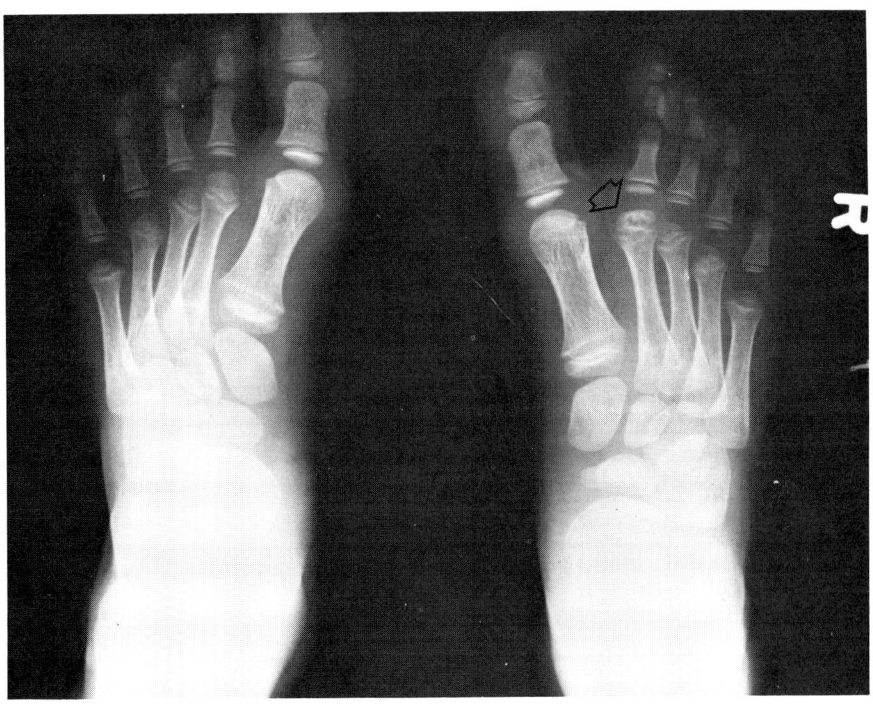

Fig. 12-21. Anteroposterior roentgenogram of a foot showing Freiberg's disease of the second metatarsal head (*arrow*).

ankle or the first metatarsophalangeal joint in an adolescent should always alert the examiner to the possibility of this disorder. Routine roentgenographic examination demonstrating the separation of the necrotic osteochondral fragment from the underlying bone substance confirms the diagnosis.

Disorders of Toe and Metatarsophalangeal Joints

Although toe deformities may be seen in childhood, these are more common in adulthood because most of the toe deformities develop gradually and are usually not bothersome in childhood. Hallux valgus and hammer toe are typical examples. However, there are congenital anomalies, such as polydactylism, syndactylism, macrodactyly, microdactyly, congenital overriding of toes, or lobster-claw foot which quickly draw the parents' attention during infancy. Once noted, one should investigate whether an anomaly is an isolated problem or part of a multiple congenital anomaly which may or may not be hereditary.

Hammer Toe

Hammer toe is essentially a proximal interphalangeal joint flexion contracture. The distal interphalangeal joint may be in flexion, neutral, or extension. The presence of a proximal interphalangeal joint flexion contracture augments the tendency of metatarsophalangeal hyperextension. The second toe is the most common location, and there is a tendency of bilateral involvement with a high familial incidence.

Claw Toe

Claw toe is a metatarsophalangeal hyperextension contracture. It is usually associated with proximal interphalangeal and distal interphalangeal flexion. When the patient stands, the tip of the toes may not be in contact with the ground. If claw toes are seen, one should always perform a complete neurological examination to rule out an underlying neurological disease. The pes cavus deformity is frequently associated with claw toes.

Mallet Toe

Mallet toe is defined as a distal interphalangeal joint flexion contracture. It usually occurs in the smaller toes and is less common than hammer toes.

Congenital Curly Toe

Congenital curly toe is a deformity in which the toe becomes bent in the plantar direction with medial deviation and lateral rotation at the distal interphalangeal joint. The involved toe curls under the adjacent toe. The third or fourth toe is the common site of involvement with a high incidence of bilateral involvement and strong familial tendency.

Congenital Overriding of the Toe

Congenital overriding of the toe is a common familial deformity and is most common in the fifth toe. The overriding is caused by dorsomedial subluxation at the metatarsophalangeal joint of the involved toe. Flexion deformity is not seen at the distal interphalangeal or proximal interphalangeal joints.

Remember most toe deformities are ignored in childhood because of lack of pain, but in later life attention is drawn to them because of pain. Hyperkeratosis is commonly seen over the prominent area where shoe contact takes place.

Morton's Neuroma (Plantar Digital Neuroma)

Morton's neuroma is a relatively common disorder in the adult. A fibroneuromatous reaction between the third and fourth metatarsal heads over the deep transverse metatarsal ligament affects the lateral terminal branch of the median plantar nerve. The impinging effect on the nerve is accentuated with

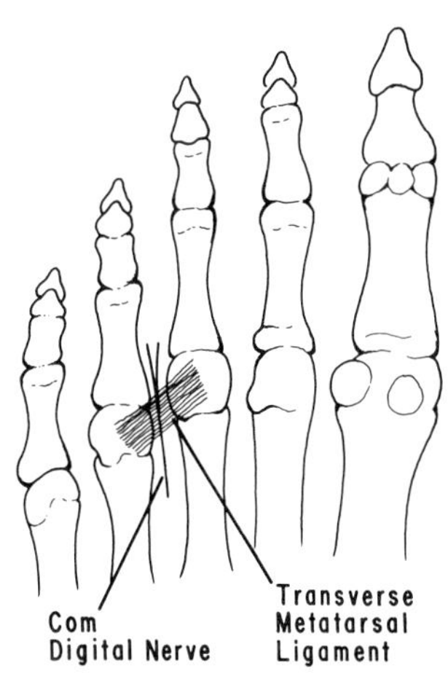

Fig. 12-22. Schematic representation of the interrelationship between the nerve and deep transverse metatarsal ligament.

weight-bearing, particularly during the push off phase of walking or when the metatarsal heads are compressed (Fig. 12-22). There is localized tenderness between the third and fourth metatarsal heads on the plantar surface. Hypesthesia over the lateral and medial side of the third and fourth toes, respectively, may be present. Morton's neuroma can occur in other web spaces involving the corresponding terminal branch of either the medial or lateral plantar nerve but less frequently.

Metatarsalgia

The term metatarsalgia denotes pain in the metatarsals and is a very common condition in the adult. It is caused by various foot deformities or arthritis of the metatarsophalangeal joints, most commonly due to rheumatoid arthritis. The term "metatarsalgia" is used in referring to a pain syndrome and is not a disease per se. It may occur as an isolated condition or occur in association with hallux valgus or rigidus. The patient complains of pain in the metatarsal heads or toes on standing during the push off phase of gait. On examination, there is localized tenderness directly under the plantar surface of the metatarsal head. The most common sites for the pain are the second and third metatarsal heads, with excessive pressure over the metatarsal heads as a cause of the pain. It is aggravated by ill-fitted shoes which squeeze the toes into a narrow toe-box. It is differentiated from Morton's neuroma by having its most severe tenderness directly under the metatarsal heads and no associated hypesthesia of the involved toes.

Hallux Valgus (Bunion)

Hallux valgus is seen in children but is much more common in the adult. The proximal phalanx of the first toe displaces laterally in relation to the first metatarsal. Metatarsus primus varus may cause hallux valgus with use of a shoe, but by far idiopathic hallux valgus is more common. Although disagreements exist, an ill-fitted shoe is probably responsible for this condition. The patient complains of pain, swelling, and tenderness at the dorsomedial aspect of the first metatarsophalangeal joint. There may be fluid accumulation due to bursitis, and the overlying skin may be hypertrophic or broken down. Excessive displacement of the great toe under the second often leads to metatarsalgia of the second and third metatarsals with development of painful calluses over the second and third toes. The first metatarsophalangeal joint itself may or may not be painful, even though there is some joint degeneration. Gout should always be considered in a differential of symptoms at the first metatarsophalangeal joint.

Hallux Varus

Hallux varus is medial deviation of the proximal phalanx of the great toe at the first metatarsophalangeal joint. It may be congenital or the postoperative result of hallux valgus. Congenital hallux varus is extremely rare and is caused by a weak adductor hallucis muscle.

Hallux Rigidus

Hallux rigidus is degenerative joint disease of the first metatarsophalangeal joint. It may or may not be associated with hallux valgus. The patient complains of pain in that joint on walking, and on examination range of motion of the first metatarsophalangeal joint is markedly limited, especially extension. Passive range of motion increases the pain. Osteophytes are palpable at the metatarsal head and base of the proximal phalanx. Roentgenographic examination reveals joint narrowing and osteophyte formation much as other degenerative joint diseases (Fig. 12-23).

Bunion of the Fifth Toe (Tailor's Bunion)

The fifth metatarsal head occasionally develops degenerative changes with osteophyte formation. This condition is common in people like tailors who sit in a cross-legged fashion placing pressure on the fifth metatarsal head. The involved joint becomes tender, and palpable osteophytes are often present.

Callus

Callus is seen in any portion of the foot where abnormal pressure or excessive friction occurs from ill-fitted shoes or well-fitted shoes with a foot deformity. It is a hyperkeratotic response of the skin to these stresses with resultant thick skin formation. The callus is most common over the toes and under the metatarsal heads.

Corns

Corns are seen more commonly over the interphalangeal joint of the fifth toe or dorsal prominence of the hammer toe. They are also seen in the web space between the fourth and fifth toes and are caused by compression of the skin between the head of the fifth proximal phalanx and the base of the fourth proximal phalanx. The web space corns are called soft corns in contrast to the hard corn seen on the dorsum of the toes. It is a hyperkeratotic response of the skin to abnormal stresses with the keratotic proliferation progressing inward with central core formation. Soft corns of the web space can be extremely painful and are often complicated by a sinus leading into the metatarsal interspace with recurrent episodes of acute infection.

Plantar Warts

Plantar warts are secondary to viral infections. Unlike calluses, they occur on nonweight-bearing surfaces, but their appearance may mimic that of a callus. On physical examination the location of the lesion becomes very important in differentiating these two lesions. Typically plantar warts are oval or round shaped and are encapsulated. They have a soft center and easily bleed on trimming. A callus is tender only to direct pressure, but a wart is also tender on lateral compression.

Ingrown Toenails

Invariably ingrown toenails occur in the great toe. The nail groove is cut into by the edge of the nail, and the groove becomes irritated often with superimposed infection. It is caused by improper pedicure and ill-fitted shoes.

Bursitis

Bursitis is an inflammation of the normal anatomical bursa. There are various superficial soft parts of the foot where the normal anatomical bursa do not exist, but localized fluid accumulation can develop which is known as adventitious bursitis. It is most common at the first and fifth metatarsophalangeal joints and under hard corns. It is also seen at the Achilles tendon insertion and the dorsum of the first metatarsophalangeal joint with or without an associated hallux valgus.

Sesamoid Disorders

The sesamoids at the first metatarsophalangeal joint often undergo pathological changes. Sesamoiditis and dislocation of the sesamoids are the most common problems encountered, with fracture, aseptic necrosis, and sesamoid degeneration being less frequent. The sesamoid on the tibial side is most prone to these changes because it supports most of the weight transferred from the first metatarsal head. Pain and tenderness are aggravated by weight-bearing on the toes. A dislocation of the sesamoid is invariably associated with hallux valgus.

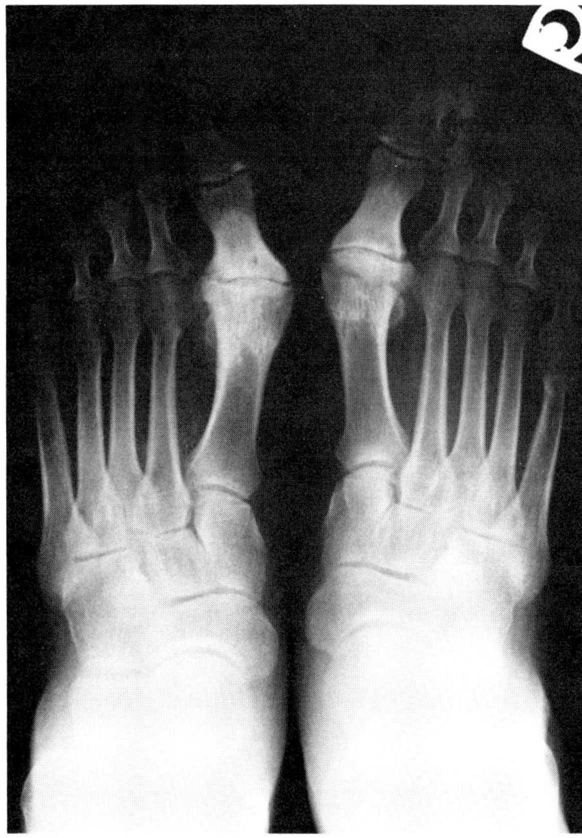

Fig. 12-23. Anteroposterior roentgenograms of bilateral hallux rigidus.

Gout

Although any joint in the body can be involved by this systemic disease, the first metatarsophalangeal joint is the most common site for its clinical manifestation. The dorsum of any of the tarsal joints is another common site of the foot. It classically has a predilection for middle-aged males. It is characterized by the deposition of sodium urate crystals in both the tissues and joints, with hyperuricemia in the blood. An acute attack of gout characteristically occurs suddenly in the morning or at night without any precipitating cause, but it can be seen following trauma or even after wearing ill-fitting shoes. Gouty arthritis is usually monoarticular, with the involved joint swollen, exquisitely painful, and the overlying skin tense, warm, and dusky red in appearance. If the disease becomes chronic, tophaceous material is deposited in the juxtaarticular tissue, and the overlying skin may undergo ulceration. Roentgenograms may be normal early in the disease, but later punched out lytic areas are seen in the juxtaarticular osseous structure.

Rheumatoid Arthritis

Like gout, rheumatoid arthritis can involve any joint in the body including the metatarsophalangeal joint. Usually, symptoms at the metatarsophalangeal joint do not occur in the acute phase of the disease, but in the chronic phase when metatarsalgia develops with toe deformities. The clinical findings of metatarsalgia are present, but the hyperextension tendency of the metatarsophalangeal joint with overlying skin change in the ball are more characteristic of rheumatoid arthritis. Atrophy of the intrinsic muscles, loss of the plantar fat pad, and hallux valgus are also seen in rheumatoid arthritis. Roentgenograms reveal destruction of the articular cartilage of the metatarsophalangeal joint and dorsal subluxation or dislocation of the metatarsophalangeal joint.

Painful Disorders Around the Heel

Calcaneal Spur

A calcaneal spur develops as a result of osteophyte formation in the calcaneal tubercle at the origin of the plantar fasciae. It is a common disorder in adults and is thought to be caused by strain on the plantar fascia. When symptomatic, there is pain and tenderness in the heel which is aggravated by weight-bearing and relieved by rest. The tenderness may be generalized to the entire plantar surface of the heel, but the point of maximum tenderness is at the osteophyte. It is usually an isolated condition, but is often seen as a local manifestation of Reiter's syndrome, ankylosing spondylitis, and Forestier's disease. A lateral roentgenogram best depicts the osteophyte formation of a calcaneal spur (Fig. 12-24). In the differential diagnosis, it is often confused with plantar fasciitis with which a spur may or may not be associated. Plantar fasciitis is a nonspecific inflammation of the plantar fascia and is generally thought to be secondary to strain of the plantar fascia.

Panniculitis

Panniculitis is a nonspecific inflammation of the elastic adipose tissue in the heel pad and is common in adults. The etiology is not known, but the condition is thought to be caused by degeneration of fibroseptum in the elastic adipose tissue brought on by weight-bearing stress or sudden impacts. Heel pain is most severe on standing or walking and particularly on heel strike. Maximum tenderness is at the posterior weight-bearing portion of the heel in contrast to the anterior portion which is most tender in calcaneal spur. Sever's disease which occurs in the calcaneal apophysis may be confused with panniculitis but is differentiated by its location over the apophysis instead of the heel and its characteristic increased density of the apophysis on the lateral roentgenogram. Panniculitis on routine lateral roent-

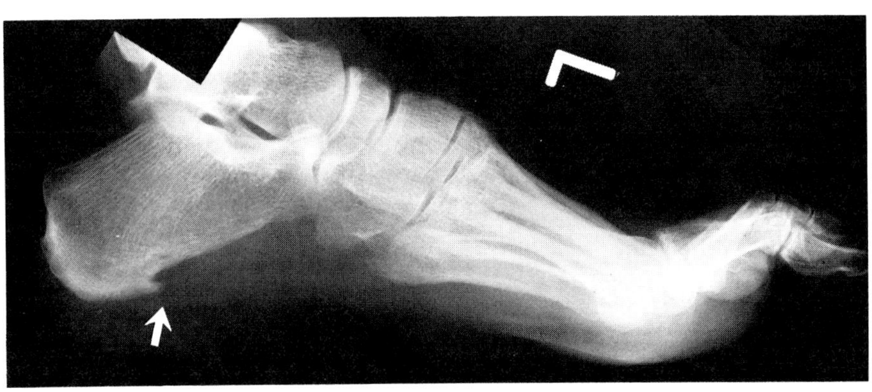

Fig. 12-24. Lateral roentgenogram of a foot, depicting a calcaneal spur (*arrow*).

genogram may be negative, but a roentgenogram taken for soft tissue exposure may reveal the disruption of the fibroseptum and decreased density of the fibrous tissue.

Achilles Tendinitis

Achilles tendinitis is a nonspecific inflammation of the tenosynovium of the Achilles tendon caused by excessive use of the triceps surae occurring in children and adults. There is pain, swelling, and tenderness over the Achilles tendon with the pain increasing on passive dorsiflexion of the ankle joint. Occasionally, crepitation can be felt over the tendon with active ankle motion.

Tendo Achilles Bursitis

Tendo Achilles bursitis is a subdermal enlargement immediately above the Achilles tendon insertion and is more common in adults than in children. It does not represent inflammation of the normal anatomical bursa, which is called retrocalcaneal bursitis, although retrocalcaneal bursitis may occur as a secondary infection to tendo Achilles bursitis. It is caused by constant pressure and friction over the area immediately above the Achilles tendon from the upper margin of the shoe counter. An excessively prominent posterosuperior border of the calcaneus predisposes to the problem. Swelling and hyperkeratotic changes are apparent over the involved area, and palpation reveals tenderness.

Retrocalcaneal Bursitis

Retrocalcaneal bursitis is an inflammation of the normal anatomical bursa located on the undersurface of the Achilles tendon at its insertion. The inflammation due to infection or nonspecific inflammatory reaction is usually acute but may become chronic. If caused by infection, the swelling, pain, and tenderness are severe, and systemic symptoms may be present. Pain increases with passive dorsiflexion of the ankle joint. Tenderness is located behind the Achilles tendon at the tendon insertion.

Exostosis of the Calcaneus

Osteochondroma (exostosis) occurring in the calcaneus causes an abnormal bony prominence which ultimately sustains excessive friction from shoes. Its growth subsides with skeletal maturation. A compression fracture of the calcaneus can produce a bony prominence at the lateral aspect known also as an exostosis. These prominences can impinge against the lateral malleolus during eversion and are painful during both standing and walking. Palpation reveals tenderness just below the lateral malleolus. Subtalar joint arthritis and lateral ligament injury are often confused with this condition. They are differentiated roentgenographically by an axial view of the calcaneus demonstrating the bony prominence facing against the lateral malleolus.

Ossification of the Achilles Tendon

Although this condition is rare and its cause is unknown, it is a distinctive entity. Of all the tendons of the foot and ankle, ossification only occurs in the Achilles tendon. It is usually at the tendon insertion but may occur in the body of the tendon. Except for limited range of ankle joint motion, the patient may be asymptomatic. The degree of motion loss is dependent on the extent of ossification. If pain is present, ankle joint motion is severely limited.

Xanthoma of the Achilles Tendon

Xanthoma is most commonly seen in the extensor tendons of the hand but may be seen in the Achilles tendon. It only develops in patients with the hereditary form of hypercholesterolemia. The Achilles tendon has a hypertrophied appearance, and, on palpation, nodules may be discernible. Xanthoma develops insidiously, usually without pain and tenderness, and the range of motion of the ankle joint is usually not impaired.

Osteomyelitis of Calcaneus

The calcaneus is a common site of osteomyelitis. Although any organism can cause the disease, Staphylococcus aureus is the most common infectious agent except for Hemophilus influenzae in infants. It is usually due to extension of a surrounding soft tissue infection, but it may be hematogenous. If acute, systemic toxicity symptoms are present plus the local findings of pain, swelling, tenderness, and local heat in the involved area. Pain and tenderness are severe in osteomyelitis of the calcaneus because pus tends to be contained in the fibroseptum of the elastic adipose tissue in the heel. Systemic symptoms are absent in chronic osteomyelitis and local symptoms are milder, but a draining sinus or chronic induration of the soft tissue may be present.

Ulcers and Gangrene of the Foot

Ulcers and gangrene are symptoms of various disease entities, and the foot is the most common site for both. *Ulcers* are caused by circulatory disorders of various causes and/or excessive local pressure. The common entities are: 1) any deformity which causes excessive pressure to result in hyperkeratosis; 2) venous congestion due to such disorders as varicose veins, thrombophlebitis, phlebothrombosis, or pregnancy; 3) lymphatic obstruction due to diseases such as lymphangitis, postirradiation therapy, postsurgical procedures, or parasite infestation; 4) arterial obstruction such as arteriosclerosis, thromboangiitis obliterans (Buerger's disease), Raynaud's disease, and Raynaud's phenomenon; 5) neuropathy, especially those conditions which affect the peripheral circulation, for example, alcoholism, syphilis, diabetes, spina bifida, and pernicious anemia, and 6) malignant tumors, such as basal cell carcinoma.

The most common site for ulceration is on the sole, particularly at the metatarsophalangeal joint. Ulcers caused by arterial obstruction are common in toes. Venous congestion ulcers are most common around the malleoli. Ulceration secondary to diabetes is complicated because both the arterial and venous vessels as well as the nervous system are involved. Often infection is superimposed on the diabetic ulcer, further complicating the clinical picture with osteomyelitis and septic arthritis.

Gangrene is a necrosis of the deep soft tissue due to arterial insufficiency. The disease entities in the differential diagnosis are tabulated in Table 12-2. Gangrene almost always first manifests itself in the toes and migrates proximally.

Painful Disorders Around the Ankle and Subtalar Joint

Arthritis of Various Etiologies

The ankle joint is a common site for various types of arthritis, especially rheumatoid and degenerative,

Table 12-2. Differential Diagnosis of Main Vascular Diseases Causing Gangrene of the Foot and Toes*

	Arterio-sclerosis Obliterans	*Thrombo-angiitis Obliterans*	*Raynaud's Disease*	*Embolism*	*Diabetes*
Age	Usually over 60 years	Usually under 40 years	Usually under 40 years	Any age	Any age
Sex	Male or female	Usually male	Usually female	Male or female	Male or female
History	Sometimes intermittent claudication	Often intermittent claudication, heavy smoker	Attacks of pallor, cyanosis, and erythema due to temperature changes	Septicemia or heart failure	Diabetes
Onset of Symptoms	Usually gradual	Usually gradual	Gradual	Sudden	Gradual
Type of Gangrene	Dry	Moderately moist	Dry with blebs	Dry	Dry or wet
Distribution of Gangrene	One or more toes or a foot; often unilateral	One or more toes or part of a foot; usually bilateral	Finger or toes or both; symmetrical	Any portion of one extremity; sometimes bilateral	One or more toes or foot; often bilateral
Degree of Pain	Moderate	Severe	Moderate	Often severe, sometimes moderate, rarely absent	Moderate
Vascular Changes	Dorsalis pedis and/or posterior tibial may not pulsate	Dorsalis pedis and posterior tibial may not pulsate	Vessels pulsate	Affected vessel does not pulsate	Dorsalis pedis and/or posterior tibial may not pulsate
X-Ray Appearance	Calcification of artery	Negative	Negative	Negative	Calcification of artery may be present
Associated Conditions	Frequently other arteriosclerotic manifestations and diabetes mellitus	Often none	Often none	Bacterial endocarditis or chronic heart disease	Systemic diabetic complications, i.e., nephropathy, retinopathy

*Modified from Yater, W. M.: Fundamentals of Internal Medicine. New York, Appleton-Century-Crofts, Inc., 1954.

with the clear exception of gout. Although rheumatoid arthritis and psoriatic arthritis commonly involve the ankle joint, the metatarsophalangeal joint is involved more frequently. Juvenile rheumatoid arthritis is especially common in the ankle joint, but other types of autoimmune related arthritis which can occur in the ankle and subtalar joints are systemic lupus erythematosus, Reiter's syndrome, scleroderma, and polymyositis. Numerous miscellaneous collagen-related diseases, such as ulcerative colitis, regional enteritis, Sjogren's syndrome, Behcet's syndrome, erythema nodosum, and erythema multiforme, may manifest arthritic symptoms in the ankle.

Primary osteoarthritis in the ankle joint itself is relatively infrequent, but degenerative joint disease secondary to fracture-dislocation or malalignment of the ankle joint secondary to a tibial fracture are common. Septic arthritis due to various organisms in the ankle joint is also common. It may be secondary to local extension of the infection from the surrounding soft tissue or hematogenous dissemination. The most frequent pathogen in infants is Hemophilus influenzae, and Staphylococcus aureus is usually the infecting agent in other age groups, although other organisms such as gonococcus, meningococcus, and streptococcus are also common. There is increased pain with weight-bearing, and an antalgic limp is present. The joint is swollen, tender, erythematous with local heat, and there is a limited range of motion which is very painful. Systemic symptoms may also be present. It is essential to aspirate joint fluid for identification of the organism. A blood cell count will reveal a leukocytosis with a predominence of neutrophils, and the erythrocyte sedimentation rate is accelerated. Blood culture may or may not grow the offending organism.

Granulomatous diseases, such as tuberculosis, coccidioidomycosis, and histoplasmosis, may occur in the ankle joint. When granulomatous diseases are suspected, skin tests should be performed to identify the possible organisms, but a synovial biopsy may be necessary for a definitive diagnosis.

Hemophilic Arthropathy

Hemophilia is a collective designation for a group of congenital blood clotting-disorders. The majority of hemophilic disorders are secondary to Factor VIII or IX deficiency, which is a sex-linked recessive disorder. Repeated episodes of intraarticular bleeding lead to severe pathological changes in the joint. The knee and elbow joints are most commonly involved, but the ankle joint is afflicted frequently. The dominant feature in acute bleeding episodes is hemarthrosis, but with repeated episodes of bleeding, degenerative joint disease, chronic synovitis, pseudotumor, or flexion deformity of the ankle may become apparent.

Charcot's Joint

Charcot's joint is a descriptive term for an arthropathy caused by numerous neurogenic disorders. The major disorders include diabetes, syphilis, syringomyelia, spinal cord injury, subacute combined degeneration of pernicious anemia, peripheral nerve injury, and leprosy. Congenital indifference to pain can also be included in this group, although it was described previously because its first manifestations are in childhood. Joint destruction from neurogenic arthropathy results from loss or diminution of proprioception, pain, and temperature perception. Neuropathic joints seldom develop if a complete motor paralysis is present. Because of sensory impairment, the patient is not aware of any joint pain, so repeated traumas result in severe destruction of the joint. Any joint can be involved in the process, but those in the lower extremity are most frequently affected because of their weight-bearing function. The ankle, intertarsal, metatarsotarsal, and metatarsophalangeal joints are the common sites of involvement. The involved joint will be deformed, unstable, and swollen. Although the pain threshold of the patient is decreased, it is not uncommon for the patient to complain of pain and tenderness. Roentgenograms show severe degeneration of the joint with extensive juxtaarticular bony destruction and calcification (Fig. 12-25).

Osteomyelitis

The distal tibia, calcaneus, and talus are common sites of osteomyelitis in the foot and ankle. Osteomyelitis of the distal tibia is either local extension from a soft tissue infection or hematogenous dissemination. It is uncommon for acute osteomyelitis of the distal tibia to develop into septic arthritis of the ankle joint, particularly in children. The two conditions should be differentiated by carefully localizing the area of tenderness, evaulating passive range of motion, and examining the joint fluid if there is joint distention. Chronic osteomyelitis of the distal-

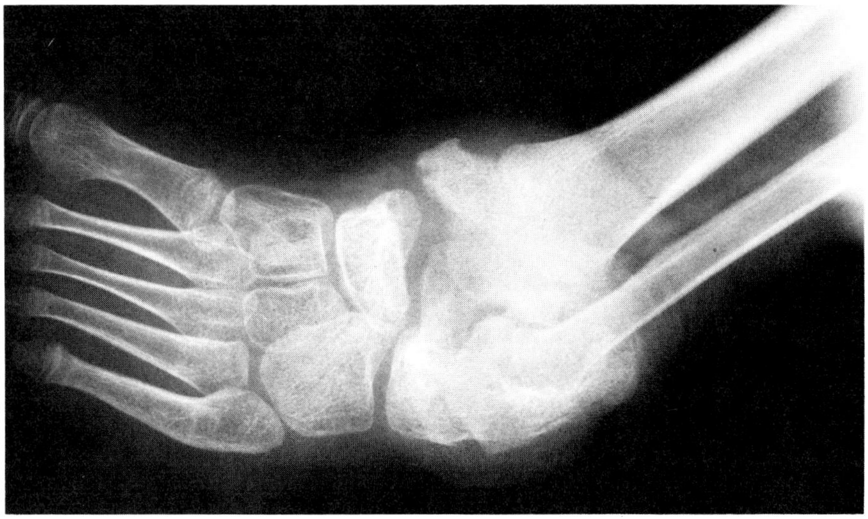

Fig. 12-25. Charcot joint of the ankle and subtalar joint with severe destruction of hindfoot bones. This is a rare case of congenital indifference to pain.

tibia presents with sinus formation, induration, and venous stasis, which develops rapidly because the surrounding soft tissue is scant.

Tarsal Tunnel Syndrome

The posterior tibial nerve sometimes is entrapped as the nerve passes through the osseofibrous tunnel between the laciniate ligament and the posterior medial malleolus (Fig. 12-26). Pain on dorsiflexion and tenderness over the posterior medial malleolus are present often with a positive Tinel's sign. It is usually the result of a fracture-dislocation of the talus or medial malleolus, but tenosynovitis of any etiology in this area and soft tissue swelling in the tunnel due to any disorder can cause the syndrome. Nerve conduction studies will show delay in conduction time of the involved nerve.

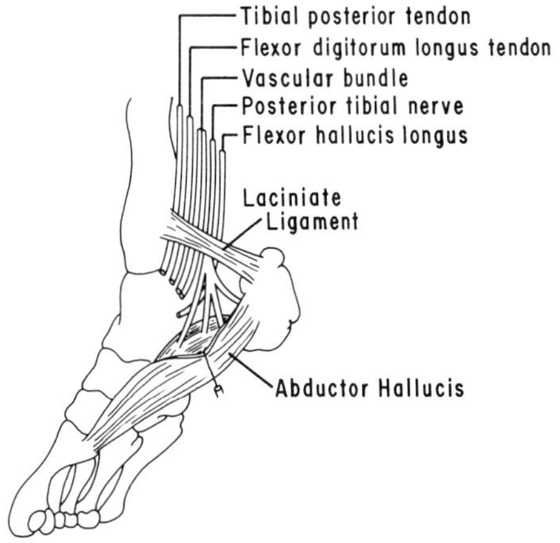

Fig. 12-26. Schematic drawing of the tarsal tunnel indicating how the nerve entrapment occurs.

Tumors

Tumors of the foot and ankle, particularly primary malignant bone tumors, are rare, although any type of bone and soft tissue tumor can occur. Metastatic lesions are also rare below the knee, but they also can involve the foot and ankle. When present, the primary complaint secondary to bone tumor is usually pain and that due to soft tissue tumor is mass, but this is not always the case. Roentgenography is the essential first step for the diagnosis of bone tumor after the clinical examination. Although tumors can occur in any part of the foot, the hindfoot and ankle are more common sites. In the foot, solitary bone cyst in the calcaneus and enchondromas in the metatarsals are more common. Other bone tumors which can occur in the foot are osteoid osteoma, osteoblastoma, osteochondroma, giant cell tumor, aneurysmal bone cyst, chondroblastoma, fibrous dysplasia, nonossifying fibroma, hemangioma, osteogenic sarcoma, chondrosarcoma, fibrosarcoma, Ewing's sarcoma, multiple myeloma, reticulum cell sarcoma, Paget's sarcoma, and the various metastatic lesions. Bone tumors occur much more frequently in the distal part of the tibia than in the foot, with the probable exception of enchondroma. The most common bone tumors in the distal tibia are nonossifying fibroma, chondromyxoid fibroma, and osteochondroma.

The majority of soft tissue tumors in the foot and ankle are benign, but malignant soft tissue tumors do occur, and one should not be lulled into a false sense of security. The common benign soft tissue lesions in the foot and ankle are ganglion, xanthoma, nodular tenosynovitis (giant cell tumor of tendon sheath), hemangioma, lymphangioma, neurofibroma, plantar fibromatosis, villonodular synovitis, and lipoma. The common malignant soft tissue tumors in the foot and ankle are squamous cell carcinoma, malignant melanoma, and synovial sarcoma. Once suspected on clinical examination, a roentgenogram is necessary as the first essential step in the evaluation of a tumor. Roentgenograms are carefully inspected for bony destruction and soft tissue detail which aid greatly in the differential diagnosis (Chap. 2). For the description and differential diagnosis of these tumors, one should consult with standard textbooks on pathology.

Fracture, Dislocation, and Ligamentous Injury of the Ankle and Foot

Fracture, dislocation, and ligamentous injury can occur in any portion of the foot and ankle. We will discuss only the more common traumatic problems unique to the foot and ankle. Standard textbooks on fracture and dislocation should be consulted for other, more specific injuries. Of all the traumatic problems below the knee, fracture, dislocation, and ligamentous injury at the ankle joint are the most common. Although described separately for convenience, it is important to be aware of the fact that they are not separate entities but are interrelated because the same abnormal stresses can produce a fracture on one side of the ankle and a ligamentous injury on the opposite side.

Fracture of the Ankle

The mechanism of fractures of the ankle are caused by external rotation, abduction, or adduction forces of the foot in relation to the tibia or vertical compression of the tibia on the talus; however, a combination of these forces is more commonly the cause. The resulting fractures from these abnormal stresses can involve one of the two malleoli, both malleoli (bimalleolar fracture), both malleoli and posterior lip of the tibia (trimalleolar fracture), or an isolated posterior or anterior lip fracture of the tibia. Bimalleolar fractures or monomalleolar fractures associated with a complete tear of the ligament on the opposite side produce an ankle joint which is grossly unstable, allowing side shift of the talus. When evaluating fractures of the ankle, one must always pay close attention to the fracture and also any concomitant ligamentous injury. Both fracture and ligament injuries present similarly with tenderness, swelling, and ecchymosis, but the location and the presence of crepitus usually can differentiate the injuries. Always remember to examine the proximal fibula in the area of the knee since this may be involved in an ankle injury because of the two-bone system.

Information regarding the mechanism of injury should be obtained from the patient, but it is not always accurate; often, roentgenograms can more reasonably estimate the mechanism of injury. The roentgenographic appearances of the fractures produced by the basic mechanisms of the ankle injury are shown in Figure 12-27. When evaluating roent-

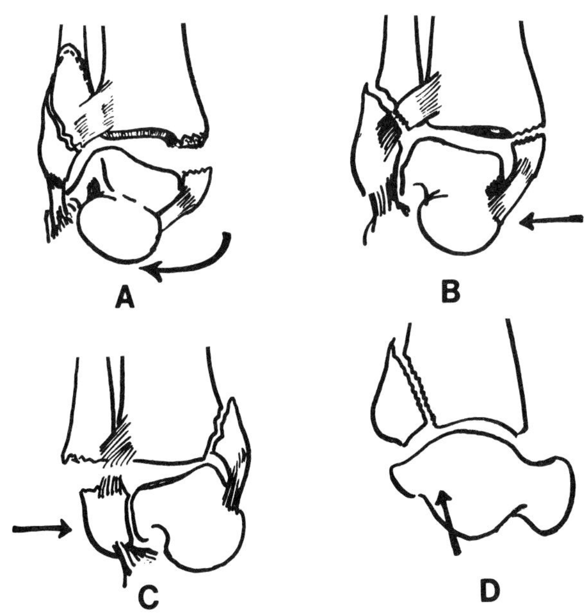

Fig. 12-27. Basic mechanisms of ankle injury. (*A*) External rotation. (*B*) Abduction. (*C*) Adduction. (*D*) Vertical compression. (Rockwood, C. A., and Green, D. P.: Fractures. Philadelphia, J. B. Lippincott, 1975)

genograms of ankle fractures, one must carefully observe the integrity of the tibiofibular syndesmosis and note any shift or tilt of the talus and correlate it with the findings on physical examination.

Ligamentous Injury of the Ankle

The ligaments involved are the deltoid ligament medially, the lateral ligament complex (anterior talofibular, posterior talofibular, and fibulocalcaneal), and the tibiofibular syndesmotic ligaments.

Deltoid ligament injury is produced by either external rotation or abduction forces. A partial tear involving the anterior portion of the deltoid ligament is the more common injury. Complete tear is usually associated with fracture of the fibula, syndesmosis separation, or both.

Injury to the lateral ligaments occurs by adduction stress usually when the ankle joint is in plantar flexion. The ligament most commonly torn is the anterior talofibular ligament. Because the anterior talofibular ligament so closely blends with the joint capsule, it also is injured simultaneously. The fibulocalcaneal ligament is involved in more severe injuries. The posterior talofibular ligament is rarely injured because it ruptures only if the ankle joint is dorsiflexed at the time of adduction stress. On physical examination, tenderness, swelling, and ecchymosis will be present over the involved ligaments. Pain is elicited with inversion. In cases of questionable stability, one should obtain stress roentgenograms under local or general anesthesia of both ankles for comparison (Fig. 12-28).

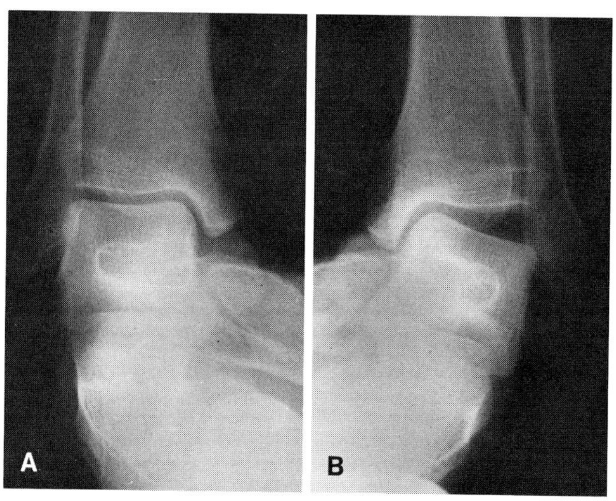

Fig. 12-28. Inversion stress roentgenograms of both ankles. Note the increased lateral talar tilt of the ankle with lateral ligament injury (*B*) compared with the uninjured side (*A*).

Injury to the syndesmotic ligaments (anteroinferior tibiofibular, posteroinferior tibiofibular, and interosseous ligaments) is usually produced by external rotation. When the anteroinferior tibiofibular ligament alone is torn, diastasis of the syndesmosis usually does not occur. If the interosseous ligament is torn in addition to the anteroinferior tibiofibular ligament, then diastasis is likely to occur. An isolated tear of the anterior tibiofibular ligament is often mistaken as an anterior talofibular ligamentous injury because of its proximity. A fibular fracture present above the tibial plafond is indicative of a tear of the tibiofibular ligament.

Dislocation of the Ankle

Subluxation or dislocation of the ankle joint is usually associated with any unstable ankle fracture. Although usually associated with fractures, an isolated anterior or posterior dislocation of the ankle without fracture can occur. Anterior dislocation is a result of posterior displacement of the tibia on a fixed foot if all the ligaments and capsular structures around the ankle are torn. On clinical examination, the foot is displaced anteriorly and assumes a slight dorsiflexed position. The normal prominence of the Achilles tendon disappears, and the dorsalis pedis pulse may be absent.

In posterior dislocations, the foot is displaced posteriorly in plantar flexion with all the ligament and capsular structures torn, except those of the posterior area. The anterior edge of the distal tibia is abnormally prominent, and the dorsalis pedis pulse may not be palpable.

Epiphyseal Separation at the Distal Tibia

The same forces producing fracture-dislocations of the ankle in the adult can produce epiphyseal plate injury in the growing child. In this age group, the epiphyseal growth plate is structurally weaker than the bone or ligaments, and the previous mechanisms described cause injury at the growth plate. Depending on the type and timing of the epiphyseal growth plate damage, the growth retardation or development of the deformity may become a potential problem in the future.

Fracture and Dislocation of the Talus

Fracture of the neck of the talus is a relatively common injury produced by hyperextension of the ankle joint. It may or may not be associated with subtalar dislocation or displacement of the body of the talus. The arterial supply to the talus is derived from the arteries from sinus tarsi (the branches of peroneal and posterior tibial arteries) and the branches from anterior tibial artery which perforates at the dorsum of the neck. If the blood supply to the talus is interrupted, which happens often with its severe displacement, the body of the talus becomes avascular.

Fracture of the body of the talus also occurs with hyperextension of the ankle but often together with compression forces. The tendency for development of aseptic necrosis of the body is even higher than in neck fractures.

Osteochondral fracture of the dome of the talus occurs with inversion or eversion forces with the foot in plantar flexion. The involvement can be either in the medial or lateral trochlea, and differentiation from osteochondritis dissecans becomes necessary in the adolescent patient.

Subtalar dislocation may occur without fracture, and the terminology is misleading because it also involves the calcaneocuboid and talonavicular joints. Medial dislocation with medial displacement of the forefoot occurs with an inversion force on the plantar flexed foot, and lateral dislocation with eversion forces on the plantar flexed foot. The deformities at the intertarsal joints are readily apparent.

Fracture of the Calcaneus

Fracture of the calcaneus is the most common tarsal bone injury. *A fracture involving the body of the calcaneus* is the most common calcaneal fracture. It often extends into the subtalar joint, with the posterior portion of the body displaced upward (Fig. 12-29). It is caused by a direct vertical force onto the calcaneus, usually a fall from a height. The spine should always be carefully examined sincc compression fracture of the spine in the dorsolumbar area is frequently associated with calcaneal fractures.

The other types of calcaneal fractures, such as *avulsion fracture of the Achilles tendon insertion* and *fracture of the sustentaculum tali* or *anterior process,* are seen less frequently. Anteroposterior and lateral roentgenograms of the foot are necessary to evaluate involvement of the subtalar joint. Fracture of the sustentaculum tali is demonstrable only in axial views.

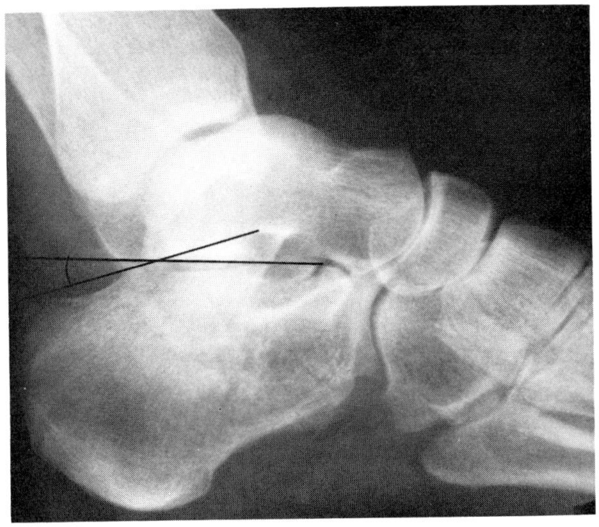

Fig. 12-29. Lateral roentgenogram of a calcaneal fracture. Note the decreased Bohler's angle (calcaneal tuber angle).

Fractures of the Metatarsals

The fractures of the metatarsal shafts invariably are the result of a heavy object falling on the dorsum of the foot, and they may have associated phalangeal fractures. The most common fracture, however, is that involving the base of the fifth metatarsal caused by adduction and plantar flexion stress on the forefoot. The sudden contraction of the peroneus brevis results in an avulsion fracture at the base of the fifth metatarsal. Local tenderness in the area plus the history and the pain with inversion-plantar flexion stress is sufficient evidence to suggest this injury.

Stress fracture in the foot is almost always seen somewhere in the metatarsals, especially in the second and third metatarsals. This condition is also called a march fracture since it is noted commonly in soldiers who give a history of a long march or cross-country run. Pain in the area is aggravated with weight-bearing, with point tenderness and swelling over the fracture. Roentgenograms usually can confirm the diagnosis, but those taken within a week of the pain may be normal (Fig. 12-30).

Rupture of the Achilles Tendon

Rupture of the Achilles tendon results from a sudden stress on the Achilles tendon, such as in

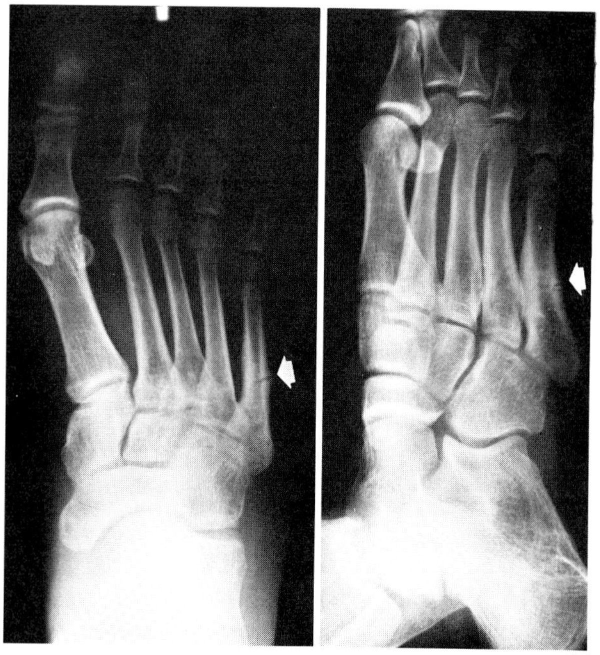

Fig. 12-30. Anteroposterior and oblique roentgenograms of a foot with a stress fracture of the fifth metatarsal bone (*arrow*).

jumping, or a sudden contraction from running. It is usually found in those males over age 30 who occasionally engage in sports. Rupture occurs in that portion of the tendon where some degeneration is present, usually near the insertion but often at the musculotendinous junction. A history of sudden onset of pain in the Achilles tendon while participating in sports is the clue. On examination, the patient will limp and be unable to stand on the toes. If the rupture is near the insertion, an area of tendon discontinuity is discernible on palpation. This may not be the case with a higher rupture at the musculotendinous junction. Thompson's test is positive regardless of the level.

SUGGESTED READINGS

Anatomy

1. Barnett, C. H., and Napier, J. R.: Axis of rotation at ankle joint in man. Its influence upon form of talus and mobility of fibula. J. Anat. *86:*1, 1952.
2. Cahill, D. R.: The anatomy and function of the contents of the human tarsal sinus and canal. Anat. Rec. *153:*1, 1965.
3. Camp, J. D., and Cilley, E. I. L.: Diagrammatic chart showing time of appearance of the various centers of ossification and period of union. Am. J. Roentgenol. *26:*905, 1931.
4. Champetier, J.: Innervation de l'articulation tibio-tarsienne (articulation talocruralis). Acta Anat. *77:*398, 1970.
5. Gardner, E., Gray, D. J., and O'Rahilly, R.: The prenatal development of the skeleton and joints of the human foot. J. Bone Joint Surg. *41-A:*847, 1959.
6. Gardner, E., and Gray, D. J.: The innervation of the joints of the foot. Anat. Rec. *161:*141, 1968.
7. Gardner, E., Gray, D. J., and O'Rahilly, R.: Anatomy: A Regional Study of Human Structure. ed. 4. Philadelphia, W. B. Saunders, 1975.
8. Gray, H.: Anatomy of the Human Body. (C. M. Goss, ed.) ed. 28. Philadelphia, Lea and Febiger, 1966.
9. Hardy, R. H.: Observations on the structure and properties of the plantar calcaneo-navicular ligament in man. J. Anat. *85:*135, 1951.
10. Hicks, J. H.: The mechanics of the foot. I. The joints. J. Anat. *87:*345, 1953.
11. Hicks, J. H.: The mechanics of the foot. II. The plantar aponeurosis and the arch. J. Anat. *88:*25, 1954.
12. Hoerr, N. L., Pyle, S. I., and Francis, C. C.: Radiographic Atlas of Skeletal Development of the Foot and Ankle. A Standard of Reference. Springfield, Ill., Charles C Thomas, 1962.
13. Hollinshead, W. H.: Anatomy for Surgeons. ed. 2. New York, Harper & Row, 1968.
14. Hubay, C. A.: Sesamoid bone of the hands and feet. Am. J. Roentgenol. Radium Ther. Nucl. Med. *61:*493, 1949.
15. Isman, R. E., and Inman, V. T.: Anthropometric studies of the human foot and ankle. Bull. Prosth. Res. *10:*97, 1969.
16. Mann, R., and Inman, V. T.: Phasic activity of intrinsic muscles of the foot. J. Bone Joint Surg. *46-A:*469, 1964.
17. Morton, D. J.: Biomechanics of the Human Foot. American Academy of Orthopaedic Surgeons Instructional Course Lectures. vol. II. pp. 92–99. Ann Arbor, Mich., J. W. Edwards, 1944.
18. Mulfinger, G. L., and Trueta, J.: The blood supply of the talus. J. Bone Joint Surg. *52-B:*160, 1970.
19. Sammarco, G. J., Burstein, A. H., and Frankel, V. H.: Biomechanics of the ankle: A kinematic study. Orthop. Clin. North. Am. *4:*75, 1973.
20. Smith, J. W.: Observations on the postural mechanism of the human knee joint. J. Anat. *90:*236, 1956.
21. University of California, Prosthetic Devices Research Project: The Pattern of Muscular Activity in the Lower Extremity During Walking; A Presentation of Summarized Data. Berkeley, 1953. (Technical Report 25, Advisory Committee on Artificial Limbs, National Research Council. Issued as Series II, Issue 25.)
22. Wright, D. G., Desai, S. M., and Henderson, W. H.: Action of the subtalar and ankle-joint complex during the stance phase of walking. J. Bone Joint Surg. *46-A:*361, 1964.

Regional Examination

23. American Academy of Orthopaedic Surgeons: Joint Motion; Method of Measuring and Recording. Edinburgh, British Orthopaedic Association, 1965.
24. Dejong, R. N.: The Neurological Examination Incorporating the Fundamentals of Neuroanatomy and Neurophysiology. ed. 3. New York, Harper & Row, 1967.
25. Duthie, R. B., and Ferguson, Jr., A. B.: Mercer's Orthopedic Surgery. ed. 7. Baltimore, Williams & Wilkins Co., 1973.
26. DuVries, H. L.: Surgery of the Foot. ed. 2. St. Louis, C. V. Mosby, 1965.
27. Farmer, T. W.: Pediatric Neurology. New York, Harper and Row, 1964.

28. Giannestras, N. J.: Foot Disorders: Medical and Surgical Management. Philadelphia, Lea & Febiger, 1967.
29. Kendall, H. O., Kendall, F. P., and Wadsworth, G. E.: Muscles, Testing and Function. Baltimore, Williams & Wilkins, 1949.
30. Tachdjian, M. O.: Pediatric Orthopaedics. Philadelphia, W. B. Saunders, 1972.
31. Thomas, A., Chesni, Y., and Saint-Anna, D.: The Neurological Examination of the Infant. London, Medical Advisory Committee of the National Spastics Society, 1960.
32. Thompson, T. C., and Doherty, J. H.: Spontaneous Rupture of Tendon of Achilles: A New Clinical Diagnostic Test. J. Trauma *2*:126, 1962.

Differential Diagnosis

33. Barrett, J. P., and Mooney, V.: Neuropathy and diabetic pressure lesions. Orthop. Clin. North Am. *4*:43, 1973.
34. Barton, N. J.: Arthroplasty of the forefoot in rheumatoid arthritis. J. Bone Joint Surg. *55-B*:126, 1973.
35. Basmajian, J. V., and Stecko, G.: The role of muscles in arch support of the foot. An electromyographic study. J. Bone Joint Surg. *45-A*:1184, 1963.
36. Brahms, M. A.: Common foot problems. J. Bone Joint Surg. *49-A*:1653, 1967.
37. Buckingham, W. W., Jr., and LeFlore, I.: Subtalar dislocation of the foot. J. Trauma *13*:753, 1973.
38. Carr, C. R., and Boyd, B. M.: Correctional osteotomy for metatarsus primus varus and hallux valgus. J. Bone Joint Surg. *50-A*:1353, 1968.
39. Coleman, S., Stelling, F. H., and Jarrett, J.: Pathomechanics and treatment of congenital vertical talus. Clin. Orthop. *70*:62, 1970.
40. Conway, J. J., and Cowell, H. R.: Tarsal coalition: Clinical significance and roentgenographic demonstration. Radiology *92*:799, 1969.
41. Cowell, H. R.: Diagnosis and Management of Peroneal Spastic Flat Foot. pp. 94–103. American Academy of Orthopaedic Surgeons Instructional Course Lecture XXIV. St. Louis, C. V. Mosby, 1975.
42. Fahey, J. J., Stark, H. H., Donovan, W. F., and Drennan, D. B.: Xanthoma of the Achilles tendon. Seven cases with familial hyperbetalipoproteinemia. J. Bone Joint Surg. *55-A*:49, 1973.
43. Giannestras, N. J.: The congenital rigid flatfoot. Its recognition and treatment in infants. Orthop. Clin. North Am. *4*:49, 1973.
44. Gibson, D. A., and Urs, N. D. K.: Arthrogryposis multiplex congenita. J. Bone Joint Surg. *52-B*:483, 1970.
45. Hall, J. E., Salter, R. B., and Bhalla, S. K.: Congenital short tendo calcaneus. J. Bone Joint Surg. *49-B*:695, 1967.
46. Harrold, A. J.: The problem of congenital vertical talus. Clin. Orthop. 97:133, 1973.
47. Herold, H. Z., and Torok, G.: Surgical correction of neglected clubfoot in the older child and adult. J. Bone Joint Surg. *55-A*:1385, 1973.
48. Hersh, A.: The role of surgery in treatment of club feet. J. Bone Joint Surg. *49-A*:1684, 1967.
49. Heyman, C. H., Herndon, C. H., and Strong, J. M.: Mobilization of the tarsometatarsal and intermetatarsal joints for the correction of resistant adduction of the fore part of the foot in congenital club-foot or congenital metatarsus varus. J. Bone Joint Surg. *40-A*:299, 1958.
50. Hollander, J. L.: Arthritis and Allied Conditions. ed. 8. Philadelphia, Lea & Febiger, 1972.
51. Kelikian, H.: Hallux valgus, allied deformities of the forefoot and metatarsalgia. Philadelphia, W. B. Saunders, 1965.
52. Kite, J. H.: Congenital metatarsus varus. J. Bone Joint Surg. *49-A*:388, 1967.
53. Kite, J. H.: Errors and complications in treating foot conditions in children. Clin. Orthop. *53*:31, 1967.
54. Levitt, R. L., Canale, S. T., Cooke, A. J., Jr., and Gartland, J.: The role of foot surgery in progressive neuromuscular disorders in children. J. Bone Joint Surg. *55-A*:1396, 1973.
55. Linscheid, R. L., Burton, R. C., and Fredericks, E. J.: Tarsal-tunnel syndrome. South. Med. J. *63*:1313, 1970.
56. Lloyd-Roberts, G. C., and Clark, R. C.: Ball and socket ankle joint in metatarsus adductus varus (s-shaped or serpentine foot). J. Bone Joint Surg. *55-B*:193, 1973.
57. Mann, R. A., and DuVries, H. L.: Intractable plantar keratosis. Orthop. Clin. North Am. *4*:67, 1973.
58. Milgram, J. E.: Office measure for relief of painful foot. J. Bone Joint Surg. *46-A*:1095, 1964.
59. Murray, R. O.: Congenital indifference to pain with special reference to skeletal changes. Br. J. Radiol. *30*:2, 1957.
60. Parrish, T. F.: Dynamic correction of clawtoes. Orthop. Clin. North Am. *4*:97, 1973.
61. Poznanski, A. K., and LaLowe, P. C.: Radiographic manifestations of the arthrogryposis syndrome. Radiology *95*:353, 1970.
62. Rockwood, C. A., Jr., and Green, D. P.: Fractures. Philadelphia, J. B. Lippincott, 1975.
63. Salter, R. B., and Harris, W. R.: Injuries involving the epiphyseal plate. J. Bone Joint Surg. *45-A*:587, 1963.
64. Seymour, N., and Evans, D. K.: A modification of the Grice subtalar arthrodesis. J. Bone Joint Surg. *50-B*:372, 1968.
65. Thornhill, H. L., Richter, R. W., Shelton, M. L., and Johnson, C. A.: Neuropathic arthropathy (Charcot forefeet) in alcoholics. Orthop. Clin. North Am. *4*:7, 1973.
66. Turco, V. J.: Surgical correction of the resistant clubfoot; One-stage posteromedial release with internal fixation: A preliminary report. J. Bone Joint Surg. *53-A*:477, 1971.
67. Waisbrod, H.: Congenital club foot. An anatomical study. J. Bone Joint Surg. *55-B*:796, 1973.
68. Waugh, W.: The ossification and vascularization of the tarsal navicular and their relation to Kohler's disease. J. Bone Joint Surg. *40-B*:765, 1958.

Index

Numbers in *italics* indicate a figure or table.